CONSUMER HEALTH USA

Volume 2

Edited by Alan M. Rees

Oryx Press
1997

© 1997 by The Oryx Press
4041 North Central at Indian School Road
Phoenix, Arizona 85012-3397

Library of Congress Cataloging-in-Publication Data

Consumer health USA / edited by Alan M. Rees.
    p.   cm.
    Includes index.
    ISBN 1-57356-068-5 (acid-free paper)
    1. Medicine, Popular. 2. Consumer education. I. Rees, Alan M.
RC81.C725 1997   94-37594
616—dc20   CIP

CONTENTS

■ ■ ■

PREFACE

■ ■ ■

Introduction

This is the second volume of *Consumer Health USA,* the first volume of which was published in 1995. *Consumer Health USA, Volume 2* captures new information made available since that time. During the interim, momentous changes in the financing, delivery, and quality of health care have transformed the landscape for medical consumers. Some 150 million Americans are now enrolled in some form of managed care. New and complex relationships linking consumers, employers, health plans, and physicians complicate and restrict consumer choice. The health care marketplace is undergoing even more dramatic reshaping than that proposed in the early years of the Clinton administration.

At the same time, there has been an explosive growth of the Internet as a means of popular communication. The availability of consumer health information in both print and electronic form has multiplied to the point that there are more than 200,000 cancer-related documents on the Internet. A variegated mix of publishers, government health agencies, academic institutions, pharmaceutical companies, promoters of dietary supplements and weight loss diets, peddlers of exercise machines, advocacy groups, professional societies, health associations, insurance companies, HMOs, hospitals, and clinics all offer health information scattered far and wide over the electronic landscape of cyberspace. If you have a medical problem, take two web sites and call your doctor in the morning! Yet the quality of many of these information sources is mixed, ranging from reliable peer-reviewed documents reporting frontline research to the dubious and outright fraudulent. In the face of this information avalanche, the consumer is confronted with the great challenge of sifting out reliable, relevant, timely, and understandable information.

Medical Consumerism and Managed Care

Consumers demand concise, accurate and meaningful information about their physical well-being and the many diseases and medical conditions experienced in their everyday lives. There is a need to confront the unknown, allay fear, and to explain, verify, or even deny the often fragmentary and contradictory information gleaned from their health care providers. Illness produces a sense of vulnerability and helplessness and a dependence on others for help with even the most routine activities of daily living. To make intelligent health care decisions,

consumers seek information through a variety of information-seeking strategies—visiting libraries; surfing the Internet; calling toll-free hotlines, clearinghouses, and Ask-a-Nurse; and consulting books, magazines, newsletters, textbooks, online services, and CD-ROM databases. Acquiring a mass of information is only too easy. The major problem confronting consumers lies rather in the evaluation and interpretation of this abundance of information in terms of its reliability and relevance.

Squeezed by managed care plans, consumers are increasingly restricted in the choice of both plans and physicians. Changes in the access and delivery of health care has introduced a major source of stress in the physician-patient relationship. The amount of time spent with the physician is likewise constrained. *Patients* have become *customers, clients, subscribers.* In this transition, the disparity in knowledge and influence between providers (producers) and consumers is widening. Third-party payers, managed care plans, hospitals, and physicians are organized to assert their interests. Consumers, on the other hand, are unorganized and lack the ability to exert their influence, and consumer advocacy remains fragmented and uncoordinated.

Yet, informed consumers can assert themselves and play a more active and productive role. Educated consumers can, for example, bring much to the patient-physician relationship facilitating communication during an ever-shrinking time allocation. This ability is well expressed by C. Everett Koop:

> In the near future, one thing seems certain: the economics of health care will mean that patients are going to have less time with their doctors. In such circumstances, it is the informed patient who will get the most from a consultation with a physician. And information technology—television, videos, print media and the Internet—can inform and empower patients by providing them with the information and vocabulary they need to work along with their physicians in taking charge of their own health. [*Time*, Fall 1996]

As managed care restricts the choice of providers and hospitals, the incentive on the part of physicians under fee-for-service to do more is shifting dramatically to the incentive to do less. Physician gatekeepers are offered financial incentives to minimize care, sometimes with "gag rules" that prohibit them from mentioning procedures not covered by the patient's insurer. The complaints against managed care plans continue to escalate with protests against early hospital discharge (some say that HMO means "Heave Mother Out"), refusal to pay for investigational drugs, restricted access to specialists, lack of continuity in care, use of a formulary of approved drugs, and denial of costly medications. In this environment, consumers must critically explore the options presented to, and withheld from, them. Informed consumers can more intelligently discuss treatment options and can more accurately determine whether information on more expensive options is being withheld from them.

The Purpose of this Book

The purpose of *Consumer Health USA, Volume 2* is to provide consumers with accurate and authoritative information derived from prestigious and reliable health organizations. The book brings together in one place nearly 150 consumer health publications selected from those currently available on topics of major concern to medical consumers. The book is almost entirely new, with only four documents carried over from the previous edition. The second volume is intended to supplement the first edition and the two volumes can be used in tandem.

The publication is designed to facilitate easy identification and photocopying, thereby eliminating the considerable time and effort involved in physically locating and acquiring elusive documents. This volume will lessen the librarian's task by permitting customer self-service at the same time as maintaining an intact collection and minimizing the risk of vandalism and loss.

It is our hope that medical consumers, exposed to market forces produced by the sweeping changes in the health care industry, will be more successful in negotiating the best health care for themselves. Consumers need now more than ever information relating to diagnosis, treatment, outcomes, and the quality of their care.

Selection of Publications

The selection of publications for inclusion reflects heavy emphasis on areas of critical contemporary interest such as heart disease, stroke, cancer, AIDS, and mental health, and other common concerns such as arthritis, obesity, osteoporosis, diabetes, eye diseases, contraception, and neurological and musculoskeletal disorders.

Most of the documents selected are derived from key agencies of the federal government. The information published by these agencies represents a condensation and digest of the findings of the United States' investment in health-related research. All of the publications have been carefully edited by government researchers for scientific accuracy and intelligibility. Of particular value are the PDQ statements and other publications of the National Cancer Institute which provide information on specific cancer sites, standard and investigational treatment protocols, clinical trials, and current research. The Agency for Health Care Policy and Research has translated for consumers the current state of the art in many areas of clinical practice. Patient versions of clinical practice guidelines are now available on cardiac rehabilitation, living with heart disease, acute low-back pain problems, quality mammograms,

managing cancer pain, post-stroke rehabilitation, urinary incontinence, and so on. Few would argue with the quality, value, or relevance of such publications.

Agencies represented in this volume include the National Institutes of Health; Food and Drug Administration; Agency for Health Care Policy and Research; National Institute on Aging; National Cancer Institute; National Eye Institute; National Heart, Blood, and Lung Institute; Centers for Disease Control and Prevention; National Institute of Diabetes and Digestive and Kidney Diseases; National Institute of Neurological Disorders and Stroke; and the National Institute of Mental Health.

An innovative feature of this current volume is the inclusion of a number of valuable documents published by health associations. We thank the following organizations for permission to reprint their publications:

- Alzheimer's Association
- American Academy of Otolaryngology—Head and Neck Surgery
- American College of Surgeons
- American Liver Foundation
- American Lupus Society
- American Social Health Association
- Aplastic Anemia Foundation
- Leukemia Society of America
- Myasthenia Gravis Foundation of America
- National Multiple Sclerosis Society
- National Osteoporosis Foundation
- National Parkinson's Foundation
- National Psoriasis Foundation
- National Reye's Syndrome Foundation
- National Sleep Foundation
- National Stroke Association
- Tourette Syndrome Association

Most of the publications included in this, and the previous volume, deal with the signs, symptoms, diagnosis, coping, treatment, and outcomes of specific diseases and medical conditions. It is, however, very likely that an increasing number of future publications selected will focus on quality and value issues such as evaluating and choosing health plans, criteria for evaluating HMOs, "report cards" on physicians and other providers, comparisons of cost and access to health care, and comparative outcomes of alternative treatments.

An initiative of the Agency for Health Care Policy and Research is aimed at extending consumer choice in the health care marketplace and to provide consumers with the tools they need to make more informed choices about their health care. The Consumer Assessments of Health Plans Study (CAHPS), now underway, is seeking information from the viewpoint of consumers on the quality of plans and services, including access to care, technical quality of care, and communication skills of providers and staffs. These research activities will doubtless be translated into valuable consumer publications.

Arrangement

The arrangement of publications is again primarily by body system, bringing together publications relating, for example, to infectious diseases, skin diseases and disorders, nutrition and weight control, and musculoskeletal and connective tissue diseases and disorders. Within body system chapters, documents are arranged alphabetically by title. Cross references to related documents in this book are located at the end of each item, and a subject index assists the reader in locating information.

A few modifications have been introduced: a separate chapter is now devoted to stroke; Genitourinary System Disorders now includes content formerly under Urogenital System Disorders; and Musculoskeletal and Connective Tissue Diseases and Disorders is a new chapter containing material on lupus, scoliosis, gout, osteoporosis, and back pain. Documents on gynecological cancers are located in the chapter on women's health concerns.

My thanks and appreciation are due to Jennifer Ashley and Anne Thompson of The Oryx Press for their talent and skill in processing a large collection of documents in print, fax, and electronic form into a well-organized and easy-to-use book.

Alan M. Rees
Cleveland Heights, Ohio
March 1997

AIDS/SEXUALLY TRANSMITTED DISEASES (STDS)

■ ■ ■

FACTS ABOUT CONDOMS AND THEIR USE IN PREVENTING HIV INFECTION AND OTHER STDS

With approximately more than one million Americans infected with HIV, most of them through sexual transmission, and an estimated 12 million other sexually transmitted diseases occurring each year in the United States, effective strategies for preventing these diseases are critical.

Refraining from sexual intercourse with an infected partner is the best way to prevent transmission of HIV and other STDs. But for those who have sexual intercourse, latex condoms are highly effective when used consistently and correctly.

The correct and consistent use of latex condoms when engaging in sexual intercourse—vaginal, anal, or oral—can greatly reduce a person's risk of acquiring or transmitting STDs, including HIV infection. In fact, recent studies provide compelling evidence that latex condoms are highly effective in protecting against HIV infection when used properly for every act of intercourse.

This protection is most evident from studies of couples in which one member is infected with HIV and the other is not, i.e., "discordant couples." In a two-year study of discordant couples in Europe, among 124 couples who reported consistent use of latex condoms, none of the uninfected partners became infected. In contrast, among the 121 couples who used condoms inconsistently, 12 (10 percent) of the uninfected partners became infected.

In another study, among a group of 134 discordant couples who did not use condoms at all or did not use them consistently, 16 partners (12 percent) became infected. This contrasts markedly with infections occurring in only 3 partners (2 percent) of the 171 couples in this study who reported consistently using condoms over the two-year period.

Condoms must be used consistently and correctly to provide maximum protection. Consistent use means using a condom from start to finish with each act of intercourse. Correct condom use should include the following steps:

- Use a new condom for each act of intercourse.
- Put on the condom as soon as erection occurs and before any sexual contact (vaginal, anal, or oral).
- Hold the tip of the condom and unroll it onto the erect penis, leaving space at the tip of the condom, yet ensuring that no air is trapped in the condom's tip.
- Adequate lubrication is important, but use only water-based lubricants, such as glycerine or lubricating jellies (which can be purchased at any pharmacy). Oil-based lubricants, such as petroleum jelly, cold cream, hand lotion, or baby oil, can weaken the condom.
- Withdraw from the partner immediately after ejaculation, holding the condom firmly to keep it from slipping off.

Myths About Condoms

Misinformation and misunderstanding persist about condom effectiveness. The Centers for Disease Control and Prevention (CDC) provides the following updated information to address some common myths about condoms. This information is based on findings from recent epidemiologic, laboratory, and clinical studies.

Myth #1: Condoms don't work.

Some persons have expressed concern about studies that report failure rates among couples using condoms for pregnancy prevention. Analysis of these studies indicates that the large range of efficacy rates is related to incorrect or inconsistent use. The fact is: latex condoms are highly effective for pregnancy prevention, but only when they are used properly. Research indicates that only 30 to 60 percent of men who claim to use condoms for contraception actually use them for every act of intercourse. Further, even people who use condoms every time may not use them correctly. Incorrect use contributes to the possibility that the condom could leak from the base or break.

Myth #2: Condoms frequently break.

Some have questioned the quality of latex condoms. Condoms are classified as medical devices and are regulated by the Food and Drug Administration. Every latex condom manufactured in the United States is tested for defects before it is packaged. During the manufacturing process, condoms are double-dipped in latex and undergo stringent quality control procedures. Several studies clearly show that condom breakage rates in this country are less than 2 percent. Most of the breakage is due to incorrect usage rather than poor condom quality. Using oil-based lubricants can weaken latex, causing the condom to break. In addition, condoms can be weakened by exposure to heat or sunlight or by age, or they can be torn by teeth or fingernails.

Myth #3: HIV can pass through condoms.

A commonly held misperception is that latex condoms contain "holes" that allow passage of HIV. Although this may be true for natural membrane condoms, laboratory studies show that intact latex condoms provide a continuous barrier to microorganisms, including HIV, as well as sperm.

Myth #4: Education about condom efficacy promotes sexual activity.

Five US studies of specific sex education programs have demonstrated that HIV education and sex education which included condom information either had no effect upon the initiation of intercourse or resulted in delayed onset of intercourse; four studies of specific programs found that HIV/sex education did not increase frequency of intercourse, and a program that included resistance skills actually resulted in a decrease in the number of youth who initiated sex. In addition, a World Health Organization (WHO) review cited 19 studies of sex education programs that found no evidence that sex education leads to earlier or increased sexual activity in young people. In fact, five of the studies cited by WHO showed that such programs can lead to a delay or decrease in sexual activity.

In a recent study of youth in Switzerland, an AIDS prevention program focusing on condom use did not increase sexual activity or the number of sex partners. But condom use did increase among those who were already sexually active. A 1987 study of young U.S. men who were sent a pamphlet discussing STDs with an offer of free condoms did not find any increase in the youths' reported sexual activity.

Preventing HIV Infection and Other STDs

Recommended Prevention Strategies

Abstaining from sexual activity is the most effective HIV prevention strategy. However, for individuals who choose to be sexually active, the following are highly effective:

- Engaging in sexual activities that do not involve vaginal, anal, or oral intercourse
- Having intercourse only with one uninfected partner

- Using latex condoms correctly from start to finish with each act of intercourse

Other HIV Prevention Strategies

Condoms for Women

The female condom or vaginal pouch has recently become available in the United States. A small study on this condom as a contraceptive indicates a failure rate of 21-26 percent in one year among typical users; for those who use the female condom correctly and consistently, the rate was approximately five percent. Although laboratory studies indicate that the device serves as a mechanical barrier to viruses, further clinical research is necessary to determine its effectiveness in preventing transmission of HIV. If a male condom cannot be used, consider using a female condom.

Plastic Condoms

A polyurethane male condom was approved by the FDA in 1991 and is now available in the United States. It is made of the same type of plastic as the female condom. The lab studies show that the new polyurethane condoms have the same barrier qualities as latex. Lab testing has shown that particles as small as sperm and HIV cannot pass through this polyurethane material. A study of the effectiveness of this polyurethane condom for prevention of pregnancy and STDs is underway. The new Polyurethane condoms offer an alternative for condom users who are allergic to latex. Also, polyurethane condoms can be made thinner than latex, have no odor, and are safe to use with oil-based lubricants.

Spermicides

Although studies indicate that nonoxynol-9, a spermicide, inactivates HIV in laboratory testing, it is not clear whether spermicides used alone or with condoms during intercourse provide protection against HIV. Therefore, latex condoms with or without spermicides should be used to prevent sexual transmission of HIV.

Making Responsible Choices

In summary, sexually transmitted diseases, including HIV infection, are preventable. The effectiveness of responsible prevention strategies depends largely on the individual. Whatever strategy one chooses, its effectiveness will depend primarily on consistent adherence to that choice.

For further information contact

CDC National AIDS Hotline: 1-800-342-2437 (AIDS)
Spanish: 1-800-344-SIDA
Deaf: 1-800-234-7889

CDC National AIDS Clearinghouse
PO Box 6003
Rockville, MD 20849-6003

■ Document Source:
U.S. Department of Health and Human Services, Public Health Service
Centers for Disease Control and Prevention
January 1995

See also: Facts About the Human Immunodeficiency Virus and its Transmission (page 3)

FACTS ABOUT THE HUMAN IMMUNODEFICIENCY VIRUS AND ITS TRANSMISSION

Research has revealed a great deal of valuable medical, scientific, and public health information about the human immunodeficiency virus (HIV) and acquired immunodeficiency syndrome (AIDS). The ways in which HIV can be transmitted have been clearly identified. Unfortunately, some materials that conflict with the scientific findings have been widely dispersed. The Centers for Disease Control and Prevention (CDC) provides the following information to correct a few misperceptions about HIV.

Transmission

HIV is spread by sexual contact with an infected person, by sharing needles and/or syringes (primarily for drug injection) with someone who is infected, or, less commonly (and now very rarely in countries where blood is screened for HIV antibodies), through transfusions of infected blood or blood clotting factors. Babies born to HIV-infected women may become infected before or during birth, or through breast-feeding after birth.

In the health care setting, workers have been infected with HIV after being stuck with needles containing HIV-infected blood or, less frequently, after infected blood contacts the worker's open cut or splashes into a mucous membrane (e.g., eyes or inside of the nose). There has been only one demonstrated instance of patients being infected by a health care worker; this involved HIV transmission from an infected dentist to six patients. Investigations have been completed involving more than 22,000 patients of 63 HIV-infected physicians, surgeons, and dentists, and no other cases of this type of transmission have been identified.

Some people fear that HIV might be transmitted in other ways; however, no scientific evidence to support any of these fears has been found. If HIV were being transmitted through other routes (for example, through air, food, water, animals, or insects), the pattern of reported AIDS cases would be much different from what has been observed, and cases would be occurring much more frequently in persons who report no identified risk for infection. All reported cases suggesting new or potentially unknown routes of transmission are thoroughly investigated by state and local health departments with the assistance, guidance, and laboratory support from CDC; *no additional routes of transmission have been recorded*, despite a national sentinel system designed to detect just such an occurrence.

The following paragraphs specifically address some of the more common misperceptions about HIV transmission.

HIV in the Environment

Scientists and medical authorities agree that HIV does not survive well in the environment, making the possibility of environmental transmission remote. HIV is found in varying concentrations or amount of blood, semen, vaginal fluid, breast milk, saliva, and tears. (See *Saliva, Tears, and Sweat*). To obtain data on the survival of HIV, laboratory studies have required the use of artificially high concentrations of laboratory-grown virus. Although these unnatural concentrations of HIV can be kept alive for days or even weeks under precisely controlled and limited laboratory conditions, CDC studies have shown that drying of even these high concentrations of HIV reduces the amount of infectious virus by 90 to 99 percent within several hours. Since the HIV concentrations used in laboratory studies are much higher than those actually found in blood or other specimens, drying of HIV-infected human blood or other body fluids reduces the theoretical risk of environmental transmission to that which has been observed—essentially zero. Incorrect interpretation of conclusions drawn from laboratory studies have unnecessarily alarmed some people.

Results from laboratory studies should not be used to assess specific personal risk of infection because (1) the amount of virus studied is not found in human specimens or elsewhere in nature, and (2) no one has been identified as infected with HIV due to contact with an environmental surface. Additionally, HIV is unable to reproduce outside its living host (unlike many bacteria or fungi, which may do so under suitable conditions), except under laboratory conditions, therefore, it does not spread or maintain infectiousness outside its host.

Households and Other Settings

Although HIV has been transmitted between family members in a household setting, this type of transmission is very rare. These transmissions are believed to have resulted from contact between skin or mucous membranes and infected blood. To prevent even such rare occurrences, precautions, as described in previously published guidelines, should be taken in all settings—including the home—to prevent exposures to the blood of persons who are HIV infected, at risk for HIV infection, or whose infection and risk status are unknown. For example, gloves should be worn during contact with blood or other body fluids that could possibly contain blood, such as urine, feces, or vomit. Cuts, sores, or breaks on both the care giver's and patient's exposed skin should be covered with bandages. Hands and other parts of the body should be washed immediately after contact with blood or other body fluids, and surfaces soiled with blood should be disinfected appropriately. Practices that increase the likelihood of blood contact, such as sharing of razors and toothbrushes, should be avoided. Needles and other sharp instruments should be used only when medically necessary and handled according to recommendations for health care settings. (Do not put caps back on needles by hand or remove needles from syringes. Dispose of needles in puncture-proof containers out of the reach of children and visitors.)

There is no known risk of HIV transmission to coworkers, clients, or consumers from contact in industries such as food-service establishments (see information on survival of HIV in the environment). Food-service workers known to be infected with HIV need not be restricted from work unless they have other infections or illnesses (such as diarrhea or hepatitis A) for which any food-service worker, regardless of HIV infection status, should be restricted. The Public Health Service recommends that all food-service workers follow recommended standards and practices of good personal hygiene and food sanitation.

In 1985, CDC issued routine precautions that all personal-service workers (e.g., hairdressers, barbers, cosmetologists, massage therapists) should follow, even though there is no evidence of transmission from a personal-service worker to a client or vice versa. Instruments that are intended to penetrate the skin (e.g., tattooing and acupuncture needles, ear piercing devices) should be used once and disposed of or thoroughly cleaned and sterilized. Instruments not intended to penetrate the skin but which may become contaminated with blood (e.g., razors) should be used for only one client and disposed of or thoroughly cleaned and disinfected after each use. Personal-service workers can use the same cleaning procedures that are recommended for health care institutions.

Kissing

Casual contact through closed-mouth or "social" kissing is not a risk for transmission of HIV. Because of the theoretical potential for contact with blood during "French" or open-mouth kissing, CDC recommends against engaging in this activity with an infected person. However, no case of AIDS reported to CDC can be attributed to transmission through any kind of kissing.

Biting

Recently, a state health department conducted an investigation of an incident that suggested blood-to-blood transmission of HIV by a human bite. There have been other reports in the medical literature in which HIV appeared to have been transmitted by a bite. Severe trauma with extensive tissue tearing and damage and presence of blood were reported in each of these instances. Biting is not a common way of transmitting HIV. In fact, there are numerous reports of bites that did not result in HIV infection.

Saliva, Tears, and Sweat

HIV has been found in saliva and tears in very low quantities from some AIDS patients. It is important to understand that finding a small amount of HIV in a body fluid does not necessarily mean that HIV can be *transmitted* by that body fluid. HIV has *not* been recovered from the sweat of HIV-infected persons. Contact with saliva, tears, or sweat has never been shown to result in transmission of HIV.

Insects

From the onset of the HIV epidemic, there has been concern about transmission of the virus by biting and bloodsucking insects. However, studies conducted by researchers at CDC and elsewhere have shown no evidence of HIV transmission through insects—even in areas where there are many cases of AIDS and large populations of insects such as mosquitoes. Lack of such outbreaks, despite intense efforts to detect them, supports the conclusion that HIV is not transmitted by insects.

The results of experiments and observations of insect biting behavior indicate that when an insect bites a person, it does not inject its own or a previously bitten person's or animal's blood into the next person bitten. Rather, it injects saliva, which acts as a lubricant or anticoagulant so the insect can feed efficiently. Such diseases as yellow fever and malaria are transmitted through the saliva of specific species of mosquitoes. However, HIV lives for only a short time inside an insect and, unlike organisms that are transmitted via insect bites, HIV does not reproduce (and does not survive) in insects. Thus, even if the virus enters a mosquito or another sucking or biting insect, the insect does not become infected and cannot transmit HIV to the next human it feeds on or bites. HIV is not found in insect feces.

There is also no reason to fear that a biting or bloodsucking insect, such as a mosquito, could transmit HIV from one person to another through HIV-infected blood left on its mouth parts. Two factors serve to explain why this is so—first, infected people do not have constant, high levels of HIV in their bloodstreams and, second, insect mouth parts do not retain large amounts of blood on their surfaces. Further, scientists who study insects have determined that biting insects normally do not travel from one person to the next immediately after ingesting blood. Rather, they fly to a resting place to digest this blood meal.

Effectiveness of Condoms

The proper and consistent use of latex condoms when engaging in sexual intercourse—vaginal, anal, or oral—can greatly reduce a person's risk of acquiring or transmitting sexually transmitted diseases, including HIV infection.

Under laboratory conditions, viruses occasionally have been shown to pass through natural membrane ("skin" or lambskin) condoms, which may contain natural pores and are therefore not recommended for disease prevention (they are documented to be effective for contraception). On the other hand, laboratory studies have consistently demonstrated that *latex condoms provide a highly effective mechanical barrier to HIV*.

In order for condoms to provide maximum protection, they must be used *consistently* (every time) and *correctly*. Incorrect use contributes to the possibility that the condom could leak or break.

When condoms are used reliably, they have been shown to prevent pregnancy up to 98 percent of the time among couples using them as their only method of contraception. Similarly, numerous studies among sexually active people have demonstrated that a properly used latex condom provides a high degree of protection against a variety of sexually transmitted diseases, including HIV infection.

Condoms are classified as medical devices and are regulated by the Food and Drug Administration. Condom manufacturers in the United States test each latex condom for defects, including holes, before it is packaged. Several studies of correct and consistent condom use clearly show that condom breakage rates in this country are less than 2 percent. Even when condoms do break, one study showed that more than half of such breaks occurred prior to ejaculation.

Latex condoms are highly effective in preventing pregnancy and most sexually transmitted diseases, including HIV infection, but only if they are used consistently and correctly.

For more detailed information about condoms, see *Facts about Condoms and Their Use in Preventing HIV Infection and Other STDS.*

The Public Health Service Response

The U.S. Public Health Service is committed to providing the scientific community and the public with accurate and objective information about HIV infection and AIDS. It is vital that clear information on HIV infection and AIDS be readily available to help prevent further transmission of the virus and to allay fears and prejudices caused by misinformation. For a complete description of CDC's HIV/AIDS prevention programs, see *Facts About The Centers for Disease Control and Prevention's (CDC) HIV/AIDS Prevention Activities.*
For more information:

CDC National AIDS Hotline:1-800-342-AIDS (2437)
Spanish: 1-800-344-SIDA (7432)
Deaf: 1-800-243-7889

CDC National AIDS Clearinghouse
PO Box 6003
Rockville, MD 20849-6003

■ **Document Source:**
   U.S. Department of Health and Human Services, Public Health Service
   Centers for Disease Control and Prevention
   August 1995

See also: Facts About Condoms and Their Use in Preventing HIV Infection (page 1)

Information from PDQ for Patients

KAPOSI'S SARCOMA

Description

What is Kaposi's sarcoma?

Kaposi's sarcoma (KS) is a disease in which cancer (malignant) cells are found in the tissues under the skin or mucous membranes that line the mouth, nose, and anus. KS causes red or purple patches (lesions) on the skin and/or mucous membranes and spreads to other organs in the body, such as the lungs, liver, or intestinal tract.

Until the early 1980s, Kaposi's sarcoma was a very rare disease that was found mainly in older men, patients who had organ transplants, or African men. With the acquired immunodeficiency syndrome (AIDS) epidemic in the early 1980s, doctors began to notice more cases of Kaposi's sarcoma in Africa and in gay men with AIDS. Kaposi's sarcoma usually spreads more quickly in these patients.

If you have signs of KS, your doctor will examine your skin and lymph nodes carefully (lymph nodes are small bean-shaped structures that are found throughout the body; they produce and store infection-fighting cells). Your doctor also may order other tests to see if you have other diseases.

Your chance of recovery (prognosis) depends on what type of Kaposi's sarcoma you have, your age, your general health, and whether or not you have AIDS.

Stage Explanation

Stages of Kaposi's Sarcoma

There is no accepted staging system for Kaposi's sarcoma. Patients are grouped depending on which type of Kaposi's sarcoma they have. There are three types of Kaposi's sarcoma:

Classic

Classic Kaposi's sarcoma usually occurs in older men of Jewish, Italian, or Mediterranean heritage. This type of Kaposi's sarcoma progresses slowly, sometimes over 10 to 15 years. As the disease gets worse, the lower legs may swell and the blood may not be able to flow properly. After some time, the disease may spread to other organs. Many patients with classic Kaposi's sarcoma may develop another type of cancer later on in their lives.

Immunosuppressive Treatment Related

Kaposi's sarcoma may occur in people who are taking drugs to make their immune systems weaker (immunosuppressants). The immune system helps the body fight off infection. People who have had an organ transplant (such as a liver or kidney transplant) have to take drugs to prevent their immune system from attacking the new organ.

Epidemic

Kaposi's sarcoma in patients who have acquired immunodeficiency syndrome (AIDS) is called epidemic Kaposi's sarcoma. AIDS is caused by a virus called the human immunodeficiency virus (HIV), which attacks and weakens the immune system. Infections and other diseases can then invade the body, and the immune system cannot fight against them. Kaposi's sarcoma in people with AIDS usually spreads more quickly than other kinds of Kaposi's sarcoma and often is found in many parts of the body.

Recurrent

Recurrent disease means that the KS has come back (recurred) after it has been treated. It may come back in the area where it first started or in another part of the body.

Treatment Option Overview

How Kaposi's Sarcoma is Treated

There are treatments for all patients with Kaposi's sarcoma. Four kinds of treatment are used:

- surgery (taking out the cancer)
- chemotherapy (using drugs to kill cancer cells)
- radiation therapy (using high-dose x-rays to kill cancer cells)
- biological therapy (using the body's immune system to fight cancer)

Radiation therapy is a common treatment for Kaposi's sarcoma. Radiation therapy uses high-dose x-rays or other high-energy rays to kill cancer cells and shrink tumors. Radiation for Kaposi's sarcoma comes from a machine outside the body (external beam radiation therapy).

Surgery means taking out the cancer. Your doctor may remove the cancer using one of the following:

- Local excision cuts out the lesion and some of the tissue around it.
- Electrodesiccation and curettage burns the lesion and removes it with a sharp instrument.
- Cryotherapy freezes the tumor and kills it.

Chemotherapy uses drugs to kill cancer cells. Chemotherapy may be taken by pill, or it may be put into the body by a needle in a vein or muscle. Chemotherapy is called a systemic treatment because the drug enters the bloodstream, travels through the body, and can kill cancer cells outside the original site. Chemotherapy for Kaposi's sarcoma also may be injected into the lesion (intralesional chemotherapy).

Biological therapy tries to get your own body to fight cancer. It uses materials made by your own body or made in a laboratory to boost, direct, or restore your body's natural defenses against disease. Biological therapy is sometimes called biological response modifier (BRM) therapy or immunotherapy.

Treatment by Stage

Treatment for Kaposi's sarcoma depends on the type of Kaposi's sarcoma you have, your age, and your general health.

You may receive treatment that is considered standard based on its effectiveness in a number of patients in past studies, or you may choose to go into a clinical trial. Not all patients are cured with standard therapy and some standard treatments may have more side effects than are desired. For these reasons, clinical trials are designed to find better ways to treat cancer patients and are based on the most up-to-date information. Clinical trials are going on in most parts of the country for most stages of Kaposi's sarcoma. If you want

more information, call the Cancer Information Service at 1-800-4-CANCER (1-800-422-6237).

Classic Kaposi's Sarcoma

Your treatment may be one of the following:

1. Radiation therapy.
2. Local excision.
3. Systemic or intralesional chemotherapy.
4. Chemotherapy plus radiation therapy.

Immunosuppressive Treatment Related Kaposi's Sarcoma

Depending on your condition, the cancer may be controlled if you stop taking immunosuppressive drugs. If you cannot stop taking the drugs or if this does not work, your treatment may be one of the following:

1. Radiation therapy.
2. A clinical trial of chemotherapy.

Epidemic Kaposi's Sarcoma

Your treatment may be one of the following:

1. Surgery (local excision, electrodesiccation and curettage, or cryotherapy).
2. Intralesional chemotherapy.
3. Systemic chemotherapy. Clinical trials are testing new drugs and drug combinations.
4. A clinical trial of biological therapy.

Recurrent Kaposi's Sarcoma

Treatment for recurrent Kaposi's sarcoma depends on your type of Kaposi's sarcoma, your general health, and your response to earlier treatments. You may want to take part in a clinical trial.

To Learn More

To learn more about Kaposi's sarcoma, call the National Cancer Institute's Cancer Information Service at 1-800-4-CANCER (1-800-422-6237). By dialing this toll-free number, you can speak with someone who can answer your questions.

The Cancer Information Service can also send you free booklets. The following general booklets on questions related to cancer may be helpful:

- What You Need to Know About Cancer
- Taking Time: Support for People with Cancer and the People Who Care About Them
- What Are Clinical Trials All About?
- Chemotherapy and You: A Guide to Self-Help During Treatment
- Radiation Therapy and You: A Guide to Self-Help During Treatment
- Eating Hints for Cancer Patients
- Advanced Cancer: Living Each Day
- When Cancer Recurs: Meeting the Challenge Again

There are other places where you can get material about cancer treatment and information about services to help you. You can check the social service office at your hospital for local and national agencies that help with your finances, getting to and from treatment, care at home, and dealing with your problems. The American Cancer Society, for example, has many free services. Their local offices are listed in the white pages of the telephone book.

You can also write to the National Cancer Institute at this address:

National Cancer Institute
Office of Cancer Communications
31 Center Drive, MSC 2580
Bethesda, MD 20892-2580

If you have AIDS, you can get information about services for AIDS patients by calling the AIDS hotline at 1-800-342-AIDS (1-800-342-2437). Additional information on clinical trials for AIDS patients can be obtained by calling the AIDS Clinical Trials Information Service at 1-800-TRIALS-A (1-800-874-2572) or by writing to the service at the following address:

AIDS Clinical Trials Information Service
PO Box 6421
Rockville, MD 20850

■ **Document Source:**
U.S. Department of Health and Human Services, Public Health Service
National Institutes of Health
National Cancer Institute
February 1996

QUESTIONS AND ANSWERS ABOUT HERPES

What is herpes?

Herpes is a common and usually mild infection. It can cause "cold sores" or "fever blisters" on the mouth or face (known as "oral herpes") and similar signs and symptoms in the genital area ("genital herpes").

What causes herpes?

Herpes is caused by one of two viruses: herpes simplex type 1 (HSV-1) and herpes-simplex type 2 (HSV-2). Herpes is different from many other common viral infections in several ways. Most importantly, herpes sets up a lifelong presence in the body, called "latency." The virus can travel the nerve pathways in a particular part of the body and hide away—virtually sleeping—in the nerve roots for long periods of time. This means that even though HSV may not be causing "cold sores" or genital signs and symptoms at a given time, it can still cause symptoms later.

What happens when you first get genital herpes?

When a person is first infected with HSV-1 or HSV-2, the immune response is not well-developed, and the virus is able to multiply more rapidly and in more places than it can later. Signs and symptoms during a first episode, therefore, can be quite pronounced. First episodes of herpes usually occur within two weeks after the virus is transmitted.

On the other hand, some people have a first episode so mild they don't even notice it. It may be a later episode, or "reactivation," that is first noticed months or years later.

How long does a 'first episode' last?

Many people experience their most dramatic signs and symptoms of HSV shortly after becoming infected. This "first episode" frequently causes small pimples or blisters that eventually crust over and scab like a small cut. But the signs of herpes come in a wide variety. They may be obvious or hard to see, painful or easily ignored.

First episodes may take from two to four weeks to heal fully. During this time, some people will experience a second crop of lesions, and some will have flu-like symptoms, including fever and swollen glands, particularly in the lymph nodes near the groin.

Treatment with antiviral drugs is standard during first episodes and can speed healing significantly.

What are the signs and symptoms of recurrent genital herpes?

Signs and symptoms of genital herpes vary greatly from one episode to the next, and from one person to the next. Breaks or irregularities in the skin ("lesions") are often found in recurrent episodes. Some will notice small sores, others will have so-called "classic" blister-like lesions that crust over. In recurrent herpes, however, this process usually takes less than half the time a first episode does.

In addition, many people have very subtle forms of recurrent herpes that can heal up in a matter of days. These can be mistaken for insect bites, abrasions, yeast, "jock itch," hemorrhoids, and other conditions. Also, they can be found not only on the penis and vulva, but near the anus, on the thigh, on the buttocks—anywhere in or around the genital area.

It's worth noting that early in the phase of reactivation many people experience an itching, tingling, or painful feeling in the area where their recurrent lesions will develop. This sort of warning symptom—called a "prodrome"—often precedes lesions by a day or two. In some people, prodrome will involve pain in the buttocks, the back of the legs, or even lower back.

Does everyone with herpes have symptoms eventually?

Some people who have latent infection never experience herpes prodrome or genital lesions. In addition, many people have such mild symptoms that they may not recognize the infection for many years.

All in all, about one in four adults in the Untied States has latent genital herpes infection. Less than a third of these individuals, however, have been diagnosed or would report a history of herpes lesions.

Can herpes be active without causing signs and symptoms?

It used to be thought that all of HSV's active times were marked by "outbreaks"—a sore, blister, or else some kind of symptom like an itch. Then researchers learned that the virus could become active without causing signs or symptoms. This phenomenon has been called a number of things, including "asymptomatic shedding" and "subclinical shedding." But the best term for it might simply be "unrecognized" herpes.

The term "unrecognized" is especially apt for three reasons: (1) some lesions are overlooked because they occur in places we simply never look; (2) some are mistaken for something else—an ingrown hair, for example; and (3) some can't be seen at all with the naked eye.

Even if you're a person with recurring signs and symptoms that you can usually recognize as herpes, there are almost certainly days when you won't be aware that the virus has reactivated and traveled to the skin or mucous membranes.

How often is herpes active?

Research suggests that reactivation is influenced by HSV type and by how long one has been infected.

HSV-2

People with a marked first episode caused by HSV-2 can expect to have several symptomatic recurrences a year. The average is four or five. In addition, people with HSV-2 also can expect to have recurrences that do not cause recognizable signs and symptoms. These probably occur less frequently than symptomatic outbreaks but account for about a third of all reactivation. In most cases, the first year has the most viral activity.

HSV-1

HSV-1 behaves quite differently in the genital area. With type 1 infection, people may have a marked first episode, but they are much less likely to have out-breaks in the first year. Their average number of symptomatic recurrences is closer to one per year, and their rates of unrecognized reactivation are lower as well.

What causes recurrences?

Herpes's triggers are poorly understood by scientists but appear to be highly individual. Research shows that prolonged exposure to strong sunlight can trigger oral herpes (as on a beach trip or skiing weekend). Known triggers for genital herpes include surgical trauma and excessive friction in the genital area. With time, many people come to recognize whatever physical or psychological stressor seems to trigger HSV in their own bodies.

How is herpes spread?

Herpes is spread by direct skin-to-skin contact. For example, if you have a cold sore and kiss someone, you can transfer the virus from your mouth to theirs. If you have active genital herpes and have vaginal or anal intercourse, you can transfer the virus from your genitals to your partner's. Finally, if you have a cold sore and put your mouth on your partner's genitals (oral sex), you can give your partner genital herpes.

Herpes also can be spread through sexual contact at times when there are no obvious signs or symptoms. Herpes is often transmitted by people who are unaware that they are infected or by people who simply don't recognize that their herpes infection is in its active phase.

How can one reduce the risk of spreading herpes to a sexual partner?

1. **Tell your partner:** Ideally, both partners will understand the basics of herpes prevention and make decisions together about which precautions are right for them.
2. **Abstain from sex when signs and symptoms are present:** Having sex during a recognized outbreak puts an uninfected partner at risk.
3. **Use condoms between outbreaks:** Condoms offer useful protection against unrecognized herpes by protecting or covering the mucous membranes that are the most likely sites of transmission. They can also help protect you from acquiring another sexually transmitted infection.

    Condoms do not provide 100 percent protection because a lesion may be in a place the condom doesn't cover. But, used consistently, they are the best available form of prevention.
4. **Microbicides/spermicides?** The spermicides used in contraceptive foams, films, and gels kill or neutralize HSV in lab tests, and more studies are under way. Spermicides may provide some protection when used in the vagina at the recommended dose for contraception. Spermicides should be used along with condoms—not in place of them.

What about treatment?

There is no treatment that can cure herpes, but there are medications which help to keep the virus in check. The prescription drugs listed below are worth discussing with your health care provider.

Dear Friends:

"Your test results show you have herpes simplex."

For tens of thousands of people every year, these words raise a number of questions and concerns about how to manage a chronic infection and its impact on intimate relationships.

With time, and with an effort to understand herpes, most people are able to resolve their concerns and lead lives in which herpes is only a minor and occasional aggravation. But the transition is not always easy.

Helping people make this transition is one major purpose of the Herpes Resource Center, a service of the American Social Health Association. A unique program for people with herpes, the HRC seeks to provide accurate, practical, non-judgmental information; to help educate the media and medical community; and to encourage and fund research on herpes.

Herpes Resource Center programs and services include:

The National Herpes Hotline (919) 361-8488

The National Herpes Hotline operates Monday through Friday, 9 a.m. to 7 p.m., eastern time. Trained health educators answer questions about transmission, prevention, and treatment of herpes. The hotline also counsels people regarding emotional issues, such as telling a partner. Callers can receive a free packet of information.

(To ensure that confidentiality and privacy are strictly protected, all educational materials are mailed in plain envelopes.)

the helper

This quarterly journal covers the medical and social impact of herpes. A special introductory issue, *Understanding Herpes,* gives an overview of herpes simplex and what you can do to manage an infection. Each issue updates readers on new clinical research and also provides a forum for personal perspectives on herpes.

Managing Herpes: How to Live and Love with a Chronic STD

This comprehensive book by Charles Ebel brings a reassuring, balanced perspective to the medical and emotional issues surrounding herpes. Topics include: recurrences, treatment options, transmission, pregnancy, telling your partner, impact on sexuality, and new research. Includes a resource list and glossary.

Additional pamphlets and audio and video tapes on herpes are available. The HRC also maintains local support groups that offer the opportunity to approach problems with the help of others.

For more information, or to order other educational materials about herpes, please fill out the form on the back of this panel or call the ASHA Resource Center at 1-800-230-6039.

You are also encouraged to make an additional, tax-deductible gift to help the HRC continue our work of helping tens of thousands of people each year understand herpes.

Best wishes,
The Staff of the Herpes Resource Center

Acyclovir

Acyclovir, sold under the brand name Zovirax®, has been available for over a decade in both a topical and capsule form. Taken by mouth several times a day, acyclovir attacks the virus by disrupting its ability to make copies of itself. The drug is safe and has virtually no side effects.

Patients can choose between two kinds of treatment.

Acute Therapy: A patient begins taking acyclovir capsules at the first sign of prodrome and continues with several capsules a day for five days. Acute therapy for first episodes can bring about a dramatic reduction in healing times. With recurrences, it can take one to two days off the healing time.

Suppressive Therapy: This means taking acyclovir every day to hold HSV in check, so that it's less likely to flare up and cause symptoms. The usual dose is 400 mg taken twice a day. Suppressive therapy brings about roughly an 80 percent reduction in the frequency of symptomatic outbreaks and can halt symptoms altogether in some patients.

Valacyclovir

Sold under the brand name Valtrex®, valacyclovir uses acyclovir as its active ingredient. Valacyclovir, however, is better absorbed by the body. The result is that valacyclovir gives symptomatic relief equal to acyclovir with less frequent dosing. It is approved for recurrent herpes at a dose of 500 mg twice daily, and it's being tested for suppressive and first episode treatment.

Famciclovir

Sold under the name Famvir®, famciclovir is a newer compound that works much the same way acyclovir does but is better absorbed and can be taken less often. Famciclovir is approved already for acute treatment of recurrent genital herpes, with a dose of 125 mg twice a day. This can reduce time to healing, as well as the period of viral multiplication. The drug is also being tested for use in first episodes and suppressive therapy.

What if I think I have genital herpes?

See a doctor while symptoms are still present. The doctor will look at the area, take a sample from the sore(s), and test to see if the herpes virus is present. The test you should request is a specific culture for HSV. This will tell you whether you have HSV-1 or HSV-2. The test will not work if the sores have healed and might not work if they're more than a few days old.

Will herpes spread to other places on my body?

During a first episode, it's possible to move virus from the location of an outbreak to other places on the body by touching the sore(s). The fingers, eyes, and other body areas can accidentally become infected in this way. Preventing self-infection is simple: Do not touch the sores during an outbreak—especially the first outbreak. If you do, wash your hands as soon as possible. The herpes virus is easily killed with soap and water.

What about pregnancy?

The spread of herpes to newborns is rare, and most mothers with a history of herpes have normal vaginal deliveries. However, an infant who contracts herpes can become very ill, so some precautions are advisable. When a woman has active herpes at the time of delivery, a cesarean-section is usually performed.

If you have a history of herpes, it's advisable to talk with your health care provider about it during a prenatal care visit. This is important even if you've never had symptoms or haven't had a recurrence in a long time. You should be examined to see if you have herpes symptoms at labor and should notify the doctor if you think you have active symptoms at that time.

If a woman has no history of herpes but has a sexual partner who does, it's important that she avoid contracting herpes during pregnancy. A first episode during pregnancy creates a more significant risk of transmission to the newborn.

ASHA's Herpes Resource Center provides up-to-date, sensitive, and accurate information about all aspects of herpes.

Telephone hotlines you can call for information and referrals in your area:

Herpes Resource Center
1-800-230-6039
Monday-Friday
9 a.m. to 7 p.m. (eastern)

National Herpes Hotline
1-919-361-8488
Monday-Friday
9 a.m. to 7 p.m. (eastern)

National STD Hotline
1-800-227-8922
Monday-Friday
8 a.m. to 11 p.m. (eastern)

For more information, or to order pamphlets, write:

American Social Health Association
PO Box 13827
Research Triangle Park, NC 27709

■ Document Source:
   American Social Health Association
   PO Box 13827
   Research Triangle Park, NC 27709
   1996

STD (VD): QUESTIONS/ANSWERS

What are STDs?

Sexually transmitted diseases (STDs), sometimes called venereal diseases (VD), are infections you get from sexual contact with an infected person. More than 25 diseases are spread through sexual contact. STDs are among the most common contagious diseases in the United States. About one in four adults in the United States has an STD. Every year, there are about 12 million new cases.

What are the dangers?

Most STDs can be cured if treated early. STDs frequently cause problems with reproductive health, making it difficult or impossible for a woman to get pregnant. They also can cause disease in newborns. Without proper medical attention, some STDs can lead to severe and permanent damage such as blindness, cancers, heart disease, or even death.

How do you get STDs?

All STDs have one thing in common. They are spread during sex—vaginal, oral, or anal. If a person is infected, he or she can pass the STD to a partner through body fluids, such as semen, vaginal fluids, and blood. Some STDs are spread through contact with these fluids. Some, like herpes and genital warts, are spread by direct contact with infected skin. STDs can be passed from woman to man and vice versa, as well as from man to man or woman to woman.

Who gets STDs?

Anyone who has sex can get an STD—men and women, homosexual or heterosexual, young and old, and people of all colors and races. No one is immune.

How do you prevent STDs?

There are many ways of lowering your risk of getting an STD. Some have to do with choice of partners. Some have to do with choice of sexual practices—the idea of "safer sex."

You have no risk if you do not have sex (abstinence). There are many ways to give and get pleasure without having sex. These include hugging, kissing, fantasizing, touching, and massage.

In general, the more people you have sex with, the greater your risk becomes. You have no risk if you have sex with only one person who is free of infection and has no other sex partners.

But it may be hard to know if your partner is free of infection. Even when you have sex with only one other person, that person could have an STD and not know it. And if your partner has sex with others but does not tell you, you are at increased risk for STDs.

It's also important to know that some STDs, like the AIDS virus (HIV), can be spread through intravenous drug needles.

How can I make sex safer?

If you have more than one partner or you are having sex with someone who might have more than one partner, here's what you can do to lower your chances of getting STDs.

- Protect yourself and others by using condoms every time you have sex, including oral and anal sex. Women and men should carry condoms and insist they be used.
- If you use latex condoms, do not use oil-based lubricants such as Vaseline® or hand lotion. Oil-based products can damage latex. Use only water-based lubricants, such as K-Y® Jelly. If you use plastic (polyurethane) condoms, you can use any type of lubricant.
- For vaginal intercourse, the condom alone is very good protection, but birth control foam, jelly, or cream can provide an extra measure of safety when used along with condoms. Read the label and make sure it contains a spermicide, because spermicide kills some kinds of STD germs. Apply the spermicide inside the vagina according to directions.
- If you're having sex with several different partners, ask your doctor to check you for STDs every six months, even if you don't have symptoms. This is particularly important for women.

Do STDs cause special problems for women?

Yes. STDs can be harder to diagnose in women. Some STD infections have no signs or symptoms at all. And some do their damage inside a woman's sex organs, where symptoms are not easily seen. Frequently, a woman has no idea that she has an STD until the infection has been active for a long time.

Untreated STDs can cause lasting damage to the female reproductive organs, leading to ectopic (tubal) pregnancies, miscarriages, and infertility. Between 100,000 and 150,000 American women become infertile each year because of STD-related infections.

Also, STDs can be passed from an infected mother to her baby during pregnancy or at birth. If the disease is detected soon enough, precautions can be taken with many STDs so that the disease is not spread to the baby. If the mother is untreated, the baby could suffer permanent damage or even death.

What are some of the more common STDs?

STD	Approximate # Affected Each Year in the U.S.
Chlamydial infections	4 million
Trichomoniasis ("trich")	3 million
Gonorrhea ("clap")	1.1 million
Genital warts (venereal warts)	750,000

STD	Approximate # Affected Each Year in the U.S.
Genital herpes	40 million affected, with as many as 500,000 new cases each year
Hepatitis B	100,000-200,000
Syphilis ("syph")	120,000
HIV infection	1 million affected, with 45,000 new AIDS cases reported each year

What are the signs and symptoms of STDs?

Often there are no signs or symptoms. So if you've had sex with someone you think is infected with an STD, a test from the doctor may be the only sure way to tell if you're infected.

Because STDs can affect anyone, it's important to know what to look for in yourself and others. Be alert to body changes in the genital area. These warning signs might appear right away, or they might not show up for weeks or even months. Or they might come and go. Even if the signs and symptoms do disappear, the disease might still be active. STDs usually do not go away on their own.

Here are some signs or symptoms that may mean you have an STD:

Both Men and Women:

- sores, bumps, or blisters near your sex organs, rectum, or mouth
- burning or pain when you urinate
- swelling or redness in your throat
- swelling in the area around your sexual organs

Women:

- unusual discharge or smell from your vagina
- pain in your pelvic (lower belly) area or deep inside your vagina during sex
- burning or itching around your vagina
- bleeding from your vagina other than your regular menstrual periods.

Men:

- a drip or discharge from your penis
- pain in the testicles

AIDS: A Special Case?

AIDS (acquired immune deficiency syndrome) is the most serious STD because so many people with AIDS have died. There is no cure and no vaccine. AIDS is the most serious stage of a viral infection caused by human immunodeficiency virus (HIV). This virus attacks the body's immune system and leaves the person with AIDS unable to fight off many kinds of infections and cancers.

The U.S. Public Health Service estimates that as many as one million are now infected with HIV in this country. Most of them have no symptoms yet, but many will someday develop AIDS.

AIDS is different from most other STDs in several ways.

How You Get HIV

HIV lives in blood, semen, and vaginal fluids. If infected blood, semen, or vaginal fluid gets into your body, the virus might infect you, too. Most of the people with AIDS became infected from having sex with a person who carried HIV or from sharing needles used to shoot drugs. HIV also can be passed from an infected mother to her baby during pregnancy or at birth.

In the past, HIV sometimes was spread to people who received contaminated blood through transfusions. But, as of March 1985, all blood supplies are screened for the virus. So the risk is now extremely low.

The most important thing you need to know about HIV infection is that in most cases there are no symptoms for months or even years. But once infected with the virus, even before any symptoms, individuals can transmit it to others. That means that most people who have the virus are spreading it without even knowing it.

What to Watch For

There are no easy clues. Because HIV makes you vulnerable to all kinds of illnesses, there are many different symptoms. And some of them have nothing to do with the genital region.

How You Don't Get It

You don't get HIV from touching, kissing, food, coughs, mosquitoes, toilet seats, donating blood, or swimming in public pools.

How to Protect Yourself

To prevent HIV infection, avoid unprotected sex with infected persons and the sharing of needles or syringes.

You can protect yourself from HIV by following the safer sex guidelines used for other STDs. Use condoms every time you have sex, no matter what kind of sex it is. For vaginal sex, spermicides can be used in addition to condoms.

Remember, the virus is most easily spread through blood. So anal sex, which causes bleeding, is very risky. So is the sharing of needles to shoot drugs into the bloodstream.

Where You Can Get Help

If you think you've been exposed to the AIDS virus and have persistent signs of illness, consult a doctor, or call your local STD clinic run by the health department.

For general AIDS information and referrals, call the National AIDS Hotline (1-800-342-AIDS). The call is free, and no one will ask your name.

Do STDs lead to AIDS?

No. STDs do not directly cause AIDS. But recent studies have shown that HIV is more easily transmitted among people who have certain other STDs—especially STDs that cause genital sores. People with herpes, syphilis, chancroid, or other infections that cause breaks in the skin should consider themselves at a greater risk for infection with HIV. People who have an STD should talk to their health care provider about the risk of HIV and the possible need for an HIV antibody test, which is a special blood test.

How do I get medical treatment?

STDs usually do not go away without treatment. Instead, they may well get worse. So it's important to get help from your doctor or from an STD clinic as soon as possible. Tests are safe and private.

If you want to learn more about STDs or want to know where to go in your area for confidential, free treatment, call the National STD Hotline at the number listed below.

What is treatment like?

Examination and testing for STDs is easy. Treatment often involves taking pills (specific antibiotics) to kill the organisms causing the disease. And with the exception of herpes, genital warts, and HIV, most STDs can be readily cured. Herpes can be treated to reduce the frequency and duration of outbreaks, but it cannot yet be cured. Genital warts can be removed, but often the virus that causes them remains present on the skin.

What if I am diagnosed with an STD?

- Inform the person(s) you have had sex with so they know they might be infected and should be tested. (Your local health department can help with this.)
- Avoid having sex while you're being treated.
- Finish taking all of your medication and get a check-up as many times as your health care provider suggests. The infection can stay active even after symptoms go away.

Where can I get more information?

For more information on STDs:

- Contact the STD clinic in your local health department.
- Check with your own doctor.
- Call the National STD Hotline (1-800-227-8922). It's toll-free and open to calls from 8:00 a.m. to 11:00 p.m. eastern time, Monday through Friday.
- Call the National AIDS Hotline (1-800-342-AIDS). It's open to calls 24 hours a day, seven days a week. Spanish-language callers can dial 1-800-344-SIDA. Deaf callers needing TTY/TTD service can dial 1-800-AIDS-TTY.

This brochure is published by the American Social Health Association (ASHA). ASHA is a private, nonprofit organization dedicated to stopping all STDs and their harmful consequences to individuals, families, and communities.

ASHA produces educational materials on sexual health; operates national hotlines for AIDS, STDs, and herpes; advocates for strong public health programs to prevent the spread of STDs; and funds research to find better treatments.

For more information on our programs or other materials, please write to us at the address below.

■ **Document Source:**
American Social Health Association
PO Box 13827
Research Triangle Park, NC 27709
1994

SURGEON GENERAL'S REPORT TO THE AMERICAN PUBLIC ON HIV INFECTION AND AIDS

HIV Infection and AIDS—A Status Report

Infection with human immunodeficiency virus (HIV), the virus that causes acquired immunodeficiency syndrome (AIDS), is one of our country's greatest health challenges. Today one million Americans—one in every 250—are infected with HIV. About one in 100 men and one in 800 women are now infected with HIV. Most of them look and feel healthy, since it takes an average of 10 years before a person with HIV develops AIDS. For infants and some adults, this time may be much shorter.

The first cases of AIDS were reported in 1981. By the end of 1992, more than 250,000 Americans had developed AIDS and more than 170,000 had died—nearly three times more Americans than those who died in the Vietnam War. In 1993 alone, from 47,000 to 66,000 more Americans may die of AIDS; an estimated 40,000 to 80,000 will get infected with HIV.

In this second decade of the AIDS epidemic, gay men still account for the majority of AIDS cases reported each year and continue to suffer an enormous burden.

However, AIDS is becoming more prominent in the young and in heterosexual men and women. AIDS is now one of the three main causes of death for women and men 25 to 44 years old in this country. It is among the top 10 causes of death for children one to four years old. AIDS is now becoming a disease of families.

Today, most of the people with AIDS are young adults. Although survival times have improved greatly for people who are diagnosed early and receive medical treatment, the disease is usually fatal. Survival times today are about the same for men and women when they find out about their infection early and receive comparable medical treatment.

Heterosexual Spread of AIDS

Although most reported AIDS cases continue to be among men who have sex with men and among injecting drug users, cases due to heterosexual contact have been increasing over the last several years. In 1992, 9 percent of the total AIDS cases and 39 percent of reported AIDS cases in women were attributable to heterosexual contact, an increase of nearly 42 percent from 1990 to 1992.

AIDS is increasing among racial and ethnic minority populations.

People of ALL races and ethnic groups have been infected with HIV, but racial and ethnic minority populations have been most disproportionately affected. Through 1992, 47 percent of all reported AIDS cases were among blacks and Hispanics, while these two population groups represent only 21 percent of the total U.S. population. Asians and Pacific Islanders and American Indians and Alaska Natives account for a small percentage of all reported AIDS cases.

AIDS is increasing outside big cities.

Most people with HIV infection and AIDS live in big cities, but the number of people developing AIDS in smaller cities, towns, and rural areas is growing. The highest U.S. rates are in the Northeast and in Puerto Rico, but the rest of the country has been catching up. Before 1985, more than half of the children with AIDS were from New York City, Newark, and Miami; since then, the majority of children with AIDS have come from outside these cities.

More women are becoming infected.

The Centers for Disease Control and Prevention (CDC) estimates that about 100,000 women in the United States are infected with HIV. They comprise 11 percent of all AIDS cases, and the percentage increases each year. Almost half of the cases of AIDS in women have been reported in the last two years.

Women can get HIV infection by having sex with somebody infected with HIV or using "contaminated" needles (previously used by an HIV-infected person) to inject drugs. While nearly half of the women with AIDS today got infected by using contaminated needles to inject drugs, more and more women are becoming infected through unprotected sex with infected men.

There is evidence that, like other sexually transmitted diseases (STDs), women may be more likely to get HIV during sex from an infected man than a man is to get it from an infected woman. However, women infected with HIV can transmit the virus to men. Cases among women who have sex only with women have been reported, although the number of cases is small: only four cases of possible female-to-female HIV sexual transmission have been reported in the medical literature.

Children of the Epidemic

An added tragedy to the growing AIDS epidemic is the children infected with HIV and the thousands of others who will be orphaned when their mothers or fathers die from AIDS. Through December 1992, more than 4,000 children were reported with AIDS—most of them were infected through contact between the infected mother and her child before it is born or during birth. However, she can also infect her baby through breastfeeding.

There are also many more children who are infected with HIV but have not been diagnosed with AIDS. About one of every four babies born to infected women will have HIV infection. In addition, a small number of children with AIDS were infected through blood transfusions and blood products received before testing of blood began in 1985.

By 1994, an estimated 7,500 children in the United States will have developed AIDS from being infected before or during birth, or from breastfeeding after birth. During the next decade, at least 125,000 children will become orphans of this epidemic and will need to be cared for by family members, caring adults, or extended family members—or placed in foster care. These orphaned children, three-fourths of them not infected with HIV, will require our care, financially and socially.

Teenagers are getting infected.

The teen years are often a time of experimentation with alcohol, drugs, and sex. Some teenagers don't believe they can become infected with HIV because they rarely see people their own age who have AIDS. Teens need to understand this discrepancy. Because the time between getting infected with HIV and developing AIDS can be 10 years or more, many people with AIDS who are in their 20s (currently one of five reported with AIDS) were infected while they were teenagers.

Teenagers who share needles to inject drugs (including steroids) or who have sex without a latex condom are getting infected. However, most won't show any symptoms of HIV infection or AIDS until they are in their 20s, even though they can still transmit the infection to others.

We now have treatments for HIV infection.

We now have medical treatments that can delay many of the illnesses associated with AIDS, and more treatments are on the way. There is hope for a vaccine in the future. However, unless many Americans change some of their behaviors, hundreds of thousands more Americans will become infected before the year 2000.

Know the facts about HIV.

HIV is the virus that causes AIDS.

After a person is infected with HIV, the virus gradually weakens the disease-fighting immune system of that person. A weakened immune system lets other diseases successfully attack the body. When a person's immune system is so weakened by HIV that his or her body can no longer fight off serious infections and some types of cancer, that person develops AIDS.

Early symptoms are hard to spot.

Most people do not have any symptoms when they are first infected with HIV. Because they look and feel healthy, most people with HIV infection don't know they are infected until they have an HIV test. However, HIV is in their bodies and they can infect other people.

Symptoms of AIDS or HIV disease eventually appear.

It may take anywhere from a few weeks to many years for symptoms to appear. Symptoms of AIDS or HIV disease can take many forms, but the symptoms usually include fever, diarrhea, weight loss, tiredness, and enlarged lymph glands. Since HIV destroys the immune system, a person with AIDS often gets many types of infections, and those infections happen more often and get worse. Some infections that may occur include yeast infections in the mouth or throat and serious infections caused by the herpes viruses.

Other common problems that occur when the person develops AIDS are certain pneumonias (*Pneumocystis carinii*) that cause coughing, fever, and difficult breathing, and a form of cancer (Kaposi's sarcoma) that produces purple blotches on the skin. Tuberculosis is also a common problem in some areas of the country. Some of these illnesses may not get better even with medication or they may come back again and again. HIV can also affect the brain, causing loss of memory or other nervous system or mental symptoms.

Other Symptoms of HIV Infection in Women

In women, the first signs of HIV infection may be any of the ones listed above or repeated serious yeast infections of the vagina. Vaginal yeast infections are common in women for many reasons other than HIV infection and can be treated with over-the-counter medications. Women with yeast infections that do not readily go away with treatment, however, or that happen over and over again, should be tested for HIV, especially if their behaviors place them at risk. Women with HIV infection may also be at increased risk of cancer of the cervix, and other conditions such as pelvic inflammatory disease. In HIV-infected women, these conditions may be more severe or difficult to treat. All such women should get PAP smears at least once a year.

How You Get HIV, and How You Don't

HIV is everyone's concern.

Your age doesn't matter. Neither does your race, religion, hometown, or gender. No matter who you are or where you live, it's possible you know somebody who has HIV infection or AIDS or may be at risk. It may be a friend or coworker. It may be a member of your family. It may be you.

How HIV Spreads

HIV is in the blood, semen, or vaginal secretions of an infected person. The two main ways of spreading HIV are having sex and using contaminated needles to inject drugs. In addition, infected women can pass HIV infection to their newborns.

Unprotected sex is dangerous.

"Unprotected sex" is sex without a latex condom. HIV can be in semen (including the first drop of fluid, even before ejaculation) and in vaginal fluids. HIV can enter the body through the vagina, penis, rectum, and, when engaging in oral sex, through the mouth. Anal sex is especially risky for both men and women. Any form of unprotected sex is risky, including oral sex. Although condoms are not perfect, they are highly effective in preventing HIV and other STDs when used consistently and correctly. Condom failure is usually due to a person not using the condom correctly, rather than flaws in the condom itself.

Oral sex can spread HIV.

Getting semen, vaginal secretions, or blood from an infected person in your mouth puts you at risk of HIV infection. The risk of getting HIV from oral sex is not as high as from anal or vaginal sex, but there is a risk. Sores or cuts anywhere in your mouth would make oral sex even more risky.

Sexually transmitted diseases (STDs) increase your chances of getting HIV.

Some STDs, such as herpes or syphilis, produce open sores or blisters on the genitals. These sores or blisters make it easier for HIV to be transmitted during sex. Other STDs, including gonorrhea and chlamydia, place a person at higher risk of getting HIV infection.

Sex with multiple partners increases your risk.

If you have sex with more than one person, you increase your odds of having sex with someone infected with HIV or other STDs. The more people you have sex with, the greater your risk of getting infected. In a sense, you are also "having sex" with all the people your partner has had sex with.

Contraceptives other than condoms do not protect you.

Birth control pills, sponges, foams, diaphragms, intrauterine devices (IUDs), or being sterilized do not protect you from HIV. Having sex during your period or while pregnant does not protect you either. No matter what method you use for birth control, a latex condom—when used correctly and consistently—offers the best protection against HIV and other STDs.

Using contaminated needles to inject drugs is very risky.

When a person injects drugs into his/her body, some of that person's blood remains in the needle or syringe. If someone else then uses the same needle or syringe ("works") to inject drugs, he/she could be shooting HIV directly into the bloodstream. This makes using needles or syringes that have been used by someone else one of the riskiest things you can do.

Any drug use may increase your risk of unsafe behaviors.

When you are under the influence of alcohol, cocaine, heroin, or other drugs, you are not thinking clearly. This can lead you to take risks for HIV infection, such as having sex with people with whom you would not normally have sex or having sex without a condom. Crack and other forms of cocaine are associated with risky sexual activity. Don't mix sex with alcohol or other drugs that affect your judgment.

Pregnant women can pass HIV to their newborn babies.

Women infected with HIV can infect their newborn babies. About one of every four babies born to infected women will have HIV infection. The time from birth to the development of AIDS for these infected children varies from weeks to years. Most often, the mother passes the HIV infection to her baby before it is born or during the birth. However, a baby can also become infected by breastfeeding from an infected woman. In the United States, if the mother is infected, the baby should be given formula instead of breast milk.

A baby born to an HIV-infected woman will test positive for HIV at birth whether or not the baby itself is actually infected, since the positive antibody is transferred from the mother. If the baby is not infected, its HIV test will become negative within about a year and a half. Most of the babies born to HIV-infected mothers will not have HIV infection, but they will probably become orphans because their mothers and, often, their fathers are infected and will likely die before the child is grown.

Ways You Do Not Get HIV Infection

There are no reports of HIV transmission from saliva, tears, or human bites.

You do not get HIV from

- Being bitten by mosquitoes or other bugs
- Being bitten by an animal
- Eating food handled, prepared, or served by somebody with HIV infection
- Sharing toilets, telephones, or clothes
- Sharing forks, spoons, knives, or drinking glasses
- Touching, hugging, or kissing a person with HIV infection
- Attending school, church, shopping malls, or other public places with HIV-infected people

---

You don't get HIV from sports.

Based on current knowledge, participation in sports carries virtually no risk for getting HIV. This is because most sports do not involve contact likely to cause bleeding. If bleeding occurs, however, you should minimize contact with an injured person's blood. It is also advisable to remove the injured person from further play until bleeding is controlled. Sweat from an HIV-infected athlete will not transmit HIV infection.

You don't get HIV from kissing.

It has been known for years that a small amount of HIV may be present in the saliva of some infected people. However, the amount of HIV in saliva is much less than in blood, semen, or vaginal fluids. Even deep or "French" kissing seems to have little risk for transmitting HIV.

Going to the doctor or dentist is safe.

To date, six people are known to have been infected with HIV while getting medical or dental treatment, and all six of them were infected by one infected dentist. Even though scientists have looked carefully at over 19,000 persons treated by HIV-infected health care providers, this is the ONLY time we know of where any medical or dental patient was infected with HIV during treatment. Doctors, dentists, and hospitals have been given information about how to prevent the spread of HIV infection in health care settings. If you are worried about getting HIV or any other infection from your doctor or dentist, share your concern and talk to them about it.

Our blood supply is among the safest in the world.

Today, there is very little chance of getting HIV from a blood transfusion, certainly not enough to stop you from receiving blood if your doctor feels you need it. Clotting factors obtained from donated blood are equally safe. Nearly all people infected with HIV through blood transfusions received those transfusions before 1985, the year it became possible to test donated blood for HIV.

Since mid-1983, all blood donations in the United States have come from volunteers who are questioned about their risks for HIV infection. People at increased risk of being infected are not allowed to donate blood. Since mid-1985, all donated blood has been tested for HIV and other viruses (seven different tests are now conducted on each blood sample). Blood that tests positive for HIV is safely discarded and is not used for transfusion. Donors are confidentially told that they are infected with HIV, and they are not allowed to donate blood again.

There is NO RISK of getting infected with HIV by GIVING blood because a new, sterile needle is used for each blood donation.

Organ and Tissue Transplants

Organ and tissue transplants are becoming more common. As with blood transfusions, the Public Health Service and the American Association of Tissue Banks have recommended that attempts be made to eliminate donors at high risk, that all donors be tested, and that organs and tissues from donors testing positive for HIV not be used. Thus, there is very little chance of getting HIV from a transplant.

Artificial Insemination and HIV

To be safe, sperm banks are requested to test sperm donors for HIV at the time of the donation, freeze and quarantine the sperm, and test the donor again six months later. If both HIV tests are negative, the sperm can then be thawed and used. If you are considering artificial insemination, talk to your doctor or call your sperm bank to discuss the procedures they use to protect you from HIV infection.

Are you at risk?

If we are to stop the spread of HIV, we must talk about it openly and honestly. The following questions cover the most common risks and raise topics that you may not be used to discussing.

Assess your OWN risk

If you answer "yes" to any of the following questions, you could have HIV infection or other STDs.

Have you ever had unprotected sex (anal, vaginal, or oral) with a man or woman who

- you **know** was infected with HIV?
- injects or has injected drugs?
- shared needles with someone who was infected?
- had sex with someone who shared needles?
- had multiple sex partners?
- you normally wouldn't have sex with?

Have you used needles or syringes that were used by anyone before you?

Have you ever given or received sex for drugs or money?

Did you or any of your sex partners

- receive treatment for hemophilia between 1978 and 1985?
- have a blood transfusion or organ transplant between 1978 and 1985?

Every person is responsible for his or her actions. HIV is passed from person to person because of what people do. Not because of who they are, where they came from, or where they live. Your actions can keep you at no risk or place you at high risk of infection. Remember, these issues must be dealt with frankly and in plain language if we are to stop this epidemic.

If you answered "yes" to any of the above questions, or if you have any doubts about how to answer these questions, it does not mean that you have HIV or other STDs. It does mean you should go to your doctor or local health clinic, talk to them about your situation, get information, and then decide if you need to be tested. If you are concerned, seek counseling and get tested. You may have HIV infection and look and feel healthy. Early diagnosis and treatment can slow the development of HIV infection into AIDS and can also help you protect your sex or drug partners.

If you don't have a doctor, your medical society can refer you to one. Or, you can find a clinic or community health center that provides both counseling and testing. At some sites, you don't even have to give your name to be tested, because testing is done anonymously. Some sites will test you for free; others will charge a fee. To find a testing site near you, call your local or state public health department or the CDC National AIDS Hotline (1-800-342-AIDS).

Facts About the HIV Tests

To know for certain if you are infected with HIV, you must have your blood tested specifically for HIV infection, not just a "routine" blood test. The tests available today to detect HIV infection are among the most accurate medical tests known. Two separate tests for HIV (called ELISA and Western blot), when used together, are correct more than 99.9 percent of the time.

When you become infected with HIV, your body makes substances called antibodies. These HIV antibodies usually show up in the test within three months after you become infected, and almost all people who are infected will show antibodies in their blood within six months. The tests detect these antibodies, not the virus itself. If your HIV test is negative, it means no antibodies were found and you probably are not infected with HIV. However, if you did something risky less than six months before the test, you may need to be tested again later just to be sure you are not infected.

Remember, testing negative today does not mean you can't get infected in the future if you use contaminated needles or have sex with an infected person. Even after a previous negative test, if you do something that puts you at risk for HIV infection, you could get infected.

Most people who test negative feel a sense of relief. If you test negative, *this is the perfect time to stop doing things that may put you at risk again.*

If you test positive, the sooner you take steps to protect your health and the health of others, the better. Early treatment, a healthy lifestyle, and a positive attitude can help you stay well.

What has your sex partner done?

It's hard to be absolutely sure what risks your sex partner has taken. Don't take someone's word for whether or not they might be infected, no matter how well you know them. Remember, you can't tell just by looking at someone whether they are or are not infected. Some people don't understand that something they did might have infected them. Some people don't know if they are infected because they haven't been tested. Some people deny that they might be infected. Some people don't tell the truth. If you're not sure whether your sex partner is infected, ask your doctor or someone at your clinic whether you need to be tested. In the meantime, the safest thing to do is to avoid having sex with your partners until you are sure they are not infected, or to use a latex condom correctly each time you have sex.

What about a blood transfusion?

From 1978 through 1985, a small proportion of the blood used for transfusion or blood clotting factor concentrates (used by people with hemophilia or "bleeding disorder") was infected with HIV. If you received blood or clotting factors between 1978 through 1985, you could have been infected with HIV and should be tested.

How to Protect Yourself from HIV Infection

HIV and Sex

The surest way to protect yourself against HIV infection and STDs is not to have sex at all, or to have sex only with one steady, uninfected partner. It is best for you to wait to have sex until you and your partner are committed to a relationship. If you are not in such a relationship, and engage in sex, you should use a latex condom correctly every time you have sex. It's not a matter of how much you trust someone, or how well you know him or her, or how healthy he or she looks—condoms help protect both of you.

Latex condoms can prevent HIV infection.

A latex condom, used properly, helps protect you and your partner from HIV and other infections spread through having sex. When used correctly and consistently, latex condoms are highly effective in preventing HIV infection and other STDs. The latex condom, correctly used, stops semen or vaginal fluids, which might have HIV in them, from passing from one person to another. This is only true for latex condoms; natural membrane (lamb skin) condoms will not provide protection against HIV because they contain tiny pores or holes. Always look for the words "latex condom" on the package when you purchase your condoms.

"Female condoms" (pouches that fit into the vagina) are being evaluated; one has been approved by the Food and Drug Administration (FDA). Because they have not been fully tested, how well they protect against HIV infection is uncertain.

You and your partner should agree to use condoms before you start having sex. You should not expose condoms to heat or sunlight, and you should make sure to check the manufacturer's expiration date on the package before use. If you have questions about selecting or using condoms, talk to your doctor, pharmacist, or counselor at your health department or AIDS service organization, or call the CDC National AIDS Hotline (1-800-342-AIDS).

Spermicides

Studies show that some spermicides kill HIV in test tubes. However, the ability of a spermicide to kill HIV in the vagina during sex is uncertain. Spermicides alone should not be used for HIV prevention. When used with a condom, the spermicide (gel, foam, film, or suppository) should be put directly inside the vagina according to the directions on the package. The amount of spermicide in a spermicide-lubricated condom is not enough to provide protection against HIV.

Adding spermicide to the inside of a condom does not help. If the condom were to break, the semen (and any HIV) would reach the vagina before the spermicide could spread out and cover the inside of the vagina. In addition, spermicides may cause vaginal sores or irritation in some women and irritation of the penis in some men. These sores or irritations, like any sore or irritation of the vagina or penis, may make it easier for HIV to get into the bloodstream.

The Proper Use of Condoms

Proper use of a new latex condom every time you have sex—from start to finish—is an effective way of protecting yourself from HIV and other STDs. Always have more than one condom available.

- Be careful when opening the condom. Do not use your teeth, fingernails, or other sharp object to open the condom wrapper because you might tear or nick the condom inside.
- Put the condom on as soon as the penis becomes erect, roll it to the base of the penis, keep the condom on throughout intercourse, and be sure it stays on until the penis is fully withdrawn.
- If you use a lubricant for vaginal or anal sex, use one that is water-based. Water-based lubricants are for sale at any pharmacy. DO NOT use oil or grease, such as petroleum jelly, cold cream, baby oil, or cooking shortening, as a lubricant; they weaken latex and make the condoms break more easily.
- Never re-use a condom.
- Never continue using a condom if it breaks during sex—stop and put on a new condom.

HIV and Drug Use

Injecting drugs, including steroids, can spread HIV from one person to another when injection equipment is shared or re-used by another person. HIV may be found in a variety of items used for drug injection, including needles, syringes, cotton, and "cookers."

- If you use drugs, stop using them for your sake and for the sake of others. Seek drug abuse treatment to help you stop.
- If you can't stop injecting drugs, never share your equipment with anyone or re-use equipment used by someone else. Don't share, borrow, or rent injection equipment ("works").
- If you share or re-use injection equipment, clean and disinfect it between uses. To do the best cleaning job possible, flush needles and syringes with water until the equipment is at least visibly clear of blood and debris. You should then completely fill the equipment SEVERAL TIMES with full-strength household bleach. The longer the syringe is completely full of fresh bleach, the more likely that HIV will be killed (some suggest that the syringe should be full of bleach for at least 30 seconds). After each bleach filling, rinse the syringe and needle by filling several times with clean water.
- Remember, however, that cleaning injection equipment with cleaners, such as bleach, does not guarantee that HIV is killed. If you cannot stop injecting drugs, use only sterile needles and syringes.

For more information call the CDC National AIDS Hotline (1-800-342-AIDS).

How to Protect Others

If you have HIV infection, you must take steps against infecting others. The safest way not to transmit HIV is not to use drugs, not to share drug injecting equipment, and not to have sex. Don't let anyone else use your needles or syringes, and don't use anybody else's. If you do have sex, your sex partner needs to know that you are infected with HIV, and a latex condom should be used every time you have sex.

If you have HIV infection, you should tell anyone with whom you've had sex or shared needles. People that you may have infected, or who may have infected you, may not know they have been exposed to HIV. They may be infected and can continue to infect others without knowing it. Let them know about your test results so they can talk to their doctor and be counseled and tested. If you are uncomfortable talking to your present or past sex or drug-use partners, ask a counselor from your health department to help you, or even to speak for you. Health department counselors are trained to do this carefully, without revealing your name.

Health care workers can reduce their risk.

A small number of health care workers have been infected on the job, usually by being stuck with a needle already used on an HIV-infected patient. This risk can be reduced if health care workers follow "universal precautions," treating all blood, semen, or vaginal secretions, no matter whom the fluid comes from, as if it contained HIV. Health care workers must wash their hands between patients; wear gloves, masks, gowns, and eye-wear when doing some procedures; dispose of used needles and other sharp medical tools by putting them in special containers; and disinfect or sterilize appropriate equipment.

New medical devices that reduce the chances of cuts or needle sticks are being developed. These precautions are for your own protection. You should support all health care workers in taking these precautions with everyone.

Research advances are promising.

We have learned a lot about HIV and AIDS since 1981. We know that HIV causes AIDS by weakening the immune system and how HIV is, and is not, passed from one person to another.

People are living longer.

Because of what we have learned, people with HIV infection and AIDS are living longer. They are also healthier and able to live active lives for a longer period. Although we still do not have a cure for HIV infection, three medicines (AZT, ddI, and ddC) that fight HIV are already available. Other medicines that prevent or treat many of the illnesses which accompany AIDS are also available. Antibiotics and other newer medicines can be used both to prevent and to treat several of the common illnesses seen with HIV infection and AIDS. Additional medicines are being developed and tested.

Drug approvals are faster.

The Food and Drug Administration (FDA) has made the review process faster for AIDS drugs. The FDA now makes available some promising drugs, still being tested, to those who have no other drugs to take. Many of the changes made to speed up the review of AIDS drugs are also being used to speed the approval of drugs for other serious diseases. For more information call 1-800-TRIALS-A.

Early treatment helps.

Doctors can diagnose many illnesses that occur in people with HIV infection. Treatments can be started early in the illness, when they are most effective. By monitoring the immune system, doctors can give medicines that help prevent persons with HIV from getting severe infections. Researchers are also working on ways to strengthen the immune systems of people with HIV infection, delaying or preventing many illnesses. Because early diagnosis, counseling, and treatment can improve the length and quality of life of AIDS patients, it is important for persons who might be infected to be evaluated by their doctor long before they become sick.

Drugs, such as AZT, for HIV infection or its complications, work just as well for blacks and Hispanics as they do for whites. In addition, these drugs work as well for women as they do for men. How well these medicines work does not depend on race or gender but on such things as the physical condition you are in when you start taking the drug, how soon treatment is begun, and how well you follow the course of treatment.

Vaccines are being tested.

Steps are being taken to find vaccines to prevent HIV infection. More than a dozen potential HIV vaccines are in the early stages of human testing right now. If these small-scale tests show promise, we can begin tests involving larger numbers of people.

Two ways of using HIV vaccines are being tested. One use is to prevent infection or disease in a person not already infected, as measles and polio vaccines have done for those illnesses. Early trials of vaccines have begun, but much more research must be done before we will know if any of them will work.

The other possible use of a vaccine is in treatment for people already infected with HIV. Use of such vaccines may strengthen the immune system and help the body defend itself against HIV. Although several vaccines of this type are being tested now, we do not yet know if any of those being tested today will be of benefit for those infected. If you are interested in participating in a clinical trial, please call 1-800-TRIALS-A.

Living with HIV Infection and AIDS

You can still lead an active life.

Life does not end with HIV infection. Many people with HIV have received early treatment, have continued to stay healthy, and are able to lead productive lives. Even if you are infected, you are still an important member of your family and your community, and you can still contribute to society.

You have much living yet to do, many things to enjoy. Knowing you are infected with HIV is not easy, but many people in national, state, and local organizations are working to make things better for you. There are many people who care about you and are working to combat HIV infection. In the meantime, you need to help us by taking care of yourself physically, spiritually, and emotionally.

Understanding the Immune System

CD4+ cells (also called T-helper cells or T4 cells) are very important in fighting infection. Unfortunately, HIV attacks these cells. In a person not infected with HIV, the number of CD4+ cells remains constant over time. In an HIV-infected person, as months and years go by, the number of CD4+ cells drops. Your CD4+ cell count is a measure of the damage to your immune system by HIV and of your body's ability to fight infection. Your doctor uses your CD4+ cell count to help decide what medical treatments are best for you.

Get treatment.

There are several medicines approved by the FDA for the treatment of HIV infection. Some of these medications may help slow the development of HIV infection to AIDS. Some have serious side effects. You should discuss all medications with your doctor or pharmacist before taking them. Other medicines may prevent or delay some of the diseases that attack your body as your immune system gets weaker. More medicines are being tested. Research is also going on to find the best doses and combinations of medicines.

Many new medicines and some old ones used for other diseases are being tested to see if they can safely kill or control HIV, boost the immune system, or help fight other illnesses. Some of these experimental medicines may be available to you. Talk to your doctor and call the AIDS Clinical Trials Information Service (1-800-TRIALS-A) if you need more information or are interested in participating in a clinical trial.

Get checked for TB.

Tuberculosis (TB) is a serious infection of the lungs (and sometimes other organs such as the brain or spine). TB germs are spread from people with active TB of the lungs or airways to other people, usually during close contact that lasts for a long time. TB germs can be spread through the air when a person with TB coughs or sneezes. TB can be both prevented and treated.

Not everybody infected with TB germs gets sick with active tuberculosis. In most people who become infected, the TB germs remain inactive and do not cause sickness. However, due to damage to their immune system, people with both HIV infection and TB germs are much more likely to get sick with active TB than people with TB germs who are not infected with HIV. For this reason, people with HIV need to be evaluated regularly for TB.

If TB is recognized early, you can be given medications to prevent you from getting sick with TB and spreading it to others. Active TB can usually be cured, but it takes a long time, at least six months. If you are infected with both HIV and TB, you may have to take medications for a longer time. Without treatment, HIV and TB work together to shorten your life. For more information call the CDC National AIDS Hotline (1-800-342-AIDS).

You can help stop HIV/AIDS.

When people work together, they can do almost anything. When people step forward, and communities work together to change the behaviors that spread HIV, their actions speak louder than words.

All of us have a job to do in stopping the spread of HIV and in caring for those infected and their families and friends. We need to learn how to prevent HIV infection and then teach others. We need to help each other stay healthy. And we need to reach out to those who are affected by, and infected with, HIV—to men, women, children, entire families—to all in need of help. No matter who you are, where you come from, where you live, you can help stop HIV and AIDS.

Help prevent discrimination.

You can help by treating people with HIV infection or AIDS the same way you would want to be treated if you were in their place. Because this problem is a very personal, emotional one, you need to understand that what you think and feel makes a difference to people around you. If you understand HIV and AIDS and help others understand, it will make a real difference. People with HIV infection and AIDS need to be protected from discrimination on the job, in housing, in schools, or in getting health care.

If people feel they will be treated badly if others know about their infection, they may try to keep it a secret or even avoid finding out if they are infected. These actions only let HIV spread faster.

However, if people feel they will be treated with respect and understanding, they will be more willing to get tested, seek medical care, and tell their sex and drug-use partners about their infection. These actions will help slow the spread of HIV.

The new Americans with Disabilities Act (Public Law 101-596) helps fight discrimination against people with disabilities and can protect people who are infected with HIV or are believed to be infected with HIV. Businesses and employers have been made aware of this law. For more information, call the CDC National AIDS Hotline (1-800-342-AIDS).

The Family and HIV

Families play an important role in stopping HIV. Families nurture children, provide a supportive environment, and teach values and discipline. Parents should teach their children how to protect themselves against HIV infection and other STDs as soon as their children are able to understand. There is no substitute for the concerned attention of a parent, caring adult, or extended family member. For a free brochure on how to talk to children about HIV infection and AIDS, call the CDC National AIDS Hotline (1-800-342-AIDS).

Schools can help prevent HIV infection.

Many schools have excellent AIDS education programs that also teach children how to protect themselves against HIV infection.

The most effective programs support and reinforce the AIDS prevention messages given at home. They are part of a comprehensive health curriculum for every grade. Schools must ensure that students receive AIDS/HIV education appropriate to their age and their needs. They must not discriminate against children with HIV and must support the right of HIV-infected children to attend school.

Talk openly about HIV and AIDS.

Social injustice and social intolerance help spread HIV infection. Respect, understanding, tolerance, and compassion make it possible for those infected or at risk to cooperate with those who would help them. This approach helps all of us prevent the spread of HIV infection.

Do you have relatives, friends, or coworkers who may be at risk? Talk to them about HIV infection and AIDS. Even people who have difficulty listening to loved ones or authorities often will listen to friends. Get them to call the CDC National AIDS Hotline (1-800-342-AIDS) or a local AIDS hotline for more information.

Communities can stop HIV.

Community action is a very powerful weapon. The strongest educational and prevention efforts are those that involve all parts of the community: businesses, schools, civic and volunteer groups, religious organizations, and individuals. Community-based organizations in many areas are already actively involved in HIV education, services, and health care—and in raising money to pay for these activities.

The CDC has started a program called "Business Responds to AIDS" to provide businesses and workers with information about how to prevent work disruptions and new HIV infections among their employees, their families, and their community.

What can you do?

Does your community, club, organization, or religious group have a program to teach HIV prevention and help people with AIDS? Does your employer have an HIV education program? If so, support those programs. If not, start a program or talk to somebody who can.

There are many things you can do. You can make time to talk to people about HIV infection. You can help someone with AIDS. You can run errands for someone sick with AIDS. You can cuddle an HIV-infected baby with no parents. Even if all you do is improve the way you talk about people living with AIDS, you are taking a step in the right direction.

Summary of Centers for Disease Control and Prevention (CDC) AIDS Case Reports

Through December 1992, CDC had received 253,448 reports of AIDS cases. These included

- 221,714 cases in men, 27,485 cases in women, and 4,249 cases in children.
- 132,625 cases in non-Hispanic whites; 75,997 cases in non-Hispanic blacks; 42,199 cases in Hispanics; 1,610 cases in Asians/Pacific Islanders; and 448 cases in American Indians/Alaska Natives (race/ethnicity is unknown for 569 persons).

Racial and ethnic minority populations have been heavily affected by HIV infection and AIDS. Through 1992, 47 percent of all reported AIDS cases were among blacks and Hispanics, while these two population groups represent only 21 percent of the total U.S. population.

Although black and Hispanic women are 16 percent of all U.S. women, they are 74 percent of U.S. women reported with AIDS since 1981. Nearly 84 percent of children with AIDS who were infected before, during, or after birth are black or Hispanic. In New York State, AIDS has been the leading cause of death since 1988 for Hispanic children one to four years of age, and the second leading cause of death for black children in the same age group.

Through 1992, a total of 946 cases of AIDS among adolescents (13-19 years of age) were reported. In 1990, HIV infection and AIDS was the sixth leading cause of death among 15- to 24-year-olds in the United States.

Among adolescents reported with AIDS, older teens, males, and racial and ethnic minorities are heavily affected. Among adolescents with AIDS, the proportion of women has increased from 18 percent of all cases in adolescents in 1987 to 29 percent in 1992.

In recent years, the fastest growing groups of persons reported with AIDS in the United States have been women and men who acquired HIV through heterosexual contact. The new cases reported annually in these population groups have more than doubled since 1989 (women—1,172 in 1989, 2,437 in 1992), (men—782 in 1989, 1,677 in 1992). New AIDS cases reported annually in men who have sex with men have increased 22 percent over the same period (homosexual/bisexual men—19,652 in 1989, 23,936 in 1992).

Through December 1992, 27,485 AIDS cases were reported among U.S. adult and adolescent women. Nearly three-fourths of those cases were directly or indirectly associated with drug injection—50 percent (13,626) of these women reported injecting drugs themselves, and another 21 percent (5,896) reported having sex with men who injected drugs.

Although most women reported with AIDS were infected through shared needles and syringes, women who were infected through heterosexual contact have the highest rate of increase. HIV has been transmitted both from men to women and from women to men and has occurred mainly through vaginal intercourse. AIDS cases among U.S. women increased 17 percent between 1990 and 1991; among men, the increase during the same time period was 4 percent.

Need More Information?

In addition to this report, there are many other publications on HIV and AIDS, including guides for teaching HIV prevention and caring for AIDS patients. Many of them are available at no charge. To get copies, to find out what programs are available in your local area, or just to ask questions about HIV or AIDS, call the CDC National AIDS Hotline. The call is free and confidential, and you do not have to give your name to get your questions answered.

CDC National AIDS Hotline:

- English service (seven days a week, 24 hours a day) 1-800-342-AIDS (2437)
- Spanish service (seven days a week, 8 a.m. till 2 a.m. eastern time) 1-800-344-7432
- TDD service for the deaf (10 a.m. till 10 p.m. eastern time, Monday through Friday) 1-800-243-7889

National Institute on Drug Abuse Hotline:

- English service 1-800-662-HELP (4357)
- Spanish service 1-800-66-AYUDA (662-9832)

CDC National Clearinghouse for Alcohol and Drug Information:

- 1-800-SAY-NO-TO (1-800-729-6686)
- AIDS Clinical Trials Information Service (ACTIS): 1-800-874-2572 or 1-800-TRIALS-A

If you need more information about programs and services in your area, you can also call your local American Red Cross chapter or your state or local health department. Further information can also be obtained from:

CDC National AIDS Clearinghouse
PO Box 6003
Rockville, MD 20849-6003

■ Document Source:
Centers for Disease Control and Prevention
Health Resources and Services Administration
National Institutes of Health
June 1994

See also: Facts About the Human Immunodeficiency Virus and Its Transmission (page 3); Understanding HIV (page 21)

UNDERSTANDING HIV

The Immune System and HIV

The body's health is defended by its immune system. White blood cells called lymphocytes (B cells and T cells) protect the body from "germs" such as viruses, bacteria, parasites, and fungi. When germs are detected, B cells and T cells are activated to defend the body.

This process is hindered in the case of the acquired immunodeficiency syndrome (AIDS). AIDS is a disease in which the body's immune system breaks down. AIDS is caused by the human immunodeficiency virus (HIV).

When HIV enters the body, it infects special T cells, where the virus grows. The virus kills these cells slowly. As more and more of the T cells die, the body's ability to fight infection weakens.

A person with HIV infection may remain healthy for many years. People with HIV infection are said to have AIDS when they are sick with serious illnesses and infections that can occur with HIV. The illnesses tend to occur late in HIV infection, when few T cells remain.

Where did HIV and AIDS come from?

We may never know where or how HIV and AIDS began. Many experts believe that AIDS was present in the United States, Europe, and Africa for several decades or longer before the earliest cases appeared in 1980 and 1981.

HIV was first identified in 1984 by French and American scientists, but the human immunodeficiency virus did not get its name until 1986.

Purpose of this Booklet

Even before HIV causes AIDS, it can cause health problems. Learning about how the virus can affect your body and getting care early, before health problems worsen, can help you live longer and have fewer health problems.

This booklet is a guide to understanding HIV and getting the right care as soon as you can. You can also share this booklet with family members and friends so they can learn more about HIV.

The booklet will tell you about some of the problems you will probably have to face and suggests questions you may want to ask your doctor, nurse, or other health care provider. Asking these questions will help you get the information you need to make decisions about your own health care.

First Steps

Learn as much as you can about HIV. Finding out you have HIV infection can be frightening and confusing. Here are some questions you may want to ask your health care provider:

- What will HIV do to my health?
- Will I need to change the way I live?
- How will HIV affect my relationships with family, friends, sex partners, and people at work or school
- What types of health care or other services will I need, now and in the future?

Having HIV means that you can give HIV infection to someone else through unprotected (unsafe) sex or sharing needles or works if you inject drugs. Be sure to ask your health care provider how you can keep from spreading HIV.

Talking about Your HIV Status

Your HIV status is very personal, and telling other people that you have HIV infection may be one of the hardest things you will ever have to do.

When you first find out you have the virus that causes AIDS, you may feel sad, depressed, ashamed, or afraid. Telling other people about your HIV infection may mean that you will get more support and help from others, but it can also lead to problems.

Local or state laws may require that your health care provider report your HIV status to the health department. Otherwise, your HIV infection should be kept confidential, unless you decide to talk about it. Ask your doctor about the laws in your state.

Your health care provider can help you decide whom to tell and help you tell them once you have decided to do so. Some of the people you may want to tell include

- sex partners
- persons with whom you inject drugs
- family
- friends

You should talk with your sex partners about using condoms for safe sex and about the risks of having a baby with HIV. If you inject drugs, you will want to discuss the danger of sharing needles or works.

You may want to talk with members of your family about how your condition might affect them. You may also choose to tell your co-workers, neighbors, or members of your church, and if you are a student, people at school, such as the school nurse, administrators, teachers, and classmates.

Some people with HIV choose not to talk about their health, and that's all right too. It's your choice.

Talking about Your HIV Infection

Possible Benefits

- Support and help from family and friends
- In some states, better health and welfare benefits
- Greater chance that your sex partner or persons you have injected drugs with will get tested for HIV

Possible Risks

- Rejection by partner, family, friends, school, club, or employer
- Changes in health benefits
- Trouble finding a place to live
- Loss of child custody

Although the risks of sharing information about your HIV infection with others may seem to outweigh the benefits, remember that these are only risks and might never happen.

Taking Care of Yourself

If you have HIV infection, you may feel, look, and act just fine. But you need to take good care of yourself as soon as you find out you have HIV—this is the key to delaying the onset of more serious problems.

Try to keep a positive outlook. Hope is very important. Everyday there are new drugs and treatments for HIV that may help you. Each time you visit your doctor, be sure to ask about new treatments and clinical trials (research studies) in which you might take part.

Try not to worry. Worrying can lead to stress, and stress can weaken your immune system. Take steps to reduce stress. Activities that may relieve your stress include breathing exercises, leisure walks, reading, and community activities. Ask your health care provider about ways to cope with worry and stress.

See your doctor often. Don't wait until you get sick. The following hints may help you stay well longer:

- Get immunizations (shots) to prevent other infections.
- Avoid exposure to infection—for example, people with colds, other illnesses, and human or pet waste.
- Eat healthy foods. This will help keep you strong, keep your energy and weight up, and help your body protect itself.
- Exercise regularly to stay strong and fit.
- Get enough sleep and rest.
- Finish your medicines, even though you may feel better.

Tell your health care provider right away if you have numbness, sores in your mouth, changes in your eyesight, or shortness of breath.

Monitoring Your Immune System

One of the blood cells infected by HIV is the CD4 cell (a special T cell). Its job is to defend your body from invaders such as viruses. The number of CD4 cells in your blood shows how strong your immune system is.

A test called the "CD4 cell count" is used to check on the progress of HIV infection. Your health care provider will probably ask you to have blood tests every few months so that your CD4 cell count can be used to show when to start medicines.

As long as your CD4 count is over 600, you will need to have it tested about every six months. If your CD4 count drops below 500, your doctor may suggest testing your blood more often and may start you on medicine to slow HIV.

Starting Treatments

Your doctor should talk with you about the risks and benefits of starting treatment with drugs for HIV. AZT, now called ZDV (for zidovudine), is the most widely used drug for HIV. If ZDV does not work or causes side effects (for example, sleep problems, leg cramps, headaches, nausea, diarrhea, or anemia), your doctor may give you didanosine (ddI) or dideoxycytidine (ddC). Be sure to tell your doctor about any side effects you may have from ddI or ddC, such as belly pain or numbness in your hands or feet.

Remember, the treatments for HIV are changing rapidly, so be sure to ask your doctor if there are new treatments.

If your HIV infection worsens, you will be more likely to have other infections that take advantage of your weakened immune system. If your CD4 cell count falls below 200, or if you have had pneumonia or other symptoms, your doctor will probably recommend that you start taking trimethoprim-sulfamethoxazole or TMP-SMX (Bactrim®, Septra®, and generic products) to prevent the most common of these infections, *Pneumocystis carinii* pneumonia, or PCP. Most people have no problem with TMP-SMX, but if you develop a rash or severe stomach problems, stop taking the medicine and call your doctor right away to discuss other treatments.

HIV and HIV-related illnesses vary from person to person. Some people have been living with HIV for many years. Others become sick soon after their diagnosis. Your medical care plan will be designed especially for you and may differ somewhat from the care described in this booklet.

Here are some questions you should ask your doctor, nurse, or other health care provider:

- How often should my CD4 count be taken?
- At what CD4 count should I begin taking medicine for HIV infection?
- What about medicines to prevent other illnesses that can occur with HIV? How will these medicines help me?
- Do they have side effects?
- Are there new treatments?

Detecting and Treating Other Diseases

Tuberculosis

Because HIV weakens the body's ability to resist infections, you are at special risk for infection with the germ that causes tuberculosis (TB). Even if you become infected with this germ, proper treatment can keep it from turning into active TB. Be sure to ask your doctor, nurse, or other health care provider:

- How often should I be tested for TB infection? What kinds of tests are needed?
- How can I avoid becoming infected with TB?
- If I get TB, how can I avoid infecting others?

Tell your health care provider if you think you have been exposed to someone with TB.

If you become infected with the bacteria that causes TB, your doctor may give you the medicine, isoniazid (INH), which you will need to take once a day, every day, for a full year, even if you feel fine. Your doctor may also recommend that you take pyridoxine, a form of vitamin B6, each day to help reduce side effects from isoniazid. Be sure to tell your doctor about any side effects you may have from the medicine, such as nausea, vomiting, loss of appetite, tiredness or weakness, skin rashes, or fever.

Instructions for taking medication for TB infection can be confusing. Work closely with your health care provider to be sure you complete your treatment.

Syphilis

Syphilis is a sexually transmitted disease (STD). It often occurs with HIV infection but can be hard to recognize and treat in persons who have HIV. Untreated syphilis can cause severe nerve, heart, and blood vessel damage and even death.

You should tell your doctor about your full sexual and medical history. Some of the questions you may want to ask include:

- What are the tests for syphilis? How often should I be tested?
- How is syphilis treated?
- Will I need tests to make sure the treatment worked?
- How can I avoid passing syphilis to others?

Your doctor may give you blood tests to learn if you have syphilis and to see how far it has progressed. You also may need other tests. You should be tested for syphilis any time you think you have been exposed to an STD.

If you have syphilis, you should tell your sex partners or persons who have injected drugs with you. Your health care provider or a health department worker can help you do this and tell you whether the law in your state requires that your sex partners be notified.

Penicillin shots are the usual treatment for early syphilis. For more advanced disease, you may require intravenous (IV) penicillin and perhaps a hospital stay. If you are allergic to penicillin, you may need to see a specialist.

Mouth and Eye Problems

Mouth problems, such as candidiasis (thrush), and eye problems are some of the signs of HIV infection. Your health care provider should check your mouth and eyes at each visit. Be sure to:

- Tell your health care provider about changes in your eyes (blurry vision or infected eyes or eyelids) or mouth (sores, dryness, bleeding, difficulty swallowing, change in taste, pain, or loose teeth).
- Visit a dentist at least twice a year or more often if mouth problems develop.

Your doctor can treat most of your HIV-related mouth and eye problems. Sometimes you may also need to see a special dentist or an eye doctor.

Pap Tests for Women with HIV

Pap tests help detect cancer of the cervix (mouth of the womb) at an early stage. Women with HIV are more likely to have abnormal Pap smears.

- If you are a woman with HIV, your health care provider should check you for STDs and perform a Pap test at least once a year.
- If you have ever had cancer of the cervix, venereal warts, or an abnormal Pap test, you should have check-ups more often.

If your Pap test is abnormal, you may need to have a colposcopy. In this special type of examination, the doctor uses an instrument to get a close-up view of the cells and tissues of the vagina and cervix.

Pregnancy and HIV

If you become pregnant and decide to have your baby, the most important thing you can do is get good prenatal care. The chances of passing HIV to your baby before or during birth are about one in four, or 25 percent, for each pregnancy.

As a general rule, treatment for HIV infection in pregnant women is the same as for others who are not pregnant. You should have a Pap test during your pregnancy, and your doctor will probably recommend a CD4 count as soon as prenatal care begins. Depending on the results, you may not need another CD4 count during your pregnancy.

If you become infected with the TB germ while you are pregnant, your doctor can give you medicine, and chest x-rays may be used with proper precautions.

If you are pregnant and have syphilis, you will need special care. Babies born to women with untreated syphilis can become seriously ill or die. Here are questions to ask if you are HIV-positive and pregnant:

- Should I be tested for syphilis during pregnancy?
- What treatments are used for syphilis during pregnancy?
- Are they safe for my baby?
- Will I be cured? Will my baby be cured?

Your immune system may work differently during pregnancy, so your doctor will watch you closely. Here are some questions you may want to ask:

- Will pregnancy affect my HIV infection?
- Will the medicines I take for HIV be safe for me and my baby?
- Will my baby get sick?
- Are there special HIV drug studies for pregnant women?
- If so, how can I take part in such a study?

After birth, your baby should be tested regularly for HIV infection, whether or not HIV is present at birth. The baby also should be tested for syphilis, even if you were treated during pregnancy. Because HIV infection can be passed through breast milk, you should not breastfeed your baby.

Family Planning Decisions

If you are thinking about avoiding pregnancy or becoming pregnant, you should talk with your health care provider about the issues that are important to you, such as:

- If I choose not to get pregnant, what birth control methods would be best for me?
- Will pregnancy make my HIV infection worse? How?
- Will HIV infection mean other problems for me during pregnancy or delivery?
- Will my HIV infection and the treatments I may need cause problems for my baby?

- If I am pregnant and choose not to continue the pregnancy, where can I go to terminate the pregnancy?
- What if I am refused help because I have HIV?
- If I choose to get pregnant, what community programs and support groups can help me and my baby?
- Once I become pregnant, should I use condoms anyway? If my partner also has HIV, do we still need condoms?

Remember, although HIV-related illnesses can be treated, as yet there is no cure for HIV. This means the infection, and likely AIDS as well, will be a part of your family's future.

If you are weakened by HIV, both you and your unborn baby will be at greater risk for other serious infections. Because you have HIV, both you and your baby will need care. You will need to plan for the care of your child if you get sick.

Getting the Support You Need

A person or family living with HIV may need many kinds of support. Your health care provider and your local health and social services departments can help you find the support you need, including someone to

- answer your questions about HIV and AIDS.
- help you find health care providers, get insurance, make health care decisions, and obtain food and housing.
- provide transportation to and from health care appointments.
- assist in planning ways to meet financial and daily needs.
- refer you and your loved ones to support groups.
- arrange for home nursing care or rehabilitation services.
- represent you in legal matters.

Many people living with HIV feel better if they can talk with other people who also have HIV. Here are some ways to find others with HIV:

- Read HIV newsletters.
- Join support groups.
- Volunteer to help others.
- Be an HIV educator or public speaker, or write a newsletter.
- Attend social events to meet other people who have HIV.

Additional Resources

There are many sources of information about living with HIV. Look in the telephone book for

- Your local health department. They can tell you where to get tested for HIV and what services are available from public sources.
- Your local or state medical society to help you find a doctor.
- Your library. They may have many materials to help you learn about HIV and AIDS.

Some hospitals, churches, and the American Red Cross, as well as HIV and AIDS organizations, offer programs and sponsor support groups that may be listed in a special directory or your newspaper. Ask your librarian about newsletters and other printed materials.

Toll-free national hotlines and information clearinghouses can send you free publications and give you the latest news about drug-testing and clinical trials.

Here are some telephone numbers to help you get the information you need:

General Information

National AIDS Hotline
English (800) 342-AIDS (2437)
Spanish (800) 344-SIDA (7432)

TDD Service for the Deaf
(800) 243-7889

National AIDS Clearinghouse
(800) 458-5231

HIV/AIDS Treatment Information

American Foundation for AIDS Research
(800) 39-AMFAR (392-6327)

AIDS Treatment Data Network
(212) 268-4196
Project Inform (800) 822-7422

Clinical Trials Conducted by the National Institutes of Health or Food and Drug Administration-Approved Trials:

AIDS Clinical Trials Information Service
1-800-TRIALS-A (874-2572)

Social Security Disability Benefits

For confidential assistance in applying for social security disability benefits, call the Social Security Administration at (800) 722-1213. You also may request a personal earnings and benefit estimate statement (PEBES) to help you estimate the retirement, disability, and survivor benefits payable on your social security record.

Start your own list of services, support groups, and where to get information now.

For Further Information

The information in this booklet was taken from the *Clinical Practice Guideline on Evaluation and Management of Early HIV Infection*. The guideline was written by a panel of private-sector experts sponsored by the Agency for Health Care Policy and Research. Other guidelines on common health problems also are being developed.

To order another copy of this booklet, call the National AIDS Hotline toll-free at **(800) 342-AIDS**, or write to

AHCPR HIV Guideline
CDC National AIDS Clearinghouse
PO Box 6003
Rockville, MD 20849-6003

To order copies of AHCPR-sponsored guidelines on other topics, call **(800) 358-9295** (for callers outside the U.S.

only: (301) 495-3453) weekdays, 9 a.m. to 5 p.m., eastern time, or write to

Agency for Health Care Policy and Research
Publications Clearinghouse
PO Box 8547
Silver Spring, MD 20907

■ **Document Source:**
U.S. Department of Health and Human Services, Public Health Service
Agency for Health Care Policy and Research
Executive Office Center, Ste 501
2101 E Jefferson St
Rockville, MD 20852
AHCPR Publication No. 94-0574
January 1994

See also: Surgeon General's Report to the American Public on HIV Infection and AIDS (page 13); Voluntary HIV Counseling and Testing: Facts, Issues & Answers (page 26)

VOLUNTARY HIV COUNSELING AND TESTING: FACTS, ISSUES & ANSWERS

New Choices: HIV and AIDS medical care offers vital benefits.

There are clear benefits to early medical attention for infection with the human immunodeficiency virus (HIV), the virus that causes acquired immunodeficiency syndrome (AIDS).

If you are infected with HIV, the virus slowly weakens your ability to fight illness. But medical treatments, including medicines and earlier use of medications, can help your body resist the virus. They do this by slowing the growth of HIV and delaying or preventing certain life-threatening conditions.

For example, some medicines can prevent the type of pneumonia that is a common problem for people who have HIV or AIDS. Doctors can also find out when your immune system begins to weaken. By evaluating your immune system on a regular basis and vaccinating you against bacterial pneumonia and influenza, doctors can help you avoid illnesses related to HIV infection and treat them more effectively when they occur. Without the help of medical care your body may develop serious illnesses more quickly. For pregnant women, medical treatment with AZT (zidovudine) may reduce the chances of your baby being infected with HIV.

It is important that you consider these medical options as you decide whether to seek counseling and testing for HIV infection. Deciding whether to seek counseling and testing can be very hard. Your choice can have a major impact on your life. Medical options have increased the benefits of counseling and testing. This brochure gives you the information you need to understand these benefits and consider them with other issues important to you. Use this brochure to make the choice that is right for you.

What is HIV, and how do I become infected?

HIV, the human immunodeficiency virus, is the virus that causes AIDS. HIV is mainly transmitted by contact with the blood, semen, or vaginal fluids of infected people. The HIV-infected person can infect others, even if no symptoms are present.

HIV is transmitted by

- Having unprotected sex—vaginal, anal, or oral—with an infected person. Unprotected sex is sexual intercourse without consistent and correct condom use.
- Using or being stuck with a needle or syringe that has been used by or for an infected person.
- Giving birth. Women with HIV infection can pass the virus to their babies during pregnancy or childbirth. In some cases, they can also pass it on when breast-feeding.
- Receiving blood. Some people have been infected by receiving blood transfusions. However, the risk of infection through blood transfusions has been practically eliminated since 1985 when careful and widespread screening and testing of the blood supply for evidence of HIV became standard practice.

What happens if I become infected with HIV?

Being infected with HIV does not always mean you have AIDS. Being infected means the virus is in your body for the rest of your life. Therefore, you can infect others if you engage in behaviors that can transmit HIV. You can infect others even if you feel fine and no symptoms of illness are present. You can infect others even if you do not know you are infected.

HIV weakens your body's immune system. This means that HIV infection can make your body more and more vulnerable to other illnesses and infections over time. Early symptoms may include tiredness, fever, diarrhea, enlarged lymph nodes, loss of appetite, or night sweats. People with HIV infection can develop many different health problems. These include severe pneumonia, several forms of cancer, damage to the brain and nervous system, and extreme weight loss. These conditions signal the onset of AIDS, the most serious stage of HIV infection. Virtually all people with HIV infection will develop AIDS, but, with treatment, the HIV infection can usually be slowed and the onset of AIDS can be delayed.

How fast does HIV infection develop into AIDS? In some people, AIDS-related illnesses may develop within a few years. Without treatment, half of HIV infected people will develop an AIDS-related illness within 10 years. To stay healthy for as long as possible, it is important to learn your HIV status, obtain medical advice, monitor your health, and consider your treatment options.

The Best Way to Know Whether You Are Infected: HIV-Antibody Counseling and Testing

You cannot tell by looking at someone whether he or she has HIV infection. Someone can look and feel perfectly healthy and still be infected. Many people who have HIV infections do not know it. Neither do their sex partners.

The HIV-antibody test is the only way to tell whether you are infected. When any virus enters your body, your immune system responds by making proteins called antibodies. Different viruses cause the body to make different antibodies. You make antibodies to HIV when you have HIV infection. The HIV-antibody test detects HIV antibodies in your blood. It tells you whether you are infected with HIV. The test does not tell you if you have AIDS or when you will get AIDS. HIV antibodies are a sign of infection, but, unlike antibodies for many other infections, they do not protect your body from disease. They do not protect you from AIDS, do not make you immune, and do not prevent you from giving HIV to someone else.

The HIV-antibody test should always include before-test and after-test counseling. This counseling is to help you understand your result, how to protect your own health, and (if you are infected) how to keep from infecting other people. It is a central part of the testing process whether you are infected or not.

Should I seek HIV counseling and testing?

If you have engaged in behavior that can transmit HIV, it is very important that you consider counseling and testing. The following checklist will help you assess your degree of risk.

At Risk

There is evidence that HIV, the virus that causes AIDS, has been in the United States at least since 1978. The following are known risk factors for HIV infection. If you answer yes to any of these questions, you should definitely seek counseling and testing. You may be at increased risk of infection if any of the following apply to you since 1978.

- Have you shared needles or syringes to inject drugs or steroids?
- If you are a male, have you had unprotected sex with other males?
- Have you had unprotected sex with someone who you know or suspect was infected with HIV?
- Have you had a sexually transmitted disease (STD)?
- Have you received a blood transfusion or clotting factor between 1978 and 1985?
- Have you had unprotected sex with someone who would answer yes to any of the above questions?

If you have had sex with someone and you didn't know their risk behavior, or you have had many sex partners, then you have increased the chances that you might be HIV infected.

If you plan to become pregnant, counseling and testing is even more important. Without treatment, HIV-infected women have about a one-in-four chance of infecting their baby during pregnancy or delivery. Medical treatment can reduce this to about a one in 12 chance.

Reasons for Seeking Counseling and Testing

People consider counseling and testing for a number of reasons, some of which may apply to you:

- Knowing whether you have HIV infection would alert you to your need to seek medical care to prevent or delay life-threatening illness. Your test result (positive or negative) would also help your doctor determine the cause and best treatment of the various illnesses you may have now or in the future. For example, if you are HIV-positive, tuberculosis (TB) and syphilis are treated differently than if you are HIV-negative.
- If you find out you are infected, knowing your result would help you protect your sex partner(s) from infection and illness. If they are not infected, you can avoid infecting them.
- Knowing your result would help you assess the safety of having a child.
- Knowing your result, even if you are infected (positive test result) may be less stressful for some people than the anxiety of thinking you might be infected but not knowing. If your result indicates you are not infected (negative), you can take action to be sure you don't become infected in the future.

Reasons for Not Seeking Counseling and Testing

People may not seek counseling and testing for a number of reasons. For instance, if they are certain they have never engaged in behavior that could infect them with HIV, or had a blood transfusion, they do not need to be counseled and tested. Other reasons are less clear-cut. For instance, they think the stress of a positive test result—and the issues it would raise among family members, friends, and sex partners—would be more harmful than not knowing if they are infected. Perhaps they fear that others may find out their result without their permission. They might also be concerned about discrimination; some people have been denied housing, jobs, and insurance because they have HIV infection.

Many people are troubled by these concerns. You should decide for yourself whether these concerns outweigh the benefits of testing and early medical attention. The latest medical knowledge gives added weight to the benefits of knowing if you are infected. If you have any doubts about what you should do, get counseling. Then you can decide whether to go ahead with testing. However, if you decide NOT to be tested, you should prevent the transmission of any possible HIV in your body to sex or needle-sharing partners.

Understanding the HIV Counseling and Testing Process

It is very important that you understand the confidentiality policies of the testing center. Ask your testing counselor how they will protect your test results. Most counseling and testing centers follow one of two policies:

- Confidential testing

    The confidential testing site records your name with the test result. They will keep your record secret from everybody except medical personnel, or in some states, the state health department. You should ask who will know the result and how it will be stored. If you have your HIV-antibody test done confidentially, you can sign a release form to have your test result sent to your doctor.
- Anonymous testing (not available in all states)

    No one asks your name. You are the only one who can tell anyone else your result.

If you wish to be tested, ask your health department, doctor, or the CDC National AIDS Hotline (1-800-342-AIDS) about the location of facilities near you.

Deciding Where to Go for Counseling and Testing

Depending on the area where you live, there are different counseling and testing places from which to choose. These options include publicly funded HIV testing centers, community health clinics, sexually transmitted disease (STD) clinics, family planning clinics, hospital clinics, drug treatment facilities, TB clinics, and your doctor's office. In making your choice, you may want to consider these factors:

- If you have been to a particular place for health care before for other reasons, you may feel more comfortable with the staff who will counsel you and offer you testing.
- If the center can provide immune system monitoring and medical care if you are infected with HIV, it might speed up the beginning of your medical treatment.
- Some counseling and testing centers offer special features. For instance, if you use drugs, you can receive counseling, testing, and help for addiction at a drug treatment facility.

At some centers, such as doctor's offices or clinics, information about your test result may become part of your medical record and may be seen by health care workers, insurers, or employers. Your status may become known to your insurance company if you make a claim for health insurance benefits or apply for life insurance or disability insurance. If any health care provider proposes to test you for HIV antibodies, discuss the reasons and the potential benefits before deciding whether or not to take the test.

You can call the CDC National AIDS Hotline (1-800-342-AIDS) to get the address of places where you can get counseling and testing. Do not go to a hospital emergency room to be counseled and tested. You should go to an emergency room only if you have a health problem that demands urgent attention. Also, do not give blood at a blood donation center as a way to get tested for HIV antibodies. Blood donation centers are not HIV-antibody counseling and testing centers and should not be used as such.

The Process of Counseling and Testing

Counseling

You should be given materials to read before you enter a group or private session with a counselor or doctor. He or she might ask why you want to be tested. Your counselor should also ask about your behavior and that of your sex partner(s). This will help your counselor and you to determine whether testing is appropriate for you. If testing is appropriate, your counselor or doctor should

- describe the test and how it is done
- explain AIDS and the ways HIV infection is spread
- discuss ways to prevent the spread of HIV
- explain the confidentiality of the test results
- discuss the meaning of possible test results
- ask what impact you think the test result will have on you
- address the question of whom you might tell about your result
- discuss the importance of telling your sex and/or drug-using partner(s) if the result indicates HIV infection

If these questions are not covered, or if you have any other questions, ask them. You should come prepared with questions that have been on your mind. Also ask your doctor or counselor how you will be told of the test result. If your test result is negative, the post-test counselor will talk to you about how to avoid behaviors that will put you at risk.

Informed Consent

You have the right to refuse any medical procedure, to be fully informed about it, and to agree to it. You should be asked to read a statement saying that you have been informed about the HIV-antibody testing procedure, you understand it, and you consent to have it done.

The Blood Test

A small amount of blood will be drawn from your arm, taken to a lab, and tested. The time it takes to get results back varies in different areas. It can take anywhere from a few days to a few weeks.

The Waiting Period

This period of days or weeks can produce anxiety and tension. Some people decide during this time that they do not want to know their test result and never return to receive it. It is very important that you finish the process and find out the test result in spite of your anxiety.

It is also important that until you return for your result and post-test counseling you act as if you were infected and could transmit the virus. In other words, don't have unprotected sex or don't have sex at all and don't share needles.

When your result arrives, you may be asked to return to the counseling and testing center to receive the information in person. Everyone tested should receive counseling, whether the result is positive or negative.

Counseling after the Test

Your counselor should tell you your result and, regardless of whether it is positive or negative, how to protect your health and the health of others. He or she will review methods to prevent the spread of HIV.

If your result is negative, your counselor may discuss retesting if, during the six months before your test, you engaged in any behaviors that might have infected you. You may be infected but your body may not yet have produced enough antibodies for the test to detect. Since it takes time for your body to develop antibodies, you may need to be retested.

If your test is positive, your counselor will tell you what this means for you. Any questions you have should be answered and your counselor will refer you for follow-up health care, support services, or further counseling. Your counselor will also talk to you about telling your sex and/or drug-using partner(s).

Type of Tests

The ELISA (Enzyme-Linked Immunosorbent Assay) is a screening test that is widely used. It can be performed relatively quickly and easily. If a reactive (so called "positive") result occurs, the test is repeated to check it.

If an ELISA test yields two or more reactive results, a different test such as the Western blot is used to confirm these results as positive for HIV antibodies. The Western blot is more specific and takes longer to perform than the ELISA. Together, the two tests are more than 99.9 percent accurate. Further evaluation can be done if results of repeated ELISA and Western blot tests are unclear. Your testing facility should do the ELISA twice on the same blood sample and confirming test such as the Western blot if the ELISA tests are repeatedly reactive.

The Meaning of Your Test Result

Negative Result

A negative result means that no HIV antibodies were found in your blood. Your condition is called seronegative. This usually means you are not infected.

Testing negative does not mean you are immune to HIV. No one is immune to HIV. Even if you test negative, there are steps you should take to protect your health and the health of your sex and/or drug-using partner(s). Do not engage in behaviors that can transmit HIV. These behaviors include having sexual intercourse with an infected person or sharing needles or syringes with an infected person. Your post-test counselor will discuss these behaviors with you.

There is a small chance that you may be infected, even though you tested negative. It takes time for the body to develop HIV antibodies after infection. Almost all people develop HIV antibodies within three months, but it can take up to six months after infection for some persons. If you engaged in behavior that can transmit the virus during the six months just before your test, you may be infected but still test negative because your body may not yet have produced antibodies. To be sure, you must be retested at least six months after you last engaged in behavior that can transmit HIV.

Indeterminate Result

Once in a while, test results are unclear. The lab cannot tell whether they are positive or negative, even if the test has been performed correctly. If this happens to you, it is important that you discuss this with your counselor or doctor, and, if appropriate, be tested again. HIV-antibody test results are extremely accurate when proper procedures are followed. However, a very small number of people may test positive even though they are not infected. These are called false positive results. If you do test positive, you should discuss with your counselor or doctor whether retesting a new blood sample is appropriate.

Positive Result

A positive result means antibodies to HIV were found in your blood. This means you have HIV infection. Your condition is called HIV-positive, or seropositive. You will most likely develop AIDS, but no one can know when you will get sick. Within 10 years after infection, about half of untreated people have developed AIDS. However, prompt medical care may delay the onset of AIDS and prevent some life-threatening conditions.

If your test result is positive, there are a number of important steps you should take immediately to protect your health.

- See a doctor, even if you don't feel sick. Ask if this doctor has experience treating people with HIV infection and is familiar with AIDS and HIV-related issues. Tell the doctor your test result and discuss immune system monitoring and treatment. Monitoring and appropriate medical action are the ways to slow the growth of HIV and to delay the onset of AIDS.
- Have a tuberculosis (TB) test done. You may be unknowingly infected with TB. You could become seriously ill if your TB goes undetected. TB can be treated successfully if detected early in your HIV infection.
- Ask your doctor if you should get flu vaccine or other vaccines.
- Enroll in a program to help you stop using drugs, drinking a lot of alcoholic beverages, or smoking. This will help you reduce or stop engaging in behaviors that can weaken your body.
- Consider joining a support group for people with HIV infection. Such support can help you cope with being HIV infected.

You should take steps to protect the health of others:

- You may infect others if you engage in behaviors that can transmit the virus (unprotected sexual intercourse—vaginal, anal, or oral—or sharing drug needles or syringes).
- To reduce the risk of transmitting HIV if you have sexual intercourse, always use latex or plastic condoms. Use them from beginning to end every time you have sex and make sure to use them properly.
- There is no known risk of infection except in situations where we come in contact with blood, semen, or vaginal fluids.

- If you are a woman, you should understand the risks of pregnancy. Without medical treatment there is about a one-in-four chance that you will pass HIV to your unborn baby. With medical treatment the chance you will pass HIV to your baby can be reduced to one in 12. This treatment includes giving AZT (zidovudine) to the woman during pregnancy and labor. The baby must be given AZT for the first several weeks of life. There must be no breastfeeding by the infected mother.
- Do not donate blood, organs, sperm, corneas (eyes), or bone marrow. Revise any organ donor permissions you have given.
- Tell any doctor or dentist who treats you that you are infected.

You should tell anyone with whom you have had unprotected sex (vaginal, anal, or oral) or shared needles since 1978 that you are (and they may be) infected with HIV. It is especially important that you tell current and recent partners. Health professionals can tell your sex and/or drug-using partner(s) for you or help you tell them yourself. All of your present and past partners should be referred for counseling and testing. If they are HIV-positive, prompt medical care may delay the onset of AIDS and prevent some life-threatening conditions. Also, they may unknowingly infect others. You have an important role to play in helping stop the spread of HIV infection.

Telling people about your test result can be a very sensitive matter. You may want to discuss it with your testing counselor. They can assist you in telling your sex or drug-using partners. If you choose to tell your partners yourself, do not make accusations. Be prepared for partners to become upset or hostile. Urge them to be counseled and tested as soon as possible. You may want to give them a copy of this brochure.

How a Positive Test Result Might Affect Your Life

Being infected with HIV is not only a health matter. It raises financial and social issues as well. One of these issues is insurance. These issues should be discussed with a qualified counselor.

Your ability to pay for health care can affect your access to monitoring and treatment. If you do not have health insurance or if you depend upon Medicaid, you may need special assistance to get treatment.

As of 1994, four drugs that act to slow HIV have been approved for use in the United States. More drugs are being tested. To find out about experimental treatments, call the AIDS Clinical Trials Information Service (1-800-TRIALS-A, that is, 1-800-874-2572), Monday through Friday between 9 a.m. and 7 p.m. eastern time. Centers that offer experimental drug treatments for AIDS-related illnesses may not be available everywhere.

Some people who do not understand AIDS may avoid persons who they know are infected with HIV. Some people who are infected have been targets of discrimination in employment, housing, and insurance. Some have been deeply hurt by the reactions of friends and family members. You should be prepared to encounter uncomfortable reactions and to deal with these issues. However, the Americans with Disabilities Act (ADA) can protect you from many forms of discrimination, especially on the job, having a place to live, and getting services available to the public.

Answers to Your Questions

Here are answers to some questions you may have about HIV-antibody counseling and testing.

- Why get tested? If you know you are infected, you can take steps to protect your health and the health of others. There are clear benefits to early treatment, even though there is no cure for HIV infection. Medical options, including medications and other approaches, can help slow the infection and delay or prevent life-threatening conditions.
- I think I recently placed myself at risk of infection with HIV. Should I get counseled and tested right away? If you get infected with HIV, tests may not detect it until a few weeks after infection. The test detects HIV antibodies in your blood. If you are infected, your body takes time to make enough antibodies for the test to measure. It can take as little as two weeks. But it might take several months. Nearly all infected people develop antibodies within three months of infection. For some persons it may take up to six months. If you think you placed yourself at risk for HIV infection, you should get counseling, and until you know you are not infected, you should protect others as if you were infected.
- Does it take long to get an appointment to be counseled and tested? It depends on where you live. Some counseling and testing facilities can schedule appointments very quickly. Others may take a few weeks. Call your local health department to find out.
- How much does HIV counseling and testing cost? Most publicly funded testing sites are free or require only a minimum fee. If you go to your doctor for counseling and testing, the cost may vary. In some areas, it can be more than $200. You can ask the cost beforehand.
- When I had blood tests done for my physical, marriage license, or insurance, was I tested for HIV antibodies? Do hospitals routinely test for HIV infection? You should not assume that your blood was tested for HIV antibodies. If you are concerned, ask your health care provider specifically if your blood was or will be tested for HIV antibodies.
- If I'm pregnant or thinking about having a baby, should I be counseled and tested? If you or your sex or drug partner have engaged in behaviors that can transmit HIV, you should get counseling and testing. If you test positive, you should be aware that without treatment there is a one-in-four chance that you will pass the virus to your unborn baby. Medical treatment can reduce this to about one chance in 12. If you are already pregnant, you should tell your health care provider you tested positive. This will help your provider care for you and your baby during and after pregnancy.

- What if an insurance company wants me to take the test? An insurance company may require that you be tested for HIV infection if you apply for a health or life policy. You have the right not to take the test. You must choose whether to take the test or find an insurer who will not ask you to do so. If the test is required, either to determine if you will be covered or to set the rates, you may wish to be tested anonymously or confidentially first.

- Will my insurer find out if I test positive? Your insurer will know you took the test if you pay for the test through insurance. Insurers can find out your test RESULT only if you release it. On some insurance forms, your signature authorizes release of medical records. If you are concerned, do not sign medical release forms unless you know their purpose. You may also choose to be counseled and tested at a facility separate from your health care provider. These facilities include publicly funded testing sites, sexually transmitted disease clinics, and family planning clinics. Call your health department or the CDC National AIDS Hotline (1-800-342-AIDS) to find out the nearest facility that offers confidential counseling and testing.

- Does the Government keep track of those who test positive? The U.S. Public Health Services does not record or collect names of people who test positive. The state health departments that do collect names treat this information as highly confidential. Most states have laws against releasing confidential information without permission. Call your state or local health department to find out the laws in your state.

- Even though I tested negative, why do I have symptoms? See a doctor about your symptoms. They are most likely caused by something other than HIV infection. Early symptoms of HIV infection can be similar to the symptoms of many other diseases that occur in people who are not infected with HIV. If you test negative and still think you might be infected, consider retesting. If you test negative again, and you have not engaged in behavior that can transmit HIV in the past six months, you are probably not infected with HIV.

- My partner tested negative. That means I'm not infected, right? Your partner's test does not always tell your status. The only way to know whether you are infected is to have your own test.

- Can I continue to work if I have HIV infection? Yes, you can continue working if you have HIV infection. HIV cannot be spread by contact that does not involve blood, semen, or vaginal secretions. Many years after infection, some people still have no symptoms and continue to work productively. In the later stages of HIV infection, illness may cause you to be too sick to work. It depends on your health and your job duties.

- How can I find a doctor who will treat me? Call your local medical society. They should be able to refer you to a doctor who will help you. For additional help, you can contact a local AIDS organization. The people there may be able to help you find a doctor who is experienced with HIV and AIDS-related issues. For the telephone numbers of these organizations, call the CDC National AIDS Hotline [1-800-342-AIDS; Spanish 1-800-344-7432; Deaf access 1-800-243-7889 (TTY)].

■ **Document Source:**
U.S. Department of Health and Human Services, Public Health Service
Centers for Disease Control and Prevention

See also: Understanding HIV (page 21)

ALLERGIES/ASTHMA

■ ■ ■

ALLERGIC DISEASES

Who gets allergies?

Allergies are incredibly common. More than 50 million Americans—one out of five—suffer from allergic diseases. One out of every 11 office visits to the doctor is for an allergic disease.

Inheritance has a major influence on allergy. If one parent has allergies, the odds are that one in three of the children will have allergies. If both parents have allergies, then all the children will probably have allergies.

Aside from inheritance, it is not known why some people get allergies and others do not. Some believe that hormonal influences, viral infections, smoking, and a number of other influences affect whether one develops allergies. No one knows all the reasons why people with equal likelihood to develop allergies become allergic to different things, or why some have hay fever and others have asthma.

Second, a person has to be exposed to an allergen, a foreign protein that causes allergy. Ragweed pollen is the major cause of allergy in the United States. It is an unusual allergen that is found in high concentrations only in this country. Most people who move to the United States are exposed to ragweed for the first time. Many have never had allergies previously in their families for centuries, yet they develop allergies within two or three years of living in the United States. A large part of why they develop allergies is exposure to ragweed, which is an incredibly potent allergy-producing plant.

Each ragweed plant produces about one billion pollen grains during an average allergy season. Those pollen grains are very small—microscopic. They float in the air and may be carried out to sea as many as 300 or 400 miles. So it does not matter if people do not have ragweed plants in their backyards; they are clearly exposed to ragweed every place in the United States except for the arid southwest and southern California, where ragweed does not grow.

Other major allergens include grass pollens, tree pollens, dust, molds, and animal dander. Worldwide, however, the major allergen is the dust mite. All temperate climate areas in the world have dust mites, which live in carpeting, mattresses, and upholstery. They have to have temperatures above 60 degrees to reproduce. Most people keep the temperature in their homes above 60 degrees all year. Dust mites also need a relative humidity above 50 percent.

People are not actually allergic to the dust mite; they are allergic to its feces. The fecal balls are sticky, heavy materials that bind to carpeting or upholstery. One of the worst ways to bring dust mite allergens into the air is to vacuum the floor; this blows the dust up into the air, where it floats for a couple of hours and makes up the motes in a beam of sunlight.

How do allergies work?

There are three components to allergies: mast cells, which contain chemicals like histamine; antibodies, a specific type of protein made by the immune system, known as IgE; and allergens, which trigger the reaction. Mast cells are the allergy-causing cells and are found in every tissue throughout the body, though they are most heavily concentrated in those tissues that are exposed to the outside world—the skin, linings of the nose and lungs, gastrointestinal tract, and reproductive system.

The IgE antibody, which actually causes allergy, sits on the surface of these mast cells. A mast cell has about 1,000 histamine-containing granules in its cytoplasm, and on its surface are between 100,000 and one million receptors for IgE. When the IgE encounters the allergen, it triggers the mast cell to release granules from its cytoplasm. Those granules contain histamine and other chemicals. These mediators that are released then interact with the tissues, causing the allergic symptoms.

With ragweed, for example, the pollen grains from the plant are male gametes equivalent to sperm. They carry the male genetic code from a male ragweed plant to a female ragweed plant. Since the pollen grains are wind borne and do not have a particular way of finding a female plant, many excess pollen grains are produced in the hopes that one or another will find a female plant and fertilize it.

On the surface of a pollen grain are enzymes that help the pollen grain enter female plants. Unfortunately, people breathe in pollen grains that are floating in the air. When a pollen grain gets on the skin that lines the inside of the nose, those enzymes are released from the pollen grain and work their way through the mucus in the nose. The enzymes sensitize the person by initiating the production of IgE antibodies, which then sensitize mast cells that are in the nose. It generally takes about two to five seasons of allergen exposure before a person makes enough IgE to result in allergy symptoms.

Everyone makes some IgE. Only people with genetic predispositions toward allergies make large quantities. IgE, like other antibodies that the body produces, is part of the body's defense mechanism. Some antibodies, like IgG, get rid of Streptococcus and help cure those infected with a strep throat. Other antibodies get rid of cold viruses. The IgE antibody is directed against parasites. Its function is to protect the body against parasitic infections. There are few parasites in the United States, but the IgE antibody system reacts against the enzymes from the surface of pollen grains as if they were parasites and elicits an allergic response. The body is misdirecting an extremely important immune response at pollens, dust, dander, and molds.

Most antibodies last in the body about three weeks, but IgE may sit on its receptor on mast cells and sensitize the mast cells for years. For example, someone who had an adverse allergic reaction to penicillin as a child could still be allergic to the drug as an adult. The IgE antibody the person made as a six-year-old child would still be present in the 40-year-old adult. It is sitting on the mast cells, which are long-lived cells, and it conveys incredibly long-lived sensitivity to allergens.

In one research study, we looked at mast cell histamine release under the electron microscope. We sensitized a mast cell to IgE, making it allergic to grass, trees, ragweed, and certain breeds of cats and dogs. We then took this mast cell and exposed it to an extract of ragweed. Over a 15-minute period, many of the granules in its cytoplasm disappeared. Fifteen minutes later, the granules were all gone.

Although the mast cell had no visible secretory granules in its cytoplasm, it was alive and well; over the next six to 24 hours it would reconstitute all the granules that had disappeared. After releasing histamine from its granules, a mast cell can once again do damage to the person the next day when he or she breathes in ragweed.

The chemicals that are released from mast cells are the mediators that cause allergies. At last count, there were 28 separate chemicals released by mast cells that orchestrate allergic responses. The allergic symptoms a person experiences depend on the tissue in which the mediators are released. For example, if these chemicals are released in the nose, the person will get hay fever, allergic rhinitis. If they are released in the chest, the person will get asthma or coughing. Chemicals released in the skin will produce hives or eczema, in the intestine will produce food allergy or diarrhea, and in the brain may result in a migraine. There is a whole spectrum of problems that these mediators can cause.

Allergic reactions often take place very quickly. Those who experience allergy may go outside on a bright, sunny, windy morning during the ragweed season and within 15 minutes begin to have allergic reactions. This reaction is referred to as immediate hypersensitivity. When mast cells release their chemicals, they cause immediate reactions.

Some people also experience late-phase reactions. When mast cells release their chemicals, they cause an inflammatory response. The site of the allergic reaction gets red, swollen, hot, and tender, causing a more prolonged response. A person may go out at 8 a.m. and experience a late reaction at 4 p.m. Such reactions may last one day, two days, one week, or one month from a single allergen exposure. They are part of the underlying problem for chronic asthma, rhinitis, eczema, hives, and other allergic diseases.

How are allergies diagnosed?

Allergy is diagnosed through skin testing, which shows an immediate reaction to allergens. The procedure traditionally involves introducing a minute amount of allergen into the skin. The tip of the needle is used to puncture the skin, causing an interaction between the allergen and a mast cell.

When doctors administer skin tests, they are introducing allergen into the skin and causing the same reaction that the patients experience in their noses or lungs during the allergy season. In the past, doctors used to take small needles and inject them under the skin surface and put a minute amount of allergen in the skin. Within 15 minutes a welt formed, like a mosquito bite, if the patient had a positive reaction. That was minimally uncomfortable, but it was still uncomfortable.

Today, doctors use a needle to put a drop of allergen on the skin without breaking the skin surface. They "tent" the skin by putting the needle through the droplet and lifting up the skin without breaking the skin surface. It is essentially painless, yet it is very sensitive and specific.

Diagnosis, preferentially, is done by skin testing. Skin tests are fast; they take about 5 minutes to administer and can be read within 15 minutes. They are very sensitive, relatively cheap, cause minimal discomfort, but require some medical expertise.

A second way to diagnose allergy is with a blood test that looks for IgE antibodies. This test is relatively expensive, slightly less sensitive, requires a blood drawing, and does not require expertise. It is done frequently by non-allergists who want to see if the patient has allergies. In proper hands, both tests are equally informative.

Allergic Rhinitis

Allergic rhinitis (hay fever) is a disease of incredible proportion. Thirty-five million Americans—17 percent of the population—experience allergic rhinitis. It is the single most common chronic disease experienced by human beings. As a single entity, one out of every 40 doctor office visits (2.5 percent) are due to allergic rhinitis.

Allergic rhinitis is caused by exposure to airborne allergens. The process of allergic rhinitis takes place in the nose. Pollen grains, dust, and dander are trapped by hairs in the nose and are trapped in the mucus that lines the inside of the nose. The allergens release soluble proteins that reach the mucous membranes, causing allergic rhinitis.

The skin that lines the inside of the nose is a succulent tissue full of glands and blood vessels. The submucous glands in this living tissue produce the mucus in the nose. In fact, that is why the lining is called a mucous membrane—it specifically makes mucus. Although many people think of mucus as a bother, mucus is quite helpful.

Mucus is important because it humidifies and protects the mucous membrane. It contains antimicrobial factors that protect people from both bacterial and viral infections. When people get colds, it is despite the fact that they have mucus; if they did not have that mucus, they would have infections all the time.

What about nasal congestion? The body has cavities in the lining of the nose where blood can pool. The nose can become swollen with blood pooling in these sinusoids. When blood is diverted into these sinusoids, this tissue gets markedly enlarged and the person cannot breathe through his or her nose. Everyone experiences nasal congestion; every 45 minutes to two hours, one side of the nose congests and the other side constricts. People breathe preferentially through one side, resting the other side, and then alternating sides. One never breathes evenly through both sides of the nose because of this process of congestion. Of course, during allergic rhinitis it gets much worse and the allergy sufferer experiences more severe, chronic nasal congestion.

What can the mucous membrane do? It can congest by pooling blood in these sinusoids; it can become itchy or sneezy by stimulating some of the sensory nerves in the nose; and it can produce secretions. These are the processes that people experience when they have rhinitis—allergic rhinitis, vasomotor rhinitis, rhinitis from colds, or from eating hot and spicy foods.

The most common features of allergic rhinitis are sneezing attacks and itching of the nose, eyes, pharynx, and palate. Clicking the tongue on the top of the mouth is the way one scratches the soft palate, and the soft palate itches if one has allergic rhinitis. One also gets a runny nose or congestion of the nose.

To confirm a diagnosis of allergic rhinitis, the doctor performs a nasal examination and looks for changes in the mucous membrane. If the patient has allergic rhinitis, the mucous membrane becomes very pale because it is swollen. In fact, it takes on a whitish-blue tint. It is very wet with a watery secretion. A smear of the mucus would be loaded with a type of white blood cell known as an eosinophil, which is very characteristic of allergic diseases, and the patient would have an increase of eosinophils in his or her blood. If the doctor does a skin test or a blood test, called a RAST test, which measures an increase in the patient's IgE antibody, both would be positive.

There are two kinds of allergic rhinitis—seasonal and perennial. Seasonal allergic rhinitis characteristically occurs as spring-fall allergies. Springtime begins with tree allergies. Grass is another major springtime allergen.

In the eastern United States, there are few allergens in July and early August, and individuals with allergic rhinitis get better. Pollen from plants that bloom in the summer is spread by the insects, not by the wind, so that is a good time for most people unless they are allergic to molds. Seasonal allergies begin again when ragweed pollinates, starting from mid-August and lasting until the first frost.

Some people also have seasonal allergies to dust during the winter months when the house is closed up and the dust mite feces are richest in the air. But most people with dust allergy have year-round—perennial—symptoms.

Other things that cause year-round allergies are molds. Many people who live in humid areas have damp cellars in which molds form. These molds cause major problems for people with mold allergies.

The other common cause of year-round allergies is allergens from pets. Cats are the worst source of pet allergens, much worse than dogs. The source of allergen from cats is not their fur or skin; it is their saliva, or the proteins in their saliva. And what do cats do all day? They preen. They put saliva on their fur, the saliva dries, aerosolizes, and is the source for the allergen. Dogs—sloppy, friendly little animals that they are—only preen selected parts of their bodies and are much less likely to expose humans to salivary allergens.

Dogs are still a major source of allergy, especially if they slobber, but if one had to choose between the two, one would choose a dog over a cat. Ideally, allergy sufferers would not have any furred animals in the house because they all cause allergy. Cockroaches also are a major source of year-round allergens.

How is allergic rhinitis treated?

Seasonal allergic rhinitis generally has a better prognosis because it is not a year-round exposure. It is easier to treat and tends to be much less severe. By contrast, perennial disease tends to be much more difficult to treat and is harder to control.

When treating patients with allergic rhinitis, doctors try specifically to take away the causes of the disease. By using allergy avoidance, they get rid of the allergen and the patient is better. Other common treatments include antihistamines, allergy immmunotherapy (allergy shots), a drug called cromolyn sodium, and topical corticosteroids.

To avoid pollen allergens, one must know when the pollen counts are highest. They are generally highest early in the morning, about 6 a.m., on a bright, sunny, breezy day. That is the time allergy sufferers should try to stay inside. If they ride in a car, they should use the car air conditioner. Allergy sufferers should use their house air conditioner, too. Air conditioning filters the air very well, taking out more than 99 percent of all the pollen- and allergen-producing material in the air. If people who are very sensitive during the ragweed, grass, or tree season must go outside in the yard, they should wear nuisance masks, which are like surgical masks and available in drug stores. They are comfortable and will reduce the likelihood of inhaling allergens.

Those with dust allergy should design their bedrooms accordingly. The worst things to have in the bedroom of an allergic person are venetian blinds, which are dust traps; down-filled blankets; feather pillows; heating vents with forced hot air; carpeting; dogs; cats; and closets full of clothing.

Instead of venetian blinds, people should have shades over the windows because they cannot trap dust. If curtains are used, they should be washable curtains that are cleaned periodically in hot water to kill the dust mites. A hardwood or linoleum floor is best, but a washable throw rug is acceptable if it is cleaned in hot water regularly. The bedding should be encased within allergen-proof encasements that are airtight to keep in dust mites, along with their feces. Pillows should be hypoallergenic and replaced every one to two years because when people sleep, they sweat and the sweat makes the pillows moldy over time. Blankets and bedding should be hypoallergenic—definitely not down-filled. If at all possible, clothing should be kept in another room. Ideally, the closets would be empty in order to remain dust free. Heat registers should be covered with a filter. New products are appearing in the market that can kill dust mites in carpeting and may prove to be a boon to allergy sufferers.

Allergy shots are extremely effective. Eighty-five percent of the people who receive allergy shots to treat hay fever due to grass, ragweed, trees, and dust get better. It usually takes one to two years. Many people get better for years, and some even permanently. Allergy shots, which are the only known way to turn off allergic disease, reduce the production of IgE and cause the body to make another class of antibody called IgG, which actually protects people from allergic diseases. Shots are the only method available for long-lasting protection from allergies.

Patients with problems only two to four weeks of the year usually are treated with medications. Those with perennial disease are more likely to be put on allergy shots unless their condition can be controlled completely with allergy medications.

There are several medications available to treat allergic rhinitis. One is cromolyn sodium administered in the nose, which prevents allergic reactions from taking place. This drug actually stops the release of chemical mediators like histamine from the mast cell. It is often a very effective therapy. Unfortunately, it must be used about four times a day as a nasal spray.

A second major improvement in therapy of allergic rhinitis has been the use of topical nasal steroids. These steroids are not anabolic steroids. They are anti-inflammatory steroids that stop the late phase reaction. They reduce the number of mast cells in the nose, reduce mucus secretion and swelling, and have other beneficial actions. Because they are given topically, they have no effects elsewhere in the body—only in the nose.

The other major medication used is antihistamines. Over the last five or six years, nonsedating antihistamines have become available. These antihistamines are just as effective as older antihistamines, but they do not cause sleepiness. However, they are considerably more expensive than some of the over-the-counter antihistamines.

Antihistamines work beautifully for immediate hypersensitivity. They reduce sneezing, itching, runny nose, and partially reduce the congestion of allergic rhinitis. Unfortunately, they have no effect on late phase reactions. Antihistamines and nasal steroids are effective combinations to treat allergic rhinitis.

Asthma

Fifteen million people—seven percent of those who live in the United States—have asthma. It is the number one cause for school absenteeism among all chronic diseases. It is the number six cause for hospitalization of all diseases and the number one cause for hospitalization of children.

It is estimated that $4.5 billion is spent every year on medically related charges for the treatment of asthma. That includes hospital and doctor visits. This is an extremely important disease that kills as many as 4,000 Americans a year.

Asthma is a disease of the airways, the tubes through which people breathe. The causes of airflow obstruction in asthma are swelling of the airways, excessive mucus production, inflammation of the airways with eosinophils and neutrophils, and airway smooth muscle contraction. Asthmatic airways are full of secretions, mucus containing eosinophils and neutrophils—white blood cells—that reflect the underlying inflammation. The epithelial cells that line the airways have been lifted off and the airways are denuded. The muscles contract, closing the airways, and the glands are very reactive and produce large quantities of mucus.

Asthma is an inability to breathe out. Normally when people breathe in, they lower their diaphragms, raise their ribs, and breathe in. It is an active process. To breathe out, they stop breathing in. Breathing out is passive. They breathe out because the lungs are made of elastic tissue, like a rubber band. When a person stops breathing in, the lungs try to assume their relaxed size and do so by letting the air out—if there is no obstruction.

Asthmatic airways have excess mucus, are swollen and inflamed, and have their muscles contracted. As people with asthmatic airways breathe in, they open up their chests and their lungs get bigger. As a result, the airways get bigger and they can move air around these obstructions. They have opened up the airways. When they stop breathing in to breathe out, these obstructions close, thereby trapping the air in the lungs.

Take a deep breath to the maximum and do not let it out for the next minute. Breathe at the top of your lungs and do not let out any air. That is what it feels like to have asthma. Asthmatics trap two liters of air in their chests, which is the amount of air in a basketball. They have to breathe at the top of their lungs. It is exhausting and feels terrible.

What causes asthma?

The most common cause of asthma is allergy. Of the children under 16 years old who have asthma, 90 percent are allergic. Of the people under 30 who have asthma, 70 percent are allergic. Of the people over 30, 50 percent have allergies.

Asthma also may be caused by infections such as bronchitis, which is a wheezing disease that effects children less than two years old and is caused by a viral infection of the airways. This disease leads to asthma; more than half the children who get bronchiolitis have asthma until they are at least seven years old.

Adults with asthma also get infections that make their asthma worse. They will have colds that commonly develop into bronchitis. Because their lungs are inflamed, the lungs get irritated by a cold very readily and go into an asthmatic attack.

Drugs like aspirin cause asthma in 10 percent of asthmatics. Aspirin and aspirinlike drugs specifically cause asthma in a population of patients that have recurring sinusitis, or infections of the sinuses, and have nasal polyps.

Other drugs that may cause asthma or make it worse are beta-adrenergic blocking agents, which are used for treatment of such conditions as migraine, too rapid a heart rate, congestive heart failure, tremor, and glaucoma.

A third type of agent that may cause asthma is sulfiting agents, which are chemicals that are added to processed foods to keep them from turning brown. If a food should ordinarily turn brown and has not, it has sulfiting agents in it. This includes dried fruits, fruit juices, vegetables, and wines. As sulfites are eaten, they mix with acids in the stomach and become sulfuric acid, which is a gas. The gas travels up through the esophagus, is breathed in, and provokes asthma.

Industrial and occupational exposures also have a bad effect on asthma. On smoggy days, the air is loaded with exhaust from motor vehicles. This is a major source of pollutants, and people with asthma experience increased asthmatic symptoms as a result.

How is asthma diagnosed?

An allergist will do spirometry to measure the patient's ability to blow air out of the chest. The patient takes a deep breath and blows into a machine called a spirometer. The doctor then measures how much and how quickly air was blown out. Most people blow all the air in their chest out within three seconds; 75 percent of the air is exhaled within one second. The point of maximum expiration is called the "peak flow."

Asthmatics have trouble blowing out the air. That is because of airflow obstruction during breathing out. As a result, they have a very hard time blowing out air and it takes much longer.

Over the past few years, the availability of inexpensive and accurate peak flow meters has made life easier for doctors. Patients can measure their own peak flow in the morning and evening. The patient blows into the flow meter and it measures the peak expiratory flow rate.

For home use it is reliable and inexpensive. A patient can use it before and after taking bronchodilators. It tells the doctor how much airflow increased with the use of bronchodilators and can be used to regulate medications. It also tells the doctor when the patient is doing well, and warns when trouble is coming.

Airway hyperresponsiveness is increased reactivity of the airways, a "twitchiness" of the airways. Asthmatics have nonspecific airway responsiveness. They react when breathing in certain chemicals, including irritants and chemical mediators, or under certain physical conditions like exercise. The importance of airway hyperreactivity is that it clearly separates those who do not have hyperreactivity from asthmatics. Airway hyperreactivity actually predicts who will develop asthma. Patients who have abnormal hyperreactivity are very likely to be predisposed to developing asthma under the right conditions.

There is a range of abnormal airway hyperreactivity among people with asthma, ranging from mild to severe, and doctors can use that range of near normal to very abnormal to determine which medications are required.

Airway hyperreactivity gets worse with allergic reactions that cause late phase reactions. But airway hyperreactivity can get better if the patient avoids allergens, goes on allergy shots, and uses inhaled cromolyn or corticosteroids. Recently, it has been recognized that one of the major targets for the treatment of asthma is airway reactivity.

How is asthma treated?

In order to treat asthma and airway reactivity, doctors recommend that asthma patients avoid the allergens to which they are sensitive whenever possible. They put the patients on allergy shots if they have allergic asthma in hopes of reducing the allergic contribution to the asthma. They use inhaled cromolyn, which stops allergic reactions, and often use inhaled corticosteroids, which stop inflammation of the airways and reduce airway hyperreactivity.

With all patients, doctors also use symptomatic treatment of asthma involving agents that relax the airways. These agents include beta-adrenergic agonists, theophylline, anticholinergics, and occasionally expectorants and mucolytics. These medications are employed to try to reverse the airflow obstruction, but they do not have any effect on the underlying causes of asthma.

Until recently, the therapy of asthma was based on the drug theophylline. This drug is an excellent, time-proven, time-tested, and very reliable bronchodilator that opens up asthmatic airways. It was the foundation of asthma therapy from 1970 to 1990.

In the 1980s beta-adrenergic agents became available. These medications relax the airways and make many people better. They became very important in asthma therapy, and have become the predominant drug used to relax airways.

In 1990, asthma therapy shifted so that all asthmatics are now treated with specific therapy aimed at the underlying causes of the disease—allergy avoidance, inhaled corticosteroids, perhaps allergy shots, and perhaps inhaled cromolyn. Nearly all patients use inhaled corticosteroids or cromolyn for the treatment of their airway inflammation. For control of airway obstruction, patients use beta-adrenergic agonists, as well as theophylline and ipratropium, which is an anti-cholinergic agent. Theophylline, however, has gone from being the foundation of treatment to a second-line therapy. It is added later and taken away sooner.

What about general treatments? It is recommended that all asthmatics exercise. Some patients have exercise-induced asthma, so it sounds contradictory, but with the proper medications every asthmatic—particularly children—can and should exercise. Swimming is the preferred form of exercise; biking is the second preferred; and running is the least preferred. It is recommended that asthmatics do not smoke, and that people with asthmatic children stop smoking. Patients are advised to monitor their pulmonary function with a home peak flow meter and learn as much as possible about asthma.

Questions and Answers

Q. Nobel Laureate Linus Pauling made mention of the fact that vitamin C has some effect on allergic reactions. What is the latest on that?

A. Scientifically, it has not been proven that vitamin C has any effect, beneficial or detrimental, on allergies. It is not harmful, at least in reasonable doses, but it will not help the disease.

Q. How are food allergies effectively identified and then treated?

A. Dr. Dean Metcalfe, here at the National Institute of Allergy and Infectious Diseases, screened adults for food allergy, and he found that when people came in and said, "I'm allergic to strawberries," they were likely to be allergic to strawberries. If people came in and said, "I'm allergic to food," they were almost never allergic to food. When people come in and can identify the food to which they are sensitive, we can confirm that by skin testing. In the case of a specific allergen, the skin tests are positive almost all the time. And, if we do a double-blind food challenge, it is frequently positive.

We have many examples where people have said, "I haven't been able to eat eggs for 25 years," and we skin tested them and the tests were negative. We did a provocation challenge, and the only response was they did not care for the taste of eggs. So, the skin test plus a good history is how we screen for food allergies.

Q. Have you ever observed any ophthalmological effects from allergies such as double vision?

A. The eye is always involved in allergy, but the symptoms are generally itching, swelling, and redness. Eye movement and visual acuity are not affected.

Q. What advice would you give to parents, both of whom suffer from allergies, regarding the introduction of foods for their infant children?

A. Our instructions are very simple. We would recommend, especially if you have two allergic parents, that solids not be introduced until the children are at least six months of age. We recommend exclusive breast-feeding through at least the first six months. There is some suggestion that very allergenic foods, like cow's milk and peanuts, should be avoided by the mother during breast-feeding because she can transfer some allergens in breast milk. But the opportunity for a child to become allergic to allergens in breast milk is very limited versus drinking cow's milk. Thus, breast-feeding is highly recommended.

Q. I have two questions. First, what are the possible side effects of allergy medications and how often do they occur? Second, I read that in some cases either asthma or hay fever, or some combination, can be due to emotional problems. Is there any information about that?

A. It has often been claimed that asthma is a psychological disease. That is not the case. Asthma is a real, very important disease that can kill you. It may be worsened by psychological stresses, but it is not caused by stress. It is not psychological. The parents of asthmatics often feel very guilty that their child has asthma, and they wonder if it is their fault in some way that influenced their child's asthma. That is not the case.

The side effects for drugs is a very broad question, very hard to answer, but I can tell you that the agents that we use today have been selected from many others because of their efficacy versus their very limited side effects. And the reason that theophylline is being used less today is because it has some side effects we wish to avoid.

Q. I would like your comment on sinusitis. Is it associated with allergies?

A. Sinusitis is an infection of the sinus areas of the skull, which are between the eyes, on either side of the cheeks, in the forehead, and center of the head. They are frequently associated with allergies and the development of sinus congestion; sinus infections are frequent accompaniments of allergy.

Q. What about the long-term effects of corticosteroids? Did I understand you to say that that was no problem?

A. Corticosteroids have major complications associated with them. In the past, we balanced the use of oral corticosteroids, which have systemic side effects, with the effects of the disease. When the disease was bad enough, we gave oral steroids and accepted the side effects if we had to. Now, with topical, inhaled steroids, we have little or no systemic effects, so we get all the beneficial capabilities of steroids with none of the unwanted side effects.

Q. Why do some medications like Benadryl, which you might give a child for hives, say, "Do not give to a child with asthma"? Is it dangerous to give a child Benadryl when he or she has hives and not asthma?

A. That is an interesting and good question. The classical (older) antihistamines, like Benadryl, if you read the label, are not supposed to be used in asthma. Testing in the early 1950s suggested that antihistamines made asthma worse. So there is a label insert that says they should not be used in asthma. We do not use any of the classical or older antihistamines for the treatment of asthma because they do not work very well. Despite the labeling, however, we do not believe they have any danger for people with asthma.

Some of the new, nonsedating antihistamines do have some efficacy in asthma, and they are being used cautiously for asthma treatment. These new antihistamines have no limitations on their use in asthma and may, indeed, be useful.

Q. I wondered if there has ever been a program to eradicate ragweed.

A. Yes, there has been. A woman in the Pennsylvania area and her family had terrible ragweed allergies and she organized the community to eradicate ragweed. It did not make any difference because ragweed moves through the air for such a long distance.

Q. Many of the over-the-counter antihistamines say, "Do not take it for more than seven days." If I want to take them longer, should I get a prescription from a doctor?

A. Antihistamines have been available since the 1940s and many people have taken antihistamines for more than 30 years. They have been among the world's safest drugs. That does not mean that you should use an over-the-counter antihistamine without caution. By and large, we would recommend that everyone would benefit from an appropriate diagnosis and proper therapy, which might include over-the-counter drugs, but might also include prescription drugs, which are really quite a bit more potent and maybe more specific.

■ Document Source:
National Institutes of Health
Clinical Center Communications
NIH Publication No. 91-3221
April 1991

FOOD ALLERGY AND INTOLERANCES

Food allergies or food intolerances affect the lives of virtually everyone at some point. People often may have an unpleasant reaction to something they ate and wonder if they have a food allergy. Almost one out of three people either say that they themselves have a food allergy or that they modify the family diet because a family member is suspected of having a food allergy. But only about three percent of children have clinically proven allergic reactions to foods. In adults, the prevalence of food allergy drops to about one percent of the total population.

This difference between the clinically proven prevalence of food allergy and the public perception is, in part, due to reactions that are termed "food intolerances" and not food allergies. A food allergy, or hypersensitivity, is an abnormal response to a food that is triggered by the immune system. The immune system is not responsible for the symptoms of a food intolerance, even though these symptoms can resemble those of a food allergy.

It is extremely important for people who have true food allergies to identify them and prevent allergic reactions to food because these reactions can cause devastating illness and, in some cases, be fatal.

Allergy Symptoms

There is a wide range of food allergy symptoms. This variability of symptoms stems from the large number of tissues in the body which can be affected by an immune reaction to food.

Frequently the first part of the body to react to food is the gastrointestinal tract. The allergic reaction in this portion of the body can cause vomiting, abdominal pain, and diarrhea. As the immune response to food affects other areas of the body, a person may develop hives (urticaria), swelling, sneezing and a runny nose, asthma, or difficulty breathing.

The most severe food allergy reaction is anaphylaxis—a systemic, life-threatening shock that can occur minutes after a person eats a food to which they are allergic. Anaphylactic reactions to food probably result in as many as 50 deaths a year in the United States. One of the characteristic features of this kind of reaction is trouble breathing caused by edema (swelling) of the throat or bronchi; it can also cause severe asthma, hives, a drop in blood pressure and loss of consciousness, and death, if not treated immediately.

Eczema due to food allergy is a different kind of reaction in which the target organ is the skin, which becomes crusty, red, scaly, and itchy. In children, eczema is frequently due to foods, but it can also be a preexisting condition made worse by certain foods. Probably fewer than one in twenty adults with eczema has an associated food allergy.

How Allergic Reactions Work

The mechanism behind an allergic reaction involves two features of the human immune response. One is the production of immunoglobulin E (IgE), a type of protein called an antibody that circulates through the blood. The other feature of the immune response is the mast cell, a specific cell that occurs in all body tissues but is especially common in areas of the body that are typical sites of allergic reactions, including the nose and throat, lungs, skin, and gastrointestinal tract.

The ability of a given individual to form IgE against something as benign as food is an inherited predisposition. Generally, such people come from families in which allergies are common, not necessarily food allergies but perhaps hay fever, asthma, or hives. Someone with two allergic parents is more likely to develop food allergies than someone with one allergic parent.

Before an allergic reaction can occur, a person who is predisposed to form IgE to foods first has to be exposed to the food. As this food is digested, it triggers certain cells to produce specific IgE in large amounts. The IgE is then released and attaches to the surface of mast cells. The next time the person eats that food, it interacts with specific IgE on the surface of the mast cells and triggers the cells to release chemicals such as histamine. Depending upon the tissue in which they are released, these chemicals will cause a person to have various symptoms of food allergy.

If the mast cells release chemicals in the ears, nose, and throat, a person may feel an itching in the mouth, and may have trouble breathing or swallowing. If the affected mast cells are in the gastrointestinal tract, the person may have abdominal pain or diarrhea. The chemicals released by skin mast cells, in contrast, can prompt hives.

Food allergens (the food fragments responsible for an allergic reaction) are proteins within the food that usually are not broken down by the heat of cooking or by stomach acids or enzymes that digest food. As a result, they survive to cross the gastrointestinal lining, enter the bloodstream, and go to target organs, causing allergic reactions throughout the body.

The complex process of digestion affects the timing and the location of a reaction. If people are allergic to a particular food, for example, they may first experience itching in the mouth as they start to eat the food. After the food is digested in the stomach, abdominal symptoms such as vomiting, diarrhea, or pain may start. When the food allergens enter and travel through the bloodstream, they can cause a drop in blood pressure. As the allergens reach the skin, finally, they can induce hives or eczema. All of this takes place within a few minutes to an hour.

Common Food Allergies

In adults, the most common foods to cause allergic reactions include: shellfish, such as shrimp, crayfish, lobster, and crab; peanuts, which is one of the chief foods to cause severe anaphylactic reactions; tree nuts, such as walnuts; fish; and egg.

In children, the pattern is somewhat different. The most common food allergens that cause problems in children are egg, milk, and peanuts.

The foods that adults or children react to are those foods they eat often. In Japan, for example, rice allergy is more frequent. In Scandinavia, codfish allergy is common.

Cross Reactivity

If someone has a life-threatening reaction to a certain food, the doctor will counsel the patient to avoid similar foods that might trigger this reaction. For example, if someone has a history of allergy to shrimp, testing will usually show that the person is not only allergic to shrimp, but also to crab, lobster, and crayfish, as well. This is called cross reactivity.

Another interesting example of cross reactivity occurs in people who are highly sensitive to ragweed. During ragweed pollination season, these people sometimes find that when they try to eat melons, in particular cantaloupe, they have itching in their mouth and they simply cannot eat the melon. Similarly, people who have severe birch pollen allergy also may react to the peels of apples.

Adults usually do not lose their allergies, but children can sometimes outgrow them. Children are more likely to outgrow allergies to milk or soy than allergies to peanuts, fish, or shrimp.

Differential Diagnoses

A differential diagnosis means distinguishing food allergy from food intolerance or other illnesses. If a patient goes to the doctor's office and says, "I think I have a food allergy," the doctor has to consider the list of other possibilities that may lead to symptoms that could be confused with food allergy.

One possibility is the contamination of foods with microorganisms, such as bacteria, and their products, such as toxins. Contaminated meat sometimes mimics a food reaction when it is really a type of food poisoning.

There are also natural substances, such as histamine, that can occur in foods and stimulate a reaction similar to an allergic reaction. For example, histamine can reach high levels in cheese, some wines, and in certain kinds of fish, particularly tuna and mackerel. In fish, histamine is believed to stem from bacterial contamination, particularly in fish that hasn't been refrigerated properly. If someone eats one of these foods with a high level of histamine, that person may have a reaction that strongly resembles an allergic reaction to food. This reaction is called histamine toxicity.

Another cause of food intolerance that is often confused with a food allergy is lactase deficiency. This most common food intolerance affects at least one out of ten people. Lactase is an enzyme that is in the lining of the gut. This enzyme degrades lactose, which is in milk. If a person does not have enough lactase, the body cannot digest the lactose in most milk products. Instead, the lactose is used by bacteria, gas is formed, and the person experiences bloating, abdominal pain, and sometimes diarrhea.

Another type of food intolerance is an adverse reaction to certain products that are added to food to enhance taste, provide color, or protect against growth of microorganisms. Compounds that are most frequently tied to adverse reactions that can be confused with food allergy are yellow dye number 5, monosodium glutamate, and sulfites. Yellow dye number 5 can cause hives, although rarely. Monosodium glutamate (MSG) is a flavor enhancer, and, when consumed in large amounts, can cause flushing, sensations of warmth, headache, facial pressure, chest pain, or feelings of detachment in some people. These transient reactions occur rapidly after eating large amounts of food to which MSG has been added.

Sulfites can occur naturally in foods or are added to enhance crispness or prevent mold growth. Sulfites in high concentrations sometimes pose problems for people with severe asthma. Sulfites can give off a gas called sulfur dioxide, which the asthmatic inhales while eating the sulfited food. This irritates the lungs and can send an asthmatic into severe bronchospasm, a constriction of the lungs. Such reactions led the U.S. Food and Drug Administration (FDA) to ban sulfites as spray-on preservatives in fresh fruits and vegetables. But they are still used in some foods and are made naturally during the fermentation of wine, for example.

There are a number of other diseases that share symptoms with food allergies including ulcers and cancers of the gastrointestinal tract. These disorders can be associated with vomiting, diarrhea, or cramping abdominal pain exacerbated by eating.

Some people may have a food intolerance that has a psychological trigger. In selected cases, a careful psychiatric evaluation may identify an unpleasant event in that person's life, often during childhood, tied to eating a particular food. The eating of that food years later, even as an adult, is associated with a rush of unpleasant sensations that can resemble an allergic reaction to food.

Diagnosis

To diagnose food allergy a doctor must first determine if the patient is having an adverse reaction to specific foods. This assessment is made with the help of a detailed patient history, the patient's diet diary, or an elimination diet.

The first of these techniques is the most valuable. The physician sits down with the person suspected of having a food allergy and takes a history to determine if the facts are consistent with a food allergy. The doctor asks such questions as

- What was the timing of the reaction? Did the reaction come on quickly, usually within an hour after eating the food?

- Was allergy treatment successful? (Antihistamines should relieve hives, for example, if they stem from a food allergy.)
- Is the reaction always associated with a certain food?
- Did anyone else get sick? For example, if the person has eaten fish contaminated with histamine, everybody who ate the fish should be sick. However, in an allergic reaction, only the person allergic to the fish becomes ill.
- How much did the patient eat before experiencing a reaction? The doctor will want to know how much you ate each time and try to relate it to the severity of the reaction.
- How was the food prepared? Some people will have a violent allergic reaction only to raw or undercooked fish. Complete cooking of the fish destroys those allergens in the fish to which they react. If the fish is cooked thoroughly, they can eat it with no allergic reaction.
- Were other foods ingested at the same time of the allergic reaction? Some foods may delay digestion and thus delay the onset of the allergic reaction.

Sometimes a diagnosis cannot be made solely on the basis of history. The doctor may also ask the patient to go back and keep a record of the contents of each meal and whether he or she had a reaction. This gives more detail from which the doctor and the patient can determine if there is consistency in the reactions.

The next step some doctors use is an elimination diet. Under the doctor's direction, the patient does not eat a food suspected of causing the allergy, like eggs, and substitutes another food, in this case another source of protein. If the patient removes the food and the symptoms go away, a diagnosis can almost be made. If the patient then eats the food (under the doctor's direction) and the symptoms come back, then the diagnosis is confirmed. This technique cannot be used, however, if the reactions are severe (in which case the patient should not resume eating the food) or infrequent.

If the patient's history, diet diary, or elimination diet suggest a specific food allergy is likely, the doctor will then use tests that can more objectively measure an allergic response to food. One of these is a scratch skin test, during which a dilute extract of the food is placed on the skin of the forearm or back. This portion of the skin is then scratched with a needle and observed for swelling or redness that would indicate a local allergic reaction. If the scratch test is positive, the patient has IgE on the skin's mast cells that is specific to the food being tested.

Skin tests are rapid, simple, and relatively safe. But a patient can have a positive skin test to a food allergen without experiencing allergic reactions to that food. A diagnosis of food allergy is made only when a patient has a positive skin test to a specific allergen and the history of their reactions also suggests an allergy to the same food.

In some extremely allergic patients who have severe anaphylactic reactions, skin testing can't be used because it could evoke a dangerous reaction. Skin testing also cannot be done on patients with extensive eczema.

For these patients a doctor may use one of two blood tests called RAST and ELISA. These tests measure the presence of food-specific IgE in the blood of patients. These tests may cost more than skin tests and results are not immediately available. As with skin testing, positive tests do not necessarily make the diagnosis.

The final method used to objectively diagnose food allergy is double-blind food challenge. This testing has come into vogue over the last few years as the "gold standard" of allergy testing. For this food challenge, various foods, some of which are suspected of inducing an allergic reaction, are each placed in individual opaque capsules. The patient is asked to swallow a capsule and is then watched to see if a reaction occurs. This process is repeated until all the capsules have been swallowed. In a true double-blind test, the doctor is also "blinded," the capsules having been made up by some other medical person, so that neither the patient nor the doctor knows which capsule contains the allergen.

The one strong advantage of such a challenge is that, if the patient has a reaction only to suspected foods and not to other foods tested, it confirms the diagnosis. However, someone with a history of severe reactions cannot be tested this way. In addition, this testing is expensive because it takes a lot of time to perform. Multiple food allergies are also difficult to evaluate with this procedure. Consequently, double-blind food challenges are not done often. This type of testing is most commonly used when the doctor believes that the reaction a person is describing is not due to a specific food and wishes to obtain evidence to support this judgment so that additional efforts may be directed at finding the real cause of the reaction.

Exercise-Induced Food Allergy

There is at least one situation where more than the simple ingestion of a food to which a person is sensitive is required to provoke a reaction, and that is in exercise-induced food allergy. People who experience this reaction eat a specific food before exercising. As they exercise and their body temperature goes up, they begin to itch, get light-headed, and soon have a full-blown allergic reaction such as hives. The cure for exercise-induced food allergy is simple—not eating for a couple of hours before exercising.

Treatment

Food allergy is treated by dietary avoidance. Once a patient and the patient's doctor have identified the food to which the patient is sensitive, the food must be removed from the patient's diet. To do this, patients must read lengthy, detailed ingredient lists on each food they are considering eating. Many allergy-producing foods such as peanuts, eggs, and milk, appear in foods one normally wouldn't associate them with. Peanuts, for example, are often used as a protein source and eggs are used in some salad dressings. The FDA requires ingredients in a food to appear on its label. People can avoid most of the things to which they are sensitive, consequently, if they read food labels carefully and avoid restaurant-prepared foods that might have ingredients to which they are allergic.

In highly allergic people even minuscule amounts of a food allergen (1/44,000 of a peanut kernel for example) can prompt an allergic reaction. Other less sensitive people may be able to tolerate small amounts of a food to which they're allergic.

Patients with severe food allergies must be prepared to treat an inadvertent exposure. Even people who are very knowledgeable about what they are sensitive to occasionally make a mistake. In order to protect themselves, people who have had anaphylactic reactions to a food should wear medical alert bracelets or necklaces stating that they have a food allergy and that they are subject to severe reactions. Such people also should always carry a syringe of adrenaline (epinephrine), obtained by prescription from their doctors, and be prepared to self-administer it if they think they are getting a food allergic reaction. They should then immediately seek medical help by either calling the rescue squad or by having themselves transported to an emergency room. Anaphylactic allergic reactions can be fatal even when they start off with mild symptoms such as a tingling in the mouth and throat or gastrointestinal discomfort.

There are several medications that can be taken to relieve food allergy symptoms that aren't part of an anaphylactic reaction. These include antihistamines to relieve gastrointestinal symptoms, hives, or sneezing and a runny nose. Bronchodilators can relieve asthma symptoms. These medications are taken after people have inadvertently ingested a food to which they are allergic but are not effective in preventing an allergic reaction when taken prior to eating the food. No medication in any form can be taken before eating a certain food that will reliably prevent an allergic reaction to that food.

There are a few unproven treatments for food allergics. One involves injections containing small quantities of the food extracts, to which the patient is allergic. These shots are given on a regular basis for a long period of time with the aim of "desensitizing" the patient to the food allergen. Allergy shots have not yet been proven to relieve food allergies.

Infants and Children

Milk and soy allergies are particularly common in infants and children. These allergies sometimes do not involve hives and asthma, but rather lead to colic, and perhaps blood in the stool or poor growth. Infants and children are thought to be particularly susceptible to this allergic syndrome because of the immaturity of their immune and digestive systems.

Milk or soy allergies in infants can develop within days to months of birth. Sometimes there is a family history of allergies or feeding problems. The clinical picture is one of a very unhappy colicky child who may not sleep well at night. The diagnosis is based in part on changing the child's diet. Rarely, food challenge is used.

If the baby is on cow's milk, the doctor may suggest a change to soy formula or exclusive breast milk, if possible. If soy formula causes an allergic reaction, parents should try feeding the baby with elemental formulas, which are processed proteins (basically sugars and amino acids). There are few if any allergens within these materials. Corticosteroids are also sometimes used to treat infants with severe food

allergies. Fortunately, time usually heals this particular gastrointestinal disease. It tends to resolve within the first few years of life.

Exclusive breast-feeding (excluding all other foods) of infants for the first six to 12 months of life is often suggested to avoid milk or soy allergies from developing within that time frame. Such breast-feeding often allows parents to avoid infant-feeding problems, especially if the parents are allergic (and the infant therefore is likely to be allergic). There are some children who are so sensitive to a certain food, however, that if the food is eaten by the mother, sufficient quantities enter the breast milk to cause a food reaction in the child. Mothers sometimes must themselves avoid eating those foods to which the baby is allergic.

There is no conclusive evidence that breast feeding prevents the development of allergies later in life. It does, however, delay the onset of food allergies by delaying the infant's exposure to those foods that can prompt allergies and may avoid altogether those feeding problems seen in infants. By delaying the introduction of solid foods until the infant is six months old or older, parents can also prolong the child's allergy-free period.

Controversial Issues

There are several disorders thought by some to be caused by food allergies, but the evidence is currently insufficient or contrary to such claims. It is controversial, for example, whether migraine headaches can be caused by food allergies. There are studies showing that people who are prone to migraines can have their headaches brought on by histamines and other substances in foods. The more difficult issue is whether food allergies actually cause migraines in such people. There is virtually no evidence that rheumatoid arthritis or osteoarthritis can be made worse by foods, despite claims to the contrary.

There is also no evidence that food allergies can cause a disorder called the allergic tension fatigue syndrome, in which people are tired, nervous, and may have problems concentrating, or have headaches.

Cerebral allergy is a term that has been applied to people who have trouble concentrating and have headaches, as well as other complaints. This is sometimes attributed to mast cells degranulating in the brain but no other place in the body. There is no evidence that such a scenario can happen, and cerebral allergy is not currently recognized by allergists.

Another controversial topic is environmental illness. In a seemingly pristine environment, some people have many non-specific complaints such as problems concentrating or depression. Sometimes this is attributed to small amounts of allergens or toxins in the environment. There is no evidence that such problems are due to food allergies.

Some people believe hyperactivity in children is caused by food allergies. But this behavioral disorder has only been suggested to be associated with food additives occasionally in children, and then only when such additives are consumed in large amounts. There is no evidence that a true food allergy can affect a child's activity except for the proviso that if a child itches and sneezes and wheezes a lot, the child may be miserable and therefore more difficult to control. Also, children who are on anti-allergy medicines that can cause drowsiness may get sleepy in school or at home.

Controversial Diagnostic Techniques

Just as there are controversial food allergy syndromes and treatments, there are also controversial ways of diagnosing food allergies. One of these is cytotoxicity testing, in which a food allergen is added to a patient's blood sample. A technician then examines the sample under the microscope to see if white cells in the blood "die." This technique has been evaluated in a number of studies and has not been found to effectively diagnose food allergy.

Another controversial approach is called sublingual or, if it is injected under the skin, subcutaneous provocative challenge. In this procedure, dilute food allergen is administered under the tongue of the person who may feel that his or her arthritis, for instance, is due to foods. The technician then asks the patient if the food allergen has aggravated the arthritis symptoms. In clinical studies, this procedure has not been shown to effectively diagnose food allergies.

An immune complex assay is sometimes done on patients suspected of having food allergies to see if there are complexes of certain antibodies bound to the food allergen in the bloodstream. It is said that these immune complexes correlate with food allergies. But the formation of such immune complexes is a normal offshoot of food digestion and everyone, if tested with a sensitive enough measurement, has them. To date, no one has conclusively shown that this test correlates with allergies to foods.

Another test is the IgG subclass assay, which looks specifically for certain kinds of IgG antibody. Again, there is no evidence that this diagnoses food allergy.

Controversial Treatments

Controversial treatments include putting a dilute solution of a particular food under the tongue about a half hour before the patient eats that food. This is an attempt to "neutralize" the subsequent exposure to the food that the patient believes is harmful. As the results of a well-conducted clinical study show, this procedure is not effective in preventing an allergic reaction.

Summary

Food allergies are caused by immunologic reactions to foods. There actually are several discrete diseases under this category and a number of foods that can cause these problems.

A medical evaluation after one suspects a food allergy is the key to proper management. Treatment is basically avoidance of the food(s) after they are identified. People with food allergies should become knowledgeable about allergies and how they are treated and should work with their physicians.

The National Institutes of Health supports research on food allergies through grants that it provides to research institutions throughout the world. Understanding the cause of immune system dysfunction in allergy will ultimately lead to better methods of diagnosing, treating, and preventing allergic diseases.

Questions and Answers

Q. Would you discuss what common substances are in both peanuts and other kinds of nuts? The response I often get when I tell people that I am severely allergic to both peanuts and nuts is that I cannot be because peanuts are a legume, unlike nuts.

A. First of all, it is possible to be allergic to two distinct foods. It is interesting that both peanuts and nuts are concentrated sources of protein, which is probably one reason why reactions to both these foods are so frequent. But you can have cross reactions between tree nuts and peanuts, or you could develop allergies to both.

Q. I would like to ask about diet during pregnancy. I have heard some talk about avoiding certain foods during your last trimester.

A. There is no evidence that avoidance of foods in the last trimester can prevent food allergies. In fact, some experimental evidence suggests this is harmful.

Q. Would gross swelling of the lips be indicative of a food allergy?

A. Well, it can be, but you can also have something called idiopathic angioedema, which can cause swelling of the lips. This disorder is not caused by food allergies. If you have such a problem, talk it over with your doctor. If there is any chance that it might be a food allergy, the doctor can place you on an elemental diet for 10 days. If the problem does not go away, you have ruled out food allergy.

Q. Is intolerance a disease entity?

A. Food intolerance is not a distinct entity. It is a term used to cover any adverse reaction to a food that doesn't have an immunologic basis.

Q. I have a 14-year-old daughter who has developed chronic hives in the past nine months. She has swelling and hives on the bottom of her feet to the point where she cannot walk; her fingers swell, and she cannot write. She has been skin tested for food allergies, and it was negative. We are going through the elimination diet process now and seeing some improvement, but not a whole lot. The only thing that controls it is prednisone. What would you suggest as the next step?

A. Sometimes there is a non-specific improvement as you manipulate the diet. But chronic hives and angioedema, especially of that duration, are almost never due to food allergies. Unfortunately, no cause is usually found. There is hope that they will resolve with time. I'd advise you to limit the use of steroids because steroids can do more damage than if you just use antihistamines.

Q. Is there any hope of better management of lactose intolerance than chewing tablets that help dissolve lactose during the meal?

A. Probably not, other than avoidance of foods that have lactose.

Q. What is the best way to diagnose lactose deficiency?

A. There are a couple of tests that involve ingesting a specific amount of lactose and then measuring the body's response. Such blood tests are done by physicians.

Q. Can you tell us anything about gluten intolerance?

A. Gluten intolerance is associated with the disease called gluten-sensitive enteropathy or celiac disease. It is due to an abnormal immune response to gluten, which is a component of wheat and some other grains.

Q. Is it possible that many people who were given the diagnosis of irritable bowel syndrome in the past are turning out to actually have allergies?

A. There is no good evidence that irritable bowel syndrome is due to food allergies in most instances.

Q. This summer I had lunch at a fast food restaurant for the first time and I broke out in hives. The doctor seemed to think maybe it was the sulfites in the food. Now you said there had been regulations for salad bars and sulfites, but in the whole food industry are there regulations for the use of sulfites?

A. Yes, there are industry-wide regulations covering the use of sulfites. Now I do not know anything about the restaurant you ate at, but it is more likely that you ate something else you are allergic to because sulfites rarely cause hives.

■ Document Source:
U.S. Department of Health and Human Services, Public Health Service
National Institutes of Health
NIH Publication No. 93-3469
April 1993

BLOOD DISEASES AND DISORDERS

■ ■ ■

APLASTIC ANEMIA ANSWER BOOK

Aplastic Anemia—The Disease

Aplastic anemia is a rare but extremely serious disorder that results from the unexplained failure of the bone marrow to produce blood cells. In all probability you had never heard of this disease until the time of diagnosis. We hope that this pamphlet helps you deal with your situation by providing basic information about aplastic anemia and the various treatment options. This pamphlet is not intended as a substitute for the advice of a physician. It is important that you ask questions and learn as much as you can about this disease. By contacting the Aplastic Anemia Foundation of America, you can be connected with others in your same situation and receive information free of charge. There are AAFA chapters around the country. You do not need to be alone in dealing with aplastic anemia.

Normal Bone Marrow Function

The central portion of bones is filled with a spongy red tissue called bone marrow. The bone marrow is essentially a factory producing the cells of the blood: red cells that carry oxygen from the lungs to all areas of the body, white cells that fight infection by attacking and destroying germs, and platelets that control bleeding by forming blood clots in areas of injury.

Continuous production of blood cells is necessary all through life because each cell has a finite life span once it leaves the bone marrow and enters the blood: red cells—120 days, platelets—six days, and white cells—one day or less!

Fortunately, the bone marrow is a superb blood cell factory and ordinarily supplies as many cells as needed, increasing production of red cells and platelets when bleeding occurs and of white cells when infection threatens.

Bone Marrow Stem Cells and Environment

The bone marrow contains a small number of precious stem cells. Just as plant seeds give rise to both mature plants and new seeds for the next generation of plants, so do the bone marrow stem cells produce blood cells and new stem cells in a lifelong cycle of production and self-renewal. Bone marrow stem cells require a proper environment for normal function. Just as a seed cannot grow in poor soil, bone marrow stem cells cannot survive and multiply in a poor environment.

Failure of the bone marrow cell production can result from damage to the stem cells or to the environment. The result is aplastic anemia.

Bone Marrow Failure

When the bone marrow cell production fails, normal blood levels of red cells, white cells, and platelets begin to fall. Symptoms of anemia, bleeding, and infection develop when blood cell levels fall to dangerously low levels.

The Diagnosis

The diagnosis of aplastic anemia begins with a blood test. Blood cell levels are normally maintained within certain ranges. The diagnosis of aplastic anemia is suspected when all three blood cell levels are very low. Confirmation of the diagnosis requires examination of a small sample of bone marrow under the microscope. Aspiration and biopsy of the bone marrow is easily carried out in the examining room or hospital bed by inserting a sturdy needle into the large pelvic bone just beneath the belt line on either side of the spine. This procedure is made more tolerable by the use of Novocain-like drugs to "numb up" the skin and bone. In aplastic anemia, the bone marrow biopsy shows a great reduction in the number of cells in the bone marrow, with a normal appearance of the few remaining cells. The diagnosis of aplastic anemia is usually made or confirmed by a hematologist—a specialist in blood disorders.

Initial Treatment

Aplastic anemia is a medical emergency. Patients with severe aplastic anemia require immediate hospital treatment.

Blood transfusion: Aplastic anemia patients are often given transfusions. Anemia is corrected by red cell transfusions. Since anemia in itself is not an emergency, red cell transfusions are usually given only when symptoms are not relieved by restriction of activity. By contrast, bleeding due to low platelets is an acute medical emergency which should be treated with platelet transfusions to prevent fatal hemorrhage. You may be asked to provide platelet donors. Do not ask close family members to donate platelets until after a bone marrow transplant has been done or ruled out since this may interfere with the effectiveness of a bone marrow transplant if a family member donor is found.

Platelets are collected from donors through a process called hemapheresis. Donating usually takes three hours. Platelets are collected from a vein in the donor's arm, passed through a blood-separating machine and returned to the donor. The platelets that are removed are then given to the aplastic anemia patient. The donor's body replaces the platelets within a day or two.

Antibiotics: Because of their extremely short life span, white cells cannot be effectively replaced by a transfusion. Therefore, control of infection depends on prompt, appropriate intravenous antibiotic therapy as soon as fever or other signs of infection appear.

Isolation: To prevent transfer of infection to aplastic anemia patients, they must often be isolated from even healthy people ("reverse quarantine"). Necessary visitors may have to wear masks and gowns and must always thoroughly wash hands before touching the patient.

Activity: Activity must be restricted to reduce symptoms of anemia. Avoid falls or accidents that could provoke bleeding and reduce contact with other people.

What You Can Do

1. Take charge of your illness!
2. Research all you can about aplastic anemia and treatment options.
3. Gather information from as many people as possible: health professionals and other patients.
4. Don't be afraid to ask questions from different sources until you fully understand the answers.
5. Record information in a notebook. Take a tape recorder to appointments and meetings.
6. Encourage friends and family to become platelet and bone marrow donors.
7. Join a support group and read about ways to cope.
8. Check with the doctor about what things to avoid.

Bone Marrow Transplantation

Bone marrow transplantation is now being used more and more frequently for aplastic anemia patients who are good candidates and who have a matched donor. Identical twins or perfectly matched siblings are the best choices for bone marrow donors for patients. If a patient does not have a perfect match within the family, a search of existing bone marrow registries may be undertaken to find a matched, unrelated donor. When a suitable donor is identified, he or she will be "harvested"—having between to 1-1½ quarts of marrow drawn out through a large needle. The filtered bone marrow cells are then transfused by IV into the patient. Production of new blood cells should be seen in two to four weeks as the patients' counts begin to recover. Immunosup-

pressive drugs, such as cyclosporin, play an important role in suppressing the transplanted donor white cells from fighting against those of the patient. Graft-versus-host disease (GVHD) is a reaction of the donor marrow against the body of the patient; donor white cells cause skin thickening, rashes, liver disease, jaundice, drying out of the eyes and mouth, weight loss, and diarrhea. Graft-versus-host disease, while it can be quite serious, can be successfully treated in most patients.

For young patients in relatively good health prior to transplant, and who have a matched donor, more than 75% are successfully cured by bone marrow transplantation. For patients who do not have a matched donor, who are over 50 years of age or who are not good candidates for bone marrow transplantation, other forms of therapy are being used.

Drug Therapies

Doctors may recommend that the patient start on drug therapy while searching for a donor, or drug therapy may be the best choice for treatment for that patient. New therapies are being developed all the time. Be sure to talk with the doctor about what is available. Immunosuppressive therapies work with a patient's immune system. One theory about aplastic anemia is that the patient's immune system is fighting against itself, thereby interfering with production of blood cells. These drugs are believed to work by stimulating the bone marrow to produce cells or by reducing the patient's immune response and thereby allowing the bone marrow to work. ATG, antithymocyte globulin, or ALG, antilymphocyte globulin, are two types of immunosuppressive therapies that have been used for treating aplastic anemia.

Another immunosuppressive drug is cyclosporin, which may be given alone or in combination with androgens, antilymphocyte globulin or serum. It is thought that cyclosporin plus androgens may stimulate blood cell production.

Hematopoetic growth factors are products of the new genetic engineering. These are copies of substances which occur naturally in the human body, but produced in larger quantities in the laboratory. Colony stimulating factors (CSFs) act to stimulate colonies of cells, such as red cells. Erythropoetin (EPO) stimulates production of red cells. Interleukin-3 (IL-3) stimulates production of other cells. It is thought that a combination of the growth factors might work in treating aplastic anemia.

Other drug therapies are being developed; your doctor will be able to help you explore these options.

Frequently Asked Questions

Who gets aplastic anemia?

Aplastic anemia can strike down literally anyone: men and women, children as well as adults, any race or socio-economic status.

Don't blood transfusions replace the cells needed by aplastic anemia patients?

Unfortunately, blood transfusions are only a temporary solution to some of the problems of aplastic anemia patients. Consider each type of cell in turn:

1. Red Cells—Red cells are the easiest to replace by transfusion. There are only four major blood types, so "matching" is usually easy, and transfused cells may remain in the body for a month or longer. However, after years of regular red cell transfusions, patients begin to accumulate toxic amounts of iron (carried inside the red cells) in critical body organs, such as the liver or heart. Iron overload from transfusions is eventually fatal.
2. Platelets—Successful long-term platelet transfusion therapy is a challenge. Since the normal life span of a platelet is so short, transfused platelets may only survive a few days; thus regular platelet transfusions several times a week may be needed. In addition, platelets carry tissue-type "markers" that are almost unique for each person. Patients "learn" to recognize foreign platelets and produce antibodies that destroy the transfused platelets instantly. Thus, aplastic anemia patients rapidly develop a need for "matched" platelets, that is, platelets from donors whose tissue-type markers resemble the patient's own markers. To support one small child with matched platelets for a year, 20 matched donors may be needed.
3. White Cells—White cells cannot be effectively supplied by transfusion. The life-span of white cells obtained from donors is so short (a few hours) that routine white cell transfusion is technically impossible.

What are the causes of aplastic anemia?

Aplastic anemia has been clearly linked to radiation, environmental toxins, insecticides, and drugs in much the same fashion that cancer has been linked to these agents. Benzene-based compounds, airplane glue, and drugs such as chloramphenicol have been linked to aplastic anemia. In some individuals, aplastic anemia is believed to be caused by a virus. To date, the exact cause of the disease in over half the cases is unknown, or idiopathic.

Are there any experimental treatments available for those who do not respond to ATG and do not have a bone marrow transplant match?

Yes. There are several alternative therapies that can be tried and some are successful to some extent. These include the use of cytokines (growth factors) or granulocyte monocyte colony stimulating factor (GM-CSF) or erythropoietin (EPO). These are approved and commercially available cytokines that are available to all physicians. In addition, several experimental cytokines are being evaluated and could potentially be useful in some aplastic anemia patients. These include interleukin 3, monocyte colony stimulating factor, stem cell factor (SCF or C-kit ligand) and IL-6. Several newer cytokines are being developed and will be available for study in the near future.

How do I find out where in my area there is experimental research going on?

In the United States of America, nearly all experimental therapy for aplastic anemia is being carried out at hospitals associated with either one of the medical schools, or one of the NIH-designated cancer centers. In addition, experimental therapies are being carried out at the National Institutes of Health in Bethesda, Maryland. A letter or call to the Hematology Division (either pediatric or adult) of the nearest medical school or designated cancer center should result in information concerning the availability of experimental therapy.

What activities should I avoid?

Patients with low red cell counts should avoid excessive exercise, going to high altitudes, or any activity that brings on a fast heart rate, any chest pain, or severe shortness of breath. Patients with low white counts may be more susceptible to infection with bacteria, not viruses. These are usually acquired from cuts in the skin or lining of the mouth or throat which might result from dental work, burns from hot food, etc. Patients with low platelets should avoid activities that result in trauma, especially head trauma.

GLOSSARY

aplastic anemia: bone marrow failure; for unknown reasons, production of blood cells slows or stops.

antibody: a complex molecule produced by lymph tissue in response to the presence of an antigen; antibodies neutralize the effect of the antigen.

antigen: foreign substance which is not usually part of the body's makeup and that stimulates antibody production; this antibody reacts specifically with a particular antigen to destroy or weaken it.

bacteria: organism that can cause infection.

bone marrow: soft tissue within the bones where blood cells are manufactured.

bone marrow aspiration: test in which a sample of bone marrow cells is removed with a needle and examined under a microscope.

bone marrow biopsy: procedure in which a small piece of bone marrow tissue is removed with a needle; sample is processed by softening the bone and examining thin slices of the softened bone under a microscope.

bone marrow transplant: procedure in which bone marrow filled with disease is destroyed by radiation or chemotherapy and then replaced with healthy cells from a donor.

chromosome: a rodlike structure that appears in the nucleus of a cell during division; contains the genes responsible for heredity.

complete blood count: CBC; amount or level of blood cells: white cells, red cells, and platelets.

cross match: type and cross; test in which the blood cells of a donor and a recipient are mixed together to determine if they are compatible.

culture: procedure used to identify the source of infection; specimen of blood, urine, sputum, or stool is taken and tested to determine the type of infection and the appropriate antibiotic.

differential: percent of different types of blood cells in the blood.

erythroblast: an immature red blood cell.

erythrocyte: a mature red blood cell that carries oxygen.

granulocyte: a white blood cell produced in the bone marrow that engulfs and destroys invading organisms.

hematocrit: the percentage of blood that is made up of cells. Normal values for men range from 42-52%, and for females, 38-48%.

hemoglobin: Hg; iron-containing coloring in the red cells that combines with oxygen from the lungs and carries it to the body's cells. Normal values for men are 13-16 gms/100 ml and 12-14 gms/100 ml for women.

histocompatibility antigens: HLA; a group of DNA substances in chromosomes that determine whether certain tissues can be transplanted; also can be used to determine the most compatible platelet donors.

human leukocyte antigen: HLA; the tissue typing test done on white cells to determine if a donor and recipient are compatible.

immunoglobulins: kill microbes directly or make it easier for white cells to kill them.

immunosuppression: decrease in the ability of the body's normal immune response to the invasion of foreign material.

leukocyte: a white blood cell.

leukopenia: a low number of white blood cells.

lymphocyte: a type of white cell that fights infection by producing antibodies and other defense substances; occurs in two forms: B cells that recognize specific antigens and produce antibodies against them, and T cells that are agents of the immune system.

megakaryocyte: a cell in the bone marrow that produces platelets.

neutropenia: low neutrophil (poly) count.

pancytopenia: low number of blood cells.

petechiae: tiny red dots on the skin due to bleeding under the skin caused by low platelet counts.

peripheral blood: blood in the bloodstream.

phagocytosis: "cell eating," the engulfment and destruction of dangerous microorganisms or cells by certain white blood cells.

platelet: blood cell that prevents bleeding and bruising.

red blood cell: oxygen-carrying cell in the blood which contains the pigment hemoglobin, produced in the bone marrow; erythrocyte.

refractory (to platelets): the immune system's response to platelet transfusions; platelets are recognized as foreign and destroyed.

reticulocyte: an immature red blood cell.

stem cell: cell from which platelets, red blood cells, and white blood cells grow in the one marrow.

thrombocytopenia: a low number of platelets in the blood. When the platelet level falls below five (or 5,000/cu.mm), it is considered a life-threatening emergency and may be corrected by a platelet transfusion.

thymocytes: (T cells) white blood cells that have travelled through the thymus.

white blood cells: blood cells which fight infection.

Blood counts: Adult normal value ranges	
White blood cells	3.5-10.6 (1000/cu.mm)
Red blood cells	4.27-5.69 (million/cu.mm)
Platelets	150.0-450.0 (1000/cu.mm)
Hemoglobin	13.3-17.1 (grams/100 ml.)
Hematocrit	38.9-49.7%

The Aplastic Anemia Foundation of America, Inc. (AAFA) is solely supported through individual contributions and is a tax exempt organization as described under the Internal Revenue Code, section 501(c)(3).

The AAFA offers free educational materials on aplastic anemia and myelodysplastic syndromes. The AAFA serves as a resource directory for patient assistance and emotional support through the volunteer efforts of patients, family members, and health care professionals throughout the World. Major research studies to find effective prevention and cure for aplastic anemia and myelodysplastic syndromes are also financially supported by the AAFA. Patients can participate in the AAFA National Registry which collects data for statistical analysis.

Contact the AAFA to receive a free information packet and to learn more about aplastic anemia, myelodysplastic syndromes, and the AAFA National Registry.

Original text was written by Dr. Robert K. Stuart, updates and edits by Linda B. Kaufman and Dr. Lyle L. Sensenbrenner.

■ Document Source:
**Aplastic Anemia Foundation of America, Inc.
PO Box 613
Annapolis, MD 21404
1-800-747-2820
September 1995**

See also: Bone Marrow Transplantation: Questions & Answers (page 47)

BONE MARROW TRANSPLANTATION: QUESTIONS & ANSWERS

Introduction

During the last decade, bone marrow transplantation has evolved from a last-resort, desperate experiment to a well-established treatment option for a variety of life-threatening diseases.

In 1977, a total of 169 patients received bone marrow transplants worldwide; by 1993, 10,000 patients had received transplants carried out in more than 250 centers in 40 countries. Currently, patients with leukemia, lymphoma, advanced or resistant solid tumors, severe aplastic anemia, and selected immune deficiency disorders and genetic errors now have another possible treatment that offers meaningful chances for cure.

As a direct result of the burgeoning interest and treatment possibilities in the field of bone marrow transplantation, the

Leukemia Society of America has developed this brochure to explain the procedure and many related questions.

Q. What is "Bone Marrow Transplantation?"

A. A bone marrow "transplant" (BMT) is best viewed not as a surgical procedure or operation, but as a transfusion of marrow, not blood, from one individual to another or to the same individual. Bone marrow is the spongy tissue inside bones which manufactures various components of blood and the immune system: red blood cells, white blood cells, and platelets. Each of these different cells has a vital role to perform in keeping the body healthy and free of disease.

In the case of leukemia, the white blood cells are the usual malignant target. Since restraints on their growth are lost, leukemic white blood cells usually overproduce. Such overproduction hinders the process of normal blood cell development in the bone marrow. Thus there is

1. decreased red blood cell production, leading to anemia.
2. decreased platelet production, leading to bleeding either internally, externally, or into the skin (bruises and purpura).
3. decreased production of normal white blood cells, leading to greater risk of infections. If untreated, leukemia can lead to progressive disease and death.

Chemotherapeutic agents (drugs and other biological material) can destroy these malignant cells but are destructive to the normal marrow cells as well. Standard treatments for leukemia usually limit the drug dosages so they are not too damaging to the bone marrow and elsewhere. Very large doses of drugs are given during a bone marrow transplant to potentially eradicate the disease. The patient's bone marrow is restored to grow as "normal," with balanced production of all blood cell components. Transplantation takes place after chemotherapy, radiation, and other treatments have eradicated the malignant cells from the patient's system, the latter designed to prohibit an intact immune system from rejecting the "foreign" or donor marrow. The patient's bone marrow is then replaced by an infusion of bone marrow from a donor (allogeneic) or from the patient him- or herself (autologous).

The transplanted bone marrow cells migrate to the marrow space and actually begin the process of repopulation. When the marrow is successfully accepted (i.e., engrafts) and the leukemic cells do not recur, the patient has a chance for leukemia-free survival, leading to cure.

In lymphoma, the cells which make up the lymph node tissue become malignant. In malignant solid tumors, the cells which make up muscle, bone, glands, i.e., all tissues, become malignant. Standard chemotherapy destroys the malignant cells but is also toxic to normal marrow cells, thus limiting the dose of drugs that can safely be given. Bone marrow transplantation is used to counter the destructive effects of chemotherapy on the normal marrow cells so that massive doses of chemotherapy can be given to eliminate cancer in patients who do not respond to standard drug dosages.

It is also known that following allogeneic transplantation, a subset of the infused cells have a beneficial anti-leukemic effect, which enhances the marrow transplant, per se, by an ongoing onslaught against residual "drug resistant" cancer cells.

Q. When is a bone marrow transplantation indicated as treatment?

A. Bone marrow transplantation is currently considered the treatment of choice for severe aplastic anemia, specific immune deficiency states (e.g., severe combined immune deficiency or SCID), chronic myeloid leukemia (CML), and in a sub-group of patients with acute lymphocytic and nonlymphocytic leukemias who have specific chromosomal markers which are known to predict a poor outcome (e.g., Philadelphia chromosome) or other factors (e.g., high tumor burden at onset). It is also indicated for those patients who have failed standard methods of treatment, primarily chemotherapy and radiation therapy. These include patients with acute lymphocytic leukemia (ALL) in second or subsequent remissions, acute myelogenous leukemia (AML) in second or subsequent remissions, resistant forms of lymphoma, as well as advanced or resistant solid tumors.

Among the considerations that determine transplant eligibility are age (usually, but not always, under 55 years of age), general physical health, condition of specific organs (heart, lungs, liver, etc.), prior chemotherapy treatment, and transfusion history. Patients should inquire about the possibilities for bone marrow transplantation soon after diagnosis. Contacts with institutions specializing in bone marrow transplantation are best directed through the patients' physician, who is familiar with the details of personal medical and psychological histories.

Q. Who can act as a donor for a bone marrow transplant?

A. The ideal donor is a tissue-matched family member, usually a sibling. Identical twins are not ideal as donors in the leukemias because of the failure to induce controlled graft-versus-host disease (GVHD) and its attendant anti-leukemic effect. Unfortunately, only one out of every four who need transplantation have genetically matched siblings.

For those who do not have a family donor, other options include autologous or unrelated donor transplants. In the autologous setting, patients act as their own donors. Patients receive back their own marrow, which had been previously removed at an earlier stage of illness or when the disease was in remission. It is then treated, frozen and stored until needed. Sometimes an unrelated donor may be identified through donor bank searches. Matched unrelated donors offer an additional 10 to 15 percent chance for transplantation.

Peripheral blood also contains marrow-like stem cells. A technique, called peripheral stem cell pheresis, is performed after priming the patient's bone marrow with substances known as growth factors during a crucial period after certain chemotherapy courses. The "turned on" bone marrow "spills" some of its cells into the peripheral bloodstream that can then be collected and isolated. Because the ratio of the stem cells in the bloodstream is generally about 10 percent of those in the marrow itself, usually three or four phereses are needed to obtain a proper number of engraftable cells.

Q. How is the bone marrow "treated" to rid it of unwanted cells?

A. Once the marrow cells are aspirated, treatment in the laboratory with specific agents is carried out in the following situations:

1. If the source of the bone marrow is the patient and if the cancer has already involved the bone marrow, the contaminating malignant cells can be removed (i.e., purged) using special advanced techniques. These may involve the use of either chemotherapy agents in the laboratory (e.g., vincristine, dexamethasone, etc.) or of microspheres attached to markers called monoclonal antibodies (e.g., cALLA, or "common acute lymphoblastic leukemia antigens"). These markers attract malignant cells. The spheres with the attached malignant cells are then eliminated using magnets. This technique is called immunomagnetic purging. Complement, a natural anticancer product, can also be used with the antibodies.

2. If the donor is not a perfect match, graft-versus-host disease (GVHD) is a serious and potentially fatal complication. Under these circumstances, to decrease the incidence and the severity of this complication, the donor bone marrow cells are cleansed of a particular population of cells (known as T cells) that are thought to cause GVHD.

Q. What determines if a donor/recipient "match" will be successful?

A. The body's immune defense system consists of white cells which travel continuously throughout the body in surveillance of foreign substances or cells. They destroy what they perceive as "non-self."

Therefore, when donor bone marrow cells are transplanted into a new host, a spectrum of donor-host interactions occurs. On one end of the spectrum, the recipient's immune system may reject the donor's cells (i.e., graft rejection or failure). On the other end, the donor's cells may attack (reject) the recipient's tissues in what is called graft-versus-host reaction. The closer the match is between the patient and the donor, the less these complications are likely to occur. Preparatory treatments that are currently used before transplantation and which suppress the patient's immune system make graft rejection a rare event. Also, current technology is now able to remove or suppress the T cells which are responsible for GVHD, thus making bone marrow transplants between genetically unmatched individuals possible. However, transplants between genetically matched individuals still have the best chance for success.

Q. How is a potentially successful bone marrow match identified?

A. Bone marrow cells have surface structures which can recognize and reject foreign tissues. These are called human leukocyte antigens, or HLAs. Four sets of HLA antigens have so far been identified: A, B, C, D. To insure the best possible acceptance of donor bone marrow, it is best to match all of the four HLA sites. The D-antigen set is closely scrutinized, since it determines the level of immune response and rejection of foreign tissues.

Two blood tests are done to determine how good the match is between donor and patient cells. They are referred to as HLA typing and MLC assay. All that is needed to determine if an individual is a possible donor is a small sample of blood. Donor and patient samples are compared by mixing small samples of white blood cells with small amounts of blood sera positive for specific HLA-A, -B, -C, and -D. If cells are destroyed, this indicates that the cells carry the particular HLA set being tested. Then, blood cells from the donor are mixed with blood cells from the patient in a radioactive assay. If there is a high amount of cross-reactivity between them, or radioactivity, the donor cells are incompatible despite the apparent match. The blood assay is called MLC, or mixed leukocyte culture assay.

A more sensitive method to detect subtle differences between the HLA typing of both the donor and the recipient is DNA typing. It is far more effective in identifying those patients at risk for development of GVHD.

Q. What is the procedure for donating bone marrow?

A. Marrow is withdrawn (harvested) from the donor's hip bone using a special syringe and needle in the operating room under a general anesthesia. A bone marrow cell count is performed to determine if the recommended cell dose of 1-2 x 10^8 nucleated cells/kg (200-600 million cell/kg) of patient weight has been achieved. The needle puncture sites may be tender for less than a week and leave essentially no scars. Some mild stiffness and tenderness will last for a day or so, but this discomfort can be lessened through exercise and low dose pain medication. Donors are usually discharged from the hospital the next day.

The relatively small amounts of marrow and blood taken from the donor (based on the volume needed by the recipient which varies from a few ounces to one to two pints) does not result in any bad effects. Marrow cells are quickly produced by the donor and the amount which is removed will be manufactured in two or three weeks. Often, blood is taken before the marrow donation and may be returned to donors to restore their blood volume.

The procedures involved in blood and bone marrow donation are simple, but they still can be new and unsettling experiences. Most centers which specialize in bone marrow transplants are aware of this, and their hospital staff are supportive. They recognize that donors are very special people.

Q. How is the marrow transplant carried out?

A. When the marrow has been taken from the donor (in some cases the patient himself), it is strained through closed plastic filters and containers to remove fat, small pieces of bone and other particles, and to break up large clumps of cells. Sometimes, the marrow is processed further to remove the previously described additional unwanted disease or immune system cells. If patients are their own donors, the marrow is preserved and frozen until the patient needs it. If the bone marrow cells are to be frozen, a protective agent called dimethyl sulfoxide (DMSO) is used to maintain the integrity of the cells in the frozen state. This substance has a strong, garlic-like odor that may be excreted into the patient's breath for one to three days. If the marrow is not stored after processing, it is packaged in plastic bags and brought to the patient's bedside. Much like a transfusion, the purified marrow enters the patient's bloodstream through an intravenous line. It finds its way to the proper place in the interior of the major bones of the body, "homes" in, and begins to produce new and normal blood cells. This process is called engraftment and usually takes two to three weeks. (The exact body mechanisms controlling the homing effect of marrow are not fully understood.)

The infusion of donor bone marrow usually takes about two hours. Marrow recipients suffer no special discomfort from the transplant, although an allergic type of reaction may develop: hives, chills, and a rapid pulse or heartbeat. Antihistamines and other allergy medication are given as a precaution.

Q. How long is it from the time patients enter the hospital until they receive the donated bone marrow?
A. The average time from admission to transplant is about two weeks. Ideally, patients should be in remission from their leukemia in order for bone marrow transplant to be considered appropriate treatment. Prior to admission, the patient's disease status and physical condition are evaluated in order to see if they will benefit from such a procedure. A series of tests which are all familiar procedures for cancer patients will take place at this time. They include bone marrow aspiration and biopsy, x-rays, blood tests, tests of heart, liver, lungs, and kidney function.

Before admission, patients receive a Hickman or Broviac catheter, a hollow tube much like an intravenous line, placed in between the neck and shoulder, leading into a vein. This special catheter allows blood samples to be taken and medications given without the use of needles and painful injections.

During the first few days after admission, chemotherapy with or without total body radiation is administered in doses large enough to destroy the patient's own bone marrow and blood cells as well as the cancer cells. This process is known as "conditioning" and serves three different purposes: (1) it creates space in the bone marrow to allow for the expansion of the new marrow cells, (2) it helps to prevent graft rejection, and (3) it eradicates malignant cells. The infusion of new marrow will rescue the patient from the cell-depleting effects of the chemotherapy and radiation.

Q. What happens after the transplant?
A. Within about two weeks, the transplanted marrow will begin to engraft and to repopulate the patient's body with healthy cells. However, not until three to four weeks after the transplant will a patient's new bone marrow have developed enough to produce sufficient mature cells. Early on, within the first three weeks after transplantation, patients will be given donated blood products as replacement for their developing cells. About six to eight weeks after the actual transplant, patients may leave the hospital if they are able to eat, have no fevers, and otherwise are well. Patients are followed for approximately three months, with visits during this time. Many hospitals, through the social work department, assist patients and families in finding living accommodations close to the transplant center.

Three to four months after the transplant, patients may be discharged back to their homes and to their referring physicians. It is not unusual for patients to remain in the hospital longer or to be readmitted for observation or further treatment of infection or graft-versus-host disease. Patients should not plan to return to work or school for six months after the transplant. Even though blood tests may be normal, the immune system takes that long to recover. Convalescence, both physical and psychological, takes up to one year.

The first two weeks after the transplant are the most physically draining for patients. Many patients develop infections. Antibiotic and antifungal medications are usually administered in order to prevent infections like pneumonia. Diarrhea and skin rash can be early effects of graft-versus-host disease. Many patients cannot eat much during this time due to the treatment-related mouth or gut sores and are given nutrients and fluids through the Hickman catheter.

Patients, staff, and visitors are often required to take some germ-free precautions, including antiseptic washing and wearing of a protective mask or sterile garments. Patients are confined to isolation. However, family members and friends may visit and be allowed to help with patients' care during this time.

Q. What is graft-versus-leukemia effect?
A. As previously mentioned, the donor marrow cells contain some active immune cells (T cells) which are responsible for the complication known as GVHD. However, another subgroup is also contained in this population of cells that fights cancer cells and causes the beneficial effect known as "graft-versus-leukemia," or GVL. Scientists are now working on methods to dissect this T cell population into its subgroups. Therefore, the harmful group that causes GVHD can be eliminated or suppressed, while the beneficial group that causes GVL is preserved.

Q. What are growth factors and why are they used?
A. Growth factors are certain substances that are produced in minute quantities in our bodies to stimulate our bone marrow to produce more cells when needed. Investigators have found that when these substances are given to patients with low blood counts, the time period for counts to return to normal is shortened. This also shortens the period during which infectious complications are most likely to occur. Two of the more commonly used factors are termed G-CSF and GM-CSF, i.e., granulocyte (type of white cell)-colony stimulating factor.

Q. What help can patients and families expect from staff of the bone marrow transplant unit?
A. Transplant teams are extensively prepared to support the patient and family throughout the stressful transplantation time. Many centers offer social services and financial advice/planning as soon as an individual is referred to the bone marrow transplant unit as a potential candidate.

Physicians receive extra education to serve on these units. Psychiatrists or psychologists, along with team physicians, provide support for patient, family, and donor. Nurses are prepared to care for the special needs of hospitalized bone marrow transplant patients. Social workers, dietitians, pharmacists, and physical and occupational therapists are all part of the transplant team and work closely with the physicians and nurses in attending to the transplant patients' social, nutritional, and medication needs. Patients and their families should not hesitate to draw upon the expertise and support of the transplant team during all stages of the transplantation and convalescent periods.

Q. Are there any side effects of the bone marrow transplantation procedure?
A. The regimen of total body irradiation and high dose chemotherapy is given to help eradicate leukemia or malignant cells and help prevent graft rejection. High dose radiation

usually affects the sexual organs which cannot be shielded because of fear of missing "hiding" leukemia cells. Sterility is a permanent side effect. Bone marrow patients are unable to conceive children. However, sexual function will not be affected. A sperm bank is usually available for male patients who wish to store sperm for future use. Radiation can cause a transient skin rash or burn, nausea, vomiting, swelling of the parotid glands (located near the ears), temporary hair loss, and mouth sores. With high-dose cytoxan, patients can develop nausea, vomiting, water retention, irritation or bleeding of the bladder, temporary air loss, and a weakening of the muscles of the heart called cardiomyopathy.

Another common drug used in bone marrow transplantation is called Ara-C. Ara-C interrupts production of blood cells in the bone marrow and causes nausea, vomiting, loss of appetite, and pain and swelling of tissues lining the esophagus and stomach. When taking this drug, patients may have difficulty in walking and experience photophobia (burning pain in their eyes looking at light). Their livers may not work normally.

Some other drugs used include: VP-16 and busulfan which can bring about a decrease in all blood cell production and which can cause skin darkening, cataracts, hair loss, and lung damage. A loss of muscle control (seizure) may also occur during treatment with high dosages of busulfan. This can be prevented by using a drug called dilantin.

Q. What are other possible complications of bone marrow transplantation?
A. Bone marrow transplants are done for high-risk patients. In spite of the great strides made, bone marrow transplantation is still a drastic procedure that may make patients ill and can be fatal. Before a transplant is done, patients' general health, and the condition of certain organs which may have been damaged by earlier treatments, are examined. However, complications may still occur and these include

1. Infections: Antimicrobial agents are used to prevent certain bacterial, viral, and fungal infections. However, due to decreased immunity following transplantation, the patient may still contract an infection which can be serious, and sometimes even fatal.
2. GVHD: As previously described, the donor bone marrow cells can attack the patient's tissues, particularly the skin (rashes, pain, itching), gastrointestinal tract (diarrhea, bleeding), or the liver (jaundice and liver dysfunction). As previously mentioned, the bone marrow may be treated in special ways to remove the cells responsible for this complication. In the meantime, medications (e.g., methotrexate, cyclosporin A, and corticosteroids) may be used to prevent and/or treat this complication.
3. Veno-occlusive disease: Blood vessels in the liver, kidneys, and less commonly in the lungs may get occluded (blocked). This leads to water retention, increased weight gain, and abnormal liver function.
4. Late complications: These may include some hormonal disturbances (e.g., decreased thyroid function, sterility, infertility, sexual dysfunction, etc.), and cataracts, lung damage, second malignancies, and chronic graft-versus-host disease.

Q. How has the Leukemia Society of America supported bone marrow transplantation research? What have been some of the major contributions? What is in store for the future?
A. Since 1955, the Leukemia Society of America has committed approximately five million dollars to pioneer the development of bone marrow transplantation. Bone marrow transplantation has become a standard treatment for aplastic anemia, leukemia, and other malignant and genetic diseases.

Use of bone marrow transplantation has increased dramatically in the 1980s. There were fewer than 200 allogeneic transplants worldwide in 1977. In 1992, 10,000 transplants were performed in over 250 centers located in 40 countries. More than 70 percent of the transplants were for leukemia. For this reason, research concerning the best methods of carrying out such treatment must be continued. There are some promising research developments in ways to prevent and to treat graft-versus-host disease which is the single largest complication of bone marrow transplantation. New drugs which control rejection and graft-versus-host disease have also widened the field by allowing the successful transplantation from unrelated donors. More potent chemotherapy drugs, newer methods, of administering current drugs, and new schedules, methods and doses of total body irradiation are being investigated so that it becomes easier to destroy the last remaining malignant cells and prevent the disease from recurring. Hopefully, methods will be found to reduce the massive doses of cell-killing drugs and total body radiation that are today's only effective treatment. As the function of malignant cells is better understood, transplantation techniques could be greatly refined.

In the future, bone marrow transplants may well be used to treat other diseases of the immune system, such as lupus erythematosus and arthritis. Transplants have already been used to correct genetic abnormalities of the immune system, such as severe combined immunodeficiency disease (SCID), and inborn abnormalities of the blood, such as sickle cell anemia and thalassemia. Exciting research is now being conducted to correct and insert missing genes into bone marrow cells which are then reinfused to correct genetic defects using patients' own bone marrow cells (e.g., sickle cell anemia and fatal enzyme deficiencies).

Q. How can I support marrow donations and transplants?
A. Of the thousands who could benefit from a marrow transplant, nearly 70 percent cannot find a suitable match within their families. These patients need to find unrelated donors—people willing to come to the assistance of someone they likely will never meet. Hundreds, perhaps thousands, of lives could be saved if more people added their names to the list of potential marrow donors.

The requirements to be a marrow donor are few. Unrelated donors must be between 18 and 55 years of age and be able to pass a thorough physical examination, according to the National Marrow Donor Program.

Q. How can I add my name to the list of potential marrow donors or contact a marrow donor registry?
A. There are two registries for unrelated marrow donors in the United States: the National Marrow Donor Program and the

American Bone Marrow Donor Registry. The National Marrow Donor Program recruits marrow donor volunteers and maintains a central registry of possible bone marrow donors through their toll-free number 1-800-654-1247. Because this organization represents the largest pool of volunteer donors, it is recommended by the Leukemia Society.

The American Bone Marrow Donor Registry is an association of independent, nonprofit donor registries throughout the United States. Individuals wishing to act as marrow donors for this group can call the American Registry at 1-800-7-DONATE. Persons wishing access to the American Bone Marrow Donor Registry on behalf of a patient should contact the Caitlin Raymond International Registry of Bone Marrow Donor Banks at 1-800-7-AMATCH.

Readings in Bone Marrow Transplantation

Non-Technical Books

Mann, Bruce W. *Leukemia: A Family's Challenge.* Traverse City, Michigan: Prism Publications Inc, 1987.

Thompson, Francesca Morosoni, MD. *Going for the Cure.* New York: St. Martin's Press, 1989.

Zumwalt, Elmo. *My Father, My Son.* New York: Macmillan Publishing Company, 1986.

Non-Technical Articles

Schmeck, Harold M. Jr. "Marrow: A Powerful New Tool." *New York Times*, January 10, 1984.

Steens, R. "Childhood Bone Marrow Transplantation." *Practitioner* 1512: 280-285, 1992.

Technical Books

Whedon, M (ed). *Bone Marrow Transplantation: Principles, Practice and Nursing Care.* Monterey, CA: Jones and Bartlett Publishers, 1991.

Techical Articles

Armitage, James O and Gale, RP. "Bone Marrow Autotransplantation." *American Journal of Medicine* 86: 203-206, 1989.

Ball, ED and Rybka, WB. "Autologous Bone Marrow Transplantation for the Treatment of Adult Acute Leukemia." *Hematology Oncology Clinics of North America* 7 (#1): 201-231, 1993.

Beatty, PG. "Results of Allogeneic Bone Marrow Transplantation with Unrelated or Mismatched Donors." *Seminars in Oncology* 19 (#3, Supplement 7): 7-12, 1992.

Bernstein, SH. "Growth Factor in the Management of Adult Acute Leukemia." *Hematology Oncology Clinics of North America* 7 (#1): 255-274, 1993.

Bortin, MM, Horowitz, MM, Gale, RP et al. "Changing Trends in Allogeneic Bone Marrow Transplantation for Leukemia in the 1980s." *Journal of the American Medical Association.* 268 (#5): 607-612, 1992.

Christiansen, NP. "Allogeneic Bone Marrow Transplantation for the Treatment of Adult Acute Leukemia." *Hematology Oncology Clinics of North America.* 7 (#1): 177-200, 1993.

Herzig, RH. "The Role of Autologous Bone Marrow Transplantation in the Treatment of Solid Tumors." *Seminars in Oncology* 19 (#3, Supplement 7): 7-12, 1992.

Lenarsky, C and Parkman, R. "Bone Marrow Transplantation for the Treatment of Immune Deficiency States." *Bone Marrow Transplantation* 6: 361-369, 1990.

Lesko, LM. "Bone Marrow Transplantation." *Psychooncology: the Psychological Care of the Patient with Cancer.* New York: Oxford University Press, 1989.

Parr, MD, Messino, MJ and McIntyre, W. "Allogeneic Bone Marrow Transplantation: Procedures and Complications." *American Journal of Hospital Pharmacy* 48: 127-137, 1991.

Singer, JW. "Role of Colony Stimulating Factors in Bone Marrow Transplantation." *Seminars in Oncology* 19 (#3, Supplement 7): 27-31, 1992.

Thomas, ED. "Bone Marrow Transplantation: Past Experiences and Future Prospects." *Seminars in Oncology* 19 (#3, Supplement 7): 3-6, 1992.

Vega, RA, Franco, CM, Abdel-Mageed, AS and Ragabe, AH. "Bone Marrow Transplantation in the Treatment of Children with Cancer: Current Status." *Hematology Oncology Clinics of North America* 1 (#4): 777-800, 1987.

Glossary

Blood typing and cross matching: Blood cells contain certain factors which can differ from person to person. Before a blood transfusion can be given safely, blood samples from the donor and recipient are typed or classified according to these blood factors (A, B, AB, or O). After typing, the blood samples are cross matched to see if they are compatible. Red cells of the donor are placed in a sample of the recipient's serum and red cells of the recipient in a sample of the donor's serum. If the blood does not form clumps, or agglutinate, the two bloods are compatible. Techniques for typing white blood cells and platelets are similar but more complicated.

Bone marrow: Marrow is the spongy tissue inside the bones which produces many of the elements of the blood.

Bone marrow transplant: A procedure in which a patient's bone marrow is destroyed by high doses of chemotherapy or radiation therapy and replaced with new bone marrow from a donor, usually a sibling with HLA typing identical to the patient's.

CBC (complete blood count): A series of tests which examines the various components of the blood, including white cells, red cells, and platelets. The tests help determine a patient's general condition and the results of treatments, including regeneration of the bone marrow after transplant.

Chemotherapy: Treatment with drugs that combat malignant disease. Usually a combination of several drugs is administered to bring a patient into a remission or abatement of disease symptoms.

Granulocytes: One type of white blood cell. It destroys invading bacteria which can cause disease.

HLA: Human leukocyte antigens; structures which appear on white blood cells as well as cells of almost all other tissues. By typing for HLA antigens, donors and recipients of white blood cells, platelets, and bone marrow can be "matched" to insure survival of transfused and transplanted cells.

Hyperalimentation: Intravenous administration of nutrients. It is also called total parenteral nutrition (TPN).

Immune response: The body's defense against disease and foreign substances, including transplanted bone marrow. During the immune system response, a substance can be ingested by a cell, recognized as "foreign," and then "killed' by other cells or a substance specifically formed against it.

Infection: The invasion and multiplication of disease-producing organisms within the body.

Intravenous: The administration of a drug or fluid substance directly to the vein.

Leukemia: A malignant disease of the blood-forming tissues, including the bone marrow. Leukemia results in the uncontrolled production and growth of abnormal white blood cells.

Leukocytes: White blood cells. They play a major part in the body's defense against infection and disease. These cells are divided into three main subgroups: granulocytes, lymphocytes, and monocytes.

Lymphatic system: Tissues found throughout the body which contain the infection-fighting white blood cells.

Lymphoma: The name of a group of malignant disorders affecting lymphatic tissues.

Malignant: Cancerous; characterized by an abnormal growth of cells.

Platelet: One of the main components of blood that produces clots to seal up injuries and prevent excessive bleeding.

Radiation therapy: Treatment using high energy radiation, as from x-ray machines.

Red blood cells: Cells that carry oxygen to all parts of the body; also called erythrocytes.

Relapse: The reappearance of a disease after a period in which symptoms of the disease had lessened or disappeared.

Remission: The disappearance of symptoms of a disease. Also, the period during which no evidence of disease is present.

Toxicity: The state of being poisonous or causing ill effects.

This publication is designed to provide accurate and authoritative information in regard to the subject matter covered. It is distributed as a public service by the Leukemia Society of America, Inc., with the understanding that the Leukemia Society of America, Inc., is not engaged in rendering medical or other professional services.

■ Document Source:
Leukemia Society of America
National Headquarters
600 Third Ave
New York, NY 10016
(212) 573-8484; (800) 955-4LSA
P-41 30 M
April 1994

See also: Aplastic Anemia Answer Book (page 44); What Everyone Should Know About Leukemia (page 78); Bone Marrow Transplantation and Peripheral Blood Stem Cell Transplantation (page 82)

Information from PDQ for Patients

CHILDHOOD ACUTE LYMPHOCYTIC LEUKEMIA

Description

What is childhood acute lymphocytic leukemia?

Childhood acute lymphocytic leukemia (also called acute lymphoblastic leukemia or ALL) is a disease in which too many underdeveloped infection-fighting white blood cells called lymphocytes are found in your child's blood and bone marrow. ALL is the most common form of leukemia in children and the most common kind of childhood cancer.

Lymphocytes are made by the bone marrow and by other organs of the lymph system. The bone marrow is the spongy tissue inside the large bones in the body. The bone marrow makes red blood cells (which carry oxygen and other materials to all tissues of the body), white blood cells (which fight infection), and platelets (which make the blood clot). Normally, the bone marrow makes cells called blasts that develop (mature) into several different types of blood cells that have specific jobs to do in the body.

The lymph system is made up of thin tubes that branch, like blood vessels, into all parts of the body. Lymph vessels carry lymph, a colorless, watery fluid that contains lymphocytes. Along the network of vessels are groups of small, bean-shaped organs called lymph nodes. Clusters of lymph nodes are found in the underarm, pelvis, neck, and abdomen. The spleen (an organ in the upper abdomen that makes lymphocytes and filters old blood cells from the blood), the thymus (a small organ beneath the breastbone), and the tonsils (an organ in your throat) are also part of the lymph system.

Lymphocytes fight infection by making substances called antibodies, which attack germs and other harmful bacteria in your child's body. In ALL, the developing lymphocytes do not mature and become too numerous. These immature lymphocytes are then found in the blood and the bone marrow. They also collect in the lymph tissues and make them swell. Lymphocytes may crowd out other blood cells in the blood and bone marrow. If your child's bone marrow cannot make enough red blood cells to carry oxygen, your child may have anemia. If your child's bone marrow cannot make enough platelets to make the blood clot normally, your child may bleed or bruise easily. The cancerous lymphocytes can also invade other organs, the spinal cord, and the brain.

Leukemia can be acute (progressing quickly with many immature cancer cells) or chronic (progressing slowly with more mature-looking leukemia cells). Acute lymphocytic leukemia progresses quickly. ALL can occur in children and adults. Treatment is different for adults than it is for children. If you want information on adult ALL, see the PDQ patient information statement on adult acute lymphocytic leukemia. Separate PDQ patient information statements are also available for chronic lymphocytic leukemia, chronic myelogenous leukemia, adult or childhood acute myeloid leukemia, and hairy cell leukemia.

If your child has symptoms of leukemia, your child's doctor may order blood tests to count the number of each of the different kind of blood cells. If the results of the blood test are not normal, your doctor may do a bone marrow aspirate. During this test, a needle is inserted into a bone in the hip and a small amount of bone marrow is taken out and looked at under the microscope. Your child's doctor can then tell what kind of leukemia your child has and plan the best treatment.

Your child's doctor may also do a spinal tap in which a needle is inserted through the back to take a sample of the fluid that surrounds your child's brain and spine. The fluid is then looked at under a microscope to see if leukemia cells are present.

Your child's chance of recovery (prognosis) depends on various features of the leukemia cells, your child's age, and the number of white blood cells in the blood (the white cell count) at diagnosis.

Stage Explanation

Stages of Childhood Acute Lymphocytic Leukemia

There is no staging for childhood acute lymphocytic leukemia. The treatment depends on whether your child has been treated or not.

Untreated

Untreated ALL means no treatment has been given except to treat symptoms. There are too many white blood cells in the blood and bone marrow, and there may be other signs and symptoms of leukemia.

In Remission

Treatment has been given and the number of white blood cells and other blood cells in the blood and bone marrow is normal. There are no signs or symptoms of leukemia.

Recurrent/refractory

Recurrent disease means the leukemia has come back (recurred) after going into remission. Refractory disease means the leukemia never went into remission after being treated.

Treatment Option Overview

How Childhood Acute Lymphocytic Leukemia is Treated

There are treatments for all patients with childhood ALL. The primary treatment for ALL is chemotherapy. Radiation therapy may be used in certain cases. Bone marrow transplantation is being studied in clinical trials.

Chemotherapy uses drugs to kill cancer cells. Chemotherapy may be taken by mouth, or it may be put into the body by a needle in a vein or muscle. Chemotherapy is called a systemic treatment because the drug enters the bloodstream, travels through the body, and can kill cancer cells throughout the body. Chemotherapy may sometimes be put into the fluid that surrounds the brain through a needle in the back (intrathecal chemotherapy).

Radiation therapy uses x-rays or other high-energy rays to kill cancer cells and shrink tumors. Radiation for ALL usually comes from a machine outside the body (external beam radiation therapy).

There are three phases of treatment for ALL. The first phase is called induction therapy. The purpose of induction therapy is to kill as many of the leukemia cells as possible and make your child go into remission. Once your child goes into remission and there are no signs of leukemia, a second phase of treatment is given (called consolidation therapy), which tries to kill any remaining leukemia cells. A third phase of treatment called maintenance therapy may be given for up to several years to keep your child in remission.

If the leukemia cells have spread to the brain, your child will receive chemotherapy with radiation therapy to the brain. During induction and maintenance, your child may also receive therapy to prevent leukemia cells from growing in the brain. This type of preventive therapy is called central nervous system (CNS) prophylaxis.

Bone marrow transplantation is a newer type of treatment. First, high doses of chemotherapy with or without radiation therapy are given to destroy all of the bone marrow in the body. Healthy marrow is then taken from another person (a donor) whose tissue is the same as or almost the same as the patient's. The donor may be a twin (the best match), a brother or sister, or another person not related. The healthy marrow from the donor is given to the patient through a needle in a vein, and the marrow replaces the marrow that was destroyed. A bone marrow transplant using marrow from a relative or person not related is called an allogeneic bone marrow transplant.

An even newer type of bone marrow transplant, called autologous bone marrow transplant, is being studied in clinical trials. During this transplant, bone marrow is taken from the patient and may be treated with drugs to kill any cancer cells. The marrow is frozen to save it. The patient is then given high-dose chemotherapy with or without radiation therapy to destroy all of the remaining marrow. The frozen marrow that was saved is thawed and given through a needle in a vein to replace the marrow that was destroyed.

Treatment by Stage

Treatment for childhood acute lymphocytic leukemia depends on the prognostic group your child is assigned to, based on your child's age, white cell count, and other factors.

Your child may receive treatment that is considered standard based on its effectiveness in a number of patients in past studies, or you may choose to have your child take part in a clinical trial. Not all patients are cured with standard therapy and some standard treatments may have more side effects than are desired. For these reasons, clinical trials are designed to test new treatments and to find better ways to treat cancer patients. Clinical trials are going on in most parts of the country for most stages of childhood ALL. If you want more information, call the Cancer Information Service at 1-800-4-CANCER (1-800-422-6237).

Untreated Childhood Acute Lymphocytic Leukemia

Your child's treatment will probably be systemic chemotherapy. Your child will also receive some type of therapy to treat or prevent leukemia in the brain. This therapy may be intrathecal chemotherapy with or without radiation therapy to the brain, or high doses of systemic chemotherapy with intrathecal chemotherapy. Clinical trials are testing new drugs and new ways of treating and preventing leukemia in the brain.

Childhood Acute Lymphocytic Leukemia in Remission

Your child's treatment will probably be systemic chemotherapy. Intrathecal and/or high doses of systemic chemotherapy is given to prevent leukemia cells from growing in the brain.

Recurrent Childhood Acute Lymphocytic Leukemia

Your child's treatment depends on the type of treatment your child received before, how soon the cancer came back following treatment, and whether the leukemia cells are found outside the bone marrow. Your child's treatment will probably be systemic chemotherapy. You may want to consider a clinical trial of new chemotherapy drugs or bone marrow transplantation for your child.

To Learn More

To learn more about childhood acute lymphocytic leukemia, call the National Cancer Institute's Cancer Information Service at 1-800-4-CANCER (1-800-422-6237). By dialing this toll-free number, you can speak with someone who can answer your questions.

The Cancer Information Service can also send you free booklets. The following booklets about leukemia may be helpful to you:

- What You Need to Know About Leukemia
- Research Report: Bone Marrow Transplantation

The following booklets on childhood cancer may also be helpful to you:

- Young People with Cancer: A Handbook for Parents
- Talking with Your Child About Cancer
- When Someone in Your Family Has Cancer
- Managing Your Child's Eating Problems During Cancer Treatment

The following general booklets related to questions on cancer may also be helpful:

- What You Need to Know About Cancer
- Taking Time: Support for People with Cancer and the People Who Care About Them
- What Are Clinical Trials All About?
- Chemotherapy and You: A Guide to Self-Help During Treatment
- Radiation Therapy and You: A Guide to Self-Help During Treatment

There are many other places you can get material about cancer treatment and services to help you. You can check the social service office at your hospital for local and national agencies that help with your finances, getting to and from treatment, care at home, and dealing with your problems. The American Cancer Society and the Leukemia Society of America have information and services for leukemia patients. Candlelighters Childhood Cancer Foundation (1-800-366-2223) has free services and publications including newsletters, bibliographies, and information for parents and brothers and sisters of children with cancer. It can also refer you to a local parent peer support group in the United States or abroad.

Local offices for these organizations are listed in the white pages of the telephone book.

You can also write to the National Cancer Institute at this address:

National Cancer Institute
Office of Cancer Communications
31 Center Drive, MSC 2580
Bethesda, MD 20892-2580

■ **Document Source:**
   U.S. Department of Health and Human Services, Public Health Service
   National Institutes of Health
   National Cancer Institute
   February 1996

Information from PDQ for Patients

CHRONIC LYMPHOCYTIC LEUKEMIA

Description

What is chronic lymphocytic leukemia?

Chronic lymphocytic leukemia (CLL) is a disease in which too many infection-fighting white blood cells called lymphocytes are found in the body. Lymphocytes are made in the bone marrow and by other organs of the lymph system. Your bone marrow is the spongy tissue inside the large bones in your body. The bone marrow makes red blood cells (which carry oxygen and other materials to all tissues of the body), white blood cells (which fight infection), and platelets (which make your blood clot). Normally, bone marrow cells called blasts develop (mature) into several different types of blood cells that have specific jobs to do in the body.

The lymph system is made up of thin tubes that branch, like blood vessels, into all parts of the body. Lymph vessels carry lymph, a colorless, watery fluid that contains lymphocytes. Along the network of vessels are groups of small, bean-shaped organs called lymph nodes. Clusters of lymph nodes are found in the underarm, pelvis, neck, and abdomen. The spleen (an organ in the upper abdomen that makes lymphocytes and filters old blood cells from the blood), the thymus (a small organ beneath the breastbone), and the tonsils (an organ in your throat) are also part of the lymph system.

Lymphocytes fight infection by making substances called antibodies, which attack germs and other harmful things in your body. In CLL, the developing lymphocytes do not mature correctly and too many are made. The lymphocytes may look normal, but they cannot fight infection as well as they should. These immature lymphocytes are then found in the blood and the bone marrow. They also collect in the lymph tissues and make them swell. Lymphocytes may crowd out other blood cells in the blood and bone marrow. If your bone marrow cannot make enough red blood cells to carry oxygen, you may have anemia. If your bone marrow cannot make enough platelets to make your blood clot normally, you may bleed or bruise easily.

Leukemia can be acute (progressing quickly with many immature cells) or chronic (progressing slowly with more mature, normal-looking cells). Chronic lymphocytic leukemia progresses slowly and usually occurs in people 60 years of age or older. In the first stages of the disease there are often no symptoms. As time goes on, more and more lymphocytes are made and symptoms begin to appear. You should see a doctor if your lymph nodes swell, your spleen or liver becomes larger than normal, you feel tired all the time, or you bleed easily.

If you have symptoms, your doctor will examine you and may order blood tests to count the number of each of the different kind of blood cells. If the results of the blood test are not normal, you may have more blood tests. Your doctor also may do a bone marrow biopsy. During this test, a needle is inserted into a bone and a small amount of bone marrow is taken out and looked at under the microscope. Your doctor can then tell what kind of leukemia you have and plan the best treatment.

Your chance of recovery (prognosis) depends on the stage of your disease, your age, and your general health.

There are separate PDQ patient information statements on acute lymphocytic leukemia (adult and childhood), acute myeloid leukemia (adult and childhood), chronic myelogenous leukemia, and hairy cell leukemia.

Stage Explanation

Stages of Chronic Lymphocytic Leukemia

Once chronic lymphocytic leukemia has been found (diagnosed), more tests may be done to find out if leukemia cells have spread to other parts of the body. This is called staging. Your doctor needs to know the stage of your disease to plan treatment. The following stages are used for chronic lymphocytic leukemia:

Stage 0

There are too many lymphocytes in the blood, but there are usually no other symptoms of leukemia. Lymph nodes and the spleen and liver are not swollen, and the number of red blood cells and platelets is normal.

Stage I

There are too many lymphocytes in the blood, and lymph nodes are swollen. The spleen and liver are not swollen and the number of blood cells and platelets is normal.

Stage II

There are too many lymphocytes in the blood, and lymph nodes and the liver and spleen are swollen.

Stage III

There are too many lymphocytes in the blood, and there are too few red blood cells (anemia). Lymph nodes and the liver or spleen may be swollen.

Stage IV

There are too many lymphocytes in the blood and too few platelets, which make it hard for the blood to clot. The lymph nodes, liver, or spleen may be swollen, and there may be too few red blood cells (anemia).

Refractory

Refractory means that the leukemia does not respond to treatment.

Treatment Option Overview

How Chronic Lymphocytic Leukemia is Treated

There are treatments for all patients with chronic lymphocytic leukemia. Three kinds of treatment are used:

- chemotherapy (using drugs to kill cancer cells)
- radiation therapy (using high-dose x-rays or other high-energy rays to kill cancer cells)
- treatment for complications of the leukemia, such as infection

The use of biological therapy (using your body's immune system to fight cancer) is being tested in clinical trials. Surgery may be used in certain cases.

Chemotherapy uses drugs to kill cancer cells. Chemotherapy may be taken by pill, or it may be put into the body by a needle in the vein or muscle.

Chemotherapy is called a systemic treatment because the drug enters the bloodstream, travels through the body, and can kill cancer cells throughout the body.

Radiation therapy uses x-rays or other high-energy rays to kill cancer cells and shrink tumors. Radiation for CLL usually comes from a machine outside the body (external radiation therapy).

If your spleen is swollen, your doctor may take out the spleen in an operation called a splenectomy. This is only done in rare cases.

Biological therapy tries to get your own body to fight cancer. It uses materials made by your own body or made in a laboratory to boost, direct, or restore your body's natural defenses against disease. Biological therapy is sometimes called biological response modifier (BRM) therapy or immunotherapy.

Because infection often occurs in patients with CLL, a special substance called immunoglobulin, which contains antibodies, may be given to prevent infections.

Sometimes a special machine is used to filter the blood to take out extra lymphocytes. This is called leukapheresis.

Bone marrow transplantation is used to replace your bone marrow with healthy bone marrow. First, all of the bone marrow in your body is destroyed with high doses of chemotherapy with or without radiation therapy. Healthy marrow is then taken from another person (a donor) whose tissue is the same as or almost the same as yours. The donor may be a twin (the best match), a brother or sister, or another person not related. The healthy marrow from the donor is given to you through a needle in the vein, and the marrow replaces the marrow that was destroyed. A bone marrow transplant using marrow from a relative or person not related to you is called an allogeneic bone marrow transplant.

Another type of bone marrow transplant, called autologous bone marrow transplant, is being studied in clinical trials. To do this type of transplant, bone marrow is taken from you and treated with drugs to kill any cancer cells. The marrow is frozen to save it. Next, you are given high-dose chemotherapy, with or without radiation therapy, to destroy all of your remaining marrow. The frozen marrow that was saved for you is then thawed and given to you through a needle in a vein to replace the marrow that was destroyed.

Treatment by Stage

Treatment for chronic lymphocytic leukemia depends on the stage of your disease, your age, and your overall health.

You may receive treatment that is considered standard based on its effectiveness in a number of patients in past studies, or you may choose to go into a clinical trial. Most patients with chronic lymphocytic leukemia are not cured with standard therapy and some standard treatments may have more side effects than are desired. For these reasons, clinical trials are designed to find better ways to treat cancer patients and are based on the most up-to-date information. Clinical trials are going on in most parts of the country for most stages of chronic lymphocytic leukemia. If you want more information, call the Cancer Information Service at 1-800-4-CANCER (1-800-422-6237).

Stage 0 Chronic Lymphocytic Leukemia

If you have stage 0 CLL, you usually do not need treatment or you may receive chemotherapy. Your doctor will follow you closely so you can be treated if the leukemia gets worse.

Stage I Chronic Lymphocytic Leukemia

Your treatment may be one of the following:

1. If you have no symptoms, you may need no treatment. Your doctor will follow you closely so you can be treated if the leukemia gets worse.
2. External radiation therapy to swollen lymph nodes.
3. Chemotherapy.

Stage II Chronic Lymphocytic Leukemia

Your treatment may be one of the following:

1. If you have few or no symptoms, you may need no treatment. Your doctor will follow you closely so you can be treated if the leukemia gets worse.
2. Chemotherapy.
3. Clinical trials of biological therapy.
4. External radiation therapy to the spleen.

Stage III Chronic Lymphocytic Leukemia

Your treatment may be one of the following:

1. Chemotherapy.
2. Clinical trials of bone marrow transplantation.
3. Surgery to remove the spleen (splenectomy).
4. External radiation therapy to the spleen.
5. External radiation therapy to the whole body (whole body radiation).
6. Clinical trials of biological therapy.

Stage IV Chronic Lymphocytic Leukemia

Your treatment may be one of the following:

1. Chemotherapy.
2. Clinical trials of bone marrow transplantation.
3. Surgery to remove the spleen (splenectomy).
4. External radiation therapy to the spleen.
5. External radiation therapy to the whole body (whole body radiation).
6. Clinical trials of biological therapy.

Refractory Chronic Lymphocytic Leukemia

Your treatment depends on many factors; you may wish to consider entering a clinical trial of new chemotherapy drugs and bone marrow transplantation.

To Learn More

To learn more about chronic lymphocytic leukemia, call the National Cancer Institute's Cancer Information Service at 1-800-4-CANCER (1-800-422-6237). By dialing this toll-free number, you can speak with someone who can answer your questions.

The Cancer Information Service can also send you free booklets. The following booklets about leukemia may be helpful to you:

- What You Need to Know About Leukemia
- Research Report: Bone Marrow Transplantation

The following general booklets on questions related to cancer may also be helpful:

- What You Need to Know About Cancer
- Taking Time: Support for People with Cancer and the People Who Care About Them
- What Are Clinical Trials All About?
- Chemotherapy and You: A Guide to Self-Help During Treatment
- Radiation Therapy and You: A Guide to Self-Help During Treatment
- Eating Hints for Cancer Patients
- Advanced Cancer: Living Each Day
- When Cancer Recurs: Meeting the Challenge Again

There are many other places you can get information about cancer treatment and services to help you. You can check the social service office at your hospital for local and national agencies that help with your finances, getting to and from treatment, care at home, and dealing with your problems. The American Cancer Society and the Leukemia Society of America have information and services for leukemia patients. Their local offices are listed in the white pages of the telephone book.

You can also write to the National Cancer Institute at this address:

National Cancer Institute
Office of Cancer Communications
31 Center Drive, MSC 2580
Bethesda, MD 20892-2580

■ **Document Source:**
U.S. Department of Health and Human Services, Public Health Service
National Institutes of Health
National Cancer Institute
February 1996

HODGKIN'S DISEASE AND THE NON-HODGKIN'S LYMPHOMAS

Hodgkin's disease and the non-Hodgkin's lymphomas are now considered among the most treatable forms of cancer.

As a group, they are diagnosed in approximately 52,900 people—about 20 out of every 100,000—in the United States annually. Lymphomas account for about 6 percent of all cancers in the United States. Their incidence is increasing at a rate of 3 to 4 percent annually.

Hodgkin's disease represents about 15 percent of all reported cases of lymphoma, striking 7,900 Americans each year. It can occur in people of any age, but most often is found in individuals between their mid-teens and mid-30s and, less frequently, in those over 50. The other forms of lymphoma are known as non-Hodgkin's lymphomas. They, too, can occur at any age but most often affect people between 40 and 70 years old.

Introduction

The aim of this booklet from the Leukemia Society of America is to provide information about *lymphomas* to patients and their families and friends. The diagnosis of lymphoma may trigger many questions about the illness and its treatment. Though these questions can best be answered by your health care providers, it is often helpful to have written information as well. Topics covered in this booklet include: the incidence of lymphomas; a description of the illness and its symptoms; procedures used to diagnose lymphomas and the treatment of lymphomas; general side effects of treatment; the use of BMT in treating lymphomas and, finally, future directions in the treatment of lymphomas. A glossary of commonly used terms is also provided in addition to a reading list with selections from the medical and lay literature. Italicized words in the text are defined in the glossary at the end of the booklet.

What They Are

Lymphomas are cancers that start in the *tissues* of the *lymph system.* The lymph system comprises the body's defense system against the infections. The system acts as the site for development, storage, and deployment of the white blood cells, called *lymphocytes,* that play a major role in protection against disease.

There are various types of lymphomas. The best way to explain the disorders is to start with a brief review of both the blood and lymph systems to see how normal blood cells grow and function within these two systems, and go over general information common to all the lymphomas.

The Blood System

The *blood* supplies oxygen, essential nutrients, growth factors, and chemicals to cells throughout the body. It plays an important part in protecting the body from infection. Blood also helps the body remove toxins and other waste materials.

Whole blood is made up of many components, including the *red cells,* clotting cells called *platelets,* and the white blood cells.

White blood cells play a major role in defending the body against infections and disease. A shortage of normally functioning white blood cells can cause increased susceptibility to bacteria, viruses, fungi, and other agents that cause infections and disease.

There are three main types of white blood cells.

- Monocytes protect the body from bacteria such as tuberculosis.
- Granulocytes also combat infection by quickly increasing in number, then by surrounding and killing foreign disease substances. They then return to their original (preinfection) numbers.
- Lymphocytes are divided into two cell types that work with our *immune system.* T cells attack viruses and cancer cells and control the function of other *white cells.*

The Lymph System

The lymph system provides the body's defense against infection and disease and, therefore, is referred to as the immune system. It is a complex network of cells and channels that runs throughout the body. A milky-colored fluid, called *lymph,* circulates throughout the lymph system.

The lymph system and lymph mainly consist of lymphocytes. These lymphocytes are either arranged in clusters—called *lymph nodes*—or they circulate through the bloodstream and the lymphatic channels to all parts of the body.

Hundreds of lymph nodes—tiny bean-shaped glands that trap and help destroy disease-producing agents—are situated along this network. Clusters of lymph nodes are found in the underarm, pelvis, neck, and abdomen. As the lymph passes through the nodes, foreign particles and cells containing toxic substances are filtered out, and other cells are picked up. It is also thought that lymph nodes are an important site for the production of antibodies and for the maturation and development of B cells. This important activity takes place in a specialized area of the node, called the *follicle,* where many different kinds of normal B cells can be seen clumped together in a small cluster, or nodule.

Other organs that make up the lymph system are the bone marrow, spleen, and thymus. These organs, known as lymphoid organs, are also responsible for the production, storage, and development of the lymphocytes.

Circulating lymphocytes may spend a good deal of time—several hours or longer—in a particular lymphoid organ, especially the spleen (an organ in the upper abdomen). Not all lymphocytes circulate. Some are resident cells that form different parts of the lymphatic tissues. These tissues make up portions of other lymphoid organs including the thymus (a small organ underneath the breastbone) and the tonsils (an organ in your throat).

Organs that are not part of the lymph system are considered nonlymphoid. However, certain nonlymphoid organs may contain lymph tissues and/or circulating lymphocytes. These related organs include the lungs, liver, kidneys, stomach, small intestine, and skin.

The Lymphomas

The word "oma" in Greek refers to tumor: therefore, a lymphoma is a tumor of the lymph system. Because lymph tissues are present in many parts of the body, lymphomas can start in almost any part of the body.

The cause of most lymphomas is unclear but is most likely related to genetic or chromosomal abnormality developing in a single normal lymphocyte in the body. The unchecked production of abnormal or cancerous lymphoma cells results.

When lymphoma occurs, cancer develops in the lymph system wherever lymphocytes are normally found. In patients with lymphomas, malignant lymphocytes multiply uncontrollably. Excessive production of these malignant lymphocytes impairs normal cell function and the body's ability to fight infection. If left untreated, lymphoma cells overcrowd the bone marrow (somewhat like leukemia) and prevent normal production of red cells, white cells, and platelets. Depending on the extent of involvement, the lymphoma cells may infiltrate major organs of the body, causing these organs to malfunction or fail. Persons with lymphoma become increasingly *susceptible* to *fatigue,* anemia, excessive bleeding, and infections.

The exact course of these disorders, and the speed with which they take it, varies from type to type. The specific types of lymphoma and their treatment are determined by a number of factors.

Types of Lymphomas

The lymphomas are divided into two distinct groups: Hodgkin's disease and the non-Hodgkin's lymphomas, based upon the natural course of disease and cells affected by disease.

Hodgkin's Disease (HD)

Hodgkin's disease is distinguished from other types of lymphoma by the presence of one characteristic type of cell, known as the Reed-Sternberg cell (named for the scientists who discovered it). Although they are found within the lymph nodes, Reed-Sternberg cells may not be lymphocytes.

Hodgkin's disease has other characteristic features that distinguish it from all other cancers of the lymph system. One of its unique features is its pattern of spread. Hodgkin's disease usually begins in the lymph nodes in one region of the body. As the disease progresses, it tends to spread in a fairly predictable manner, moving from one part of the lymph system to the next. Hodgkin's disease then moves into organs including the lungs, liver, bone, and bone marrow.

There are four stages of Hodgkin's disease, based on the pattern of spread of the disease. Stage I represents local early-stage disease, while Stage IV means that the disease has spread to various organs distant from the original site of the disease. The histology, or pathologic interpretation under the microscope, may be nodular sclerosis, mixed cellularity, lymphocyte predominant, or lymphocyte depleted. Because of the overall success of therapy, these subtypes are generally not important to the *prognosis* of HD.

Non-Hodgkin's Lymphoma (NHL)

In contrast, while the non-Hodgkin's lymphomas may begin in the lymph nodes, in about 20 percent of the cases, they start in sites outside of the nodes, such as the lungs, liver, and gastrointestinal tract.

These lymphomas usually progress in a far less systematic and predictable manner than Hodgkin's disease. Cells in different organs can be affected at the same time and, quite frequently, they spread through the lymph and blood during the early stages of abnormal production.

Also, unlike Hodgkin's disease, these disorders cannot be identified by the consistent presence of one particular type of cell. Most non-Hodgkin's lymphomas consist of malignant B cells. T cells can also become malignant and can disrupt the production of other cells as well.

There are many kinds of non-Hodgkin's lymphomas involving various cell subsets, growth patterns, and rates of progress. Multiple systems of identification have been used in the past to classify these diseases. The most common classification system, the International Working Formulation, translates and consolidates the terms from all these systems. Currently, scientists are developing a new classification that will take into account recent advances in the understanding of the biology and behavior of these diseases. However, the International Working Formulation remains a great advance in our understanding of these malignancies.

The non-Hodgkin's lymphomas are first broken down into two main categories, depending upon the growth pattern within the lymph node affected by the disease when viewed under a microscope (which is called the histology).

- **Follicular Lymphomas** attempt to maintain the normal follicle pattern seen in lymph nodes. For this reason, this type of disease, where the cells are clumped together, is called follicular lymphoma. This pattern of cell distribution is usually only seen in lymph nodes affected by the disease. Occasionally, follicular patterns can be seen in tissues that are not of lymphoid origin.
- **Diffuse Lymphomas** involve the lymph node diffusely, and no follicular pattern can be identified. When biopsies of tissue that are not of lymphoid origin are

obtained, the disease is usually diagnosed as diffuse lymphoma, since follicular patterns are not often identified outside of nodes.

The lymphomas are further defined by the cell size and the appearance of the cell nucleus, the center of the cell which contains the cell's *chromosomes* and DNA. Based upon the size of the lymphoma cell (large or small compared to a normal red blood cell) and whether the nucleus has a cleft in it (a large indentation seen underneath the microscope), pathologists identify follicular and diffuse lymphomas as being small or large cleaved, or small or large noncleaved, cell subtypes.

Once the histology is identified, it is identified as either low-grade, intermediate-grade, or high-grade lymphoma. These grades are based upon knowledge of the natural histories of these diseases, and how fast each one spreads.

NHL Classifications

There are 10 different types of non-Hodgkin's lymphomas recognized in the International Working Formulation. The following is a complete set of classifications, including a description of the three grades and the types which they include.

Low-grade Lymphomas are commonly referred to as indolent, or slowly growing, because they often take years to develop into aggressive disease. Median survival can be six years or longer even without active treatment. Their natural course is considered "favorable." The low-grade lymphomas are

- Small lymphocytic
- Follicular, predominantly small cleaved cell
- Follicular, mixed, small cleaved and large cell

Intermediate-grade Lymphomas progress much faster than low-grade disorders. Based upon their natural history, the average survival rate is only 2.5 years without treatment and, consequently, their prognosis is considered "unfavorable." The forms including in this group are

- Follicular, predominantly large cell
- Diffuse, small cleaved cell
- Diffuse, mixed, small and large cell
- Diffuse, large cell, cleaved or noncleaved

High-grade Lymphomas are very aggressive and spread rapidly. Left untreated, these lymphomas prove fatal within six months to one year, and their natural course is also considered "unfavorable." The following forms are classified as aggressive or high-grade:

- Large cell, immunoblastic
- Lymphoblastic
- Small noncleaved cell, Burkitt's or non-Burkitt's lymphoma

Two of the high-grade disorders occur more frequently in children and adolescents than they do in adults. The non-Hodgkin's lymphomas are comparatively rare in young people but, as a group, they do represent about 10 percent of all malignant childhood disorders. Of the various forms, lymphoblastic lymphoma and small noncleaved cell lymphoma are the most common in children and deserve special mention. They always appear with diffuse patterns in the lymph nodes.

Lymphoblastic Lymphoma most frequently occurs during the teenage years, although it does occur in children, as well as in adults. It usually consists of very immature malignant T cells, or blasts, first produced in the thymus. When the development of these cells is interrupted, they continue to produce immature, mostly useless blast cells. They accumulate quickly, outgrow their area of containment, and spread through the body. Abnormal masses of tissue form in the lymph nodes in the neck and the area of the upper chest, causing respiratory problems, swelling, and unusual congestion in the head and face.

Somall, noncleaved cell lymphoma, also known as **Burkitt's Lymphoma,** is a common childhood disorder in tropical Africa, but it is also seen in the United States. Named for the scientist who discovered it, rather than the main cell involved, it usually affects B cells. In Africans, tumors first form in the jaw, ovaries, and kidneys. In Americans, however, the first signs of disease often appear in the lymph nodes of the neck and digestive system.

Miscellaneous Categories of Lymphomas

There is also a "miscellaneous" category listed in the working formulation. It includes lymphomas that show cellular features and clinical presentations that do not fit into the standard classifications, and those that are extremely rare. Within this group is the disorder called mycosis fungoides and Sezary Syndrome.

Mycosis Fungoides (and Sezary Syndrome) is a lymphoma of the skin that scientists believe is caused by the uncontrolled growth of malignant lymphocytes derived from the T4 or T helper subset. It is often preceded by a long history of skin disorders that may mimic eczema and psoriasis. At first, this lymphoma may progress slowly, but eventually it spreads to other areas and organs throughout the body and can behave as an aggressive large cell lymphoma. In some cases a leukemic phase called Sezary Syndrome can occur when T lymphocytes appear in the blood.

The other disorders that fall into the miscellaneous category are composite lymphoma, "true" histiocytic lymphoma, extramedullary plasmacytoma, and unclassifiable—or U-cell—lymphomas. Unclassifiable lymphomas involve cells with such primitive features that they cannot be defined, called null cells.

As a group, the disorders listed under this miscellaneous heading represent only a very small number of non-Hodgkin's lymphomas. However, their course, *symptoms,* and treatment are generally similar to those of the other lymphomas, and much of the information presented in this booklet applies to these disorders as well.

Symptoms

In most cases, patients seek attention because of the appearance of swollen glands in the neck, armpits, or groin. These swollen lymph nodes are mostly painless. They may be present for several weeks before attention is directed toward them. They are unresponsive to treatment with antibiotics.

Patients may experience loss of appetite and weight loss, along with nausea, vomiting, indigestion, and abdominal pain or bloating. Sometimes a feeling of fullness may be present, the result of an enlarged liver, spleen, or abdominal lymph nodes. Pressure or pain in the lower back, often extending down one or both legs, is another fairly common symptom. Other symptoms include itching, bone pain, headaches, constant coughing, and abnormal pressure and congestion in the face, neck, and upper chest.

General symptoms may include feeling tired, having a flu-like syndrome, or aching all over. Fatigue may be the result of anemia. Others experience night sweats and some may have recurring high-grade or constant low-grade fevers. Like most cancers, non-Hodgkin's lymphoma is best treated when it's found early. You should see your doctor if symptoms occur for more than two weeks.

Since all these symptoms are common to many illnesses, from minor ailments to serious disorders, the correct diagnostic procedures must be performed in order to confirm or rule out the diagnosis of lymphoma.

Diagnosis

The medical history provides strong clues to the diagnosis of lymphoma. In a thorough physical examination the lymphoma reveals itself by node or liver and/or spleen enlargement. Blood samples are also taken to determine overall disease composition, cell count, and how well the kidneys and liver are functioning.

The diagnosis is confirmed following biopsy of the suspected site. The biopsy is a relatively minor surgical procedure in which a local area is *anesthetized,* then a small incision is made for removal and inspection of a small tissue sample. It may require an exploratory procedure if the tumor is deeper within the body. Once the material is obtained, it is appropriately fixed, stained, and the material analyzed to define the type, structural characteristics, arrangement, and pattern of growth within the organ and the immunologic features (the latter via fluorescent cell sorting). With such multiple diagnostic approaches, a physician can then determine major biological features of Hodgkin's disease or the non-Hodgkin's lymphomas. These biological features of the lymphoma cell are important prognostic factors. With this prognostic information, the physician can draw up a treatment plan.

If an initial examination indicates the possibility of lymphoma, treatment should be provided by an appropriate physician, usually a hematologist-oncologist specializing in the diagnosis and care of the broad spectrum of malignant blood and related diseases.

The choice of treatment and your chances of recovery (prognosis) depend on the stage of your lymphoma (whether it is just in one area or has spread throughout the body), your age, and your overall condition.

Once the exact form of lymphoma has been identified the disease is "staged" to see if, and how far, it has progressed. As a general statement, *staging* is essential to establishing an appropriate treatment plan. The extent of this spread, or stage, helps define the treatment of Hodgkin's disease because this disorder usually progresses in an orderly and predictable manner.

Staging

Staging requires that a second series of tests be performed that can include any or all of the following:

Imaging

- X-rays, or computerized axial tomography *(CT) scans,* and abdominal *ultrasound.*
- Lymphangiograms, or x-rays, of the lymphatic system that are obtained through a process called lymphangiography. During this procedure, a special dye that allows the lymphatic system to stand out is inserted into lymphatic channels through a small incision in each foot. These channels are fragile, so the dye is injected slowly, over a period of about two to four hours. The skin and urine often develop a bluish cast until the dye is completely gone from the body, which normally takes from one to two weeks.
- In many instances, CT scans may be effectively used in place of lymphangiography.

Biopsy

- Additional surgical or deep-needle biopsies of glands and organs. Tissue is often removed from certain organs, for instance the liver and bone marrow, by needle. An anesthetic is used to deaden a localized area. Then, a needle is inserted into the organ or bone, and a small amount of tissue or marrow is withdrawn through a syringe for analysis.

Blood and Other Tests

- Additional blood work.
- In cases thought to involve the meninges, or covering of the *central nervous system,* a lumbar puncture, or spinal tap, is performed. The procedure involves the insertion of a needle between the vertebrae at the base of the spine and withdrawal of cerebrospinal fluid, which is examined under the microscope in order to determine if malignant cells are present.

Staging Laparotomy

Exploratory surgery of the organs in the abdomen and pelvic regions (staging laparotomy) may also be done for Hodgkin's disease. It allows surgeons to get a first-hand look at suspicious areas and to take biopsies of lymph nodes and tissues that would otherwise be hard to reach.

The value of staging by laparotomy with modern treatment is currently debated among lymphoma experts. Every case must be individualized. It is usually done only when it is needed to help your doctor plan your treatment. The procedure is not performed for the non-Hodgkin's lymphomas.

The spleen is also examined. It is sometimes important to know if the cells in this organ are affected because it is often the first indication that the illness has spread below the diaphragm (the thin muscle under the lungs that helps you breathe).

If the results of the tests taken on other organs below the diaphragm show that they are already affected, or if this becomes apparent during surgery, it usually means the spleen is involved as well. In this case, since the illness has obviously spread, treatment is usually chemotherapy.

Unfortunately, it is very difficult to accurately assess splenic involvement. Scans of the spleen are often unclear. Even during exploratory surgery, its appearance may be of little help. An enlarged spleen with a mottled surface can be functioning perfectly well and a normal-looking spleen can be diseased.

Removal of the spleen (splenectomy) is rarely, if ever, performed on children under the age of six because they are very susceptible to post-splenectomy infections caused by certain types of bacteria. Therefore, most physicians prefer to treat the disease more aggressively rather than remove the spleen. This threat lessens with age, and anyone older than six is immunized prior to undergoing the surgery, which further reduces the risk of post-splenectomy infections in older children and adults. Any patient who is splenectomized, irrespective of age, must receive a pneumococcal vaccine.

The results of this second series of tests are then analyzed and, based upon the extent of spread, one of the following stages is used:

Stage I

The disease is found in one lymph node area or in only one organ or area outside of the lymph nodes.

Stage II

The disease is found in two or more node areas on the same side of the diaphragm, or in one area or organ outside of the lymph nodes and in the lymph nodes around it, on the same side of the diaphragm.

Stage III

The disease has spread to nodes on both sides of the diaphragm. The lymphoma may also have spread to an area or organ near the lymph node areas and/or to the spleen.

Stage IV

The disease has spread in more than one spot to an organ or organs outside of the lymph system. Lymphoma cells may or may not be found in nodes near these organs. The disease may have also spread to only one organ outside of the lymph system, but lymph nodes far away from that organ are involved.

Each of these stages may be accompanied by one of the following letters:

B indicates the presence of a specific symptom, including unexplained fever above 101 degrees F, night sweats, and weight loss greater than 10 percent of normal body weight.

A means the absence of specific symptoms.

E is used when the disease involves sites outside to the lymph nodes (extranodal). Another letter may be added to **E** to define exactly which organ or site is involved. These letters include:

- **N** = nodes
- **S** = spleen
- **H** = liver
- **P** = pleura
- **L** = lungs
- **O** = bone
- **M** = bone marrow
- **D** = skin

Relapse

This term means that the disease has come back after it has been treated. It may come back in the area where it first started or in another part of the body.

Treatment

Before 1970, very few people diagnosed with any of the lymphomas actually recovered from their illness, and most with advanced disease died within two years. Since that time, the progress made in treating these disorders has been dramatic, particularly within the last decade. Many lymphomas are now potentially curable. Some forms still do not completely respond to treatment, but more and more, people are enjoying longer periods of life and are free of disease.

Treatment of most lymphomas starts soon after diagnosis and consists of chemotherapy, radiotherapy, or a combination of the two methods.

Chemotherapy

Chemotherapy consists of the use of specific drug preparations to stop the growth of rapidly dividing cells. Treatment involves a combination of drugs, called combination chemotherapy.

There are a number of combinations, or *regimens*, that can be effective in combating these disorders. These regimens are made up of various mixtures of agents and dosage levels, and generally include some drugs that are taken *orally*, as well as some that are administered *intravenously*, or by vein. Hodgkin's disease and the non-Hodgkin's lymphomas have been treated with various combinations. The regimens most often used in the treatment of Hodgkin's disease are:

- MOPP—mechlorethamine + oncovin (vincristine) + procarbazine + prednisone
- ABVD—adriamycin (doxorubicin) + bleomycin + vinblastine + dacarbazine

For the non-Hodgkin's lymphomas, the following combinations are among the most frequently given:

- CHOP—cyclophosphamide (cytoxan) + adriamycin (doxorubicin) + oncovin (vincristine) + prednisone
- COMP—cyclophosphamide (cytoxan) + oncovin (vincristine) + methotrexate + prednisone

- COPP—cyclophosphamide (cytoxan) + oncovine (vincristine) + procarbazine + prednisone
- COPBLAM III—cyclophosphamide (cytoxan) + oncovin (vincristine) + prednisone + bleomycin + adriamycin (doxorubicin) + procarbazine. The oncovin and bleomycin are given as injections.
- CVP—cyclophosphamide (cytoxan) + vincristine (oncovin) + prednisone
- MACOP-B—methotrexate with leucoverin rescue + adriamycin (doxorubicin) + cyclophosphamide (cytoxan) + oncovin (vincristine) + dexamethasone
- m-BACOD—methotrexate + bleomycin + adriamycin (doxorubicin) + cyclophosphamide (cytoxan) + oncovin (vincristine) + dexamethasone
- ProMACE-MOPP—prednisone + methotrexate + adriamycin (doxorubicin) + cyclophosphamide (cytoxan) + etoposide (VP-16) + mechlorethamine + oncovine (vincristine) + procarbazine
- ProMACE-CytoBom—prednisone + methotrexate + adramycin (doxorubicin) + cyclophosphamide (cytoxan) + etoposide (VP-16) + cytarabine (Cytosar) + bleomycin + oncovin (vincristine) + methotrexate

Treatment with combination chemotherapy lasts about six months, but in some cases may last as long as 12 months. Different drug regimens have different schedules of administration, but generally, chemotherapy is dispensed in 21 or 28-day cycles that are broken down into two periods. During the first interval, specific drugs are administered on appointed days. For instance, one drug may be given on days one through seven, and another only on days one and/or eight. This is followed by a period of rest, and the cycle begins again. If two drug regimens are used together, they may be administered in alternating cycles. Each combination may be given for three months at a time. At the current time, it is not clear which of these combinations is the best therapy.

Radiotherapy

In radiotherapy, doses of high-energy radiation are directed at specific portions of the body called *fields:* for example, the abdominal field, the pelvic field, or the mantle field, which includes the upper chest and neck.

Even when a lymphoma appears locally, research shows that it is more effective to irradiate a site containing diseased nodes, as well as the surrounding area or field, rather than just the site itself. In certain cases, treatment may consist of total nodal radiation that involves nodes in the entire trunk of the body, or, in other words, all the fields. When people are treated with radiotherapy, shields are used to protect various organs and with modern equipment, radiation can be quickly delivered to a targeted area with little or no scattering to other parts of the body.

Side Effects of Therapy

Both chemotherapy and radiotherapy are generally administered on an outpatient basis, and for most people, hospitalization is kept to a minimum. Obviously, patients who need exploratory surgery have to spend some time in the hospital to recuperate, especially if the spleen is removed. Also, people undergoing intensive therapy may occasionally require hospitalization. Some drug regimens include a few short hospital stays for in-patient treatment. In addition, therapy depresses bone marrow functioning and, therefore, reduces normal blood cell production. Sometimes patients may have to be kept in a sterile environment to protect them from infection, or they may need other support treatment such as antibiotics, growth factors, and blood transfusions to replace depleted cells. These hospital visits are usually brief, lasting anywhere from one to five days.

The aim of treatment is to destroy as many malignant cells as possible and bring the disease into *remission*—a state in which there is no evidence of residual disease. In order to do this, high doses of chemotherapy and radiotherapy are often necessary. Treatment is always toxic to some normal cells as well as the targeted malignant cells.

Toxic side effects depend upon the intensity of treatment. Since both forms of therapy decrease blood cell production, all patients should be aware that they are more prone to infection, hemorrhage, fatigue, and other symptoms of anemia. Such effects may be diminished by treatment with blood cell growth factors. Future studies will determine if such treatment minimizes complications.

Other short-term complications may include a dry mouth and throat, nausea and vomiting, gastrointestinal upsets such as diarrhea and constipation, hair loss, muscle weakness and nerve damage, i.e., tingling sensations in the fingers and toes (hyperarthrias), loss of reflexes, and a temporary paralysis or pain.

Certain drugs may cause high blood pressure or hypertension. Others may cause blood sugar levels to fluctuate, accelerating any underlying tendencies toward high blood sugar (hyperglycemia).

Some patients may notice an increase in appetite or water retention that causes a bloated or puffy appearance, especially around the face.

Urine may take on a red or orange cast. Occasionally, patients may see blood, usually a sign of cystitis, which is a local irritation in the wall of the bladder. Prevention includes adequate fluid intake. If bloody urine does occur, the physician needs to be notified immediately.

In addition, men may experience temporary periods of impotence, and women may notice a change in their menstrual cycles as well as a temporary loss of sexual interest.

Although these side effects are anything but pleasant, they are reasonably short-term. Most of these conditions can be treated or disappear once therapy is discontinued.

There are also some longer range complications associated with treatment. For example, some people may develop pneumonia within one to three months after radiotherapy. Symptoms include a dry cough and abnormal shortness of breath during periods of exertion. In a small percentage of patients, radiotherapy can cause an inflammation of the sac that surrounds the heart or heart muscle itself. This condition usually occurs within one year after treatment but has been reported to occur as many as four years later. Most often, these complications resolve themselves, but additional medical attention may be required.

Radiotheapy to the neck and chest is also thought to cause a condition called hypothyroidism, which is an underactive thyroid gland, in a significant number of people. The rate of incidence appears to increase with time. If and when hypothyroidism does develop, it is easily treated with thyroid extract.

Certain chemotherapeutic drugs may damage the heart muscle, producing CHF (congestive heart failure). Chemotherapeutic agents may produce long-term sterility in men and infertility in women.

Furthermore, several studies have shown a possible link between intensive treatment and the development of leukemia, or another form of lymphoma, about five to 10 years later. This risk (estimated at about 5 to 10 percent) seems highest among patients 40 and older treated with both chemotherapy and radiotherapy, or with prolonged courses of certain chemotherapeutic drugs. Also the rates of lung cancer and other solid tumors are slightly higher among people who have undergone high-dose radiation. Individuals who have undergone such treatment are encouraged not to smoke.

Treatment Options

While the treatment programs outlined here are fairly standard, therapies and their side effects vary from disorder to disorder, as well as from person to person. It is extremely important that patients discuss their individual program thoroughly with their physician. This discussion should include the type of treatment to be prescribed, any precautions to be taken during therapy, and ways to lessen the severity of impact. Patients are also encouraged to report any unusual or unexpected developments to their health care provider immediately.

Bone marrow transplantation represents a new area of hope for patients whose illness is resistant to standard forms of treatment, or who repeatedly relapse. This procedure will be explored later in the book.

Hodgkin's Disease

Hodgkin's disease is mostly curable. The overall cure rate is now estimated at 75 percent. Ninety percent of all people diagnosed with early-state illness, and over 50 percent of those with a more advanced stage, are now living longer than 10 years with no sign of recurrence.

As previously noted, treatment for Hodgkin's disease is primarily based on the extent to which the illness has spread, or, in other words, its stage.

Radiation therapy is often the only treatment necessary for Stages I and II. Patients with B symptoms or large masses, particularly in the chest, are often treated with both chemotherapy and radiation. Stage IIIA may be treated with radiotherapy or chemotherapy, or a combination of the two.

Combination chemotherapy with or without radiotherapy is the most effective treatment for Stages IIIB and IVA and B. Patients are usually treated with ABVD alone or in combination with MOPP.

While most people with Hodgkin's disease achieve long-term remission, a small percentage of patients develop relapse. There are a number of options available to those who experience a recurrence. People who have been treated with

radiation can often be brought back into remission with additional radiotherapy or with chemotherapy, usually MOPP or ABVD. Those who have already received one drug regimen can be treated again with the same combination or with an alternate regimen. For instance, MOPP patients may respond to ABVD and vice versa. Or they may be given both combinations. There are also a number of other combinations, containing different drugs and dosage levels, that have been successful in combating recurrent disease.

Bone marrow transplantation offers an opportunity for prolonged disease-free survival, and this approach should be considered for every patient with disease recurrent after chemotherapy.

The Non-Hodgkin's Lymphomas

The exhaustive research conducted on the non-Hodgkin's lymphomas over the last decade has yielded more effective treatment methods, and the results are very encouraging. Overall, 50 to 60 percent of patients are now living five years or longer with no sign of recurrent disease.

While there are a number of factors used to determine the best treatment for these disorders, the most significant consideration is histologic classification, followed by stage of spread.

Actually, very few people are diagnosed with "true" Stage I or II non-Hodgkin's lymphoma, even among those who have fairly minor or localized symptoms. By nature, these disorders usually spread very early in the course of disease. By the time most people seek medical attention, tests show that the disorder has progressed to Stage III or IV. Of course, there are some patients who really do have early-stage disease. This booklet covers treatment for those cases where it applies.

In reading about treatment for the non-Hodgkin's lymphomas, it is important not to confuse the stage of spread with the histologic grade, because often the two do not equate. This is a very pertinent point and it is important to review the difference between stage and histologic grade again.

The stage of spread is determined by how many organs contain diseased cells. The histologic grade is based on the appearance under the microscope and biologic behavior of the cells. Consequently, whether a disorder is staged at a level of I or IV, it can either be indolent or aggressive. Therefore, although the stage is important to treatment and its success, the deciding factor is whether a disorder is classified as low-, intermediate-, or high-grade.

The Low-grade Lymphomas

The low-grade lymphomas grow so slowly that people can live for many years mostly without symptoms. While some patients do experience periods of mild discomfort, very often the only outward evidence of disease is the painless enlargement of the lymph nodes in the neck, armpit, or groin. Somewhere between five and 10 years, however, these disorders usually begin to progress rapidly. At this point, they can become quite aggressive or high-grade, producing more severe and *systemic* symptoms such as fever, night sweats, and weight loss.

People with Stage I or II disorder are generally treated with radiotherapy. Radiation successfully induces remission and, it is now believed, possibly even long-term cure in many patients with early-stage disease.

As we have already discussed, though, most people do not have Stage I or II lymphoma. When tested, most patients are found to have Stage III or IV disease. Unfortunately, there is currently no known standard curative therapy for a low-grade disorder that has spread.

Again, it is important to remember that the stage is different than the grade. A Stage III or IV lymphoma can still be in its chronic or indolent phase, and treatment does prolong the lives of many people with a late-stage illness.

There are two schools of thought regarding the best way to treat Stage III or IV low-grade disorders. One is to begin intensive therapy right after diagnosis, whether a patient has symptoms or not, in an effort to achieve and maintain a complete remission. Treatment generally consists of high-dose radiotherapy, chemotherapy, or a combination of the two. Studies are still being conducted on this approach, but so far it appears that although initial remission is achieved with different standard chemotherapy regimens, most people eventually develop relapse, sometimes with a more aggressive or drug-resistant disorder.

Intensive treatment is in itself dangerous, but recent studies have suggested that such treatment may induce high rates of remission. Further evaluation of new intensive treatment programs is under way at major cancer centers to assess the value of intensive therapy for low-grade lymphomas. Such treatments include combinations of multiple chemotherapy drugs, extensive radiation therapy, and even high-dose therapy followed by bone marrow transplant.

On the other hand, if it is decided that such intensive treatment is not an option for therapy, as in the case of an elderly patient, symptoms can usually be controlled with radiation or single-agent chemotherapeutic drugs such as cyclophosphamide or chlorambucil. As low-grade lymphomas become more aggressive, such patients are generally treated with combination chemotherapy.

The Intermediate-grade Lymphomas

Without treatment, the intermediate-grade lymphomas progress fairly rapidly, but there have been considerable inroads made in treating these disorders. Remission can be induced in approximately 50 to 75 percent of patients, many of whom can look forward to long-term survival. Initial treatment has been so successful that people who stay in remission for three years from diagnosis are often considered cured.

Traditionally, patients with Stage I disorder have been treated with radiotherapy and, in certain instances, radiation is still the treatment of choice. However, while most patients enter remission, relapses still occur. Proper combination chemotherapy is extremely effective in inducing and sustaining remission in more than 75 percent of patients with localized disease. In some cases, as little as three doses of chemotherapy and radiation therapy may be effective.

Stage II, III, and IV intermediate-grade lymphomas are treated with combination chemotherapy, most often with drug combinations that include cyclophosphamide and adramycin.

Recent studies have suggested that no combination of chemotherapy drugs produces better results than those expected with CHOP alone, although certain patient and treatment-related features may be more important at determining results. In selected cases, treatment may also include radiotherapy, and rarely surgery may be performed to remove tumors, especially those obstructing the gastrointestinal tract.

Occasionally, CNS prophylaxis may be indicated in order to prevent malignant cells from multiplying within the central nervous system. The human body contains a network of capillary walls, called the blood-brain barrier, that usually protects the spinal column and brain from dangerous substances. While the blood and lymph may carry abnormal cells right through this barrier, it is very difficult for most drugs to penetrate it in sufficient amounts to destroy them, creating a natural haven for disease.

CNS prophylaxis can be given in several ways, depending upon individual circumstances. High doses of drugs such as methotrexate which are administered intravenously cross the so-called blood barrier and may be included in a standard chemotherapy regimen. Treatment may involve a separate procedure such as crania irradiation, intrathecal chemotherapy, a combination of the two, or, as is often the case, all these in proper sequence. Intrathecal therapy is via lumbar puncture. Treatment is generally given weekly for a period of about eight weeks and, if it is handled as a separate procedure, it may be given at the same time as standard therapy or right after it is completed.

The High-grade Lymphomas

As in the case of intermediate-grade disorders, substantial progress has been made in the treatment of high-grade lymphomas. Fifty to 75 percent of patients enter remission, and most people who do not relapse within one year can look forward to a life free from recurrence.

High-grade disorders grow extremely rapidly and, regardless of stage, are treated very aggressively. Treatment consists of intensive combination chemotherapy which is sometimes supplemented with radiation to help reduce large masses of malignant tissue. Most patients, including children and adolescents, also receive some type of central nervous system prophylaxis. The procedures involved in CNS therapy are described in the section covering intermediate-grade lymphomas.

The drug regimens used to treat high-grade disorders are determined by a number of factors, the most important being histology.

Many of the combinations listed in this booklet can be effective in treating immunoblastic and small noncleaved cell lymphomas, but there are other regimens that can be used. In certain instances, younger patients may be treated for a longer period than adults, sometimes up to 18 months.

Lymphoblastic lymphoma is treated with very high doses of multi-drug chemotherapy similar to the treatment required for acute leukemia. A number of different regimens using different drugs and dosages of these drugs are used to treat this disorder.

Mycosis Fungoides and Sezary Syndrome

Mycosis fungoides is a special T cell lymphoma of the skin believed to be caused by the uncontrolled growth of the help subset of T cells. When this form of lymphoma is limited to the skin, including chemotherapeutic drugs, which are applied directly to the eruption, and electron-beam radiation.

The agents most frequently used in topical chemotherapy are methochlorethamine, carmustine, and cytosine arabinoside (or Ara-C). Electron beams have a limited range of penetration so the entire surface of the body can be irradiated without damaging deeper levels of tissue.

These therapies have few side effects, and remission has been induced in approximately 90 percent of patients with early-stage disease. Many people stay in remission for an extended period after only one course of treatment.

Patients with advanced disease are treated with systemic combination chemotherapy, generally with a regimen similar to those listed earlier in this booklet, and high-dose radiotherapy.

Recurrent and Drug-resistant Non-Hodgkin's Lymphomas

While increasingly higher numbers of people with non-Hodgkin's lymphoma are enjoying long-term survival, there is still a percentage who do not go into complete remission or who develop relapse.

Recurring low-grade lymphomas can be controlled with radiation or with single-agent or combination chemotherapy. Many patients go back into remission, but while it may be sustained for quite a few years, most people experience another recurrence. In some instances, a third and even a fourth remission can be induced, but each period seems shorter than the one preceding it.

Patients with relapsed intermediate- and high-grade lymphomas may be treated with more aggressive forms of chemotherapy and radiotherapy. A second remission can be achieved, but in most cases, it is generally short-lived and the illness returns.

Bone marrow transplantation offers some people with recurrent and drug-resistant disorders another opportunity for extended disease-free survival. This option should be seriously considered by patients and physicians. People for whom this procedure is not applicable, however, eventually have to spend more time in the hospital. Still, there have been many advances made in terms of supportive care, including improved methods of pain control, and prolonged physical suffering or discomfort is rarely a problem.

Bone Marrow Transplantation

Bone marrow transplantation is an area of treatment that offers hope to patients whose lymphoma does not respond to regular therapy, who have developed relapse, or who are at a high risk of recurrence. It is a procedure that enables people to receive more aggressive treatment than anything administered in standard therapy regimens.

Patients are given intensive chemotherapy and radiotherapy to destroy even the most resistant malignant cells. Such aggressive therapy effectively kills lymphoma cells. However, it also wipes out normal blood cells as well as the tissue involved in blood cell production, including the bone marrow.

Once chemotherapy is completed, a small portion of marrow, matched specifically to a patient's genetic type, is intravenously injected into the bloodstream. From there, it makes its way into the cavities of the large bones. Until this marrow begins to grow and function, though, patients are totally dependent upon supportive care, such as antibiotics and blood transfusions, to protect them from infection, hemorrhage, and anemia.

In time, the transplanted marrow produces a whole new series of healthy cells to populate the blood and lymphatic system.

There are two types of bone marrow transplants: allogeneic and autologous. Allogeneic transplants involve the infusion of *type-specific* healthy marrow from a donor, usually a sibling. It is also possible to identify a type-specific unrelated donor from the population at large.

Autologous transplants use a patient's own marrow. In this procedure marrow is taken from patients under general anesthesia, often purged to removed residual lymphoma cells, and frozen for future use. After the patient is treated with chemotherapy and radiotherapy, the marrow is thawed and reinfused.

Autologous transplantation eliminates the need for a genetically matched donor. Furthermore, since lymphoma does not usually start in the bone marrow, most patients are presumed to have "clean" marrow. This, of course, increases the probability that purging will be completed effectively and minimizes the chance of relapse.

Peripheral Stem Cell Transplantation

Peripheral stem cell transplantation is an important new treatment option for patients with lymphoma. In this treatment approach, cells from the blood are collected when the patient has normal blood counts and are saved via a process called pheresis. Investigators are learning more about these cells. It is now realized that these special *stem cells* can repopulate the bone marrow at least as well as bone marrow cells and may be as good or better at restoring bone marrow to normal function after high-dose chemotherapy or radiation.

Both bone marrow and peripheral stem cell transplantation are promising areas of treatment for people with resistant or recurrent disease. Patients are advised to discuss both types of transplantation with their physician as soon as possible. Recent studies suggest that transplants are more successful when low-grade lymphomas are still in their indolent stage, and intermediate- or high-grade disorders are in remission. This is also the time when most people feel their best. Understandably, patients are often hesitant to undergo such a major treatment procedure. However, early evidence indicates that many people who otherwise might have died are now enjoying long-term survival and, possibly, have even been cured.

Causes and Risk Factors

The exact cause, or causes, of the lymphomas and the means of preventing them are unknown.

The incidence of non-Hodgkin's lymphoma increased rapidly in recent years. Numbers of new non-Hodgkin's lymphomas grew 50 percent between 1973 and 1987. Part of the increase seems to be due to a dramatic rise in the disease among younger men, who develop it as a complication of AIDS. In the San Francisco area, hit particularly hard by the AIDS epidemic, rates of the disease in men 20 to 54 years old more than tripled between 1983 and 1987.

However, non-Hodgkin's lymphoma rates have climbed steadily in the last few decades, even without AIDS-related cases. Non-Hodgkin's lymphomas in older age groups have increased 3.4 percent per year in Americans over 65 years of age.

People exposed to herbicides or excessive amounts of radiation, for instance survivors of the atomic bomb in Hiroshima, and individuals who have undergone aggressive radiotherapy, have a slightly greater than average chance of developing some form of the disease. There is also an increased rate of incidence among people who have been treated with high doses of chemotherapy or other immunosuppressive drugs for non-malignant conditions, such as heart or kidney transplants, rheumatoid arthritis, chronic renal or bowel disease, and lupus. However, most patients do not have a history of any of these disorders or such intensive drug therapy or radiation exposure.

Researchers believe that the lymphomas involve a complex interaction of individual genetics and body chemistry. Many patients are found to have abnormalities in their immune response and in specific pairs of chromosomes, but the actual significance of these irregularities is still uncertain.

Researchers also believe that one or more viruses may possibly be involved, but a direct cause-and-effect between various micro-organisms, including viruses, and these disorders has yet to be clearly established.

Retroviruses, which are also known as RNA tumor viruses or type-C viruses, are known to cause lymphoma in animals, but there is no evidence to suggest that they play any role in human malignancies.

One virus, HTLV-1, has been connected to a very rare form of human leukemia-lymphoma. The HTLV-1 virus affects mature T cells and is most often found in people from southern Japan, Africa, South America, and the Caribbean countries. This leukemia-lymphoma is a distinctly different disease and bears no resemblance to the disorders that are more common to populations originating in the United States and Europe.

There is some evidence to link a common herpes-type virus, called the Epstein-Barr virus, to the development of Burkitt's lymphoma in African children. The exact part it plays is uncertain since other genetic and environmental factors, such as malaria, may also contribute to the onset of this disorder.

Various studies indicate that the lymphomas follow no apparent hereditary pattern. There is no data to support any specific ethnic or dietary risk factors.

Information and Support

None of the lymphomas are easy for patients and their families to live with and accept. A confirmed diagnosis can trigger any number of emotional responses, ranging from denial to devastation. It is not uncommon to feel helpless, angry and confused. Understandably, people often fear for their lives or that of their loved one. On the other hand, patients diagnosed with a low-grade lymphoma may wonder if they are really sick at all. Some people are embarrassed because they or a family member have a malignant disease. Many are concerned about the possibility of high medical expenses. Naturally, there are questions about obtaining a second opinion, treatment and its side effects, and alternative forms.

Of course, it is best for patients and their families to speak directly with their doctor regarding any specific medical questions or doubts. It can also be helpful to talk with other health professionals, patients, and family members who understand the complexity of feelings and specific ongoing needs of those living with an illness of this nature. There are a variety of programs designed to help ease the emotional and economic strain created by lymphoma. The Leukemia Society of America will be happy to provide patients and their families with further information about available programs. Just contact our national office in New York City or one of our local chapters listed at the end of this article.

Hope for the Future

There has been tremendous headway made in treating all the lymphomas due to improved diagnosis and staging techniques and the dramatic advances in chemotherapy and radiotherapy.

Today, most people with Hodgkin's disease can look forward to a life without recurrence, and many patients with non-Hodgkin's lymphoma can feel they have a good chance for a complete recovery.

Scientists are continually searching for the possible causes of these disorders and constantly refining procedures for their identification and classification. Experiments with new drugs and drug combinations, as well as with different ways to administer radiation, are yielding even safer and more effective methods of treatment.

One promising new area under investigation is immunotherapy. This involves drugs, such as interferon, that seem to slow the growth of lymphoma cells while they stimulate and strengthen the body's own natural defense against malignant disease. Another class of drugs, the colony-stimulating factors, hasten bone marrow and blood cell recovery after chemotherapy.

Bone marrow transplantation offers patients another avenue of hope. Initial findings indicate that this procedure has extended the lives of a significant number of people, many of whom appear to be cured. Extensive research is now being conducted on ways to improve pretransplant treatment, to incorporate autologous BMT as part of initial treatment, to broaden the range of compatible donors, and to develop more effective methods of purging patients' own marrow.

Other clinical studies are exploring the use of radioactively labeled antibodies in conjunction with high-dose chemotherapy and an autologous BMT to treat patients at high risk of relapse.

Research on the lymphomas is currently underway on every major continent throughout the world. As each year passes, new discoveries are made, and the odds for prolonged remission and disease-free survival continue to increase for all patients.

Glossary

anesthetize: To treat with a medicine that causes partial or total loss of sensation and prevents pain.

anemia: Having fewer than the normal number of red blood cells. Causes symptoms of tiredness, shortness of breath, and weakness.

biopsy: A procedure in which a doctor surgically removes some tissue and examines it under a microscope.

blood: Made in the bone marrow, consists of red blood cells (erythrocytes), white blood cells (leukocytes), and platelets (thrombocytes).

cell: The smallest living unit. All living tissue is composed of cells.

central nervous system (CNS): The body system made up of the brain and spinal cord. The central nervous system is a natural sanctuary site for some leukemia cells and sometimes must be treated with chemotherapy or radiation or the two in combination which is known as CNS prophylaxis.

chromosomes: A part of the cell's nucleus that contains DNA. Chromosomes carry hereditary characteristics.

fatigue: A feeling of low energy, "washed-out feeling," general tiredness.

field: The specific area of the body that receives radioactive substances from the machines that emit x-rays.

follicles: A cluster of cells.

Hodgkin's disease: A form of cancer (lymphoma) affecting the lymph and other tissues that play a part in the individual's ability to fight infection.

immune system: The body's system of defense against disease or infections.

intravenous (IV): Administration of a chemotherapy drug directly into a vein.

lymph nodes: Small, bean-shaped organs found throughout the body that are part of the immune system.

lymph system: Tissues found throughout the body that contain the infection-fighting white blood cells; the immune system.

lymphocytes: White blood cells important to the immune system's defense against disease organisms in the body, including cancer cells.

lymphoma: A cancer that originates in the body's lymphatic tissues, primarily the lymph nodes or the lymph tissue of such organs as the stomach, small intestine, or bone.

non-Hodgkin's lymphoma: A term used for all types of lymphoma other than Hodgkin's disease.

oral: By mouth.

platelets (thrombocytes:) Blood cells that seal off injuries to prevent excessive bleeding.

prognosis: The outcome of a disease. A medical prediction of how a patient's disease may progress or how a patient recovers.

red cells: Blood cells that circulate in the blood and carry oxygen to all parts of the body.

regimen: Combination of drugs and their schedule for administration.

relapse: The reappearance of a disease after a period in which symptoms of the disease had lessened or disappeared.

remission: The period during which no evidence of disease is present.

staging: The process to determine if and how far a cancer has spread.

stem cells: Refers to cells that have the ability to mature into any of the different cell types.

susceptible: Easily affected, likely to be stricken with.

symptoms: Physical signs of the disease.

systemic: Not confined to one part of the body, but affecting the body as a whole.

tissue: Cells that perform a similar function and are organized together in the body.

topical: Applied directly to the skin.

type-specific: By characterizing structures that appear on cells, donors and recipients of platelets and bone marrow can be "matched" for their specific type to aid survival of transfused and transplanted cells.

ultrasound: A medical test that uses sound wavelengths to detect a mass or determine its composition.

white cells: Cells produced by the bone marrow and lymph nodes that help the body fight infections.

Further Readings in Lymphomas

Non-technical Books

Leukemia Society of America. *Bone Marrow Transplantation.* English and Spanish versions, 1993 and 1994.

Leukemia Society of America. *Coping with Survival,* 1993.

Leukemia Society of America. *Understanding Chemotherapy,* 1993.

National Institutes of Health *Understanding the Immune System:* NIH Publication No. 92529. Revised October, 1991.

Technical Books

Benn, P. and Hoppe, R., "Cutaneous Lymphomas," De Vita V. et al. "Hodgkin's disease," Karp, J. et al. "Cancer in AIDS," Longo D. et al. "Lymphocytic Lymphomas," and Poplack, E. et al. "Leukemias and Lymphomas of Childhood" in *Cancer: Principles and Practice of Oncology,* 4th Ed. (DeVita, Vincent T. et al., eds.) Philadelphia: Lippincott, 1993.

Technical Articles

Anderson, JW and Smalley RV. "Interferon alfa plus chemotherapy for non-Hodgkin's lymphoma." *New England Journal of Medicine* 329(24): 1821-1822, 1993.

Armitage, JO. "Treatment of non-Hodgkin's lymphoma." *New England Journal of Medicine* 328(14): 1023-1030, 1993.

Beral, V et al. "AIDS-associated non-Hodgkin's lymphoma." *Lancet* 337(8745): 805-809.

DeVita, VT and Hubbard, SM. "Hodgkin's disease." *New England Journal of Medicine* 328(8): 560-565, 1993.

Fisher, RI et al. "Comparison of a standard regimen (CHOP) with three intensive chemotherapy regimens for advanced non-Hodgkin's lymphoma." *New England Journal of Medicine* 328(14): 1002-1006, 1993.

Freedman, AS et al. "Autologous bone marrow transplantation in B-cell non-Hodgkin's lymphoma." *Journal of Clinical Oncology* 8(5): 784-791, 1990.

Hochster, HS et al. "Activity of fludarabine in previously treated non-Hodgkin's low-grade lymphoma." *Journal of Clinical Oncology* 10(1): 28-32, 1992.

Kadin, ME. "Ki-1-positive anaplastic large-cell lymphoma: a clinicopathologic entity." *Journal of Clinical Oncology* 9(4): 533-536, 1991.

Kay, AC et al. "2-Chlorodeoxyadenosine treatment of low-grade lymphomas." *Journal of Clinical Oncology* 10(3): 371-377, 1992.

Lynch, DC et al. "Dose intensification with autologous bone marrow transplantation in relapsed and resistant Hodgkin's disease." *Lancet* 341(8852): 1051-1054, 1993.

Morel, P et al. "Role of early splenectomy in malignant lymphomas." *Cancer* 71(1): 207-215, 1993.

Pettengell, R et al. "Granulocyte colony-stimulating factor to prevent dose-limiting neutropenia in non-Hodgkin's lymphomas." *Blood* 80(6): 1430-1436, 1992.

Portlock, CS. "Non-Hodgkin's lymphomas." *Cancer* February 1 1990 Supplement: 718-722.

Press, OW. "Radiolabeled-antibody therapy of B-cell lymphoma with autologous bone marrow support." *New England Journal of Medicine* 329(17): 1219-1224, 1994.

Pryzant, RM et al. "Long-term reduction in sperm count after chemotherapy with and without radiation therapy for non-Hodgkin's lymphomas." *Journal of Clinical Oncology* 11(2): 239-247.

The Selected Cancers Cooperative Study Group. "The Association of Selected Cancer with Service in the US Military in Vietnam." *Archives Internal Medicine* 150:2473-2483, 1990.

Urba, WJ and Longo, D. "Hodgkin's disease." *New England Journal of Medicine* 326(10): 678-687, 1992.

Vose, JM et al. "High-dose chemotherapy and autologous hematopoietic stem-cell transplantation for aggressive non-Hodgkin's lymphoma." *Journal of Clinical Oncology* 11(10): 1846-1851.

Acknowledgments

The Leukemia Society would like to thank Fredrick B. Hagemeister Jr., MD, Associate Professor of Medicine, Department of Hematology, Lymphoma Section, the University of Texas M.D. Anderson Cancer Center, who contributed and reviewed much of the material contained in this booklet.

■ **Document Source:**
Leukemia Society of America
National Headquarters
600 Third Ave
New York, NY 10016
(212) 573-8484; (800) 955-4LSA
August 1994

MULTIPLE MYELOMA (MM)

Written by Ann Elliot

Multiple myeloma (MM) is also known as myelomatosis, plasma cell myeloma, and—in parts of eastern Europe—as Kahler's disease after the physician who first described it at the end of the last century.

Multiple myeloma (MM) is rarely curable, but it is highly treatable. The disease used to be considered a bone cancer. It is actually one of the hematologic malignancies, and thus is related to leukemias and lymphomas. It accounts for about 10 percent of all hematologic cancers. The Leukemia Society of America estimates a total of 12,800 new cases of MM (less than five cases per 100,000 people) and 9,400 deaths from the disease in the United States every year. MM strikes African Americans about twice as frequently as whites. Marginally, more men are afflicted than women, but the difference is insignificant. The disease most often occurs between the ages of 50 and 70, with the peak incidence in the 60 to 65 age group. Only 3 percent of cases are found under the age of 40. A steady increase in incidence of the disease has been noted over the past 30 years. At least in part, this is due to improved diagnosis.

Benign monoclonal gammopathy, monoclonal gammopathy of undetermined significance, isolated plasmacytoma of bone, extramedullary plasmacytoma, Waldenstrom's macroglobulinemia, and plasma cell leukemia are related conditions. They are briefly discussed at the end of this article.

What Is It?

MM is a malignant disorder of the immune system. In the healthy body, *plasma cells* are found in the bone marrow. They are responsible for the production of antibodies. Antibodies are proteins (immunoglobulins) that are released into the circulation in response to the presence of an antigen—which may be a protein on the surface of an infectious agent, or it may be a foreign chemical or substance. Normal plasma cells manufacture the antibodies to match exactly and specifically the invading antigen.

In MM, plasma cells are abnormal and are present in enormous numbers in the bone marrow. They manufacture immunoglobulins that cannot function as antibodies. The malignant plasma cells do not usually circulate in great numbers in the bloodstream as do the cancer cells in leukemia. In order to understand the disease process in MM, it is helpful to know something about the functions, composition, and growth of healthy blood and bone marrow components.

Blood Functions and Composition

The blood is a vital transportation system that carries oxygen, food, and nutrients such as vitamins, hormones, and necessary chemicals and electrolytes to all the cells of the body; it carries away waste materials and toxins; it is involved in temperature control; and it is an essential element in the body's defense against infection.

Whole blood is made up of many components. Each component has a specific role in the overall functions of the blood. Three main blood elements play roles in hematologic diseases. (The word *hematologic* means "of or relating to blood or blood-forming tissues.") These are the red cells, clotting cells, and the white cells. They circulate through the bloodstream in a clear yellowish fluid known as *plasma.*

Red Blood Cells (Erythrocytes) give the blood its red color. They carry an iron-rich protein known as hemoglobin, which picks up oxygen from the lungs, transports it, and releases it to the organs and tissues. When people are short of red blood cells, they are anemic. Anemia can cause weakness and lack of energy, dizziness, shortness of breath, headaches, and irritability.

Clotting Cells (Platelets or, sometimes, **Thrombocytes)** are tiny disk-shaped cells that are needed to make blood clot to prevent abnormal or excessive bleeding as a result of injury to blood vessels. A deficiency of platelets can cause spontaneous bleeding of mucous membranes (such as those of the gums or nose) and bleeding into other tissues. Unexplained or excessive bruising of the skin is characteristic of platelet deficiency.

White Blood Cells (Leukocytes) play the major role in the defense of the body against disease-producing bacteria, viruses, and fungi. There are three main types of leukocytes, and they have specific infection-fighting functions:

- Monocytes defend the body against bacterial infections and also ingest aging and degenerating blood cells.
- Granulocytes combat infection by rapidly increasing in number in response to the presence of bacteria or foreign substances. They congregate around, engulf, and destroy the offending object. They then die and are ingested by monocytes. When the infection is under control, their rate of production returns to normal.
- Lymphocytes patrol the bloodstream, the lymph system, and the lymphoid organs—which include the spleen, thymus, thyroid, and lymph glands. The lymph system can best be described as a filtering and drainage system, which is connected to the bloodstream. Lymph itself is a clear fluid. White blood cells suspended in it give it a milky appearance. Lymph circulates through a network of glands and vessels, picks up waste material, and deposits it into the bloodstream for removal from the body. By complex interactions, the two main types of lymphocyte—the T cells and the B cells—combine forces to regulate the immune response.
- T cells are responsible for cellular immunity. They attack and destroy virus-infected and malignant cells. There are several different kinds of T cells and they interact with each other and regulate each other. They also regulate the response of B cells.
- B cells respond to the presence of antigens by dividing and maturing into plasma cells. Plasma cells produce and release antibodies. T cells signal the B cells when to begin this process and when to stop it. Antibodies neutralize infectious agents or foreign substances so that they can be destroyed by T cells, granulocytes, or monocytes, in combination with other complex defense mechanisms of the body.

Blood Cell Growth

Blood cells grow in the same general manner as other cells of the body. The tissues or organs of the body contain a pool of immature—or *undifferentiated*—cells known as stem cells. In response to the needs of the body—such as the need to replace worn-out or damaged cells, stem cells divide and mature and become fully developed and functional, i.e., *differentiated.* When the need is satisfied, the production of new cells slows or halts.

The process of blood-cell growth and development is called *hematopoiesis.* The original cells of all the blood cells are known as *pluripotent* stem cells, and these arise in the bone marrow, which is the spongy meshwork material that fills the cavities of the large bones. The pluripotent stem cells contain the genetic information that controls the development of the characteristics of the different types of blood cell. Depending on which type of cell is needed by the body to replace old and worn-out cells, or to respond to an immediate need such as an infection, the pluripotent stem cells divide and begin to differentiate into that particular cell line. One line forms red blood cells; one line—the myeloid line—forms the monocytes and granulocytes; one line—the lymphoid line—gives rise to the lymphocytes, and this line splits quite early in the process into separate T-cell and B-cell lines. The various blood cells are not released from the marrow into the bloodstream until they are fully differentiated, mature, and ready to function efficiently. It takes many cell divisions for this to occur.

In the case of the B-cell line, the early B cells are very small. They become progressively larger with successive cell divisions. The mature, fully differentiated form is the plasma cell or plasmacyte. This is a large, distinctive-looking lymphocyte, with a nucleus set to one side of the cell. Not until the cells differentiate into plasma cells can they produce antibodies.

The entire blood-cell growth, maintenance, and destruction cycle is a very efficient and orderly process. The abnormal growth and reproduction of any cell type disrupts this process and affects the body's general health and well-being.

Cancer

Cancer is the uncontrolled and abnormal growth of a particular cell type. In the healthy body, dividing cells are under internal control of their own genetic material (their DNA) and under external control from surrounding cells and other systems of the body. When the need to divide and make new cells is fulfilled, cell division ceases. If cellular DNA is damaged in some way—for example, by environmental poisons, by ionizing radiation, or even by simple wear and tear—the healthy body either sends T cells to destroy the damaged and potentially cancerous cell, or it fixes the damage. Sometimes, however, the damage is such that the cell somehow slips by the avenging T cells, and ceases to respond to normal controls. If the resulting tumor has a relatively low rate of growth and remains localized, it is often quite easily removed in its entirety, and will not recur. Such tumors are called *benign.* If the tumor grows rapidly and spreads to other parts of the body, it is called a *malignant* tumor, or a cancer.

Multiple Myeloma

In MM, at some time early in the process of lymphoid hematopoiesis, a pre-B cell or a B-stem cell incurs DNA damage. It divides uncontrollably and develops into plasma cells that are abnormal. These infiltrate the bone marrow, spreading into the cavities of all the large bones of the body.

In 70 percent of MM cases, the bones develop multiple holes. This is the explanation for the "multiple" part of the name of the disease and the reason that it used to be considered a cancer of the bone. The holes—*osteolytic lesions*—cause the bones to be fragile and subject to fractures. They are caused partly by the rapid growth of the myeloma cells, which mechanically shoulder aside normal bone-forming cells, preventing them from repairing general wear and tear of the bone; and partly by the secretion from the plasma cells of *osteoclast activating factor* (OAF), a substance that stimulates cells called osteoclasts. The normal function of osteoclasts is to destroy dead and dying bone. This function is speeded up and distorted by the secretion of OAF by the large clumps of plasma cells. The severe pain suffered by many untreated MM patients is thought to be caused by microfractures resulting from the fragility of damaged bones.

Many MM patients develop *hypercalcemia.* This is an increased level of calcium in the bloodstream. It results from the destruction of bone, from osteolytic lesions, or sometimes from the development of generalized *osteoporosis,* in which all the bones are soft and porous and have lost calcium.

In almost all cases of MM (93 percent), the malignant plasma cells retain the ability to produce immunoglobulin (Ig), but the mass of Ig released into the circulation is nonfunctional. It is known as *paraprotein,* i.e., abnormal protein. It does not form competent antibodies to combat antigens.

The malignant cells produce one specific protein—which can vary from patient to patient but is always the same in one patient—and is called a *monoclonal* protein (M protein) because it is produced by a clone of the original cell that became malignant. In most patients, the cells secrete a type of Ig known as IgG; the next most frequent type is IgA. When blood serum is subjected to a process called *electrophoresis,* the various proteins suspended in it are pulled by an electric current at different speeds depending upon the size of their molecules and their charge. When the proteins are charted, the M protein shows up as a "spike," because its molecules are identical and are numerous in comparison to other proteins in the serum.

In 75 percent of patients, the plasma cells also produce monoclonal incomplete immonoglobulins, called light chains. These are excreted in the urine and are the so-called *Bence Jones* proteins; they are named after a British physician, Henry Bence Jones (1813-1873), who first discovered them. Bence Jones proteins may deposit in the kidney, clogging the microscopic tubules. Ultimately, this damages the kidney and can cause renal failure. Hypercalcemia may exacerbate kidney problems, because excess calcium in the bloodstream causes excessive fluid loss and dehydration.

The multiplication of the malignant cells in the bone marrow crowds out and suppresses other hematopoietic cells. This may cause a significant decrease in red blood cells, causing anemia; and in platelets, causing abnormal bleeding.

The depletion of normal white blood cells compromises the patient's immunity in several ways. First, the numbers of monocytes and granulocytes are greatly reduced so that the patient is at risk from bacterial infections. Second, the delicate and complex balance between the different types of T cells is distorted, and their interaction with B cells is disrupted. The reduced number of normal B cells mature into plasma cells that produce functional Ig in response to infection, but for some reason that is not yet fully understood, this Ig breaks down more quickly than in a healthy person. In a healthy person, also, normal plasma cells signal the body when enough antibody has been made, and there is a short-lived shutdown of Ig production. This is apparently exaggerated in MM, so that the immunosuppression is prolonged.

Symptoms

A common early symptom of MM is *pain* in the lower back or in the ribs. Typically, the pain goes away if the patient stays quite still and is made worse by movement. It may be mistaken for arthritis or muscle spasm; or it may be confused with the aching back that accompanies the type of osteoporosis—which has nothing to do with MM—suffered by many older patients, particularly women. Typically, also, the pain is controlled for limited time periods by mild non-aspirin pain killers such as Tylenol®.

Unusual *tiredness and pallor* may be an indication of anemia and could be due to MM.

Frequent recurrent infections, such as bacterial pneumonia, urinary-tract infections, and shingles are signs of a malfunctioning immune system and may also indicate MM.

Symptoms of hypercalcemia are *weakness and fatigue, confusion* and difficulty with thought processes, *constipation,* increased *thirst, increased urine output,* and *nausea* or *vomiting.* If a patient has hypercalcemia, MM is a possibility.

Kidney failure—with or without kidney pain, with or without disturbances in urination such as the production of very small amounts of urine—may also be an indication of the disease.

It is important to note that not all MM patients suffer all or even any of these common symptoms of the disease. Sometimes MM is discovered when electrophoresis is done during routine blood tests for the other conditions, and the typical M-protein spike turns up.

Much less frequent symptoms accompanying MM are those related to certain complications of the disease. These are *hyperviscosity syndrome, cryoglobulinemia,* and *amyloidosis.*

Hyperviscosity syndrome occurs when the blood becomes very thick and sticky because of the abnormally large quantities of protein suspended in it. It is difficult for it to get through the small capillaries, and this may cause visual disturbances and other neurological troubles; it sometimes leads to strokes. In addition, the red blood cells tend to stick together in clumps or *rouleaux.* If blood is drawn from a patient with this syndrome, it tends to flow very slowly.

Cryoglobulinemia is a condition in which the paraprotein is of a specific type that precipitates out in the cold. Patients will suffer unusual pain and numbness in the fingers and toes in cold weather because the small blood vessels in their extremities are blocked.

Amyloidosis is a rare complication that occurs more often in patients whose plasma cells produce only light chains. Amyloid protein is a starch-like substance formed by the combination of light chains and other serum proteins; it infiltrates tissues and organs—particularly the kidneys, but also the liver and heart—disrupting their normal functions. It also infiltrates the walls of blood vessels so that they become inelastic and cannot maintain blood pressure. Thus, symptoms of amyloid disease may include low blood pressure and kidney, heart, and liver failure. Soreness and weakness of the muscles of the fingers and hand—a condition known as carpal tunnel syndrome—is sometimes caused by amyloid deposits exerting pressure on the nerve that goes through the carpal tunnel of the wrist. Amyloidosis, however, is also a disease and may occur completely independent of MM.

Diagnosis

Several diseases, especially in older patients, mimic MM. These include certain rheumatic diseases, in which a monoclonal (M) protein in the serum and a plasma cell reaction in the bone marrow are sometimes present; and metastatic carcinoma (a type of solid tumor that has spread to other sites in the body), which frequently produces osteolytic lesions. If MM is suspected, several tests are performed to confirm the diagnosis.

First, a bone marrow *aspiration* or *biopsy* is taken. The physician numbs an area—usually at the top of the hip, or over the breast bone—and uses a syringe with a long fine needle to aspirate (suck out) a small amount of bone marrow. A pathologist examines the marrow sample under the microscope for the presence of plasma cells. MM is probable if more than 10 percent of the cells seen in the sample are plasma cells.

Blood samples are drawn and electrophoresis performed to determine the presence or absence of a spike of M protein. Electrophoresis is also performed on a urine sample to find out if Bence Jones proteins are present.

The diagnosis of MM usually is confirmed by the presence of both excessive plasma cells in the bone marrow biopsy and a large M-protein spike in serum and/or urine. If a positive diagnosis is made, several further tests are done to assess the extent of the disease, to plan therapy, and to establish a baseline so that the effectiveness of treatment can be measured.

A complete blood count is done. This includes a determination of hemoglobin present, which is a measure of the degree of anemia, and a count of the number of platelets and white blood cells in the blood.

The level of calcium in the serum is determined to ascertain whether the patient is hypercalcemic.

Levels of creatinine and blood urea nitrogen (BUN) in the serum are measured; raised creatinine or BUN levels indicate decreased kidney function.

A serum protein shed by B cells, *beta-2 microglobulin*, is measured. The level of this protein is an indication of the severity of the disease.

Bone x-rays of the whole skeleton are taken to see if osteolytic lesions or osteoporosis are present. Sometimes the body is scanned by computer-assisted tomography—a CAT or CT scan. The CAT scanner is able to "see" lesions in soft tissues as well as in bone. Occasionally, magnetic resonance imaging (MRI) is used to obtain a detailed picture of a particular bone or area of the body.

Prognosis

Although MM has only rarely been cured, it is a highly treatable disease. Before the advent of chemotherapy, median survival after diagnosis was about seven months. Nowadays, median survival is 30 to 40 months—which means that many people live much longer than that, and treatment ensures a reasonable quality of life. A few patients (3 percent) have apparently achieved a true and complete remission and have survived at least 10 years after treatment.

To assess the prognosis of individual patients, it is necessary to know the extent or *stage* of the disease. Physicians divide MM into three stages:

- Stage I: Low tumor mass: 25 to 40 percent of patients survive at least five years.
- Stage II: Intermediate tumor mass: 15 to 30 percent of patients survive at least five years.
- Stage III: High tumor mass: 10 to 25 percent of patients survive at least five years.

Physicians have established certain criteria to classify the stages. The criteria reflect the tumor mass present in the patient. The numbers are somewhat arbitrary and vary—although insignificantly—among medical centers. Representative numbers, as supplied by the National Cancer Institute, are as follows:

- Stage I.
  - Hemoglobin more than 10.0gm/100 ml serum
  - Normal serum calcium
  - Normal bone structure
  - Low M-protein production:
    IgG less than 5.0 gm/100 ml serum
    IgA less than 3.0 gm/100 ml serum
    Urinary Bence Jones protein less than 4 gm excreted in 24 hours.
- Stage II. This is the intermediate state and includes all patients whose numbers fall between those of Stages I and III.
- Stage III.
  - Hemoglobin less than 8.5 gm/100 ml serum
  - Serum calcium more than 12.0 gm/100 ml serum
  - More than three lytic bone lesions
  - High M-protein production:
    IgG more than 7.0 gm/100 ml serum
    IgA more than 5.0 gm/100 ml serum
    Urinary Bence Jones protein more than 12.0 gm excreted in 24 hours.

Impaired renal function, as measured by creatinine in serum, worsens the prognosis whatever the stage of the disease. If the patient has a serum creatinine level of more than 2.0 mg/100 ml serum, renal function is considered impaired.

Other factors sometimes used to help stage the disease are as follows:

- *Beta-2 microglobulin* levels in serum; a raised level indicates a poorer prognosis.
- *Plasma-cell labeling index:* this is a measure of the rate at which the malignant cells are multiplying; the higher the rate of multiplication, the poorer the prognosis.

Treatment

Stage I MM is often *smoldering* or, as it is alternatively called, *indolent.* This means the disease is progressing very slowly, if at all. Although the patient has a significant M-protein spike and abnormal numbers of plasma cells in the bone marrow, he or she has no symptoms and may have none for several years. Every few months, the physician will recommend tests of blood and urine for any increase in paraprotein; levels of serum creatinine and calcium will be checked and skeletal x-rays taken. No treatment is indicated unless the disease becomes symptomatic or shows obvious signs of progression.

When active MM is present at diagnosis, or develops from the smoldering disease, chemotherapy is indicated. Patients are recommended to seek help from an oncologist (cancer specialist) or hematologist (specialist in blood disorders) at a medical center with the experience and resources to support treatment services. Usually, after a treatment regimen has been planned by the oncologist, the patient can, if he or she wishes, continue therapy under the supervision of their own primary care doctor.

Chemotherapy

Chemotherapeutic drugs are medications or chemicals with cancer-fighting abilities. Cells that are actively multiplying absorb them and are killed, or prevented from dividing to form new cells. The drugs are usually not taken up by cells that are "resting," i.e., not actively dividing, and therefore courses of chemotherapy must be spread over time to "catch" those cells that were not susceptible first time around. Unfortunately, the drugs are also toxic to normal cells that are multiplying. To a large extent, this explains the side effects of chemotherapy. Cells of the bone marrow are normally actively dividing, as are cells lining the stomach and intestines, and the cells of hair follicles; therefore, the patient's blood counts will drop, and he or she may lose their hair and experience some nausea, vomiting, and diarrhea.

Some physicians advocate aggressive therapy as soon as MM is positively diagnosed; usually, however, as chemotherapy goes, initial treatments for MM are mild. They are almost always on an outpatient basis, and patients are able to live and function normally while in treatment. The chemically induced immunosuppression (evidence by the decreased white blood cell counts) somewhat increases the risk of infection. However, MM patients should always avoid exposure to bacteria or viruses, since the risk of infection is inherent in the disease itself.

A number of alkylating agents, antineoplastic antibiotics, mitotic inhibitors, and glucocoritcoids are used in the treatment of MM. These drugs are used in various combinations. They include melphalan (Alkeran), cyclophosphamide (Cytoxan), carmustine (BCNU), vincristine (Oncovin), and doxorubicin (Adriamycin), prednisone, methyl prednisolone (both of which have several different trade names); and dexamethasone (Decadron). Cancer centers differ in which combination they prefer; some centers are now using high-dose glucocorticoids alone as primary therapy. So far, no regimen stands out as being significantly better or worse than another. Dosage and toxic reactions to the agents vary with each individual and with each drug or combination of drugs.

Complete responses (i.e., disappearance of paraprotein from blood and urine, and disappearance of abnormal numbers of plasma cells from the bone marrow) are rare, but the majority of patients (between 60 and 70 percent) will show measurable and clinically meaningful improvement (an objective response) to initial chemotherapy. Most patients reach a point of maximum response (usually after about twelve months of treatment), after which further therapy makes no difference to their condition. Treatment is then halted. About every two months while in this *plateau* phase, the patient is monitored (serum, urine, blood counts, and x-rays) to check that the disease is not progressing.

However, after some months or sometimes years, the disease almost always reactivates. If the response to the initial treatment was very good, the same therapy may be repeated. If this does not work, a different regimen is used. Unfortunately, the usual pattern is for the response to the drugs to decrease and of the MM to become refractory.

For the 30 to 40 percent of patients whose disease is resistant to the conventional initial therapies, and for those whose disease has become refractory, more aggressive regimens are appropriate. Reactions to these so-called "salvage" therapies are much more severe, and usually the patients are hospitalized for the treatments. About 40 percent will achieve an objective response.

Recently, some encouraging results have been achieved with the use of *interferon.* This is a *biological response modifier* produced by several different types of cells in the healthy body to fight cancer and viral infections. For therapy, recombinant interferon alpha-2, produced by genetic engineering, is administered. It is used after the patient has achieved maximum response to chemotherapy and has been found to prolong the plateau phase.

Bone Marrow Transplantation

Until quite recently, bone marrow transplantation (BMT) was considered an experimental procedure. Before 1969, only about 200 transplants had been undertaken. With expanded knowledge and improved techniques, particularly to protect the patient from post-transplant complications, the number of transplants performed has increased steadily. Now, in the 1990s, more than 3,000 transplantations per year are performed worldwide and, for some diseases, the procedure is considered to be standard.

The rationale behind bone marrow transplantation is that the patient's diseased marrow is destroyed and then replaced by healthy marrow. Very high-dose aggressive chemotherapy, usually in conjunction with total body irradiation (TBI), is employed to destroy the patient's marrow. Cancer-free marrow is then infused into the veins in the same manner as a blood transfusion. It makes its way into the bones, engrafts, and starts to grow. Within a few weeks, the new marrow reproduces a whole new population of healthy blood cells. However, until the new marrow is established and functional, the patient is dependent upon supportive care to defend against anemia and bleeding, and must spend several weeks in a highly sophisticated protective environment to avoid infection. Air, food, and drink are all sterilized before reaching the patient. Visitors are strictly limited and must observe certain precautions; for instance, they must wear masks and sterile clothing. Even after release from the hospital, a BMT recipient must continue to exercise great care to avoid infection for several months. Because young children tend to carry infection, some physicians recommend that patients avoid close contact with children under the age of 12 for about half a year.

In *allogeneic transplantation*, marrow is donated by a healthy individual whose bone marrow genetically "matches" that of the recipient as closely as possible. Usually the donor is a sibling. The cells of the body, including the white blood cells, have proteins on their surfaces called human leukocyte antigens (HLA). These are inherited in groups by classical Mendelian inheritance, which means a sibling has a one-in-four chance of carrying the same HLA antigens as the patient.

Depending upon which particular antigen groups are present on a patient's cells—some groups are more common and therefore less difficult to match— the chances of finding a nonrelated donor with a compatible marrow is between one in one hundred, and one in one million. The National Marrow Donor Program and the American Association of Bone Marrow Registries both maintain extensive lists of typed donors who can be called upon. The match must be as close to perfect as possible because any antigenic difference is capable of causing the immune cells of the new marrow to cry "foreign," triggering *graft-versus-host disease* (GVHD), a serious complication in which the T cells of the graft attack the cells of the host. To minimize this threat, cyclosporin is administered to suppress the immune response of the grafted marrow. After about six months, the engrafted cells achieve tolerance and cease to consider the cells of the host as "not self."

Syngeneic transplantation is the ideal form of BMT. The donor in this case is an identical twin; by definition, identical twins share identical antigens. If the patient is lucky enough to have a healthy identical twin able to donate marrow, there is no danger of GVHD and no danger of reinfusing cancerous cells.

In *autologous* marrow transplantation, the patient's own marrow is used. The marrow is harvested when the patient is as disease-free as possible; courses of chemotherapy are given until the marrow—in the case of MM—is virtually free of abnormal plasma cells and the M-protein spike is at a minimum. The harvested marrow is frozen until after the patient's residual marrow has been destroyed by chemotherapy (usually Cytoxan) and TBI. It is then thawed and reinfused.

BMT is an option for some younger MM patients. Thus far, the upper age limit is about 50 for allogeneic BMT and

670 for autologous BMT. It must be emphasized that the only patients eligible are those whose general health status—aside from their cancer—is very good. This means that heart, lungs, kidney function, etc. must be unimpaired. Prospective candidates for the procedure should be aware that transplantation is a drastic procedure and should consider the risks before going ahead.

That said, the results of BMT for MM patients have been very encouraging and—again, to emphasize—for younger patients in good physical condition, it offers at present the best chance of a cure. Worldwide, many centers are doing both allogeneic and autologous BMT for MM. Several patients have achieved complete responses after allogeneic BMT and, at the time of writing, the longest disease-free survival is seven years. One patient who received a syngeneic transplant has been alive and healthy for 11 years. The problem with BMT in this disease is the difficulty of eradicating every last malignant cell from the body.

In autologous BMT, this difficulty is compounded by the need to ensure that no malignant cell survives in the grafted marrow. Therefore, autologous BMT is usually reserved for those patients who have no compatible sibling match and who have refractory disease and, therefore, no other options. It is, however, possible to do autologous transplantation on slightly older patients since the recovery period is not quite so difficult as in allogeneic BMT.

The techniques for BMT are well established. The toxicity of the treatment can usually be well handled by the patients. What remains as problematic is the durability of the responses after the treatment. There are more and more successes, but still no guarantees.

Treatment of Symptoms

The best treatment for all the symptoms of MM is chemotherapy. In particular, bone pain subsides rapidly, even in those patients who have apparently achieved little objective response.

Mild persistent pain can be controlled with nonaspirin analgesics. For more severe "hot spots" of pain, associated with stubborn accumulations of plasma cells, radiation therapy is prescribed. When the numbers of infiltrating malignant cells have been reduced, bone can to some extent heal its microfractures. However, large lytic lesions and osteoporosis remain, and the bones continue to be fragile. Exercise is very helpful to keep them from becoming more so and to build up muscle tone to support them. Walking, swimming, cycling, and water-walking are fine forms of exercise. Running or lifting heavy objects—even pulling or pushing heavy doors—should be avoided, and any other activity that involves jarring or straining. Custom-designed corsets may be prescribed to provide support for the spine.

Exercise also helps alleviate the symptoms of hypercalcemia and some urinary problems; physical activity must be accompanied by increased fluid intake. Patients should drink three to four quarts of liquid per day.

Anemia and low platelet counts can be temporarily corrected with blood transfusions until the patient's own marrow has recovered its ability to produce red blood cells and clotting cells.

Nausea from chemotherapy can be controlled by a variety of drugs. Some of these, such as compazine, are effective but may make the patient fell very sleepy or "out of it." If this occurs, other compounds and/or dosages should be tried. The patient is the only one who can decide a reasonable compromise between nausea and the ability to function mentally.

Causes and Risk Factors

The causes of MM are obscure. People exposed to excessive radiation and those who have worked in industries involving heavy metals or chemicals used in the manufacture of plastics or wood paper pulp are statistically at a somewhat higher risk than the general populace. However, these are risk factors that are not limited to MM. They also apply to several other malignant diseases. No convincing hereditary pattern has been demonstrated. MM is not contagious.

Emotional Aspects

The psychological trauma of learning that one has an incurable disease is like an overwhelming physical blow. No easy generalizations can be made as to how any one patient will react. Life to most people—even older people—is a ribbon stretching to infinity. To suddenly be told the ribbon is not endless, that somewhere in the not too distant future it will be cut, is very hard to accept.

The word "cancer" is loaded. People react with denial, anger, panic, numbness, depression. They may feel alone and cut off from the rest of the human race by their condition. They may be very afraid: afraid of pain, of death, of loss of freedom and independence, of becoming unattractive to their mates, of being unable to work. People feel estranged by the new world of hospitals and the new vocabulary pertaining to their disease. Often people are appalled at the financial burden their illness is likely to put on their family. Some feel devastating sadness as they realize they will not see their children or grandchildren grow up.

Sometimes people have so much hope as each new treatment begins that they are almost euphoric—only to be dashed to despair if the magic does not happen. People bargain with God or fate: "If I do such and such, I shall be allowed to get better. . . ." Some people, looking for reasons for their disease, are stricken with guilt. "I would not now have MM if I had eaten more vegetables . . . not smoked . . . not enjoyed my life so much." Or they are told a good attitude is a way to a cure, and they are miserably guilty when they feel their attitude is not adequate.

Such reactions are common and normal. It usually helps patients if they have someone to talk with about their feelings, fears, and miseries. Of course, they should feel free to talk with their doctor or oncologist. Especially, they should feel free to question treatments and feel empowered to ask for changes to be made. Thus empowered, patients feel some measure of control over their lies and may not feel so helpless and so dependent upon the doctor.

But a spouse, or special friends and relatives, are usually even more important in helping the patient deal with psycho-logical stress. Professional counselors, psychologists, and psychiatrists attached to the hospital may also be of help.

Support groups, which are organized by the hospital or cancer center, by service organizations like the Leukemia Society, or by members of the clergy, are valuable. Since the groups consist of people who are similarly afflicted, they help to dispel feelings of isolation, and most patients feel great relief in being able to discuss their disease with people in the same situation. The groups are run by professionals, either for the patient alone or for the patients and their families.

It should be remembered that members of a patient's family also suffer a crippling psychological blow and often need as much help to handle the situation as the patient.

To many patients, the worst of having the disease is the reaction of others. Some people still think the word "cancer" is akin to the word "leprosy." Sometimes close friends and relatives draw back—usually because they don't know how to behave in the situation, but also because many people are still in terror of cancer, feeling it may be contagious.

Cancer is not contagious. A spouse, a child, a grandchild, a friend, or a lover can all be closely embraced, with no danger to them. The patient is the only one at any risk. MM poses an increased risk of infection, particularly when the patient is in therapy and the blood counts are at their lowest; common sense should be used to avoid needless exposure to viruses at those times.

It seems absurd to talk of good that can come out of having cancer, but many patients report that they learn for the first time to use their time to the full. The senses are awakened to reach for every emotion and experience. Many patients feel: "I'm going to use every minute of every day, and if I do beat this disease, I shall be way ahead." And the days seem more full, colors are brighter, sounds sweeter.

Some patients also experience companionship and closeness with particular friends or relatives—or with people in support groups—that they might have missed had they not had cancer. At such crisis times of life, many people find themselves enabled to express feelings and emotions that might otherwise never have been aired.

It should also be said that most physicians have a new attitude to treatment of cancer. The realization has come that the quality of life is now as important as its length. Patients are now considered as human beings and not simply as the hosts of a disease.

The Leukemia Society of America is a valuable resource. The Society and representatives from local chapters are ready to help ease the emotional and economic strain on MM patients and their families.

Research and Hope for the Future

Clinical trials are the means by which researchers learn which approaches are more effective than others. After much painstaking preliminary laboratory research, a network of physicians and scientists across the country test a new regimen in hundreds of volunteer patients. These patients are carefully monitored during the trial and followed up afterwards by a team of specialists in the forefront of the field. If the new treatment proves to be efficacious, these patients are the first to benefit. There are criteria that may bar a patient from such a trial. However, patients who are eligible should feel encouraged to enter. Before starting treatment, patients are fully informed of the nature and rationale of the new regimen and of the risks and possible side effects. They are free at that time to decline to enter and, at any time during the study, are free to leave the trial.

Chemotherapy has given MM patients many months and often years of life with little or no disability. The frustration of relapses has kept scientists and physicians busy studying compounds already available, varying dosages and timing of different combinations of drugs in an effort to improve the response and to extend the durability of the plateau phase.

Because interferon has proven effective in prolonging the response phase after conventional chemotherapy, efforts to capitalize on this property are under way. Different regimens are being tried. In one trial, high-dose combinations of conventional MM drugs are alternated with courses of interferon. The results are encouraging. Several complete responses have been noted. It is still too early to say how long these responses will last.

Research also continues into improving the quality of life of MM patients. Positive results have been obtained from a recent study using recombinant, genetically engineered *erythropoietin* that stimulates the growth of red blood cells to control anemia resulting from MM.

Research in the encouraging field of bone marrow transplantation continues in cancer centers all over the world. To destroy the patient's diseased bone marrow, a combination of very high-dose chemotherapy and total body irradiation (TBI) has been the conventional treatment. But TBI is hard on the patient. TBI exerts a bad effect on the microenvironment of the bone marrow; this consists of the supporting cells of the marrow not directly involved with hematopoiesis, and is also known as the bone marrow *stroma*. Damage to the stoma means the engraftment is delayed.

Busulfan is an alkylating agent that specifically attacks stem cells. Many doctors believe that busulfan does the same job as TBI, without as much physical hardship to the patient. The question is whether busulfan is as effective as TBI. To answer the question, careful and extensive studies are under way. If busulfan indeed proves better, it is possible that more and somewhat older patients will be eligible for BMT.

Some autologous transplants are being done using peripheral stem cells. These cells can be separated from the blood and concentrated and then treated just as the marrow is treated. They will re-engraft as effectively as bone marrow and are used either to augment the marrow transplant or as a substitute. This opens the door to transplant therapy for those patients whose marrow has been too battered by chemotherapy to be useful.

If it can be guaranteed that every malignant cell is wiped out in the patient's marrow harvest—or the peripheral stem-cell harvest—before it is reinfused, autologous BMT offers advantages over allogeneic BMT. Many studies are under way to test methods of purging the harvested marrow. Antibodies (known as monoclonal antibodies) that are specific for early pre-B cells—the precursors of myeloma cells—have been developed. Antibodies by themselves do not kill cells; they just attach themselves to their appropriate antigens on the cell surface. In the healthy body, mechanisms exist to destroy these "marked" cells. These mechanisms break down in MM patients, so it does no good simply to treat the patient with the monoclonal antibodies. However, outside the body, natural mechanisms can be employed. The marrow harvest is treated with the monoclonal antibodies; the marked cells are then lysed (burst) by treating them with a natural substance called *complement*. It has been shown that this treatment in no way damages the ability of the marrow to re-engraft.

Other methods of purging include treating the marrow with chemotherapy and also linking the monoclonal antibody to various poisons to form *immunotoxins* to kill the malignant cells. Some scientists believe that the malignant cells do not survive freezing so that purging the marrow may even be repugnant.

Tests are also under way to use the monoclonal antibodies to carry poisons directly to the malignant cells in the body. One poison being linked to the antibody is *ricin*, a very potent plant alkaloid. The antibodies ignore healthy cells and it is hoped the treatment will prove not only effective but reasonably free of side effects.

Chromosome analysis of myeloma cells is being done to try and establish which particular gene changes affect the prognosis of the patient. Again, to know more about the hows and whys will ultimately lead to specific and rational therapies.

The composition and function of many different proteins that are manufactured by cells—such as enzymes, hormones, and cytokines—have been determined. Through mechanisms of genetic engineering and recombinant DNA, these chemicals can be produced in pure form. Their effects in tissue culture (in which cells of different types are gown outside the body) as well as in the body can be studied. Factors that stimulate and factors that inhibit growth and cell division have been isolated.

An important growth factor for myeloma cells has been identified. This is interleukin 6 (IL-6). IL-6 is necessary for the growth, at least in tissue culture, of some malignant plasma cells. It is now believed that cells of the bone marrow stroma supply the IL-6 to keep the MM plasma cells multiplying. Some of the plasma cells acquire the ability to produce it themselves so that after a time they do not need the stroma. It has been postulated that in plasma cell leukemia, a severe form of MM, the cells can be free in the circulation because they have learned to do without IL-6 from the bone marrow stroma. IL-6 has stimulated a lot of interest. Scientists are trying to find ways to chemically block it so that it cannot exert its influence on myeloma cells.

A monoclonal antibody specific for IL-6 has been developed. A small number of plasma cell leukemia patients in Italy were entered in a clinical trial using this antibody. A definite improvement was noted in most of the patients but, unfortunately, the response was transitory and all patients relapsed. Although this test did not succeed, useful knowledge has been gained. It is now certain that blocking IL-6 has an effect.

Another phenomenon of great interest in MM is multidrug resistance. As has been noted in most patients, the disease responds to one or more courses of chemotherapy and then it becomes resistant. Research has shown that a protein—P-glycoprotein—is present in resistant cells. This is a natural substance, occurring in cells of the body that normally are concerned with excretion, such as cells of the liver or of the kidney. It works by pumping toxins out of the cell. Therefore, when a resistant malignant cell is attacked by a chemotherapuetic drug, it pumps it out, and the cell survives to multiply. It is believed that among the trillions of cell divisions that occur in a cancer, a genetic change or mutation gives rise to a cell with this property. This cell and its progeny survive all courses of therapy, and ultimately take over the cancer. Patients whose MM is refractory from the beginning probably suffer tumors that have always had the P-glycoprotein. Research is being done to find ways of "side-stepping" or blocking P-glycoprotein so that all the cancer cells remain susceptible to chemotherapy.

MM is a cancer that has recently attracted a lot of scientific interest. Each new discovery adds to the hope of a longer life or of a cure for its victims.

Related Plasma Cell Disorders

Benign Monoclonal Gammopathy

In this condition, patients have more than 10 percent plasma cells in the bone marrow and large M-protein spikes, but have no anemia, and normal calcium and creatinine. The large protein spike and the high number of plasma cells usually would indicate active MM. If there is any doubt as to whether full-blown active MM is present, the patient is not given chemotherapy until serial blood and urine tests confirm that the disease is active. Ultimately, this usually happens.

Monoclonal Gammopathy of Undetermined Significance (MGUS)

Patients with MGUS have an M protein in the serum without any of the other symptoms or findings of MM, macroglobulinemia, amyloidosis, or lymphoma. In time, many patients will develop one of these malignancies and so are kept under regular observation to detect changes in M protein or other signs of disease progression. Some physicians consider MGUS and benign monoclonal gammopathy to be different phases of the same condition.

Isolated Plasmactyoma of Bone

This is a solitary lytic lesion of plasma cells, usually found on a skeletal X-ray survey or CAT scan. If the patient has no other symptoms, and if a bone marrow biopsy from an uninvolved site shows fewer than 5 percent plasma cells, and no M protein is present in serum or urine, the outlook for the patient is better than for disseminated MM. Fifty percent of such patients will survive 10 years. The isolated lesion is treated with radiation therapy. Most patients ultimately develop disseminated MM.

Extramedullary Plasmacytoma

Some patients develop isolated plasma cell tumors of soft tissues, mostly occurring in the tonsils, sinuses, or nasopharynx. No lesions are present in the skeleton, no excess plasma cells are found on bone marrow biopsy, and no M protein is present in serum or urine. Radiation therapy and sometimes surgical removal are the standard treatments. Seventy percent of patients are cured. The rest ultimately develop disseminated MM.

Waldenstom's Macroglobulinemia

In this disease, the plasma cells are larger than in MM, and the paraprotein produced is a much larger molecule. Patients with this disease are much more likely to develop hyperviscosity syndrome than those with regular MM. As with MM, the disease is studied for evidence of progression before therapy is started. Standard therapy is with chlorambucil. *Plasmapheresis* is the treatment for hyperviscosity: the blood is removed from the body, centrifuged to remove the cellular components, and the plasma replaced with a physiological saline solution. The blood is then returned to the patient.

Plasma Cell Leukemia

This is a severe form of MM in which the plasma cells are present in large numbers in the peripheral circulation. The treatment is the same as for MM, but the prognosis is poor.

Sources

Non-technical Publications

Geier, M.A. *Cancer: What's It Doing in My Life?* Hope Publishing House, Pasadena CA, 1985. A very well-written book by a woman with lymphoma: it deals with how she copes with her disease, and how she deals with other people handling her disease. Includes appendices with practical advice on how to organize one's affairs when cancer strikes, and sources for help.

Leukemia Society of America. *Coping with Survival: Support for People Living with Adult Leukemia and Lymphoma,* 1990. A useful and practical booklet on psychological aspects of cancer. Written for people with leukemia and lymphoma, but applies equally to those with multiple myeloma.

Thompson, F.M. *Going for the Cure.* St. Martin's Press, New York, 1989. A young orthopedic surgeon is diagnosed with multiple myeloma. She is the first patient at Dana-Farber Cancer Institute to have an autologous bone marrow transplant for multiple myeloma. She tells her own story in this gripping, moving, and very readable book.

Winningham, M.L. et al. *Rhythmic Walking: Exercise for People Living with Cancer,* 1990. James Cancer Hospital, Columbus, OH. A booklet written by an exercise physiologist and two oncology nurses at the Arthur G. James Cancer Hospital and Research Institute, the Ohio State University; a program to help cancer patients develop a safe, regular exercise program.

Technical Publications

Anderson, K.C., et al. Monoclonal antibody-purged bone marrow transplantation therapy for multiple myeloma. *Blood* 77, 4:712-720, 1991.

Blattner, W. Epidemiology of multiple myeloma and related plasma cell disorders: an analytic review. In *Progress in Myeloma,* Potter M., ed., Elsevier/North Holland, Inc., pp 1-52, 1980.

Broder, S., Waldmann, T.A. Characteristics of multiple myeloma as an immonodeficiency disease. In *Progress in Myeloma,* Potter M., ed., Elsevier/North Holland, Inc., pp 151-169, 1980.

Cline, M.J., Haskell, C.M. Multiple myeloma and macroglobulinemia. In *Cancer Chemotherapy*, W.B. Saunders Co., Philadelphia, PA, pp 264-280, 1975.

Cooper, E.H. Biochemical and immunologic disorders in disease of the lymphoid tissue. In *Diseases of the Lymphatic System: Diagnosis and Therapy*, Molander, D.W., ed., Springer-Verlag, New York, Inc., New York, pp 157-180, 1984.

Feinstein, D.I., Multiple myeloma. *Cancer Center Report; Kenneth Norris Jr. Comprehensive Cancer Center, University of Southern California*, p 11, March 1991.

Forbes, I.J., Leong, A.S-Y., *Essential Oncology of the Lymphocyte*, Springer-Verlag, New York, Inc., New York, 1987.

Grayson, R.W., Psychological care of patients with cancer. Diseases of the Lymphatic System: Diagnosis and Therapy, Molander, D.W., ed., Springer-Verlag, New York, Inc., New York, pp 306-332, 1984.

Kartner, N. Ling V. Multidrug resistance in cancer. *Scientific American*, pp. 44-51, March 1989.

Ludwig, H. et al. Erythropoietin treatment for anemia associated with multiple myeloma. *NEJM* 322,24: 1693-1699, 1990.

Mandelli, F., et al. Maintenance treatment with recombinant interferon Alfa-2b in patients with multiple myeloma responding to conventional induction chemotherapy. *NEJM* 322,24: 1430-1434, 1990.

Salmon, S.E., Immunoglobulin synthesis and tumor kinetics of multiple myeloma. *Sem Hematol* 10:135-147, 1973.

Schechter, G.P., Wahl, L.M., Horton, J.E. *In vitro* bone resorption by human myeloma cells. In *Progress in Myeloma*, Potter M., ed., Elsevier/North Holland, Inc., pp 67-80, 1980.

Zolla-Pazner, S. Immunodeficiency induced by plasma cell tumors; comparison of finding in human and murine hosts. In *Progress in Myeloma*, Potter M., ed., Elsevier/North Holland, Inc., pp 171-184, 1980.

Acknowledgments

Grateful thanks are due to the following individuals: Eric Draut, MD, Peter Tutschka, MD, and David Yohn, PhD, of the Ohio State University Comprehensive Cancer Center, Columbus, OH; Kenneth Anderson, MD, Jerome Ritz, MD, and Ms. Bernadette Miner of Dana-Farber Cancer Institute, Boston, MA; Meletios Dimopoulos, MD, and Ms. Kay B. Delasalle of M.D. Anderson Cancer Center, Houston, TX; and Bernard Futscher, PhD, and Raymond Taetle, MD, of Arizona Cancer Center, Tucson, AZ.

■ **Leukemia Society of America**
  National Headquarters
  600 Third Ave
  New York 10016
  212-573-8484
  1-800-955-4LSA Hotline for information
  July 1993

WHAT EVERYONE SHOULD KNOW ABOUT LEUKEMIA

What is leukemia?

It's a disease of the parts of the body that **make blood.**

In leukemia the body makes too many *abnormal* cells, causing—

Infections

Leukemic cells lack the infection-fighting ability of normal white blood cells.

Anemia

Production of red blood cells drops as leukemic cells flood the system.

Excessive Bleeding

Clotting ability decreases as number of platelets (tiny disks needed for clotting) drops.

- Without treatment, 90 percent of acute leukemia victims would die within a year.

Why should I know more about leukemia?

Because

It kills more children between the ages of two and 15 than any other disease. (Only accidents kill more children).

It kills more adults than children. People over 60 are most often affected, and men more often than women.

Over 90,000 Americans will contract leukemia or related blood diseases this year. More than 50,000 others will die from these diseases.

There is no known way to prevent leukemia, but it can be treated effectively.

Today, modern treatments offer more hope than ever before to people who have leukemia.[*]

There are two main types of leukemia.

—and several varieties of each type.

Lympohocytic Leukemia

—marked by an increased number of white blood cells called lymphocytes. These cells are made in the lymph glands and bone marrow. In lymphocytic leukemia, most lymphocytes produced are abnormal or immature.

---

[*] This article is *not* a substitute for an informed discussion between a patient and his or her health-care provider of the procedures or medications described in this article.

Granulocytic Leukemia[*]

—marked by an increase in white blood cells called granulocytes. These are usually made in the bone marrow but may also arise from other tissue, such as in the liver or spleen. Normal granulocytes play a crucial role in the body's defense against infection, but leukemic granulocytes lack this ability.

Leukemia can occur in either of 2 forms.

Acute progresses rapidly.

Life expectancy is short without treatment (a few weeks to a few months). But drugs and/or bone marrow transplants have extended life expectancy for children with acute leukemia and cured about 72 percent. (A smaller proportion of adults with acute leukemia are also cured.)

- The type most often seen in children, it can occur at any age. Accounts for about ½ of leukemia cases.

Chronic progresses slowly.

With proper treatment, life expectancy is three to 20 years or more from onset of illness.

- Occurs most often in adults but can occur at any age. Accounts for about ½ of leukemia cases.

What happens in leukemia?

In both acute and chronic leukemia, an extremely high number of abnormal white blood cells are produced, flooding the bone marrow.

Acute leukemia affects

Red Blood Cells

These essential cells carry oxygen to all parts of the body. Made in the bone marrow, they number several million in each drop of blood.

- In leukemia, red blood cell count drops as red blood cells are replaced by abnormal cells.

  The result: Anemia from lack of oxygen causes pallor, weakness, fatigue, etc.

Platelets

These tiny blood cells, formed in the bone marrow, are essential for clotting. They collect around a wound and form a "plug" (clot) to stop bleeding.

- In leukemia, platelet production goes down.

  The result: Excessive bleeding, bruising, and hemorrhaging occur when blood won't clot.

White Blood Cells

Normal white cells fight infections by destroying bacteria, viruses, and foreign matter in the blood, and help build immunity to disease.

- In leukemia, white cells are replaced by abnormal cells and/or function poorly.

  The result: Infections occur repeatedly because the leukemic cells, are unable to fight off bacteria or viruses.

Blood Forming Tissue

Normally these tissues produce red cells, several kinds of white cells, and platelets.

- In leukemia, abnormal white cells invade the blood-forming tissues—especially the bone marrow—and disrupt normal production of blood cells.

  The result: Swelling occurs in lymph nodes, spleen, liver, and kidneys.

Chronic leukemia has less dramatic effects.

In lymphocytic leukemia

the main effect may be simply an increase in lymphocytes circulating in the blood and bone marrow. Multiple lymph node tumors may also develop.

It may go on for many years with few or no ill effects, but infections and hemorrhaging eventually develop.

In granulocytic leukemia

overgrowth and overproduction of abnormal bone marrow often causes an increase in platelets as well as white cells.

It can be controlled for several years, but most cases eventually convert to an acute phase.

What causes leukemia?

It's believed that a change in gene^{**} structure causes the abnormalities and uncontrolled multiplication of white cells in leukemia.

The cause of this change is unknown, but several factors are suspected:

- Environmental factors may make certain people more susceptible. For example, a leukemic's twin is more likely to get the disease. It's not clear whether this is environmental or genetic.
- Certain birth defects (not inherited)—such as Down syndrome—are associated with higher risk of leukemia.
- X-rays may increase susceptibility to leukemia in some cases.

---

* This type is also called "myeloid" or "myelocytic" leukemia.
**Genes are the "blueprints" for cell growth. They are located on the chromosomes, inside the nucleus of every cell.

- Other forms of radiation—such as that released by atomic bombs—are related to higher incidence of leukemia.
- Viruses are suspected because viruses have been linked to certain leukemias in animals. Viruses can cause genetic change.
- Chemical irritants—such as benzol vapors—are suspected of causing a variety of blood disorders, including leukemia.

Studies indicate leukemia is

- **NOT** inherited.
- **NOT** contagious.

What are the symptoms of leukemia?

Symptoms are similar to those of many common ailments but eventually become more persistent and severe:

- Anemia, pale compression
- Weakness
- Chronic fatigue
- High fever
- Bleeding without clotting
- Bruising easily
- Recurrent infection
- Pain in joints and bones
- Swelling of lymph nodes, spleen, liver

See your physician if any of these symptoms persist or recur. You should have a complete physical exam, including blood tests. If leukemia is suspected, a bone marrow test is done. The sooner treatment begins, the more effective it can be.

How is leukemia treated?

In recent years, tremendous advances in treatment have been made. Treatment may include

Chemotherapy

This involves the use of powerful drugs in various combinations to kill abnormal cells and/or slow their growth, giving normal cells a chance. In some cases, the drugs are given intravenously over a period of days.

Bone Marrow Transplant

Healthy bone marrow is injected into the patient's bloodstream, enters the bones, and, if all goes well, starts producing healthy cells and platelets. If a suitable donor can't be found, the patient's own marrow may be used after the diseased cells have been removed.

Radiation

Usually used in combination with chemotherapy, it can be an effective treatment for organs damaged by diseased cells.

Today, leukemia has an average cure rate of 40 percent. A cure is defined as a relapse-free five-year remission (disappearance of symptoms). But some types of leukemia are harder to treat than others.

The Three Stages of Treatment

Initial Treatment

Drugs are given daily to induce remission. Usually within four weeks, the patient is free from any signs of disease.

Maintenance Therapy

Long-term treatment usually lasts two to three years. Selected drugs are used in combination to extend and maintain remission.

Supportive Therapy

This is used when the disease is active. It may include

- blood transfusions
- platelet transfusions
- antibiotics

The best chance for a long-term remission is treatment

- in specially equipped medical facilities
- by a team of specially trained physicians, nurses and paramedics

Leukemia patients now have a longer life expectancy than ever!

Is help available to leukemia patients?

Yes! Many sources offer assistance to leukemia patients and their families. For example—

The Leukemia Society of America

A national health agency with local chapters all over the United States (57 chapters in 31 states and DC), it's ready to assist with the high cost of treatment on an outpatient basis (up to $750 per patient per year).

Patient-aid programs offered by local LSA chapters include

- Drugs for care, treatment, and/or control of leukemia.
- Transfusions of blood and certain blood components, and some related services.
- Transportations to and from doctor's office, treatment center, hospital within approved limits.
- Cranial radiation for certain patients.
- X-ray therapy in certain stages of Hodgkin's disease.
- Counseling to help patients and families adjust to the medical crisis.
- Referrals to other resources for services not covered by LSA.

An application form may be obtained from your local chapter.

Special Clinics and Hospitals

Those which specialize in the treatment of leukemia and allied diseases offer the best treatment available. Some are especially for children. They are supported by state and federal funds.

Community Services

Financial support and counseling may be available from

- voluntary health agencies
- hospital social service departments
- state welfare departments
- state child service programs

Emergency Transportation may be available to transport acute patients. For example:

- State Air National Guard
- USAF, US Army
- Private industry

   Help with sending messages or establishing phone-patches may be available, too. Check with

- American Red Cross
- American Amateur Radio Relay League (ham radio)

Cancer Chemotherapy Cooperative Groups

They offer experimental anticancer therapy and limited help with hospital costs and other drugs.

   They're organized and financially supported by the federal government and are located throughout the United States.

What about the future?

There's reason to expect new and better treatments for leukemia.

Research continues on—

Cell Growth and Structure

What changes make leukemic cells behave as they do? How can they be made more susceptible to antileukemic drugs? How do they differ from normal cells?

Possible Causes of Leukemia

including—

- viruses
- chemicals
- radiation
- defects in body chemistry

New Treatments

such as—

- Safer, more effective drugs which will kill leukemic cells with minimal damage to normal ones
- Better supportive therapy to counteract the complications of chemotherapy and radiation

Immunotherapy

—the study of the body's natural defense system. Is leukemia partly a result of a defect in this system? How can the body's immunity be strengthened so it would destroy any leukemic cells not killed by drug therapy?

Your help is needed in the fight against leukemia.

- **Learn about leukemia—what it does, what its symptoms are.**
- **See your physician** if any suspicious symptoms occur.
- **Help inform others** so they will know about leukemia.
- **Support leukemia research** local patient aid and education.

For further information contact

Leukemia Society of America
600 Third Ave
New York, NY 10016
1-212-573-8484
1-800-955-4LSA Hotline for information

■ **Document Source:**
   Leukemia Society of America
   National Headquarters
   600 Third Ave
   New York, NY 10016
   July 1995

See also: Childhood Acute Lymphocytic Leukemia (page 53); Chronic Lymphocytic Leukemia (page 55); Hodgkins Disease and the Non-Hodgkins Lymphomas (page 58); Multiple Myeloma (page 69)

CANCER (GENERAL)

■■■

BONE MARROW TRANSPLANTATION AND PERIPHERAL BLOOD STEM CELL TRANSPLANTATION

Research Report

This *Research Report* discusses bone marrow transplantation (BMT) procedures, the diseases that can be treated with BMT or peripheral blood stem cell transplantation (PBSCT), and current research on these treatments. Less than two decades ago, BMT was strictly an investigational procedure. Today, it is recognized as an effective treatment for some types of cancer and certain other diseases.

This booklet is designed to help people better understand this method of treatment. Patients and their families who want detailed information about these procedures, health care workers, and those with a strong interest in the topic will find it helpful. The booklet contains some technical information that assumes that the reader has a basic knowledge of cancer [see Glossary].

Information presented here was gathered from medical textbooks; recent articles in scientific literature; PDQ, the cancer information database developed by the National Cancer Institute (NCI); NCI researchers; and other scientists. Knowledge about BMT and PBSCT is increasing steadily. Up-to-date information on these and other cancer-related subjects is available from the NCI-supported Cancer Information Service (CIS). The toll-free number of the CIS is 1-800-4-CANCER.

Description and Function of Bone Marrow

Bone marrow is the soft, spongy material found inside bones. The bone marrow contains a network of blood vessels and fibers surrounded by fat and by cells that give rise to white blood cells (WBCs), red blood cells (RBCs), and platelets. The production of blood cells is the chief function of the bone marrow. In children, the cells that give rise to blood cells can be found throughout the marrow. In adults, these cells are found mostly in the marrow of the bones of the chest, hips, back, skull, and of the upper arms and legs.

All blood cells develop from very immature cells called *stem cells*. Most stem cells are found in the bone marrow, although some, called *peripheral blood stem cells,* circulate in blood vessels throughout the body. Stem cells can divide to form more stem cells, or they can go through a series of cell division by which they become fully mature blood cells. Most blood cells mature in the bone marrow. However, some white blood cells (also called lymphocytes) complete their maturation in the thymus, spleen, or lymph nodes.

White Blood Cells

White blood cells (also called leukocytes) are principal components of the *immune system,* the organs and cells that act together to defend the body against infection and other diseases. WBCs function by destroying "foreign" substances such as bacteria and viruses. When an infection is present, the production of WBCs increases. If the number of leukocytes is abnormally low (a condition known as *leukopenia*), infection is more likely to occur, and it is more difficult for the body to get rid of the infection.

There are several major types of WBCs—neutrophils, eosinophils, basophils, lymphocytes, and monocytes. Each has a different function.

- Neutrophils are a primary defense against bacterial infection. These cells can leave the bloodstream and migrate to the site of the infection. Neutrophils perform their function partially through *phagocytosis,* and *foreign substances.*
- Eosinophils are important in phagocytosis as well as in allergic and inflammatory reactions.
- Basophils play a special role in allergic reactions.
- Lymphocytes are found in the blood as well as in many other parts of the body. The three main types of lymphocytes—*B cells, T cells,* and *NK cells*—interact in complex ways as part of the *immune response.* Special B cells produce specific *antibodies,* proteins that help destroy foreign substances. T cells attack virus-infected cells, foreign tissue, and cancer cells. They also produce a number of substances that regulate the immune response. Among other functions, NK cells destroy can-

cer cells and virus-infected cells through phagocytosis and by producing substances that can kill such cells.

- Monocytes migrate into tissues and develop into *macrophages* when they are needed as part of the immune response. Monocytes and macrophages play a key role in phagocytosis.

As a group, neutrophils, eosinophils, and basophils may be referred to by names that describe how they look under the microscope. They are called granulocytes because of their dotted, or granular, appearance; the granules in these cells are filled with chemicals that can destroy foreign substances in the body. They also are called polymorphonuclear leukocytes (PMNs, or "polys"). Monocytes are referred to as agranulocytes or mononuclear cells.

Red Blood Cells

Red blood cells (also called erythrocytes) serve two important functions. With the help of an iron-containing protein called *hemoglobin,* they carry oxygen from the lungs to cells in all parts of the body. Oxygen helps cells obtain energy from the nutrients we eat. RBCs also take carbon dioxide back to the lungs from the cells; carbon dioxide is released as a waste product of cell processes. Too few RBCs or too little hemoglobin is a condition known as *anemia.* It can cause weakness, lack of energy, dizziness, shortness of breath, headache, and irritability.

Platelets

Platelets help prevent bleeding by causing blood clots to form at the site of an injury. An abnormally low number of platelets (a condition known as *thrombocytopenia)* may result in easy bruising and excessive bleeding from wounds or in mucous membranes and other tissues.

Purposes and Use of Transplantation

In bone marrow transplantation (BMT), marrow is removed from a bone with a needle. Bone marrow transplants can be divided into three groups according to where the marrow for transplantation comes from: the patient, an identical twin, or another person. In peripheral blood stem cell transplantation (PBSCT), the stem cells usually come from the patient. After treatment, the patient receives the marrow intravenously (by injection into a vein). In peripheral blood stem cell transplantation, stem cells are removed from the patient's circulating blood before treatment and then returned after treatment. The main purpose of these procedures in cancer treatment is to make it possible for patients to receive very high doses of *chemotherapy* and, in many cases, *radiation therapy* as well. To understand more about why BMT and PBSCT are used, it may be helpful to know more about how chemotherapy and radiation therapy work.

Chemotherapy and radiation therapy generally affect cells that are dividing. They are used to treat cancer because cancer cells divide more often than most other cells. Chemotherapeutic drugs and radiation are given in high doses to increase their effectiveness. However, high-dose treatment can severely damage or destroy the patient's bone marrow so that the patient is no longer able to produce needed blood cells. Destroying the marrow may be a part of treatment for diseases that affect the bone marrow (leukemias and other diseases) or it may simply be a side effect of treatment for cancers that affect other parts of the body. In any case, BMT and PBSCT allow stem cells that were damaged by treatment to be replaced with healthy stem cells that can produce the blood cells the patient needs.

BMT has been thoroughly tested in patients with certain types of cancer—among them *neuroblastoma* (an uncommon cancer that occurs most frequently in children) and certain types of *leukemia* and *lymphoma.* Many physicians consider it the best available treatment option for these diseases under specific circumstances. BMT also is being evaluated in the treatment of other types of cancer, including cancers of the breast, lung, ovary; *germ cell tumors; multiple myeloma;* certain other childhood cancers; and some primary brain tumors in both adults and children. BMT has also been used in the treatment of cancers that have spread, are not responding to other treatment, or cannot be removed by surgery (such as some that affect the head and neck). PBSCT, with or without BMT, is being studied for its usefulness in treating some of the same diseases. Patients who have cancer cells in their bone marrow or who do not have enough stem cells in their marrow may be considered for PBSCT. National Cancer Institute materials on many types of cancer are available through the Cancer Information Service (CIS) at 1-800-4-CANCER. CIS staff members also can provide information about current clinical trials (research studies) of BMT and PBSCT.

Several noncancerous disorders also are being treated with BMT. These include *aplastic anemia; severe combined immunodeficiency disease* (SCID), *thalassemia,* and *myelodyplastic syndromes.*

Types of Transplantation

As mentioned previously, there are three groups of bone marrow transplantation. The type of transplant a patient receives depends upon a number of factors, including the type of disease and the availability of a suitable donor.

Syngeneic Transplantation

In *syngeneic transplantation,* bone marrow is taken from an identical twin. Different people usually have different sets of proteins called *human leukocyte-associated* (HLA) *antigens* on the surface of their cells that allow white blood cells to distinguish the body's own cells from those of another person. However, because identical twins have the same genes, they also have the same set of HLA antigens (they are said to be a perfect HLA match). As a result, the patient's body usually accepts the *graft* (transplant). Given that identical twins represent only 0.3 percent of all births (1 birth out of every 270), syngeneic transplantation is rare.

Allogeneic Transplantation

Allogeneic transplantation, in which bone marrow comes from a person other than the patient or an identical twin, is much more common. Usually the patient's sibling or parent serves as the donor, but unrelated donors are sometimes used. (In rare cases, a child may donate marrow for a parent.)

The success of allogeneic transplantation depends largely on how closely the HLA antigens of the donor's marrow match those of the recipient's marrow, which is determined by special blood tests. (The matching of bone marrow is a much more complicated process than is the matching of blood types. Scientists look at six HLA antigens, and most institutions require a match on a least five of these proteins.) The higher the number of matches, the greater the chance that a patient's body will accept the graft. A good HLA match also reduces the chance that the transplanted bone marrow will react against the patient's body. This reaction, called *graft-versus-host disease* (GVHD), is a potentially serious complication of BMT.

Close relatives, especially brothers and sisters, are more likely than unrelated people to have HLA-matched bone marrow. However, only 30 to 40 percent of patients have an HLA-matched sibling or parent. The odds of obtaining HLA-compatible marrow from an unrelated donor are slim. Nevertheless, recent years have seen an increase in the use of marrow from unrelated donors. In 1988, for example, unrelated donor marrow was used for just 5 percent of all allogeneic transplantation; by 1990 this number had doubled to 10 percent. This increase has been possible in part through the existence of large bone marrow registries, such as the National Marrow Donor Program (NMDP) and the American Bone Marrow Donor Registry (ABMDR) (see Resources).

The NMDP is a federally funded program that was created in 1986 to improve a patient's chance of finding a suitable donor. The NMDP coordinates searches among donor and transplant centers throughout the United States and other countries. It receives requests for bone marrow donors from these centers, searches a central computer file (which currently contains more than 1,442,000 names) for a match, coordinates additional testing of donors, and helps with transplantation arrangements. The NMDP works in association with the American Red Cross, whose local chapters may be helpful in locating bone marrow donors.

The ABMDR is a privately funded registry of more than 500,000 potential marrow donors. Like NMDP, its function is to identify allogeneic matches by coordinating international searches among donor banks. The ABMDR also can provide information and assistance to physicians, transplant coordinators, and patients throughout the search process.

Because the likelihood of HLA matching is highest among people of similar racial and ethnic backgrounds, it is important that registries have a diverse population of potential donors so that all BMT candidates have a good chance of finding a match. Through recruitment programs for minority donors, which are in place throughout the country, NMDP and ABMDR hope to expand the donor pool for minority patients.

Autologous Transplantation

In *autologous transplantation,* patients receive their own marrow or peripheral stem cells. Because the patient is the donor, HLA matching is not necessary; moreover, there is virtually no risk of GVHD.

For autologous transplantation to be successful, the patient's marrow must be relatively free of disease when it is harvested (removed). In some patients, autologous transplantation is feasible because the cancer does not involve the bone marrow. (A sample of the bone marrow, removed in a procedure called *bone marrow aspiration,* is checked for the presence of cancer cells.) In other patients, such as leukemia and lymphoma patients, initial treatment to induce *remission* (the disappearance of the signs of cancer) is necessary before bone marrow harvesting. Depending on their disease and other factors, patients may then either proceed immediately with the high-dose treatment and transplantation procedure or store their marrow and proceed with high-dose treatment and transplantation only if their disease returns.

In an effort to protect the patient from relapse caused by undetected cancer cells in the autologous marrow, the marrow often is treated before storage or transplantation. Treatment to remove or destroy cancer cells in the harvested marrow, known as *purging,* can be accomplished in a number of ways. These include the use of drugs to kill cancer cells or of *monoclonal antibodies* to kill or remove cancer cells; various methods also may be used to separate healthy cells from cancer cells. Although cancer cells may be less likely to be in the peripheral blood than in the marrow, peripheral stem cell harvests also may be purged.

Not all patients undergoing autologous BMT receive purged marrow because it is not clear whether purging truly reduces the risk of relapse after transplantation. Purging does not necessarily remove all cancer cells from the harvested marrow. Patients with solid tumors who relapse often do so at the site of the original tumor, indicating that the transplanted marrow may not be responsible for the recurrence. Moreover, purging with the anticancer drugs may result in delayed recovery of bone marrow function after transplantation because stem cells in the harvested marrow may be destroyed along with cancer cells. The value of purging in BMT and PBSCT continues to be studied.

Transplantation Procedures

Transplantation of bone marrow or peripheral blood stem cells involves potentially serious risks, and patients require the care of skilled medical staff and state-of-the-art support services. For this reason, BMT and PBSCT should be performed at established transplant centers whenever possible.

The steps involved in transplantation vary from one medical center to another and with the type of transplantation done. Also, as research advances, the procedures are changing. General transplantation procedures are discussed below.

Patient Selection and Consent

When considering transplantation, physicians carefully evaluate a patient's medical history to be sure this procedure is the most appropriate treatment option. The potential complications of BMT and PBSCT, which are discussed later in the *Report,* are given significant consideration because they can be severe and, in some cases, fatal. Patient and physician must work closely together to weigh the potential benefits against the risks.

If allogeneic BMT is determined to be an appropriate and desirable treatment, a suitable donor must be identified. As noted earlier, many resources exist for finding a donor. The number of donors is increasing constantly, and the success rate of finding a donor has increased greatly in recent years. However, there is still a very real possibility that a person without a twin will not find a donor with enough matching antigens for the treatment to proceed.

After reviewing the transplantation process, the patient is asked to sign hospital consent forms authorizing the procedure. Signing the consent forms means that the patient has been given enough information to make an informed decision about treatment and to understand what the treatment involves. Patients should be made fully aware of the risks, benefits, and costs of transplantation as well as possible treatment alternatives.

Some specific questions that patients may want to ask their physicians before signing the consent form are:

- What are the benefits of this treatment?
- What are the risks and side effects?
- How long will I be in the hospital and unable to work or go to school?
- How will I have to change my normal activities?
- How much will the treatment cost?
- Will my insurance pay for this treatment? If not, is financial help available?
- Will I have to be far from home? If so, how soon can I return home?
- How often will I need checkups?

Pretreatment Procedures

Before the actual transplantation, the patient undergoes several days of laboratory and diagnostic tests. Doctors check the patient's general medical condition, looking for signs of infection or damage to organs from previous treatment. A dental exam generally is recommended to make sure the mouth is as healthy as possible before treatment begins, because treatment will likely cause it to become sensitive and easily infected.

An *intravenous catheter* usually is surgically placed in one of the large veins in the chest. The catheter is used for drawing blood samples; for giving the patient blood or blood products, antibiotics, other drugs, and nutritional support; and for transplanting the new marrow. Many medical centers use Hickman or Broviac catheters, which are thin, flexible tubes similar to regular intravenous tubing. One end of the catheter remains outside the chest and must be kept very clean to prevent infection. Catheters generally can remain in place for many months. (Before they leave the hospital, patients are taught how to care for the catheter at home.) Implantable ports, in which the end of the catheter remains under the skin, are sometimes used as an alternative to Hickman or Broviac

catheters. With these ports, a needle is inserted through the skin and into the catheter.

Procedures for Allogeneic or Syngeneic Donors

Donors for allogeneic or syngeneic transplants need not make changes in diet, work, or social activities before bone marrow donation. Typically, the donor enters the hospital the day before or the day of the donation. Donors normally stay in the hospital for one or two nights because most receive general anesthesia, which puts them to sleep. The use of newer anesthetics has made bone marrow donation possible as an outpatient procedure at some centers. Sometimes, local anesthesia is used instead to numb the area of the body where the marrow will be removed.

Bone marrow is removed from the pelvic (hip) bones and, in rare cases, from the sternum (breastbone) as well. Generally, four to eight small incisions (not requiring stitches) are make in the pelvic area, and a large needle is inserted through these incisions 20 to 30 times to draw the marrow out of the bones. Usually, 500 to 1,000 milliliters (one to two pints) of the donor's marrow is taken. This marrow contains 3 to 5 percent of all the donor's developing blood cells. Typically, the extraction process lasts about one hour.

Harvested bone marrow is then processed to remove blood and bone fragments. Allogeneic marrow may be treated to remove T lymphocytes in a process known as *T-cell depletion.* Marrow that is to be stored may be combined with dimethyl sulfoxide (a preservative, often referred to as DMSO) and placed in a liquid nitrogen freezer to keep stem cells alive until the day of transplantation. Using this technique, known as *cryopreservation,* bone marrow can be preserved for three years or more.

Because only a small amount of marrow is removed, donating usually does not pose any significant problems for the donor. Within a few weeks, the donor's body will have replaced the donated marrow. Soreness around the incisions may linger for a few days, and donors often feel tired for some time. The time required for a donor to recover varies from person to person. Some are back to their usual routine in a day or two. Others may take several days or as long as a week, but rarely longer.

Although donor complications are uncommon and much effort is devoted to their prevention, they sometimes occur. Complications are easily treated with proper medical attention. Because incisions are made to extract the marrow, infection is a possibility. Blood loss also can occur. For this reason, allogeneic and syngeneic donors routinely store two units of their own blood beforehand to be given during and after the procedure.

Harvesting Marrow or Peripheral Blood Stem Cells for Autologous Transplantation

When autologous transplantation is planned, the procedures for harvesting marrow differ, depending on factors such as the patient's physical condition and the time between harvesting and transplantation. In general, harvesting procedures are similar to those for allogeneic and syngeneic donors. However, if purging is to be done, up to 2,000 milliliters (two quarts) may be taken so that an adequate amount of marrow remains after purging. Removal of a larger amount of marrow requires a greater number of needle punctures and a longer period of time to collect the marrow. Any problems with bleeding are treated with transfusions of blood products from a blood bank. The marrow is stored until the time of transplantation.

Peripheral stem cells are harvested in a process called apheresis or leukapheresis. In this procedure, blood is removed through an intravenous catheter or through a large vein in the arm and is run through a machine that removes stem cells. The rest of the blood is returned to the patient. Typically, apheresis takes two to four hours and is repeated an average of six times. There usually is no need for hospitalization or anesthesia. Stem cells collected by apheresis are cryopreserved in the same way as is bone marrow.

Because the concentration of stem cells circulating in blood is at least 10 times lower than that found in the marrow, researchers are exploring ways to "mobilize" the stem cells—that is, to increase the number that can be harvested. One way is to collect them during the recovery period after chemotherapy, when the number of circulating stem cells may be as much as 25 times higher than usual. Another way is to treat the patient with *hematopoietic growth factors*. Normally produced by the body to stimulate blood cell production, these substances also can be made in the laboratory in large quantities. The most studied hematopoietic factors are the *colony-stimulating factors* and *interleukins*, which increase the production of white blood cells and can enhance the yield of peripheral blood stem cells. The effectiveness of mobilization may be increased through a combination of approaches.

Conditioning Regimens

Conditioning—treatment with high-dose chemotherapy with or without radiation therapy—is critical to the success of the transplantation. Conditioning serves a number of functions for cancer patients. Its primary purpose is to destroy cancer cells throughout the body more effectively than may be possible through conventional treatment. In addition, cells in the marrow are destroyed, creating space for the new marrow. Conditioning serves a third purpose in patients undergoing allogeneic transplantation: Because it destroys the cells of the immune system, it reduces the risk that the recipient will reject the graft.

Conditioning regimens for transplantation vary according to the patient's disease and medical condition and according to the medical center performing the procedure. The anticancer drugs used in high-dose chemotherapy may be given over the course of two to six days. If total body irradiation (TBI) is used, it may be given in one dose or in multiple doses over the course of several days (*fractionated radiation therapy*). Fractionated schedules appear to minimize the risk of side effects and are generally preferred over single doses.

Marrow or Stem Cell Infusion

Shortly after the high-dose treatment is completed, the patient receives the donated or autologous marrow through the intravenous catheter. Peripheral blood stem cells for autologous transplantation are infused in the same way. The *infusion* of marrow or peripheral blood stem cells is called the *rescue process*. The stem cells travel through the bloodstream to the bone marrow, where they begin to produce new WBCs, RBCs, and platelets. *Engraftment* (blood cell production from transplanted stem cells) usually occurs within about two to four weeks following transplantation. Complete recovery of immune function takes much longer, however—up to several months for autologous transplant recipients and one to two years for patients receiving allogeneic transplants. Physicians evaluate results of various blood tests to confirm that new blood cells are being produced and that the cancer has not returned. Bone marrow aspiration also can help doctors determine how well new marrow components are forming.

Supportive Care

Supportive care is an essential aspect of transplantation. The goal of supportive care is to prevent or manage the side effects of high-dose chemotherapy and/or radiation therapy. Side effects requiring supportive care include *immunosuppression*, anemia, and bleeding (all of which are caused by low numbers of blood cells); nausea, vomiting, and loss of appetite (caused by irritation of the gastrointestinal tract); and malfunction of the lungs, liver, kidneys, and heart (caused by damage to these organs).

One of the most serious effects of high-dose cancer treatment is immunosuppression, in which the patient's body is unable to defend itself against infection. Supportive care for immunosuppression usually includes protective isolation: Patients must stay in a hospital room, where it is easier to keep the environment free of infectious agents. Depending on the institution, medical staff and visitors entering the patient's room may be required to go through some preventive measures ranging from thorough hand washing to putting on masks and gowns. Generally, patients also may start receiving antibiotics, antiviral agents, and antifungal agents just before or soon after chemotherapy radiation therapy in an effort to prevent infection. Intravenous *immunoglobulin therapy* also is used by some centers as a preventive measure against infection. In this treatment, antibodies are isolated from donor blood and administered to the patient. Protective isolation and infection-fighting substances are continued from the time the patient's own marrow is destroyed until the transplanted marrow or peripheral blood stem cells produce enough white blood cells to fight infection.

To reduce the severity of immunosuppression, many patients receive hematopoietic growth factors. Growth factors administered after BMT or PBSCT can speed engraftment, decrease the risk of infection, and reduce the likelihood of graft failure.

Because chemotherapy and radiation therapy damage the bone marrow's ability to produce RBCs and platelets, patients usually need periodic blood transfusions to treat anemia and thrombocytopenia. To reduce the risk of GVHD, all donated blood products given to transplantation patients are treated with radiation. This destroys lymphocytes that might otherwise attack the patient's cells and cause GVHD.

Adequate nutrition is vitally important for BMT patients. Chemotherapy and radiation therapy often cause nausea, vomiting, and mouth sores, which may make eating difficult for several weeks. In addition, some treatment plans require a period of time when the patient is not permitted to eat; this allows the gastrointestinal tract to heal following chemotherapy. Patients who are unable to eat can receive all necessary nutrients through the intravenous catheter, a process called *total parenteral nutrition*.

Convalescence and Followup Care

Most patients stay in the hospital for one to two months after BMT. This is necessary to monitor whether engraftment has been successful and to treat any potential complications, such as infection and acute GVHD. Hospitalization time may be reduced when PBSCT is done alone or with BMT because engraftment time tends to be faster. The use of hematopoietic growth factors also can shorten the time many patients must spend in the hospital.

Generally, a patient is discharged from the hospital after the neutrophil count is greater than 500 in a standard measure of blood for at least two consecutive days. Other considerations are the RBC and platelet counts, the presence or absence of recurrent infections, and the patient's general physical condition. Patients may need frequent platelet and blood transfusions even after discharge; for this reason, the catheter is left in place for as long as three to six months after transplantation.

Some patients will need to return to the hospital's outpatient department daily for the first two weeks, while others can be seen less frequently. Followup visits to the transplant clinic continue every one to two weeks for the first several months to ensure that blood counts are normal and that the cancer has not returned. Patients are then seen every month for about six months. Later, the schedule of checkups is based on each patient's need. Generally, checkups are done every two to six months. Most followup visits include bone marrow aspiration to determine the condition of the marrow.

Many patients need a full year to recover physically and psychologically from transplantation. Even after that period, life may not return to "normal"—the way it was before the illness: Medication may be necessary indefinitely, and the patient's lifestyle may have to be changed to help prevent fatigue, avoid infectious diseases, and cope with the long-term effects of treatment.

There are physical changes to deal with, such as dry eyes, skin sensitivity, and, for some patients, reproductive disorders. In addition, changes in liver function may require alterations in diet. Some patients also experience changes in their self-image because they have received part of their body from someone else. On the other hand, some people think of their transplantation date as a new "birthday."

Complications for the Recipient

Patients experience a number of complications after transplantation. Some are temporary and relatively minor, but others can be life threatening. The likelihood that serious complications will develop is affected by, among other factors, a patient's age and general physical condition before transplantation.

Temporary side effects that are common among patients receiving chemotherapy and/or radiation therapy include hair loss, nausea and vomiting, fatigue, loss of appetite, mouth sores, and skin reactions. Additional information about these and other side effects of cancer treatment is available in the NCI booklets *Chemotherapy and You* and *Radiation Therapy and You.*

Some patients also experience temporary side effects that are caused by drugs given to prevent or treat the more severe complications of transplantation. These side effects depend on the drugs that are used, but they include gastrointestinal problems, high blood pressure, and, in some cases, seizures and problems with vision. Hematopoietic growth factors also may produce temporary side effects such as bone pain, muscle aches, and flu-like symptoms.

Serious side effects that are related to high-dose treatment or the transplantation itself are discussed below. The seriousness of these complications is different for each person.

Infections

Patients undergoing BMT are at significant risk of developing infections for several months after transplantation. Cytomegaloviruses, *Aspergillus* (a type of fungus), and *Pneumocystis carinii* (a protozoan) are among the most important causes of life-threatening infections, including pneumonia. Many patients develop herpes zoster virus infections (shingles), and herpes simplex virus infections (cold sores and genital herpes) often become reactivated in patients who were previously infected with this virus. *Mucositis,* an inflammation of the mouth and gastrointestinal tract, also is common after BMT.

Some infections may be prevented by the administration of antiviral agents, antibiotics, and antifungal agents before and after transplantation. These drugs also may be used to treat infections. Patients must be watched closely just after BMT, before engraftment occurs, because this is the period in which they are at highest risk for infection. In addition, patients have routine lab work, chest x-rays, and other exams to check for signs and symptoms of infection during the entire treatment process. Because of improvements in prevention strategies, fewer patients die of infection after transplantation than did in previous years. Infections also are a potential complication for patients undergoing PBSCT. However, because engraftment tends to occur earlier than for BMT, the period of highest risk is shortened. Often, infections that do occur are related to catheter use.

Graft-versus-host Disease

Graft-versus-host disease is one of the most serious potential complications of allogeneic BMT. It occurs when T cells in the donated marrow (the graft) identify the recipient's body (the host) as foreign and attack it. This situation is different from other types of organ transplantation (such as kidney or heart transplantation), in which the donated organ is rejected by the patient's immune system. Although the donated marrow can be rejected by whatever remains of the patient's original immune system, more often, it is the T lymphocytes produced by the new marrow that launch an attack against the patient. Without preventive measures, most patients undergoing allogeneic BMT would develop GVHD.

Symptoms of GVHD can develop within days or as long as three years after transplantation. Generally, GVHD that develops within three months following transplantation is known as acute GVHD; when it develops later, it is called chronic GVHD. Because the time periods in which acute and chronic GVHD can develop overlap, these diseases are better identified by their symptoms, which are somewhat different for each type.

Common symptoms of acute GVHD are skin rashes, jaundice, liver disease, and diarrhea. Because recovery of immune function after BMT is delayed, patients also have persistent susceptibility to infections. Patients with mild forms of acute GVHD are likely to recover completely, but those with severe forms may die of complications of the disease. Chronic GVHD produces temporary darkening of the skin and hardening and thickening of patches of skin and the layers of tissues under it. Occasionally, the liver, esophagus, and other parts of the gastrointestinal tract are affected. Mucous membranes may become dry, and hair loss may occur. Bacterial infections and weight loss are common. As with acute GVHD, severe cases of chronic GVHD may be fatal.

Several factors affect a patient's risk of developing GVHD. The most important is the degree of HLA matching: The more antigens that match, the lower the risk of GVHD. About 70 percent of patients who receive donor marrow with two mismatched antigens develop significant acute GVHD, versus 40 percent of patients receiving HLA-identical marrow. (Mild GVHD occasionally develops after autologous BMT or PBSCT; it usually is related to the presence of T lymphocytes in transfused blood products from another person.) Age also affects the risk of GVHD, with older patients being more susceptible to the disease than are younger ones. In addition, a recipient whose donor is of the opposite sex is more likely to develop GVHD than a recipient whose donor is of the same sex. Chronic GVHD, which affects at least one-third of allogeneic BMT patients, develops most often in those who have had acute GVHD.

To reduce the risk of GVHD after transplantation, most patients routinely receive immunosuppressive therapy with cyclosporine and/or methotrexate, drugs that help suppress T lymphocytes. Combinations of drugs appear to be most effective. Another technique for preventing GVHD is T-cell depletion, which involves eliminating lymphocytes in the donated marrow before it is given to the patient. The T cells are removed or destroyed by means of monoclonal antibodies or other processes. Although T-cell depletion appears to reduce the chance that a patient will develop severe GVHD, this technique has other associated risks: Graft failure may be more likely when T-cell depleted marrow is used, and leukemia patients may be more likely to have a relapse.

Should GVHD occur despite efforts to prevent it, high-dose *corticosteroids* (such as prednisone) are given to relieve symptoms of the disease and to suppress T-cell activity. Patients may receive *antithymocyte globulin,* which acts against immature T cells (thymocytes), or monoclonal antibodies that are directed against T cells. Higher doses of cyclosporine also can be helpful.

Interestingly, many studies have shown that mild GVHD may be beneficial over the long term, perhaps because the activated graft cells may be better able to kill cancer cells (a so-called "graft-versus-cancer" effect). Leukemia and lymphoma patients who develop mild GVHD are less likely to have a relapse than are patients who never have the reaction. For this reason, researchers are studying ways to introduce "graft-versus-cancer" effects in autologous BMT.

Bleeding

Bleeding may be a problem, especially during the first four weeks after BMT, when platelet production is greatly reduced. Bleeding most often occurs in the mucous membranes of the nose and mouth; it also may develop under the skin or in the gastrointestinal tract. Platelet transfusions are given if there is any evidence of bleeding and/or to maintain the platelet count at the minimum needed to prevent bleeding. Platelets may be donated by the marrow donor or another closely HLA-matched individual.

Organ Complications

Patients may develop complications in the liver, kidneys, lungs, and/or heart. Because these vital organs are susceptible to serious damage, only patients without preexisting problems are considered for transplantation.

Several factors may contribute to the development of liver disease in patients undergoing BMT or PBSCT. Chemotherapy and radiation treatments may cause deposits of fibrous material to form in the small veins of the liver, which obstruct blood flow out of it. This obstruction is known as venocclusive disease (VOD). VOD is an important and sometimes severe complication in BMT. Symptoms of VOD include swelling of the liver, abdominal pain, weight gain, and poor liver function. Other conditions that may cause liver damage are viral hepatitis, fungal and bacterial infections, and GVHD. In addition, some drugs used to treat infection may cause liver problems. Liver disease is difficult to treat, and medical care is generally directed at controlling the patient's symptoms. Some medical centers are investigating whether certain drugs can prevent liver disease.

Chemotherapy, radiation therapy, antibiotics, and immunosuppressive agents (especially cyclosporine) also may cause kidney failure. When this happens, urine production decreases, waste products accumulate in the blood, and the patient becomes more susceptible to infection, bleeding, and drug toxicity. Should kidney problems develop, the patient's fluid balance is carefully controlled. Dietary modifications, including total parenteral nutrition, may be necessary, and drug doses may need to be changed. Some patients may need *dialysis.* As with liver disease, the likelihood of kidney failure may be reduced by certain drugs.

Complications also may develop in the lungs after transplantation. Often, infections are the cause of these problems. However, radiation therapy and chemotherapy also may be damaging, causing pneumonitis, an inflammation of the lungs. Some patients develop pulmonary fibrosis, a condition that may result in shortness of breath. Measures to prevent lung problems include antibiotic therapy and the use of lung shields during total body irradiation (TBI).

Chemotherapy—in particular, doxirubicin—can damage the heart and produce a number of complications that affect its function. Certain complications can be life threatening. However, only a small percentage of patients undergoing transplantation experience heart complications.

Graft Failure

Grafting is considered a failure when bone marrow function does not return or when it is lost after a period of recovery. Unsuccessful transplantations usually result from one of two main situations. In one case, graft rejection, the recipient's body rejects the donated marrow; in the other, engraftment does not occur or doesn't continue—that is, the transplanted stem cells simply fail to grow and produce new blood cells. Graft rejection is a problem that is exclusive to allogeneic transplant recipients, whereas other types of graft failure may occur in patients receiving any type of transplant.

A number of factors may contribute to the risk of graft rejection. One of the most significant is the use of marrow with an imperfect HLA match. Graft rejection is more common among patients who have not had TBI because such patients are more likely to retain some immune activity after pretransplantation conditioning. The use of T-cell depleted donor marrow also is associated with an increased risk of graft rejection.

Engraftment is less likely to occur in patients with extensive *marrow fibrosis* before transplantation. Unsuccessful transplantation also may result from a viral illness or from the use of drugs that suppress the immune system (such as methotrexate). In leukemia patients, graft failure often is associated with a recurrence of leukemia; the leukemic cells may inhibit the growth of the transplanted cells. In some cases, the reasons for graft failure are not known.

Long-Term Effects

Long-term effects of transplantation are largely related to pretransplantation conditioning regimens. Some of these problems are discussed below.

Infertility

Chemotherapy and radiation therapy often cause temporary or permanent reproductive difficulties. The extent of these problems depends on the patient's age and sex and on the dosage and duration of treatment. Most patients who receive TBI as part of their conditioning treatment become sterile. However, sexual desire and function usually return to normal after transplantation. Infertility is common among men who are treated with chemotherapy or radiation therapy. For this reason, men are usually encouraged to consider sperm banking before treatment begins, if they wish to father children after transplantation.

Menstrual irregularities often develop in women who have received high-dose chemotherapy. Although periods may return up to two years after transplantation in younger women, patients over the age of 25 are likely to develop early menopause. Hormone replacement therapy can help relieve the symptoms of menopause and may be recommended for other medical reasons. (However, this treatment may not be appropriate for women who have had breast cancer.) Cryopreservation of fertilized or unfertilized eggs before cancer therapy is possible for some women. Women who wish to become pregnant after they have undergone transplantation should speak with their doctor; pregnancy may not be advisable for health reasons.

Sterility can be a psychologically distressing side effect. This important issue should be addressed by the patient, partner, family, and health care provider care team before and after transplantation.

Growth Problems

Studies have shown that some children treated with TBI may have impaired growth, particularly when single-dose TBI is given. The radiation can cause a reduction in growth hormone production and can damage children's bones. The result may be a delay in growth of about two years.

Cataracts

Cataracts may occur three to six years after TBI. Roughly three-quarters of patients who receive single-dose TBI develop cataracts. The number is reduced to about 20 percent in patients who receive fractionated radiation doses or in those who do not receive TBI. Patients who develop cataracts generally need corrective surgery, which often restores normal vision.

Secondary Cancers

Because BMT has been done for only a few decades, not all of the long-term effects of the procedure are known. There is some concern that high-dose chemotherapy, irradiation, immunosuppression, stem cell mobilization, or other unknown factors related to the procedure may increase the risk for secondary cancers. Studies have shown that the risk varies considerably depending on the patient's age, general health, menopausal status (for women), and previous history of radiation. The dosage and type of drug given also affect the likelihood that a second cancer may develop.

Financial Considerations

Because it is a highly technical procedure that requires extensive hospitalization, BMT is very expensive. Advances in treatment methods, including the use of PBSCT, have reduced the time many patients must spend in the hospital by speeding recovery; this shorter recovery time has brought about a reduction in cost. Still, transplantation expenses often exceed $100,000. Most centers require a guarantee of funds in advance to cover these costs. However, some health care provider insurance plans now cover some costs of transplantation for specific diseases.

Costs are incurred not only in the hospital, but outside as well. Patients and their families may need to stay near the transplant center for several months so that the patient can receive follow-up care. This can involve a considerable amount of money, particularly if accommodations are far from home. After the patient returns home, other expenses may arise. No patient is able to function independently immediately after discharge from the hospital, and convalescence at home takes a significant amount of time. Family members may need to call on home helpers or visiting nurses to assist them with the care of the patient. In some cases, insurers cover a portion of these costs. In other cases, local service organizations may be able to help.

There are some options for relieving the financial burden associated with BMT. A hospital social worker can be a valuable resource in planning for these financial needs. Patients and their families may use an existing charitable fund from a church or service group (Kiwanis, Lions, Rotary, Masons, etc.); contributions to these funds are tax deductible.

Families can also contact the Leukemia Society of America and the American Cancer Society (listed in the white pages of the telephone directory). These organizations may be able to help with costs of transportation and other expenses.

Organizations such as the Corporate Angel Network (CAN) will sometimes help with air transportation. This organization's member companies share their scheduled executive jet flights with cancer patients needing to travel to obtain medical care.

Government programs such as Medicaid and Social Security also may provide financial assistance for health care provider expenses and disability. Medicaid is a program for people of low income; information about coverage is available from a local public health or social services office or from a State Medicaid office. Supplemental Security Income is available to disabled people of low income and Social Security disability to certain disabled workers. A local Social Security office (listed in the Government section of the telephone directory) can explain eligibility criteria and benefits.

Income tax deductions can be claimed for some BMT expenses. Families should check with an accountant or attorney regarding such deductions. The local Internal Revenue Service office and possibly the hospital's social services staff also can provide guidance on tax considerations.

The NCI's Cancer Information Service (1-800-4-CANCER) can provide patients and their families with additional information about financial assistance.

Psychosocial Considerations

BMT causes tremendous stress for patients and their families, who must struggle physically, emotionally, and financially with the therapy and the disruption it may bring to their lives. Families often must travel a long distance to a treatment center and arrange to live away from home for an extended period of time. (The number of treatment centers that can perform BMT has grown considerably in recent years, but they still tend to be clustered in major metropolitan areas.) For many people, this means a lengthy separation from other family members. Making these adjustments can be very dif-

ficult; patients and their families may find it helpful to use support services offered through the hospital or another organization, such as the American Cancer Society.

The energy required during and after transplantation is considerable. Fatigue is a common complaint: Patients tire of the rigors of treatment, and both they and their families often feel the pressure of not knowing what will happen.

During the BMT process, medical problems are likely to take priority over psychological needs. However, the psychological stresses of BMT are considerable and should not be minimized. For many reasons, both families and patients may experience guilt, relief, fear, anger, depression, and anxiety. At any time during treatment or followup, members of the health care provider team may help patients and families deal with these issues. Patients and their families are encouraged to consult with a social worker, a member of the clergy, or a counselor.

The Future of Transplantation

An estimated 12,000 BMTs were performed in 1992, approximately half of which were allogeneic and half autologous. The use of autologous transplantation (including PBSCT) has grown significantly during the past several years as improvements in the procedure have been made. The number of patients who receive allogeneic transplants also is rising, in part because large donor registries have increased the number of available donors. Advances in transplantation techniques likely will further expand the use of BMT and PBSCT in the coming years.

The use of hematopoietic growth factors is one of the most promising areas of research. Other growth factors are under investigation in addition to the well-studied GM-CSF, G-CSF, and the interleukins. Erythropoietin (a red blood cell growth factor) can increase peripheral blood stem cell yield before transplantation and can reduce the need for RBC transfusions afterward. Researchers have discovered a growth factor that stimulates the production of platelets, which has been named thrombopoietin. In the future, treatment with this growth factor may be able to complement or replace transfusions with platelets. Stem cell factor, which stimulates the maturation of stem cells, may be useful for speeding engraftment. Researchers also are investigating whether growth factors can be applied to harvested stem cells *in vitro* (in the laboratory) to increase the number of stem cells available for transplantation.

Other *biological response modifiers* under investigation include *interferons* and monoclonal antibodies. Interferons may stop the growth of cancer cells when used before or after BMT for chronic myelogenous leukemia. Monoclonal antibodies can be bound to *radioisotopes* or anticancer drugs and targeted to cancer cells. In this way, drugs or radiation can be delivered directly to cancer cells without damaging healthy cells.

Because even small numbers of cancer cells can grow and cause a relapse after transplantation, researchers are exploring ways to detect cancer in patients who otherwise appear to be in remission. Once technique involved the use of monoclonal antibodies linked to radioisotopes or special dyes that allow the cancer to be seen. Another technique, known as polymer-agse chain reaction (or PCR), magnifies the genetic abnormalities of some types of cancer so that they can be detected. Researchers also are trying to identify other factors that may indicate a high risk of relapse.

A new approach under study in allogenic transplantation involves using umbilical cord blood, which generally contains high levels of stem cells. The feasibility of cord blood cell banking is under investigation.

Many issues surrounding BMT and PBSCT in cancer treatment are being addressed in current *clinical trials;* others are still under study in the laboratory. Marrow transplant technology is also being evaluated for treatment of other disorders in which the immune system's ability to function has been affected.

Clinical Trials and PDQ

To improve the outcome of treatment for patients with cancers, NCI supports clinical trials at many hospitals throughout the United States. Volunteers who take part in this research make an important contribution to medical science and may have the first chance to benefit from improved treatment methods. Physicians are encouraged to tell their patients about the option of participating in such trials. To help patients and doctors learn about current methods of treatment and clinical trials, NCI has developed PDQ, a database designed to give physicians and patients quick and easy access to

- descriptions of ongoing clinical trials, including information about the objectives of the studies, medical eligibility requirements, details of the treatment programs, and the names and addresses of physicians and facilities conducting the studies
- the latest treatment information for most types of cancer
- names and addresses of physicians and organizations involved in cancer care

Information specialists at the Cancer Information Service (CIS) use a variety of resources, including PDQ, to answer questions about cancer prevention, diagnosis, treatment, rehabilitation, and research. To obtain information from the PDQ database, physicians, patients, and the public may call the CIS toll free at 1-800-4-CANCER. Staff members also can tell doctors how to obtain regular access to the database.

In addition, PDQ statements containing up-to-date treatment information are available by fax machine through the CancerFax service. Those wanting to use this service should dial (301) 402-5874 from a fax machine telephone and follow instructions to obtain a list of the CancerFax contents and the corresponding code numbers. Users then can call the service again and enter the code numbers of the printout they wish to receive by fax.

PDQ statements, fact sheets on various cancer topics, and citations and abstracts on selected topics from the CANCER-LIT database can be obtained through CancerNet. This service allows users to access cancer information through electronic mail. It is available through a number of different networks including BITNET and Internet.

Glossary

Allogeneic transplantation: A procedure in which a patient receives bone marrow from another person other than an identical twin.

Anemia: A condition in which the number of red cells or the amount of hemoglobin in the blood is abnormally low.

Antibodies: Proteins produced by certain white blood cells in response to a foreign substance (antigen). Each antibody can bind only to one specific antigen. The purpose of this binding is to help destroy the antigen.

Antigen: Any foreign or "nonself" substance that, when introduced into the body, activates the immune system.

Antithymocyte globulin: A protein preparation used to prevent and treat graft-versus-host disease.

Aplastic anemia: A deficiency of certain types of blood cells caused by poor bone marrow function.

Autologous transplantation: A procedure in which bone marrow or peripheral blood stem cells are removed from a patient, stored as the patient receives high-dose therapy, and reinfused into the same patient.

B cells: Lymphocytes that are thought to develop in the bone marrow. In response to antigens, B cells produce antibodies. Also known as B lymphocytes.

Biological response modifier (BRM): A substance that boosts, directs, or restores the body's normal immune (defense) system. BRMs are produced naturally in the body and also can be manufactured in the laboratory.

Bone marrow aspiration: A procedure in which a needle is inserted into the center of a bone, usually the hip, to remove a sample of bone marrow for examination under a microscope.

Cataract: A condition in which the lens of the eye becomes clouded, resulting in painless loss of vision that often can be relieved surgically.

Chemotherapy: Treatment with anticancer drugs.

Clinical trial: Medical research conducted with volunteers. Each trial is designed to answer scientific questions and to find better ways to treat patients or prevent disease.

Colony-stimulating factors (CSFs): Proteins that stimulate the development of cells in the bone marrow; also called hematopoietic growth factors.

Conditioning: Treatment with high-dose chemotherapy, and sometimes with high-dose radiation therapy as well, to prepare a patient for bone marrow transplantation or peripheral blood stem cell transplantation.

Corticosteroids: Natural or synthetic hormones that influence or control key functions of the body, including the immune response. Corticosteroids can be used to prevent and treat graft-versus-host disease.

Cryopreservation: The freezing of cells for use at a later time.

Dialysis: The removal of certain elements from the blood by a filtering process. This word is most often used to refer to a filtering process that is done when the kidneys are not functioning normally.

Engraftment: The process in which transplanted bone marrow or peripheral blood stem cells begin to grow in the bone marrow of the host and to manufacture new white blood cells, red blood cells, and platelets.

Fractionated radiation therapy: Treatment in which radiation is given in several small doses.

Germ cell tumor: A tumor arising from cells that give rise to sperm or eggs or that resemble the cells that give rise to sperm or eggs. As a result of normal development, germ cells are found in the ovaries and testes and along the midline of the body, such as in the center of the chest and the center back area of the wall of the abdominal cavity.

Graft: Tissue taken from one person (donor) and transferred to another person (recipient), or taken from one part of a person's body and transferred to another part of that same person's body.

Graft-versus-host disease: A reaction of white blood cells in transplanted tissue (the graft) against the tissues of the recipient (the host).

Hematopoietic growth factors: Proteins that stimulate the development of blood cells from stem cells; also called colony-stimulating factors.

Hemoglobin: A protein in red blood cells that carries oxygen from the lungs to all cells of the body. Hemoglobin gives blood its red color.

Human leukocyte-associated (HLA) antigens: A series of proteins on the surface of cells that are important in transplantation and transfusion. When bone marrow transplantation is being considered, the HLAs on white blood cells (leukocytes) of the patient and the potential donor are compared. HLAs on platelets are matched when platelets are being transfused. A perfect HLA match occurs only between identical twins.

Immune response: The activity of the immune system against foreign substances (antigens).

Immune system: the complex group of organs and cells that defends the body against infection or other diseases.

Immunoglobulin therapy: Treatment with antibodies to prevent infection.

Immunosuppression: An extreme weakening of the immune response caused by drugs or other means.

Infusion: The introduction of a fluid into a vein.

Interferons: Proteins, produced by the body, that help the immune system function in a number of ways. Large quantities of different interferons may be produced in the laboratory and used to treat some forms of cancer.

Interleukins: Proteins that carry regulatory signals between blood-forming cells. Large quantities of interleukins can be produced in the laboratory and used to treat some forms of cancer. Interleukins are biological response modifiers.

Intravenous catheter: A thin plastic tube that is inserted into a vein to allow the addition of substances to the blood.

Leukemia: Cancer that begins in developing blood cells in the bone marrow. As a result, large numbers of immature blood cells are produced and released into the bloodstream, and the cancer cells in the marrow crowd out normal developing blood cells

Leukopenia: An abnormally low number of white blood cells.

Lymphoma: Cancer of the lymphatic system, which is composed of the tissues and organs that produce and store cells that fight infection and disease. The lymphatic system includes the bone marrow, spleen, thymus, lymph nodes, and a network of vessels that carry fluid and infection-fighting cells.

Macrophages: Cells found at the site of infection or injury that are capable of "eating" cells or particles that the body wants to eliminate. Monocytes, a type of white blood cells, develop into macrophages when they leave the bloodstream and enter other tissue.

Marrow fibrosis: The development of fibrous tissue in the bone marrow. Marrow fibrosis interferes with blood cell production.

Metastasis: The spread of cancer cells to distant areas of the body through the lymphatic system or bloodstream.

Monoclonal antibodies: Laboratory-produced identical antibodies that can target a specific antigen. They can be made in large quantities in the laboratory and are being studied to determine their effectiveness in the detection and treatment of cancer.

Mucositis: Inflammation and irritation of the mucous membranes.

Multiple myeloma: Cancer that affects antibody-producing B cells. The disease causes the growth of many tumors in the bone marrow and in the hard, outer portion of the bones.

Myelodysplastic syndromes: Disorders of bone marrow function. They are characterized by blood cells that look abnormal and by low numbers of certain blood cells.

Neuroblastoma: Cancer that begins in immature nerve cells. This disease most often occurs in infants and children and tends to be found in the center of the chest and the center back area of the wall of the abdominal cavity.

NK (natural killer) cells: Large lymphocytes that attack certain cells on contact and probably help regulate the immune system.

Peripheral blood stem cells: Stem cells that circulate in the blood.

Phagocytosis: The process by which certain cells surround and destroy organisms and break down products of other cells.

Purging: Removal of tumor cells from harvested marrow or blood before autologous transplantation.

Radiation therapy: Treatment with high-energy rays to kill cancer cells. Also called radiotherapy.

Radioisotope: A substance that emits radiation. Radioisotopes can be used in both cancer detection and treatment.

Refractory: Not responding to treatment.

Remission: Complete or partial disappearance of the signs and symptoms of disease in response to treatment. The period during which a disease is under control.

Rescue process: The infusion of harvested bone marrow or peripheral blood stem cells into a patient who has undergone high-dose therapy.

Severe combined immunodeficiency disease (SCID): A disorder characterized by the complete absence or a marked deficiency of B cells and T cells. SCID leaves an individual with little or no protection against infection.

Soft tissue sarcoma: A type of cancer that begins in connective tissue (tissue that connects, supports, and surrounds other tissue and organs). Muscles, tendons, fibrous tissue, fat, nerves, tissue around joints, blood vessels, and lymph vessels are kinds of connective tissue.

Stem cells: The immature cells from which all blood cells develop.

Syngeneic transplantation: A procedure in which a patient receives bone marrow from a genetically identical individual (identical twin).

T cells: White blood cells that mature in the thymus and perform several important functions in the immune response. Also known as T lymphocytes.

T-cell depletion: Treatment to get rid of T cells, which play an important role in the immune response. Elimination of T cells from an allogeneic bone marrow graft may reduce the chance of graft-versus-host disease.

Thalassemia: A disease in which hemoglobin production is abnormal. It often results in severe anemia.

Thrombocytopenia: An abnormally low number of platelets in the blood.

Total parenteral nutrition: The intravenous infusion of essential nutrients to patients who are unable to eat.

Resources

American Cancer Society
1599 Clifton Rd, NE
Atlanta, GA 30329-4251
1-800-ACS-2345

The American Cancer Society (ACS) is a national voluntary organization. It offers a wide range of services to patients and their families and carries out programs of research and education. It is financed through donations from individuals and private groups. Local chapters of the ACS may be listed in the telephone directory; information is also available by dialing the toll-free number listed above.

Leukemia Society of America
Fourth Fl
600 Third Ave
New York, NY 10016
1-800-955-4LSA (1-800-955-4572)

The Leukemia Society of America is a voluntary organization that offers educational materials and information to leukemia and lymphoma patients and their families. It has many local chapters whose addresses may be listed in the telephone directory. Information is also available by dialing the toll-free number listed above.

National Marrow Donor Program
Suite 400
3433 Broadway St, NE
Minneapolis, MN 55413
Donor Information: 1-800-654-1247
Patient Search Information: 1-800-526-7809

The National Marrow Donor Program (NMDP) is funded by a Federal contract with the American Red Cross, the American Association of Blood Banks, and the Council of Community Blood Centers. It was created to improve the efficiency and effectiveness of the donor search so that a larger number of unrelated bone marrow transplantations can be carried out. Businesses interested in setting up corporate recruitment programs should contact NMDP at 1-800-526-7809.

American Red Cross
430 17th St, NW
Washington, DC 20006
202-737-8300

The American Red Cross collects and distributes blood and blood products and provides a range of services for emergency situations and people in need of social service support. It coordinates bone marrow testing and donation in association with the National Marrow Donor Program. Local chapters are listed in the white pages of the telephone directory.

American Bone Marrow Donor Registry, Search Coordinating Center
Caitlin Raymond International Registry of Bone Marrow Donor Banks
University of Massachusetts Medical Center
55 Lake Ave N
Worcester, MA 01655
Donor Information: 1-800-7-DONATE (1-800-736-6283)
Patient Search Information: 1-800-7-A-MATC (1-800-726-2824)

The American Bone Marrow Donor Registry is a nonprofit organization that coordinates donor searches among participating donor centers in the United States and throughout the world.

International Bone Marrow Transplant Registry
Medical College of Wisconsin
PO Box 26509
8701 Watertown Plank Rd
Milwaukee, WI 53226
414-456-8325

This research organization collects and analyzes data about allogeneic bone marrow transplantations performed at BMT centers throughout the world and autologous transplantations done in North America. (It does not make donor matches.) Staff are available to answer questions about the procedure.

Selected References

Available from Libraries

Bortin, MM, et al. "Changing Trends in Allogeneic Bone Marrow Transplantation for Leukemia in the 1980s," *Journal of the American Medical Association,* Vol. 268(5), 1992, pp. 607–612.

Bortin, MM, et al. "Increasing Utilization of Allogeneic Bone Marrow Transplantation: Results of the 1988–1990 Survey," *Annals of Internal Medicine,* Vol. 116(6), 1992, pp. 505–512.

Champlin, R. "T-cell Depletion To Prevent Graft-Versus-Host-Disease After Bone Marrow Transplantation," *Hematology/Oncology Clinics of North America,* Vol. 4(3), 1990, pp. 687–698.

DeVita, VT, Jr, Hellman, S, and Rosenberg, SA, eds. *Cancer: Principles and Practices of Oncology.* Philadelphia, J.B. Lippincott Company, 1993.

Ferrara, JLM and Deeg, HJ. "Mechanisms of Disease: Graft-Versus-Host Disease," *The New England Journal of Medicine,* Vol. 324(10), 1991, pp. 667–674.

Holland, JC and Rowland, JH. *Handbook of Psychooncology: Psychological Care of the Patient with Cancer.* New York, Oxford University Press, 1989.

Kernan, NA, et al. "Analysis of 462 Transplantations from Unrelated Donors Facilitated by the National Marrow Donor Program," *The New England Journal of Medicine,* Vol. 328(9), 1993, pp. 593–602.

Kessinger, A and Armitage, J. "The Use of Peripheral Stem Cell Support of High-Dose Chemotherapy," in *Important Advances in Oncology 1993.* DeVita, VT Jr, et al., eds. Philadelphia, J.B. Lippincott Co., 1993.

Meropol, NJ, et al. "High-Dose Chemotherapy with Autologous Stem Cell Support for Breast Cancer," *Oncology,* Vol. 6(12), 1992, pp. 53–63.

Thorne, AC, et al. "Harvesting Bone Marrow in an Outpatient Setting Using Newer Anesthetic Agents," *Journal of Clinical Oncology,* Vol. 11(2), 1993, pp. 320–323.

Treleaven, J and Barrett, J. *Bone Marrow Transplantation in Practice.* Edinburgh, Churchill Livingstone, 1992.

Available from the National Cancer Institute

Chemotherapy and You: A Guide to Self-Help During Treatment. Office of Cancer Communications, National Cancer Institute. NIH Publication No. 94-1136.

Radiation Therapy and You: A Guide to Self-Help During Treatment. Office of Cancer Communications, National Cancer Institute. NIH Publication No. 94-2227.

Research Report: Leukemia. Office of Cancer Communications, National Cancer Institute. NIH Publication No. 93-329.

The Immune System—How It Works. National Cancer Institute, National Institute of Allergy and Infectious Diseases. NIH Publication No. 92-3229.

What Are Clinical Trials All About? Office of Cancer Communications, National Cancer Institute. NIH Publication No. 92-2706.

Additional Information

To obtain information on this subject and to order other NCI publications, call the toll-free Cancer Information Service (CIS) at

1-800-4-CANCER

■ **Document Source:**
   U.S. Department of Health and Human Services, Public Health Service
   National Institutes of Health
   National Cancer Institute
   NIH Publication Number 95-1178
   Revised November 1994

See also: Bone Marrow Transplantation: Questions & Answers (page 47)

CHEMOTHERAPY AND YOU: A GUIDE TO SELF-HELP DURING TREATMENT

About this Booklet

This booklet will help you, your family, and your friends understand chemotherapy, the use of drugs to treat cancer. It will answer many of the questions you may have about this method of cancer treatment. It will also show you how you can help yourself during chemotherapy.

Taking care of yourself during chemotherapy is important for several reasons. For one thing, it can lessen some of the physical side effects you may have from your treatment. As you will see, some simple tips can make a big difference in how you feel. But the benefits of self-help aren't just physical; they're psychological, too. Knowing some ways to take care of yourself can give your emotions a boost at a time when you may be feeling that much of what's happening to you is out of your control. This feeling can be easier to deal with when you discover how much you can contribute to your own well-being, in partnership with your doctors and nurses.

Chemotherapy and You will help you become an informed partner in your care. Remember, though, it is only a guide. Self-help is never a substitute for professional medical care. Be sure to ask your doctor and nurse any questions you may have about chemotherapy, and tell them about any side effects you may have.

You will find several helpful sections at the end of this booklet. The section *Paying for Chemotherapy* gives you information about insurance and other payment methods. The section called *Resources* tells you how to get more information about cancer and how to find many services available to cancer patients and their families. The glossary explains many terms related to cancer and chemotherapy. Additionally, you can get a free series of fact sheets on anticancer drugs from the National Cancer Institute.

Understanding Chemotherapy

What is chemotherapy?

Chemotherapy is the use of drugs to treat cancer. The drugs often are called anticancer drugs.

How does chemotherapy work?

Normal cells grow and die in a controlled way. But cancer occurs when cells become abnormal and keep dividing and forming more cells without control or order. Anticancer drugs destroy cancer cells by stopping them from growing or multiplying at one or more points in their life cycle. Because some drugs work better together than alone, chemotherapy often may consist of more than one drug. This is called combination chemotherapy.

In addition to chemotherapy, other methods sometimes are used to treat cancer. For example, your doctor may recommend that you have surgery to remove a tumor or to relieve certain symptoms that may be caused by your cancer. You also may receive radiation therapy to treat your cancer or its symptoms. Sometimes, as described below, your doctor may suggest a combination of chemotherapy, surgery, and/or radiation therapy.

Other types of drugs may be used to treat your cancer. These may include certain drugs that can block the effect of hormones. Doctors may also use biological therapy to boost the body's natural defenses against cancer.

What can chemotherapy achieve?

Depending on the type of cancer and its stage of development, chemotherapy can be used

- To cure cancer.
- To keep the cancer from spreading.
- To slow the cancer's growth.
- To kill cancer cells that may have spread to other parts of the body from the original tumor.
- To relieve symptoms that may be caused by the cancer.

Chemotherapy also can help people live more comfortably; this is known as palliative care.

Will chemotherapy be my only treatment for cancer?

Sometimes chemotherapy is the only therapy a patient receives. More often, however, chemotherapy is used in addition to surgery and/or radiation therapy; when it is used for this purpose it is called adjuvant therapy. There are several reasons why chemotherapy may be given in addition to other treatment methods. For instance, chemotherapy may be used to shrink a tumor before surgery or radiation therapy. It also may be used after surgery and/or radiation therapy to help destroy any cancer cells that may remain.

Which drugs will I get?

Your doctor decides which drug or drugs will work best for you. The decision depends on what kind of cancer you have, where it is, the extent of its growth, how it is affecting your normal body functions, and your general health.

Your doctor also may suggest that you join a clinical trial for chemotherapy, or you may want to bring up this option with your doctor. Clinical trials are carefully designed research studies that test promising new cancer treatments. Patients who take part in research may be the first to benefit from improved treatment methods. These patients also can make an important contribution to medical care because the results of the studies may help many people. Patients participate in clinical trials only if they choose to and are free to withdraw at any time.

To learn more about clinical trials, call the National Cancer Institute's Cancer Information Service and ask for the booklet *What Are Clinical Trials All About?* You also may want to ask about the video *Patient to Patient: Cancer Clinical Trials and You.* This videotape can put to rest fears you may have about taking part in clinical trials. The Cancer Information Service can be reached by dialing 1-800-4-CANCER (1-800-422-6237).

Where will I get chemotherapy?

You may get your chemotherapy at home, in your doctor's office, in a clinic, in your hospital's outpatient department, or in a hospital. The choice of where you get chemotherapy depends on which drug or drugs you are getting, your hospital's policies, and your doctor's preferences. When you first start chemotherapy, you may need to stay at the hospital for a short time so that your doctor can watch the medicine's effects closely and make any adjustments that are needed.

How often will I get chemotherapy, and how long will I get it?

How often—and for how long—you get chemotherapy depends on the kind of cancer you have, the goals of the treatment, the drugs that are used, and how your body responds to them. You may get chemotherapy every day, every week, or every month. Chemotherapy is often given in on-and-off cycles that include rest periods so that your body has a chance to build healthy new cells and regain its strength. Your doctor should be able to estimate how long you will be getting chemotherapy.

Whatever schedule your doctor prescribes, it is very important to stay with it. Otherwise, the anticancer drugs might not have their desired effect. If you miss a treatment session or skip a dose of medication, contact your doctor for instructions about what to do.

Sometimes, your doctor may delay a treatment based on the results of certain blood tests. Your doctor will let you know what to do during this time and when it's okay to start your treatment sessions again.

How will I get chemotherapy?

Depending on the type of cancer you have and the drug or drugs you are getting, your chemotherapy may be given in one or more of the following ways:

- Into a vein (intravenously, or IV). You will get the drug through a thin needle inserted into a vein, usually on your hand or lower arm. Another way to get IV chemotherapy is by means of a catheter, a thin tube that is placed into a large vein in your body and remains there as long as it is needed. This type of catheter is known as a central venous catheter. Sometimes, a central venous catheter is attached to a port, a small plastic or metal container placed surgically under the skin.
- By mouth (orally, or PO) in pill, capsule, or liquid form. You will swallow the drug, just as you do many other medications.
- Into a muscle (intramuscularly, or IM), under the skin (subcutaneously, or SQ, or SC), or directly into a cancerous area in the skin (intralesionally, or IL). You will get an injection with a needle.
- Topically. The medication will be applied onto the skin.

Chemotherapy also may be delivered to specific areas of the body using a catheter. Catheters may be placed into the spinal fluid, abdominal cavity, bladder, or liver. Your doctor or nurse may use specific terms when talking about certain types of catheters. For example, an intrathecal (IT) catheter is used to deliver drugs into the spinal fluid. Intracavitary (IC) catheters can be placed in the abdomen, pelvis, or chest.

Two kinds of pumps—external and internal—may be used to control the rate of delivery of chemotherapy. External pumps remain outside of the body. Some are portable and allow a person to move around while the pump is in use. Other external pumps are not portable and may restrict activity. Internal pumps are placed surgically inside the body, usually right under the skin. They contain a small reservoir (storage area) that delivers the drugs into the catheter. Internal pumps allow people to go about most of their daily activities.

Does chemotherapy hurt?

Getting chemotherapy by mouth, on the skin, or by injection generally feels the same as taking other medications by these methods. Having an IV usually feels like having blood drawn for a blood test. Some people feel a coolness or other unusual sensation in the area of the injection when the IV is started. Report these feelings to your doctor or nurse. Be sure that you also report any pain, burning, or discomfort that occurs during or after an IV treatment.

Many people have little or no trouble having the IV needle in their hand or lower arm. However, if a person has a hard time for any reason, or if it becomes difficult to insert the needle into a vein for each treatment, it may be possible to use a central venous catheter or port. This avoids repeated insertion of the needle into the vein.

Central venous catheters and ports cause no pain or discomfort if they are properly placed and cared for, although a person usually is aware that they are there. It is important to report any pain or discomfort with a catheter or port to your doctor or nurse.

Can I take other medicines while I am getting chemotherapy?

Some medicines may interfere with the effects of your chemotherapy. That is why you should take a list of all your medications to your doctor before you start chemotherapy. Your list should include the name of each drug, how often you take it, the reason you take it, and the dose. Remember to include over-the-counter drugs such as laxatives, cold pills, pain relievers, and vitamins. Your doctor will tell you if you should stop taking any of these medications before you start chemotherapy. After your treatments begin, be sure to check with your doctor before taking any new medicines or stopping the ones you already are taking.

Will I be able to work during chemotherapy?

Most people are able to continue working while they are being treated with anticancer drugs. It may be possible to schedule your treatments late in the day or right before the weekend, so they interfere with work as little as possible.

If your chemotherapy makes you very tired, you might want to think about adjusting your work schedule for a while. Speak with your employer about your needs and wishes at this time. You may be able to agree on a part-time schedule, or perhaps you can do some of your work at home.

Under Federal and state laws, some employers may be required to allow you to work a flexible schedule to meet your treatment needs. To find out about your on-the-job protections, check with your local American Cancer Society, a social worker, or your congressional or state representative. The National Cancer Institute's publication *Facing Forward: A Guide for Cancer Survivors* also has information on work-related concerns.

How will I know if my chemotherapy is working?

Your doctor and nurse will use several methods to measure how well your treatments are working. You will have frequent physical exams, blood tests, scans, and x-rays. Don't hesitate to ask the doctor about the test results and what they show about your progress.

While tests and exams can tell a lot about how chemotherapy is working, side effects tell very little. (Side effects— such as nausea or hair loss—occur because chemotherapy harms some normal cells as well as cancer cells.) Sometimes people think that if they don't have side effects, the drugs aren't working, or that, if they do have side effects, the drugs are not working well. But side effects vary so much from person to person, and from drug to drug, that having them or not having them usually isn't a sign of whether the treatment is effective.

If you do have side effects, there is a lot you can do to help relieve them. The next section of this booklet describes some of the most common side effects of chemotherapy and gives you some hints for coping with them.

Coping with Side Effects

If you have questions about side effects, you are not alone. Before chemotherapy starts, most people are concerned about whether they will have side effects and, if so, what they will be like. Once treatments begin, people who have side effects want to know the best ways to cope with them. This section will answer some of your questions.

If you are reading this section before you start chemotherapy, you may feel overwhelmed by the wide range of side effects it describes. But remember: Every person doesn't get every side effect, and some people get few, if any. In addition, the severity of side effects varies greatly from person to person. Whether you have a particular side effect, and how severe it will be, depends on the kind of chemotherapy you get and how your body reacts. Be sure to talk to your doctor and nurse about which side effects are most likely to occur with your chemotherapy, how long they might last, how serious they might be, and when you should seek medical attention for them.

What causes side effects?

Because cancer cells grow and divide rapidly, anticancer drugs are made to kill fast-growing cells. But certain normal, healthy cells also multiply quickly, and chemotherapy can affect these cells, too. When it does, side effects may result. The fast-growing, normal cells most likely to be affected are blood cells forming in the bone marrow and cells in the digestive tract, reproductive system, and hair follicles. Anticancer drugs can also damage cells of the heart, kidney, bladder, lungs, and nervous system. The most common side effects of chemotherapy include nausea and vomiting, hair loss, and fatigue. Other common side effects include an increased chance of bleeding, getting an infection, or developing anemia. These side effects result from changes in blood cells during chemotherapy.

How long do side effects last?

Most normal cells recover quickly when chemotherapy is over, so most side effects gradually disappear after treatment ends, and the healthy cells have a chance to grow normally. The time it takes to get over some side effects and regain energy varies from person to person. How soon you will feel better depends on many factors, including your overall health and the kinds of drugs you have been taking.

While many side effects go away fairly rapidly, certain ones may take months or years to disappear completely. Sometimes, the side effects can last a lifetime, as when chemotherapy causes permanent damage to the heart, lungs, kidneys, or reproductive organs. And certain types of chemotherapy occasionally may cause delayed effects, such as a second cancer, that show up many years later.

It is important to remember that many people have no long-term problems due to chemotherapy. It also is reassuring to know that doctors are making great progress in preventing some of chemotherapy's more serious side effects. For instance, they are using many new drugs and techniques that increase chemotherapy's powerful effects on cancer cells while decreasing its harmful effects on the body's healthy cells.

The side effects of chemotherapy can be unpleasant, but they must be measured against the treatment's ability to destroy cancer. People getting chemotherapy sometimes become discouraged about the length of time their treatment is taking or the side effects they are having. If that happens to you, talk to your doctor. It may be that your medication or the treatment schedule can be changed. Or your doctor may be able to suggest ways to reduce side effects or make them easier to tolerate. Remember though, your doctor will not ask you to continue treatments unless the expected benefits outweigh any problems you might have.

On the pages that follow, you will find suggestions for dealing with some of the more common side effects of chemotherapy.

Nausea and Vomiting

Chemotherapy can cause nausea and vomiting by affecting the stomach, the area of the brain that controls vomiting, or both. This reaction to chemotherapy varies from person to person and from drug to drug. For example, some people never vomit or feel nauseous. Others feel mildly nauseated most of the time, while some become severely nauseated for a limited time during or after a treatment. Their symptoms may start soon after a treatment or hours later. They may feel sick for a few hours or for about a day. Be sure to tell your doctor or nurse if you are very nauseated and/or have vomited for more than a day or if your nausea is so bad that you cannot even keep liquids down.

Nausea and vomiting can almost always be controlled or at least lessened. If you experience this side effect, your doctor can choose from a range of drugs known as antiemetics, which help curb nausea and vomiting. Different drugs work for different people, and it may be necessary to use more than one drug to get relief. Don't give up. Continue to work with your doctor and nurse to find the drug or drugs that work best for you.

You can also try the following ideas:

- Avoid big meals so your stomach won't feel too full. Eat small meals throughout the day, instead of one, two, or three large meals.
- Drink liquids at least an hour before or after mealtime, instead of with your meals.
- Eat and drink slowly.
- Stay away from sweet, fried, or fatty foods.
- Eat foods cold or at room temperature so you won't be bothered by strong smells.
- Chew your food well for easier digestion.
- If nausea is a problem in the morning, try eating dry foods like cereal, toast, or crackers before getting up. (Don't try this if you have mouth or throat sores or if you are troubled by a lack of saliva.)
- Drink cool, clear, unsweetened fruit juices, such as apple or grape juice, or light-colored sodas, such as ginger ale, that have lost their fizz.
- Suck on ice cubes, mints, or tart candies. (Don't use tart candies if you have mouth or throat sores.)

- Try to avoid odors that bother you, such as cooking smells, smoke, or perfume.
- Prepare and freeze meals in advance for days when you don't feel like cooking.
- Rest in a chair after eating, but don't lie flat for at least two hours after you've finished your meal.
- Wear loose-fitting clothes.
- Breathe deeply and slowly when you feel nauseated.
- Distract yourself by chatting with friends or family members, listening to music, or watching a movie or TV show.
- Use relaxation techniques.
- Avoid eating for at least a few hours before treatment if nausea usually occurs during chemotherapy.

Hair Loss

Hair loss (alopecia) is a common side effect of chemotherapy, but it doesn't always happen. Your doctor can tell you whether hair loss is likely to occur with the drug or drugs you are taking. When hair loss does occur, the hair may become thinner or may fall out entirely. The hair usually grows back after the treatments are over. Some people even start to get their hair back while they are still having treatments. In some cases, hair may grow back in a different color or texture.

Hair loss can occur on all parts of the body, not just the head. Facial hair, arm and leg hair, underarm hair, and pubic hair all may be affected.

Hair loss usually doesn't happen right away; more often, it begins after a few treatments. At that point, hair may fall out gradually or in clumps. Any hair that is still growing may become dull and dry.

To care for your scalp and hair during chemotherapy

- Use mild shampoos.
- Use soft hair brushes.
- Use low heat when drying your hair.
- Don't use brush rollers to set your hair.
- Don't dye your hair or get a permanent.
- Have your hair cut short. A shorter style will make your hair look thicker and fuller. It will also make hair loss easier to manage if it occurs.
- Use a sunscreen, sunblock, hat, or scarf to protect your scalp from the sun if you lose a lot of the hair on your head. Some people who lose all or most of their hair choose to wear turbans, scarves, caps, wigs, or hairpieces. Others leave their head uncovered. Still others switch back and forth, depending on whether they are in public or at home with friends and family members. There are no right or wrong choices; do whatever feels comfortable for you.

Here are some tips if you choose to cover your head

- Get your wig or hairpiece before you lose a lot of hair. That way, you can match your natural color and current hair style if you wish. You may be able to buy a wig or hairpiece at a specialty shop just for cancer patients. Someone even may come to your home to help you. You also can buy a wig or hairpiece through a catalog or by phone. Call the American Cancer Society for more information.

- Consider borrowing a wig or hairpiece, rather than buying one. Check with the local chapter of the American Cancer Society or with the social work department at your hospital.
- Remember that a hairpiece needed because of cancer treatment is a tax-deductible expense and may be at least partially covered by your health insurance. Be sure to check your policy.

Losing hair from your head, face, or body can be hard to accept. It's common—and perfectly all right—to feel angry or depressed about this loss. Talking about your feelings can help.

Fatigue/Anemia

Chemotherapy can reduce the bone marrow's ability to make red blood cells, which carry oxygen to all parts of your body. When there are too few red blood cells, body tissues don't get enough oxygen to do their work. This condition is called anemia.

Anemia can make you feel very weak and tired. Other symptoms of anemia include dizziness, chills, or shortness of breath. Be sure to report any of these symptoms to your doctor.

Your doctor will check your blood cell count often during your treatment. If your red count falls too low, you may need a blood transfusion to increase the number of red blood cells in your body.

Here are some things you can do to help yourself feel better if you develop anemia:

- Get plenty of rest. Sleep more at night and take naps during the day if you can.
- Limit your activities. Do only the things that are most important to you.
- Don't be afraid to get help when you need it. Ask family and friends to pitch in with things like child care, shopping, housework, or driving.
- Eat a well-balanced diet.
- When sitting or lying down, get up slowly. This will help prevent dizziness.

Infection

Chemotherapy can make you more likely to get infections. This happens because most anticancer drugs affect the bone marrow and decrease its ability to produce white blood cells, the cells that fight many types of infections. An infection can begin in almost any part of your body including your mouth, skin, lungs, urinary tract, rectum, and reproductive tract.

Your doctor will check your blood cell count often while you are getting chemotherapy. Your doctor also may add colony stimulating factors to your treatment to keep your blood count from getting too far below normal. In spite of these extra steps, however, your white blood cell count still may drop. If this happens, your doctor may postpone your next treatment or give you a lower dose of drugs for a while.

When your white count is lower than normal, it is very important to try to prevent infections by taking the following steps:

- Wash your hands often during the day. Be sure to wash them extra well before you eat and before and after you use the bathroom.
- Clean your rectal area gently but thoroughly after each bowel movement. Ask your doctor or nurse for advice if the area becomes irritated or if you have hemorrhoids. Also, check with your doctor before using enemas or suppositories.
- Stay away from people who have diseases you can catch, such as a cold, the flu, measles, or chickenpox. Also try to avoid crowds.
- Stay away from children who recently have received immunizations, such as vaccines for polio, measles, mumps, and rubella (German measles).
- Don't cut or tear the cuticles of your nails.
- Be careful not to cut or nick yourself when using scissors, needles, or knives.
- Use an electric shaver instead of a razor to prevent breaks or cuts in your skin.
- Use a soft toothbrush that won't hurt your gums.
- Don't squeeze or scratch pimples.
- Take a warm (not hot) bath, shower, or sponge bath every day. Pat your skin dry using a light touch. Don't rub.
- Use lotion or oil to soften and heal your skin if it becomes dry and cracked.
- Clean cuts and scrapes right away with warm water, soap, and an antiseptic.
- Wear protective gloves when gardening or cleaning up after animals and others, especially small children.
- Do not get any immunization shots without checking first with your doctor to see if it's all right.

Most infections come from the bacteria normally found on the skin and in the intestines and genital tract. In some cases, the cause of an infection may not be known. When your white blood cell count is low, your body may not be able to fight off infections. So, even if you take extra care, you still may get an infection.

Be alert to the signs that you might have an infection and check your body regularly for its signs, paying special attention to your eyes, nose, mouth, and genital and rectal areas. The symptoms of infection include

- Fever over 100 degrees F.
- Chills.
- Sweating.
- Loose bowels (this can also be a side effect of chemotherapy).
- A burning feeling when you urinate.
- A severe cough or sore throat.
- Unusual vaginal discharge or itching.
- Redness or swelling, especially around a wound, sore, pimple, or intravenous catheter sites.

Report any signs of infection to your doctor right away. This is especially important when your white blood cell count is low. If you have a fever, don't use aspirin, acetaminophen, or any other medicine to bring your temperature down without first checking with your doctor.

Blood Clotting Problem

Anticancer drugs can affect the bone marrow's ability to make platelets, the blood cells that help stop bleeding by making your blood clot. If your blood does not have enough platelets, you may bleed or bruise more easily than usual, even from a minor injury.

Be sure to let your doctor know if you have unexplained bruising, small red spots under the skin, reddish or pinkish urine, or black or bloody bowel movements. Also report any bleeding from your gums or nose. Your doctor will check your platelet count often while you are having chemotherapy. If your platelet count falls too low, the doctor may give you a transfusion to build up the count.

Here are some ways to avoid problems if your platelet count is low:

- Don't take any medicine without first checking with your doctor or nurse. This includes aspirin or aspirin-free pain relievers, including acetaminophen, ibuprofen, and any other medicines you can buy without a prescription. These drugs may affect platelet function.
- Don't drink any alcoholic beverages unless your doctor says it's all right.
- Use a very soft toothbrush to clean your teeth.
- Clean your nose by blowing gently into a soft tissue.
- Take care not to cut or nick yourself when using scissors, needles, knives, or tools.
- Be careful not to burn yourself when ironing or cooking. Use a padded glove when you reach into the oven.
- Avoid contact sports and other activities that might result in injury.

Mouth, Gum, and Throat Problems

Good oral care is important during cancer treatment. Anticancer drugs can cause sores in the mouth and throat. They can also make these tissues dry and irritated or cause them to bleed. In addition to being painful, mouth sores can become infected by the many germs that live in the mouth. Because infections can be hard to fight during chemotherapy and can lead to serious problems, it's important to take every possible step to prevent them.

Here are some suggestions for keeping your mouth, gums, and throat healthy:

- If possible, see your dentist before you start chemotherapy to have your teeth cleaned and to take care of any problems such as cavities, abscesses, gum disease, or poorly fitting dentures. Ask your dentist to show you the best ways to brush and floss your teeth during chemotherapy. Chemotherapy can make you more likely to get cavities, so your dentist may suggest using a fluoride rinse or gel each day to help prevent tooth decay.
- Brush your teeth and gums after every meal. Use a soft toothbrush and a gentle touch; brushing too hard can damage soft mouth tissues. Ask your doctor, nurse, or dentist to suggest a special type of toothbrush and/or toothpaste if your gums are very sensitive.
- Rinse your toothbrush well after each use and store it in a dry place.
- Avoid commercial mouthwashes that contain a large amount of salt or alcohol. Ask you doctor or nurse about a mild mouthwash that you might use.

If you develop sores in your mouth, be sure to contact your doctor or nurse because you may need medical treatment for the sores. If the sores are painful or keep you from eating, you also can try these ideas:

- Ask your doctor if there is anything you can apply directly to the sores. You also may ask your doctor to prescribe a medicine you can use to ease the pain.
- Eat foods cold or at room temperature. Hot and warm foods can irritate a tender mouth and throat.
- Choose soft, soothing foods, such as ice cream, milkshakes, baby food, soft fruits (bananas and applesauce), mashed potatoes, cooked cereals, soft-boiled or scrambled eggs, cottage cheese, macaroni and cheese, custards, puddings, and gelatin. You also can puree cooked foods in the blender to make them smoother and easier to eat.
- Avoid irritating, acidic foods, such as tomatoes, citrus fruit, and fruit juice (orange, grapefruit, and lemon); spicy or salty foods; and rough, coarse, or dry foods such as raw vegetables, granola, and toast.

If mouth dryness bothers you or makes it hard for you to eat, try these tips:

- Ask your doctor if you should use an artificial saliva product to moisten your mouth.
- Drink plenty of liquids.
- Suck on ice cubes, popsicles, or sugarless hard candy. You can also chew sugarless gum.
- Moisten dry foods with butter, margarine, gravy, sauces, or broth.
- Dunk crisp, dry foods in mild liquids.
- Eat soft and pureed foods like those listed above.
- Use lip balm if your lips become dry.

Diarrhea

When chemotherapy affects the cells lining the intestine, the result can be diarrhea (loose stools). If you have diarrhea that continues for more than 24 hours, or if you have pain and cramping along with the diarrhea, call your doctor. In severe cases, the doctor may prescribe an antidiarrheal medicine. However, you should not take any over-the-counter antidiarrheal medicines without asking your doctor first.

You can also try these ideas to help control diarrhea:

- Eat smaller amounts of food, but eat more often.
- Avoid high-fiber foods, which can lead to diarrhea and cramping. High-fiber foods include whole-grain breads and cereals, raw vegetables, beans, nuts, seeds, popcorn, and fresh and dried fruit. Eat low-fiber foods, instead. Low-fiber foods include white bread, white

rice or noodles, creamed cereals, ripe bananas, canned or cooked fruit without skins, cottage cheese, yogurt, eggs, mashed or baked potatoes without the skin, pureed vegetables, chicken or turkey without the skin, and fish.

- Avoid coffee, tea, alcohol, and sweets. Stay away from fried, greasy, or highly spiced foods, too. They are all irritating and can cause diarrhea and cramping.
- Avoid milk and milk products if they make your diarrhea worse.
- Unless your doctor has told you otherwise, eat more potassium-rich foods because diarrhea can cause you to lose this important mineral. Bananas, oranges, potatoes, and peach and apricot nectars are good sources of potassium.
- Drink plenty of fluids to replace those you have lost through diarrhea. Mild, clear liquids, such as apple juice, water, weak tea, clear broth, or ginger ale are best. Drink them slowly, and make sure they are at room temperature. Let carbonated drinks lose their fizz before you drink them.
- If your diarrhea is severe, it is important to let your doctor know. Ask your doctor if you should try a clear liquid diet to give your bowels time to rest. As you feel better, you gradually can add the low-fiber foods listed above. A clear liquid diet doesn't provide all the nutrients you need, so don't follow one for more than three to five days.
- If your diarrhea is very severe, you may need to get intravenous fluids to replace the water and nutrients you have lost.

Constipation

Some people who get chemotherapy become constipated because of the drugs they are taking. Others may become constipated because they are less active or less nourished than usual. Tell your doctor if you have not had a bowel movement for more than a day or two. You may need to take a laxative or stool softener or use an enema, but don't use these remedies unless you have checked with your doctor, especially if your white blood cell count is low.

You also can try these ideas to deal with constipation:

- Drink plenty of fluids to help loosen the bowels. Warm and hot fluids work especially well.
- Eat a lot of high-fiber foods. High-fiber foods include bran, whole-wheat breads and cereals, raw or cooked vegetables, fresh and dried fruit, nuts, and popcorn.
- Get some exercise. Simply getting out for a walk can help, as can a more structured exercise program. Be sure to check with your doctor before becoming more active.

Nerve and Muscle Effects

Your nervous system affects just about all your body's organs and tissues. So it's not surprising that when chemotherapy affects the cells of the nervous system—as the drugs sometimes do—a wide range of side effects can result. For example, certain drugs can cause peripheral neuropathy, a condition that may make you feel a tingling, burning, weakness, or numbness in the hands and/or feet. Other nerve-related symptoms include loss of balance, clumsiness, difficulty picking up objects and buttoning clothing, walking problems, jaw pain, hearing loss, stomach pain, and constipation. In addition to affecting the nerves, certain anticancer drugs also can affect the muscles and make them weak, tired, or sore.

In some cases, nerve and muscle effects—though annoying—may not be serious. In other cases, nerve and muscle symptoms may indicate serious problems that need medical attention. Be sure to report any suspected nerve or muscle symptoms to your doctor.

Caution and common sense can help you deal with nerve and muscle problems. For example, if your fingers become numb, be very careful when grasping objects that are sharp, hot, or otherwise dangerous. If your sense of balance or muscle strength is affected, avoid falls by moving carefully, using handrails when going up or down stairs and using bathmats in the bathtub or shower. Do not wear slippery shoes.

Effects on Skin and Nails

You may have minor skin problems while you are having chemotherapy. Possible side effects include redness, itching, peeling, dryness, and acne. Your nails may become brittle, darkened, or cracked. They also may develop vertical lines or bands.

You will be able to take care of most of these problems yourself. If you develop acne, try to keep your face clean and dry and use over-the-counter medicated creams or soaps. For itching, apply cornstarch as you would a dusting powder. To help avoid dryness, take quick showers or sponge baths rather than long, hot baths. Apply cream and lotion while your skin is still moist and avoid perfume, cologne, or aftershave lotion that contains alcohol. You can strengthen your nails with the remedies sold for this purpose, but be alert to signs of a worsening problem because these products can be irritating to some people. Protect your nails by wearing gloves when washing dishes, gardening, or performing other work around the house. Get further advice from your doctor if these skin and nail problems don't respond to your efforts. Be sure to let your doctor know if you have redness, pain, or changes around the cuticles.

Certain anticancer drugs, when given intravenously, may produce a fairly dramatic darkening of the skin all along the vein. Some people use makeup to cover the area, but this can become difficult and time-consuming if several veins are affected, which sometimes happens. The darkened areas usually will fade on their own a few months after treatment ends.

Exposure to the sun may increase the effects some anticancer drugs have on your skin. Check with your doctor or nurse about using a sunscreen lotion with a skin protection factor of 15 to protect against the sun's effects. They may even suggest that you avoid being in direct sunlight or that you use a product, such as zinc oxide, that blocks the sun's rays completely. Long-sleeve cotton shirts, hats, and pants also will block the sun.

Some people who have had radiation therapy develop "radiation recall" during their chemotherapy. During or shortly after anticancer drugs are given, the skin over the area that was treated with radiation turns red—a shade anywhere from light to very bright—and may itch or burn. This reaction may last hours or even days. You can soothe the itching and burning by putting a cool, wet compress over the affected area. Radiation recall reactions should be reported to your doctor or nurse.

Most skin problems are not serious, but a few demand immediate attention. For example, certain drugs given intravenously can cause serious and permanent tissue damage if they leak out of the vein. Tell your doctor or nurse right away if you feel any burning or pain when you are getting IV drugs. These symptoms don't always mean there's a problem but they always must be checked out at once.

You also should let your doctor or nurse know right away if you develop sudden or severe itching, if your skin breaks out in a rash or hives, or if you have wheezing or any other trouble breathing. These symptoms may mean you are having an allergic reaction that may need to be treated at once.

Kidney and Bladder Effects

Some anticancer drugs can irritate the bladder or cause temporary or permanent damage to the kidneys. Be sure to ask your doctor if your anticancer drugs are among the ones that have this effect, and notify the doctor if you have any symptoms that might indicate a problem. Signs to watch for include

- Pain or burning when you urinate
- Frequent urination
- A feeling that you must urinate right away (urgency)
- Reddish or bloody urine
- Fever
- Chills

In general, it's a good idea to drink plenty of fluids to ensure good urine flow and help prevent problems; this is especially important if your drugs are among those that affect the kidney and bladder. Water, juice, coffee, tea, soup, soft drinks, broth, ice cream, soup, popsicles, and gelatin are all considered fluids. Your doctor will let you know if you must increase your fluid intake.

You also should be aware that some anticancer drugs cause the urine to change color (orange, red, or yellow) or to take on a strong or medicinelike odor. The color and odor of semen may be affected, as well. Check with your doctor to see if the drugs you are taking have this effect.

Flu-Like Syndrome

Some people report feeling as though they have the flu a few hours to a few days after chemotherapy. Flu-like symptoms—muscle aches, headache, tiredness, nausea, slight fever, chills, and poor appetite—may last from one to three days. These symptoms also can be caused by an infection or by the cancer itself, so it's important to check with your doctor if you have flulike symptoms.

Fluid Retention

Your body may retain fluid when you are having chemotherapy. This may be due to hormonal changes from your therapy, to the effects of the drugs themselves, or to your cancer. Check with your doctor or nurse if you notice swelling or puffiness in your face, hands, feet, or abdomen. You may need to avoid table salt and foods with a high sodium content. If the problem is severe, your doctor may prescribe diuretics, medicine to help your body get rid of excess fluids. However, don't take any over-the-counter diuretics without asking your doctor first.

Sexual Effects: Physical and Psychological

Chemotherapy may—but does not always—affect sexual organs and functioning in both men and women. The side effects that might occur depend on the drugs used and the person's age and general health.

Men

Chemotherapy drugs may lower the number of sperm cells, reduce their ability to move, or cause other abnormalities. These changes can result in infertility, which may be temporary or permanent. Infertility affects a man's ability to father a child but does not affect his ability to have sexual intercourse.

Because permanent sterility may occur, it's important to discuss this issue with your doctor before you begin chemotherapy. If you wish, you might consider sperm banking, a procedure that freezes sperm for future use.

Men undergoing chemotherapy should use an effective means of birth control with their partners during treatment because of the harmful effects of the drugs on chromosomes. Ask your doctor when you can stop using birth control for this purpose.

Women

Anticancer drugs can damage the ovaries and reduce the amount of hormones they produce. As a result, some women find that their menstrual periods become irregular or stop completely while they are having chemotherapy.

The hormonal effects of chemotherapy also may cause menopause-like symptoms such as hot flashes and itching, burning, or dryness of vaginal tissues. These tissue changes can make intercourse uncomfortable, but the symptoms often can be relieved by using a water-based vaginal lubricant. The tissue changes also can make a woman more likely to get vaginal infections. To help prevent infection, avoid oil-based lubricants such as petroleum jelly, wear cotton underwear and pantyhose with a ventilated cotton lining, and don't wear tight slacks or shorts. Your doctor also may prescribe a vaginal cream or suppository to reduce the chances of infection. If infection does occur, it should be treated right away.

Damage to the ovaries may result in infertility, the inability to become pregnant. In some cases, the infertility is a temporary condition; in other cases, it may be permanent. Whether infertility occurs, and how long it lasts, depends on many factors, including the type of drug, the dosage given, and the woman's age.

Although pregnancy may be possible during chemotherapy, it still is not advisable because some anticancer drugs may cause birth defects. Doctors advise women of childbearing age—from the teens through the end of menopause—to use birth control throughout their treatment.

If a woman is pregnant when her cancer is discovered, it may be possible to delay chemotherapy until after the baby is born. For a woman who needs treatment sooner, the doctor may suggest starting chemotherapy after the 12th week of pregnancy, when the fetus is beyond the stage of greatest risk. In some cases, termination of the pregnancy may be considered.

Sexuality

Sexual feelings and attitudes vary among people during chemotherapy. Some people find that they feel closer than ever to their partners and have an increased desire for sexual activity. Others experience little or no change in their sexual desire and energy level. Still others find that their sexual interest declines because of the physical and emotional stresses of having cancer and getting chemotherapy. These stresses may include worries about changes in appearance; anxiety about health, family, or finances; or side effects, including fatigue and hormonal changes.

A partner's concerns or fears can also affect the sexual relationship. Some may worry that physical intimacy will harm the person who has cancer; others may fear that they might "catch" the cancer or be affected by the drugs. Many of these issues can be cleared up by talking about misunderstandings. Both you and your partner should feel free to discuss sexual concerns with your doctor, nurse, or other counselor who can give you the information and the reassurance you need.

You and your partner also should try to share your feelings with one another. If it's difficult for you to talk to each other about sex, or cancer, or both, you may want to speak to a counselor who can help you communicate more openly. People who can help include psychiatrists, psychologists, social workers, marriage counselors, sex therapists, and members of the clergy.

If you were comfortable with and enjoyed sexual relations before starting therapy, chances are you will still find pleasure in physical intimacy during your treatment. You may discover, however, that intimacy takes on a new meaning and character. Hugging, touching, holding, and cuddling may become more important, while sexual intercourse may become less important. Remember that what was true before you started chemotherapy remains true now: There is no one right way to express your sexuality. It's up to you and your partner to determine together what is pleasurable and satisfying to you both.

The American Cancer Society has two free booklets on sexuality that may be helpful—one for women and one for men. Contact your local unit or the national office for copies.

Eating Well during Chemotherapy

It is very important to eat as well as you can while you are undergoing treatment. People who eat well can cope with side effects better and are able to fight infection more easily. In addition, their bodies can rebuild healthy tissues faster.

Eating well during chemotherapy means choosing a balanced diet that contains all the nutrients the body needs. A good way to do this is to eat foods from each of the following food groups: fruits and vegetables; poultry, fish, and meat; cereals and breads; and dairy products. Eating well also means having a diet high enough in calories to keep your weight up and, most important, high enough in protein to build and repair skin, hair, muscles, and organs.

You may also need to drink extra amounts of fluid to protect your bladder and kidneys during your treatment.

What if I don't feel like eating?

Even when you know it's important to eat well, there may be days when you feel you just can't. This may happen because side effects such as nausea or mouth and throat problems make it difficult or painful to eat. You also can lose your appetite if you feel depressed or tired. If this is the case, be sure to read the sections in this article on your particular discomforts. They will give you tips that can make it easier for you to eat.

When a poor appetite is the problem, try these hints:

- Eat small meals or snacks whenever you want. You don't have to eat three regular meals each day.
- Vary your diet and try new foods and recipes.
- When possible, take a walk before meals; this makes you feel hungrier.
- Try changing your mealtime routine. For example, eat by candlelight or in a different location.
- Eat with friends or family members. When eating alone, listen to the radio or watch TV.
- If you live alone, you might want to arrange for Meals on Wheels or a similar program to bring food to you. Ask your doctor, nurse, local American Cancer Society office, or the Cancer Information Service about these programs, which are provided in many communities.

The National Cancer Institute's booklet *Eating Hints* provides more tips about how to make eating easier and more enjoyable. It also gives many ideas about how to eat well and increase your protein and calorie intake during cancer treatment. For a free copy of *Eating Hints,* call the Cancer Information Service at 1-800-4-CANCER.

Can I drink alcoholic beverages?

Small amounts of alcohol can help you relax and increase your appetite. On the other hand, alcohol may interact with some drugs to reduce their effectiveness or worsen their side effects. For this reason, some people must drink less alcohol or avoid alcohol completely during chemotherapy. Be sure to ask your doctor if it's okay for you to drink beer, wine, or other alcoholic beverages.

Should I take vitamin or mineral supplements?

There is no single answer to this question, but one thing is clear: No diet or nutritional plan can cure cancer, and taking vitamin and mineral supplements should never be considered a substitute for medical care. You should not take any supplements without your doctor's knowledge and consent.

Talking with Your Doctor and Nurse

Some people with cancer want to know every detail about their condition and their treatment. Others prefer only general information. The choice of how much information to seek is yours, but there are questions that every person getting chemotherapy should ask. These include

- Why do I need chemotherapy?
- What are the benefits of chemotherapy?
- What are the risks of chemotherapy?
- What drug or drugs will I be taking?
- How will the drugs be given?
- Where will I get my treatments?
- How long will my treatment last?
- What are the possible side effects?
- Are there any side effects that I should report right away?
- Are there any other possible treatment methods for my type of cancer?

This list is just a start. You always should feel free to ask your doctor, nurse, and pharmacist as many questions as you want. If you don't understand their answers, keep asking until you do. Remember, when it comes to cancer and cancer treatment there is no such thing as a stupid question. To make sure you get all the answers you want, you may find it helpful to draw up a list of questions before your appointment. Some people even keep a running list and jot down each new question as it occurs to them.

To help remember your doctor's answers, you may want to take notes during your appointment. Don't feel shy about asking your doctor to slow down when you need more time to write. You may also ask if you can use a tape recorder during your visit. That way, you can review your conversation later as many times as you wish. Some doctors like this idea and others don't, so be sure to check before you try it. Another way to help you remember is to bring a friend or family member to sit with you while you talk to your doctor. This person can help you understand what your doctor says during your visit and help refresh your memory afterward.

Chemotherapy and Your Emotions

Chemotherapy can bring major changes to a person's life. It can affect overall health, threaten a sense of well-being, disrupt day-to-day schedules, and put a strain on personal relationships. No wonder, then, that many people feel fearful, anxious, angry, or depressed at some point during their chemotherapy.

These emotions are perfectly normal and understandable, but they also can be disturbing. Fortunately, there are ways to cope with these emotional "side effects," just as there are ways to cope with the physical side effects of chemotherapy.

How can I get the support I need?

There are many sources of support you can draw on. Here are some of the most important:

- Doctors and nurses. If you have questions or worries about your cancer treatment, talk with members of your health care team.
- Counseling professionals. There are many kinds of counselors who can help you express, understand, and cope with the emotions cancer treatment can cause. Depending on your preferences and needs, you might want to talk with a psychiatrist, psychologist, social worker, sex therapist, or member of the clergy.
- Friends and family members. Talking with friends or family members can help you feel a lot better. Often, they can comfort and reassure you in ways that no one else can. You may find, though, that you'll need to help them help you. At a time when you might expect that others will rush to your aid, you may have to make the first move.

    Many people do not understand cancer, and they may withdraw from you because they're afraid of your illness. Others may worry that they will upset you by saying the wrong thing.

    You can help relieve these fears by being open in talking with others about your illness, your treatment, your needs, and your feelings. By talking openly, you can correct mistaken ideas about cancer. You can also let people know that there's no single right thing to say, so long as their caring comes through loud and clear. Once people know they can talk with you honestly, they may be more willing and able to open up and lend their support.

    The National Cancer Institute's booklet *Taking Time* offers useful advice to help cancer patients and their families and friends communicate with one another.
- Support groups. Support groups are made up of people who are going through the same kinds of experiences as you. Many people with cancer find they can share thoughts and feelings with group members that they don't feel comfortable sharing with anyone else. Support groups also can serve as an important source of practical information about living with cancer.

Support can also be found in one-to-one programs that put you in touch with another person very similar to you in terms of age, sex, type of cancer, and so forth. In some programs, this person comes to visit you. In others, a hotline puts you in touch with someone you can talk with on the telephone.

Sources for information about support programs include your hospital's social work department, the local office of your American Cancer Society, and the National Cancer Institute's Cancer Information Service.

How can I make my daily life easier?

Here are some tips to help you while you are getting chemotherapy:

- Try to keep your treatment goals in mind. This will help you keep a positive attitude on days when the going gets rough.
- Remember that eating well is very important. Your body needs food to rebuild tissues and regain strength.
- Learn as much as you want to know about your disease and its treatment. This can lessen your fear of the unknown and increase your feeling of control.
- Keep a journal or diary while you're in treatment. A record of your activities and thoughts can help you understand the feelings you have as you go through treatment, and highlight questions you need to ask your doctor or nurse. You also can use your journal to record the steps you take to cope with side effects and how well those steps work. That way, you'll know which methods worked best for you in case you have the same side effects again.
- Set realistic goals and don't be too hard on yourself. You may not have as much energy as usual, so try to get as much rest as you can, let the small stuff slide, and only do the things that are most important to you.
- Try new hobbies and learn new skills. Exercise if you can. Using your body can make you feel better about yourself, help you get rid of tension or anger, and build your appetite. Ask your doctor or nurse about a safe and practical exercise program.

How can I relieve stress?

You can use a number of methods to cope with the stresses of cancer and its treatment. The techniques described here can help you relax. Try some of these methods to find the one (or ones) that work best for you. You may want to check with your doctor before using these techniques, especially if you have lung problems.

- Muscle tension and release. Lie down in a quiet room. Take a slow, deep breath. As you breathe in, tense a particular muscle or group of muscles. For example, you can squeeze your eyes shut, frown, clench your teeth, make a fist, or stiffen your arms or legs. Hold your breath and keep your muscles tense for a second or two. Then breathe out, release the tension, and let your body relax completely. Repeat the process with another muscle or muscle group.

    You also can try a variation of this method, called *progressive relaxation.* Start with the toes of one foot and, working upward, progressively tense and relax all the muscles of one leg. Next, do the same with the other leg. Then tense and relax the rest of the muscle groups in your body, including those in your scalp. Remember to hold your breath while tensing your muscles and to breathe out when releasing the tension.

- Rhythmic breathing. Get into a comfortable position and relax all your muscles. If you keep your eyes open, focus on a distant object. If you close your eyes, imagine a peaceful scene or simply clear your mind and focus on your breathing.

    Breathe in and out slowly and comfortably through your nose. If you like, you can keep the rhythm steady by saying to yourself, "In, one two; Out, one two." Feel yourself relax and go limp each time you breathe out.

    You can do this technique for just a few seconds or for up to 10 minutes. End your rhythmic breathing by counting slowly and silently to three.

- Biofeedback. With training in biofeedback, you can control body functions such as heart rate, blood pressure, and muscle tension. A machine will sense when your body shows signs of tension and will let you know in some way such as making a sound or flashing a light. The machine will also give you feedback when you relax your body. Eventually, you will be able to control your relaxation responses without having to depend on feedback from the machine. Your doctor or nurse can refer you to someone trained in teaching biofeedback.

- Imagery. Imagery is a way of daydreaming that uses all your senses. It is usually done with your eyes closed. To begin, breathe slowly and feel yourself relax. Imagine a ball of healing energy—perhaps a white light—forming somewhere in your body. When you can "see" the ball of energy, imagine that as you breathe in you can blow the ball to any part of the body where you feel pain, tension, or discomfort such as nausea. When you breathe out, picture the air moving the ball away from your body, taking with it any painful or uncomfortable feelings. (Be sure to breathe naturally; don't blow.) Continue to picture the ball moving toward you and away from you each time you breathe in and out. You may see the ball getting bigger and bigger as it takes away more and more tension and discomfort.

    To end the imagery, count slowly to three, breathe in deeply, open your eyes, and say to yourself, "I feel alert and relaxed." If you choose to use imagery as a relaxation technique, please be sure to read the caution in the following section.

- Visualization. Visualization is a method that is similar to imagery. With visualization, you create an inner picture that represents your fight against cancer. Some people getting chemotherapy use images of rockets blasting away their cancer cells or of knights in armor battling their cancer cells. Others create an image of their white blood cells or their drugs attacking the cancer cells.

    Visualization and imagery may help to relieve stress and to increase your sense of self-control. But it is very important to remember that they can never take the place of the medical care your doctor prescribes to treat your cancer.

- Hypnosis. Hypnosis puts you in a trance-like state that can reduce discomfort and anxiety. You can be hypnotized by a qualified person, or you can learn how to hypnotize yourself. If you are interested in learning more, ask your doctor or nurse to refer you to someone trained in the technique.

- Distraction. You use distraction any time an activity takes your mind off your worries or discomforts. Try watching TV, listening to the radio, reading, going to the movies, or working with your hands by doing needlework or puzzles, building models, or painting. You may be surprised how comfortably the time passes.

Paying for Chemotherapy

The cost of chemotherapy varies with the kinds and dose of drugs used, how long and how often they are given, and whether you get them at home, in a clinic or office, or in the hospital. Most health insurance policies (including Medicare Part B, which helps pay for doctors' bills and many other medical services) cover at least part of the cost of many kinds of chemotherapy.

Sometimes, however, an insurer may not pay for the use of certain drugs for certain kinds of cancers—at least not at first. If your insurer denies payment for your treatment, don't give up. Most people do get payment eventually.

Teamwork with your doctor and the office staff is important. Be sure to let them know if you have been denied payment. They can consult with your insurer and help answer any questions your insurer may have. They also can consult with the company that makes the drug or drugs you are taking. Often, these companies can provide information or other services that will help you get payment.

In some states, Medicaid (which makes health care services available for people with financial need) may help pay for certain treatments. Contact the office that handles social services in your city or county to find out whether you are eligible for Medicaid and whether your chemotherapy is a covered expense.

If you need help paying for treatments, contact your hospital's social service office, the Cancer Information Service, or the local office of the American Cancer Society. They may be able to direct you to other sources of help. Another possibility is the Leukemia Society of America; to find a chapter near you, check the white pages of your local telephone book.

A Final Word

The National Cancer Institute hopes *Chemotherapy and You* helps you and your family, whether you are waiting to begin chemotherapy or already have begun your treatment. Discuss the information in this booklet with your doctor and nurse, and take good care of yourself during your chemotherapy. By working together, you, your family, and your health care providers will make the strongest possible team in your fight against cancer.

Resources

Information about cancer is available from many sources, including the ones listed below. You may want to check for additional information at your local library or bookstore and from support groups in your community.

Cancer Information Service
1-800-4-CANCER

The Cancer Information Service, a program of the National Cancer Institute, is a nationwide telephone service for cancer patients and their families and friends, the public, and health care professionals. The staff can answer any questions in English or Spanish and can send free National Cancer Institute booklets about cancer. They also know about local resources and services. One toll-free number, 1-800-4-CANCER (1-800-422-6237), connects callers with the office that serves their area.

PDQ

People who have cancer, those who care about them, and doctors need up-to-date and accurate information about cancer treatment. To meet these needs, PDQ was developed by NCI. PDQ contains an up-to-date list of clinical trials all over the country. The Cancer Information Service, at 1-800-4-CANCER, can provide PDQ information to doctors, patients, and the public.

American Cancer Society
1599 Clifton Rd, NE
Atlanta, GA 30329
1-800-ACS-2345

The American Cancer Society is a voluntary organization with a national office (at the above address) and local units all over the country. To obtain further information about services and activities in local areas, call the Society's toll-free number, 1-800-ACS-2345 (1-800-227-2345), or the number listed under American Cancer Society in the white pages of the telephone book.

Other Booklets

National Cancer Institute printed materials, including the booklets listed below, are available from the Cancer Information Service free of charge by calling 1-800-4-CANCER.

- Advanced Cancer: Living Each Day
- Eating Hints: Recipes and Tips for Better Nutrition During Cancer Treatment
- Facing Forward: A Guide for Cancer Survivors
- Questions and Answers About Pain Control (also available from the American Cancer Society)
- Radiation Therapy and You: A Guide to Self-Help During Treatment
- Taking Time: Support for People with Cancer and the People Who Care About Them
- What Are Clinical Trials All About?
- What You Need to Know About Cancer. A series of booklets about different types of cancer.
- When Cancer Recurs: Meeting the Challenge Again

Glossary

This glossary reviews the meaning of some words used in *Chemotherapy and You*. It also explains some words related to chemotherapy that are not mentioned in this booklet but that you may hear from your doctor or nurse.

Adjuvant therapy: Anticancer drugs or hormones given after surgery and/or radiation to help prevent the cancer from coming back.

Alopecia: Hair loss.

Anemia: Having too few red blood cells. Symptoms of anemia include feeling tired, weak, and short of breath.

Anorexia: Poor appetite.

Antiemetic: A medicine that prevents or controls nausea and vomiting.

Benign: A term used to describe a tumor that is not cancerous.

Biological therapy: Treatment to stimulate or restore the ability of the immune system to fight infection and disease. Also called **immunotherapy.**

Blood count: The number of red blood cells, white blood cells, and platelets in a sample of blood. This is also called the complete blood count (CBC).

Bone marrow: The inner, spongy tissue of bones where red blood cells and white blood cells are formed.

Cancer: A general name for more than 100 diseases in which abnormal cells grow out of control; a malignant tumor.

Catheter: A thin flexible tube through which fluids can enter or leave the body.

Central venous catheter: A special thin, flexible tube placed in a large vein. It remains there for as long as it is needed to deliver and withdraw fluids.

Chemotherapy: The use of drugs to treat cancer.

Chromosomes: Threadlike bodies found in the nucleus, or center part, of a cell and that carry the information of heredity.

Clinical Trials: Medical research studies conducted with volunteers. Each study is designed to answer scientific questions and to find better ways to prevent or treat cancer.

Colony-stimulating factors: Substances that stimulate the production of blood cells. Treatment with colony-stimulating factors (CSF) can help the blood-forming tissue recover from the effects of chemotherapy and radiation therapy. These include granulocyte colony-stimulating factors (G-CSF) and granulocyte-macrophage colony-stimulating factors (GM-CSF).

Combination chemotherapy: The use of more than one drug to treat cancer.

Diuretics: Drugs that help the body get rid of excess water and salt.

Gastrointestinal: Having to do with the digestive tract, which includes the mouth, esophagus, stomach, and intestines.

Hormones: Natural substances released by an organ that can influence the function of other organs in the body.

Infusion: Slow and/or prolonged intravenous delivery of a drug or fluids.

Injection: Using a syringe and needle to push fluids or drugs into the body; often called a shot.

Intra-arterial (IA): Into an artery.

Intracavitary (IC): Into a cavity, or space, specifically the abdomen, pelvis, or the chest.

Intralesional (IL): Into the cancerous area in the skin.

Intramuscular (IM): Into a muscle.

Intrathecal (IT): Into the spinal fluid.

Intravenous (IV): Into a vein.

Malignant: Used to describe a cancerous tumor.

Metastasis: When cancer cells break away from their original site and spread to other parts of the body.

Palliative care: Treatment to relieve, rather than cure, symptoms caused by cancer. Palliative care can help people live more comfortably.

Peripheral neuropathy: A condition of the nervous system that usually begins in the hands and/or feet with symptoms of numbness, tingling, burning, and/or weakness. Can be caused by certain anticancer drugs.

Per os (PO): By mouth, orally.

Platelets: Special blood cells that help stop bleeding.

Port: A small plastic or metal container surgically placed under the skin and attached to a central venous catheter inside the body. Blood and fluids can enter or leave the body through the port using a special needle.

Radiation therapy: Cancer treatment with radiation (high-energy rays).

Red blood cells: Cells that supply oxygen to tissues throughout the body.

Remission: The disappearance of signs and symptoms of disease.

Stomatitis: Sores on the inside lining of the mouth.

Subcutaneous (SQ or SC): Under the skin.

Tumor: An abnormal growth of cells or tissues. Tumors may be benign (noncancerous) or malignant (cancerous).

White blood cells: The blood cells that fight infection.

The NCI is the U.S. Government's main agency for cancer research and information about cancer. The NCI's publications are free. They may be copied or reproduced without written permission.

■ Document Source:
**U.S. Department of Health and Human Services, Public Health Service
National Institutes of Health
National Cancer Institute
Bethesda, Maryland 20892
NIH Publication No. 94-1136
June 16, 1994**

Information from PDQ for Patients

THYROID CANCER

Description

What is cancer of the thyroid?

Cancer of the thyroid is a disease in which cancer (malignant) cells are found in the tissues of the thyroid gland. Your thyroid gland is at the base of your throat. It has two lobes, one on the right side and one on the left. Your thyroid gland makes important hormones that help your body to function normally.

Cancer of the thyroid is more common in women than in men. Most patients are between 25 and 65 years old. People who have been exposed to large amounts of radiation, or who have had radiation treatment for medical problems in the head and neck, have a higher chance of getting thyroid cancer. The cancer may not occur until 20 years or longer after radiation treatment.

Like most cancers, cancer of the thyroid is best treated when it is found (diagnosed) early. You should see your doctor if you have a lump or swelling in the front of your neck or in other parts of your neck.

If you have symptoms, your doctor will feel your thyroid and check for lumps in your neck. Your doctor may order blood tests and special scans to see whether a lump in your thyroid is making too many hormones. Your doctor may want to take a small amount of tissue from your thyroid. This is called a biopsy. To do this, a small needle is inserted into your thyroid at the base of your throat, and some tissue is drawn out. The tissue is then looked at under a microscope to see whether it contains cancer.

There are four main types of cancer of the thyroid (based on how the cancer cells look under a microscope): papillary, follicular, medullary, and anaplastic. Your chance of recovery (prognosis) depends on the type of thyroid cancer you have, whether it is just in the thyroid or has spread to other parts of the body (stage), your age, and your overall health. Some types of thyroid cancer grow much faster than others.

The genes in our cells carry the hereditary information from our parents. An abnormal gene has been found in patients with some forms of thyroid cancer. If you have medullary thyroid cancer, you may have been born with a certain abnormal gene which may have led to your cancer. Some of your family members may have also inherited this abnormal gene. Tests have been developed to determine who has the genetic defect long before any cancer appears. It is important that you and your family members (children, grandchildren, parents, brothers, sisters, nieces, and nephews) see a doctor about tests that will show if you or they have this abnormal gene. These tests are confidential and can help your doctor to help you and your family. Family members, including young children, who don't have cancer, but do have this abnormal gene, may reduce the chance of developing medullary thyroid cancer by having surgery to safely remove their thyroids (thyroidectomy).

Stage Explanation

Stages of Cancer of the Thyroid

Once cancer of the thyroid is found (diagnosed), more tests will be done to find out if cancer cells have spread to other parts of the body. This is called staging. Your doctor needs to know the stage of your disease to plan treatment.

The following stages are used for papillary cancers of the thyroid:

Stage I Papillary

Cancer is only in the thyroid and may be found in one or both lobes.

Stage II Papillary

In patients younger than 45 years of age:
    Cancer has spread beyond the thyroid.
In patients older than 45 years of age:
    Cancer is only in the thyroid and larger than one centimeter (about 1/2 inch).

Stage III Papillary

Cancer is found in patients older than 45 years of age and has spread outside the thyroid (but not outside of the neck) or has spread to the lymph nodes.

Stage IV Papillary

Cancer is found in patients older than 45 years of age and has spread to other parts of the body, such as the lungs and bones.

The following stages are used for follicular cancers of the thyroid:

Stage I Follicular

Cancer is only in the thyroid and may be found in one or both lobes.

Stage II Follicular

In patients younger than 45 years of age:
    Cancer has spread beyond the thyroid.
In patients older than 45 years of age:
    Cancer is only in the thyroid and larger than one centimeter (about 1/2 inch).

Stage III Follicular

Cancer is found in patients older than 45 years of age and has spread outside the thyroid (but not outside of the neck) or to the lymph nodes.

Stage IV Follicular

Cancer is found in patients older than 45 years of age and has spread to other parts of the body, such as the lungs and bones.

Other types or stages of thyroid cancer include the following:

Stage I Medullary

Cancer is less than one centimeter (about 1/2 inch) in size.

Stage II Medullary

Cancer is between one and four centimeters (about 1/2 to one 1/2 inches) in size.

Stage III Medullary

Cancer has spread to the lymph nodes.

Stage IV Medullary

Cancer has spread to other parts of the body.

Anaplastic

There is no staging system for anaplastic cancer of the thyroid. This type of cancer of the thyroid grows faster than the other types.

Recurrent

Recurrent disease means that the cancer has come back (recurred) after it has been treated. It may come back in the thyroid or in another part of the body.

Treatment Option Overview

How Cancer of the Thyroid Is Treated

There are treatments for all patients with cancer of the thyroid. Four types of treatment are used:

- surgery (taking out the cancer)
- radiation therapy (using high-dose x-rays or other high-energy rays to kill cancer cells)
- hormone therapy (using hormones to stop cancer cells from growing)
- chemotherapy (using drugs to kill cancer cells)

Surgery is the most common treatment for cancer of the thyroid. Your doctor may remove the cancer using one of the following operations:

- Lobectomy removes only the side of the thyroid where the cancer is found. Lymph nodes in the area may be taken out (biopsied) to see if they contain cancer.
- Near-total thyroidectomy removes all of the thyroid except for a small part.
- Total thyroidectomy removes the entire thyroid.
- Lymph node dissection removes lymph nodes in the neck that contain cancer.

Radiation therapy uses high-energy x-rays to kill cancer cells and shrink tumors. Radiation for cancer of the thyroid may come from a machine outside the body (external radiation therapy) or from drinking a liquid that contains radioactive iodine. Because the thyroid takes up iodine, the radioactive iodine collects in any thyroid tissue remaining in the body and kills the cancer cells.

Hormone therapy uses hormones to stop cancer cells from growing. In treating cancer of the thyroid, hormones can be used to stop the body from making other hormones that might make cancer cells grow. Hormones are usually given as pills.

Chemotherapy uses drugs to kill cancer cells. Chemotherapy may be taken by pill, or it may be put into the body by a needle in the vein or muscle. Chemotherapy is called a systemic treatment because the drug enters the bloodstream, travels through the body, and can kill cancer cells outside the thyroid.

Treatment by Stage

Treatment for cancer of the thyroid depends on the type and stage of your disease, your age, and your overall health.

You may receive treatment that is considered standard based on its effectiveness in a number of patients in past studies, or you may choose to go into a clinical trial. Not all patients are cured with standard therapy and some standard treatments may have more side effects than are desired. For these reasons, clinical trials are designed to find better ways to treat cancer patients and are based on the most up-to-date information. Clinical trials are going on in many parts of the country for some patients with cancer of the thyroid. If you want more information, call the Cancer Information Service at 1-800-4-CANCER (1-800-422-6237).

Stage I Papillary Thyroid Cancer

Your treatment may be one of the following:

1. Surgery to remove one lobe of the thyroid (lobectomy), followed by hormone therapy. Radioactive iodine also may be given following surgery.
2. Surgery to remove the thyroid (total thyroidectomy).

Stage I Follicular Thyroid Cancer

Your treatment may be one of the following:

1. Surgery to remove the thyroid (total thyroidectomy).
2. Surgery to remove one lobe of the thyroid (lobectomy), followed by hormone therapy. Radioactive iodine also may be given following surgery.

Stage II Papillary Thyroid Cancer

Your treatment may be one of the following:

1. Surgery to remove one lobe of the thyroid (lobectomy) and lymph nodes that contain cancer, followed by hormone therapy. Radioactive iodine also may be given following surgery.
2. Surgery to remove the thyroid (total thyroidectomy).

Stage II Follicular Thyroid Cancer

Your treatment may be one of the following:

1. Surgery to remove the thyroid (total thyroidectomy).
2. Surgery to remove one lobe of the thyroid (lobectomy) and lymph nodes that contain cancer, followed by hormone therapy. Radioactive iodine also may be given following surgery.

Stage III Papillary Thyroid Cancer

Your treatment may be one of the following:

1. Surgery to remove the entire thyroid (total thyroidectomy) and lymph nodes where cancer has spread.
2. Total thyroidectomy followed by radiation therapy with radioactive iodine or external beam radiation therapy.

Stage III Follicular Thyroid Cancer

Your treatment may be one of the following:

1. Surgery to remove the entire thyroid (total thyroidectomy) and lymph nodes or other tissues around the thyroid where the cancer has spread.
2. Total thyroidectomy followed by radioactive iodine or external beam radiation therapy.

Stage IV Papillary Thyroid Cancer

Your treatment may be one of the following:

1. Radioactive iodine.
2. External beam radiation therapy.
3. Hormone therapy.
4. A clinical trial of chemotherapy.

Stage IV Follicular Thyroid Cancer

Your treatment may be one of the following:

1. Radioactive iodine.
2. External beam radiation therapy.
3. Hormone therapy.
4. A clinical trial of chemotherapy.

Medullary Thyroid Cancer

Your treatment will probably be surgery to remove the entire thyroid (total thyroidectomy) unless the cancer has spread to other parts of the body. If lymph nodes in the neck contain cancer, the lymph nodes in the neck will be removed (lymph node dissection). If the cancer has spread to other parts of the body, chemotherapy may be given.

Anaplastic Thyroid Cancer

Your treatment may be one of the following:

1. Surgery to remove the thyroid and the tissues around it. Because this cancer often spreads very quickly to other tissues, your doctor may have to take out part of the tube through which you breath. Your doctor will then make an airway in the throat so you can breath. This is called a tracheotomy.
2. Total thyroidectomy to reduce symptoms if the disease remains in the area of the thyroid.
3. External beam radiation therapy.
4. Chemotherapy.
5. Clinical trials studying new methods of treatment for thyroid cancer.

Recurrent Thyroid Cancer

Your choice of treatment depends on the type of thyroid cancer you have, the kind of treatment you had before, and where the cancer comes back. Your treatment may be one of the following:

1. Surgery with or without radioactive iodine.
2. External beam radiation therapy to relieve symptoms caused by the cancer.
3. Chemotherapy.
4. Radioactive iodine.
5. Radiation therapy given during surgery.
6. Clinical trials.

To Learn More

To learn more about cancer of the thyroid, call the National Cancer Institute's Cancer Information Service at 1-800-4-CANCER (1-800-422-6237). By dialing this toll-free number, you can speak with someone who can answer your questions.

The Cancer Information Service can also send you free booklets. The following booklet about thyroid cancer may be helpful to you:

- In Answer to Your Questions About Thyroid Cancer

The following general booklets on questions related to cancer may be helpful:

- What You Need To Know About Cancer
- Taking Time: Support for People with Cancer and the People Who Care About Them
- What Are Clinical Trials All About?
- Chemotherapy and You: A Guide to Self-Help During Treatment
- Radiation Therapy and You: A Guide to Self-Help During Treatment
- Eating Hints for Cancer Patients
- Advanced Cancer: Living Each Day
- When Cancer Recurs: Meeting the Challenge Again

There are other places where you can get material about cancer treatment and information about services to help you. You can check the social service office at your hospital for local and national agencies that help with your finances, getting to and from treatment, care at home, and dealing with your problems. The American Cancer Society, for example, has many free services. Their local offices are listed in the white pages of the telephone book.

You can also write to the National Cancer Institute at this address:

National Cancer Institute
Office of Cancer Communications
31 Center Drive, MSC 2580
Bethesda, MD 20892-2580

■ **Document Source:**
U.S. Department of Health and Human Services, Public Health Service
National Institutes of Health
National Cancer Institute

WHAT YOU NEED TO KNOW ABOUT CANCERS OF THE BONE

Each year, more than 2,000 people in the United States learn that they have bone cancer. This National Cancer Institute (NCI) booklet will help you learn about this disease. It describes the symptoms, diagnosis, and treatment of bone cancer. It also has information about rehabilitation and about living with this disease.

Other NCI booklets are listed at the end of the article. We know that booklets like these cannot answer every question you may have about bone cancer. They cannot take the place of talks with doctors, nurses, and other members of the health care team. We hope our booklets will help with those talks.

Throughout this booklet, words that may be new to readers are printed in *italics*. Definitions of these and other terms related to bone cancer are listed at the end of the article. For some words, a "sounds-like" spelling is also given.

Our knowledge about bone cancer keeps increasing. For up-to-date information, call the NCI-supported Cancer Information Service (CIS) toll free at 1-800-4-CANCER (1-800-422-6237).

Bones

The 206 bones in the body serve several purposes. They support and protect internal organs (for example, the skull protects the brain and the ribs protect the lungs). Muscles pull against bones to make the body move. *Bone marrow,* the soft, spongy tissue in the center of many bones, makes and stores blood cells.

What is cancer?

Cancer is a group of diseases. More than 100 different types of cancer are known. They all have one thing in common: cells become abnormal. These abnormal cells grow and destroy body tissue and can spread to other parts of the body.

Healthy cells that make up the body's tissues grow, divide, and replace themselves in an orderly way. This process keeps the body in good repair. If cells lose the ability to control their growth, they grow too rapidly and without any order. They form too much tissue. The mass of extra tissue is called a *tumor.* Tumors can be *benign* or *malignant.*

- Benign tumors are not cancer. They do not spread to other parts of the body and are seldom a threat to life. Benign tumors can usually be removed. Although benign bone tumors sometimes return, they usually can be removed with additional surgery.
- Malignant tumors are cancer. They can invade and destroy nearby healthy tissues and organs. Cancer cells also can break away from the tumor and enter the bloodstream. That is how bone cancer can spread to other parts of the body. This spread is called *metastasis.*

Cancer that begins in the bone is called primary bone cancer. It is found most often in the arms and legs, but it can occur in any bone in the body. Children and young people are more likely than adults to have bone cancers.

Primary bone cancers are called *sarcomas.* There are several types of sarcoma. Each type begins in a different kind of bone tissue. The most common are *osteosarcoma, Ewing's sarcoma,* and *chondrosarcoma.*

- Osteosarcoma is the most common type of bone cancer in young people. It usually occurs between ages 10 and 25. Males are affected more often than females. Osteosarcoma often starts in the ends of bones, where new bone tissue forms as a young person grows. It usually affects the long bones of the arms or legs.
- Ewing's sarcoma usually is found in people between 10 and 25 years old; teenagers are most often affected. This cancer forms in the middle part (shaft) of large bones. It most often affects the hipbones and the long bones in the thigh and upper arm. It also occurs in the ribs.
- Chondrosarcoma is found mainly in adults. This type of tumor forms in cartilage, the rubbery tissue around joints.

Other types of bone cancer include *fibrosarcoma, malignant giant cell tumor,* and *chordoma.* These rare cancers most often affect people over 30.

Cancers that begin in the bone are quite rare. On the other hand, it is not unusual for cancer to spread to the bones from other parts of the body. When this happens, the disease is not called bone cancer. Each type of cancer is named for the organ or the tissue in which it begins. Cancer that spreads is the same disease and has the same name as the original, or primary, cancer. Treatment for cancer that has spread to the bones depends on where the cancer started and the extent of the spread.

Cancers that begin in muscles, fat, nerves, blood vessels, and other types of connective or supporting tissues in the body are called *soft tissue sarcomas.* They can affect both children and adults. They are not discussed in this booklet.

Leukemia, multiple myeloma, and lymphoma are cancers that arise in cells produced in the bone marrow. These are different diseases, not types of bone cancer. The *What You Need to Know* series includes booklets on each of these types of cancer.

Symptoms

Symptoms of bone cancer tend to develop slowly. They depend on the type, location, and size of the tumor.

Pain is the most frequent symptom of bone cancer. Sometimes a firm, slightly tender lump on the bone can be felt through the skin. In some cases, bone cancer interferes with normal movements. Bone cancer can also cause bones to break.

These symptoms are not sure signs of cancer. They may also be caused by other, less serious problems. Only a doctor can tell for sure.

Diagnosis

To diagnose bone cancer, the doctor asks about the patient's personal and family medical history and does a complete physical exam. In addition to checking the general signs of health, the doctor usually orders blood tests and *x-rays.* X-rays can show the location, size, and shape of a bone tumor. On x-rays, benign tumors usually look round and smooth, with distinct edges. Bone cancers generally have odd shapes and irregular edges.

If x-rays show that the tumor is possible cancer, some of the following special tests may be done. These tests also may show whether the cancer has begun to spread.

- *Bone scans* outline the size, shape, and location of abnormal areas in the bone. A small amount of radioactive material is injected into the bloodstream. This material collects in the bones and is detected by a special instrument called a scanner.
- *CT* or *CAT scan* is an x-ray procedure that gives detailed pictures of cross sections of the body. The pictures are created by a computer.
- *MRI (magnetic resonance imaging)* also creates detailed pictures of cross sections of the body. MRI uses a very strong magnet linked to a computer.
- *Angiograms* are special x-rays of blood vessels. A dye that shows up on x-rays is injected into the bloodstream

so that the vessels can be seen in detail. This test is also done to help plan surgery.

A *biopsy* is the only sure way to tell whether cancer is present. Biopsies are best done at a hospital where doctors are experienced in the diagnosis of bone cancers. The doctor removes a sample of tissue from the bone tumor. A *pathologist* looks at the tissue under a microscope. If cancer is found, the pathologist can tell the type of sarcoma and whether it is likely to grow slowly or quickly.

If a diagnosis of bone cancer is made, it is important for the doctor to know exactly where the cancer is located and whether it has spread from its original location. This information is very important for planning treatment. The results of exams, tests, x-rays, scans, and the biopsy are all used in *staging* the cancer. The stage indicates whether the disease has spread and how much tissue is affected.

Treatment

Doctors consider a number of factors to decide on the best treatment for bone cancer. Among these are the type, location, size, and extent of the tumor as well as the patient's age and general health. The doctor will develop a treatment plan to fit each patient's needs.

Planning Treatment

Before starting treatment, the patient might want a second doctor to review the diagnosis and treatment plan. A second opinion may take one or two weeks. This short delay will not reduce the chance that treatment will be successful. There are a number of ways to get a second opinion:

- The patient's doctor may suggest a specialist who treats bone cancer or one who treats children with cancer.
- The Cancer Information Service, at 1-800-4-CANCER, can tell callers about cancer centers and other NCI-supported programs in their area.
- Patients can get the names of doctors from their local medical society, a nearby hospital, or a medical school.

Treatment Methods

Bone cancer is treated with *surgery, radiation therapy,* and/or *chemotherapy.* The doctor often uses a combination of treatment methods, depending on the patient's needs. Patients may be referred to doctors who specialize in different kinds of cancer treatment. Often, the specialists work together as a team. The team may include a surgeon, a pediatric oncologist, and a radiation oncologist.

Surgery is part of the treatment for most bone cancers. Because the disease may recur near the original site, the surgeon removes the tumor and some healthy bone and other tissue around the tumor.

When bone cancer occurs in an arm or leg, the surgeon tries, whenever possible, to remove just the tumor and an area of healthy tissue around it. Sometimes, the surgeon can use a metal device to replace bone that is removed. In some children, the surgeon may replace the bone with a metal device that can be lengthened as the child grows. This limb-sparing

procedure will require additional operations to keep expanding the artificial bone.

Sometimes, however, when the tumor is large, *amputation* may be necessary. If the limb is removed, a *prosthesis* (artificial part) can be made. The artificial part takes the place of a leg, arm, hand, or foot.

Chemotherapy uses drugs to kill cancer cells. Often the doctor uses a combination of three or more drugs. Chemotherapy may be given by mouth or by injection into a muscle or blood vessel. The drugs travel through the body in the bloodstream. Chemotherapy is given in cycles: a treatment period followed by a recovery period, then another treatment and recovery period, and so on.

Some patients have chemotherapy as an outpatient at the hospital, clinic, or doctor's office or at home. Depending on which drugs are given, however, the patient may need to stay in the hospital for a short while.

Chemotherapy is almost always used in combination with surgery for cancers of the bone. Sometimes chemotherapy is used to shrink a tumor before surgery. It is also used as an *adjuvant therapy* after surgery to kill cancer cells that may remain in the body and to prevent the disease from recurring. In some cases, a patient may have chemotherapy both before and after surgery. For some bone cancers, chemotherapy is combined with radiation therapy. Chemotherapy also may be used to control bone cancer that has spread.

Radiation therapy (also called radiotherapy) uses high-energy rays to damage cancer cells and stop them from growing. In some cases, radiation therapy is used instead of surgery to destroy the tumor. This form of treatment can also be used to destroy cancer cells that remain in the area after surgery.

The patient goes to the hospital or clinic each day for radiation treatments. Usually, treatments are given five days a week for five to eight weeks.

Side Effects of Treatment

The methods used to treat bone cancer are very powerful. It is hard to limit the effects of treatment so that only cancer cells are destroyed; healthy tissue may also be damaged. That's why treatment often causes side effects. Side effects depend on the type of treatment and on the part of the body being treated.

Surgery for cancer of the bone is a major operation. The area must be carefully watched for infection. Rehabilitation is an important part of post-surgery treatment.

The side effects of chemotherapy depend on the drugs that are given. In addition, each person reacts differently. Chemotherapy affects rapidly growing cells, such as blood-forming cells and those that line the digestive tract. As a result, patients may have side effects such as lower resistance to infection, loss of appetite, nausea, vomiting, or mouth sores. They may also have less energy and may lose their hair. These are short-term side effects; they usually end after treatment stops.

During radiation therapy, patients may become very tired as treatment continues. Resting as much as possible is important. Skin reactions such as redness or dryness in the area being treated are common, and the skin should be protected from the sun. Good skin care is important at this time, but the patient should not use any lotion or cream on the skin without the doctor's advice.

For some patients, it may be important to have a complete dental exam before treatment begins. Because cancer treatment may make the mouth sensitive and easily infected, doctors often advise patients to see a dentist so that their mouths are as healthy as possible.

Loss of appetite can be a problem for patients during their treatment for cancer. Patients who eat well may be better able to withstand the side effects of their treatment, so good nutrition is important. Eating well means getting enough calories to prevent weight loss and having enough protein to regain strength and rebuild normal tissues. Many patients find that eating several small meals and snacks during the day works better than trying to have three large meals.

The side effects that patients have during cancer treatment vary for each person. They may even be different from one treatment to the next. Doctors try to plan treatment to keep problems to a minimum. Fortunately, most side effects are temporary. Doctors, nurses, and dietitians can explain the side effects of cancer treatment and can suggest ways to deal with them. Helpful information about cancer treatment and coping with side effects is given in the NCI publications *Chemotherapy and You, Radiation Therapy and You,* and *Eating Hints.*

Researchers are concerned about the possibility of long-term effects in young people who are treated with chemotherapy and radiation therapy. These depend on the location of the tumor and the way it was treated. Some types of chemotherapy may affect a patient's *fertility.* When this side effect is permanent, it is not possible for the person to have children. This may be true for both men and women. Radiation therapy may increase the possibility that a second tumor will later develop in the area that was treated. The doctor can tell patients and their families more about these possible effects.

Follow-up Care

Regular followup is very important after treatment for bone cancer. The doctor will continue to check the patient closely for several years. It is important to be sure that cancer has not come back or to find and treat it promptly if it does. Checkups may include a physical exam, x-rays, scans, blood tests, and other laboratory tests.

Cancer treatment may cause side effects many years later. For this reason, patients should continue to have checkups and should report any problem as soon as it appears.

Patients who have had part or all of a limb removed will need physical therapy. Physical therapists and doctors who specialize in rehabilitation help patients learn to do their regular activities in new ways. Physical therapists also help patients learn to use their prostheses.

Living with Cancer

The diagnosis of cancer can change the lives of patients and the people close to them. These changes can be difficult to handle. It's natural for patients and their families and friends to have many different and sometimes confusing emotions.

At times, patients and their loved ones may feel frightened, angry, or depressed. These are normal reactions when people face a serious health problem. Patients, including children and teenagers, usually are better able to cope with their emotions if they can talk openly about their illness and their feelings with family members and friends.

Sharing feelings with others can help everyone feel more at ease, opening the way for others to show their concern and offer their support. *Young People with Cancer* may help parents understand and respond to their children's questions and concerns. Cancer patients and their families can also find helpful information in *Taking Time: Support for People with Cancer and the People Who Care About Them.*

Concerns about what the future holds—as well as worries about tests, treatments, hospital stays, and medical bills—are common. Talking with doctors, nurses, or other members of the health care team may help to calm fears and ease confusion. Patients can take an active part in decisions about their medical care by asking questions about bone cancer and their treatment choices. Patients, family, or friends often find it helpful to write down questions to ask the doctor as they think of them. Taking notes during visits to the doctor can help them remember what was said. Patients should ask the doctor to explain anything that is not clear.

Patients and families have many important questions, and the doctor is the best person to answer them. Most people ask about the extent of their cancer, how it can be treated, and how successful the treatment is likely to be.

These are other important questions to ask the doctor:

- What are my treatment choices?
- What are the benefits of treatment?
- What are the risks and side effects of treatment?
- If I have pain, how will you help me?
- Will I need to change my normal activities? For how long?
- How often will I need to have checkups?

Sometimes patients use statistics to try to figure out their chance of being cured. It is important to remember, however, that statistics are averages. They are based on the experience of large numbers of people, and no two cancer patients are alike. Only the doctor who takes care of a patient knows enough about his or her case to discuss the chance of recovery *(prognosis).* Doctors often talk about "surviving" bone cancer, or they may use the term "remission" rather than "cure." Even though many bone cancer patients recover completely, doctors use these terms because the disease can recur.

People who have had bone cancer may worry that removal of a limb or other surgery will affect not only how they look but how other people feel about them. Parents may worry about whether their children will be able to take part in normal school and social activities. Adults who have had extensive surgery may be concerned about working, taking part in social activities, caring for their families, or starting new relationships.

The doctor can give advice about treatment, working, going to school, or other activities. Patients may also want to discuss concerns about the future, family relationships, and finances. If it is hard to talk with the doctor about feelings or other personal matters, it may be helpful to speak with a nurse, social worker, counselor, or member of the clergy.

A physical or vocational therapist can help patients get used to new ways of doing things. This is especially important for those who have lost all or part of a limb and are learning to use a prosthesis. Therapists also understand and can help patients deal with the feelings that come with these changes.

Learning to live with the changes that are brought about by bone cancer is easier for patients and those who care about them when they have helpful information and support services. Many patients feel that it helps to talk with others who are facing problems like theirs. They can meet other cancer patients through self-help and support groups. Some hospitals have special support groups for youngsters with cancer and their families. Often, a social worker at the hospital or clinic can suggest local and national groups that will help with rehabilitation, emotional support, financial aid, transportation, or home care.

The American Cancer Society (ACS), for example, is a nonprofit organization that has many services for patients and their families. Local ACS offices are listed in the telephone book. The address and telephone number of the national ACS office are at the end of this article.

Information about other programs and services is available through the Cancer Information Service. The toll-free number is 1-800-4-CANCER.

Living with any serious illness can be difficult and challenging. The public library is a good source of books and articles on living with cancer. Cancer patients and their families can also find helpful suggestions in the NCI booklets listed at the end of this article.

The Promise of Cancer Research

At this time, little is known about the causes of bone cancer. Doctors can seldom explain why one person gets this rare type of cancer and another doesn't. We do know, however, that bone cancer is not contagious; no one can "catch" cancer from another person.

Scientists at hospitals and medical centers all across the country are studying bone cancer. They are trying to learn what causes this disease and how to prevent it. They are also looking for better ways to diagnose and treat it.

The NCI is supporting many studies of new treatments for bone cancer. When laboratory research shows that a new treatment method has promise, it is used to treat cancer patients in clinical trials. These trials are designed to answer scientific questions and to find out whether a new treatment is safe and effective. Patients who take part in clinical trials make an important contribution to medical science and may have the first chance to benefit from improved treatment methods. Researchers are exploring new drugs and drug combinations and new ways of giving radiation therapy and chemotherapy. They are also looking for ways to use surgery more effectively in combination with other forms of treatment.

Cancer patients and their family members may want to read an NCI booklet called *What Are Clinical Trials All About?*, which explains some of the possible benefits and risks of treatment studies. Those who are interested in taking part in a trial should discuss this option with their doctor.

One way to learn about clinical trials is through PDQ, a computerized resource of cancer treatment information. Developed by NCI, PDQ contains an up-to-date list of trials all over the country. The Cancer Information Service, at 1-800-4-CANCER, can provide PDQ information to doctors, patients, and the public.

Medical Terms

Adjuvant therapy (AD-ju-vant THER-a-pee): Treatment given in addition to the primary treatment.

Amputation (am-pyoo-TAY-shun): Surgery to remove all or part of an arm or leg.

Angiogram (AN-jee-o-gram): An x-ray of blood vessels. The vessels can be seen following the injection of a dye that shows up in the x-ray pictures.

Benign (bee-NINE): Not cancer; does not spread to other parts of the body.

Biopsy (BY-op-see): Removal of a sample of tissue for examination under a microscope. This tells the doctor whether cancer cells are present.

Bone marrow: The soft, spongy tissue in the center of many bones; it produces blood cells (white blood cells, red blood cells, and platelets).

Bone scan: A technique to create images of bones on a computer screen or on film. A small amount of radioactive material is injected and travels through the bloodstream. It collects in the bones, especially in abnormal areas of the bones, and is detected by a scanner.

Cancer: A term for more than 100 diseases that have uncontrolled growth of abnormal cells. Cancer cells can spread through the bloodstream and lymphatic system to other parts of the body.

Cartilage (CAR-ti-lij): Firm, rubbery tissue that cushions bones at joints.

Chemotherapy (kee-mo-THER-a-pee): Treatment with anti-cancer drugs.

Chondrosarcoma (KON-dro-sar-KO-ma): A cancer that forms in cartilage.

Chordoma (kor-DO-ma): A form of bone cancer that usually starts in the lower spinal column.

Clinical trials: Studies of new cancer treatments. Each study is designed to answer scientific questions and to find better ways to treat patients.

CT or CAT scan: An x-ray procedure that uses a computer to produce detailed pictures of cross sections of the body.

Ewing's sarcoma (YOO-ingz sar-KO-ma): A bone cancer that forms in the middle (shaft) of large bones. It most often affects the hipbones and the bones of the upper arm and thigh.

Fertility: The ability to produce children.

Fibrosarcoma (FY-bro-sar-KO-ma): A form of bone cancer that occurs mainly in middle-aged and elderly people. It usually starts in the pelvis.

Graft: Healthy skin, bone, or other tissue taken from one part of the body to replace diseased or injured tissue removed from another part of the body.

Malignant (ma-LIG-nant): Cancerous; can spread to other parts of the body.

Malignant giant cell tumor: A type of bone tumor.

Metastasis (me-TAS-ta-sis): The spread of cancer from one part of the body to another. Cells in the metastatic (second) tumor are like those in the original (primary) cancer.

MRI (magnetic resonance imaging) (mag-NET-ik REZ-o-nans IM-a-jing): A diagnostic technique that uses a huge magnet linked to a computer to create pictures of cross sections of the body.

Oncologist (on-KOL-o-jist): A doctor who specializes in treating cancer. A pediatric oncologist specializes in treating children with cancer.

Osteosarcoma (OSS-tee-o-sar-KO-ma): A cancer of the bone that is most common in children. Also called osteogenic sarcoma.

Pathologist (path-OL-o-jist): A doctor who identifies disease by studying cells and tissues under a microscope.

Prognosis (prog-NO-sis): The probable outcome of a disease; the prospect of recovery.

Prosthesis (pros-THEE-sis): An artificial replacement for a missing body part.

Radiation therapy (ray-dee-AY-shun THER-a-pee): Treatment with high-energy rays from x-rays or other sources to kill cancer cells.

Sarcoma (sar-KO-ma): A type of cancer that starts in bone or connective tissue.

Soft tissue sarcoma: A sarcoma that begins in the muscle, fat, fibrous tissue, blood vessels, or other supporting tissue of the body. Not a type of bone cancer.

Staging: The process of learning the extent of a tumor and whether the disease has spread from its original site to other parts of the body.

Surgery: An operation.

Tumor (TOO-mer): An abnormal mass of tissue.

X-ray: High-energy radiation. It is used in low doses to diagnose diseases and in high doses to treat cancer.

Resources

Information about cancer is available from several sources, including the ones listed below. You may wish to check for additional information at your local library or bookstore or from support groups in your community.

Cancer Information Service (CIS) 1-800-4-CANCER

The Cancer Information Service, a program of the National Cancer Institute, provides a nationwide telephone service for cancer patients and their families and friends, the public, and health professionals. The staff can answer questions and can send booklets about cancer. They also know about local resources and services. One toll-free number, 1-800-4-CANCER (1-800-422-6237), connects callers all over the country to the office that serves their area. Spanish-speaking staff members are available.

American Cancer Society (ACS)
1599 Clifton Road, NE
Atlanta, GA 30329
1-800-ACS-2345

The American Cancer Society is a voluntary organization with a national office (at the above address) and local units all over the country. It supports research, conducts educational programs, provides free booklets, and offers many services to patients and their families. To obtain booklets or to learn about services and activities in local areas, call the Society's toll-free number, 1-800-ACS-2345 (1-800-227-2345), or the number listed under American Cancer Society in the white pages of the local telephone book.

Candlelighters Childhood Cancer Foundation (CCCF)
Suite 460
7910 Woodmont Avenue
Bethesda, MD 20814
301-657-8401
1-800-366-CCCF

Candlelighters is a national organization of parents whose children have or have had cancer. It operates a patient information service and publishes newsletters for parents and young people. Local chapters sponsor family support groups.

Other Booklets

The National Cancer Institute booklets listed below are available free of charge. You may request them by calling 1-800-4-CANCER.

Booklets About Cancer Treatment

- Chemotherapy and You: A Guide to Self-Help During Treatment
- Radiation Therapy and You: A Guide to Self-Help During Treatment
- Eating Hints: Recipes and Tips for Better Nutrition During Cancer Treatment
- Questions and Answers About Pain Control (also available from the American Cancer Society)
- Young People with Cancer: A Handbook for Parents
- What Are Clinical Trials All About?

Booklets About Living with Cancer

- Taking Time: Support for People with Cancer and the People Who Care About Them
- Facing Forward: A Guide for Cancer Survivors
- When Cancer Recurs: Meeting the Challenge Again
- Advanced Cancer: Living Each Day

This booklet was written and published by the National Cancer Institute (NCI). The NCI is the U.S. Government's main agency for cancer research and information about cancer. The NCI's headquarters is at 9000 Rockville Pike, Bethesda, MD 20892.

■ **Document Source:**
U.S. Department of Health and Human Services, Public Health Service
National Institutes of Health
National Cancer Institute
NIH Publication No. 93-1571
March 1993

CONTRACEPTION AND REPRODUCTION

■ ■ ■

CHOOSING A CONTRACEPTIVE

by Merle S. Goldberg

Choosing a method of birth control is a highly personal decision, based on individual preferences, medical history, lifestyle, and other factors. Each method carries with it a number of risks and benefits of which the user should be aware.

Each method of birth control has a failure rate—an inability to prevent pregnancy over a one-year period. Sometimes the failure rate is due to the method, and sometimes it is due to human error, such as incorrect use or not using it at all. Each method has possible side effects, some minor and some serious. Some methods require lifestyle modifications, such as remembering to use the method with each and every sexual intercourse. Some cannot be used by individuals with certain medical problems.

Spermicides Used Alone

Spermicides, which come in many forms—foams, jellies, gels, and suppositories—work by forming a physical and chemical barrier to sperm. They should be inserted into the vagina within an hour before intercourse. If intercourse is repeated, more spermicide should be inserted. The active ingredient in most spermicides is the chemical nonoxynol-9. The failure rate for spermicides in preventing pregnancy when used alone is from 20 to 30 percent.

Spermicides are available without a prescription. People who experience burning or irritation with these products should not use them.

Barrier Methods

There are five barrier methods of contraception: male condoms, female condoms, diaphragm, sponge, and cervical cap. In each instance, the method works by keeping the sperm and egg apart. Usually, these methods have only minor side effects. The main possible side effect is an allergic reaction either to the material of the barrier or the spermicides that should be used with them. Using the methods correctly for each and every sexual intercourse gives the best protection.

Male Condom

A male condom is a sheath that covers the penis during sex. Condoms are made of either latex rubber or natural skin (also called "lambskin" but actually made from sheep intestines). Only latex condoms have been shown to be highly effective in helping to prevent STDs. Latex provides a good barrier to even small viruses such as human immunodeficiency virus and hepatitis B. Each condom can only be used once. Condoms have a birth control failure rate of about 15 percent. Most of the failures can be traced to improper use.

Some condoms have spermicide added. This may give some additional contraceptive protection. Vaginal spermicides may also be added before sexual intercourse.

Some condoms have lubricants added. These do not improve birth control or STD protection. Non-oil-based lubricants can also be used with condoms. However, oil-based lubricants such as petroleum jelly (Vaseline) should not be used because they weaken the latex. Condoms are available without a prescription.

Female Condom

The Reality Female Condom was approved by FDA in April 1993. It consists of a lubricated polyurethane sheath with a flexible polyurethane ring on each end. One ring is inserted into the vagina much like a diaphragm, while the other remains outside, partially covering the labia. The female condom may offer some protection against STDs, but for highly effective protection, male latex condoms must be used.

FDA Commissioner David A. Kessler, MD, in announcing the approval, said, "I have to stress that the male latex condom remains the best shield against AIDS and other sexually transmitted diseases. Couples should go on using the male latex condom."

In a six-month trial, the pregnancy rate for the Reality Female Condom was about 13 percent. The estimated yearly

Birth Control Guide

Type	Male Condom	Female Condom	Spermicides Used Alone	Sponge	Diaphragm with Spermicide	Cervical Cap with Spermicide	Birth Control Pills	Implant (Norplant)	Injection (Depo-Provera)	IUD	Periodic Abstinence (NFP)	Surgical Sterilization
Estimated Effectiveness	About 85%	An estimated 74–79%	70–80%	72–82%	82–94%	At least 82%	97–99%	99%	99%	95–96%	Very variable, perhaps 53–86%	Over 99%
Risks	Rarely, irritation and allergic reactions	Rarely, irritation and allergic reactions	Rarely, irritation and allergic reactions	Rarely, irritation and allergic reactions; difficulty in removal; very rarely, toxic shock syndrome	Rarely, irritation and allergic reactions; bladder infection; very rarely, toxic shock syndrome	Abnormal pap test; vaginal or cervical infections; very rarely, toxic shock syndrome	Blood clots, heart attacks and strokes, gallbladder disease, liver tumors, water retention, hypertension, mood changes, dizziness and nausea; not for smokers	Menstrual cycle irregularity; headaches, nervousness, depression, nausea, dizziness, change of appetite, breast tenderness, weight gain, enlargement of ovaries and/or fallopian tubes, excessive growth of body and facial hair; may subside after first year	Amenorrhea, weight gain, and other side effects similar to those with Norplant	Cramps, bleeding, pelvic inflammatory disease, infertility; rarely, perforation of the uterus	None	Pain, infection, and, for female tubal ligation, possible surgical complications
STD Protection	Latex condoms help protect against sexually transmitted diseases, including herpes and AIDS	May give some protection against sexually transmitted diseases, including herpes and AIDS; not as effective as male latex condom	Unknown	None	None	None	None	None	None	None	None	None
Convenience	Applied immediately before intercourse; used only once and discarded	Applied immediately before intercourse; used only once and discarded	Applied more than one hour before intercourse	Can be inserted hours before intercourse and left in place up to 24 hours; used only once and discarded	Inserted before intercourse; can be left in place 24 hours, but additional spermicide must be inserted if intercourse is repeated	Can remain in place for 48 hours; not necessary to reapply spermicide upon repeated intercourse; may be difficult to insert	Pill must be taken on daily schedule, regardless of the frequency of intercourse	Effective 24 hours after implantation for approximately five years; can be removed by physician at any time	One injection every three months	After insertion stays in place until physician removes it	Requires frequent monitoring of body functions and periods of abstinence	Vasectomy is a one-time procedure usually performed in a doctor's office; tubal ligation is a one-time procedure performed in an operating room
Availability	Nonprescription	Nonprescription	Nonprescription	Nonprescription	Rx	Rx	Rx	Rx; minor outpatient surgical procedure	Rx	Rx	Instructions from physician or clinic	

Efficacy rates given in this chart are estimates based on a number of different studies. They should be understood as yearly estimates, with those dependent on conscientious use subject to a greater chance of human error and reduced effectiveness. For comparison, 60 to 85 percent of sexually active women using no contraception would be expected to become pregnant in a year. This chart should not be used alone, but only as a summary of information in the accompanying article.

failure rate ranges from 21 to 26 percent. This means that about one in four women who use Reality may become pregnant during a year.

Sponge

The contraceptive sponge, approved by FDA in 1983, is made of white polyurethane foam. The sponge, shaped like a small doughnut, contains the spermicide nonoxynol-9. Like the diaphragm, it is inserted into the vagina to cover the cervix during and after intercourse. It does not require fitting by a health professional and is available without prescription. It is to be used only once and then discarded. The failure rate is between 18 and 28 percent. An extremely rare side effect is toxic shock syndrome (TSS), a potentially fatal infection caused by a strain of the bacterium *Staphylococcus aureus* and more commonly associated with tampon use.

Diaphragm

The diaphragm is a flexible rubber disk with a rigid rim. Diaphragms range in size from two to four inches in diameter and are designed to cover the cervix during and after intercourse so that sperm cannot reach the uterus. Spermicidal jelly or cream must be placed inside the diaphragm for it to be effective.

The diaphragm must be fitted by a health professional and the correct size prescribed to ensure a snug seal with the vaginal wall. If intercourse is repeated, additional spermicide should be added with the diaphragm still in place. The diaphragm should be left in place for at least six hours after intercourse. The diaphragm used with spermicide has a failure rate of from 6 to 18 percent.

In addition to the possible allergic reactions or irritation common to all barrier methods, there have been some reports of bladder infections with this method. As with the contraceptive sponge, TSS is an extremely rare side effect.

Cervical Cap

The cervical cap, approved for contraceptive use in the United States in 1988, is a dome-shaped rubber cap in various sizes that fits snugly over the cervix. Like the diaphragm it is used with a spermicide and must be fitted by a health professional. It is more difficult to insert than the diaphragm, but may be left in place for up to 48 hours. In addition to the allergic reactions that can occur with any barrier method, 5.2 to 27 percent of users in various studies have reported an unpleasant odor and/or discharge. There also appears to be an increased incidence of irregular Pap tests in the first six months of using the cap, and TSS is an extremely rare side effect. The cap has a failure rate of about 18 percent.

Hormonal Contraception

Hormonal contraception involves ways of delivering forms of two female reproductive hormones—estrogen and progestogen—that help regulate ovulation (release of an egg), the condition of the uterine lining, and other parts of the menstrual cycle. Unlike barrier methods, hormones are not inert,

do interact with the body, and have the potential for serious side effects, though this is rare. When properly used, hormonal methods are also extremely effective. Hormonal methods are available only by prescription.

Birth Control Pills

There are two types of birth control pills: combination pills, which contain both estrogen and a progestin (a natural or synthetic progesterone), and "mini-pills," which contain only progestin. The combination pill prevents ovulation, while the mini-pill reduces cervical mucus and causes it to thicken. This prevents the sperm from reaching the egg. Also, progestins keep the endometrium (uterine lining) from thickening. This prevents the fertilized egg from implanting in the uterus. The failure rate for the mini-pill is 1 to 3 percent; for the combination pill it is 1 to 2 percent.

Combination oral contraceptives offer significant protection against ovarian cancer, endometrial cancer, iron-deficiency anemia, pelvic inflammatory disease (PID), and fibrocystic breast disease. Women who take combination pills have a lower risk of functional ovarian cysts.

The decision about whether to take an oral contraceptive should be made only after consultation with a health professional. Smokers and women with certain medical conditions should not take the pill. These conditions include: a history of blood clots in the legs, eyes, or deep veins of the legs; heart attacks, strokes, or angina; cancer of the breast, vagina, cervix, or uterus; any undiagnosed, abnormal vaginal bleeding; liver tumors; or jaundice due to pregnancy or use of birth control pills.

Women with the following conditions should discuss with a health professional whether the benefits of the pill outweigh its risks for them:

- high blood pressure
- heart, kidney, or gallbladder disease
- a family history of heart attack or stroke
- severe headaches or depression
- elevated cholesterol or triglycerides
- epilepsy
- diabetes

Serious side effects of the pill include blood clots that can lead to stroke, heart attack, pulmonary embolism, or death. A clot may, on rare occasions, occur in the blood vessel of the eye, causing impaired vision or even blindness. The pills may also cause high blood pressure that returns to normal after oral contraceptives are stopped. Minor side effects, which usually subside after a few months' use, include: nausea, headaches, breast swelling, fluid retention, weight gain, irregular bleeding, and depression. Sometimes taking a pill with a lower dose of hormones can reduce these effects.

The effectiveness of birth control pills may be reduced by a few other medications, including some antibiotics, barbiturates, and antifungal medications. On the other hand, birth control pills may prolong the effects of theophylline and caffeine. They also may prolong the effects of benzodiazepines such as Librium (chlordiazepodide), Valium (diazepam), and Xanax (alprazolam). Because of the variety of these drug interactions, women should always tell their health professionals when they are taking birth control pills.

Norplant

Norplant—the first contraceptive implant—was approved by FDA in 1990. In a minor surgical procedure, six matchstick-sized rubber capsules containing progestin are placed just underneath the skin of the upper arm. The implant is effective within 24 hours and provides progestin for up to five years or until it is removed. Both the insertion and the removal must be performed by a qualified professional.

Because contraception is automatic and does not depend on the user, the failure rate for Norplant is less than 1 percent for women who weigh less than 150 pounds. Women who weigh more have a higher pregnancy rate after the first two years.

Women who cannot take birth control pills for medical reasons should not consider Norplant a contraceptive option. The potential side effects of the implant include: irregular menstrual bleeding, headaches, nervousness, depression, nausea, dizziness, skin rash, acne, change of appetite, breast tenderness, weight gain, enlargement of the ovaries or fallopian tubes, and excessive growth of body and facial hair. These side effects may subside after the first year.

Depo-Provera

Depo-Provera is an injectable form of a progestin. It was approved by FDA in 1992 for contraceptive use. Previously, it was approved for treating endometrial and renal cancers. Depo-Provera has a failure rate of only 1 percent. Each injection provides contraceptive protection for 14 weeks. It is injected every three months into a muscle in the buttocks or arm by a trained professional. The side effects are the same as those for Norplant and progestin-only pills. In addition, there may be irregular bleeding and spotting during the first months followed by periods of amenorrhea (no menstrual period). About 50 percent of the women who use Depo-Provera for one year or longer report amenorrhea. Other side effects, such as weight gain and others described for Norplant, may occur.

Intrauterine Devices

IUDs are small, plastic, flexible devices that are inserted into the uterus through the cervix by a trained clinician. Only two IUDs are presently marketed in the United States: ParaGard T380A, a T-shaped device partially covered by copper and effective for eight years; and Progestasert, which is also T-shaped but contains a progestin released over a one-year period. After that time, the IUD should be replaced. Both IUDs have a 4 to 5 percent failure rate.

It is not known exactly how IUDs work. At one time it was thought that the IUD affected the uterus so that it would be inhospitable to implantation. New evidence, however, suggests that uterine and tubal fluids are altered, particularly in the case of copper-bearing IUDs, inhibiting the transport of sperm through the cervical mucus and uterus.

The risk of PID with IUD use is highest in those with multiple sex partners or with a history of previous PID. Therefore, the IUD is recommended primarily for women in mutually monogamous relationships.

In addition to PID, other complications include perforation of the uterus (usually at the time of insertion), septic abortion, or ectopic (tubal) pregnancy. Women may also experience some short-term side effects—cramping and dizziness at the time of insertion; bleeding, cramps and backache that may continue for a few days after the insertion; spotting between periods; and longer and heavier menstruation during the first few periods after insertion.

Periodic Abstinence

Periodic abstinence entails not having sexual intercourse during the woman's fertile period. Sometimes this method is called natural family planning (NFP) or "rhythm." Using periodic abstinence is dependent on the ability to identify the approximately 10 days in each menstrual cycle that a woman is fertile. Methods to help determine this include

- The basal body temperature method is based on the knowledge that just before ovulation a woman's basal body temperature drops several tenths of a degree and after ovulation it returns to normal. The method requires that the woman take her temperature each morning before she gets out of bed.
- The cervical mucus method, also called the Billings method, depends on a woman recognizing the changes in cervical mucus that indicate ovulation is occurring or has occurred. There are now electronic thermometers with memories and electrical resistance meters that can more accurately pinpoint a woman's fertile period. The method has a failure rate of 14 to 47 percent.

Periodic abstinence has none of the side effects of artificial methods of contraception.

Surgical Sterilization

Surgical sterilization must be considered permanent. Tubal ligation seals a woman's fallopian tubes so that an egg cannot travel to the uterus. Vasectomy involves closing off a man's vas deferens so that sperm will not be carried to the penis.

Vasectomy is considered safer than female sterilization. It is a minor surgical procedure, most often performed in a doctor's office under local anesthesia. The procedure usually takes less than 30 minutes. Minor post-surgical complications may occur.

Tubal ligation is an operating-room procedure performed under general anesthesia. The fallopian tubes can be reached by a number of surgical techniques, and, depending on the technique, the operation is sometimes an outpatient procedure or requires only an overnight stay. In a minilaparotomy, a two-inch incision is made in the abdomen. The surgeon, using special instruments, lifts the fallopian tubes and, using clips, a plastic ring, or an electric current, seals the tubes. Another method, laparoscopy, involves making a small incision above the navel and distending the abdominal cavity so that the intestine separates from the uterus and fallopian tubes. Then a laparoscope—a miniaturized, flexible telescope—is used to visualize the fallopian tubes while closing them off.

Both of these methods are replacing the traditional laparotomy.

Major complications, which are rare in female sterilization, include: infection, hemorrhage, and problems associated with the use of general anesthesia. It is estimated that major complications occur in 1.7 percent of the cases, while the overall complication rate has been reported to be between 0.1 and 15.3 percent.

The failure rate of laparoscopy and minilaparotomy procedures as well as vasectomy, is less than 1 percent. Although there has been some success in reopening the fallopian tubes or the vas deferens, the success rate is low, and sterilization should be considered irreversible.

■ **Document Source:**
U.S. Department of Health and Human Services, Public Health Service
Food and Drug Administration
FDA Consumer
September 1993

See also: Facts About Oral Contraceptives (page 119)

FACTS ABOUT ORAL CONTRACEPTIVES

When oral contraceptives were introduced in the United States in 1960, many women believed they had found the answer to the need for convenient, safe, and reliable birth control. By 1965, "the pill" was America's leading contraceptive.

With the 1970s came disillusionment: The pill was not perfect. While it was highly effective and convenient, it had many minor side effects and a few serious ones. Though severe complications were rare, "pill scare" reports created an aura of danger. Pill use dropped in the mid-70s.

Today the pill has been put into perspective. It is not for everyone, but recent studies show it to be safe for most young, healthy, nonsmoking users. Despite widespread publicity on the pill's drawbacks, its benefits must be substantial. It is still the most popular reversible birth control method in America, with more than seven million women taking it daily.

Two Decades of Research

Oral contraceptives are probably the most extensively studied medication in history, yet they are not fully understood. Twenty years of research has, however, brought much safer pills and a long list of guidelines to help doctors screen out women most likely to develop serious complications.

The most important outcome of recent research is that groups of women with a high risk of developing pill complications have been identified. These include smokers, older women (the risks start to rise at 30), and those with a history of certain illnesses. While current knowledge is not precise enough to predict exactly which individuals will suffer serious pill complications, it is continually improving.

New studies also show benefits of pill use, besides contraception, such as protection from pelvic inflammatory disease and other conditions. Many doctors today stress that women should be made aware of these benefits, as well as the possible problems, so they can make informed decisions about the pill.

Research on oral contraceptives continues. Each year the National Institute of Child Health and Human Development (NICHD), a part of the National Institutes of Health, spends millions of dollars to evaluate current pills and develop better ones. This brochure, prepared by staff of the NICHD, describes the latest news on oral contraceptives.

Today's Pills

The most popular oral contraceptives are "combined" pills. These contain two synthetic hormones (an estrogen and a progestogen) similar to the hormones the ovary normally produces.

When studies linked the amount of estrogen in birth control pills with serious side effects—including blood clots, heart attacks, and strokes—researchers developed new pill formulas with less estrogen. They also developed a progestogen-only pill known as the "mini-pill."

Ten years ago, doctors often prescribed combined pills with 100 to 150 micrograms of estrogen. Today the Food and Drug Administration urges physicians to start patients on combined pills with no more than 50 micrograms of estrogen and, if possible, one of the newer "low dose" combined pills with only 30 or 35 micrograms of estrogen.

Major studies have concluded that switching from higher doses to pills with 50 micrograms of estrogen cuts the blood clot risk substantially. Recent research suggests that pills with less than 50 micrograms of estrogen cut the risk even further.

Progestogen levels in pills have also dropped over the years. Mini-pills contain even less progestogen than low-dose combined pills, which may make the mini-pill the safest oral contraceptive known.

How they work. Combined birth-control pills, including the newer low-dose forms, work by suppressing ovulation, the release of an egg from the ovary. Without a released egg, pregnancy cannot occur. Though rare, it is possible for women using combined pills to ovulate. Then other mechanisms work to prevent pregnancy.

Both kinds of pills make the cervical mucus thick and "inhospitable" to sperm, discouraging entry to the uterus. In addition, they make it difficult for a fertilized egg to implant by causing changes in fallopian tube contractions and in the uterine lining. These actions explain why the mini-pill works, as it generally does not suppress ovulation.

Effectiveness. Taken properly, the combined pills are better than 99 percent effective. Some formulas with less estrogen may be slightly less effective, about 98 to 99 percent.

Mini-pills are comparable in effectiveness to the IUD, at around 98 percent. But they must be taken without fail every day—ideally at the same time. Missing just one mini-pill can undo the contraceptive protection. Also, because mini-pills do not generally suppress ovulation, many doctors recommend a backup method, such as a diaphragm or condoms, at mid-cycle.

Why Pills Fail

If you take oral contraceptives, you should be prepared to use an additional form of birth control, because there are times the pill's effectiveness can be diminished.

Skipping pills. This is probably the main reason for reduced effectiveness. Directions for what to do after missing a dose vary with the pill formula and are included in the package insert that comes with all pills. Using a backup method for the rest of the cycle (while continuing to take the pill) will increase protection from pregnancy.

Illness. If you become sick with vomiting or diarrhea, your oral contraceptives may not be fully absorbed. It is safest to use an additional method for the rest of the cycle.

Drug interaction. Some medications can diminish the pill's effectiveness, including certain antibiotics (rifampin, and perhaps ampicillin and tetracycline); epilepsy drugs (Dilantin); anti-inflammatory or antiarthritic drugs (phenylbutazone); and barbiturates (phenobarbital). If you are treated for any ailment, even one that seems totally unrelated to pill use, be sure to inform your physician if you take birth control pills.

Should you take the Pill?

Many women are attracted by the advantages of the pill but are also concerned by the list of possible complications. Keep in mind that the process of weighing the benefits and risks is a highly individual one. No two women have exactly the same medical history or birth control needs. A doctor will help you make the best decision for *you.*

For some women the pill is ruled out altogether. Using pills with estrogen is too risky for women who have had blood clots, heart attack, or stroke; chest pain caused by angina pectoris; known or suspected breast cancer or cancer of the uterine lining; undiagnosed abnormal vaginal bleeding (which may indicate cancer and must be checked out); liver tumors; or jaundice during pregnancy.

Other health problems may also forbid pill use. These include fibroid uterine growths, diabetes, high cholesterol levels, high blood pressure, obesity, depression, gall bladder disease, and exposure to DES before birth.

In addition, because the pill tends to cause the body to retain water, women with a history of migraine headaches, asthma, epilepsy, or kidney and heart diseases may find the pill worsens their condition. If they choose to take it, they must be monitored closely by their doctors. Cigarette smoking and age also add to the chances of a woman developing serious pill-related complications.

But what about a woman without any of these risk factors? Once a woman's doctor has found that she has no detectable physical reason for avoiding the pill, the decision is in her hands. The pill carries a relatively small risk of serious complications even to the safest group of users—young,

healthy nonsmokers. Therefore it is important that the decision be an informed one.

Understanding the risks. The "patient leaflet" that comes with all pills contains a complete list of potential complications. Women should remember, though

- The pill affects all body cells, so the potential complications linked with it are many. But the chances of most young, healthy, nonsmoking women developing a particular complication are slim.
- The most serious side effects are also the most rare.
- Many of the risks known today were estimated through studies of *older* women using the *higher* dose pills. Therefore some experts believe that these studies may overstate the likelihood of complications in *younger* women using the newer *low-dose* pills or mini-pills.
- Knowledge of the health risks associated with childbirth can help to place in perspective the problems associated with pill use. The chances of dying from a childbirth complication exceed the chances of dying from a pill complication, *except* for smoking pill users aged 35 and over. As shown in the chart below, in either event, death is very rare. (Many women die each year for other reasons, including accidents and other health problems, as shown by the overall death rate included below for comparison.)

Estimated Annual Deaths per 100,000 Women

Cause of Death	Ages 15-19	20-24	25-29	30-34	35-39	40-44
Childbirth	5	6	7	13	21	22
Pill complications, smokers	2	4	6	12	31	61
Pill complications, non-smokers	1	1	2	3	9	18
All causes, including accidents	54	67	74	98	146	237

Other considerations: minor side effects. The pill also causes many minor side effects. Although they are not life threatening, they are nuisances and many women stop taking the pill because of them.

A minority of women on the pill experience nausea or vomiting (usually only in the first few cycles), weight changes, breast tenderness, abdominal cramps, or skin discoloration. Bladder and vaginal infections may also occur more frequently with pill use. In addition, some women report changes in sex drive (either increased or decreased), a loss of scalp hair, or an intolerance to contact lenses (because of water retention).

Many of these complaints disappear after the first few cycles of pill use. They may occur less often with low-dose pills and mini-pills. The newer formulas, however, are more likely to cause menstrual irregularities, such as spotting, breakthrough bleeding (which should be reported to a doctor), or, rarely, a lack of periods altogether. Menstrual irregularities are much more common with mini-pills than with combined pills, but cycles often become regular with time.

Knowing the benefits, too. The combined pill, when taken properly, is unmatched in effectiveness. And the pill in general allows more spontaneity in sexual relations than barrier methods that must be applied at the time of intercourse.

These benefits have long been known. But we are now learning that the pill protects women from some relatively common and potentially serious disorders that have nothing to do with its use as a contraceptive. According to recent estimates, each year, the pill prevents

- 51,000 cases of pelvic inflammatory disease, 13,300 of which would have required hospitalization,
- 20,000 hospitalizations for certain types of noncancerous breast disease,
- 9,900 hospitalizations for ectopic pregnancy,
- 3,000 hospitalizations for ovarian cysts,
- 27,000 cases of iron deficiency anemia, and
- 2,700 cases of rheumatoid arthritis.

The protection against pelvic inflammatory disease (PID) may be the most important noncontraceptive benefit of the pill. PID—a bacterial infection of the uterus, fallopian tubes, or ovaries—affects an estimated 850,000 U.S. women yearly. It can lead to infertility or, in rare cases, death. Studies have shown that women on the pill have half the chance of developing PID compared to women using no form of birth control. (Women using barrier devices also have half the chance.)

Other advantages of the pill include less menstrual cramping, lighter blood flow, and for those using combined pills, very regular periods. Some women using oral contraceptives also have diminished premenstrual tension. And women with acne often find the pill improves their complexion.

The Major Risk

The most serious side effect of oral contraceptive use is an increased risk of cardiovascular disease—specifically blood clots, heart attacks, and strokes. But even these complications are occurring less frequently, according to Bruce Stadel, MD (NICHD), as a result of lower hormone content in pills, better screening of women who might be at high risk, and, perhaps most importantly, the recent drop in pill use among women over 35.

What are the odds? Pill-related heart attacks are very rare. They occur in an estimated one in 14,000 users between the ages of 30 and 39. Between the ages of 40 and 44 the risk rises to about one case in 1,500 women on the pill.

Strokes occur five times more frequently among women taking oral contraceptives. But they are a rare event, too, affecting about one in 2,700 women on the pill.

Although clots in the veins occur more often than heart attacks or strokes, they are still uncommon, affecting about one in 500 previously healthy women on the pill. Hormone changes in pregnancy cause clots far more frequently than pills do.

Who are the high-risk women? The vast majority of heart attacks and strokes among pill users occur in women who smoke, women over 35, and women with other health conditions, such as high blood pressure, that ordinarily contribute to cardiovascular risk. Women with a combination of two or more of these factors carry the greatest risk of all. (See "Compounding the Risks.")

Some research shows that the length of pill use can affect the chances of having a cardiovascular complication. A recent study found that women aged 40 to 49 who had taken the pill for five or more years had twice the average heart attack risk—even years after they stopped taking the pill. Heavy smoking adds far more to the chances of having a heart attack, however.

Perhaps surprisingly, age and smoking habits do not seem to increase the chances of developing blood clots in the veins. But women with certain blood types—A, B, or AB—are twice as likely to develop clots as women with type O. This is true whether a woman is on the pill or not.

NICHD-funded research has shown that women who experience clotting disorders may lack the ability to produce extra amounts of a certain anticlotting blood protein that women on the pill need. Unfortunately, it is not yet possible to predict who will have this problem. But researchers have found evidence suggesting that women may counteract it through regular exercise, which may spur the body to produce more of the anticlotting protein.

Because oral contraceptives double the chances of developing blood clots after surgery, doctors advise women taking the pill to stop, if possible, at least four weeks before any scheduled operation. And all women on the pill should know the symptoms that indicate a possible blood clot—sharp pain in the chest, coughing blood, or sudden shortness of breath; pain in the calf; or sudden partial or complete loss of vision—and notify their doctors immediately if they experience any of them.

High blood pressure. Although many women experience a mild elevation in blood pressure when they are taking oral contraceptives, it usually remains within the normal range and returns to "pre-pill" levels when they stop. Studies several years ago found that pill users have three to six times the average risk of developing high blood pressure. It has been estimated to occur in one to four percent of women who take the pill and is usually confined to those over 35. Newer studies show that high blood pressure is not a common problem for today's younger pill takers. But *all* women on the pill should have their blood pressure checked every six to 12 months.

Compounding the Risks

Factors such as smoking, increasing age, or high blood pressure add to the chances of developing cardiovascular disorders—problems in the heart or blood vessels. Combine any of these factors with oral contraceptive use, and the risks multiply. And when a woman has more than one risk factor, her chances of a serious pill complication skyrocket.

Smoking. Most of the women who have a heart attack or stroke while using the pill are smokers. The mechanism is not understood, but the pill somehow intensifies the adverse effects of smoking on the circulatory system.

To illustrate: One study found that either using oral contraceptives or smoking increased the odds of having a stroke by about six times. In women who both smoked *and* took the pill, the risks did not just add together. Instead, they jumped to 22 times the risk of stroke in women who neither smoked nor took the pill.

All smokers using the pill are at greater risk than non-smokers. The likelihood of heart attack or stroke rises sharply for those who smoke more than 15 cigarettes per day. From the standpoint of safety, doctors now advise pill users not to just cut back, but to quit smoking altogether.

Age. The natural aging process also increases the chances of developing cardiovascular disorders, and birth control pills accentuate the risk. An example: In women who *don't* use the pill, those aged 40 to 44 are about five times as likely to have a heart attack as those aged 30 to 39. But in pill users, the older age group is about nine times as likely to have a heart attack.

The cardiovascular risks of the pill begin to rise substantially around age 30, particularly in smokers. However, there is no definite cutoff age for pill use. Some doctors believe that regardless of smoking habits, women should consider other forms of contraception starting at age 30. Others feel that at age 30, women *who smoke* and take the pill should choose between the two, while *nonsmokers* are relatively safe until age 35. Still others hold that the new low-dose pills and mini-pills may be safe options for women over 35 who do not smoke or have other unfavorable health conditions.

Obviously, the final word is not yet in. Over the next few years, NICHD-supported studies should help clarify the pill's risks to women over 30.

Health conditions. Women at any age with health problems that ordinarily increase the chances of cardiovascular disease are even more at risk when using the pill. The conditions include

- high blood pressure,
- a history of high blood pressure in pregnancy,
- obesity,
- diabetes mellitus, and
- elevated cholesterol.

Combined risk factors. When more than one of the above risk factors are present, the chances of a serious pill complication increase dramatically. A recent study found that the odds of having a heart attack are increased by

- 3 times among pill users,
- 5 times among smokers,
- 8 times among people with high blood pressure, and
- 170 times among pill users with high blood pressure who smoke.

An expert on oral contraceptives at the Centers for Disease Control (CDC), Dr. Howard Ory, stresses that "the most serious adverse effect of pill use—death from cardiovascular disease—is also the *most preventable.*"

"If women who use the pill would not smoke," he states, "at least *half* of all deaths associated with pill use could be avoided. If, in addition, women with other predisposing factors for cardiovascular disease, such as high blood pressure, high cholesterol, and diabetes mellitus would not use the pill, deaths could be further reduced."

The Pill and Cancer

Probably the question women ask most frequently about oral contraceptives is, "Does the pill cause cancer?"

Because most kinds of cancer take so long to develop, the answer must still be tentative, but it is reassuring: There is no firm evidence that the pill causes cancer.

The NICHD and the CDC are currently cosponsoring a long-term project to analyze the pill's relationship to breast cancer and cancer of the reproductive tract. Although final results will not be available until the mid-1980s, the preliminary results are encouraging, showing no association between the pill and breast cancer. Early results also suggest that women who have used the pill for at least one year have *half* the average risk of developing cancer of the ovary and of the endometrium (the lining of the uterus).

No clear cause-and-effect relationship has been established between the pill and cancer of the cervix, but most doctors still feel it is very important for women on the pill to have yearly Pap smears.

One kind of potentially life-threatening cell growth that is linked with the pill is an extremely rare liver tumor known as hepatic adenoma. Although it is not cancerous, it can cause internal bleeding. It occurs in about one in 33,000 pill users per year, mostly women who have taken the pill for about five years or more. Early detection of the condition can make a difference. Make sure that your checkups include a physical exam of the abdomen.

The Pill and Body Chemistry

Studies of women taking combined pills with at least 50 micrograms of estrogen show changes in the levels of sugars, fats, and proteins in the blood, and alterations in the way the body uses certain nutrients. These and other metabolic changes can cause slightly altered thyroid, liver, and blood tests, though results usually remain within the normal range.

While it appears that metabolic changes are lessened with the newer formulas, the long-range effects of even small changes in body chemistry in pill users are unknown. Current studies supported by the NICHD are expected to define these changes more precisely and to determine whether they affect the risk of cardiovascular disease in pill users.

Nutritional changes. Oral contraceptives can affect nutritional status, but studies of this topic often have conflicting results. This is because many variables, such as hormone shifts throughout a menstrual cycle, can also change the body's nutritional needs.

In women taking the combined pill, studies have found increased levels of vitamin A and iron; decreased levels of vitamins B-6, B-12, C, and riboflavin; and both increases and decreases in levels of folic acid and zinc.

A lowered level of vitamin B-6 is the most consistently reported nutritional change in pill users. One NICHD-funded study found that lowered levels of B-6 during pregnancy and lactation were more common in women who used the pill for a long time (more than 30 months) and became pregnant within four months after stopping the pill. Nevertheless, it is uncertain whether pill use is a cause of true vitamin B-6 deficiency, which is linked with depression. Other symptoms of vitamin deficiency include weakness, lethargy, dizziness, skin and gum irritations, and an increased susceptibility to infection.

Next to vitamin B-6, folic acid is the nutrient most significantly affected by the pill. Changes in folic acid metabolism have been reported in connection with two conditions in pill users. A few women using oral contraceptives have developed a rare but serious anemia which responds to treatment with folic acid supplements. In addition, the pill is linked with changes in folic acid metabolism in cells around the cervix, which may be related to a kind of abnormal cell growth called cervical dysplasia. An NICHD-supported study found that cervical dysplasia sometimes improves with folic acid supplements.

For pill users, a balanced diet is often recommended over routine vitamin and mineral supplements for two reasons. First, overdosing on supplements can be toxic, and second, people taking supplements often do not try as hard to get a balanced diet. Vitamin supplements cannot take the place of a balanced diet; in fact, they need to have proper foods present to work right. But when medical tests show a vitamin deficiency, vitamin supplement therapy may be in order.

Recent studies on oral contraceptives and metabolism found that pill users do not eliminate caffeine or valium as efficiently as nonusers. This means that either substance can accumulate in the body. As a result, women using the pill may be more prone to caffeine side effects such as nervousness and insomnia. Those using valium could become oversedated if the dosage is not carefully watched.

Depression

Oral contraceptives alleviate depression in some women and worsen it in others. Symptoms of depression related to pill use include pessimism, dissatisfaction, listlessness, tension, crying, and perhaps anxiety or a loss of sex drive. Although many of the reports of pill-related depression came when higher doses of estrogen were widely used, it is not clear whether depression is less common with the newer low-dose pills or mini-pills.

Depression can be a symptom of vitamin B-6 deficiency. The pill can affect the body's use of B-6 and other vitamins and minerals, and studies have found that some depressed pill users are B-6 deficient. These women may respond to vitamin B-6 therapy. Women who become seriously depressed while on the pill should discuss it with their physicians and consider switching to another form of birth control.

The Pill and Childbearing

Many women taking birth control pills are planning to have children at some time. For them, the news is good: There appears to be little risk that use of the pill leads to sterility. In fact, because the pill protects many women from pelvic inflammatory disease, which can damage the fallopian tubes, it guards against a leading cause of infertility.

Fertility. Former pill users may take a few months longer to conceive than other women, but an estimated 80 percent of women resume normal reproductive functions within three months after stopping the pill and more than 95 percent are ovulating within a year.

Women who do not regain normal periods within six months should see a doctor for a complete evaluation. Most women who have menstrual problems after stopping the pill had irregular periods before they started taking it. But some studies suggest that there is a very slim chance that the pill itself causes a condition known as "post-pill amenorrhea"—a lack of periods. Though the cause of the problem is a matter of much debate among researchers, infertility after stopping the pill generally is temporary and responds to treatment.

Pregnancy. Many doctors recommend that women who wish to become pregnant use traditional barrier contraceptives for at least three months after stopping the pill. Usually, a woman's menstrual cycle will become regular during this time, which permits the doctor to accurately date the start of the pregnancy. When former pill users do become pregnant, they have no greater risk of complications than other women.

Although it happens extremely rarely, oral contraceptives can fail even when a woman has been conscientious about taking them every day. In addition to causing an unplanned pregnancy, pill failure can lead to inadvertent exposure of a developing fetus to extra hormones. Some studies show a slightly increased risk of birth defects in infants exposed before birth to oral contraceptive hormones; other studies have found no risk. Experts generally agree that the risks, if they exist at all, are very small.

But for absolute safety, if you even suspect you might be pregnant, immediately stop taking the pill, switch to another form of contraception, and have a pregnancy test as soon as possible. Studies have shown no added risk of birth defects when conception occurs one month after stopping the pill.

Breastfeeding. Physicians often recommend methods other than the pill for women who are nursing babies. For one thing, the estrogen in combined pills can suppress milk production. Also, very small quantities of hormones pass from the mother to her nursing infant. Although no long-term effects of this ingestion have been reported, the possibility of risk to the baby has not been extensively studied. For women who want to breastfeed and use an oral contraceptive, doctors frequently suggest the mini-pill, since it does not suppress lactation.

How to Minimize the Risks

Both doctors and the women for whom they prescribe birth control pills have a role in reducing the chances of pill-related complications. Doctors must screen patients carefully, follow up conscientiously, and prescribe the lowest possible dose that is compatible with an individual woman's needs. Yet as recently as 1978, one-fourth of the women taking the pill in the United States were still using formulas with more than 50 micrograms of estrogen. Check your prescription: If it contains more than 50 micrograms, you might ask your physician if you can try a lower dose.

Women must be open with their doctors, informing them of any health problems. They must also know the signs that indicate a possibly serious complication of pill use and call their doctors immediately. In addition, women on the pill should exercise regularly. Above all, they should have medical checkups at least yearly (more frequently if their doctors advise).

Twenty years ago, there was hope that the pill would prove to be the perfect form of birth control: effective, convenient, and safe for all women. Ten years ago, reports of side effects brought disillusionment. Today, we know that the pill, though imperfect, is an option many women can use safely. We now have better formulas, better screening of women, and a better informed public. And as these trends continue, we can look forward to even safer use of the pill.

Warning Signals

Women taking oral contraceptives should be alert to any physical or mental change that may warrant a visit to the doctor. If you experience any of the following symptoms, notify your physician at once and remind him or her that you are on the pill.

- Severe abdominal pain
- Chest pain, coughing, shortness of breath
- Pain or tenderness in calf or thigh
- Severe headache, dizziness, or faintness
- Muscle weakness or numbness
- Speech disturbance
- Eye problems: blurred vision, flashing lights, blindness
- Breast lump
- Severe depression
- Yellowing of skin

"Facts About Oral Contraceptives" was written by Maureen B. Gardner, Office of Research Reporting, National Institute of Child Health and Human Development (NICHD). It is reprinted from the June 1983 issue of *Good Housekeeping* magazine with permission of the publisher.

The NICHD, part of the Federal Government's National Institutes of Health, conducts and supports research on the various processes that determine the health of children, adults, families, and populations. For more copies of this fact sheet or others in this series, write to NICHD, PO Box 29111, Washington, DC 20040.

Other Publications in This Series:

- *Facts About Anorexia Nervosa*
- *Facts About Cesarean Childbirth*
- *Facts About Childhood Hyperactivity*
- *Facts About Down Syndrome*
- *Facts About Dyslexia*
- *Facts About Dysmenorrhea and Premenstrual Syndrome*
- *Facts About Precocious Puberty*
- *Facts About Pregnancy and Smoking*
- *Facts About Premature Birth*
- *Facts About Vasectomy Safety*

■ Document Source:
U.S. Department of Health and Human Services, Public Health Service
National Institutes of Health
National Institute of Child Health and Human Development

DENTAL CARE AND ORAL HEALTH

■ ■ ■

TAKING CARE OF YOUR TEETH AND MOUTH

A healthy smile is a bonus at any age. Too often, older people-especially those who wear false teeth (or dentures)—feel they no longer need dental checkups. If you haven't learned the basics of oral health care, it is not too late to start. And even if you have, it's a good time to review.

Tooth Decay (Cavities)

Tooth decay is not just a children's disease; it can happen as long as natural teeth are in the mouth. Tooth decay is caused by bacteria that normally live in the mouth. The bacteria cling to teeth and form a sticky, colorless film called dental plaque. The bacteria in plaque live on sugars and produce decay-causing acids that dissolve minerals on tooth surfaces. Tooth decay can also develop on the exposed roots of the teeth if you have gum disease or receding gums (where gums pull away from the teeth, exposing the roots).

Just as with children, fluoride is important for adult teeth. Research has shown that adding fluoride to the water supply is the best and least costly way to prevent tooth decay. In addition, using fluoride toothpastes and mouthrinses can add protection. Daily fluoride rinses can be bought at most drug stores without a prescription. If you have a problem with cavities, your dentist or dental hygienist may give you a fluoride treatment during the office visit. The dentist may prescribe a fluoride gel or mouthrinse for you to use at home.

Gum (Periodontal) Disease

A common cause of tooth loss after age 35 is gum (periodontal) disease. These are infections of the gum and bone that hold the teeth in place. Gum diseases are also caused by dental plaque. The bacteria in plaque causes the gums to become inflamed and bleed easily. If left untreated, the disease gets worse as pockets of infection form between the teeth and gums. This causes receding gums and loss of supporting bone. You may lose enough bone to cause your teeth to become loose and fall out.

You can prevent gum disease by removing plaque. Thoroughly brush and floss your teeth each day. Carefully check your mouth for early signs of disease such as red, swollen, or bleeding gums. See your dentist regularly every six-12 months—or at once if these signs are present.

Cleaning Your Teeth and Gums

An important part of good oral health is knowing how to brush and floss correctly. Thorough brushing each day removes plaque. Gently brush the teeth on all sides with a soft bristle brush using a fluoride toothpaste. Circular and short back-and-forth strokes work best. Take the time to brush carefully along the gum line. Lightly brushing your tongue also helps to remove plaque and food debris and makes your mouth feel fresh.

In addition to brushing, using dental floss is necessary to keep the gums healthy. Proper flossing is important because it removes plaque and leftover food that a toothbrush cannot reach. Your dentist or dental hygienist can show you the best way to brush and floss your teeth. If brushing or flossing results in bleeding gums, pain, or irritation, see your dentist at once.

An antibacterial mouthrinse, approved for the control of plaque and swollen gums, may be prescribed by your dentist. The mouthrinse is used in addition to careful daily brushing and flossing.

Some people (with arthritis or other conditions that limit motion) may find it hard to hold a toothbrush. To overcome this, the toothbrush handle can be attached to the hand with a wide elastic band or may be enlarged by attaching it to a sponge, styrofoam ball, or similar object. People with limited shoulder movement may find brushing easier if the handle of the brush is lengthened by attaching a long piece of wood or plastic. Electric toothbrushes are helpful to many.

Other Conditions of the Mouth

Dry mouth (xerostomia) is common in many adults and may make it hard to eat, swallow, taste, and speak. The condition happens when salivary glands fail to work properly as a result of various diseases or medical treatments, such as chemotherapy or radiation therapy to the head and neck area. Dry mouth is also a side effect of more than 400 commonly used medicines, including drugs for high blood pressure, antidepressants, and antihistamines. Dry mouth can affect oral health by adding to tooth decay and infection.

Until recently, dry mouth was regarded as a normal part of aging. We now know that healthy older adults produce as much saliva as younger adults. So, if you think you have dry mouth, talk with your dentist or doctor. To relieve the dryness, drink extra water and avoid sugary snacks, beverages with caffeine, tobacco, and alcohol—all of which increase dryness in the mouth.

Cancer therapies, such as radiation to the head and neck or chemotherapy, can cause oral problems, including dry mouth, tooth decay, painful mouth sores, and cracked and peeling lips. Before starting cancer treatment, it is important to see a dentist and take care of any necessary dental work. Your dentist will also show you how to care for your teeth and mouth before, during, and after your cancer treatment to prevent or reduce the oral problems that can occur.

Oral cancer (mouth cancer) most often occurs in people over age 40. The disease frequently goes unnoticed in its early, curable stages. This is true in part because many older people, particularly those wearing full dentures, do not visit their dentists often enough and because pain is usually not an early symptom of the disease. People who smoke cigarettes, use other tobacco products, or drink excessive amounts of alcohol are at increased risk for oral cancer.

It is important to spot oral cancer as early as possible, since treatment works best before the disease has spread. If you notice any red or white patches on the gums or tongue, sores that do not heal within two weeks, or if you have difficulty chewing or swallowing, be sure to see a dentist.

A head and neck exam, which should be a part of every dental check-up, will allow your dentist to detect early signs of oral cancer.

Dentures

If you wear false teeth (dentures), keep them clean and free from food that can cause stains, bad breath, and gum irritation. Once a day, brush all surfaces of the dentures with a denture care product. Remove your dentures from your mouth and place them in water or a denture-cleansing liquid while you sleep. It is also helpful to rinse your mouth with a warm salt water solution in the morning, after meals, and at bedtime.

Partial dentures should be cared for in the same way as full dentures. Because bacteria tend to collect under the clasps of partial dentures, it is especially important to clean this area.

Dentures will seem awkward at first. When learning to eat with false teeth, select soft nonsticky food, cut food into small pieces, and chew slowly using both sides of the mouth. Dentures may make your mouth less sensitive to hot foods and liquids, and lower your ability to detect harmful objects such as bones. If problems in eating, talking, or simply wearing dentures continue after the first few weeks, see your dentist about making adjustments.

In time, dentures need to be replaced or readjusted because of changes that occur in tissues of your mouth. Do not try to repair dentures at home since this may damage the dentures which in turn may further hurt your mouth.

Dental Implants

Dental implants are anchors that permanently hold replacement teeth. There are several different types of implants, but the most popular are metal screws surgically placed into the jaw bones. If there isn't enough bone, a separate surgical procedure to add bone may be needed. Because bone heals slowly, treatment with implants can often take longer (four months to one year or more) than bridges or dentures. If you are considering dental implants, it is important to select an experienced dentist with whom you can discuss your concerns frankly beforehand to be certain the procedure is right for you.

Professional Care

In addition to practicing good oral hygiene, it is important to have regular checkups by the dentist whether you have natural teeth or dentures. It is also important to follow through with any special treatments that are necessary to ensure good oral health. For instance, if you have sensitive teeth caused by receding gums, your dentist may suggest using a special toothpaste for a few months. Teeth are meant to last a lifetime. By taking good care of your teeth and gums, you can protect them for years to come.

Additional Dental Health Information

More information about general dental care is available from:

National Institute of Dental Research (NIDR)
Building 31, Room 2C35
31 Center Dr MSC 2290
Bethesda, MD 20892-2290
301-496-4261

NIDR publishes information on oral research and general dental care. Some publications available are:

- Fever Blisters and Canker Sores
- Fluoride to Protect the Teeth of Adults
- Rx for Sound Teeth
- What You Need to Know About Periodontal (Gum) Disease

National Oral Health Information Clearinghouse
1 Nohic Way
Bethesda, MD 20892-3500
301-402-7364

NIDR also offers publications on oral health for special care patients through the National Oral Health Information Clearinghouse. Special care patients are people whose medical conditions or treatments affect oral health. Publications available include:

- Dry Mouth (Xerostomia)
- Chemotherapy and Oral Health
- Periodontal Disease and Diabetes—A Guide for Patients
- Radiation Therapy and Oral Health
- TMD (Temporomandibular Disorders)
- What You Need to Know About Oral Cancer

American Dental Association (ADA)

211 East Chicago Avenue
Chicago, IL 60611
1-800-621-8099

ADA distributes educational materials on dental health and sponsors the National Senior Smile Week.

National Agricultural Library Food & Nutrition Information Center
Room 304
10301 Baltimore Blvd
Beltsville, MD 20705-2351
310-504-5719

The Food and Nutrition Center offers the bibliography *Nutri-Topics Series: Nutrition and Dental Health*. This bibliography lists information available to consumers.

The National Institute on Aging Information Center
PO Box 8057
Gaithersburg, MD 20898-8057
1-800-222-2225
1-800-222-4225 (TTY)

NIA publishes fact sheets on various health related topics of interest to older people and their families. For a complete listing of publications, call or write to the above address.

■ **Document Source:**
U.S. Department of Health and Human Services, Public Health Service
National Institutes of Health
National Institute on Aging
1994

TMD: TEMPOROMANDIBULAR DISORDERS

You may have read articles in newspapers and magazines about "TMD"—temporomandibular (jaw) disorders, also called "TMJ syndrome." Perhaps you have even felt pain sometimes in your jaw area, or maybe your dentist or physician has told you that you have TMD.

If you have questions about TMD, you are not alone. Researchers, too, are looking for answers to what causes TMD, what are the best treatments, and how we can prevent these disorders. The National Institute of Dental Research has written this pamphlet to share with you what we have learned about TMD.

TMD is not just one disorder, but a group of conditions, often painful, that affect the jaw joint (temporomandibular joint or TMJ) and the muscles that control chewing. Although we don't know how many people actually have TMD, the disorders appear to affect about twice as many women as men.

The good news is that for most people, pain in the area of the jaw joint or muscles is not a signal that a serious problem is developing. Generally, discomfort from TMD is occasional and temporary, often occurring in cycles. The pain eventually goes away with little or no treatment. Only a small percentage of people with TMD pain develop significant, long-term symptoms.

What is the temporomandibular joint?

The temporomandibular joint connects the lower jaw, called the mandible, to the temporal bone at the side of the head. If you place your fingers just in front of your ears and open your mouth, you can feel the joint on each side of your head. Because these joints are flexible, the jaw can move smoothly up and down and side to side, enabling us to talk, chew and yawn. Muscles attached to and surrounding the jaw joint control its position and movement.

When we open our mouths, the rounded ends of the lower jaw, called condyles, glide along the joint socket of the temporal bone. The condyles slide back to their original position when we close our mouths. To keep this motion smooth, a soft disc lies between the condyle and the temporal bone. This disc absorbs shocks to the TMJ from chewing and other movements.

What are temporomandibular disorders?

Today, researchers generally agree that temporomandibular disorders fall into three main categories:

- myofascial pain, the most common form of TMD, which is discomfort or pain in the muscles that control jaw function and the neck and shoulder muscles;
- internal derangement of the joint, meaning a dislocated jaw or displaced disc, or injury to the condyle;
- degenerative joint disease, such as osteoarthritis or rheumatoid arthritis in the jaw joint.

A person may have one or more of these conditions at the same time.

What causes TMD?

We know that severe injury to the jaw or temporomandibular joint can cause TMD. A heavy blow, for example, can fracture the bones of the joint or damage the disc, disrupting the smooth motion of the jaw and causing pain or locking. Arthritis in the jaw joint may also result from injury.

Other causes of TMD are less clear. Some suggest, for example, that a bad bite (malocclusion) can trigger TMD, but recent research disputes that view. Orthodontic treatment, such as braces and the use of headgear, has also been blamed for some forms of TMD, but studies now show that this is unlikely.

And there is no scientific proof that gum chewing causes clicking sounds in the jaw joint, or that jaw clicking leads to serious TMJ problems. In fact, jaw clicking is fairly common in the general population. If there are no other symptoms, such as pain or locking, jaw clicking usually does not need treatment.

Researchers believe that most people with clicking or popping in the jaw joint likely have a displaced disc—the soft, shock-absorbing disc is not in a normal position. As long as the displaced disc causes no pain or problems with jaw movement, no treatment is needed.

Some experts suggest that stress, either mental or physical, may cause or aggravate TMD. People with TMD often clench or grind their teeth at night, which can tire the jaw muscles and lead to pain. It is not clear, however, whether stress is the cause of the clenching/grinding and subsequent jaw pain, or the result of dealing with chronic jaw pain or dysfunction. Scientists are exploring how behavioral, psychological and physical factors may combine to cause TMD.

TMD Signs and Symptoms

A variety of symptoms may be linked to TMD. Pain, particularly in the chewing muscles and/or jaw joint, is the most common symptom. Other likely symptoms include

- limited movement or locking of the jaw,
- radiating pain in the face, neck, or shoulders,
- painful clicking, popping, or grating sounds in the jaw joint when opening or closing the mouth,
- a sudden, major change in the way the upper and lower teeth fit together.

Symptoms such as headaches, earaches, dizziness, and hearing problems may sometimes be related to TMD. It is important to keep in mind, however, that occasional discomfort in the jaw joint or chewing muscles is quite common and is generally not a cause for concern. Researchers are working to clarify TMD symptoms, with the goal of developing easier and better methods of diagnosis and improved treatment.

Diagnosis

Because the exact causes and symptoms of TMD are not clear, diagnosing these disorders can be confusing. At present, there is no widely accepted, standard test to correctly identify TMD. In about 90 percent of cases, however, the patient's description of symptoms, combined with a simple physical examination of the face and jaw, provides information useful for diagnosing these disorders.

The examination includes feeling the jaw joints and chewing muscles for pain or tenderness; listening for clicking, popping, or grating sounds during jaw movement; and examining for limited motion or locking of the jaw while opening or closing the mouth. Checking the patient's dental and medical history is very important. In most cases, this evaluation provides enough information to locate the pain or jaw problem, to make a diagnosis, and to start treatment to relieve pain or jaw locking.

Regular dental x-rays and TMJ x-rays (transcranial radiographs) are not generally useful in diagnosing TMD. Other x-ray techniques, such as arthrography (joint x-rays using dye); magnetic resonance imaging (MRI), which pictures the soft tissues; and tomography (a special type of x-ray) are usually needed only when the practitioner strongly suspects a condition such as arthritis or when significant pain persists over time and symptoms do not improve with treatment. Before undergoing any expensive diagnostic test, it is always wise to get another independent opinion.

One of the most important areas of TMD research is developing clear guidelines for diagnosing these disorders. Once scientists agree on what these guidelines should be, it will be easier for practitioners to correctly identify temporomandibular disorders and to decide what treatment, if any, is needed.

Treatment

The key words to keep in mind about TMD treatment are "conservative" and "reversible." Conservative treatments are as simple as possible and are used most often because most patients do not have severe, degenerative TMD. Conservative treatments do not invade the tissues of the face, jaw, or joint. Reversible treatments do not cause permanent, or irreversible, changes in the structure or position of the jaw or teeth.

Because most TMD problems are temporary and do not get worse, simple treatment is all that is usually needed to relieve discomfort. Self-care practices, for example, eating soft foods, applying heat or ice packs, and avoiding extreme jaw movements (such as wide yawning, loud singing, and gum chewing), are useful in easing TMD symptoms. Learning special techniques for relaxing and reducing stress may also help patients deal with pain that often comes with TMD problems.

Other conservative, reversible treatments include physical therapy you can do at home, which focuses on gentle muscle stretching and relaxing exercises, and short-term use of muscle-relaxing and anti-inflammatory drugs.

The health care provider may recommend an oral appliance, also called a splint or bite plate, which is a plastic guard that fits over the upper or lower teeth. The splint can help reduce clenching or grinding, which eases muscle tension. An oral splint should be used only for a short time and should not cause permanent changes in the bite. If a splint causes or increases pain, stop using it and see your practitioner.

The conservative, reversible treatments described are useful for temporary relief of pain and muscle spasm—they are not "cures" for TMD. If symptoms continue over time or come back often, check with your doctor.

There are other types of TMD treatment, such as surgery or injections, that invade the tissues. Some involve injecting pain relieving medications into painful muscle sites, often called "trigger points." Researchers are studying this type of treatment to see if these injections are helpful over time.

Surgical treatments are often irreversible and should be avoided where possible. When such treatment is necessary, be sure to have the doctor explain to you, in words you can understand, the reason for the treatment, the risks involved, and other types of treatment that may be available.

Scientists have learned that certain irreversible treatments, such as surgical replacement of jaw joints with artificial implants, may cause severe pain and permanent jaw damage. Some of these devices may fail to function properly or may break apart in the jaw over time. *Before undergoing any surgery on the jaw joint, it is very important to get other independent opinions.*

The Food and Drug Administration has recalled artificial jaw joint implants made by Vitek, Inc., which may break down and damage surrounding bone. If you have these implants, see your oral surgeon or dentist. If there are problems with your implants, the devices may need to be removed. Persons who have Vitek implants should call Medic Alert at 1-800-554-5297 for more information.

Other irreversible treatments that are of little value—and may make the problem worse—include orthodontics to change the bite; restorative dentistry, which uses crown and bridge work to balance the bite; and occlusal adjustment, grinding down teeth to bring the bite into balance.

Although more studies are needed on the safety and effectiveness of most TMD treatments, scientists strongly recommend using the most conservative, reversible treatments possible before considering invasive treatments. Even when the TMD problem has become chronic, most patients still do not need aggressive types of treatment.

If you think you have TMD . . .

Keep in mind that for most people, discomfort from TMD will eventually go away whether treated or not. Simple self-care practices are often effective in easing TMD symptoms.

If more treatment is needed, it should be conservative and reversible. Avoid, if at all possible, treatments that cause permanent changes in the bite or jaw. If irreversible treatments are recommended, be sure to get a reliable second opinion.

Many practitioners, especially dentists, are familiar with the conservative treatment of TMD. Because TMD is usually painful, pain clinics in hospitals and universities are also a good source of advice and second opinions for these disorders. Specially trained facial pain experts can often be helpful in diagnosing and treating TMD.

Research

The National Institute of Dental Research supports an active research program on TMD. Developing reliable guidelines for diagnosing these disorders is a top priority. Studies are also under way on the causes, treatments, and prevention of TMD. Through continued research, pieces of the TMD puzzle are falling slowly but steadily into place.

■ Document Source:
National Institutes of Health
National Institute of Dental Research
NIH Publication No. 94-3487

DIABETES AND OTHER ENDOCRINE DISORDERS

■ ■ ■

DIABETES OVERVIEW

Who has diabetes?

Almost everyone knows someone who has diabetes. About 14 million people in the United States have diabetes mellitus, a serious, life-long disorder that is, as yet, incurable. Almost half of these people do not know they have diabetes and are not under medical care. Each year, 500,000 to 700,000 people are diagnosed with diabetes.

Although diabetes occurs most often in older adults, it is one of the most common chronic disorders in U.S. children. Each year, 11,000 to 12,000 children and teenagers are diagnosed with diabetes.

What is diabetes?

Diabetes is a disorder of metabolism, the way the body uses digested food for growth and energy. Most of the food we eat is broken down by the digestive juices into chemicals, including a simple sugar called glucose. After digestion, the glucose passes into the bloodstream where it is available for body cells to use for growth and energy.

For the glucose to get into the cells, insulin must be present. Insulin is a hormone produced by the pancreas.

When most people eat, the pancreas automatically produces the right amount of insulin to take care of the glucose. In people with diabetes, however, the pancreas either produces little or no insulin, or the body's cells do not respond to the insulin that is produced. As a result, glucose builds up in the blood, overflows into the urine, and passes out of the body. Thus, the body loses its main source of fuel even though the blood contains large amounts.

There are two major types of diabetes. Type I, known as insulin-dependent diabetes (IDDM), is considered an autoimmune disease because the pancreatic cells that produce insulin, the beta cells, are destroyed by the body's own immune system. The pancreas then produces little or no insulin. To live, the person with IDDM needs daily injections of insulin.

At present, scientists do not know exactly what causes the body's immune system to attack the beta cells, but they believe that both genetic factors and viruses may be involved. IDDM accounts for 5 to 10 percent of diagnosed diabetes in the United States.

IDDM develops most often in children or young adults, although the disorder can appear at any age. Symptoms of IDDM usually develop over a short period, although beta cell destruction can begin months, or even years, earlier. Symptoms include increased thirst and urination, constant hunger, weight loss, blurred vision, and great tiredness. If not diagnosed and treated with insulin, the person can lapse into a life-threatening coma.

The most common form of diabetes is Type II, called noninsulin-dependent diabetes (NIDDM). Ninety to 95 percent of people with diabetes have NIDDM. This form of diabetes usually develops in adults over the age of 40, and it is most common among adults over 55. About 80 percent of people with NIDDM are overweight.

In NIDDM, the pancreas usually produces insulin, but for some reason, the body cannot use the insulin effectively. The end result is the same as for IDDM—an unhealthy buildup of glucose in the blood and an inability of the body to make efficient use of its main source of fuel.

The symptoms of NIDDM appear to develop gradually, and they tend to be vague and not as noticeable as in IDDM. Symptoms include feelings of tiredness or illness, frequent urination, especially at night, unusual thirst, weight loss, blurred vision, frequent infections, and slow healing of sores.

A third form of diabetes, called gestational diabetes, develops or is discovered during pregnancy. The diabetes usually disappears when the pregnancy is over, but women who have had gestational diabetes have an increased risk of developing NIDDM later in their lives.

Diabetes is not contagious. It cannot be "caught" from another person. However, having a family history of diabetes places a person at higher risk for diabetes, especially NIDDM. Other risk factors for NIDDM include being overweight, older, and of black, Hispanic, or Native American origin.

Scope and Impact of Diabetes

Diabetes is widely recognized as one of the leading causes of death and disability in the United States. In 1991, diabetes caused or contributed to more than 200,000 deaths. The true toll is probably much higher because diabetes was not listed on half of the death certificates for people who had diabetes. Diabetes is associated with long-term complications that affect almost every major part of the body. It can cause blindness, heart disease, strokes, kidney failure, amputations, nerve damage, and birth defects in babies born to women with diabetes.

In terms of medical care, treatment supplies, hospitalizations, time lost from work, disability payments, and premature death, diabetes cost this country $92 billion in 1992.

Who gets diabetes?

Diabetes can develop in people of any age or ethnic background, although some groups appear to be at higher risk for certain types of diabetes. IDDM occurs equally among males and females, and it is more common in the white, non-Hispanic population. Although worldwide statistics are not available, it appears that IDDM is unknown or rare in some ethnic groups, including some Asian, African, and Native American populations. On the other hand, some northern European countries, including Finland and Sweden, have very high rates of IDDM. The reasons for these differences are not known.

NIDDM is more common in older people, especially older women, and it occurs more often among blacks, Hispanics, and Native Americans. Compared with non-Hispanic whites, diabetes rates are 60 percent higher in U.S. blacks and 110 to 120 percent higher in Mexican Americans and Puerto Ricans. Native Americans have the highest rates of diabetes in the world. In one tribe, the Pima Indians, half of all adults have NIDDM. The rate of diabetes is likely to increase because older people, Hispanics, and other minority people make up the fastest growing parts of the U.S. population.

Treatment of Diabetes

Before the discovery of insulin in 1921, all people with IDDM died within a few years of the onset of their disease. Although insulin is not considered a cure for diabetes, its discovery was the first major breakthrough in diabetes treatment. Today, daily injections of insulin are the basic therapy for IDDM. Insulin injections must be balanced with diet and mealtimes, exercise, and daily testing of blood glucose levels, with insulin dosage levels adjusted as needed. Diet, exercise, and blood or urine testing for glucose form the basis for management of NIDDM. In addition, some people with NIDDM take oral drugs or insulin to lower their blood glucose levels.

However, people with diabetes try to avoid having blood glucose levels that are too low. This condition is known as hypoglycemia. When blood glucose levels drop too low, the person may become nervous and shaky, judgment may be impaired, and eventually the person could pass out. The treatment for hypoglycemia is to eat or drink something with sugar in it. When the opposite happens and blood glucose levels rise too high, a condition known as hyperglycemia, the body may form ketones and the person becomes very ill. Hypoglycemia and hyperglycemia, which can occur in people with IDDM or NIDDM, are potentially life-threatening emergencies.

People with diabetes are responsible for their day-to-day care. They should also be under the general care of a doctor who monitors their diabetes control and checks for diabetes complications. Doctors that specialize in diabetes are called endocrinologists or diabetologists. In addition, people with diabetes often see other specialists such as ophthalmologists for eye examinations, podiatrists for foot care, dietitians for meal planning guidance, and diabetes educators for instruction in day-to-day care.

The goal of diabetes management is to keep blood glucose levels as close to the normal (nondiabetic) range as possible. A recent Government study, sponsored by the National Institute of Diabetes and Digestive and Kidney Diseases (NIDDK), has proved that lowering blood glucose levels to the normal range reduces the risk of developing major complications of diabetes.

The 10-year study, called the Diabetes Control and Complications Trial (DCCT), was completed in 1993 and included 1,441 individuals with IDDM. The DCCT compared two treatment approaches: conventional management, which aims mainly to avoid extremely high or low blood glucose levels, and intensive management, which focuses on keeping blood glucose levels as close to normal as possible. The purpose of the study was to determine whether intensive management of diabetes affects the development and severity of eye, kidney, and nerve complications of diabetes. The study findings showed that persons in the intensively managed group had significantly lower rates of these complications. Researchers believe that DCCT findings have important implications for the treatment of NIDDM, as well as IDDM.

Research on Diabetes

The DCCT is one of many research programs being carried out by the Federal Government and by nongovernment organizations to improve the health and well-being of people with diabetes and to find ways to prevent and cure the disorder.

The NIDDK supports basic and clinical research in its own laboratories, in research centers, and at hospitals throughout the United States. The NIDDK also gathers and analyzes statistics about diabetes. Other NIH Institutes carry out research on diabetes-related eye diseases, heart and vascular complications, pregnancy, and dental problems. Other Government agencies that sponsor diabetes programs are the Centers for Disease Control and Prevention, the Indian Health Service, the Health Resources and Services Administration, and the Department of Veterans Affairs.

Many organizations outside of the Government support diabetes research and education activities. These organizations include the American Diabetes Association, the Juvenile Diabetes Foundation International, the American Association of Diabetes Educators, the Joslin Diabetes Center, the International Diabetes Center, the Barbara Davis Center for Childhood Diabetes, drug companies that develop diabetes products, and many other groups.

In the past 15 years, advances in diabetes research have led to better ways to manage diabetes and treat its complications. Major advances include

- New forms of purified insulin such as human insulin produced through genetic engineering.
- Development of better ways for doctors to monitor blood glucose levels and for people with diabetes to test their own blood glucose levels at home.
- Development of external and implantable insulin pumps that deliver appropriate amounts of insulin, replacing daily injections.
- The use of laser treatment for diabetic eye disease, reducing the risk of blindness.
- Successful transplantation of kidneys in people whose own kidneys failed because of diabetes.
- Better ways of managing diabetic pregnancies, improving chances of a successful outcome.
- Development of new drugs to treat NIDDM and better ways to manage this form of diabetes through weight control.
- Proof that intensive management of blood glucose levels reduces and may prevent development of microvascular complications of diabetes.
- Firm evidence that antihypertensive drugs called ACE-inhibitors prevent or delay kidney failure in people with diabetes.

In the future, insulin may be administered through nasal sprays or taken in the form of a pill. Devices to "read" blood glucose levels without having to prick a finger to get a blood sample are also being developed.

Research is ongoing to find the cause or causes of diabetes and ways to prevent and cure the disorder. Scientists are searching for genes that may be involved in NIDDM and IDDM. Some genetic markers for IDDM have been identified, and it is now possible to screen relatives of people with IDDM to see if they are at risk for diabetes. Studies are now under way using drugs that stop the immune system from attacking the beta cells to try to prevent IDDM from developing in people who are at high risk for the disorder. One substance currently under study as a preventive is glutamic acid decarboxylase, also called GAD.

Transplantation of the pancreas or insulin-producing beta cells offers the best hope of cure for people with IDDM. Some successful pancreas transplants have been performed. However, people who have transplants must take powerful drugs that prevent rejection of the transplanted organ. These drugs are costly and may eventually cause serious health problems. Scientists are working to develop less harmful drugs and better methods of transplanting pancreatic tissue to prevent rejection by the body.

Some methods under study include encapsulating the beta cells in a semi-permeable membrane to protect them from immune attack; implanting the cells in the thymus gland as a way of inducing tolerance by the immune system; and

using techniques of bioengineering to create artificial beta cells that secrete insulin in response to glucose.

For NIDDM, the focus is on ways to prevent diabetes. Preventive approaches include identifying people at high risk for the disorder and encouraging them to lose weight, exercise more, and follow a healthy diet.

Additional Resources About Diabetes

More information about diabetes, including pamphlets about IDDM, NIDDM, gestational diabetes, diabetes research, statistics about diabetes, and diabetes education, is available from

National Diabetes Information Clearinghouse
1 Information Way
Bethesda, Maryland 20892-3560

The following organizations also distribute materials and support programs for people with diabetes and their families and friends:

American Association of Diabetes Educators
444 N Michigan Avenue, Suite 1240
Chicago, IL 60611
(800) 832-6874
(312) 644-2233

American Diabetes Association
ADA National Service Center
1660 Duke Street
Alexandria, VA 22314
(800) 232-3472
(703) 549-1500

Juvenile Diabetes Foundation International
432 Park Avenue South
New York, NY 10016-8013
(800) 223-1138
(212) 889-7575

■ **Document Source:**
U.S. Department of Health and Human Services, Public Health Service
National Institutes of Health
National Institute of Diabetes and Digestive and Kidney Diseases
NIH Publication No. 94-3235
April 1994

See also: Diabetic Neuropathy: The Nerve Damage of Diabetes (page 132); Hypoglycemia (page 138); Insulin-Dependent Diabetes (page 140); Kidney Disease of Diabetes (page 150); Diabetic Retinopathy (page 167)

DIABETIC NEUROPATHY: THE NERVE DAMAGE OF DIABETES

What is diabetic neuropathy?

Diabetic neuropathy is a nerve disorder caused by diabetes. Symptoms of neuropathy include numbness and sometimes pain in the hands, feet, or legs. Nerve damage caused by diabetes can also lead to problems with internal organs such as the digestive tract, heart, and sexual organs causing indigestion, diarrhea or constipation, dizziness, bladder infections, and impotence. In some cases, neuropathy can flare up suddenly, causing weakness and weight loss. Depression may follow. While some treatments are available, a great deal of research is still needed to understand how diabetes affects the nerves and to find more effective treatments for this complication.

How common is diabetic neuropathy?

People with diabetes can develop nerve problems at any time. Significant clinical neuropathy can develop within the first 10 years after diagnosis of diabetes and the risk of developing neuropathy increases the longer a person has diabetes. Some recent studies have reported that

- 60 percent of patients with diabetes have some form of neuropathy, but in most cases (30 to 40 percent), there are no symptoms.
- 30 to 40 percent of patients with diabetes have symptoms suggesting neuropathy, compared with 10 percent of people without diabetes.

Diabetic neuropathy appears to be more common in smokers, people over 40 years of age, and those who have had problems controlling their blood glucose levels.

What causes diabetic neuropathy?

Scientists do not know what causes diabetic neuropathy, but several factors are likely to contribute to the disorder. High blood glucose, a condition associated with diabetes, causes chemical changes in nerves. These changes impair the nerves' ability to transmit signals. High blood glucose also damages blood vessels that carry oxygen and nutrients to the nerves. In addition, inherited factors probably unrelated to diabetes may make some people more susceptible to nerve disease than others.

How high blood glucose leads to nerve damage is a subject of intense research. The precise mechanism is not known. Researchers have discovered that high glucose levels affect many metabolic pathways in the nerves, leading to an accumulation of a sugar called sorbitol and depletion of a substance called myoinositol. However, studies in humans have not shown convincingly that these changes are the mechanism that causes nerve damage.

More recently, researchers have focused on the effects of excessive glucose metabolism on the amount of nitrous oxide in nerves. Nitrous oxide dilates blood vessels. In a person with diabetes, low levels of nitrous oxide may lead to constriction of blood vessels supplying the nerve, contributing to nerve damage. Another promising area of research centers on the effect of high glucose attaching to proteins, altering the structure and function of the proteins and affecting vascular function.

Scientists are studying how these changes occur, how they are connected, how they cause nerve damage, and how to prevent and treat damage.

What are the symptoms of diabetic neuropathy?

The symptoms of diabetic neuropathy vary. Numbness and tingling in feet are often the first sign. Some people notice no symptoms, while others are severely disabled. Neuropathy may cause both pain and insensitivity to pain in the same person. Often, symptoms are slight at first, and since most nerve damage occurs over a period of years, mild cases may go unnoticed for a long time. In some people, mainly those afflicted by focal neuropathy, the onset of pain may be sudden and severe.

What are the major types of neuropathy?

The symptoms of neuropathy also depend on which nerves and what part of the body is affected. Neuropathy may be diffuse, affecting many parts of the body, or focal, affecting a single, specific nerve and part of the body.

Diffuse Neuropathy

The two categories of diffuse neuropathy are peripheral neuropathy affecting the feet and hands and autonomic neuropathy affecting the internal organs.

Peripheral Neuropathy

The most common type of peripheral neuropathy damages the nerves of the limbs, especially the feet. Nerves on both sides of the body are affected. Common symptoms of this kind of neuropathy are

- Numbness or insensitivity to pain or temperature
- Tingling, burning, or prickling
- Sharp pains or cramps
- Extreme sensitivity to touch, even light touch
- Loss of balance and coordination

These symptoms are often worse at night.

The damage to nerves often results in loss of reflexes and muscle weakness. The foot often becomes wider and shorter, the gait changes, and foot ulcers appear as pressure is put on parts of the foot that are less protected. Because of the loss of sensation, injuries may go unnoticed and often become infected. If ulcers or foot injuries are not treated in time, the infection may involve the bone and require amputation. However, problems caused by minor injuries can usually be controlled if they are caught in time. Avoiding foot injury by wearing well-fitted shoes and examining the feet daily can help prevent amputations.

Autonomic Neuropathy

(Also called visceral neuropathy)
Autonomic neuropathy is another form of diffuse neuropathy. It affects the nerves that serve the heart and internal organs and produces changes in many processes and systems.

Urination and Sexual Response

Autonomic neuropathy most often affects the organs that control urination and sexual function. Nerve damage can prevent the bladder from emptying completely, so bacteria grow more easily in the urinary tract (bladder and kidneys). When the nerves of the bladder are damaged, a person may have difficulty knowing when the bladder is full or controlling it, resulting in urinary incontinence.

The nerve damage and circulatory problems of diabetes can also lead to a gradual loss of sexual response in both men and women, although sex drive is unchanged. A man may be unable to have erections or may reach sexual climax without ejaculating normally.

Digestion

Autonomic neuropathy can affect digestion. Nerve damage can cause the stomach to empty too slowly, a disorder called gastric stasis. When the condition is severe (gastroparesis), a person can have persistent nausea and vomiting, bloating, and loss of appetite. Blood glucose levels tend to fluctuate greatly with this condition.

If nerves in the esophagus are involved, swallowing may be difficult. Nerve damage to the bowels can cause constipation or frequent diarrhea, especially at night. Problems with the digestive system often lead to weight loss.

Cardiovascular System

Autonomic neuropathy can affect the cardiovascular system, which controls the circulation of blood throughout the body. Damage to this system interferes with the nerve impulses from various parts of the body that signal the need for blood and regulate blood pressure and heart rate. As a result, blood pressure may drop sharply after sitting or standing, causing a person to feel dizzy or light-headed, or even to faint (orthostatic hypotension).

Neuropathy that affects the cardiovascular system may also affect the perception of pain from heart disease. People may not experience angina as a warning sign of heart disease or may suffer painless heart attacks. It may also raise the risk of a heart attack during general anesthesia.

Hypoglycemia

Autonomic neuropathy can hinder the body's normal response to low blood sugar or hypoglycemia, which makes it difficult to recognize and treat an insulin reaction.

Sweating

Autonomic neuropathy can affect the nerves that control sweating. Sometimes, nerve damage interferes with the activity of the sweat glands, making it difficult for the body to regulate its temperature. Other times, the result can be profuse sweating at night or while eating (gustatory sweating).

Focal Neuropathy

(Including multiplex neuropathy)
Occasionally, diabetic neuropathy appears suddenly and affects specific nerves, most often in the torso, leg, or head. Focal neuropathy may cause

- Pain in the front of a thigh
- Severe pain in the lower back or pelvis
- Pain in the chest, stomach, or flank
- Chest or abdominal pain sometimes mistaken for angina, heart attack, or appendicitis
- Aching behind an eye
- Inability to focus the eye
- Double vision
- Paralysis on one side of the face (Bell's palsy)
- Problems with hearing

This kind of neuropathy is unpredictable and occurs most often in older people who have mild diabetes. Although focal neuropathy can be painful, it tends to improve by itself after a period of weeks or months without causing long-term damage.

People with diabetes are also prone to developing compression neuropathies. The most common form of compression neuropathy is carpal tunnel syndrome. Asymptomatic carpal tunnel syndrome occurs in 20 to 30 percent of people with diabetes, and symptomatic carpal tunnel syndrome occurs in 6 to 11 percent. Numbness and tingling of the hand are the most common symptoms. Muscle weakness may also develop.

How do doctors diagnose diabetic neuropathy?

A doctor diagnoses neuropathy based on symptoms and a physical exam. During the exam, the doctor may check muscle strength, reflexes, and sensitivity to position, vibration, temperature, and light touch. Sometimes special tests are also used to help determine the cause of symptoms and to suggest treatment.

A simple screening test to check point sensation in the feet can be done in the doctor's office. The test uses a nylon filament mounted on a small wand. The filament delivers a standardized 10-gram force when touched to areas of the foot. Patients who cannot sense pressure from the filament have lost protective sensation and are at risk for developing neuropathic foot ulcers. Physicians may order the filament (with instructions for use) free from the Gillis W. Long Hansen's Disease Center, LEAP Program, 5445 Point Clair Road, Carville, Louisiana 70721; telephone 504-642-4714.

Nerve conduction studies check the flow of electrical current through a nerve. With this test, an image of the nerve impulse is projected on a screen as it transmits an electrical signal. Impulses that seem slower or weaker than usual indicate possible damage to the nerve. This test allows the doctor to assess the condition of all the nerves in the arms and legs.

Electromyography (EMG) is used to see how well muscles respond to electrical impulses transmitted by nearby nerves. The electrical activity of the muscle is displayed on a screen. A response that is slower or weaker than usual suggests damage to the nerve or muscle. This test is often done at the same time as nerve conduction studies.

Ultrasound employs sound waves. The sound waves are too high to hear, but they produce an image showing how well the bladder and other parts of the urinary tract are functioning.

Nerve biopsy involves removing a sample of nerve tissue for examination. This test is most often used in research settings.

If your doctor suspects autonomic neuropathy, you may also be referred to a physician who specializes in digestive disorders (gastroenterologist) for additional tests.

How is diabetic neuropathy usually treated?

Treatment aims to relieve discomfort and prevent further tissue damage. The first step is to bring blood sugar under control by diet and oral drugs or insulin injections, if needed, and by careful monitoring of blood sugar levels. Although symptoms can sometimes worsen at first as blood sugar is brought under control, maintaining lower blood sugar levels helps reverse the pain or loss of sensation that neuropathy can cause. Good control of blood sugar may also help prevent or delay the onset of further problems.

Another important part of treatment involves special care of the feet, which are prone to problems.

A number of medications and other approaches are used to relieve the symptoms of diabetic neuropathy.

Relief of Pain

For relief of pain, burning, tingling, or numbness, the doctor may suggest an analgesic such as aspirin or acetaminophen or anti-inflammatory drugs containing ibuprofen. Nonsteroidal anti-inflammatory drugs should be used with caution in people with renal disease. Antidepressant medications such as amitriptyline (sometimes used with fluphenazine) or nerve medications such as carbamazepine or phenytoin sodium may be helpful. Codeine is sometimes prescribed for short-term use to relieve severe pain. In addition, a topical cream, capsaicin, is now available to help relieve the pain of neuropathy.

The doctor may also prescribe a therapy known as transcutaneous electronic nerve stimulations (TENS). In this treatment, small amounts of electricity block pain signals as they pass through a patient's skin. Other treatments include hypnosis, relaxation training, biofeedback, and acupuncture. Some people find that walking regularly or using elastic stockings helps relieve leg pain. Warm (not hot) baths, massage, or an analgesic ointment such as Ben Gay may also help.

Gastrointestinal Problems

Indigestion, belching, nausea or vomiting are symptoms of gastroparesis. For patients with mild symptoms of slow stomach emptying, doctors suggest eating small, frequent meals and avoiding fats. Eating less fiber may also relieve symptoms. For patients with severe gastroparesis, the doctor may prescribe metoclopramide, which speeds digestion and helps relieve nausea. Other drugs that help regulate digestion or reduce stomach acid secretion may also be used or erythromycine may be prescribed. In each case, the potential benefits of these drugs need to be weighed against their side effects.

To relieve diarrhea or other bowel problems, antibiotics or clonidine HCl, a drug used to treat high blood pressure, are sometimes prescribed. The antibiotic tetracycline may be prescribed. A wheat-free diet may also bring relief since the gluten in flour sometimes causes diarrhea.

Neurological problems affecting the urinary tract can result in infections or incontinence. The doctor may prescribe an antibiotic to clear up an infection and suggest drinking more fluids to prevent further infections. If incontinence is a problem, patients may be advised to urinate at regular times (every three hours, for example) since they may not be able to tell when the bladder is full.

Dizziness, Weakness

Sitting or standing slowly may help prevent light-headedness, dizziness, or fainting, which are symptoms that may be associated with some forms of autonomic neuropathy. Raising the head of the bed and wearing elastic stockings may also help. Increased salt in the diet and treatment with salt-retaining hormones such as fludrocortisone are other possible approaches. In certain patients, drugs used to treat hypertension can instead raise blood pressure, although predicting which patients will have this paradoxical reaction is difficult.

Muscle weakness or loss of coordination caused by diabetic neuropathy can often be helped by physical therapy.

Urinary and Sexual Problems

Nerve and circulatory problems of diabetes can disrupt normal male sexual function, resulting in impotence. After ruling out a hormonal cause of impotence, the doctor can provide information about methods available to treat impotence caused by neuropathy. Short-term solutions involve using a mechanical vacuum device or injecting a drug called a vasodilator into the penis before sex. Both methods raise blood flow to the penis, making it easier to have and maintain an erection. Surgical procedures, in which an inflatable or semirigid device is implanted in the penis, offer a more permanent solution. For some people, counseling may help relieve the stress caused by neuropathy and thereby help restore sexual function.

In women who feel their sexual life is not satisfactory, the role of diabetic neuropathy is less clear. Illness, vaginal or urinary tract infections, and anxiety about pregnancy complicated by diabetes can interfere with a woman's ability to enjoy intimacy. Infections can be reduced by good blood glucose control. Counseling may also help a woman identify and cope with sexual concerns.

Why is good foot care important for people with diabetic neuropathy?

People with diabetes need to take special care of their feet. Neuropathy and blood vessel disease both increase the risk of foot ulcers. The nerves to the feet are the longest in the body and are most often affected by neuropathy. Because of the loss of sensation caused by neuropathy, sores or injuries to the feet may not be noticed and may become ulcerated.

At least 15 percent of all people with diabetes eventually have a foot ulcer, and 6 out of every 1,000 people with diabetes have an amputation. However, doctors estimate that nearly three quarters of all amputations caused by neuropathy and poor circulation could be prevented with careful foot care.

To prevent foot problems from developing, people with diabetes should follow these rules for foot care:

- Check your feet and toes daily for any cuts, sores, bruises, bumps, or infections—using a mirror if necessary.
- Wash your feet daily, using warm (not hot) water and a mild soap. If you have neuropathy, you should test the water temperature with your wrist before putting your feet in the water. Doctors do not advise soaking your feet for long periods, since you may lose protective calluses. Dry your feet carefully with a soft towel, especially between the toes.
- Cover your feet (except for the skin between the toes) with petroleum jelly, a lotion containing lanolin, or cold cream before putting on shoes and socks. In people with diabetes, the feet tend to sweat less than normal. Using a moisturizer helps prevent dry, cracked skin.
- Wear thick, soft socks and avoid wearing slippery stockings, mended stockings, or stockings with seams.
- Wear shoes that fit your feet well and allow your toes to move. Break in new shoes gradually, wearing them for only an hour at a time at first. After years of neuropathy, as reflexes are lost, the feet are likely to become wider and flatter. If you have difficulty finding shoes that fit, ask your doctor to refer you to a specialist, called a pedorthist, who can provide you with corrective shoes or inserts.
- Examine your shoes before putting them on to make sure they have no tears, sharp edges, or objects in them that might injure your feet.
- Never go barefoot, especially on the beach, hot sand, or rocks.
- Cut your toenails straight across, but be careful not to leave any sharp corners that could cut the next toe.
- Use an emery board or pumice stone to file away dead skin, but do not remove calluses, which act as protective padding. Do not try to cut off any growths yourself, and avoid using harsh chemicals such as wart remover on your feet.
- Test the water temperature with your elbow before stepping in a bath.
- If your feet are cold at night, wear socks. (Do not use heating pads or hot water bottles.)
- Avoid sitting with your legs crossed. Crossing your legs can reduce the flow of blood to the feet.
- Ask your doctor to check your feet at every visit, and call your doctor if you notice that a sore is not healing well.
- If you are not able to take care of your own feet, ask your doctor to recommend a podiatrist (specialist in the care and treatment of feet) who can help.

Are there any experimental treatments for diabetic neuropathy?

Several new drugs under study may eventually prevent or reverse diabetic neuropathy. However, extensive testing is required by the U.S. Food and Drug Administration to establish the safety and efficacy of drugs before they are approved for widespread use.

Researchers are exploring treatment with a compound called myoinositol. Early findings have shown that nerves in diabetic animals and humans have less than normal amounts of this substance. Myoinositol supplements increase the levels of this substance in tissues of diabetic animals, but research is still needed to show any concrete lasting benefits from this treatment.

Another area of research concerns the drug amino-guanidine. In animals, this drug blocks cross-linking of proteins that occurs more quickly than normal in tissues exposed to high levels of glucose. Early clinical tests are under way to determine the effects of aminoguanidine in humans.

One approach that appeared promising involved the use of aldose reductase inhibitors (ARIs). ARIs are a class of drugs that block the formation of the sugar alcohol sorbitol, which is thought to damage nerves. Scientists hoped these drugs would prevent and might even repair nerve damage. But so far, clinical trials have shown that these drugs have major side effects and, consequently, they are not available for clinical use.

Some General Hints

- Ask your doctor to suggest an exercise routine that is right for you. Many people who exercise regularly find the pain of neuropathy less severe. Aside from helping you reach and maintain a healthy weight, exercise also improves the body's use of insulin, helps improve circulation, and strengthens muscles. Check with your doctor before starting exercise that can be hard on your feet, such as running or aerobics.
- If you smoke, try to stop because smoking makes circulatory problems worse and increases the risk of neuropathy and heart disease.
- Reduce the amount of alcohol you drink. Recent research has indicated that as few as four drinks per week can worsen neuropathy.
- Take special care of your feet.

What resources are available for people with diabetic neuropathy?

American Association of Diabetes Educators
444 N Michigan Avenue, Suite 1240
Chicago, IL 60611
(800) 832-6874 or (312) 644-2233

A professional organization that can help individuals locate a diabetes educator in their community.

American Diabetes Association National Service Center
1660 Duke Street
Alexandria, VA 22314
(800) 232-3472 or (703) 549-1500

A private, voluntary organization that fosters public awareness of diabetes and supports and promotes diabetes research and education. The association has printed information on many aspects of diabetes, and local affiliates sponsor community programs. Local affiliates can be found in the telephone directory or through the national office.

American Dietetic Association
216 W Jackson Boulevard
Chicago, IL 60606-6995
(800) 877-1600 or (312) 899-0040

A professional organization that can help individuals locate a registered dietitian in their community.

American Heart Association
7320 Greenville Avenue
Dallas, TX 75231
(800) 242-1793

A private, voluntary organization that distributes literature on heart disease and how to prevent it. Local affiliates can be found in the telephone directory.

Juvenile Diabetes Foundation International
381 Park Avenue South, Suite 507
New York, NY 10016-8013
(212) 689-2860 or (800) 223-1138

A private, voluntary organization that funds research on diabetes and promotes public awareness. Local chapters located across the country sponsor programs and fund-raising activities. Information about local groups is available in telephone directories or from the national office.

National Diabetes Information Clearinghouse
1 Information Way
Bethesda, MD 20892-3560
(301) 654-3327

A program of the National Institute of Diabetes and Digestive and Kidney Diseases, the Federal Government's lead agency for diabetes research. The clearinghouse distributes a variety of publications to the public and to health professionals.

Additional Reading

For more information about diabetic neuropathy and diabetes research:

Albert, L., Restraining pain: What's available for easing the pain of diabetic neuropathy, Diabetes Forecast, January 1988, pp. 39-41.

American Diabetes Association and the American Academy of Neurology, Report and recommendations of the San Antonio Conference on Diabetic Neuropathy, Diabetes Care, July/August 1988, pp. 592-597.

Bell, D. & Clements, R., Diabetes and the digestive system, Diabetes Forecast, December 1987, pp. 43-46.

Clark, C.M., & Lee, D.A., Prevention and treatment of the complications of diabetes mellitus, The New England Journal of Medicine, May 4, 1995, pp. 1210-1218.

Cohen, M. et al., Managing diabetes complications, Patient Care, December 15, 1988, pp. 28-39.

Dyck, P. J., Aldose reductase inhibitors and diabetic neuropathy, Diabetes Forecast, May 1989, pp. 41-43.

Dyck, P. J., Resolvable problems in diabetic neuropathy, The Journal of NIH Research, June 1990, pp. 57-62.

Dyck, P. J., Thomas, P.K., and Asbury, A.K., Diabetic Neuropathy, Saunders, W.B., Company, 1987.

Gerding, D. et al., Problems in diabetic foot care, Patient Care, August 15, 1988, pp.102-118.

Greene, D., & Stevens, M., Diabetic peripheral neuropathy: New approaches to treatment, classification, and staging, Diabetes Spectrum, July/August 1993, pp. 223-257.

Haase, G. et al., Neuropathy: Diabetic? Nutritional?, Patient Care, May 15, 1990, pp. 112-134.

Jaspan, J. et al., GI complications of diabetes, Patient Care, January 15, 1990, pp.108-128.

Mills, P., Drugs that block complications, Diabetes Self-Management, September/October 1988, pp. 14-16.

National Institute of Diabetes and Digestive and Kidney Diseases. Diabetes Special Report, 1994 (NIH Publication No. 94-3422). Bethesda, MD.

Vinik, A., et al., Diabetic neuropathies, Diabetes Care, December 1992, pp. 1926-1975.

Wakelee-Lynch, J., Relieving pain with peppers, Diabetes Forecast, June 1992, pp. 34-37.

Weiss, R., Behind the pain: Causes and treatment of diabetic neuropathy, Diabetes Interview, November 1993, pp. 1, 12-13.

■ Document Source:
U.S. Department of Health and Human Services, Public Health Service
National Institutes of Health
National Institute of Diabetes and Digestive and Kidney Diseases
NIH Publication No. 95-3185
July 1995

HYPOGLYCEMIA

What is hypoglycemia?

Glucose, a form of sugar, is the body's main fuel. Hypoglycemia, or low blood sugar, occurs when blood levels of glucose drop too low to fuel the body's activity.

Carbohydrates (sugars and starches) are the body's main dietary sources of glucose. During digestion, the glucose is absorbed into the blood stream (hence the term "blood sugar"), which carries it to every cell in the body. Unused glucose is stored in the liver as glycogen.

Hypoglycemia can occur as a complication of diabetes, as a condition in itself, or in association with other disorders.

How does the body control glucose?

The amount of glucose in the blood is controlled mainly by the hormones insulin and glucagon. Too much or too little of these hormones can cause blood sugar levels to fall too low (hypoglycemia) or rise too high (hyperglycemia). Other hormones that influence blood sugar levels are cortisol, growth hormone, and catecholamines (epinephrine and norepinephrine).

The pancreas, a gland in the upper abdomen, produces insulin and glucagon. The pancreas is dotted with hormone-producing tissue called the islets of Langerhans, which contain alpha and beta cells. When blood sugar rises after a meal, the beta cells release insulin. The insulin helps glucose enter body cells, lowering blood levels of glucose to the normal range. When blood sugar drops too low, the alpha cells secrete glucagon. This signals the liver to release stored glycogen and change it back to glucose, raising blood sugar levels to the normal range. Muscles also store glycogen that can be converted to glucose.

Blood Sugar Range

The normal range for blood sugar is about 60 mg/dl (milligrams of glucose per deciliter of blood) to 120 mg/dl, depending on when a person last ate. In the fasting state, blood sugar can occasionally fall below 60 mg/dl and even to below 50 mg/dl and not indicate a serious abnormality or disease. This can be seen in healthy women, particularly after prolonged fasting. Blood sugar levels below 45 mg/dl are almost always associated with a serious abnormality.

What are the symptoms of hypoglycemia?

A person with hypoglycemia may feel weak, drowsy, confused, hungry, and dizzy. Paleness, headache, irritability, trembling, sweating, rapid heart beat, and a cold, clammy feeling are also signs of low blood sugar. In severe cases, a person can lose consciousness and even lapse into a coma.

The symptoms associated with hypoglycemia are sometimes mistaken for symptoms caused by conditions not related to blood sugar. For example, unusual stress and anxiety can cause excess production of catecholamines, resulting in symptoms similar to those caused by hypoglycemia but having no relation to blood sugar levels.

Hypoglycemia in Diabetes

The most common cause of hypoglycemia is as a complication of diabetes. Diabetes occurs when the body cannot use glucose for fuel because either the pancreas is not able to make enough insulin or the insulin that is available is not effective. As a result, glucose builds up in the blood instead of getting into body cells.

The aim of treatment in diabetes is to lower high blood sugar levels. To do this, people with diabetes may use insulin or oral drugs, depending on the type of diabetes they have or the severity of their condition. Hypoglycemia occurs most often in people who use insulin to lower their blood sugar. All people with insulin-dependent diabetes (IDDM or Type I) and some people with noninsulin-dependent diabetes (NIDDM or Type II) use insulin. People with Type II diabetes who take oral drugs called sulfonylureas are also vulnerable to low blood sugar episodes.

Conditions that can lead to hypoglycemia in people with diabetes include taking too much medication, missing or delaying a meal, eating too little food for the amount of insulin taken, exercising too strenuously, drinking too much alcohol, or any combination of these factors. People who have diabetes often refer to hypoglycemia as an "insulin reaction."

Managing Hypoglycemia in Diabetes

People with diabetes should consult their health care providers for individual guidelines on target blood sugar ranges that are best for them. The lowest safe blood sugar level for an individual varies, depending on the person's age, medical condition, and ability to sense hypoglycemic symptoms. A target range that is safe for a young adult with no diabetes complications, for example, may be too low for a young child or an older person who may have other medical problems.

Because they are attuned to the symptoms, people with diabetes can usually recognize when their blood sugar levels are dropping too low. They can treat the condition quickly by eating or drinking something with sugar in it such as candy, juice, or nondiet soda. Taking glucose tablets or gels (available in drug stores) is another convenient and quick way to treat hypoglycemia.

People with IDDM are most vulnerable to severe insulin reactions, which can cause loss of consciousness. A few patients with long-standing insulin-dependent diabetes may develop a condition known as hypoglycemia unawareness, in which they have difficulty recognizing the symptoms of low blood sugar. For emergency use in patients with IDDM, physicians often prescribe an injectable form of the hormone glucagon. A glucagon injection (given by another person) quickly eases the symptoms of low blood sugar, releasing a burst of glucose into the blood.

Emergency medical help may be needed if the person does not recover in a few minutes after treatment for hypoglycemia. A person suffering a severe insulin reaction may be admitted to the hospital so that blood sugar can be stabilized.

People with diabetes can reduce or prevent episodes of hypoglycemia by monitoring their blood sugar levels frequently and learning to recognize the symptoms of low blood sugar and the situations that may trigger it. They should consult their health care providers for advice about the best way to treat low blood sugar. Friends and relatives should know about the symptoms of hypoglycemia and how to treat it in case of emergency.

Episodes of hypoglycemia in people with IDDM may become more common now that research has shown that carefully controlled blood sugar helps prevent the complications of diabetes. Keeping blood sugar in a close-to-normal range requires multiple injections of insulin each day or use of an insulin pump, frequent testing of blood glucose, a diet and exercise plan, and guidance from health care professionals.

Other Causes of Hypoglycemia

Hypoglycemia in people who do not have diabetes is far less common than once believed. However, it can occur in some people under certain conditions such as early pregnancy, prolonged fasting, and long periods of strenuous exercise. People on beta blocker medications who exercise are at higher risk of hypoglycemia, and aspirin can induce hypoglycemia in some children. Drinking alcohol can cause blood sugar to drop in some sensitive individuals, and hypoglycemia has been well documented in chronic alcoholics and binge drinkers. Eating unripe ackee fruit from Jamaica is a rare cause of low blood sugar.

Diagnosis

To diagnose hypoglycemia in people who do not have diabetes, the doctor looks for the following three conditions:

- The patient complains of symptoms of hypoglycemia
- Blood glucose levels are measured while the person is experiencing those symptoms and found to be 45 mg/dl or less in a woman or 55 mg/dl or less in a man
- The symptoms are promptly relieved upon ingestion of sugar

For many years, the oral glucose tolerance test (OGTT) was used to diagnose hypoglycemia. Experts now realize that the OGTT can actually trigger hypoglycemic symptoms in people with no signs of the disorder. For a more accurate diagnosis, experts now recommend that blood sugar be tested at the same time a person is experiencing hypoglycemic

symptoms. The doctor will also check the patient for health conditions such as diabetes, obtain a medication history, and assess the degree and severity of the patient's symptoms. Laboratory tests to measure insulin production and levels of C-peptide (a substance that the pancreas releases into the bloodstream in equal amounts to insulin) may be performed.

Reactive Hypoglycemia

A diagnosis of reactive hypoglycemia is considered only after other possible causes of low blood sugar have been ruled out. Reactive hypoglycemia with no known cause is a condition in which the symptoms of low blood sugar appear two to five hours after eating foods high in glucose.

Ten to 20 years ago, hypoglycemia was a popular diagnosis. However, studies now show that this condition is actually quite rare. In these studies, most patients who experienced the symptoms of hypoglycemia after eating glucose-rich foods consistently had normal levels of blood sugar—above 60 mg/dl. Some researchers have suggested that some people may be extra sensitive to the body's normal release of the hormone epinephrine after a meal.

People with symptoms of reactive hypoglycemia unrelated to other medical conditions or problems are usually advised to follow a healthy eating plan. The doctor or dietitian may suggest that such a person avoid foods high in carbohydrates; eat small, frequent meals and snacks throughout the day; exercise regularly; and eat a variety of foods, including whole grains, vegetables, and fruits.

Rare Causes of Hypoglycemia

Fasting hypoglycemia occurs when the stomach is empty. It usually develops in the early morning when a person awakens. As with other forms of hypoglycemia, the symptoms include headache, lack of energy, and an inability to concentrate. Fasting hypoglycemia may be caused by a variety of conditions such as hereditary enzyme or hormone deficiencies, liver disease, and insulin-producing tumors.

In hereditary fructose intolerance, a disorder usually seen in children, the body is unable to metabolize the natural sugar fructose. Attacks of hypoglycemia, marked by seizures, vomiting, and unconsciousness, are treated by giving glucose and eliminating fructose from the diet.

Galactosemia, a rare genetic disorder, hampers the body's ability to process the sugar galactose. An infant with this disorder may appear normal at birth, but after a few days or weeks of drinking milk (which contains galactose), the child may begin to vomit, lose weight, and develop cataracts. The liver may fail to release stored glycogen into the blood, triggering hypoglycemia. Removing milk from the diet is the usual treatment.

A deficiency of growth hormone causes increased sensitivity to insulin. This sensitivity occurs because growth hormone opposes the action of insulin on muscle and fat cells. For this reason, children with growth hormone deficiency sometimes suffer from hypoglycemia, which goes away after treatment.

People with insulin-producing tumors, which arise in the islet cells of the pancreas, suffer from severe episodes of hypoglycemia.

To diagnose these tumors, called insulinomas, a doctor will put the patient on a 24- to 72-hour fast while measuring blood levels of glucose, insulin, and proinsulin. High levels of insulin and proinsulin in the presence of low levels of glucose strongly suggest an insulin-producing tumor. These tumors are usually benign and can be surgically removed.

In rare cases, some cancers such as breast cancer and adrenal cancer may cause hypoglycemia through secretion of a hormone called insulin-like growth factor II. The treatment is removal of the tumor, if possible.

Research

The National Institute of Diabetes and Digestive and Kidney Diseases (NIDDK) was established by Congress in 1950 as one of the National Institutes of Health, the research arm of the Public Health Service under the U.S. Department of Health and Human Services.

The NIDDK conducts and supports research in diabetes, glucose metabolism, insulin action, and the hormonal controls of blood sugar. Current studies also focus on fasting hypoglycemia, obesity, and insulin resistance.

Resources on Hypoglycemia

American Diabetes Association (ADA)
National Service Center
1660 Duke Street
Alexandria, VA 22314
(800) 232-3472 or (703) 549-1500

The ADA is a private, voluntary organization that fosters public awareness of diabetes and supports and promotes diabetes research and education. The ADA distributes printed information on many aspects of diabetes, and local affiliates sponsor community programs. Local affiliates, located in every state, are listed in telephone directories or can be located by contacting the national office.

The American Dietetic Association
National Center for Nutrition and Dietetics
216 West Jackson Boulevard
Chicago, IL 60606-6995
(800) 366-1655 or (312) 899-0040

The American Dietetic Association is a professional organization for registered dietitians. It publishes a variety of materials for patient and professional education and supports an information and referral service for the general public.

Juvenile Diabetes Foundation (JDF) International
432 Park Avenue, South
New York, NY 10016
(800) 223-1138 or (212) 889-7575

The JDF is a private, voluntary organization that promotes research and public education in diabetes, primarily insulin-dependent diabetes. Local chapters, located across the country, are listed in telephone directories or can be found by contacting the national office.

National Diabetes Information Clearinghouse (NDIC)
1 Information Way
Bethesda, MD 20892-3560

The NDIC is a service of NIDDK. The clearinghouse distributes a variety of diabetes-related materials to the public and to health professionals, including a literature search listing publications and articles about hypoglycemia in diabetes.

Additional Readings

Bennion, Lynn J., "Hypoglycemia: A diagnostic challenge," Clinical Diabetes, July/August 1985, pp. 85-90.

DCCT Research Group, "Epidemiology of severe hypoglycemia in the diabetes control and complications trial," The American Journal of Medicine, vol. 90, April 1991, pp. 450-459.

Field, James B., "Hypoglycemia: Definition, clinical presentations, classifications and laboratory tests," in Endocrinology and Metabolism Clinics of North America, vol. 18, no. 1, March 1989.

Foster, Daniel & Rubenstein, Arthur, "Hypoglycemia, insulinoma, and other hormone-secreting tumors of the pancreas" in Principles of Internal Medicine. Ed. E. Braunwald et al [K. J. Isselbacher, R. G. Petersdorf, J. D. Wilson, J. B. Martin, & A. S. Fauci] McGraw-Hill Book Company, 1987, pp. 1800-1807.

Metz, Robert J., "Is the problem hypoglycemia?" Patient Care, Oct. 15, 1983, pp. 61-89.

Nelson, Roger L., "Oral glucose tolerance test: Indications and limitations," Mayo Clinic Proceedings, vol. 63, 1988, pp. 263-269.

Palardy, Jean et al., "Blood glucose measurements during symptomatic episodes in patients with suspected postprandial hypoglycemia," New England Journal of Medicine, Nov. 23, 1989, pp. 1421-1425.

Service, F. John, "Hypoglycemic Disorders," New England Journal of Medicine, April 27, 1995, pp. 1144-1152.

Service, F. John, "Hypoglycemia," in Cecil's Textbook of Medicine. James B. Wyngaarden & Lloyd H. Smith, Jr. (Eds). W. B. Saunders Company, 1988, pp. 1381-1387.

Service, F. John, "Hypoglycemia and the postprandial syndrome," New England Journal of Medicine, (Editorial), Nov. 23, 1989, pp. 1472-1474.

■ **Document Source:**
U.S. Department of Health and Human Services, Public Health Service
National Institutes of Health
National Institute of Diabetes and Digestive and Kidney Diseases
NIH Publication No. 95-3926
May 1995

INSULIN-DEPENDENT DIABETES

What is diabetes?

Diabetes is a group of conditions in which glucose (sugar) levels are abnormally high. Diabetes occurs when the pancreas stops making enough insulin, which is necessary for the proper metabolism of digested foods.

About 14 million people in the United States have some form of diabetes, although only half are diagnosed. The three main types of diabetes are insulin-dependent, also known as Type I diabetes; noninsulin-dependent, also called Type II diabetes; and gestational diabetes, which occurs during pregnancy.

Insulin-dependent diabetes mellitus (IDDM) most often develops in children and young adults. Sometimes people over age 40 get IDDM, but it usually begins at younger ages. For this reason, IDDM used to be known as "juvenile" diabetes. IDDM is one of the most common chronic disorders in U.S. children. Each year, from 11,000 to 12,000 children are diagnosed with IDDM. Among the more than 7 million people in the United States who are being treated for diabetes, about 5 to 10 percent have IDDM.

Noninsulin-dependent diabetes mellitus (NIDDM) is the most common type of diabetes. It accounts for 90 to 95 percent of diagnosed diabetes and almost all of undiagnosed diabetes. NIDDM usually develops in adults over age 40 and is most common in those who are overweight. People with NIDDM usually produce some insulin, but the body cells cannot use it efficiently because the cells are resistant to the insulin. By losing weight, exercising, or taking oral medications, most people with NIDDM can overcome this resistance to insulin. However, some people with NIDDM require daily insulin injections.

Gestational diabetes occurs in some women during pregnancy. It usually ends after the baby is born, but women with gestational diabetes may develop NIDDM when they get older. Gestational diabetes results from the body's resistance to the action of insulin. This resistance is caused by hormones the placenta produces during pregnancy. The condition develops about midway through the pregnancy. Gestational diabetes is usually treated with diet. Some women may need insulin. Gestational diabetes cannot be treated with pills that lower blood glucose as these medicines can cause harm to the baby.

This booklet is about insulin-dependent diabetes, or IDDM for short. The word "diabetes" in the text refers to insulin-dependent diabetes unless otherwise noted. This booklet does not replace the advice of a doctor. However, it can help you learn about diabetes and suggest questions to ask a doctor. Local diabetes organizations and clinics that sponsor meetings and educational programs about diabetes can also be helpful. See **Other Resources** for names of groups that have information about diabetes programs.

What causes diabetes?

When we eat, foods containing proteins, fats, and carbohydrates are broken down into simpler, easily absorbed chemicals. One of these is a form of simple sugar called glucose. Glucose circulates in the blood stream where it is available for body cells to use. The body relies on glucose as a source of fuel for important organs such as the brain.

The pancreas, a large gland located behind the stomach, produces the hormone insulin. In people without diabetes, the pancreas makes the correct amount of insulin needed to allow glucose to enter body cells. In people with diabetes, however, not enough insulin is produced. As a result, glucose builds up in blood, overflows into the urine, and passes out of the body unused. Thus, the body loses an important source of fuel—even though the blood contains large amounts of glucose.

Insulin also allows the body to store excess glucose as fat, proteins as muscle protein, and important enzymes that control metabolism. A severe deficiency of insulin causes excess breakdown of stored fats and proteins.

What are the causes and symptoms of IDDM?

Causes of IDDM

In people with insulin-dependent diabetes (IDDM), the pancreas produces too little or no insulin at all. The pancreas is not able to produce insulin because the body's immune system has destroyed the insulin-producing cells.

Scientists do not know why the body's immune system, which allows it to fight disease and other "foreign" substances that may invade the body, attacks and destroys insulin-producing cells. A combination of factors may be involved, including exposure to common viruses or other substances early in life, as well as an inherited risk for IDDM.

Researchers can now test family members of people with IDDM to identify those at increased risk for diabetes. Scientists hope to find a way to prevent the disease through a study called the Diabetes Prevention Trial-Type 1. This study is described in the research section of this text.

Early Symptoms of IDDM

The early symptoms of IDDM can be gradual or sudden. They include frequent urination (particularly at night), increased thirst, unexplained weight loss (in spite of increased appetite), and extreme tiredness. These symptoms are caused by the build-up of sugar in the blood and its loss in the urine.

To eliminate sugar in the urine, the kidney "borrows" water from the body. The loss of this extra sugar and water in the urine results in dehydration, which causes increased thirst. In addition to causing high blood glucose, the lack of insulin causes the body to break down stored fats and proteins. As fats are broken down, the body can convert these fats into waste products called ketones. If ketone production is excessive, abnormal amounts of ketones in the blood can spill into the urine. If blood ketone levels rise too high, a life-threatening condition called ketoacidosis can develop, which requires immediate medical attention. Symptoms of ketoacidosis include abdominal pain, vomiting, rapid breathing, extreme tiredness, and drowsiness.

Points to Remember

The symptoms of IDDM include

- Frequent urination
- Increased thirst
- Increased hunger
- Unexplained weight loss
- Extreme tiredness

Michael is 10 years old. During his summer break from school he noticed he was always thirsty. He drank many glasses of water, milk, juice, or soda after playing baseball, while he watched TV, and with meals. As a result, Michael needed to urinate constantly. He also complained of being very hungry all the time. Michael's parents took him to the doctor. After learning of his symptoms and performing appropriate tests, Michael's doctor said he had insulin-dependent diabetes and would need to begin taking insulin injections, monitoring his blood sugar levels, and watching his diet.

How does a person live with diabetes?

Diabetes requires constant attention and daily care to keep blood sugar levels in balance. Injecting insulin, following a diet, exercising, and testing blood sugar are some of the day-to-day requirements. To feel good and stay healthy, a person with IDDM must follow a daily management routine. For this reason, diabetes is often referred to as a "24-hour" disease. This section provides general guidelines for diabetes management and explains the roles of various health care professionals who can help you manage your diabetes. The treatment recommendations are based on a 10-year study recently completed by the Federal Government called the Diabetes Control and Complications Trial (DCCT).

The Diabetes Control and Complications Trial

Diabetes can affect many parts of the body. Over time, it can damage a person's kidneys, eyes, nerves, and heart. These long-term complications can result in kidney disease, vision loss, nerve damage, heart attack, and other problems. The DCCT proved that lowering blood sugar levels delayed or prevented diabetes complications by 50 to 80 percent.

The DCCT compared two approaches to managing IDDM: intensive and standard treatment. People in the intensive treatment group learned how to adjust their insulin according to food intake and exercise. They injected insulin three to four times a day or used an insulin pump and tested their blood sugar at least four times a day and once a week at three a.m. They also followed a diet and exercise plan and met once a month with a health care team composed of a physician, nurse educator, dietitian, and mental health professional.

People in the standard treatment group followed a plan that was not as strict. They took one or two insulin injections a day, tested sugar levels once or twice a day, and met with the doctor or nurse every three months.

At the end of the DCCT, volunteers on intensive treatment had lower rates of kidney, eye, and nerve damage than volunteers in the standard treatment group. The study showed that efforts to improve control of blood sugar made a major difference. In fact, the study found that any long-term lowering of blood sugar levels will reduce the risk of complications, even in people with poor control of their diabetes and early complications of diabetes. For this reason, people with IDDM are encouraged to do the best they can to keep their blood sugar levels as close to the normal range as possible.

However, intensive treatment does increase the risk of low blood sugar episodes, or hypoglycemia, and is not recommended for everyone, particularly older adults, children under age 13, people with heart problems or advanced complications, and people with a history of frequent severe hypoglycemia. Your doctor should help you decide if intensive control is right for you. There is more information about hypoglycemia here.

Points to Remember

The DCCT showed that intensive control of blood sugar levels can help reduce the risk of complications associated with diabetes. The study showed that any sustained lowering of blood sugar levels is helpful.

Health Care Providers

Diabetes requires daily attention, and you need to learn how to care for your diabetes. A number of people can help you:

A Doctor Experienced in Treating Diabetes

These doctors are called endocrinologists or diabetologists. They will work with you to develop an individualized management routine and help you determine your ideal blood sugar range and ways to stay within that range.

"People with IDDM should be under the care of, or have regular contact with, a diabetes specialist who is up to date on diabetes and its management," advises Dr. Julio Santiago, an endocrinologist with the DCCT Center at Washington University in St. Louis. "During the last 10 years, diabetes care has greatly improved and become more complex. Services offered by diabetes specialists help people with IDDM learn the nuts and bolts of modern care and its benefits," he says.

A Diabetes Educator

Diabetes educators specialize in teaching people how to manage their diabetes. Most are registered nurses, pharmacists, dietitians, or physician assistants with advanced training and experience. They help you and your physician develop a management plan based on your age, school or work schedule, daily activities, and eating habits. They can teach you the importance of good nutrition, exercising regularly, and testing your blood sugar. These professionals can also help you adjust to having diabetes. Diabetes educators who use the initials CDE (Certified Diabetes Educator) after their names have passed an examination qualifying them to provide health education to people with diabetes.

A Nutritionist or Dietitian

Nutritionists or dietitians trained in diabetes care provide diet guidelines and meal planning advice. They can teach you how to balance food intake and insulin requirements and how to handle special situations such as low blood sugar (hypoglycemia) and sick days. Some dietitians are also CDEs.

A Mental Health Professional

A person with diabetes can never take a vacation from daily management chores. For this and other reasons, diabetes can affect the way a person feels. If you need advice on managing diabetes during stressful or difficult times, or if having diabetes makes you feel sad or depressed, talking to a social worker, psychologist, or psychiatrist may be helpful.

"These professionals are trained to help people cope with chronic conditions that require constant care," says Dr. Alan Jacobson, a psychiatrist at the Joslin Diabetes Center in Boston. Dr. Jacobson, who counseled volunteers at the DCCT center at Joslin, says "Discussing their problems and anxieties with a professional helped DCCT volunteers feel emotionally and physically in control."

If a mental health professional is not available to you, Dr. Jacobson suggests joining a local diabetes support group. "Talking with someone else who has IDDM may help," he advises. Information about support groups is available from your physician or CDE and local offices of the American Diabetes Association (ADA) and Juvenile Diabetes Foundation (JDF) International. These organizations also can provide suggestions on how to form a support group if one does not exist in your community. The addresses of these organizations are located here.

Daily Insulin

People with IDDM must give themselves insulin every day. Insulin cannot be taken in pill form. It can be injected, which involves use of a needle and syringe, or it can be given by an insulin pump. Insulin pumps are worn outside the body on a belt or in a pocket. They deliver a steady supply of insulin through a tube that connects to a needle placed under the skin. Extra amounts of insulin are taken before meals, depending on the blood glucose level and food to be eaten.

Another injection aid is an insulin pen. This device contains a replaceable insulin cartridge and a sterile, disposable needle. Insulin pens are handy because they eliminate the need for carrying extra syringes and insulin bottles. Jet injectors can also be used to give insulin, but these devices are expensive. A jet injector uses high pressure rather than a needle to propel insulin through the skin and into the tissue. Researchers are exploring the use of implantable pumps and other devices for giving insulin. Talk to your doctor about the insulin delivery system that is best for you.

The amount of insulin you need depends on your height, weight, age, food intake, and activity level. Insulin doses must be balanced with meal times and activities, and dosage levels can be affected by illness, stress, or unexpected events. Your doctor or diabetes educator will calculate how much insulin you should take each day to keep your blood sugar levels from rising too high or falling too low. They also will advise you about handling special situations. Most people with newly diagnosed IDDM can begin to inject their own insulin and estimate their insulin dosage needs within the first few days after instruction by a diabetes educator.

Points to Remember

All people with IDDM need insulin. Ways to give insulin include

- A needle and syringe
- An insulin pump
- An insulin pen
- A jet injector

Blood Glucose Monitoring

Since the early 1980s, self-monitoring of blood glucose (SMBG) has been shown to be the best way to determine if the blood sugar levels of a person with IDDM are too high or too low. The measurement helps you monitor your diabetes control to determine if adjustments in diet, insulin, or exercise are needed. Although SMBG may at first seem difficult and adds to the expense of treatment, diabetes management has improved greatly since this testing method became widely available.

SMBG involves taking a drop of blood, usually from the tip of a finger, and placing it on a specially coated strip. Strips are "read" either visually or by a meter. Visually read strips change color according to the amount of sugar in the blood. The color is then compared to a color chart provided with the strips. To use a glucose meter, you insert the strip into the meter and it gives a digital reading of your blood sugar level, usually within a minute.

Using a blood glucose meter is a more accurate way to test blood sugar. SMBG meters available since the early 1990s offer many features. Some are small and lightweight, and some can store blood sugar readings for a few days or weeks. Meters are sold in drug stores or in diabetes supply stores. You should consult your diabetes educator about which meter would be most appropriate for your lifestyle. Before using a meter, you should receive instructions from a health care professional on how to operate and maintain the device. Correct use of the meter is necessary to obtain accurate readings.

It is important to follow the manufacturer's recommendations for testing the accuracy of your meter (called calibrating the meter). Failure to do so could cause inaccurate test readings, leading to errors in management.

Results of blood sugar measurements should be recorded in a diabetes diary available through pharmacies and doctors' offices. The books have space for recording events such as extra activities or sickness that may affect blood sugar levels. This information will help you and your doctor adjust insulin doses or make other changes in care, if necessary. Sometimes the diary may show patterns in blood sugar levels that indicate a need to contact a health professional between office visits.

Frequent SMBG was an important tool in the DCCT. "For volunteers in the intensive management group, blood glucose testing results served as a guidepost to making decisions about food intake and insulin doses in order to achieve better control," says Ms. Patricia Callahan, a DCCT diabetes nurse educator at the International Diabetes Center in Minneapolis. "Blood glucose testing should be done at least four times a day or as often as necessary to achieve optimal control," she advises. "The idea is to use your SMBG to make adjustments in your food, exercise, and insulin so that your blood sugar stays in a range that is best for you." Another blood test, the hemoglobin A1c test, shows the average level of blood sugar for the past two to three months. Your blood sample is sent to a laboratory for analysis. You should have a hemoglobin A1c test at least every three months. Based on the results, you and your physician will know how well you have been doing in controlling your diabetes over the last few months.

Meal Plans

Like everyone else, people with IDDM should follow a healthy eating plan. Your meal plan should be low in fat and cholesterol because these foods have been linked to heart disease, a common problem in people with diabetes. Children and pregnant women with diabetes may have additional nutritional needs. Guidelines for nutrition are available from your dietitian, diabetes educator, or the ADA. Organizations that can help you find resources for nutritional guidance are listed at the end of this article.

Different foods have different effects on blood sugar. Therefore, you should try to be as consistent as possible in your food choices and eating times. Some foods raise blood sugar quickly; others have a more gradual effect. By testing your blood sugar after eating, you can learn how particular foods affect your blood sugar levels.

Points to Remember

Blood glucose testing is very important for monitoring daily care.

- SMBG shows current blood sugar levels.
- Hemoglobin A1c tests average blood sugar levels over the past two to three months.

Robert is a 38-year-old father and construction worker. He has IDDM and understands the need to test his blood sugar levels often. When Robert wakes up in the morning, he tests his blood sugar level before injecting his insulin and eating breakfast. He also tests his blood sugar level before lunch, dinner, bedtime, and at other times, as necessary. Robert carries his blood glucose meter with him at all times. Daily, he writes down the results of his blood glucose tests and insulin doses. He brings these records to his doctor so they can discuss the results and make any necessary changes.

Timing of meals and coordinating them according to your insulin injections is important. Regular insulin, for example, has its peak glucose-lowering effect approximately two hours after injection and acts for four to six hours. It is usually given before meals. Other insulin preparations are absorbed more slowly and have a longer duration of action.

Insulin regimens should be designed to fit a person's eating habits and lifestyle and should be as consistent as possible on a day-to-day basis. A dietitian can personalize a meal plan to include foods you like. Your physician and diabetes educator can also help.

The DCCT volunteers on intensive treatment learned about the relationship between food choices and blood sugar levels. "Each individual's insulin needs were adjusted to fit his or her lifestyle and diet, rather than trying to match the diet to fit the insulin," says Ms. Linda Delahanty, a dietitian with the DCCT Center at Massachusetts General Hospital in Boston. By understanding the relationship between food choices and blood sugar levels, she notes, volunteers in the intensive therapy group had more flexibility in their daily lives and could adjust their insulin doses to changes in their food intake and activity levels.

Exercise

People with IDDM are encouraged to exercise for the same reasons as people without diabetes. Exercise keeps the body in tone and is good for the heart and lungs. Before exercising you should check your blood sugar levels because exercise tends to lower blood sugar. If your blood sugar is too low or if some time has passed since you ate, you should eat a snack before exercising. Sometimes exercise can cause very high blood sugar to rise even higher. If your blood sugar is over 300 mg/dl (before eating), you should give yourself insulin or wait until your blood sugar level falls before beginning to exercise.

"Exercise is an important part of the patient's management plan. Participation in sports and regular exercise helps to improve overall physical fitness," says Dr. Santiago. An exercise program should be planned with the help of a doctor or an experienced physical therapist or trainer.

Points to Remember

- Consult with a dietitian to develop a meal plan for you.
- Learn how different foods affect your blood sugar levels.
- Try to keep insulin injections, meals, and activities as consistent as possible on a day-to-day basis.

Jake has IDDM and is getting ready to go to college. He is planning to live off campus. For the first time, Jake will have to cook his own meals and shop for food. He consulted a dietitian to learn how to choose healthy foods and prepare balanced meals. His dietitian taught him how different foods could affect his blood sugar levels and gave him tips for preparing nutritious meals that fit into his busy schedule.

How should diabetic emergencies be handled?

People with diabetes must always balance food, exercise, and insulin to control blood sugar levels. When this balance is disrupted, certain emergency conditions, including low blood sugar (hypoglycemia) or high blood sugar (hyperglycemia), may result. People with IDDM should always wear a medical identification bracelet, necklace, or watch band. These tags state that the wearer has IDDM and list a telephone number to call for help.

Points to Remember

Exercise can lower blood sugar levels quickly. Before beginning exercise

- Check your blood sugar levels.
- If your blood sugar is on the low side, eat a snack.
- If your blood sugar is very high, you should bring it under control before beginning to exercise.
- It may also be necessary to lower your insulin dose before planned exercise.

Sally, an eight-year-old with IDDM, loves to do gymnastics with her friends in the youth gymnastics league. She practices at the local gym every day for an hour. Before Sally exercises, she checks her blood sugar level to make sure it is okay to start her workout. If her blood sugar level is too low, she eats a snack before beginning her gymnastics routine.

Hypoglycemia

Very low blood sugar, called hypoglycemia, is sometimes referred to as an "insulin reaction." This condition can be caused by too much insulin, too little or delayed food, exercise, alcohol, or any combination of these factors. When hypoglycemia occurs, a person can become cranky, tired, sweaty, hungry, confused, and shaky. If blood sugar levels drop too low, a person can lose consciousness or experience a seizure.

Hypoglycemia can usually be treated quickly by eating or drinking something with sugar in it, such as a sweetened drink or orange juice. You should always carry a high-sugar snack that can be used to treat an insulin reaction. Special products to treat insulin reactions, including glucose tablets and gels, are available in drugstores.

If a person loses consciousness or cannot swallow because of hypoglycemia, medical help is necessary. Dial 911 or take the person to a hospital emergency room. An injectable medication called glucagon, available by prescription in drugstores, raises blood sugar quickly. A family member or friend should learn when and how to inject glucagon in an emergency. Your doctor, diabetes educator, or dietitian can give advice about treating hypoglycemia. In the DCCT, volunteers on intensive treatment had three times as many episodes of hypoglycemia severe enough to require help from another person as the volunteers on standard therapy. Because of this potential danger, intensive management is not recommended for everyone, particularly older adults, children under age 13, or people with heart problems or advanced complications. People who do not experience the usual symptoms of low blood sugar, a condition known as hypoglycemia unawareness, need to take extra care to avoid hypoglycemia. They should measure their blood glucose more often, particularly before driving or operating dangerous machinery.

Points to Remember

- Hypoglycemia is low blood sugar.
- Hypoglycemia can develop quickly, especially with exercise.
- Always carry a high-sugar snack to treat low blood sugar.
- Hypogycemia, if not treated in time, can lead to unconsciousness.
- Test blood sugar levels to avoid hypoglycemia, particularly before driving or exercising.

Lisa is 17 years old and has IDDM. She competes on her high school's track team. Her team practices in the late afternoon after classes. Lisa carries a book bag every day to school to hold her blood glucose meter and its supplies, extra sources of sugar, her lunch, and her books. She tests her blood sugar before lunch and before late afternoon practice.

Once when she ate a light lunch, she began to experience hypoglycemia while practicing. Lisa's coach recognized her clumsiness and confusion as symptoms of low blood sugar and quickly gave her a can of regular cola. A few minutes later, she felt better, measured her blood sugar, and finished practice. Lisa's coach was able to prevent a dangerous situation from developing because she had been taught about the symptoms and treatment of hypoglycemia.

Hyperglycemia

Hyperglycemia is the opposite of hypoglycemia. Hyperglycemia occurs when the body has too much sugar in the blood. This condition may be caused by insufficient insulin, overeating, inactivity, illness, stress, or a combination of these factors. The symptoms of hyperglycemia include extreme thirst, frequent urination, fatigue, blurred vision, vomiting, and weight loss.

If your blood sugar levels are above 250 mg/dl before meals, you should test your urine for ketones. Ketones are chemicals that the body makes when insulin levels are very low and excessive amounts of fat are being burned. Ketone buildup over several hours can lead to serious illness and coma, a condition called ketoacidosis. Ketone testing kits are available in drugstores or at doctors' offices. They should be available for you to use at home when you are ill or when your blood sugar is very high. Signs of ketoacidosis include vomiting, weakness, rapid breathing, and a sweet breath odor.

Points to Remember

- Hyperglycemia is high blood sugar.
- Hyperglycemia develops more slowly than hypoglycemia.
- Hyperglycemia can indicate that ketoacidosis may be present.
- If blood sugar is high, test urine for ketones.

How does diabetes affect your body?

Diabetes can cause damage to both large and small blood vessels, resulting in complications affecting the kidneys, eyes, nerves, heart, and gums. The DCCT showed that maintaining blood sugar levels as close to normal as possible prevents or slows the development of many of these complications.

Kidney Disease

Diabetic kidney disease, called diabetic nephropathy, can be a life-threatening complication of IDDM in about 40 percent of people who have had diabetes for 20 or more years. The kidneys are vital to good health because they serve as a filtering system to clean waste products from the blood. Diabetic nephropathy develops when the small blood vessels that filter these wastes are damaged. Sometimes this damage causes the kidneys to stop working. This condition is called kidney failure or end-stage renal disease. People with kidney failure must either have their blood cleaned by a dialysis machine or have a kidney transplant.

High blood pressure (hypertension) also increases a person's chance of developing kidney disease. People with diabetes are more likely to develop high blood pressure than people without diabetes. Therefore, keeping blood pressure under control is especially important for someone with IDDM. Your doctor should check your blood pressure at every visit.

Blood pressure tests measure how hard your heart is working to pump blood to the organs and vessels in your body. If blood pressure is too high, it can be treated with a doctor's help. Left untreated, bladder and kidney infections can also harm the kidneys. Consult your doctor if symptoms such as painful urination occur.

An early sign of kidney disease is albumin or protein in the urine. A doctor should test your urine for protein or albumin once a year. The doctor should also do an annual blood test to evaluate kidney function. More frequent tests may be necessary if findings are not normal.

The DCCT proved that intensive therapy can prevent the development and slow the progression of early diabetic kidney disease. Another recent study has shown that a type of medication called an ACE inhibitor can help protect the kidneys from damage.

> Kevin is a 35-year-old sales representative and has IDDM. He visits his endocrinologist several times a year to have his blood pressure checked and his hemoglobin A1c measured. Once a year, the doctor takes a blood test to measure Kevin's cholesterol level and his kidney function. The doctor also asks Kevin to collect his urine in a container over a 24-hour period to check for protein or albumin in his kidneys. Albumin or protein in the urine is an early sign of diabetic kidney disease.

Eye Disease

Diabetes can affect the small blood vessels in the back of the eye, a condition called diabetic retinopathy. Retinopathy means disease of the retina, the tissue at the back of the eye that is sensitive to light. Diabetes eventually causes changes in the tiny vessels that supply the retina with blood. These small changes are called background retinopathy. Most people who have had diabetes for a number of years have background retinopathy, which usually does not affect sight. Over time, the blood vessels may rupture or leak fluid. In a minority of patients, most often those with higher blood sugar, retinopathy becomes more severe and new blood vessels may grow on the retina. These vessels may bleed into the clear gel, or vitreous, that fills the eye or detach the retina from its normal position because of bleeding or scar formation.

Laser treatment can help restore vision impaired by diabetic retinopathy. If you have had IDDM for five years or more, you should see an eye doctor at least once a year for an examination through dilated pupils. An annual exam is the best way to detect and treat eye damage before the condition becomes severe. Laser treatment, as well as surgical procedures performed by eye doctors who specialize in diabetic problems, can often help preserve useful vision even in cases of advanced retinopathy.

In the DCCT, intensive management reduced the risk of diabetic eye disease by 76 percent in participants with no eye damage at the beginning of the study. In those with early retinopathy, intensive therapy slowed the progression of eye damage by 50 percent.

> Joan is a 40-year-old artist. She has had IDDM for 20 years. Every year she visits her ophthalmologist to have her eyes checked for diabetic eye disease. Her doctor dilates Joan's pupils and looks into her eyes carefully to detect any changes that may have occurred since her last visit. They discuss diabetic retinopathy and the importance of yearly check-ups to detect and treat any eye problems that may occur. Although Joan has very mild diabetic changes in her eyes, these changes do not pose a threat to her vision and are not likely to progress if she stays in excellent diabetic control.

Nerve Disease

Nerve disease caused by diabetes is called diabetic neuropathy. There are three types of nerve disease: peripheral, autonomic, and mononeuropathy. Peripheral neuropathy affects the hands, feet, legs, toes, or fingers. A person's feet, legs, and fingertips may lose feeling, burn, or become painful. To relieve the pain, doctors prescribe pain-killing drugs and sometimes antidepressant drugs. Scientists are studying other substances to help relieve pain associated with diabetic peripheral neuropathy.

Because of the loss of feeling associated with peripheral neuropathy, feet are especially vulnerable. You should check your feet carefully each day for cuts, bruises, and sores. If you notice anything unusual, see a doctor as soon as possible because foot infections and open sores can be difficult to treat in people with diabetes. Your doctor should check your feet at every visit. At least once a year, the doctor should check your neurological function by testing how well you sense temperature, pinprick, vibration in your feet, and changes of position in your toes. Your doctor may recommend that you see a foot care specialist, called a podiatrist.

Another type of nerve disease that may occur after several years of diabetes is called autonomic neuropathy. Autonomic neuropathy affects the internal organs such as the heart, stomach, sexual organs, and urinary tract. It can cause digestive problems and lead to incontinence (a loss of ability to control urine or bowel movements) and sexual impotence. A doctor can help diagnose problems associated with internal organs and may prescribe medication to help relieve pain and other problems associated with autonomic neuropathy. Mononeuropathy is a form of nerve disease that affects specific nerves, most often in the torso, leg, or head. Mononeuropathy may cause pain in the lower back, chest, abdomen, or in the front of one thigh. Sometimes, this nerve disease can cause aching in the eye, an inability to focus the eye, or double vision.

Mononeuropathy may also cause facial paralysis, a condition called Bell's palsy, or problems with hearing. Mononeuropathies occur most often in older people and can be quite painful. Usually the symptoms improve in weeks or months without causing long-term damage.

Lowering blood sugar levels may help prevent or reduce early neuropathy. DCCT study results showed the risk of significant nerve damage was reduced by 60 percent in persons on intensive treatment.

> Every time Joe, who is a 45-year-old mail carrier and has IDDM, visits his doctor, he takes off his shoes and socks so his doctor does not forget to check his feet for sores, ulcers, and wounds. The doctor also checks his nerve reflexes and sense of feeling. Joe and his doctor discuss ways to prevent foot and nerve problems. Since Joe has lost some of his ankle reflexes and toe sensation, the doctor also stresses the importance of not smoking, not going barefoot, and keeping blood sugar levels under control.

Cardiovascular Disease

As with high blood pressure, heart disease is more common in people with diabetes than in people without diabetes.

People with diabetes tend to have more fat and cholesterol in their arteries. The arteries are the large blood vessels that keep the heart beating and the blood flowing. When too much fat and cholesterol build up in the arteries, the arteries and heart must work harder. Over time, this extra work can lead to a heart attack. To help avoid heart problems, you should have your blood cholesterol and triglyceride levels checked once a year. Other risk factors that may cause the heart to become overworked include high blood pressure, smoking, age, extra weight, and lack of exercise. People with diabetes are also at greater risk for stroke and other forms of large blood vessel disease. A stroke is the result of damage to the blood vessels that circulate blood in the brain. Blockage of major blood vessels in the feet, legs, or arms is called peripheral vascular disease. Peripheral vascular disease causes poor circulation and can contribute to foot and leg ulcers.

DCCT participants were checked regularly for heart disease and related problems, although they were not expected to have many heart-related problems because of their young age. Volunteers in the intensive treatment group had fewer heart attacks and significantly lower risks of developing high blood cholesterol, which causes heart disease. The risk was 35 percent lower in these volunteers, suggesting that intensive treatment can help prevent heart disease. The DCCT volunteers on intensive therapy are being followed closely for the next 10 years to see if their risk of heart disease is reduced.

Points to Remember

To reduce the risk of heart disease:

- Do not smoke.
- Eat a diet low in fat and high in fruits and vegetables.
- Have your blood pressure checked regularly.
- Have your cholesterol checked regularly.

Periodontal (Gum) Disease

People with diabetes, especially those with poor control of their blood sugar, are at risk for developing infections of the gum and bone that hold the teeth in place. Like all infections, gum infections can cause blood sugar to rise and make diabetes harder to control.

Periodontal disease starts as gingivitis, which causes sore, bleeding gums. If not stopped, gingivitis can lead to serious periodontal disease that can damage the bone that holds the tooth in its socket. Without treatment, teeth may loosen and fall out.

Good blood sugar control lowers the risk of gum disease. People with good control have no more gum disease than people without diabetes. Good blood sugar control, daily brushing and flossing, and regular dental check-ups are the best defense against gum problems.

Points to Remember

Take special care of your teeth and gums.

- Visit your dentist every six months.
- Brush and floss teeth at least twice daily.
- Practice other dental care guidelines recommended by the dentist or dental hygienist.

How should special situations be handled?

Illness, Stress, and Surgery

Illness and stress can affect blood sugar levels in people with diabetes. Therefore, during times of illness and stress, you need to be extra careful about keeping blood sugar levels in control. If you develop an illness such as the flu or strep throat, keep in touch with your doctor, test your blood sugar levels often, and check your urine for ketones. Even if you are feeling too sick to eat or have trouble keeping food down, you should continue giving yourself some insulin. In such situations, your doctor will tell you how much insulin to take as well as liquid diets to follow.

A doctor or diabetes nurse educator can also provide guidelines on how to handle stress. If you need hospitalization for an illness or require surgery, doctors and hospital personnel should know that you have diabetes. Your diabetes doctor should also be informed about the hospitalization and should be part of the team that monitors your care. Your doctor will give you advice regarding who to call in case of illness, vomiting, or very high blood sugar levels. In many cases, an early telephone call can prevent lengthy hospitalization.

Pregnancy

Before the 1950s, most pregnant women with diabetes had little chance of having a normal baby. Since the 1960s major advances in diabetes treatment have taken place in Europe and North America. Today, with careful planning, most women with diabetes can become pregnant and deliver a healthy baby with the help of their doctors. Women with diabetes need to discuss their plans with their physicians before they become pregnant. Several studies show that excellent blood glucose control is important at the time a women becomes pregnant. Careful control during the first two months of pregnancy can reduce the risk of major birth defects. Later, during the third to ninth months of pregnancy, excellent blood glucose control is essential to protect the health of the baby and reduce complications related to premature delivery.

If you are a pregnant woman with IDDM, you should be treated by a team of doctors or at a center that specializes in the treatment of diabetic pregnancies. The center can provide guidelines for handling such pregnancy-related problems as morning sickness as well as closely monitor your baby before, during, and after delivery.

Because pregnancy sometimes can affect the eyes, kidneys, and blood pressure, your doctors will need to check your eyes, kidneys, and blood pressure before and throughout the pregnancy.

School and Social Activities

Children with IDDM can attend school, do homework, play with friends, and participate in clubs or sports. However, special attention should be paid to diabetes care while the child is in school and involved in daily activities. If old enough, children may keep a blood glucose meter at school or with the school nurse. To safeguard against hypoglycemia, the child can carry extra snacks, or snacks can be given to the teacher for use in case the child's blood sugar level drops. Teachers, friends, club leaders, school nurses, or coaches should be aware that a child has diabetes and should know the signs of low blood sugar and how to treat it in case of emergency.

Points to Remember

- Most women with IDDM can have successful pregnancies.
- Blood sugar levels should be in good control before a woman becomes pregnant.
- Women with IDDM must be under the close care of specialists experienced in diabetic pregnancies.

Maria, a 25-year-old woman who has IDDM, wanted children. She and her husband visited her doctor for guidance. Maria's doctor said that before she conceived, her blood sugar levels should be in very good control and her kidneys, eyes, and blood pressure must be checked. Maria began a strict diabetes management schedule. She checked her blood sugar levels four times a day, ate healthy meals, began a walking routine, and had numerous blood and urine tests to make sure her body was healthy enough to carry a baby.

Once Maria became pregnant, she continued watching her diabetes carefully and visiting her doctor regularly. She spent a great deal of time monitoring her diabetes to make sure she and her baby would be healthy. Maria's hard work paid off because, after nine months, she gave birth to a healthy baby boy.

Points to Remember

- Inform teachers and school staff that your child has diabetes and how to treat hypoglycemia.
- Always bring extra snacks in case hypoglycemia occurs with exercise.

Just like people without diabetes, people with diabetes can go to parties and participate in social activities. Some helpful tips are

- Call ahead to see what foods the host or hostess will serve and at approximately what time. This will help you keep track of how much food you should eat or how much insulin you will need.
- If there does not seem to be food you should eat, offer to bring a snack that everyone, including you, can enjoy.
- Make sure you bring your blood glucose meter to the party to check blood sugar levels before participating in any physical activities, such as strenuous dancing.

Adults with diabetes, even those with IDDM, can drink alcohol safely in moderation. Moderation usually means one or two occasional drinks taken with food. Drinking on an empty stomach and at bedtime can cause blood sugar levels to drop quickly, causing hypoglycemia, with symptoms of shakiness, dizziness, and confusion. People who do not know that someone has diabetes may mistake these symptoms for drunkenness. A dietitian can give guidelines about using alcohol and how to include it in a meal plan. People with nerve damage due to diabetes should avoid frequent alcohol use.

Points to Remember

- Alcohol can lower blood glucose.
- Always eat when drinking alcohol.
- Drink in moderation.
- If you have nerve damage due to diabetes, avoid regular alcohol use.

What is happening in diabetes research?

The DCCT was one of many recent research programs supported by the Federal Government and by nongovernment organizations to improve the health and well-being of people with diabetes and to find ways to prevent and cure the disorder. A 10-year follow-up to the DCCT, the Epidemiology of Diabetes Intervention and Complications Study, is focusing on the development of macrovascular and renal complications in DCCT volunteers.

The National Institute of Diabetes and Digestive and Kidney Diseases (NIDDK) conducts basic and clinical research in its own laboratories and supports research at centers and hospitals throughout the United States. Other institutes of the National Institutes of Health support studies on diabetic eye, heart, vascular, and nerve disease; pregnancy and diabetes; dental complications; and the immunological aspects of diabetes. This research has led to improved treatments for the complications of diabetes and ways to prevent complications from occurring.

Preventing Diabetes

Researchers are searching diligently for the causes of all forms of diabetes and ways to delay or prevent the disorder. Much progress has been made. Scientists have identified antibodies in the blood that make a person susceptible to IDDM, making it possible to screen relatives of people with diabetes and determine their risk for developing the disease.

A new NIDDK clinical trial, the Diabetes Prevention Trial-Type 1 (DPT-1), began in 1994. It is identifying relatives at risk for developing IDDM and treating them with low doses of insulin or with oral insulin-like agents in the hope of preventing IDDM. Similar research is being conducted at other medical centers throughout the world. These studies are based on encouraging results in laboratory animals with IDDM and on pilot studies in relatives of people with IDDM.

Advances in Managing Diabetes

In the past 15 years, many advances have improved treatment for people with diabetes:

Genetically Engineered Insulin

Because it is identical to insulin produced by the human body, genetically engineered insulin is less apt to cause skin and other allergic reactions. Supplies of genetically engineered insulin are readily available.

Self-monitoring of Blood Glucose

By testing your own blood sugar, you enable your doctor to offer you much better treatment than was available before 1980 when testing urine for glucose was the only way of estimating diabetes control.

Hemoglobin A1c Testing

Using one blood test, doctors can now monitor your average blood sugar control over a period of two to three months. This test tells you how well you are doing and whether any changes are needed in your management routine.

Insulin Pumps, Insulin Pens, and Other Aids for Administering Insulin

Insulin pumps, including implantable pumps now under development, can supply insulin in a more natural pattern, similar to the way the pancreas in a person without diabetes makes insulin. Other injection aids make giving insulin easier and more convenient than in the past, even in young children and people who are visually impaired.

Other improvements in diabetes management being developed include insulin in the form of nasal sprays, patches, or pills, and devices to test blood sugar levels without having to prick a finger to get a blood sample. Perhaps one of the most important advances has been the development of an entirely new approach to diabetes management in which IDDM patients take responsibility for much of their own care.

Curing Diabetes

Transplantation of the pancreas or of the insulin-producing islets of the pancreas offer a hope for a cure for IDDM. Many people with IDDM have had successful pancreas transplants, and a few have had islet transplants. Unfortunately, pancreas and islet transplants cannot be offered to everyone with diabetes as yet. The body's immune system rejects "foreign" or transplanted tissue, and people who have transplants must take powerful drugs to prevent rejection. These drugs are costly and may cause serious health problems. Therefore, pancreas or islet transplants are usually given only to people who have had or require a kidney transplant because of advanced complications and are already taking drugs to prevent rejection.

Researchers are working to develop less harmful drugs and better methods of transplanting pancreatic tissue to prevent rejection by the body, such as encapsulating the islet cells in a semi-permeable membrane that offers protection from immune attack, implanting the cells in the thymus gland to induce tolerance by the immune system, and using bioengineering techniques to create artificial islet cells that secrete insulin in response to increased sugar levels in the blood.

Clinical Trials

Clinical trials are one way to test new treatments that emerge from basic research. NIDDK plans and supports clinical trials related to diabetes, such as the DCCT and DPT-Type 1. For information about NIDDK-supported clinical trials, contact the National Diabetes Information Clearinghouse (NDIC), at the address and telephone number below.

Other medical centers also conduct clinical studies. The best way to find out about studies in progress is to contact a nearby university-affiliated hospital or large medical center. Additional information can also be obtained from a local chapter of the American Diabetes Association or Juvenile Diabetes Foundation.

Other Resources

The following organizations offer educational materials about diabetes and can help you find support groups and education programs in your community, including family activities and camp programs for children. Local affiliates and chapters of these organizations often can identify health professionals such as diabetologists, certified diabetes educators, and dietitians in the community. To locate affiliates and chapters of these organizations, consult your local telephone directory, or contact the following national offices:

American Association of Diabetes Educators
444 N Michigan Avenue, Suite 1240
Chicago, IL 60611
(800) 832-6874

American Diabetes Association
ADA National Service Center
1660 Duke Street
Alexandria, VA 22314
(800) 232-3472

Juvenile Diabetes Foundation International
432 Park Avenue South
New York, NY 10016-8013
(800) 223-1138

American Dietetic Association
216 W Jackson Blvd.
Chicago, IL 60606-6995
(800) 366-1655

Additional publications about diabetes are available from the National Diabetes Information Clearinghouse. The clearinghouse can also provide information about research and clinical trials supported by the National Institutes of Health.

National Diabetes Information Clearinghouse
1 Information Way
Bethesda, MD 20892-3560

For more information about improving blood sugar control, write

National Diabetes Outreach Program
1 Diabetes Way
Bethesda, MD 20892-3600

Acknowledgments: Our thanks to Julio Santiago, MD, of Washington University for his careful review of this text. We also wish to acknowledge the contributions of Patricia Callahan, RN, BS, CDE; Linda Delahanty, MS; and R.D. Alan Jacobson, MD.

■ **Document Source:**
U.S. Department of Health and Human Services, Public Health Service
National Institutes of Health
National Institute of Diabetes and Digestive and Kidney Diseases
NIH Pub. No. 94-2098
October 1994

KIDNEY DISEASE OF DIABETES

Each year in the United States, more than 50,000 people are diagnosed with end-stage renal disease (ESRD), a serious condition in which the kidneys fail to rid the body of wastes. ESRD is the final stage of a slow deterioration of the kidneys, a process known as nephropathy.

Diabetes is the most common cause of ESRD, resulting in about one-third of new ESRD cases. Even when drugs and diet are able to control diabetes, the disease can lead to nephropathy and ESRD. Most people with diabetes do not develop nephropathy that is severe enough to cause ESRD. About 15 million people in the United States have diabetes, and about 50,000 people have ESRD as a result of diabetes.

ESRD patients undergo either dialysis, which substitutes for some of the filtering functions of the kidneys, or transplantation to receive a healthy donor kidney. Most U.S. citizens who develop ESRD are eligible for federally funded care. In 1994, the Federal Government spent about $9.3 billion on care for patients with ESRD.

African Americans and Native Americans develop diabetes, nephropathy, and ESRD at rates higher than average. Scientists have not been able to explain these higher rates. Nor can they explain fully the interplay of factors leading to diabetic nephropathy—factors including heredity, diet, and other medical conditions, such as high blood pressure. They have found that high blood pressure and high levels of blood sugar increase the risk that a person with diabetes will progress to ESRD.

Primary Diagnoses (Causes) for ESRD (1991)

- 2.9 percent Interstitial Nephritis
- 2.9 percent Polycystic Kidney Disease
- 11.4 percent Glomerulonephritis
- 18.1 percent Other Causes
- 28.8 percent High Blood Pressure
- 35.9 percent Diabetes

Two Types of Diabetes

In diabetes—also called diabetes mellitus, or DM—the body does not properly process and use certain foods, especially carbohydrates. The human body normally converts carbohydrates to glucose, the simple sugar that is the main source of energy for the body's cells. To enter cells, glucose needs the help of insulin, a hormone produced by the pancreas. When a person does not make enough insulin, or the body is unable to use the insulin that is present, the body cannot process glucose, and it builds up in the bloodstream. High levels of glucose in the blood or urine lead to a diagnosis of diabetes.

NIDDM

Most people with diabetes have a form known as noninsulin-dependent diabetes (NIDDM), or Type II diabetes. Many people with NIDDM do not respond normally to their own or to injected insulin—a condition called insulin resistance. NIDDM occurs more often in people over the age of 40, and many people with NIDDM are overweight. Many also are not aware that they have the disease. Some people with NIDDM control their blood sugar with diet and an exercise program leading to weight loss. Others must take pills that stimulate production of insulin; still others require injections of insulin.

IDDM

A less common form of diabetes, known as insulin-dependent diabetes (IDDM), or Type I diabetes, tends to occur in young adults and children. In cases of IDDM, the body produces little or no insulin. People with IDDM must receive daily insulin injections.

NIDDM accounts for about 95 percent of all cases of diabetes; IDDM accounts for about 5 percent. Both types of diabetes can lead to kidney disease. IDDM is more likely to lead to ESRD. About 40 percent of people with IDDM develop severe kidney disease and ESRD by the age of 50. Some develop ESRD before the age of 30. NIDDM causes 80 percent of the ESRD in African Americans and Native Americans.

The Course of Kidney Disease

The deterioration that characterizes kidney disease of diabetes takes place in and around the glomeruli, the blood-filtering units of the kidneys. Early in the disease, the filtering efficiency diminishes, and important proteins in the blood are lost to the urine. Medical professionals gauge the presence and extent of early kidney disease by measuring protein in the urine. Later in the disease, the kidneys lose their ability to remove waste products, such as creatinine and urea, from the blood.

Symptoms related to kidney failure usually occur only in late stages of the disease, when kidney function has diminished to less than 25 percent of normal capacity. For many years before that point, kidney disease of diabetes exists as a silent process.

Five Stages

Scientists have described five stages in the progression to ESRD in people with diabetes. They are as follows:

Stage I. The flow of blood through the kidneys, and therefore through the glomeruli, increases—this is called hyperfiltration—and the kidneys are larger than normal. Some people remain in stage I indefinitely; others advance to stage II after many years.

Stage II. The rate of filtration remains elevated or at near-normal levels, and the glomeruli begin to show damage. Small amounts of a blood protein known as albumin leak into the urine—a condition known as microalbuminuria. In its earliest stages, microalbuminuria may come and go. But as the rate of albumin loss increases from 20 to 200 micrograms per minute, microalbuminuria becomes more constant. (Normal losses of albumin are less than five micrograms per minute.) A special test is required to detect microalbuminuria. People with NIDDM and IDDM may remain in stage II for many years, especially if they have normal blood pressure and good control of their blood sugar levels.

Stage III. The loss of albumin and other proteins in the urine exceeds 200 micrograms per minute. It now can be detected during routine urine tests. Because such tests often involve dipping indicator strips into the urine, they are referred to as "dipstick methods." Stage III sometimes is referred to as "dipstick-positive proteinuria" (or "clinical albuminuria" or "overt diabetic nephropathy"). Some patients develop high blood pressure. The glomeruli suffer increased damage. The kidneys progressively lose the ability to filter waste, and blood levels of creatinine and urea-nitrogen rise. People with IDDM and NIDDM may remain at stage III for many years.

Stage IV. This is referred to as "advanced clinical nephropathy." The glomerular filtration rate decreases to less than 75 milliliters per minute, large amounts of protein pass into the urine, and high blood pressure almost always occurs. Levels of creatinine and urea-nitrogen in the blood rise further.

Stage V. The final stage is ESRD. The glomerular filtration rate drops to less than 10 milliliters per minute. Symptoms of kidney failure occur.

These stages describe the progression of kidney disease for most people with IDDM who develop ESRD. For people with IDDM, the average length of time required to progress from onset of kidney disease to stage IV is 17 years. The average length of time to progress to ESRD is 23 years. Progression to ESRD may occur more rapidly (five to 10 years) in people with untreated high blood pressure. If proteinuria does not develop within 25 years, the risk of developing advanced kidney disease begins to decrease. Advancement to stages IV and V occurs less frequently in people with NIDDM than in people with IDDM. Nevertheless, about 60 percent of people with diabetes who develop ESRD have NIDDM.

Effects of High Blood Pressure

High blood pressure, or hypertension, is a major factor in the development of kidney problems in people with diabetes. Both a family history of hypertension and the presence of hypertension appear to increase chances of developing kidney disease. Hypertension also accelerates the progress of kidney disease where it already exists.

Hypertension usually is defined as blood pressure exceeding 140 millimeters of mercury-systolic and 90 millimeters of mercury-diastolic. Professionals shorten the name of this limit to "140 over 90." The terms systolic and diastolic refer to pressure in the arteries during contraction of the heart (systolic) and between heartbeats (diastolic).

Hypertension can be seen not only as a cause of kidney disease, but also as a result of damage created by the disease. As kidney disease proceeds, physical changes in the kidneys lead to increased blood pressure. Therefore, a dangerous spiral, involving rising blood pressure and factors that raise blood pressure, occurs. Early detection and treatment of even mild hypertension are essential for people with diabetes.

Preventing and Slowing Kidney Disease

Blood Pressure Medicines

Scientists have made great progress in developing methods that slow the onset and progression of kidney disease in people with diabetes. Drugs used to lower blood pressure (antihypertensive drugs) can slow the progression of kidney disease significantly. One drug, an angiotensin-converting enzyme (ACE) inhibitor, has proven effective in preventing progression to stages IV and V. Calcium channel blockers, another class of antihypertensive drugs, also show promise.

An example of an effective ACE inhibitor is captopril, which the Food and Drug Administration approved for treating kidney disease of Type I diabetes. The benefits of captopril extend beyond its ability to lower blood pressure; it may directly protect the kidney's glomeruli. ACE inhibitors have lowered proteinuria and slowed deterioration even in diabetic patients who did not have high blood pressure.

Some, but not all, calcium channel blockers may be able to decrease proteinuria and damage to kidney tissue. Researchers are investigating whether combinations of calcium channel blockers and ACE inhibitors might be more effective than either treatment used alone. Patients with even mild hypertension or persistent microalbuminuria should consult a physician about the use of antihypertensive medicines.

Low-Protein Diets

A diet containing reduced amounts of protein may benefit people with kidney disease of diabetes. In people with diabetes, excessive consumption of protein may be harmful. Experts recommend that most patients with stage III or stage IV nephropathy consume moderate amounts of protein.

Intensive Management

Antihypertensive drugs and low-protein diets can slow kidney disease when significant nephropathy is present, as in stages III and IV. A third treatment, known as intensive management or glycemic control, has shown great promise for people with IDDM, especially for those with early stages of nephropathy.

Intensive management is a treatment regimen that aims to keep blood glucose levels close to normal. The regimen includes frequently testing blood sugar, administering insulin on the basis of food intake and exercise, following a diet and exercise plan, and frequently consulting a health care team.

A number of studies have pointed to the beneficial effects of intensive management. Two such studies, funded by the National Institute of Diabetes and Digestive and Kidney Diseases (NIDDK) of the National Institutes of Health, are the Diabetes Control and Complications Trial (DCCT) and a trial led by researchers at the University of Minnesota Medical School.

The DCCT, conducted from 1983 to 1993, involved 1,441 participants who had IDDM. Researchers found a 50-percent decrease in both development and progression of early diabetic kidney disease (stages I and II) in participants who followed an intensive regimen for controlling blood sugar levels. The intensively managed patients had average blood sugar levels of 150 milligrams per deciliter—about 80 milligrams per deciliter lower than the levels observed in the conventionally managed patients.

In the Minnesota Medical School trial, researchers examined kidney tissues of long-term diabetics who received healthy kidney transplants. After five years, patients who followed an intensive regimen developed significantly fewer lesions in their glomeruli than did patients not following an intensive regimen. This result, along with findings of the DCCT and studies performed in Scandinavia, suggests that any program resulting in sustained lowering of blood glucose levels will be beneficial to patients in the early stages of diabetic nephropathy.

Dialysis and Transplantation

When people with diabetes reach ESRD, they must undergo either dialysis or a kidney transplant. As recently as the 1970s, medical experts commonly excluded people with diabetes from dialysis and transplantation, in part because the experts felt damage caused by diabetes would offset benefits of the treatments. Today, because of better control of diabetes and improved rates of survival following treatment, doctors do not hesitate to offer dialysis and kidney transplantation to people with diabetes.

Currently, the survival of kidneys transplanted into diabetes patients is about the same as survival of transplants in people without diabetes. Dialysis for people with diabetes also works well in the short run. Even so, people with diabetes who receive transplants or dialysis experience higher morbidity and mortality because of coexisting complications of the diabetes—such as damage to the heart, eyes, and nerves.

Good Care Makes a Difference

If you have diabetes:

- Ask your doctor about the DCCT and how its results might help you.
- Have your doctor measure your glycohemoglobin regularly. The HbA1c test averages your level of blood sugar for the previous one to three months.
- Follow your doctor's advice regarding insulin injections, medicines, diet, exercise, and monitoring your blood sugar.
- Have your blood pressure checked several times a year. If blood pressure is high, follow your doctor's plan for keeping it near normal levels.
- Ask your doctor whether you might benefit from receiving an ACE inhibitor.
- Have your urine checked yearly for microalbumin and protein. If there is protein in your urine, have your blood checked for elevated amounts of waste products such as creatinine.
- Ask your doctor whether you should reduce the amount of protein in your diet.

Looking to the Future

The incidences of both diabetes and ESRD caused by diabetes have been rising. Some experts predict that diabetes soon might account for half the cases of ESRD. In light of the increasing morbidity and mortality related to diabetes and ESRD, patients, researchers, and health care professionals will continue to benefit by addressing the relationship between the two diseases. The NIDDK is a leader in supporting research in this area.

Several areas of research supported by NIDDK hold great potential. Discovery of ways to predict who will develop kidney disease may lead to greater prevention, as people with diabetes who learn they are at risk institute strategies such as intensive management and blood pressure control. Discovery of better anti-rejection drugs will improve results of kidney transplantation in patients with diabetes who develop ESRD. For some people with IDDM, advances in transplantation—especially transplantation of insulin-producing cells of the pancreas—could lead to a cure for both diabetes and the kidney disease of diabetes.

References

Lewis, E.J., et al., The effect of angiotensin-converting-enzyme inhibition on diabetic nephropathy. *New England Journal of Medicine,* Vol. 329, No. 20, pp. 1456-1462, 1993.

Diabetes Control and Complications Trial [fact sheet], August 1994. National Diabetes Information Clearinghouse, 1 Information Way, Bethesda, MD 20892-3560.

Barbosa, J., et al., Effect of glycemic control on early diabetic renal lesions. *Journal of the American Medical Association,* Vol. 272, No. 8, pp. 600-606, 1994.

For More Information

National Kidney and Urologic Diseases Information Clearinghouse
3 Information Way
Bethesda, MD 20892-3580

The National Kidney and Urologic Diseases Information Clearinghouse is a service of the National Institute of Diabetes and Digestive and Kidney Diseases, part of the National Institutes of Health, under the U.S. Public Health Service. Authorized in 1987, the clearinghouse provides information about diseases of the kidneys and urologic system to people with such afflictions and to their families, health care professionals, and the public. The clearinghouse answers inquiries; develops, reviews, and distributes publications; and works closely with professional and patient organizations and government agencies to coordinate resources about kidney and urologic diseases.

Publications produced by the clearinghouse are reviewed carefully for scientific accuracy, content, and readability. Publications produced by outside sources are also reviewed carefully before being used to supplement clearinghouse materials when responding to inquiries.

■ **Document Source:**
  U.S. Department of Health and Human Services, Public Health Service
  National Institutes of Health
  National Institute of Diabetes and Digestive and Kidney Diseases
  NIH Publication No. 95-3925
  July 1995

EARS, NOSE, AND THROAT (ENT) DISORDERS

■ ■ ■

ABOUT TONSILLECTOMY AND ADENOIDECTOMY

Tonsillectomy (ton-si-lect'-tuh-me) and adenoidectomy (add-noid-ect'-tuh-me) is the surgical removal of the tonsils and adenoids. This booklet has been prepared to tell you about this operation, the conditions leading to it, and why your doctor may recommend this procedure.

It is important to remember that each individual is different, and the reasons for the outcome of any operation depend upon the patient's individual condition. This booklet is not intended to take the place of the professional opinion of a qualified surgeon who is familiar with your situation. After reading this booklet, you may have further questions; you should discuss these openly and honestly with your surgeon.

About the Tonsils and Adenoids

The tonsils are two masses of tissue embedded on either side of the back of the throat. Adenoid tissue is located high in the throat behind the nose.

Tonsils and adenoids are believed to fight infection by producing antibodies to bacteria and viruses that enter through the mouth and nose. When they become chronically infected, however, they may cause serious health problems.

Symptoms and Complications of Tonsillitis

Tonsillitis (inflammation of the tonsils) can cause fever, sore throat, painful swallowing, and swelling of the lymph nodes in the neck. The condition is diagnosed by examining the tonsils, which may be enlarged and reddened. Small patches of yellowish pus maybe seen on their surface. Recurrently infected tonsils may pose a threat to other parts of the body. Some children with frequent bouts of severe tonsillitis may develop other diseases such as rheumatic fever (heart trouble) and kidney infection. Infected adenoids may cause middle ear infections and hearing loss. Further, enlarged and inflamed tonsils and adenoids can block the nose and throat, and can interfere with normal breathing, swallowing, speaking, and the functioning of the eustachian tube, which can impair hearing.

About the Operation

In the past, before the days of antibiotics, the removal of both tonsils and adenoids was sometimes routinely recommended for many children. Today, however, the role of both the tonsils and adenoids in the body's defense mechanisms is recognized as being very important. Therefore, only the tonsils are removed (tonsillectomy) when they develop chronic or recurrent infection, and only the adenoids are removed (adenoidectomy) when they develop similar problems or are believed to cause recurrent ear infections.

Tonsillectomy or adenoidectomy is most frequently performed on children, but it may sometimes be necessary in adults as well. It is considered among the safest of all surgical procedures.

A complication occasionally associated with tonsillectomy or adenoidectomy is bleeding, either immediately after the operation, or several days later. In both of these occurrences, bleeding can usually be readily controlled by the surgeon.

Tonsillectomy or adenoidectomy is performed through the patient's mouth. With children, a general anesthetic is almost always used (that is, the patient is asleep during the operation). When tonsillectomy is performed on adults, however, the patient sometimes is awake for the operation and a local anesthetic is used to eliminate pain.

During the operation, the surgeon separates and removes the tonsils from the side of the throat; the adenoids are removed from behind the palate. Often, no stitches are required, except in a few instances where excessive bleeding occurs.

Recovery

The usual hospital stay following a tonsillectomy or adenoidectomy is eight to 10 hours, or until the patient is completely recovered from anesthesia. Many patients may be able to go home on the same day as the operation. Patients with specific problems may require an overnight hospital stay.

During the first week following the operation, the patient may experience throat and ear pain, but recovery usually occurs within 10 days to two weeks. Occasionally, some bleeding will occur several days after the operation. This is usually not a serious complication, but the surgeon should be notified immediately so that the bleeding can be controlled.

Surgery by Surgeons

A fully trained surgeon is a physician who, after medical school, has gone through years of training in an accredited residency program to learn the specialized skills of a surgeon. One good sign of a surgeon's competence is certification by a national surgical board approved by the American Board of Medical Specialties. All board-certified surgeons have satisfactorily completed an approved residency training program and have passed a rigorous specialty examination.

The letters FACS (Fellow of the American College of Surgeons) after a surgeon's name are a further indication of a physician's qualifications. Surgeons who become Fellows of the College have passed a comprehensive evaluation of their surgical training and skills; they also have demonstrated their commitment to high standards of ethical conduct. This evaluation is conducted according to national standards that were established to ensure that patients receive the best possible surgical care.

Reviewed by Jerome C. Goldstein, MD, FACS, Executive Vice-President, American Academy of Otorhinolaryngology, Alexandria, VA and Paul H. Ward, MD, FACS, Professor Emeritus, UCLA School of Medicine, Los Angeles, CA.

■ **Document Source:**
American College of Surgeons
55 East Erie St
Chicago, IL 60611

"DOCTOR, WHAT CAUSES THE NOISE IN MY EARS?" TEN COMMON QUESTIONS ABOUT TINNITUS

I sometimes hear ringing in my ears. Is this unusual?

Not at all. *Tinnitus* is the name for these head noises, and they are very common. Nearly 36 million other Americans suffer from this discomfort. Tinnitus may come and go, or you may be aware of a continuous sound. It can vary in pitch from a low roar to a high squeal or whine, and you may hear it in one or both ears. When the *ringing* is constant it can be annoying and distracting. More than seven million people are afflicted so severely that they cannot lead normal lives.

Can other people hear the noise in my ears?

Not usually, but sometimes they are able to hear a certain type of tinnitus. This is called *objective tinnitus*, and it is caused either by abnormalities in blood vessels around the outside of the ear or by muscle spasms which may sound like clicks or cracklings inside the middle ear.

What causes tinnitus?

There are many possible causes for *subjective tinnitus*, the noise only the patient can hear. Some causes are not serious. (For instance, a small plug of wax might cause temporary tinnitus.) Tinnitus can also be a symptom of more serious middle ear problems such as infection, a hole in the eardrum, an accumulation of fluid or stiffening (otosclerosis) of the middle ear bones. Tinnitus can also be a symptom of a head and neck aneurysm or acoustic neuroma, either of which can be life threatening. These problems often involve a loss of hearing. Tinnitus may also be caused by allergy, high (or low) blood pressure, a tumor, diabetes, thyroid problems, injury to the head or neck, and a variety of other specific causes including: anti-inflamatories, antibiotics, sedatives/antidepressants, and aspirin. (Aspirin can be a possible cause of tinnitus if overused, depending on the size of the patient. Talk to your doctor if you take aspirin and your ears ring.) The treatment will be quite different in each case. It is important to see a physician who specializes in ear disorders (an otolaryngologist) to attempt to determine the cause of your tinnitus and what kind of treatment, if any, may be needed.

What is the most common cause of tinnitus?

Most tinnitus comes from damage to the microscopic endings of the hearing nerve in the inner ear. The health of these nerve endings is important for acute hearing, and injury to them brings on hearing loss and often tinnitus. Advancing age is generally accompanied by a certain amount of hearing nerve impairment—and even tinnitus. Exposure to loud noises is probably the leading cause of tinnitus in today's world, and it often damages hearing as well. Unfortunately, many people are unaware of, or unconcerned about, the harmful effects of excessively loud industrial noise, firearms noise, high intensity music, and other loud noises. Stereo headsets played too loudly appear to be an increasing cause of ear damage in otherwise healthy young people.

What is the treatment of tinnitus?

In most cases, there is no specific treatment for noises in the ear or head. If an otolaryngologist finds on examination that your tinnitus has a specific cause, he may be able to remove the cause and thus eliminate the noise. This investigation may require a fairly extensive workup including x-rays, balance testing, and laboratory work. However, most causes of tinnitus cannot be identified. Occasionally, medicines may help the noise even though no cause can be identified. The medicines used are many. Frequently, the patient is requested to take a medicine to see if it helps.

When there is no identifiable cause, can something be done to lessen the tinnitus?

Yes, the following list of dos and don'ts can help lessen the severity of tinnitus. First of all, remember that the auditory (hearing) system is one of the most delicate and sensitive mechanisms of the human body. Since it is a part of the general nervous system, its responses are affected to some degree by the anxiety state of the person involved. Therefore, it is advisable to make every effort to

1. Avoid exposure to loud sounds and noises.
2. Get your blood pressure checked; if it is high, seek your doctor's help to get it under control.
3. Decrease your intake of salt (which impairs good blood circulation). Avoid salty foods and do not add salt to your food in cooking or at the table.
4. Avoid nerve stimulants such as coffee and colas (caffeine), tobacco (nicotine), and marijuana.
5. Exercise daily. It improves your circulation.
6. Get adequate rest and avoid overfatigue.
7. Stop worrying about the noise. Tinnitus will not cause you to go deaf or result in losing your mind or your life. Recognize your head noises as an annoying but minor reality, and then learn to ignore them as much as possible. This type of control can sometimes be greatly enhanced via the techniques of *biofeedback* and/or *masking*.
8. Reduce nervous anxiety, which may further stress an already tense hearing system.

What is biofeedback? Does it really work?

Biofeedback involves concentration and relaxation exercises designed to teach voluntary control of the circulation to various parts of the body and how to relax muscle groups throughout the body. When this type of control is accomplished, it may be effective in reducing the intensity of tinnitus in some patients.

What about masking? What is a tinnitus masker?

Tinnitus is usually more bothersome when the surroundings are quiet, especially when you are in bed. A competing sound such as a ticking clock or a radio may help *mask* head noises, making them less noticeable. Some physicians suggest listening to FM music at low volume. Many patients have been helped by dialing between two FM stations for the purpose of picking up subdued static, again at low volume. Such static may be extremely soothing, with a soft, rushing kind of sound known as *white noise*. Other patients prefer small electrical devices (e.g., *Sleep Mate*) which produce soothing background noise. These are sold through certain department stores and catalogs.

The tinnitus masker is a small electronic instrument built into or combined with a hearing aid. It generates a competitive but pleasant sound which for some individuals *masks* the tinnitus by reducing awareness of head noise. The result is similar to successful use of white noise—by helping a patient overcome his awareness of tinnitus before going to sleep at night.

Will hearing aids help reduce the noise?

People with impaired hearing sometimes find that their hearing aids reduce head noise and occasionally cause it to go away. Even a person with a minor hearing deficit may find that hearing aids relieve his tinnitus. However, a thorough trial before purchase is advisable if the primary purpose is the relief of tinnitus. Often, when the hearing aid is removed, the head noise returns to its former level.

Conclusion

Prior to any treatment of tinnitus or head noise, it is important that you have a thorough examination including an evaluation by your otolaryngologist. Once your doctor has completed this evaluation, an essential part of the treatment will be to help you to understand your tinnitus, what has caused it, and how best it may be treated.

Your hearing is too precious to treat carelessly. That is why this pamphlet is offered. We hope it has been helpful. If you have further questions, your otolaryngologist will be happy to try to answer them for you.

This article is published as a public service. The material may be freely used for noncommercial purposes so long as attribution is given to the American Academy of Otolaryngology—Head and Neck Surgery, Inc.

■ **Document Source:**
American Academy of Otolaryngology—Head and Neck Surgery
One Prince St
Alexandria, VA 22314-3357
1995

EARS, ALTITUDE, AND AIRPLANE TRAVEL

Have you ever wondered why your ears pop when you fly on an airplane? Or why, when they fail to pop, you get an earache? Have you ever wondered why the babies on an airplane fuss and cry so much during descent?

Ear problems are the most common medical complaint of airplane travelers, and while they are usually simple, minor annoyances, they occasionally result in temporary pain and hearing loss. This pamphlet is provided as a public service to help you understand the reasons for occasional ear problems during air travel, how to avoid them, and how to care for them.

Anatomy

Anatomists divide the ear into three parts:

1. **The outer ear** meaning the part of the ear you can see on the side of the head plus the ear canal leading down to the ear drum.
2. **The middle ear** meaning the ear drum, ear bones (ossicles), and the air spaces behind the ear drum and in the mastoid cavities.
3. **The inner ear** meaning where the nerve endings are for the organs of hearing and balance (equilibrium).

It is the middle ear that causes discomfort during air travel, and this is so because it is an air pocket inside the head that is vulnerable to changes in air pressure.

Normally, each time (or each second or third time) you swallow, your ears make a little click or popping sound. This is the moment that a small bubble of air enters your middle ear, up from the back of your nose. It passes through the Eustachian tube, a membrane-lined tube about the size of a pencil lead which connects the back of the nose with the middle ear. The air in the middle ear is constantly being absorbed by its membranous lining, but it is frequently re-supplied through the Eustachian tube during the process of swallowing. In this manner, air pressure on both sides of the eardrum stays about equal. If, and when, the air pressure is not equal, the ear feels blocked.

What causes blocked ears and Eustachian tubes?

The Eustachian tube can be blocked, or obstructed, for a variety of reasons. When that occurs, the middle ear pressure cannot be equalized. The air already there absorbs and a vacuum occurs, sucking the eardrum inward. Such an eardrum cannot vibrate naturally, so hearing sounds muffled or blocked. Also, the stretching of the eardrum can be painful. If the tube remains blocked for a period of time, fluid (like blood serum) will seep into the area from the membranes in an attempt to fill up the ear to overcome the vacuum. This is called "fluid in the ear," serous otitis or aero-otitis.

The most common cause for a blocked Eustachian tube is the common "cold." Sinus infections and nasal allergies (hayfever, etc.) are also frequently causes. This is because the membranes that line the Eustachian tube are similar to and continuous with nasal membranes. Consequently, a stuffy nose leads to stuffy ears because the swollen membranes block the opening of the Eustachian tube.

Another cause of blocked Eustachian tubes is infection of the middle ear which creates swollen membranes.

Children are especially vulnerable to blockages as their Eustachian tubes are narrower than in adults.

How can air travel cause problems?

Air travel is sometimes associated with rapid changes in air pressure. To maintain comfort, the Eustachian tube must function properly, that is, open frequently and widely enough to equalize the changes in pressure. This is especially true when the airplane is coming down for a landing, going from low atmospheric pressure down closer to earth where the air pressure is higher.

In the early days of airplanes with open cabins and cockpits, this was a major problem to flyers. Today's aircraft are pressurized so that air pressure changes are minimized. Even so, some changes in pressure are unavoidable, even in the best and most modern airplanes.

Actually, any situation in which rapid altitude or pressure changes occur creates the problem. You may have experienced it when riding in elevators of tall buildings or when diving to the bottom of a swimming pool. Deep sea divers are taught how to equalize their ear pressures; so are pilots. You can learn the tricks too.

How do you unblock your ears?

The act of swallowing activates the muscle that opens the Eustachian tube. You swallow more often when you chew gum or let mints melt in your mouth. These are good practices, especially just before and during descent. Yawning is even better. It is a stronger activator of that muscle. Be sure to avoid sleeping during descent, because you may not be swallowing often enough to keep up with the pressure changes. (The flight attendant will be happy to awaken you just before descent.)

If yawning and swallowing are not effective, the most forceful way to unblock your ears is as follows: (1) Pinch your nostrils shut; (2) Take a mouthful of air; (3) Using your cheek and throat muscles, force the air into the back of your nose as if you were trying to blow your thumb and fingers off your nostrils. When you hear a loud pop in your ears, you have succeeded. You may have to repeat this several times during descent.

Babies cannot intentionally pop their ears, but may do so if they are sucking on a bottle or pacifier. Feed your baby, and do not allow him to sleep during descent.

What precautions should you take?

When inflating your ears, you should not use force from your chest (lungs) or abdomen (diaphragm) which can create pressures that are too high. The proper technique involves only pressure created by your cheek and throat muscles.

If you have a cold, a sinus infection, or an allergy attack, it is best to postpone an airplane trip.

Also, if you recently have undergone ear surgery, consult with your surgeon on how soon you may safely fly.

What about decongestants and nose sprays?

Many experienced air travelers use a decongestant pill or nasal spray an hour or so before descent That will shrink the membranes and make the ears pop more easily. Travelers with allergy problems should take their medication at the beginning of the flight for the same reason.

Decongestant tablets and sprays can be purchased without a prescription. However, they should be avoided by persons with heart disease, high blood pressure, irregular heart rhythms, thyroid disease, or excessive nervousness. Such persons should consult their physicians before using these medicines. Pregnant women should likewise consult their physicians first.

What to Do If Your Ears Will Not Unblock

Even after landing you can continue the pressure equalizing techniques, and you may find the decongestants and nose sprays to be helpful. (However, avoid making a habit of nose sprays. After a few days, they may cause more congestion than they relieve.) If your ears fail to open, or if pain persists, you will need to seek the help of a physician who has experience in the care of ear disorders. He may need to release the pressure or fluid with a small incision in the ear drum.

This article is published as a public service. The material may be freely used for noncommercial purposes so long as attribution is given to the American Academy of Otolaryngology—Head and Neck Surgery, Inc.

■ Document Source:
American Academy of Otolaryngology—Head and Neck Surgery
One Prince St
Alexandria, VA 22314-3357
1995

HOARSENESS: PREVENTION & TREATMENT TIPS

What is hoarseness?

Hoarseness is a general term which describes abnormal voice changes. When hoarse, the voice may sound breathy, raspy, strained, or there may be changes in volume (loudness) or pitch (how high or low the voice is). The changes in sound are usually due to disorders related to the vocal folds which are the sound-producing parts of the voice box (larynx). While breathing, the vocal folds remain apart. When speaking or singing, they come together, and as air leaves the lungs, they vibrate, producing sound. The more tightly the vocal folds are held and the smaller the vocal folds, the more rapidly they vibrate. More rapid vibration makes a higher voice pitch. Swelling or lumps on the vocal folds prevent them from coming together properly, which makes a change in the voice.

What are the causes?

There are many causes of hoarseness. Fortunately, most are not serious and tend to go away in a short period of time. The most common causes are **acute laryngitis** which usually occurs due to swelling from a common cold, upper respiratory tract viral infection, or irritation caused by excessive voice use such as screaming at a sporting event or rock concert.

More prolonged hoarseness is usually due to using your voice either too much, too loudly, or improperly over extended periods of time. These habits can lead to **vocal nodules** (singers nodes), which are callous-like growths, or may lead to polyps of the vocal folds (more extensive swelling). Vocal nodules are common in children and adults who raise their voice in work or play. Uncommonly, polyps or nodules may lead to cancer.

A common cause of hoarseness in older adults is **gastroesophageal reflux,** when stomach acid comes up the swallowing tube (esophagus) and irritates the vocal folds. Many patients with reflux-related changes of voice do not have symptoms of heartburn. Usually, the voice is worse in the morning and improves during the day. These people may have a sensation of a lump in their throat, mucous sticking in their throat or an excessive desire to clear their throat.

Smoking is another cause of hoarseness. Since smoking is the major cause of throat cancer, if smokers are hoarse, they should see an otolaryngologist.

Many unusual causes for hoarseness include **allergies, thyroid problems, neurological disorders, trauma to the voice box,** and occasionally the **normal menstrual cycle.** Many people experience some hoarseness with **advanced age.**

Who can treat my hoarseness?

Hoarseness due to a cold or flu may be evaluated by family physicians, pediatricians, and internists (who have learned how to examine the larynx). When hoarseness lasts longer than two weeks or has no obvious cause, it should be evaluated by an otolaryngologist—head and neck surgeon (ear, nose, and throat doctor). Problems with the voice are best managed by a team of professionals who know and understand how the voice functions. These professionals are otolaryngology—head and neck surgeons, speech/language pathologists, and teachers of singing, acting, or public speaking. Voice disorders have many different characteristics which may give professionals a clue to the cause.

When should I see an otolaryngologist (ENT doctor)?

- If hoarseness lasts longer than two to three weeks
- If hoarseness is associated with

  - pain not from a cold or flu
  - coughing up blood
  - difficulty swallowing
  - a lump in the neck

- Complete loss or severe change in voice lasting longer than a few days

How is hoarseness evaluated?

An otolaryngologist will obtain a thorough history of the hoarseness and your general health. Your doctor will usually look at the vocal folds with a mirror placed in the back of your throat. Occasionally a very small lighted flexible scope (fiberoptic tube scope) may need to be passed through your nose (or in some cases, a rigid scope may be used which is placed in the back of your mouth) in order to view your vocal folds. Videotaping the examination may also help with the analysis.

These procedures are not uncomfortable and are well tolerated by most patients. In some cases, special tests (known as acoustic analysis) designed to evaluate the voice may be recommended. These measure voice irregularities, how the voice sounds (acoustic content), airflow, and other characteristics that are helpful in establishing a diagnosis and guiding treatment.

How are vocal disorders treated?

The treatment of hoarseness depends on the cause. Most hoarseness can be treated by simply resting the voice or modifying how it is used. The otolaryngologist may make some recommendations about voice use behavior, refer the patient to other voice team members, and in some instances recommend surgery if a discreet lesion, such as a nodule or polyp, is identified. Avoidance of smoking or exposure to secondhand smoke (passive smoking) is recommended to all patients. Drinking fluids is also helpful.

Specialists in speech/language pathology are trained to assist patients in behavior modification which may help eliminate some voice disorders. Sometimes, patients have developed bad habits, such as smoking or overuse of their voice by yelling and screaming, which may cause the voice disorder. The speech/language pathologist may teach patients to alter their method of speech production to improve the sound of the voice and to resolve problems, such as vocal nodules. When a patient's problem is specifically related to singing, a singing teacher may help improve the patients' singing techniques.

What can I do to prevent and treat mild hoarseness?

- If you smoke, quit
- Avoid agents which dehydrate the body, such as alcohol and caffeine
- Avoid secondhand smoke
- Drink plenty of water
- Humidify your home
- Watch your diet—avoid spicy foods and alcohol
- Try not to use your voice too long or too loudly
- Seek professional voice training
- Avoid speaking or singing when your voice is injured or hoarse (this is similar to not walking on a sprained ankle)

This article is published as a public service. The material may be freely used for noncommercial purposes so long as attribution is given to the American Academy of Otolaryngology—Head and Neck Surgery, Inc.

■ Document Source:
American Academy of Otolaryngology—Head and Neck Surgery
One Prince St
Alexandria, VA 22314-3357
1995

MENIERE'S DISEASE

What is Meniere's disease?

Meniere's disease, also called idiopathic endolymphatic hydrops, is a disorder of the inner ear. Although the cause is unknown, it probably results from an abnormality in the fluids of the inner ear. Meniere's disease is one of the most common causes of dizziness originating in the inner ear. In most cases only one ear is involved, but both ears may be affected in about 15 percent of patients. Meniere's disease typically starts between the ages of 20 and 50 years. Men and women are affected in equal numbers.

What are the symptoms?

The symptoms of Meniere's disease are episodic rotational vertigo (attacks of a spinning sensation), hearing loss, tinnitus (a roaring, buzzing, or ringing sound in the ear), and a sensation of fullness in the affected ear. Vertigo is usually the most troublesome symptom of Meniere's disease. It is defined as a sensation of movement when no movement is occurring. Vertigo is commonly produced by disorders of the inner ear but may also occur in central nervous system disorders. The vertigo of Meniere's disease occurs in attacks of a spinning sensation and is accompanied by dysequilibrium (an off-balance sensation), nausea, and sometimes vomiting. The vertigo lasts for 20 minutes to two hours or longer. During attacks, patients are usually unable to perform activities normal to their work or home life. Sleepiness may follow for several hours, and the off-balance sensation may last for days.

There may be an intermittent hearing loss early in the disease, especially in the low pitches, but a fixed hearing loss involving tones of all pitches commonly develops in time. Loud sounds may be uncomfortable and appear distorted in the affected ear.

The tinnitus and fullness of the ear in Meniere's disease may come and go with changes in hearing, occur during or just before attacks, or be constant.

The symptoms of Meniere's disease may be only a minor nuisance, or can become disabling, especially if the attacks of vertigo are severe, frequent, and occur without warning.

How is a diagnosis made?

The physician will take a history of the frequency, duration, severity, and character of your attacks, the duration of hearing loss or whether it has been changing, and whether you have had tinnitus or fullness in either or both ears. You may be asked whether there is a history of syphilis, mumps, or other serious infections in the past, inflammations of the eye, an autoimmune disorder or allergy, or ear surgery in the past. You may be asked questions about your general health, such as whether you have diabetes, high blood pressure, high blood cholesterol, thyroid, neurologic, or emotional disorders. Tests may be ordered to look for these problems in certain cases. The physical examination of the ears and other structures of the head and neck is usually normal, except during an attack.

An audiometric examination (hearing test) typically indicates a sensory type of hearing loss in the affected ear. Speech discrimination (the patient's ability to distinguish between words like "sit" and "fit") is often diminished in the affected ear. An ENG (electronystagmograph) may be performed to evaluate balance function. This is done in a darkened room. Recording electrodes are placed near the eyes. Wires from the electrodes are attached to a machine similar to a heart monitor. Warm and cool water or air are gently introduced into each ear canal. Since the eyes and ears work in a coordinated manner through the nervous system, measurement of eye movements can be used to test the balance system. In about 50 percent of patients, the balance function is reduced in the affected ear. Other balance tests, such as rotational testing or balance platform, may also be performed to evaluate the balance system.

Other tests may be done! Electrocochleography (ECoG) may indicate increased inner ear fluid pressure in some cases of Meniere's disease. The auditory brain stem response (ABR), a computerized test of the hearing nerves and brain pathways, computed tomography (CT), or magnetic resonance imaging (MRI) may be needed to rule out a tumor occurring on the hearing and balance nerve. Such tumors are rare, but they can cause symptoms similar to Meniere's disease.

What treatment will the physician recommend?

Diet and Medication

A low salt diet and a diuretic (water pill) may reduce the frequency of attacks of Meniere's disease in some patients. In order to receive the full benefit of the diuretic, it is important that you restrict your intake of salt and take the medication regularly as directed.

Anti-vertigo medications, e.g., Antivert® (meclizine generic), or Valium®(diazepam generic), may provide temporary relief. Anti-nausea medication is sometimes prescribed. Anti-vertigo and anti-nausea medications may cause drowsiness.

Life Style

Avoid caffeine, smoking, and alcohol. Get regular sleep and eat properly. Remain physically active, but avoid excessive fatigue. Stress may aggravate the vertigo and tinnitus of Meniere's disease. Stress avoidance or counselling may be advised.

Precautions

If you have vertigo without warning, you should not drive, because failure to control the vehicle may be hazardous to yourself and others. Safety may require you to forego ladders, scaffolds, and swimming.

When is surgery recommended?

If vertigo attacks are not controlled by conservative measures and are disabling, one of the following surgical procedures might be recommended:

1. The endolymphatic shunt or decompression procedure is an ear operation that usually preserves hearing. Attacks of vertigo are controlled in one-half to two-thirds of cases, but control is not permanent in all cases. Recovery time after this procedure is short compared to the other procedures.

2. Selective vestibular neurectomy is a procedure in which the balance nerve is cut as it leaves the inner ear and goes to the brain. Vertigo attacks are permanently cured in a high percentage of cases, and hearing is preserved in most cases.

3. Labyrinthectomy and eighth nerve section are procedures in which the balance and hearing mechanism in the inner ear are destroyed on one side. This is considered when the patient with Meniere's disease has poor hearing in the affected ear. Labyrinthectomy and eighth nerve section result in the highest rates for control of vertigo attacks.

   Other operations or treatments may be advised in some cases. If surgical treatment seems to be needed, the risks and benefits should be thoroughly discussed with your surgeon. Although there is no cure for Meniere's disease, the attacks of vertigo can be controlled in nearly all cases.

This article is published as a public service. The material may be freely used for noncommercial purposes so long as attribution is given to the American Academy of Otolaryngology—Head and Neck Surgery, Inc.

■ Document Source:
American Academy of Otolaryngology—Head and Neck Surgery
One Prince St
Alexandria, VA 22314-3357
1995

MIDDLE EAR FLUID IN YOUNG CHILDREN

About the Ear and Hearing

The ear has three parts—the outer ear, the middle ear, and the inner ear. The outer ear includes the part outside the head and the ear canal. The eardrum is a small circle of tissue about the size of a fingertip at the end of the ear canal. The middle ear is the space, usually filled with air, behind the eardrum. When a child has middle ear fluid, this is where it is found. A small tube — the eustachian tube — connects the middle ear to the back of the nose. Three tiny bones (the malleus, incus, and stapes) connect the eardrum through the middle ear to the inner ear. The inner ear is further inside the head and is important for hearing and balance.

In a healthy ear, sound waves travel through the ear canal and make the eardrum move back and forth. This makes the three bones in the middle ear move. The movement of these bones sends sound waves across the middle ear to the inner ear. The inner ear sends the sound messages to the brain. But if the middle ear has fluid in it, then the eardrum and the bones cannot move well. This could cause your child to have trouble hearing.

Purpose of this Booklet

This booklet is about middle ear fluid in children ages one through three who have no other health problems. After reading this booklet, you should know more about

- Causes of middle ear fluid.
- Tests for middle ear fluid and hearing.
- Treatments for middle ear fluid and hearing loss caused by middle ear fluid.
- How to work with your child's health care provider to find the best treatment for your child's middle ear fluid.

Another name for middle ear fluid is otitis media with effusion. Some people also call it "glue ear." Otitis media means middle ear inflammation, and effusion means fluid.

What is middle ear fluid?

If your child has middle ear fluid, it means that a watery or mucouslike fluid has collected behind the eardrum. Many children get middle ear fluid during their early years. But middle ear fluid is not the same as an ear infection.

- An **Ear Infection** usually happens in only one ear at a time. With a middle ear infection, your child may have fever and sharp ear pain. When your health care provider looks into your child's ear, they might see a bulging red eardrum and some fluid in the middle ear.

- **Middle Ear Fluid** is usually found in both ears at once. Most children do not have fever or pain with middle ear fluid. A special test is needed to look for this fluid.

What causes middle ear fluid?

Here are some things that may cause middle ear fluid to happen in your child:

- Past ear infection. It is common for children to have middle ear infections. And some children with middle ear infection later have middle ear fluid.
- Blockage of the eustachian tube.
- Cold or flu.

There is no one cause for middle ear fluid. Often, your child's health care provider will not know what caused the middle ear fluid.

You may want to use the chart at the end of this booklet to keep track of when your child has ear problems and medical treatments.

Why should I be worried about middle ear fluid?

Most health care providers and parents worry that a child who has middle ear fluid in one or both ears can have trouble hearing. Experts do not know how much middle ear fluid affects hearing. Experts are not sure if hearing loss from middle ear fluid can cause delays in learning to talk and, sometimes later on, problems with school work. They do not know for sure what the long-term effects of middle ear fluid are.

How can middle ear fluid be prevented?

Recent studies show that children who live with smokers and who spend time in group child care have more ear infections.

Because some children who have middle ear infections later get middle ear fluid, you might help prevent middle ear fluid by

- Keeping your child away from cigarette smoke.
- Trying to keep your child away from playmates who are sick.

How do I know if my child is affected by middle ear fluid?

Sometimes a child with middle ear fluid does not hear well. The most common complaint of parents whose child has middle ear fluid is that the child turns the sound up too loud or sits too close to the television set. Or sometimes the child does not seem to be paying attention.

Speak to your child's health care provider if you are concerned about your child's hearing. Often, middle ear fluid is found at a regular check-up.

Your child's health care provider may use the first two tests below to check for middle ear fluid.

- A **Pneumatic Otoscope** may be used to check for middle ear fluid. With this tool, the health care provider looks at the eardrum. The fluid in the middle ear may be seen behind the eardrum. Even when the fluid cannot be seen, the health care provider can test for fluid with this tool by blowing a puff of air onto the eardrum to see how well the eardrum moves. The child must be still for this test to work. The child will feel the otoscope in the ear, but the test does not hurt. This test does NOT measure the child's hearing level. Many health care providers feel that the pneumatic otoscope is the best test for middle ear fluid.
- **Tympanometry** is another test for middle ear fluid. Tympanometry helps the health care provider find out

how well the eardrum moves.For tympanometry, a soft plug that is about the size of a person's little fingertip is placed snugly into the ear canal. The probe is connected to a machine called a tympanometer. The child hears a low noise for a short time while the machine records how the eardrum reacts. An eardrum with fluid behind it does not move as well as a normal eardrum.

Like the first test, the child must sit still for this test and will feel the probe in the ear. The test does not hurt. Tympanometry does NOT measure hearing level.

- **Hearing Testing** may be done to see how well your child hears. Hearing testing does not test for middle ear fluid. In this case, it measures if the fluid is affecting your child's hearing level. The type of hearing test used depends on your child's age and listening ability.

How can middle ear fluid be treated?

Middle ear fluid can be treated in many ways. It is important to know that a treatment that works for one child may not work for another. If one treatment does not work, another treatment can be tried. Please discuss each of the treatments listed here with your child's health care provider. Be sure to ask about the possible advantages and disadvantages of each treatment as well. Then, decide with your child's health care provider on the treatment for middle ear fluid.

- **Observation**—Middle ear fluid often goes away without treatment. Some studies show that for most children middle ear fluid clears after three to six months without treatment.
- **Antibiotic Drug Treatment**—Studies show that middle ear fluid cleared slightly faster in some children given antibiotic drugs than those not given antibiotics. However, antibiotics have some unwanted effects, such as diarrhea, rash, and others. Also, they can be expensive, and some children have trouble taking them. For these reasons, you and your child's health care provider may want to try observation first.

  Before making a decision, ask your child's health care provider about the costs and possible unwanted effects.
- **Surgery to Put "Tubes" in the Ears**—In this minor operation, a small cut is made in the child's eardrum and fluid in the middle ear is gently sucked out. Then a small metal or plastic tube is put into the slit in the eardrum. A general anesthetic is used to put the child to sleep for this operation. When the fluid is removed from the middle ear, the child's hearing returns to its normal level.

Ask your child's health care provider about the costs and possible harms of this surgery.

The tubes are left in place until they fall out, or until your child's health care provider feels that they are no longer needed. About one third (one out of three) of children with ear tubes need to have another operation to insert new tubes within five years after the first operation.

What are the advantages and disadvantages of middle ear fluid treatments?

The advantages and disadvantages of treatments for middle ear fluid are listed in the following table. Please discuss these choices further with your child's health care provider.

Treatment	Advantages	Disadvantages
Observation	In about 60 percent of children, middle ear fluid goes away without treatment within three months; in 85 percent it goes away within six months. There is very little cost and no side effects of observation.	Middle ear fluid does not go away in about 40 percent of children in three months and in about 15 percent in six months.
Antibiotic drug	May increase chance by about 14 percent and speed of middle ear fluid going away.	Middle ear fluid may not go away. May decrease chance of middle ear infection. Unwanted drug effects (such as diarrhea, rash). Development of drug-resistant strains of bacteria. Bother of buying and giving drug. Cost of drug.
Surgery (tubes)	Middle ear fluid goes away right away. Hearing returns to normal right away.	Temporary discomfort for child. Risks of anesthesia. May need to protect ears during bathing and swimming while tubes are in place. Some children need another surgery to place new tubes in the ears. Eardrum changes possible. Time lost to take child for surgery. Most costly choice.

When should middle ear fluid be treated?

The treatment that your child gets for middle ear fluid depends on

- How long your child has had middle ear fluid.
- If the fluid is causing hearing problems for your child.

Here are some examples of how your child might best be treated for middle ear fluid.

Remember to discuss all treatments with your child's health care provider. Be sure to ask about the advantages and disadvantages of each treatment.

If your child has had *middle ear fluid for up to three months,* then your child's health care provider may recommend one of these treatments:

- Observation OR antibiotic therapy. You and your provider may choose observation because antibiotic therapy can cause some unwanted effects.
- Taking steps to prevent middle ear fluid (especially keeping your child away from cigarette smoke).

If your child has had *middle ear fluid for three months or more,* then your child's health care provider may recommend the following treatments:

- Observation OR antibiotic drugs. You and your provider may choose observation because antibiotic therapy can cause some unwanted effects.
- Taking steps to prevent middle ear fluid (especially keeping your child away from cigarette smoke).

Also

- A hearing test is recommended if your child has had middle ear fluid for 3 months or more. If this shows that your child has a hearing loss in both ears, your child's health care provider may recommend surgery to put tubes in the eardrums.
- Talk to your child's health care provider about any other concerns you have about your child's development—for example, if your child does not seem to be learning to talk on schedule.

If your child has had *middle ear fluid that has lasted from four to six months with a hearing loss in both ears,* then your child's health care provider may recommend:

- Surgery to put tubes in the eardrums. Tubes in the eardrums should clear the middle ear fluid and return your child's hearing to normal. Discuss this surgery with your child's health care provider.

Also

- Find out if your child's ears should be protected from water after the surgery and when to bring your child back for a check-up.

What treatments are not recommended for my child?

A number of medicines and surgical treatments are not recommended for young children with middle ear fluid.

The medicines not recommended are

- Decongestants and antihistamines.
- Steroids.

Most studies show that decongestants and antihistamines used together or alone did not improve or cure middle ear fluid. There are not yet enough studies to tell whether steroids can cure or improve middle ear fluid.

The surgical treatments not recommended are

- Adenoidectomy.
- Tonsillectomy.

There are not yet enough studies to tell if adenoidectomy (removing the adenoids—tissue at the back of the throat,

behind the nose) cures or improves middle ear fluid in children younger than four years old. But it does seem to help older children. Tonsillectomy (removing the tonsils at the back of the throat) has not been shown to cure or improve middle ear fluid in children.

If your child's health care provider suggests one of these surgeries, there may be another medical reason to do the surgery. Ask why your child needs the surgery. If you are still unsure, you may want to talk to another health care provider.

How do I keep track of my child's ear problems?

You may want to use a chart like this one to keep track of your child's ear problems and how they were treated. This may help your child's health care provider to find the cause of the middle ear fluid.

For *(child's name):* _____
Health care provider's name: _____
Health care provider's telephone number: _____

Date and type of middle ear problem fluid or infection	Treatment	Results

For Further Information

The information in this booklet was based on the *Clinical Practice Guideline, Otitis Media with Effusion in Young Children.* The *Guideline* was developed by a non-federal panel of experts sponsored by the Agency for Health Care Policy and Research. Other guidelines on common health problems are available, and more are being developed.

For more information about guidelines or to receive more copies of this booklet, call toll-free: 1-800-358-9295 or write to

Agency for Health Care Policy and Research
Publications Clearinghouse
PO Box 8547
Silver Spring, MD 20907

■ **Document Source:**
   U.S. Department of Health and Human Services, Public Health Service
   Agency for Health Care Policy and Research
   Executive Office Center, Ste 501
   2101 E Jefferson St
   Rockville, MD 20852
   AHCPR Publication No. 94-0624
   July 1994

SNORING: NOT FUNNY, NOT HOPELESS

> Some 45 percent of normal adults snore at least occasionally, and 25 percent are habitual snorers. Problem snoring is more frequent in males and overweight persons, and it usually grows worse with age.

More than 300 devices are registered in the U.S. Patent and Trademark Office as cures for snoring. Some are variations on the old idea of sewing a tennis ball on the pajama back—to force the snorer to sleep on his side. (Snoring is often worse when the person sleeps on his back.) Chin and head straps, neck collars, and devices inserted into the mouth are usually disappointing as snoring cures. Many electrical devices have been designed to produce painful or unpleasant stimuli when the patient snores. The presumption was that a person could be trained or conditioned not to snore. Unfortunately, snoring is not under the person's control whatsoever, and if these devices work, it is probably because they keep the snorer awake.

What causes snoring?

The noisy sounds of snoring occur when there is an obstruction to the free flow of air through the passages at the back of the mouth and nose. This is the collapsible part of the airway where the tongue and upper throat meet the soft palate and uvula (the fleshy structure that dangles from the roof of the mouth back into the throat). When these structures strike against each other and vibrate during breathing, that is snoring. Persons who snore have at least one of the following problems:

1. Poor muscle tone (lack of tightness) in the muscles of the tongue and throat. Flabby muscles allow the tongue to fall backwards into the airway or allow the throat muscles to be drawn in from the sides into the airway. This occurs when the person's muscular control is too relaxed from alcohol or from drugs which cause sleepiness. It also happens in some persons when they relax in the deep-sleep stages.
2. Excessive bulkiness of tissues of the throat. Large tonsils and adenoids, for example, commonly cause snoring in children. Overweight persons also have bulky neck tissues. Cysts or tumors could also be present, but they are rare.
3. Excessive length of the soft palate and uvula. A long palate may narrow the opening from the nose into the throat. As it dangles in the airway, it acts as a flutter valve during relaxed breathing and contributes to the noise of snoring. A long uvula makes matters even worse.
4. Obstructed nasal airways. When a person has a stuffy or blocked-up nose he must pull hard to inhale air

through it. This creates an exaggerated vacuum in his throat, in the collapsible part of the airway, and it pulls together the floppy tissues of the throat. So snoring occurs even in persons who would not snore if they could breathe through the nose properly. This explains why some people snore only during the hay fever season or when they have a cold or sinus infection. Also, deformities of the nose or nasal septum frequently cause such obstruction. "Deviated septum" is a common term for a deformity inside the nose in the wall that separates one nostril from the other.

Is snoring serious?

Socially—yes. It is disruptive to family life. It makes the snorer an object of ridicule and causes other household members sleepless nights and resentfulness. Snorers become unwelcome roommates on vacations or business trips.

And medically—yes. It disturbs the sleeping patterns of the snorer himself, so that he may not sleep restfully. Furthermore, heavy snorers tend to develop high blood pressure at a younger age than non-snorers.

The most exaggerated form of snoring is known as obstructive sleep apnea, when loud snoring is interrupted by frequent episodes of totally obstructed breathing. This is serious if the episodes last over 10 seconds each and occur more than seven times per hour. Your physician may recommend a laboratory sleep study as a way of evaluating your symptoms. Apnea patients may experience 30 to 300 obstructed events per night, and many spend as much as half their sleep time with blood oxygen levels below normal. During their obstructive episodes, the heart must pump harder to circulate the blood faster. This can cause irregular heartbeats, and after many years it leads to elevated blood pressure and heart enlargement. The immediate effect of this oxygen starvation is that the person must sleep in a lighter stage and tense his muscles enough to open his airway to get air into his lungs. Since snorers with severe sleep apnea are often unaware of it, laboratory sleep study may be the only way to discover it.

Persons with obstructive sleep apnea may spend little of their night-time hours in the deep-sleep stages that are essential for a good rest. Therefore, they awaken unrefreshed and are sleepy much of the day. They may fall asleep while driving to work or while on the job.

Can snoring be cured?

By far, the majority of snorers can be helped.

For adults who are mild or occasional snorers, the following self-help remedies are worth trying.

1. Adopt an athletic lifestyle and exercise daily to develop good muscle tone and lose weight.
2. Avoid tranquilizers, sleeping pills, and antihistamines before bedtime.
3. Avoid alcoholic beverages within four hours of retiring.

4. Avoid heavy meals within three hours of retiring.
5. Avoid getting overtired; establish regular sleeping patterns.
6. Sleep sideways rather than on the back. Consider sewing a pocket on the pajama back to hold a tennis ball. This helps to avoid sleeping on your back.
7. Tilt the entire bed with the head upwards four inches (place bricks under the bedposts at the bedhead).
8. Allow the nonsnorer to get to sleep first.

Heavy snorers, those who snore in any position they sleep in, and so-called "obnoxious snorers," need more help than the suggestions above.

When snoring becomes disruptive to the life of the snorer or his family, medical advice should be sought, especially if other household members suspect the obstructive sleep apnea problem (very loud snoring with periods when all airflow stops—even though the snorer is trying to breathe).

The heavy snorer deserves a thorough examination of the nose, mouth, palate, throat, and neck. Studies in a sleep laboratory are valuable to determine how serious the snoring is and what effects it has on the snorer's health. Treatment will depend, of course, on the diagnosis. It may be as simple as managing a nasal allergy or infection, surgically correcting a nasal deformity, or removing tonsils and adenoids. Or, snoring/apnea may respond best to surgery on the throat and palate to tighten up flabby tissues and expand the air passages, an operation called UvuloPalatoPharyngoPlasty (UPPP). To the patient, it feels like having a tonsillectomy. If surgery is too risky, unwanted, or unsuccessful, the patient may sleep every night wearing a nasal mask which delivers air pressure into the throat ("CPAP").

Every chronically snoring child should also be thoroughly examined. Medical evidence suggests a tonsillectomy and adenoidectomy will probably make an important difference in the health and well-being of the child.

Remember, snoring means obstructed breathing, and obstruction can be serious. It's not funny, and it's definitely not hopeless.

This leaflet is published as a public service. The material may be freely used for noncommercial purposes so long as attribution is given to the American Academy of Otolaryngology—Head and Neck Surgery, Inc.

■ **Document Source:**
American Academy of Otolaryngology—Head and Neck Surgery
One Prince St
Alexandria, VA 22314-3357
1995

EYE DISEASES AND DISORDERS

■■■

CATARACT IN ADULTS: A PATIENT'S GUIDE

This booklet can help you decide what to do if you have a cataract. Talk about it with your eye doctor so you can make the choices that are right for you.

What is a cataract?

A cataract is a cloudy area in the lens of the eye.

A normal lens is clear. It lets light pass to the back of the eye. A cataract blocks some of the light. As a cataract develops, it becomes harder for a person to see.

Cataract is a normal part of aging. About half of Americans ages 65 to 74 have cataract. About 70 percent of those age 75 and over have this condition.

Most people with cataract have a cataract in both eyes. However, one eye may be worse than the other because each cataract develops at a different rate.

Some people with cataract don't even know it. Their cataract may be small, or the changes in their vision may not bother them very much. Other people who have cataract cannot see well enough to do the things they need or want to do.

What are the symptoms of cataract?

Here are some signs of cataract:

- Cloudy, fuzzy, foggy, or filmy vision.
- Changes in the way you see colors.
- Problems driving at night because headlights seem too bright.
- Problems with glare from lamps or the sun.
- Frequent changes in your eyeglass prescription.
- Double vision.
- Better near vision for a while; only in farsighted people.

These symptoms also can be signs of other eye problems. **See your eye doctor to find out what you have and how it can be treated.**

How is cataract diagnosed?

A regular eye exam is all that is needed to find a cataract. Your eye doctor will ask you to read a letter chart to see how sharp your sight is. You probably will get eye drops to enlarge your pupils (the round black centers of your eyes). This helps the doctor to see the inside of your eyes. The doctor will use a bright light to see whether your lenses are clear and to check for other problems in the back of your eyes.

Other eye tests may also be used occasionally to show how poorly you see with cataract or how well you might see after surgery:

- Glare test.
- Contrast sensitivity test.
- Potential vision test.
- Specular photographic microscopy.

Only a few people need these tests.

How is cataract treated?

A change in your glasses, stronger bifocals, or the use of magnifying lenses may help improve your vision and be treatment enough. The way to surgically treat a cataract is to remove all or part of the lens and replace it with an artificial lens.

Just because you have a cataract does not mean it must be removed immediately. Cataract surgery can almost always be put off until you are unhappy with the way you see.

Your eye doctor will tell you whether you are one of a small number of people who must have surgery. For example, your doctor may need to see or treat an eye problem that is behind the cataract. Or surgery may be required because a cataract is so large that it could cause blindness.

How do I decide whether to have surgery?

Most people have plenty of time to decide about cataract surgery. Your doctor cannot make your decision for you, but talking with your doctor can help you decide.

Tell your doctor how your cataract affects your vision and your life. Check the statements below that apply to you and share this list with your doctor:

- I need to drive, but there is too much glare from the sun or headlights.
- I do not see well enough to do my best at work.
- I do not see well enough to do the things I need to do at home.
- I do not see well enough to do things I like to do (for example, read, watch TV, sew, hike, play cards, go out with friends).
- I am afraid I will bump into something or fall.
- Because of my cataract, I am not as independent as I would like to be.
- My glasses do not help me see well enough.
- My eyesight bothers me a lot.

You may also have other specific problems that you want to discuss with your eye doctor.

What should I know about surgery?

Your doctor will discuss the options with you before choosing the best kind of cataract removal and lens replacement for you. He or she will also explain how to prepare for surgery and how to take care of yourself after it is over.

Most people do not need to stay overnight in a hospital to have cataract surgery. You may go to an outpatient center or hospital, have your cataract removed, and leave when your doctor says you are fit to leave. However, you will need a friend or family member to take you home. You also will need someone to stay with you for at least a day to help you follow your doctor's instructions.

It takes a few months for an eye to heal after cataract surgery. Your eye doctor should check your progress and make sure you have the care you need until your eye recovers fully.

Removing the Lens

There are three types of surgery to remove lenses that have a cataract:

- *Extracapsular surgery.* The eye surgeon removes the lens, leaving behind the back half of the capsule (the outer covering of the lens).
- *Phacoemulsification* (pronounced FAY-co-ee-mul-sih-fih-CAY-shun). In this type of extracapsular surgery, the surgeon softens the lens with sound waves and removes it through a needle. The back half of the lens capsule is left behind.
- *Intracapsular surgery.* The surgeon removes the entire lens, including the capsule. This method is rarely used.

Replacing the Lens

A person who has cataract surgery usually gets an artificial lens at the same time. A plastic disc, called an intraocular lens, is placed in the lens capsule inside the eye. Other choices are contact lenses and cataract glasses. Your doctor will help you to decide which choice is best for you.

Can a cataract return?

A cataract cannot return because all or part of the lens has been removed. However, in about half of all people who have extracapsular surgery or phacoemulsification, the lens capsule becomes cloudy. This cloudiness of the lens capsule, if it occurs, usually develops a year or more after surgery. It causes the same vision problems as a cataract does.

The treatment for this condition is a procedure called YAG capsulotomy. The doctor uses a laser (light) beam to make a tiny hole in the capsule to let light pass. This surgery is painless and does not require a hospital stay.

Most people see better after YAG capsulotomy, but, as with cataract surgery, complications can occur. Your doctor will discuss the risks with you. *YAG capsulotomy should not be performed as a preventive measure.*

Is cataract surgery right for me?

Most people who have a cataract recover from surgery with no problems and improved vision. In fact, serious complications are not common with modern cataract surgery. This type of surgery has a success rate of 95 percent in patients with otherwise healthy eyes. But no surgery is risk free. Although serious complications are not common, when they occur they could result in loss of vision.

If you have a cataract in both eyes, experts say it is best to wait until your first eye heals before having surgery on the second eye. If the eye that has a cataract is your only working eye, you and your doctor should weigh very carefully the benefits and risks of cataract surgery.

You will be able to make the right decision for yourself if you know the facts. Ask your doctor to explain anything you do not understand. There is no such thing as a "dumb" question when it comes to your health. Here are some questions you might ask:

- Do I need surgery right away?
- If not, how long can I wait?
- What are my personal risks?
- What benefits can I expect?
- If I choose surgery, which type is best for me?
- Which lens replacement is best for me?
- What are the chances of developing cloudiness in the lens capsule after cataract surgery?
- What are the benefits and risks of YAG capsulotomy?

You may wish to write down other questions to ask your doctor to help you make an informed decision about treatment.

Benefits and Risks of Cataract Surgery

Improvements in Activities

- Everyday activities
- Driving
- Reading
- Working
- Moving around

- Social activities
- Hobbies
- Safety
- Self-confidence
- Independence

Possible Complications

- High pressure in the eye
- Blood collection inside the eye
- Infection inside the eye
- Artificial lens damage or dislocation
- Drooping eyelid
- Retinal detachment
- Severe bleeding inside the eye
- Swelling or clouding of the cornea
- Blindness
- Loss of the eye

How can I learn more about cataract?

Organizations that can provide additional information include:

American Academy of Ophthalmology
PO Box 7424
San Francisco, CA 94120-7424
Phone: (415) 561-8500

American Optometric Association
Communications Center
243 North Lindbergh Blvd
St. Louis, MO 63141-7881
Phone: (314) 991-4100

National Eye Institute
National Institutes of Health
Bethesda, MD 20892
Phone: (301) 496-5248

National Society to Prevent Blindness
500 East Remington Rd
Schaumburg, IL 60173
Phone: toll free 1-800-331-2020

For Further Information

The information in this booklet was based on the *Clinical Practice Guideline on Cataract in Adults: Management of Functional Impairment.* The guideline was developed by an expert panel sponsored by the Agency for Health Care Policy and Research. Other guidelines on common health problems are available, and more are being developed.

For more information on guidelines or to receive more copies of this booklet, call toll free 1-800-358-9295 or write to

Agency for Health Care Policy and Research
Publications Clearinghouse
PO Box 8547
Silver Spring, MD 20907

■ Document Source:
   U.S. Department of Health and Human Services, Public Health Service
   Agency for Health Care Policy and Research
   Executive Office Center, Ste 501
   2101 E Jefferson St

Rockville, MD 20852
AHCPR Publication No. 93-0544
February 1993

DIABETIC RETINOPATHY

This pamphlet has been written to help people with diabetic retinopathy and their families better understand the disease. It describes the cause, symptoms, diagnosis, and treatment of diabetic retinopathy.

Diabetic retinopathy is a potentially blinding complication of diabetes that damages the eye's retina. It affects half of the 14 million Americans with diabetes.

At first, you may notice no changes in your vision. But don't let diabetic retinopathy fool you. It could get worse over the years and threaten your good vision. With timely treatment, 90 percent of those with advanced diabetic retinopathy can be saved from going blind.

The National Eye Institute (NEI) is the Federal government's lead agency for vision research. The NEI urges all people with diabetes to have an eye examination through dilated pupils at least once a year.

1. What is the retina?

The retina is a light-sensitive tissue at the back of the eye. When light enters the eye, the retina changes the light into nerve signals. The retina then sends these signals along the optic nerve to the brain. Without a retina, the eye cannot communicate with the brain, making vision impossible.

2. How does diabetic retinopathy damage the retina?

Diabetic retinopathy occurs when diabetes damages the tiny blood vessels in the retina. At this point, most people do not notice any changes in their vision.

Some people develop a condition called **macular edema.** It occurs when the damaged blood vessels leak fluid and lipids onto the macula, the part of the retina that lets us see detail. The fluid makes the macula swell, blurring vision.

As the disease progresses, it enters its advanced, or **proliferative,** stage. Fragile, new blood vessels grow along the retina and in the clear, gel-like vitreous that fills the inside of the eye. Without timely treatment, these new blood vessels can bleed, cloud vision, and destroy the retina.

3. Who is at risk for this disease?

All people with diabetes are at risk—those with Type I diabetes (juvenile onset) and those with Type II diabetes (adult onset).

During pregnancy, diabetic retinopathy may also be a problem for women with diabetes. It is recommended that all pregnant women with diabetes have dilated eye examinations each trimester to protect their vision.

4. What are its symptoms?

Diabetic retinopathy often has no early warning signs. At some point, though, you may have macular edema. It blurs vision, making it hard to do things like read and drive. In some cases, your vision will get better or worse during the day.

As new blood vessels form at the back of the eye, they can bleed (hemorrhage) and blur vision. The first time this happens, it may not be very severe. In most cases, it will leave just a few specks of blood, or spots, floating in your vision. They often go away after a few hours.

These spots are often followed within a few days or weeks by a much greater leakage of blood. The blood will blur your vision. In extreme cases, a person will only be able to tell light from dark in that eye. It may take the blood anywhere from a few days to months or even years to clear from inside of your eye. In some cases, the blood will not clear. You should be aware that large hemorrhages tend to happen more than once, often during sleep.

5. How is it detected?

Diabetic retinopathy is detected during an eye examination that includes:

- **Visual acuity test:** This eye chart test measures how well you see at various distances.
- **Pupil dilation:** The eye care professional places drops into the eye to widen the pupil. This allows him or her to see more of the retina and look for signs of diabetic retinopathy. After the examination, close-up vision may remain blurred for several hours.
- **Ophthalmoscopy:** This is an examination of the retina in which the eye care professional (1) looks through a device with a special magnifying lens that provides a narrow view of the retina or (2), wearing a headset with a bright light, looks through a special magnifying glass and gains a wide view of the retina.
- **Tonometry:** A standard test that determines the fluid pressure inside the eye. Elevated pressure is a possible sign of glaucoma, another common eye problem in people with diabetes.

Your eye care professional will look at your retina for early signs of the disease, such as (1) leaking blood vessels, (2) retinal swelling, such as macular edema, (3) pale, fatty deposits on the retina—signs of leaking blood vessels, (4) damaged nerve tissue, and (5) any changes in the blood vessels.

Should your doctor suspect that you need treatment for macular edema, he or she may ask you to have a test called **fluorescein angiography.**

In this test, a special dye is injected into your arm. Pictures are then taken as the dye passes through the blood vessels in the retina. This test allows your doctor to find the leaking blood vessels.

6. How is it treated?

There are two treatments for diabetic retinopathy. They are very effective in reducing vision loss from this disease. In fact, even people with advanced retinopathy have a 90 percent chance of keeping their vision when they get treatment before the retina is severely damaged. These treatments are

Laser Surgery

Doctors will perform laser surgery to treat severe macular edema and proliferative retinopathy.

Macular Edema: Timely laser surgery can reduce vision loss from macular edema by half. But you may need to have laser surgery more than once to control the leaking fluid.

During the surgery, your doctor will aim a high-energy beam of light directly onto the damaged blood vessels. This is called **focal laser treatment.** This seals the vessels and stops them from leaking. Generally, laser surgery is used to stabilize vision, not necessarily to improve it.

Proliferative Retinopathy: In treating advanced diabetic retinopathy, doctors use the laser to destroy the abnormal blood vessels that form at the back of the eye.

Rather than focus the light on a single spot, your eye care professional will make hundreds of small laser burns away from the center of the retina. This is called **scatter laser treatment.** The treatment shrinks the abnormal blood vessels. You will lose some of your side vision after this surgery, to save the rest of your sight. Laser surgery may also slightly reduce your color and night vision.

Laser surgery is performed in a doctor's office or eye clinic. Before the surgery, your ophthalmologist will (1) dilate your pupil and (2) apply drops to numb the eye. In some cases, the doctor also may numb the area behind the eye to prevent any discomfort.

The lights in the office will be dim. As you sit facing the laser machine, your doctor will hold a special lens to your eye. During the procedure, you may see flashes of bright green or red light. These flashes may eventually create a stinging sensation that makes you feel a little uncomfortable.

You may leave the office once the treatment is done, but you will need someone to drive you home. Because your pupils will remain dilated for a few hours, you also should bring a pair of sunglasses.

For the rest of the day, your vision will probably be a little blurry. Your eye may also hurt a bit. This is easily controlled with drugs that your eye care professional suggests.

Vitrectomy

If you have a lot of blood in the vitreous, you may need an eye operation called a **vitrectomy** to restore sight. It involves removing the cloudy vitreous and replacing it with a salt solution. Because the vitreous is mostly water, you will notice no change between the salt solution and the normal vitreous.

Studies show that people who have a vitrectomy soon after a large hemorrhage are more likely to protect their vision than someone who waits to have the operation. Early vitrectomy is especially effective in people with insulin-dependent diabetes, who may be at greater risk of blindness from a hemorrhage into the eye.

Vitrectomy is often done under local anesthesia (using drops to numb the eye). This means that you will be awake during the operation. The doctor makes a tiny incision in the sclera, or white of the eye. Next, a small instrument is placed into the eye. It removes the vitreous and inserts the salt solution into the eye.

You may be able to return home soon after the vitrectomy. Or, you may be asked to stay in the hospital overnight. Your eye will be red and sensitive. After the operation, you will need to wear an eyepatch for a few days or weeks to protect the eye. You will also need to use medicated eye drops to protect against infection.

Although laser surgery and vitrectomy are very successful, they do not cure diabetic retinopathy. Once you have proliferative retinopathy, you will always be at risk for new bleeding. This means you may need treatment more than once to protect your sight.

7. What research is being done?

The NEI is currently supporting a number of research studies in both the laboratory and with patients to learn more about the cause of diabetic retinopathy. This research should provide better ways to detect, treat, and prevent vision loss in people with diabetes.

For example, it is likely that in the coming years researchers will develop drugs that turn off enzyme activity that has been shown to cause diabetic retinopathy. Some day, these drugs will help people to control the disease and reduce the need for laser surgery.

8. What can you do to protect your vision?

The NEI urges all people with diabetes to have an eye examination through dilated pupils at least once a year. If you have more serious retinopathy, you may need to have a dilated eye examination more often.

A recent study, the Diabetes Control and Complications Trial (DCCT), showed that better control of blood sugar level slows the onset and progression of retinopathy and lessens the need for laser surgery for severe retinopathy.

The study found that the group that tried to keep their blood sugar levels as close to normal as possible had much less eye, kidney, and nerve disease. This level of blood sugar control may not be best for everyone, including some elderly patients, children under 13, or people with heart disease. So ask your doctor if this program is right for you.

For more information about diabetic retinopathy or diabetes, you may wish to contact

American Academy of Ophthalmology
655 Beach St
PO Box 7424
San Francisco, CA 94109-7424
(415) 561-8500

American Optometric Association
243 Lindbergh Blvd

St. Louis, MO 63141
(314) 991-4100

American Diabetes Association
1660 Duke St
Alexandria, VA 22314
(703) 549-1500

Juvenile Diabetes Foundation International
432 Park Ave S
New York, NY 10016
(212) 889-7575

National Eye Institute
2020 Vision Pl
Bethesda, MD 20892-3655
(301) 496-5248

National Diabetes Outreach Program National Institute of Diabetes and Digestive and Kidney Diseases
1 Diabetes Way
Bethesda, MD 20892-3560
1-800-GET-LEVEL

■ **Document Source:**
   U.S. Department of Health and Human Services Public Health Service
   National Institutes of Health
   National Eye Institute
   NIH Publication No. 95-3252

See also: Diabetes Overview (page 130)

DON'T LOSE SIGHT OF AGE-RELATED MACULAR DEGENERATION: INFORMATION FOR PEOPLE AT RISK

1. What is age-related macular degeneration (AMD)?

AMD is a common eye disease associated with aging that gradually destroys sharp, central vision. Central vision is needed for seeing objects clearly and for common daily tasks such as reading and driving. In some people, AMD advances so slowly that it will have little effect on their vision as they age. But in others, the disease progresses faster and may lead to a loss of vision in one or both eyes.

2. How does AMD damage vision?

The retina is a paper-thin tissue that lines the back of the eye and sends visual signals to the brain. In the middle of the retina is a tiny area called the macula. The macula is made up of millions of light-sensing cells that help to produce central vision.

AMD occurs in two forms:

Dry AMD

Ninety percent of all people with AMD have this type. Scientists are still not sure what causes dry AMD. Studies suggest that an area of the retina becomes diseased, leading to the slow breakdown of the light-sensing cells in the macula and a gradual loss of central vision.

Wet AMD

Although only 10 percent of all people with AMD have this type, it accounts for 90 percent of all blindness from the disease. As dry AMD worsens, new blood vessels may begin to grow and cause wet AMD. Because these new blood vessels tend to be very fragile, they will often leak blood and fluid under the macula. This causes rapid damage to the macula that can lead to the loss of central vision in a short period of time.

3. Who is most likely to get AMD?

The greatest risk factor is age. Although AMD may occur during middle age, studies show that people over age 60 are clearly at greater risk than other age groups. For instance, a large study found that people in middle-age have about a two percent risk of getting AMD, but this risk increased to nearly 30 percent in those over age 75.

Other AMD risk factors include:

Gender

Women tend to be at greater risk for AMD than men.

Race

Whites are much more likely to lose vision from AMD than Blacks.

Smoking

Smoking may increase the risk of AMD.

Family History

Those with immediate family members who have AMD are at a higher risk of developing the disease.

4. What are the symptoms?

Both dry and wet AMD cause no pain. The most common early sign of dry AMD is blurred vision. As fewer cells in the macula are able to function, people will see details less clearly in front of them, such as faces or words in a book. Often this blurred vision will go away in brighter light. If the loss of these light-sensing cells becomes great, people may see a small—but growing—blind spot in the middle of their field of vision.

The classic early symptom of wet AMD is that straight lines appear crooked. This results when fluid from the leaking blood vessels gathers and lifts the macula, distorting vision.

A small blind spot may also appear in wet AMD, resulting in loss of one's central vision.

5. How is it detected?

Your eye care professional may suspect AMD if you are over age 60 and have had recent changes in your central vision. To look for signs of the disease, he or she will use eye drops to dilate, or enlarge, your pupils. Dilating the pupils allows your eye care professional to view the back of the eye better.

You may also be asked to view an Amsler grid, a pattern that looks like a checkerboard. Early changes in your central vision will cause the grid to appear distorted, a sign of AMD.

6. How can it be treated?

No treatment now exists for dry AMD. It has been suggested that taking certain extra vitamins and minerals may slow the progress of the disease. But this treatment needs much more research before scientists can know for sure if it's helpful.

Eye care professionals can treat some cases of wet AMD with laser surgery. This treatment involves aiming a strong light beam onto the new blood vessels to destroy them. Laser surgery is done in a doctor's office or in an eye clinic and lasts a short period of time. Although a person may go home the same day, he or she will need to return for follow-up exams.

7. What research is being done?

The National Eye Institute is funding a number of research studies to learn what causes AMD and how it can be better treated. For instance, in the Age Related Eye Diseases Study (AREDS), researchers are assessing the aging process in the eyes of thousands of older people to discover the earliest signs of AMD. The same study is also evaluating the effects of certain vitamins and minerals in preventing or slowing the progress of AMD.

At the same time, other scientists are trying to learn more about how the cells in the retina work. This knowledge will allow them some day to pinpoint the cause of the disease and design methods to prevent it.

8. What can you do to protect your vision?

Although there is no effective treatment for dry AMD at this time, it is crucial that those who progress to wet AMD and need laser surgery have it before the disease destroys central vision. For this reason, if you have dry AMD or are age 60 or older, you should have your eyes examined through dilated pupils at least once a year. You may also want to get an Amsler grid from your eye care professional to check your vision at home.

To learn more about AMD, write

National Eye Health Education Program
Box 20/20
Bethesda, MD 20892

■ Document Source:
U.S. Department of Health and Human Services, Public Health Service
National Institutes of Health
National Eye Institute
NIH Publication No. 93-3462

GUARDING AGAINST GLAUCOMA

by S.J. Ackerman

An outstanding scholar still in his 30s, John felt his "sight getting weak and dull"—occupational eyestrain, he supposed. Soon his left eye dimmed, starting from the left side. Then his right eye failed, "perceptibly and gradually over three years." By age 43, he was totally blind.

That was in 1652. John Milton triumphed over blindness, still serving the British foreign office and writing literary classics like "Paradise Lost." Yet he never ceased lamenting "how my light is spent/Ere half my days, in this dark world and wide."

What relegated him to seeing "a universal blank" was probably open-angle glaucoma, which today needlessly blinds 80,000 Americans each year. It causes another 900,000 to lose some vision. Yet now we have means Milton lacked to thwart "the sneak thief of sight" with a number of treatments approved by the Food and Drug Administration.

Glaucomas are a group of diseases sharing certain features, commonly including high intraocular pressure (IOP), damaged optic nerves, and loss of peripheral vision. Early detection can contain two glaucomas: chronic (sometimes called common) and acute.

Primary open-angle glaucoma (chronic glaucoma) affects mostly adults over age 35. This most prevalent glaucoma is the sneak-thief disease without noticeable symptoms. By the time it's detected, it has started doing damage.

The uncommon primary angle-closure glaucoma (acute glaucoma) may seem the opposite of common glaucoma, erupting in a sudden, violent attack. It's also possible to get both common and acute ("combined-mechanism") glaucoma together. The unusual low-pressure glaucoma is another variant. Regular eye examinations can help protect against the onset of open-angle and closed-angle glaucomas.

The cornea is the clear outer covering of the eye. Separating it from the iris (the colored part) is the anterior chamber, a space filled and inflated by aqueous humor. This fluid (unrelated to the tears which bathe the outside surface of the cornea) originates in the ciliary body just behind the iris. It circulates in the anterior chamber, nourishing the eye's delicate tissue and keeping it from collapsing, at a pressure usually measuring between 10 and 20 millimeters of mercury. To maintain equilibrium, the aqueous humor drains through a porous tissue in the angle in front of the iris, where it meets the cornea, called the trabecular meshwork.

If the aqueous humor cannot drain properly, either because the drainage canals become clogged (as in chronic glaucoma) or because the iris is pushing against the cornea (as in angle-closure glaucoma), it backs up, exerting pressure on the gel in the vitreous cavity at the center of the eye. Eventually, the building pressure affects the delicate optic nerve at the rear. Since the optic nerve transmits visual images to the brain, damage to parts of it correspondingly reduces vision.

Pressure over 21 millimeters may prompt concern, while pressure over 24 mm can indicate glaucoma level—but not always. These measures are not absolute. Some individuals tolerate higher pressures than others. Half the people with undiagnosed glaucoma have pressures below 22 mm, while others with higher pressures never develop glaucoma, with optic nerve damage causing loss of vision. Low-pressure glaucoma can be especially elusive. Moreover, tonometry (the measurement of eye pressure) can be affected by many factors, even by the time of day (IOP measuring highest in the morning).

Tonometry measures the force necessary to indent the eye. One method is to anesthetize the eye, then press a tonometer onto it. Another is to measure the force needed for a puff of air to indent the cornea.

While widespread eye-puff testing at health fairs detects pressure levels, a more thorough examination calls for an ophthalmoscopic test enabling doctors to see into your eye to examine the optic nerve for damage or a high ratio of its central cup to the surrounding disc. They must also take personal characteristics into account in evaluating an individual's risk of glaucoma.

Chronic Glaucoma

Physicians do not like to begin therapy prematurely in individuals identified as at risk for chronic glaucoma. Patients who are considered "pre-glaucoma" should have their eyes examined as often as their doctors think necessary.

Increasingly frequent dosages of medications may be needed as the eye develops tolerance to the medicine. Drug therapy can effectively thwart the progress of glaucoma, but it can mean taking an escalating variety of eye drops and pills, with various side effects, for life.

Topical medications for glaucoma are serious medicine, not to be confused with over-the-counter eye drops for easing common eye irritations. The most popular maintenance eye drop, Timoptic (timolol maleate), may have side effects on the nerves, digestion, vision, skin, respiration, and heart of some individuals. Timoptic is a beta-blocker eye drop. Taken usually twice daily, beta blockers decrease production of aqueous humor. Side effects may include lowered pulse rate and blood pressure, exacerbated asthma, and fatigue. In June 1995, British researchers reported that drops in this class may be related to breathing impairment in elderly people with previously unrecognized respiratory problems.

Timoptic's century-old predecessor, pilocarpine, requires more frequent use to do its job, increasing drainage of aqueous fluid in both open- and closed-angle glaucomas. Pilocarpine is a miotic, designed to increase aqueous fluid drainage. Because miotics work by making the pupil smaller, they can result in dim vision and may increase the risk of cataracts.

Another class of medications, adrenergic agonists, such as epinephrine, also increases aqueous humor drainage, with possible side effects of allergic reactions, blurred vision, headache, and increased heart rate. Alpha adrenergic agonists decrease aqueous humor production after surgery or aid patients taking maximum dosages of other medications. Side effects include red eyes, allergic reactions, and dry mouth.

Diamox carbonic anhydrase inhibitor tablets, like beta blockers, decrease production of aqueous fluid, but these drugs seem to provoke more prominent side effects in some people, including mental depression, kidney stones, tingling in the hands and feet, and sometimes anemia.

FDA's May 1995 approval of a Carbonic Anhydrase Inhibitor in eye drop form as Trusopt (dorzolamide) provides a medication that may have fewer and reduced incidence of these severe side effects.

Since reactions to medications vary so much from person to person, a drug that causes one individual problems may be easily tolerated by another. An appropriate drug regimen, therefore, needs to be worked out carefully between patient and health professional.

Glaucoma medications are potent drugs. Those who take them should consult a pharmacist to be certain that they won't interact adversely with any other prescriptions or over-the-counter drugs being taken. For example, some over-the-counter products, including decongestants, may not be suited for people at risk of glaucoma.

Acute Glaucoma

A century after Milton gradually lost his sight, composer Johann Sebastian Bach went blind in a violent flash, probably from acute (closed-angle) glaucoma. Bach thought he aggravated his weak vision by a lifetime of copying music in the dim light of church organ lofts; his portrait shows a characteristic squint. Though a surgeon claimed to have operated successfully on Bach's eyes, the composer's vision failed again in a few days. He died a few months later, after a futile—and possibly harmful—second operation.

Acute glaucoma may seem the opposite of open-angle because it erupts in violent attacks and intense pain, rather than emerging subtly. Yet patients may not notice minor preliminary episodes, which pave the way for serious seizures. People beset by a major seizure must get to an ophthalmologist, or at least a hospital emergency room, promptly to save their vision.

Monitoring can protect people prone to acute glaucoma from major attacks.

Acute glaucoma attacks are emergencies because aqueous fluid gets trapped in the angle of the eye suddenly. Having nowhere to go, its abrupt backup can damage the optic nerves, eventually squashing them irreparably.

Regular, thorough eye checkups can detect the risk of acute glaucoma. High IOP, family history, and other indicators resemble those for common glaucoma, but very far-sighted people and those of Asian descent are most vulnerable to angle-closure glaucoma. Once a major angle-closure attack

seems imminent, preventive laser surgery is advisable, since an attack can damage the eye quickly.

Risks and Responses

Elevated eye pressure and detectable damage to the optic nerves are significant risk indicators for glaucoma. To prevent needless blindness from undetected, untreated glaucoma, the American Academy of Ophthalmology offers additional guidelines for assessing risk.

The academy's guidelines include comparing the diameter of the eye's cup to that of its disc to obtain a physical gauge of the likelihood of glaucoma. Estimates are made vertically along an imaginary line drawn through the center of the disc from the 12 o'clock to the 6 o'clock position. The normal optic nerve illustrated with a small cup has a cup-to-disc ratio of less than 0.5, indicating a low probability of glaucoma. Moderately advanced cupping, with a cup-to-disc ratio of 0.6 to 0.8 and a neural rim starting to thin, increases the suspicion of glaucoma. Almost total cup-to-disc ratio of 0.9, exhibiting a very thin neural rim, creates a high level of glaucoma suspicion.

Personal history factors also enter the assessment, as shown in the chart below. The greater the number in the third column, the greater the risk.

Variable	Category	Weight
Age	younger than 50 years	0
	50-64 years	1
	65-74 years	2
	older than 75 years	3
Race	Caucasian/other	0
	African American	2
Family History	Negative or positive	
of Glaucoma	in non-first degree relatives	0
	Positive for parents	1
	Positive for siblings	2
Last Complete Eye	Within last two years	0
Examination	2-5 years ago	1
	more than 5 years ago	2

Level of Glaucoma Risk (Total Score)

High	4 or greater
Moderate	3
Low	2 or less

Other variables in risk assessment include extreme nearsightedness or farsightedness, high blood pressure, and steroid use.

People at risk of glaucoma should faithfully have eye checkups at the intervals their ophthalmologists recommend. Everyone over 40 should have a full eye examination every two years, regardless of risk factors; African Americans should be vigilant after age 30. Adult relatives of persons diagnosed with glaucoma should have regular eye checkups. Glaucoma seems to be hereditary, and even cousins may be at risk if you are.

Glaucoma treatment decisions are personalized. Even eye color may affect the rate at which a person absorbs eye medications.

Regular monitoring of people diagnosed with narrow-angle conditions looks for increased IOP or tissue damage. Telltale symptoms of an attack include blurred vision, halos around lights, and eye pain sharp enough to induce vomiting. The eye becomes reddened, feeling as if it could burst (though it can't). Persons experiencing such attacks should go immediately to an ophthalmologist or an emergency room, ideally calling in advance to ready staff to receive a case of closed-angle, acute glaucoma.

Emergency procedures use eye drops and clinical eye massage to reduce IOP and prevent the eye from hardening. Once stabilized, the patient may have laser surgery to create an artificial opening for aqueous fluid to drain. Acute glaucoma usually attacks one eye before the other, so laser surgery on the unaffected eye may be recommended at the time to forestall a second attack there.

Laser Surgery

Some patients may require traditional scalpel surgery, but in recent years laser operations have come into favor. Laser surgery can't repair existing damage, but it usually stops glaucoma, both in acute emergencies and open-angle cases. It may involve minor side effects, including restrictions on wearing contact lenses, but its risks are quite low. Sometimes, it must be repeated if its drainage openings begin to close.

Light amplification by stimulated emission of radiation—LASER—sends a uniform, focused beam of light to pin-point applications. In glaucoma surgery for angle closure, the laser creates a minute hole in the iris, just large enough to allow aqueous fluid to flow freely.

Despite its high-tech wizardry, most laser surgery for glaucoma seems quite undramatic to the patient undergoing it. (See "Light for Sight," *FDA Consumer*, July-August 1990.) An acute glaucoma patient peers into the eyepiece on one side of a boxy device while a surgeon manipulating controls peers into an eye-piece opposite. There's little or no additional pain, often not even unpleasant sensation, as the surgeon beams an intense beam of light to "burn" an escape channel for aqueous fluid, usually in the upper edge of the iris.

The Nd: YAG (neodymium: yttrium aluminum garnet crystal) laser has emerged with several advantages over the earlier argon laser, including lower energy requirement, fewer pulses, reduced obstruction, and a lower rate of subsequent closure of incisions. Its portability allows the YAG laser to serve even remote Inuit villages in Alaska previously inaccessible for sophisticated optical surgery.

No wonder that laser surgery in just 25 years has largely displaced traditional scalpel surgery, which involves hospital stays and higher risks. Its low risk allows use earlier in the course of the disease, when its potential benefit is greater.

On the Horizon

Diligence in countering early the subtle onset of glaucoma is the best protection. Research is making such diligence easier.

Ongoing research aims to simplify dosage demands while reducing side effects. For instance, the nuisance of taking preventive eye medications several times a day discourages some people from protecting themselves fully. Work is under way to perfect a once-a-week eye preparation and one-a-day eye drops to ease the use of topical eye medications.

Already, dispenser tips that measure more consistent doses of eye drops are improving their use.

Even the standard course of escalating treatment for common glaucoma is being reconsidered. The practice more common in Europe suggests that reversing this order by starting with surgery may be promising. In August 1993, the National Eye Institute announced the Collaborative Initial Glaucoma Treatment Study to compare the long-term effect of treating newly diagnosed primary open-angle glaucoma with standard treatment versus immediate laser surgery.

For More Information

For more information about glaucoma, contact

- your doctor
- American Academy of Ophthalmology's Glaucoma 2001 Campaign (for chronic open-angle glaucoma): (415) 561-8500
- Glaucoma Research Foundation: 1-800-826-6693 or (415) 986-3162
- National Eye Institute: (301) 496-5248

■ **Document Source:**
U.S. Department of Health and Human Services, Public Health Service
Food and Drug Administration
FDA Consumer
November 1995

NOT A CURE-ALL: EYE SURGERY HELPS SOME SEE BETTER

by Marian Segal

"Men seldom make passes at girls who wear glasses," Dorothy Parker observed in 1926. True or not, when the writer penned her now famous line, the only alternative to glasses was poor sight. Things are rosier—but not perfect—in 1995.

Today, growing numbers of women and men alike are opting for refractive eye surgery to correct their myopia (nearsightedness) in hopes of abandoning their glasses or contact lenses. The most common procedure is called radial keratotomy, or RK, and the National Eye Institute says about 250,000 are done each year in the United States, up from 30,000 just five years ago.

Another surgery, newly available in the United States, is photorefractive keratectomy, or PRK. The Food and Drug Administration last October approved the Summit Apex excimer laser system for use in this procedure.

A report by the American Academy of Ophthalmology published in the July 7, 1993, issue of Ophthalmology indicates that cosmetic reasons are not at the top of the list of reasons why people choose to have refractive surgery. The report states: "In two studies, approximately 75 percent of the patients who were interviewed about their reasons for seeking radial keratotomy stated that they wished to see well without physical dependence on ... spectacles or contact lenses. Patients also sought radial keratotomy to improve their performance in profession or sport, to improve cosmetic appearance, for simple convenience, or at times to meet the visual requirements for occupations such as law enforcement and firefighting."

David Euley, a 52-year-old Darnestown, MD, kitchen designer and home remodeler, began to consider RK when he found himself becoming increasingly frustrated with his glasses, particularly at work.

"It was difficult to go back and forth from blueprints to taking measurements to working on a computer," he says, adding that he needed a separate prescription for computer work.

Euley talked with several ophthalmologists before deciding to have the surgery last December. Interviewed four months later, he was delighted with the results: "This is the first time in 25 years I've been able to see the titles on television without glasses. I can read license plates. I can see the deer in my backyard. And my glasses are sitting on a shelf somewhere."

Six incisions in each cornea (the clear part of the front of the eye) left Euley with uncorrected vision improved from 20/800 in both eyes to 20/20 in the right and 20/25 in the left. (A person with 20/40 vision, for example, would see an object from 20 feet that another with perfect vision—20/20—could see at 40 feet. Some people see even better than 20/20.)

RK is often done in the doctor's office. As in Euley's case, surgeries on each eye are usually scheduled a few weeks apart, as a precaution in case there are complications. The patient is given anesthetic eye drops to numb the eye. Using a high-precision diamond blade knife, the surgeon makes from four to eight spoke-like incisions in the cornea, while the patient focuses on the light of the operating microscope. The surgery takes about 10 to 15 minutes.

I can see clearly now.

Euley can read those license plates without glasses now because the incisions changed the shape of his corneas. Normally, the cornea and lens bend light rays to focus directly on the retina—the tissue at the back of the eye that receives the image. If the cornea or lens is too rounded, or the eyeball is elongated, the light focuses in front of the retina, blurring distant objects. RK reduces or eliminates the myopia by flattening the cornea and redirecting the light to focus on the retina.

The patient may have some pain or discomfort for 24 to 48 hours after surgery, possibly requiring medication. Glare, starbursting, or a halo effect, especially at night, is common for a few months and occasionally persists a year or more. Vision also commonly fluctuates during the day, with acuity best in the morning and diminishing somewhat at night. This decreases in severity during the first year, but may last for many years.

Notwithstanding some claims to the contrary, RK is not a cure-all. (The Federal Trade Commission is investigating the problem of misleading claims in advertisements.) Repu-

table ophthalmologists will tell prospective patients the procedure is not completely risk-free, and perfect vision cannot be guaranteed.

Is RK safe and effective?

"FDA does not regulate radial keratotomy because it is a medical procedure, not a medical device," says Emma Knight, an ophthalmologist and medical reviewer with FDA's Center for Devices and Radiological Health. "The knife used in RK had been cleared by the agency for general corneal surgery."

The National Eye Institute (NEI), however, concluded from a 10-year study called "Prospective Evaluation of Radial Keratotomy (PERK)" that RK is "reasonably safe and effective . . . with serious complications being rare."

All patients in the study had -2 to -8 diopters and could be corrected to 20/20 vision or better with glasses or contact lenses. (A diopter is the unit of measurement of spectacle or contact lens power. A minus value indicates nearsightedness; plus indicates farsightedness, or hyperopia. Euley's correction was -3.25 diopters.)

Results of the NEI-sponsored multicenter trial were reported by study investigator George Waring III, MD, and colleagues in the October 1994 Archives of Ophthalmology. Among 374 patients (with 693 operated eyes) who returned for the 10-year follow-up

- 70 percent said they did not wear glasses or contact lenses for distance vision.
- 53 percent had 20/20 vision without glasses.
- 85 percent had at least 20/40 vision without glasses—the acuity most states require for driving without glasses.
- Of the total 793 eyes operated (including data from the most recent examination of those who didn't return for the 10-year follow-up), 143 lost one line of best spectacle-corrected vision on the standard eye chart, 19 lost two lines, and four lost three lines. (Best corrected vision in all but 16 eyes was 20/20—they previously had better than 20/20 corrected vision. Thirteen eyes were corrected to 20/25 and three to 20/30.) This means that, although eyesight *without* glasses was improved from pre-surgery acuity, residual nearsightedness could not be corrected with glasses to pre-surgery acuity.
- 38 percent of patients were corrected within one-half diopter of the predicted result; 60 percent were within one diopter.
- 43 percent developed "hyperopic shift"—a gradual change toward farsightedness (one or more diopters between six months and 10 years) at a younger age than would be expected.

The cornea is weakened by radial keratotomy, increasing the risk of eye rupture from physical trauma. According to the article by the American Academy of Ophthalmology, however, there have been reports of severe eye trauma without damage to the incision wounds. The report also says that potentially blinding complications, such as corneal infection or perforation, are rare.

More recent studies using newer RK techniques have achieved better optical results, says Peter Hersh, MD, director of keratorefractive surgery at Montefiore Hospital, Bronx, NY.

Surgeons have designed improved methods for calculating the number and length of incisions and the diameter of the optical zone (the central clear zone that has no cuts) that will produce the best results in a given patient, he says.

"We've had numbers reported as high as 95 percent or so for 20/40 as the procedure has evolved," Hersh says. "The most important variable is patient age. Younger patients tend to heal their incisions better and more quickly, and therefore get less of an effect. Also, patients with lower degrees of myopia do better than high myopes," he says. Some other factors that may be considered when determining surgical procedure include corneal curvature, topography and thickness, and ocular pressure.

The Laser Method

An alternative to radial keratotomy is photorefractive keratectomy, or PRK. "In countries where PRK has been available for some time, the procedure has largely replaced RK as the procedure of choice," says FDA's Knight, adding that "with FDA approval of the excimer laser, this trend is expected to follow in the United States."

In this procedure, the surgeon operates an excimer laser programmed to deliver bursts of ultraviolet light that vaporize precisely targeted corneal tissue. The effect, as in RK, is to flatten the cornea. Also like RK, PRK takes about 15 minutes and is done under topical anesthesia.

In October 1994, FDA's ophthalmic devices advisory panel recommended conditional approval of one manufacturer's excimer laser for refractive surgery, pending reformatting and reanalysis of some of the data.

"This was the first time the agency critically assessed safety and effectiveness data of any device for refractive surgery," says Knight, "and the meeting was long and full of debate."

Approval in October 1995 was based on PRK results in about 1,600 healthy myopic eyes. In most eyes, the corneal surface healed in three days, and vision took at least three months to stabilize. Most patients studied were corrected to 20/20 vision or better with glasses or contact lenses before surgery. Best corrected vision was worse in 6 percent of patients after surgery but, of those, only 1 percent had less than 20/25 acuity and fewer than 0.2 percent were worse than 20/40.

In 95 percent of eyes, vision without glasses was corrected to 20/40 or better; 65 percent achieved 20/20 or better. About 5 percent of patients continued to need glasses all the time for distance, and up to 15 percent needed glasses occasionally, such as for driving. Results were best in younger patients with lower degrees of myopia.

Some 63 percent of patients had mild corneal haze after surgery, and 10 percent experienced mild glare and halos around lights. These conditions diminished or disappeared in most patients in six months.

According to the American Academy of Ophthalmology, RK results are best in patients with low to moderate nearsightedness and generally is not recommended for people with a correction higher than -5 diopters. PRK is effective for patients with higher myopia as well and is approved for treatment of up to -7 diopters.

With approval of the laser, FDA also reviewed and approved a physician training program and a patient information booklet. The training program for surgeons covers operation and calibration of the laser, plus extensive clinical, didactic, and practical sessions. The patient booklet is provided to physicians, who in turn are required to give it to patients and discuss it with them before surgery.

Mary Taylor had her first PRK in November 1993. The highly myopic 42-year-old Winchester, VA, woman had worn glasses since second grade. Her correction was -9.5 diopters in one eye and -10 in the other.

"I tried contacts a few times, but never really got comfortable with them," she says, "and, although I didn't especially mind wearing glasses, I was bothered by how helpless I felt without them. The thought of losing them if something happened while I was driving or swimming—even if I had a spare pair—was always a worry in the back of my mind."

Taylor says she received about 700 laser bursts at periodic intervals during the procedure. Then the doctor put a soft "bandage" contact lens in her eye to be worn the next few days until the surface cells healed. She was given a nonsteroidal anti-inflammatory eyedrop for pain and a prescription for additional pain medicine, if needed.

"That first day I felt a mild discomfort, like a residual scratchiness after removing a piece of sand from the eye. It was gone when I woke up the next morning," Taylor says. Although her vision improved greatly immediately, it took about a month or two, she says, before she was seeing 20/20. Six months after the first operation, she returned for surgery in the second eye.

As of October 1994, according to Taylor's doctor, her vision was 20/25 without glasses and 20/20 with glasses, and her correction was -0.75 diopter. Taylor says she still has some trouble with night glare and needs glasses to drive at night, but she's delighted with the results. "For the first time in my life that I could remember, I could see my feet in the shower," she says.

RK vs. PRK

Jeffrey Robin, MD, has a unique perspective on RK and PRK. Head of the department of refractive surgery at the Cleveland Clinic, Robin has done both procedures on patients in clinical trials and has, himself, undergone both procedures.

"I've worn glasses since I was eight, and started wearing contact lenses when I was 17 or 18," Robin says. "I went through many pairs of lenses—tore them, slept in them. I was not a good contact lens patient and I detested wearing my glasses, basically because I didn't perceive I was seeing well with them," he says.

About five years ago, at age 35, Robin had an 8-incisional RK in his right eye. A year later, he had PRK in the left. He felt only minor, temporary discomfort after both surgeries but says that before anti-inflammatory drops were used with PRK, that procedure often produced intense post-surgery pain.

"With RK, vision is almost instantaneously improved—I went from about 20/800 to better than 20/20 the morning after surgery," Robin says. "After PRK, I had better than 20/20 after about 10 days to two weeks. The big difference with the laser is that the correction is solid—there's no visual fluctuations and really no starbursting like you get with RK. Except for the couple of weeks after my RK when I used night driving glasses, I haven't worn glasses since. I've almost forgotten I ever wore them."

Four years of follow-up with PRK has shown fewer complications, such as infection or cataract, than are seen with RK. Also, hyperopic shift has not been seen with PRK, nor is the cornea weakened as it is in RK. On the other hand, Robin says, "we have 15 or 16 years of experience with RK as opposed to about four years with PRK. Between one million and two million Americans have had RK and probably only 4,000 to 5,000 have had PRK, so we kind of know the warts—the good and bad sides—of RK whereas we don't really know all those things with our more limited experience with PRK."

Both refractive surgeries are considered cosmetic procedures and generally are not covered by insurance. Robin says that RK generally varies from $600 to $1,500 per eye and laser surgery costs around $2,000 per eye.

Prospects for 20/20 in 2020

Visions of a world entirely without glasses in the foreseeable future are probably premature; refractive surgery is not for everyone.

"From a medical standpoint, we are most concerned about people who have wound healing problems," Robin says, "because in all these procedures, the results are ultimately affected by two things—what we do as surgeons, and then how the patient's body reacts to the laser or knife wounds."

The procedures should not be done on patients with connective tissue diseases such as rheumatoid arthritis or lupus erythematosus, or on people with uncontrolled diabetes, autoimmune disease, or some eye diseases such as poorly controlled glaucoma, macular disease, retinal problems, extremely dry eyes, and certain corneal problems. Pregnant women also should not have refractive surgery, because the refraction of the eye changes during pregnancy.

Robin, Hersh, and Knight all agree that people who are not comfortable with the possibility that they may still need glasses or contact lenses at least part-time after surgery are probably not good candidates. Prospective patients should carefully weigh their hoped-for benefits against the calculated risks. After all, no surgeon can guarantee 20/20 vision except for hindsightedness.

New Progress with an Old Idea

Refractive surgery is not a new idea. Little wonder, since about one-fourth of the world's population is nearsighted—about 63 million in the United States alone. According to a report in the October 1994 Archives of Ophthalmology on the results of a 10-year study on radial keratotomy, the procedure was first described by European ophthalmologists in the late 1800s. It was further developed in Japan in the 1940s and 1950s, evolved into its modern form in Russia in the 1960s and 1970s, and was first done in the United States in 1978.

Despite RK's long history, refractive surgery is still in its "early toddlerhood," says Jeffrey Robin, MD Head of the department of refractive surgery at the Cleveland Clinic, Robin foresees a broader spectrum of procedures, pending laser approval, that will include RK, PRK, and others now under study.

"There's a growing menu of approaches that can potentially help people with a variety of refractive errors—low, moderate, and high nearsightedness, farsightedness, and even presbyopia [farsightedness associated with aging]," he says, noting that surgeons are also combining the knife and laser techniques to try to achieve better accuracy and effectiveness, especially for very nearsighted people.

For example, in an experimental procedure called laser in situ keratomileusis (LASIK), the surgeon uses a knife to cut a flap of corneal tissue, lases targeted cells beneath it, and then replaces the flap.

"Possible advantages of LASIK are better results with high myopia, less chance of scarring and haze, faster recovery, and less pain than simple PRK," says FDA's Emma Knight, MD, an ophthalmologist with the agency's Center for Devices and Radiological Health. "From FDA's standpoint, we want to know not just if LASIK is a good enough procedure, but if it is as good or better than PRK. So we've asked people to do randomized studies. We must also be sure there are not any greater risks than with standard PRK."

This article originally appeared in the July-August 1995 *FDA Consumer*. This version is from a reprint of the original article and contains revisions made in November 1995.

■ **Document Source:**
U.S. Department of Health and Human Services, Public Health Service
Food and Drug Administration
Publication No. (FDA) 96-1227

GASTROINTESTINAL SYSTEM DISORDERS

■ ■ ■

Information from PDQ for Patients

COLON CANCER

Description

What is cancer of the colon?

Cancer of the colon, a common form of cancer, is a disease in which cancer (malignant) cells are found in the tissues of the colon. The colon is part of the body's digestive system. The purpose of the digestive system is to remove nutrients (vitamins, minerals, and proteins) from the food you eat and to store the waste until it passes out of the body. The digestive system is made up of the esophagus, stomach, and the small and large intestines. The last six feet of intestine is called the large bowel or colon.

Genes are markers in cells associated with hereditary traits. Abnormal genes have been found in patients with some forms of colon and rectal cancer. Tests are being developed to determine who carries these genes long before cancer appears.

Like most cancers, cancer of the colon is best treated when it is found (diagnosed) early. Because of this, screening tests (such as a rectal exam, proctoscopy, and colonoscopy) may be done regularly in patients who are at higher risk to get cancer. These tests may be done in patients who are over age 50; who have a family history of cancer of the colon, rectum, or of the female organs; who have had small noncancerous growths (polyps) in the colon; or who have a history of ulcerative colitis (ulcers in the lining of the large intestines). Your doctor may order these tests to look for cancer if you have a change in bowel habits or if you have any bleeding from your rectum.

Your doctor will usually begin by giving you a rectal exam. In a rectal exam a doctor, wearing thin gloves, puts a greased finger into the rectum and gently feels for lumps. Your doctor may then check the material to see if there is any blood in it.

Your doctor may also want to look inside the rectum and lower colon with a special instrument called a sigmoidoscope or a proctosigmoidoscope. This exam, called a proctoscopy or procto exam, finds about half of all colon and rectal cancers. The test is usually done in a doctor's office. You may feel some pressure, but you usually do not feel pain.

Your doctor may also want to look inside the rectum and the entire colon (colonoscopy) with a special tool called a colonoscope. This test is also done in a doctor's office. You may feel some pressure but usually no pain.

If tissue that is not normal is found, the doctor will need to cut out a small piece and look at it under the microscope to see if there are any cancer cells. This is called a biopsy. Biopsies are usually done during the proctoscopy or colonoscopy, in a doctor's office. Your prognosis (chance of recovery) and choice of treatment depend on the stage of your cancer (whether it is just in the inner lining of your colon or if it has spread to other places) and your general state of health. After your treatment, you may have a blood test (to measure amounts of carcinoembryonic antigen or CEA in your blood) and x-ray tests to see if your cancer has come back.

Stage Explanation

Stages of Cancer of the Colon

Once cancer of the colon is found (diagnosed), more tests will be done to find out if cancer cells have spread to other parts of the body (staging). Your doctor needs to know the stage of your disease to plan treatment. The following stages are used for cancer of the colon:

Stage 0 or Carcinoma In Situ

Stage 0 cancer of the colon is very early cancer. The cancer is found only in the innermost lining of the colon.

Stage I

The cancer has spread beyond the innermost lining of the colon to the second and third layers and involves the inside wall of the colon, but has not spread to the outer wall of the colon or outside the colon.

Stage I colon cancer is sometimes called Dukes A colon cancer.

Stage II

Cancer has spread outside the colon to nearby tissue, but it has not gone into the lymph nodes. (Lymph nodes are small, bean-shaped structures that are found throughout the body. They produce and store cells that fight infection.)

Stage II colon cancer is sometimes called Dukes B colon cancer.

Stage III

Cancer has spread to nearby lymph nodes, but it has not spread to other parts of the body. (Lymph nodes are small, bean-shaped structures that are found throughout the body. They produce and store cells that fight infection.)

Stage III colon cancer is sometimes called Dukes C colon cancer.

Stage IV

Cancer has spread to other parts of the body.

Stage IV colon cancer is sometimes called Dukes D colon cancer.

Recurrent

Recurrent disease means that the cancer has come back (recurred) after it has been treated. It may come back in the colon or in another part of the body. Recurrent cancer of the colon is often found in the liver and/or lungs.

Treatment Option Overview

How Cancer of the Colon Is Treated

There are treatments for all patients with cancer of the colon. Three kinds of treatments are available:

- Surgery (taking out the cancer)
- Radiation therapy (using high-dose x-rays or other high-energy rays to kill cancer cells)
- Chemotherapy (using drugs to kill cancer cells).

Surgery is the most common treatment for all stages of cancer of the colon. Your doctor may take out the cancer from the colon using one of the following methods.

If your cancer is found at a very early stage, your doctor may take out the cancer without cutting into your abdomen. Instead, your doctor may put a tube through the rectum into the colon and cut the tumor out. This is called a local excision. If the cancer is found in a small bulging piece of tissue (called a polyp), the operation is called a polypectomy.

If your cancer is larger, your doctor will take out the cancer and a small amount of healthy tissue around it. The healthy parts of the colon are then sewn together (anastomosis). If only a small amount of tissue is removed, this is called a wedge resection. If a larger amount of tissue is removed, this is called a bowel resection. Your doctor will also take out lymph nodes near the intestine and look at them under the microscope to see if they contain cancer.

If your doctor is not able to sew your colon back together, he or she will make an opening (stoma) on the outside of the body for waste to pass out of the body. This is called a colostomy. Sometimes, the colostomy is only needed until the colon has healed, and then it can be reversed. However, your doctor may have to take out the entire lower colon, and the colostomy is permanent. If you have a colostomy, you will need to wear a special bag to collect body wastes. This special bag, which sticks to the skin around the stoma with a special glue, can be thrown away after it is used. This bag does not show under clothing, and most people take care of these bags themselves.

Radiation therapy uses x-rays or other high-energy rays to kill cancer cells and shrink tumors. Radiation may come from a machine outside the body (external radiation therapy) or from putting materials that contain radiation through thin plastic tubes (internal radiation therapy) in the intestine area. Radiation can be used alone or in addition to surgery and/or chemotherapy.

Chemotherapy uses drugs to kill cancer cells. Chemotherapy may be taken by pill, or it may be put into the body by a needle in a vein. You may be given chemotherapy through a tube that will be left in your vein while a small pump gives you constant treatment over a period of weeks. Chemotherapy is called a systemic treatment because the drug enters the bloodstream, travels through the body, and can kill cancer cells outside the colon. If your cancer has spread to the liver, you may be given chemotherapy directly into the artery going to the liver.

If your doctor removes all the cancer that can be seen at the time of the operation, you may be given chemotherapy after surgery to kill any cancer cells that are left. Chemotherapy given after an operation to a person who has no cancer cells that can be seen is called adjuvant chemotherapy.

Biological treatment tries to get your own body to fight cancer. It uses materials made by your own body or made in a laboratory to boost, direct, or restore your body's natural defenses against disease. Biological treatment is sometimes called biological response modifier (BRM) therapy or immunotherapy.

Treatment by Stage

Treatments for cancer of the colon depend on the stage of your disease and your general health.

You may receive treatment that is considered standard based on its effectiveness in a number of patients in past studies, or you may choose to go into a clinical trial. Not all patients are cured with standard therapy and some standard treatments may have more side effects than are desired. For these reasons, clinical trials are designed to find better ways to treat cancer patients and are based on the most up-to-date information. Clinical trials are going on in most parts of the country for most stages of cancer of the colon. If you wish to know more about clinical trials, call the Cancer Information Service at 1-800-4-CANCER (1-800-422-6237).

Stage 0 Colon Cancer

Your treatment may be one of the following:

1. Local excision or simple polypectomy
2. Wedge resection

Stage I Colon Cancer

Treatment is usually surgery (bowel resection) to remove the cancer and join the cut ends of the bowel.

Stage II Colon Cancer

Your treatment may be one of the following:

1. Treatment is usually surgery (bowel resection) to remove the cancer.
2. Clinical trials of chemotherapy, radiation therapy, or biological therapy following surgery.
3. If your tumor has spread to nearby tissue, you may also receive chemotherapy or radiotherapy following surgery.

Stage III Colon Cancer

Your treatment may be one of the following:

1. Treatment is usually surgery (bowel resection) to remove the cancer, followed by chemotherapy.
2. Clinical trials of chemotherapy, radiation therapy, and/or biological therapy following surgery.

Stage IV Colon Cancer

Your treatment may be one of the following:

1. Surgery (bowel resection) to remove the cancer or to make the colon go around the cancer so that it can still work.
2. Surgery to remove parts of other organs such as the liver, lungs, and ovaries, where the cancer may have spread.
3. Radiation therapy to relieve symptoms.
4. Chemotherapy.
5. Clinical trials of chemotherapy or biological therapy.

Recurrent Colon Cancer

If the cancer has come back (recurred) in only one part of the body, treatment may consist of an operation to take out the cancer. If the cancer has spread to several parts of the body, your doctor may give you either chemotherapy or radiation therapy. You may also choose to participate in a clinical trial testing new chemotherapy drugs or biological therapy.

To Learn More

To learn more about cancer of the colon, call the National Cancer Institute's Cancer Information Service at 1-800-4-CANCER (1-800-422-6237). By dialing this toll-free number, you can speak with someone who can answer your questions.

The Cancer Information Service can also send you free booklets. The following booklet about cancer of the colon may be helpful to you:

- What You Need to Know About Cancer of the Colon and Rectum

The following general booklets on topics related to cancer may also be helpful:

- What You Need to Know About Cancer
- Taking Time: Support for People with Cancer and the People Who Care About Them
- What Are Clinical Trials All About?
- Chemotherapy and You: A Guide to Self-Help During Treatment
- Radiation Therapy and You: A Guide to Self-Help During Treatment
- Eating Hints for Cancer Patients
- Advanced Cancer: Living Each Day
- When Cancer Recurs: Meeting the Challenge Again

There are many other places you can get information about cancer treatment and services to help you. To learn more about the care of colostomies, you may contact the United Ostomy Association, whose office is listed in the telephone book. You can check the social service office at your hospital for local and national agencies that help with your finances, getting to and from treatment, care at home, and dealing with your problems. The American Cancer Society, for example, has many free services. Their local offices are listed in the white pages of the telephone book.

You can also write to the National Cancer Institute at this address:

National Cancer Institute
Office of Cancer Communications
31 Center Dr, MSC 2580
Bethesda, MD 20892-2580

■ **Document Source:**
U.S. Department of Health and Human Services, Public Health Service
National Institutes of Health
National Cancer Institute
February 1996

CONSTIPATION

What is constipation?

Constipation is passage of small amounts of hard, dry bowel movements, usually fewer than three times a week. People who are constipated may find it difficult and painful to have a bowel movement. Other symptoms of constipation include feeling bloated, uncomfortable, and sluggish.

Many people think they are constipated when, in fact, their bowel movements are regular. For example, some people believe they are constipated, or irregular, if they do not have a bowel movement every day. However, there is no right number of daily or weekly bowel movements. Normal may be three times a day or three times a week depending on the person. In addition, some people naturally have firmer stools than others.

At one time or another almost everyone gets constipated. Poor diet and lack of exercise are usually the causes. In most cases, constipation is temporary and not serious. Understanding causes, prevention, and treatment will help most people find relief.

Who gets constipated?

According to the 1991 National Health Interview Survey, about 4-1/2 million people in the United States say they are constipated most or all of the time. Those reporting constipation most often are women, children, and adults age 65 and over. Pregnant women also complain of constipation, and it is a common problem following childbirth or surgery.

Constipation is the most common gastrointestinal complaint in the United States, resulting in about two million annual visits to the doctor. However, most people treat themselves without seeking medical help, as is evident from the $725 million Americans spend on laxatives each year.

What causes constipation?

To understand constipation, it helps to know how the colon (large intestine) works. As food moves through it, the colon absorbs water while forming waste products, or stool. Muscle contractions in the colon push the stool toward the rectum. By the time stool reaches the rectum, it is solid because most of the water has been absorbed. The hard and dry stools of constipation occur when the colon absorbs too much water. This happens because the colon's muscle contractions are slow or sluggish, causing the stool to move through the colon too slowly.

Diet

The most common cause of constipation is a diet low in fiber found in vegetables, fruits, and whole grains and high in fats found in cheese, eggs, and meats. People who eat plenty of high-fiber foods are less likely to become constipated.

Fiber—soluble and insoluble—is the part of fruits, vegetables, and grains that the body cannot digest. Soluble fiber dissolves easily in water and takes on a soft, gel-like texture in the intestines. Insoluble fiber passes almost unchanged through the intestines. The bulk and soft texture of fiber help prevent hard, dry stools that are difficult to pass.

On average, Americans eat about five to 20 grams of fiber daily, short of the 20 to 35 grams recommended by the American Dietetic Association. Both children and adults eat too many refined and processed foods in which the natural fiber is removed.

A low-fiber diet also plays a key role in constipation among older adults. They often lack interest in eating and may choose fast foods low in fiber. In addition, loss of teeth may force older people to eat soft foods that are processed and low in fiber.

Not Enough Liquids

Liquids like water and juice add fluid to the colon and bulk to stools, making bowel movements softer and easier to pass. People who have problems with constipation should drink enough of these liquids every day, about eight 8-ounce glasses. Other liquids, like coffee and soft drinks, that contain caffeine seem to have a dehydrating effect.

Lack of Exercise

Lack of exercise can lead to constipation, although doctors do not know precisely why. For example, constipation often occurs after an accident or during an illness when one must stay in bed and cannot exercise.

Medications

Pain medications (especially narcotics), antacids that contain aluminum, antispasmodics, antidepressants, iron supplements, diuretics, and anticonvulsants for epilepsy can slow passage of bowel movements.

Irritable Bowel Syndrome (IBS)

Some people with IBS, also known as spastic colon, have spasms in the colon that affect bowel movements. Constipation and diarrhea often alternate, and abdominal cramping, gassiness, and bloating are other common complaints. Although IBS can produce lifelong symptoms, it is not a life-threatening condition. It often worsens with stress, but there is no specific cause or anything unusual that the doctor can see in the colon.

Changes in Life or Routine

During pregnancy, women may be constipated because of hormonal changes or because the heavy uterus compresses the intestine. Aging may also affect bowel regularity because a slower metabolism results in less intestinal activity and muscle tone. In addition, people often become constipated when traveling because their normal diet and daily routines are disrupted.

Abuse of Laxatives

Myths about constipation have led to a serious abuse of laxatives. This is common among older adults who are preoccupied with having a daily bowel movement.

Laxatives usually are not necessary and can be habit-forming. The colon begins to rely on laxatives to bring on bowel movements. Over time, laxatives can damage nerve cells in the colon and interfere with the colon's natural ability to contract. For the same reason, regular use of enemas can also lead to a loss of normal bowel function.

Ignoring the Urge to Have a Bowel Movement

People who ignore the urge to have a bowel movement may eventually stop feeling the urge, which can lead to constipation. Some people delay having a bowel movement because they do not want to use toilets outside the home. Others ignore the urge because of emotional stress or because they are too busy. Children may postpone having a bowel movement because of stressful toilet training or because they do not want to interrupt their play.

Common Causes of Constipation

- Not enough fiber in diet
- Not enough liquids
- Lack of exercise
- Medications
- Irritable bowel syndrome
- Changes in life or routine such as pregnancy, older age, and travel
- Abuse of laxatives
- Ignoring the urge to have a bowel movement
- Specific diseases such as multiple sclerosis and lupus
- Problems with the colon and rectum
- Problems with intestinal function (chronic idiopathic constipation)

Specific Diseases

Diseases that cause constipation include neurological disorders, metabolic and endocrine disorders, and systemic conditions that affect organ systems. These disorders can slow the movement of stool through the colon, rectum, or anus.

Problems with the Colon and Rectum

Intestinal obstruction, scar tissue (adhesions), diverticulosis, tumors, colorectal stricture, Hirschsprung's disease, or cancer can compress, squeeze, or narrow the intestine and rectum and cause constipation.

Diseases That Cause Constipation

Neurological disorders that may cause constipation include

- Multiple sclerosis
- Parkinson's disease
- Chronic idiopathic intestinal pseudo-obstruction
- Stroke
- Spinal cord injuries

Metabolic and endocrine conditions include

- Diabetes
- Underactive or overactive thyroid gland
- Uremia

Systemic disorders include

- Amyloidosis
- Lupus
- Scleroderma

Problems with Intestinal Function (Chronic Idiopathic Constipation)

Also known as functional constipation, chronic idiopathic (of unknown origin) constipation is rare. However, some people are chronically constipated and do not respond to standard treatment. This chronic constipation may be related to multiple problems with hormonal control or with nerves and muscles in the colon, rectum, or anus. Functional constipation occurs in both children and adults and is most common in women.

Colonic inertia and delayed transit are two types of functional constipation caused by decreased muscle activity in the colon. These syndromes may affect the entire colon or may be confined to the left or lower (sigmoid) colon.

Functional constipation that stems from abnormalities in the structure of the anus and rectum is known as anorectal dysfunction, or anismus. These abnormalities result in an inability to relax the rectal and anal muscles that allow stool to exit.

What diagnostic tests are used?

Most people do not need extensive testing and can be treated with changes in diet and exercise. For example, in young people with mild symptoms, a medical history and physical examination may be all the doctor needs to suggest successful treatment. The tests the doctor performs depend on the duration and severity of the constipation, the person's age, and whether there is blood in stools, recent changes in bowel movements, or weight loss.

Medical History

The doctor may ask a patient to describe his or her constipation, including duration of symptoms, frequency of bowel movements, consistency of stools, presence of blood in the stool, and toilet habits (how often and where one has bowel movements). Recording eating habits, medication, and level of physical activity or exercise also helps the doctor determine the cause of constipation.

Physical Examination

A physical exam may include a digital rectal exam with a gloved, lubricated finger to evaluate the tone of the muscle that closes off the anus (anal sphincter) and to detect tenderness, obstruction, or blood. In some cases, blood and thyroid tests may be necessary.

Extensive testing usually is reserved for people with severe symptoms, for those with sudden changes in number and consistency of bowel movements or blood in the stool, and for older adults. Because of an increased risk of colorectal cancer in older adults, the doctor may use these tests to rule out a diagnosis of cancer:

- Barium enema x-ray
- Sigmoidoscopy or colonoscopy
- Colorectal transit study
- Anorectal function tests

Barium Enema X-Ray

A barium enema x-ray involves viewing the rectum, colon, and lower part of the small intestine to locate any problems. This part of the digestive tract is known as the bowel. This test may show intestinal obstruction and Hirschsprung's disease, a lack of nerves within the colon.

The night before the test, bowel cleansing, also called bowel prep, is necessary to clear the lower digestive tract. The patient drinks eight ounces of a special liquid every 15 minutes for about four hours. This liquid flushes out the bowel. A clean bowel is important, because even a small amount of stool in the colon can hide details and result in an inaccurate exam. Because the colon does not show up well on an x-ray, the doctor fills the organs with a barium enema, a chalky liquid to make the area visible. Once the mixture coats the organs, x-rays are taken that reveal their shape and condition. The patient may feel some abdominal cramping when the barium fills the colon but usually feels little discomfort after the procedure. Stools may be a whitish color for a few days after the exam.

Sigmoidoscopy or Colonoscopy

An examination of the rectum and lower colon (sigmoid) is called a sigmoidoscopy. An examination of the rectum and entire colon is called a colonoscopy.

The night before a sigmoidoscopy, the patient usually has a liquid dinner and takes an enema at bedtime. A light breakfast and a cleansing enema an hour before the test may also be necessary.

To perform a sigmoidoscopy, the doctor uses a long, flexible tube with a light on the end called a sigmoidoscope to view the rectum and lower colon. First, the doctor examines the rectum with a gloved, lubricated finger. Then, the sigmoidoscope is inserted through the anus into the rectum and lower colon. The procedure may cause a mild sensation of wanting to move the bowels and abdominal pressure. Sometimes the doctor fills the organs with air to get a better view. The air may cause mild cramping.

To perform a colonoscopy, the doctor uses a flexible tube with a light on the end called a colonoscope to view the entire colon. This tube is longer than a sigmoidoscope. The same bowel cleansing used for the barium x-ray is needed to clear the bowel of waste. The patient is lightly sedated before the exam. During the exam, the patient lies on his or her side and the doctor inserts the tube through the anus and rectum into the colon. If an abnormality is seen, the doctor can use the colonoscope to remove a small piece of tissue for examination (biopsy). The patient may feel gassy and bloated after the procedure.

Colorectal Transit Study

This test, reserved for those with chronic constipation, shows how well food moves through the colon. The patient swallows capsules containing small markers, which are visible on x-ray. The movement of the markers through the colon is monitored with abdominal x-rays taken several times three to seven days after the capsule is swallowed. The patient follows a high-fiber diet during the course of this test.

Anorectal Function Tests

These tests diagnose constipation caused by abnormal functioning of the anus or rectum (anorectal function). Anorectal manometry evaluates anal sphincter muscle function. A catheter or air-filled balloon inserted into the anus is slowly pulled back through the sphincter muscle to measure muscle tone and contractions.

Defecography is an x-ray of the anorectal area that evaluates completeness of stool elimination, identifies anorectal abnormalities, and evaluates rectal muscle contractions and relaxation. During the exam, the doctor fills the rectum with a soft paste that is the same consistency as stool. The patient sits on a toilet positioned inside an x-ray machine and then relaxes and squeezes the anus and expels the solution. The doctor studies the x-rays for anorectal problems that occurred while the patient emptied the paste.

How is constipation treated?

Although treatment depends on the cause, severity, and duration, in most cases dietary and lifestyle changes will help relieve symptoms and help prevent constipation.

Surgical removal of the colon may be an option for people with severe symptoms caused by colonic inertia. However, the benefits of this surgery must be weighed against possible complications, which include abdominal pain and diarrhea.

Can constipation be serious?

Sometimes constipation can lead to complications. These complications include hemorrhoids caused by straining to have a bowel movement or anal fissures (tears in the skin around the anus) caused when hard stool stretches the sphincter muscle. As a result, rectal bleeding may occur that appears as bright red streaks on the surface of the stool. Treatment for hemorrhoids may include warm tub baths, ice packs, and application of a cream to the affected area. Treatment for anal fissure may include stretching the sphincter muscle or surgical removal of tissue or skin in the affected area.

Sometimes straining causes a small amount of intestinal lining to push out from the anal opening. This condition is known as rectal prolapse and may lead to secretion of mucus from the anus. Usually, eliminating the cause of the prolapse such as straining or coughing is the only treatment necessary. Severe or chronic prolapse requires surgery to strengthen and tighten the anal sphincter muscle or to repair the prolapsed lining.

Constipation may also cause hard stool to pack the intestine and rectum so tightly that the normal pushing action of the colon is not enough to expel the stool. This condition, called fecal impaction, occurs most often in children and older adults. An impaction can be softened with mineral oil taken by mouth and an enema. After softening the impaction, the doctor may break up and remove part of the hardened stool by inserting one or two fingers in the anus.

Diet

A diet with enough fiber (20 to 35 grams each day) helps form soft, bulky stool. A doctor or dietitian can help plan an appropriate diet. High-fiber foods include beans; whole grains and bran cereals; fresh fruits; and vegetables such as asparagus, brussels sprouts, cabbage, and carrots. For people prone to constipation, limiting foods that have little or no fiber such as ice cream, cheese, meat, and processed foods is also important.

Points to Remember

1. Constipation affects almost everyone at one time or another.
2. Many people think they are constipated when, in fact, their bowel movements are regular.
3. The most common causes of constipation are poor diet and lack of exercise.
4. Additional causes of constipation include medications, irritable bowel syndrome, abuse of laxatives, and specific diseases.
5. A medical history and physical examination may be the only diagnostic tests needed before the doctor suggests treatment.
6. In most cases, following these simple tips will help relieve symptoms and prevent recurrence of constipation:

   - Eat a well-balanced, high-fiber diet that includes beans, bran, whole grains, fresh fruits, and vegetables.
   - Drink plenty of liquids.
   - Exercise regularly.
   - Set aside time after breakfast or dinner for undisturbed visits to the toilet.
   - Do not ignore the urge to have a bowel movement.
   - Understand that normal bowel habits vary.
   - Whenever a significant or prolonged change in bowel habits occurs, check with a doctor.

7. Most people with mild constipation do not need laxatives. However, doctors may recommend laxatives for a limited time for people with chronic constipation.

Lifestyle Changes

Other changes that can help treat and prevent constipation include drinking enough water and other liquids such as fruit and vegetable juices and clear soup, engaging in daily exercise, and reserving enough time to have a bowel movement. In addition, the urge to have a bowel movement should not be ignored.

Laxatives

Most people who are mildly constipated do not need laxatives. However, for those who have made lifestyle changes and are still constipated, doctors may recommend laxatives or enemas for a limited time. These treatments can help retrain a chronically sluggish bowel. For children, short-term treatment with laxatives, along with retraining to establish regular bowel habits, also helps prevent constipation.

A doctor should determine when a patient needs a laxative and which form is best. Laxatives taken by mouth are available in liquid, tablet, gum, powder, and granule forms. They work in various ways:

- Bulk-forming laxatives generally are considered the safest but can interfere with absorption of some medi-

cines. These laxatives, also known as fiber supplements, are taken with water. They absorb water in the intestine and make the stool softer. Brand names include Metamucil®, Citrucel®, and Serutan®.
- Stimulants cause rhythmic muscle contractions in the intestines. Brand names include Correctol®, Ex-Lax®, Dulcolax®, Purge®, Feen-A-Mint®, and Senokot®.
- Stool softeners provide moisture to the stool and prevent dehydration. These laxatives are often recommended after childbirth or surgery. Products include Colace®, Dialose®, and Surfak®.
- Lubricants grease the stool enabling it to move through the intestine more easily. Mineral oil is the most common lubricant.
- Saline laxatives act like a sponge to draw water into the colon for easier passage of stool. Laxatives in this group include Milk of Magnesia®, Citrate of Magnesia®, and Haley's M-O®.

People who are dependent on laxatives need to slowly stop using the medications. A doctor can assist in this process. In most people, this restores the colon's natural ability to contract.

Other Treatment

Treatment may be directed at a specific cause. For example, the doctor may recommend discontinuing medication or performing surgery to correct an anorectal problem such as rectal prolapse.

People with chronic constipation caused by anorectal dysfunction can use biofeedback to retrain the muscles that control release of bowel movements. Biofeedback involves using a sensor to monitor muscle activity that at the same time can be displayed on a computer screen allowing for an accurate assessment of body functions. A health care professional uses this information to help the patient learn how to use these muscles.

Additional Readings

Cummings, M. (1991). Overuse hazardous: Laxatives rarely needed. *FDA Consumer, 25* (3), 33-35. General patient information article.

Larson, D.E. (Ed.). (1990). *Mayo Clinic family health book.* New York, NY: William Morrow and Company, Inc. General medical guide that includes a section on constipation.

National Institute on Aging. (1994). *Age page: Constipation* [Brochure]. Washington, DC: U.S. Government Printing Office. General patient information brochure.

Additional Resources

International Foundation for Bowel Dysfunction
PO Box 17864
Milwaukee, WI 53217
(414) 964-1799

Intestinal Disease Foundation
1323 Forbes Ave, Ste 200
Pittsburgh, PA 15219
(412) 261-5888

■ Document Source:
U.S. Department of Health and Human Services, Public Health Service
National Institutes of Health
National Institute of Diabetes and Digestive and Kidney Diseases
NIH Publication No. 95-2754
July 1995

Information from PDQ for Patients

GASTRIC CANCER

Description

What is cancer of the stomach?

Cancer of the stomach, also called gastric cancer, is a disease in which cancer (malignant) cells are found in the tissues of the stomach. The stomach is a J-shaped organ in your upper abdomen where your food is broken down (digested). Food reaches your stomach through a tube called the esophagus that connects your mouth to your stomach. After leaving your stomach, partially digested food passes into the small intestine and then into the large intestine, called the colon.

Sometimes, cancer can be in the stomach for a long time and can grow very large before it causes symptoms. In the early stages of cancer of the stomach, you may have indigestion and stomach discomfort, a bloated feeling after eating, mild nausea, loss of appetite, or heartburn. In more advanced stages of cancer of the stomach, you may have blood in your stool, vomiting, weight loss, or pain in the stomach. Your chance of getting stomach cancer is higher if you have an infection of the stomach caused by Helicobacter pylori, if you are older, if you are a man, or if you have eaten a diet that included a lot of dry, salted foods during your life. Other things that increase your chances of getting stomach cancer are a stomach disorder called atrophic gastritis or Menetrier's disease, a disorder of your blood called pernicious anemia, or a hereditary condition of growths (called polyps) in your large intestine.

If you have symptoms, your doctor will usually order an upper gastrointestinal x-ray (also called an upper GI series). For this exam, you drink a liquid containing barium, which makes the stomach easier to see in the x-ray. This test is usually performed in a doctor's office or in a hospital radiology department.

Your doctor may also look inside your stomach with a thin, lighted tube called a gastroscope. This is called a gastroscopy, and it finds most cancers of the stomach. For this test, the gastroscope is inserted through your mouth and guided into your stomach. Your doctor may spray a local anesthetic (a drug that causes loss of feeling for a short period of time) in your throat or give you other medicine to relax you before the test so that you do not feel pain.

If your doctor sees tissue that is not normal, he or she may cut out a small piece so it can be looked at under a microscope to see if there are any cancer cells. This is called a biopsy. Biopsies are usually done during the gastroscopy.

Your chance of recovery (prognosis) and choice of treatment depend on the stage of your cancer (whether it is just in the stomach or if it has spread to other places) and your general state of health.

Stage Explanation

Stages of Cancer of the Stomach

Once cancer of the stomach is found, more tests will be done to find out if cancer cells have spread to other parts of the body. This is called staging. Your doctor needs to know the stage of your disease to plan treatment. The following stages are used for cancer of the stomach:

Stage 0

Stage 0 cancer of the stomach is very early cancer. Cancer is found only in the innermost layer of the stomach wall.

Stage I

Cancer is in the second or third layers of the stomach wall and has not spread to lymph nodes near the cancer or is in the second layer of the stomach wall and has spread to lymph nodes very close to the tumor. (Lymph nodes are small-bean-shaped structures that are found throughout the body. They produce and store infection-fighting cells.)

Stage II

Any of the following may be true:

1. Cancer is in the second layer of the stomach wall and has spread to lymph nodes further away from the tumor.
2. Cancer is only in the muscle layer (the third layer) of the stomach and has spread to lymph nodes very close to the tumor.
3. Cancer is in all four layers of the stomach wall but has not spread to lymph nodes or other organs.

Stage III

Any of the following may be true:

1. Cancer is in the third layer of the stomach wall and has spread to lymph nodes further away from the tumor.
2. Cancer is in all four layers of the stomach wall and has spread to lymph nodes either very close to the tumor or further away from the tumor.
3. Cancer is in all four layers of the stomach wall and has spread to nearby tissues. The cancer may or may not have spread to lymph nodes very close to the tumor.

Stage IV

Cancer has spread to nearby tissues and to lymph nodes further away from the tumor or has spread to other parts of the body.

Recurrent

Recurrent disease means that the cancer has come back (recurred) after it has been treated. It may come back in the stomach or in another part of the body such as the liver or lymph nodes.

Treatment Option Overview

How Cancer of the Stomach is Treated

There are treatments for most patients with cancer of the stomach. Two kinds of treatment are used:

- surgery (taking out the cancer in an operation)
- chemotherapy (using drugs to kill cancer cells)

Radiation therapy and biological therapy are being tested in clinical trials.

Surgery is a common treatment for all stages of cancer of the stomach. Your doctor may remove the cancer using one of the following operations:

- Subtotal gastrectomy removes the part of the stomach that contains cancer and parts of other tissues and organs near the tumor. Nearby lymph nodes are also removed (lymph node dissection). The spleen (an organ in the upper abdomen that filters your blood and removes old blood cells) may be removed if necessary.
- Total gastrectomy removes the entire stomach and parts of the esophagus, the small intestine, and other tissue near the tumor. The spleen is removed in some cases. Nearby lymph nodes arc also removed (lymph node dissection). The esophagus is connected to the small intestine so you can continue to eat and swallow.

If only part of the stomach is removed, you should be able to eat fairly normally. If your entire stomach is removed, you may need to eat small meals often and to eat foods low in sugar and high in fat and protein. Most patients can adjust to this new way of eating.

Chemotherapy uses drugs to kill cancer cells. Chemotherapy may be taken by pill, or it may be put into the body by a needle in the vein or muscle. Chemotherapy is called a systemic treatment because the drug enters the bloodstream, travels through the body, and can kill cancer cells outside the stomach.

Treatment given after surgery when no cancer cells can be seen is called adjuvant therapy. Adjuvant therapy for cancer of the stomach is being tested in clinical trials.

Radiation therapy uses high-energy x-rays to kill cancer cells and shrink tumors. Radiation may come from a machine outside the body (external radiation therapy) or from putting materials that produce radiation (radioisotopes) through thin plastic tubes in the area where the cancer cells are found (internal radiation therapy).

Biological therapy tries to get your own body to fight cancer. It uses materials made by your own body or made in a laboratory to boost, direct, or restore your body's natural defenses against disease. Biological therapy is sometimes called biological response modifier (BRM) therapy or immunotherapy.

Treatment by Stage

Treatment for cancer of the stomach depends on the stage of your disease, the part of the stomach where the cancer is, and your general health.

You may receive treatment that is considered standard based on its effectiveness in a number of patients in past studies, or you may choose to go into a clinical trial. Many patients with cancer of the stomach are not cured with standard therapy and some standard treatments may have more side effects than are desired. For these reasons, clinical trials are designed to find better ways to treat cancer patients and are based on the most up-to-date information. Clinical trials are going on in most parts of the country for most stages of cancer of the stomach. If you want more information, call the Cancer Information Service at 1-800-4-CANCER (1-800-422-6237).

Stage 0 Gastric Cancer

Your treatment may be one of the following:

1. Surgery to remove part of the stomach (subtotal gastrectomy).
2. Surgery to remove the entire stomach and some of the tissue around it (total gastrectomy).

Lymph nodes around the stomach may also be removed during surgery (lymph node dissection).

Stage I Gastric Cancer

Your treatment may be one of the following:

1. Surgery to remove part of the stomach (subtotal gastrectomy).
2. Surgery to remove the entire stomach and some of the tissue around it (total gastrectomy).

Lymph nodes around the stomach may also be removed (lymph node dissection).

Stage II Gastric Cancer

Your treatment may be one of the following:

1. Surgery to remove part of the stomach (subtotal gastrectomy).
2. Surgery to remove the entire stomach and some of the tissue around it (total gastrectomy).
3. A clinical trial of surgery followed by adjuvant radiation therapy and/or chemotherapy.

Lymph nodes around the stomach may also be removed (lymph node dissection).

Stage III Gastric Cancer

Your treatment may be one of the following:

1. Surgery to remove the entire stomach and some of the tissue around it (total gastrectomy). Lymph nodes may also be removed.
2. A clinical trial of surgery followed by adjuvant radiation therapy and/or chemotherapy.
3. A clinical trial of chemotherapy with or without radiation therapy.

Stage IV Gastric Cancer

Your treatment may be one of the following:

1. Surgery to relieve symptoms, reduce bleeding, or remove a tumor that is blocking the stomach.
2. Chemotherapy to relieve symptoms.

Recurrent Gastric Cancer

Your treatment may be chemotherapy to relieve symptoms. Clinical trials are testing new chemotherapy drugs and biological therapy.

To Learn More

To learn more about cancer of the stomach, call the National Cancer Institute's Cancer Information Service at 1-800-4-CANCER (1-800-422-6237). By dialing this toll-free number, you can speak with someone who can answer your questions.

The Cancer Information Service can also send you free booklets. The following booklet about cancer of the stomach may be helpful to you:

- What You Need to Know About Stomach Cancer

The following general booklets on questions related to cancer may also be helpful:

- What You Need to Know About Cancer
- Taking Time: Support for People with Cancer and the People Who Care About Them
- What Are Clinical Trials All About?
- Chemotherapy and You: A Guide to Self-Help During Treatment
- Radiation Therapy and You: A Guide to Self-Help During Treatment
- Eating Hints for Cancer Patients
- Advanced Cancer: Living Each Day
- When Cancer Recurs: Meeting the Challenge Again

There are many other places you can get information about cancer treatment and services to help you. You can check the social service office at your hospital for local and national agencies that help with your finances, getting to and from treatment, care at home, and dealing with your problems. The American Cancer Society, for example, has many free services. Their local offices are listed in the white pages of the telephone book.

You can also write to the National Cancer Institute at this address:

National Cancer Institute
Office of Cancer Communications
31 Center Dr, MSC 2580
Bethesda, MD 20892-2580

■ **Document Source:**
   U.S. Department of Health and Human Services, Public Health Service
   National Institutes of Health
   National Cancer Institute
   April 1996

GASTROESOPHAGEAL REFLUX DISEASE: HIATAL HERNIA AND HEARTBURN

Gastroesophageal reflux disease (GERD) is a digestive disorder that affects the lower esophageal sphincter (LES)—the muscle connecting the esophagus with the stomach. Many people, including pregnant women, suffer from heartburn or acid indigestion caused by GERD. Doctors believe that some people suffer from GERD due to a condition called hiatal hernia. In most cases, heartburn can be relieved through diet and lifestyle changes; however, some people may require medication or surgery. This fact sheet provides information on GERD—its causes, symptoms, treatment, and long-term complications.

What is gastroesophageal reflux?

Gastroesophageal refers to the stomach and esophagus. Reflux means to flow back or return. Therefore, gastroesophageal reflux is the return of the stomach's contents back up into the esophagus.

In normal digestion, the LES opens to allow food to pass into the stomach and closes to prevent food and acidic stomach juices from flowing back into the esophagus. Gastroesophageal reflux occurs when the LES is weak or relaxes inappropriately allowing the stomach's contents to flow up into the esophagus.

The severity of GERD depends on LES dysfunction as well as the type and amount of fluid brought up from the stomach and the neutralizing effect of saliva.

What is the role of hiatal hernia?

Some doctors believe a hiatal hernia may weaken the LES and cause reflux. Hiatal hernia occurs when the upper part of the stomach moves up into the chest through a small opening in the diaphragm (diaphragmatic hiatus). The diaphragm is the muscle separating the stomach from the chest. Recent studies show that the opening in the diaphragm acts as an additional sphincter around the lower end of the esophagus. Studies also show that hiatal hernia results in retention of acid and other contents above this opening. These substances can reflux easily into the esophagus.

Coughing, vomiting, straining, or sudden physical exertion can cause increased pressure in the abdomen resulting in hiatal hernia. Obesity and pregnancy also contribute to this condition. Many otherwise healthy people age 50 and over have a small hiatal hernia. Although considered a condition of middle age, hiatal hernias affect people of all ages.

Hiatal hernias usually do not require treatment. However, treatment may be necessary if the hernia is in danger of becoming strangulated (twisted in away that cuts off blood supply, i.e., paraesophageal hernia) or is complicated by severe GERD or esophagitis (inflammation of the esophagus).

The doctor may perform surgery to reduce the size of the hernia or to prevent strangulation.

What other factors contribute to GERD?

Dietary and lifestyle choices may contribute to GERD. Certain foods and beverages, including chocolate, peppermint, fried or fatty foods, coffee, or alcoholic beverages, may weaken the LES causing reflux and heartburn. Studies show that cigarette smoking relaxes the LES. Obesity and pregnancy can also cause GERD.

What does heartburn feel like?

Heartburn, also called acid indigestion, is the most common symptom of GERD and usually feels like a burning chest pain beginning behind the breastbone and moving upward to the neck and throat. Many people say it feels like food is coming back into the mouth leaving an acid or bitter taste.

The burning, pressure, or pain of heartburn can last as long as two hours and is often worse after eating. Lying down or bending over can also result in heartburn. Many people obtain relief by standing upright or by taking an antacid that clears acid out of the esophagus.

Heartburn pain can be mistaken for the pain associated with heart disease or a heart attack, but there are differences. Exercise may aggravate pain resulting from heart disease, and rest may relieve the pain. Heartburn pain is less likely to be associated with physical activity.

How common is heartburn?

More than 60 million American adults experience GERD and heartburn at least once a month, and about 25 million adults suffer daily from heartburn. Twenty-five percent of pregnant women experience daily heartburn, and more than 50 percent have occasional distress. Recent studies show that GERD in infants and children is more common than previously recognized and may produce recurrent vomiting, coughing and other respiratory problems, or failure to thrive.

What is the treatment for GERD?

Doctors recommend lifestyle and dietary changes for most people with GERD. Treatment aims at decreasing the amount of reflux or reducing damage to the lining of the esophagus from refluxed materials.

Avoiding foods and beverages that can weaken the LES is recommended. These foods include chocolate, peppermint, fatty foods, coffee, and alcoholic beverages. Foods and beverages that can irritate a damaged esophageal lining, such as citrus fruits and juices, tomato products, and pepper, should also be avoided.

Decreasing the size of portions at mealtime may also help control symptoms. Eating meals at least two to three hours before bedtime may lessen reflux by allowing the acid in the

stomach to decrease and the stomach to empty partially. In addition, being overweight often worsens symptoms. Many overweight people find relief when they lose weight.

Cigarette smoking weakens the LES. Therefore, stopping smoking is important to reduce GERD symptoms.

Elevating the head of the bed on six-inch blocks or sleeping on a specially designed wedge reduces heartburn by allowing gravity to minimize reflux of stomach contents into the esophagus.

Antacids taken regularly can neutralize acid in the esophagus and stomach and stop heartburn. Many people find that nonprescription antacids provide temporary or partial relief. An antacid combined with a foaming agent such as alginic acid helps some people. These compounds are believed to form a foam barrier on top of the stomach that prevents acid reflux from occurring.

Long-term use of antacids, however, can result in side effects, including diarrhea, altered calcium metabolism (a change in the way the body breaks down and uses calcium), and buildup of magnesium in the body. Too much magnesium can be serious for patients with kidney disease. If antacids are needed for more than three weeks, a doctor should be consulted.

For chronic reflux and heartburn, the doctor may prescribe medications to reduce acid in the stomach. These medicines include H2 blockers, which inhibit acid secretion in the stomach. Currently, four H2 blockers are available: cimetidine, famotidine, nizatidine, and ranitidine. Another type of drug, the proton pump (or acid pump) inhibitor omeprazole inhibits an enzyme (a protein in the acid-producing cells of the stomach) necessary for acid secretion. The acid pump inhibitor lansoprazole is currently under investigation as a new treatment for GERD.

Other approaches to therapy will increase the strength of the LES and quicken emptying of stomach contents with motility drugs that act on the upper gastrointestinal (GI) tract. These drugs include cisapride, bethanechol, and metoclopramide.

Tips to Control Heartburn

- Avoid foods and beverages that affect LES pressure or irritate the esophagus lining, including fried and fatty foods, peppermint, chocolate, alcohol, coffee, citrus fruit and juices, and tomato products.
- Lose weight if overweight.
- Stop smoking.
- Elevate the head of the bed six inches.
- Avoid lying down two to three hours after eating.
- Take an antacid.

What if symptoms persist?

People with severe, chronic esophageal reflux or with symptoms not relieved by the treatment described above may need more complete diagnostic evaluation. Doctors use a variety of tests and procedures to examine a patient with chronic heartburn.

An upper GI series may be performed during the early phase of testing. This test is a special x-ray that shows the esophagus, stomach, and duodenum (the upper part of the small intestine). While an upper GI series provides limited information about possible reflux, it is used to rule out other diagnoses, such as peptic ulcers.

Endoscopy is an important procedure for individuals with chronic GERD. By placing a small lighted tube with a tiny video camera on the end (endoscope) into the esophagus, the doctor may see inflammation or irritation of the tissue lining the esophagus (esophagitis). If the findings of the endoscopy are abnormal or questionable, biopsy (removing a small sample of tissue) from the lining of the esophagus may be helpful.

The Bernstein test (dripping a mild acid through a tube placed in the mid-esophagus) is often performed as part of a complete evaluation. This test attempts to confirm that the symptoms result from acid in the esophagus. Esophageal manometric studies—pressure measurements of the esophagus—occasionally help identify critically low pressure in the LES or abnormalities in esophageal muscle contraction.

For patients in whom diagnosis is difficult, doctors may measure the acid levels inside the esophagus through pH testing. Testing pH monitors the acidity level of the esophagus and symptoms during meals, activity, and sleep. Newer techniques of long-term pH monitoring are improving diagnostic capability in this area.

Does GERD require surgery?

A small number of people with GERD may need surgery because of severe reflux and poor response to medical treatment. Fundoplication is a surgical procedure that increases pressure in the lower esophagus. However, surgery should not be considered until all other measures have been tried.

What are the complications of long-term GERD?

Sometimes GERD results in serious complications. Esophagitis can occur as a result of too much stomach acid in the esophagus. Esophagitis may cause esophageal bleeding or ulcers. In addition, a narrowing or stricture of the esophagus may occur from chronic scarring. Some people develop a condition known as Barrett's esophagus, which is severe damage to the skin-like lining of the esophagus. Doctors believe this condition may be a precursor to esophageal cancer.

Conclusion

Although GERD can limit daily activities and productivity, it is rarely life-threatening. With an understanding of the causes and proper treatment, most people will find relief.

Additional Readings

Cramer T. A burning question: When do you need an antacid? FDA Consumer 1992; 26(1): 19-22. This article for consumers provides general information about antacids.

Larson DE, Editor-in-chief. Mayo Clinic Family Health Book. New York: William Morrow and Company, Inc., 1990. This general medical guide includes sections about esophageal reflux and hiatal hernia.

Richter JE. Why does surgery work for GERD? Practical Gastroenterology 1993; XVII(10): 10-18. This article for physicians describes antireflux surgery.

Sutherland JE. Gastroesophageal reflux disease: when antacids aren't enough. Postgraduate Medicine 1991; 89(7): 45-53. This article for primary care physicians provides guidelines to determine if a patient has reflux disease and offers treatment methods.

■ Document Source:
U.S. Department of Health and Human Services, Public Health Service
National Institutes of Health
National Institute of Diabetes and Digestive and Kidney Diseases
NIH Publication No. 94-882
September 1994

HEMORRHOIDS

What are hemorrhoids?

Hemorrhoids are swollen but normally present blood vessels in and around the anus and lower rectum that stretch under pressure, similar to varicose veins in the legs.

The increased pressure and swelling may result from straining to move the bowel. Other contributing factors include pregnancy, heredity, aging, and chronic constipation or diarrhea.

Hemorrhoids are either inside the anus (internal) or under the skin around the anus (external).

What are the symptoms of hemorrhoids?

Many anorectal problems, including fissures, fistulae, abscesses, or irritation and itching (pruritus ani), have similar symptoms and are incorrectly referred to as hemorrhoids.

Hemorrhoids usually are not dangerous or life-threatening. In most cases, hemorrhoidal symptoms will go away within a few days.

Although many people have hemorrhoids, not all experience symptoms. The most common symptom of internal hemorrhoids is bright red blood covering the stool, on toilet paper, or in the toilet bowl. However, an internal hemorrhoid may protrude through the anus outside the body, becoming irritated and painful. This is known as a protruding hemorrhoid.

Symptoms of external hemorrhoids may include painful swelling or a hard lump around the anus that results when a blood clot forms. This condition is known as a thrombosed external hemorrhoid.

In addition, excessive straining, rubbing, or cleaning around the anus may cause irritation with bleeding and/or itching, which may produce a vicious cycle of symptoms. Draining mucus may also cause itching.

How common are hemorrhoids?

Hemorrhoids are very common in men and women. About half of the population have hemorrhoids by age 50. Hemorrhoids are also common among pregnant women. The pressure of the fetus in the abdomen, as well as hormonal changes, cause the hemorrhoidal vessels to enlarge. These vessels are also placed under severe pressure during childbirth. For most women, however, hemorrhoids caused by pregnancy are a temporary problem.

How are hemorrhoids diagnosed?

A thorough evaluation and proper diagnosis by the doctor is important any time bleeding from the rectum or blood in the stool lasts more than a couple of days. Bleeding may also be a symptom of other digestive diseases, including colorectal cancer.

The doctor will examine the anus and rectum to look for swollen blood vessels that indicate hemorrhoids and will also perform a digital rectal exam with a gloved, lubricated finger to feel for abnormalities.

Closer evaluation of the rectum for hemorrhoids requires an exam with an anoscope, a hollow, lighted tube useful for viewing internal hemorrhoids, or a proctoscope, useful for more completely examining the entire rectum.

To rule out other causes of gastrointestinal bleeding, the doctor may examine the rectum and lower colon (sigmoid) with sigmoidoscopy or the entire colon with colonoscopy. Sigmoidoscopy and colonoscopy are diagnostic procedures that also involve the use of lighted, flexible tubes inserted through the rectum.

What is the treatment?

Medical treatment of hemorrhoids initially is aimed at relieving symptoms. Measures to reduce symptoms include:

- Warm tub or sitz baths several times a day in plain, warm water for about 10 minutes.
- Ice packs to help reduce swelling.
- Application of a hemorroidal cream or suppository to the affected area for a limited time.

Prevention of the recurrence of hemorrhoids is aimed at changing conditions associated with the pressure and straining of constipation. Doctors will often recommend increasing fiber and fluids in the diet. Eating the right amount of fiber and drinking six to eight glasses of fluid (not alcohol) result in softer, bulkier stools. A softer stool makes emptying the bowels easier and lessens the pressure on hemorrhoids caused by straining. Eliminating straining also helps prevent the hemorrhoids from protruding.

Good sources of fiber are fruits, vegetables, and whole grains. In addition, doctors may suggest a bulk stool softener or a fiber supplement such as psyllium (Metamucil) or methylcellulose (Citrucel).

In some cases, hemorrhoids must be treated surgically. These methods are used to shrink and destroy the hemorrhoidal tissue and are performed under anesthesia. The doctor will perform the surgery during an office or hospital visit.

A number of surgical methods may be used to remove or reduce the size of internal hemorrhoids. These techniques include:

- Rubber band ligation—A rubber band is placed around the base of the hemorrhoid inside the rectum. The band cuts off circulation, and the hemorrhoid withers away within a few days.
- Sclerotherapy—A chemical solution is injected around the blood vessel to shrink the hemorrhoid.

Techniques used to treat both internal and external hemorrhoids include:

- Electrical or laser heat (laser coagulation) or infrared light (infrared photo coagulation)—Both techniques use special devices to burn hemorrhoidal tissue.
- Hemorrhoidectomy—Occasionally, extensive or severe internal or external hemorrhoids may require removal by surgery known as hemorrhoidectomy. This is the best method for permanent removal of hemorrhoids.

How are hemorrhoids prevented?

The best way to prevent hemorrhoids is to keep stools soft so they pass easily, thus decreasing pressure and straining, and to empty bowels as soon as possible after the urge occurs. Exercise, including walking, and increased fiber in the diet help reduce constipation and straining by producing stools that are softer and easier to pass. In addition, a person should not sit on the toilet for a long period of time.

Additional Readings

Bleeding in the Digestive Tract. 1992. Fact sheet discusses many common causes of bleeding in the digestive tract and related diagnostic procedures and treatment. Available from the National Digestive Diseases Information Clearinghouse, Box NDDIC, 9000 Rockville Pike, Bethesda, MD 20892.

Cocchiara, J.L. Hemorrhoids: A practical approach to an aggravating problem. *Postgraduate Medicine* 1991; 89(1): 149-152. Article for health care professionals discusses causes, symptoms, and treatments.

Sohn, N. Hemorrhoids: Etiology, pathogenesis, classification, and medical therapy. *Practical Gastroenterology* 1991; XV(9): 21-24. General article for physicians.

Stehlin, D. No strain no pain: The bottom line in treating hemorrhoids. *FDA Consumer 1992;* 26(2): 31-33. General information article for patients and the public.

National Digestive Diseases Information Clearinghouse
2 Information Way
Bethesda, MD 20892-3570

The National Digestive Diseases Information Clearinghouse is a service of the National Institute of Diabetes and Digestive and Kidney Diseases, part of the National Institutes of Health, under the U.S. Public Health Service. The clearinghouse, authorized by Congress in 1980, is designed to increase knowledge and understanding about digestive diseases and health among people with digestive diseases and their families, health care professionals, and the public. The clearinghouse answers inquiries; develops, reviews, and distributes publications; and works closely with professional and patient organizations and government agencies to coordinate informational resources about digestive diseases.

Publications produced by the clearinghouse are reviewed carefully for scientific accuracy, content, and readability. Publications produced by sources other than the clearinghouse are also reviewed for scientific accuracy and are used, along with clearinghouse publications, to answer requests.

■ Document Source:
   U.S. Department of Health and Human Services, Public Health Service
   National Institutes of Health
   National Institute of Diabetes and Digestive and Kidney Diseases
   NIH Pub. No. 95-3021
   May 1994

Information from PDQ for Patients

PANCREATIC CANCER

Description

What is cancer of the pancreas?

Cancer of the pancreas is a disease in which cancer (malignant) cells are found in the tissues of the pancreas. The pancreas is about six inches long and is shaped something like a thin pear, wider at one end and narrowing at the other. The pancreas lies behind the stomach, inside a loop formed by part of the small intestine. The broader right end of the pancreas is called the head, the middle section is called the body, and the narrow left end is the tail.

The pancreas has two basic jobs in your body. It produces juices that help you break down (digest) your food and hormones (such as insulin) that regulate how your body stores and uses food. The area of the pancreas that produces digestive juices is called the exocrine pancreas. About 95 percent of pancreatic cancers begin in the exocrine pancreas. The hormone-producing area of the pancreas is called the endocrine pancreas. Only about 5 percent of pancreatic cancers start here. This statement has information on cancer of the exocrine pancreas.

Cancer of the pancreas is hard to find (diagnose) because the organ is hidden behind other organs. Organs around the pancreas include the stomach, small intestine, bile ducts (tubes through which bile, a digestive juice made by the liver, flows from the liver to the small intestine), gallbladder (the small sac below the liver that stores bile), the liver, and the spleen (the organ that stores red blood cells and filters blood to remove excess blood cells). The signs of pancreatic cancer are like many other illnesses, and there may be no signs in the first stages. You should see your doctor if you have any of the following: nausea, loss of appetite, weight loss without trying to lose weight, pain in the upper or middle of your abdomen, or yellowing of your skin (jaundice).

If you have symptoms, your doctor will examine you and order tests to see if you have cancer and what your treatment should be. You may have an ultrasound, a test that uses sound waves to find tumors. A CT scan, a special type of x-ray that uses a computer to make a picture of the inside of your abdomen, may also be done. Another special scan called magnetic resonance imaging (MRI), which uses magnetic waves to make a picture of the inside of your abdomen, may be done as well.

A test called an ERCP (endoscopic retrograde cholangiopancreatography) may also be done. During this test, a flexible tube is put down the throat, through the stomach, and into the small intestine. Your doctor can see through the tube and inject dye into the drainage tube (duct) of the pancreas so that the area can be seen more clearly on an x-ray. During ERCP, your doctor may also put a fine needle into the pancreas to take out some cells. This is called a biopsy. The cells can then be looked at under a microscope to see if they contain cancer.

PTC (percutaneous transhepatic cholangiography) is another test that can help find cancer of the pancreas. During this test, a thin needle is put into the liver through your right side. Dye is injected into the bile ducts in the liver so that blockages can be seen on x-rays.

In some cases, a needle can be inserted into the pancreas during an x-ray or ultrasound so that cells can be taken out to see if they contain cancer. You may need surgery to see if you have cancer of the pancreas. If this is the case, your doctor will cut into the abdomen and look at the pancreas and the tissues around it for cancer. If you have cancer and it looks like it has not spread to other tissues, your doctor may remove the cancer or relieve blockages caused by the tumor.

Stage Explanation

Stages of Cancer of the Pancreas

Once cancer of the pancreas is found, more tests will be done to find out if the cancer has spread from the pancreas to the tissues around it or to other parts of the body. This is called staging. The following stages are used for cancer of the pancreas:

Stage I

Cancer is found only in the pancreas itself, or has started to spread just to the tissues next to the pancreas, such as the small intestine, the stomach, or the bile duct.

Stage II

Cancer has spread to nearby organs such as the stomach, spleen, or colon, but has not entered the lymph nodes. (Lymph nodes are small, bean-shaped structures that are found throughout the body; they produce and store infection-fighting cells).

Stage III

Cancer has spread to lymph nodes near the pancreas. The cancer may or may not have spread to nearby organs.

Stage IV

Cancer has spread to places far away from the pancreas, such as the liver or lungs.

Recurrent

Recurrent disease means that the cancer has come back (recurred) after it has been treated. It may come back in the pancreas or in another part of the body.

Treatment Option Overview

How Cancer of the Pancreas Is Treated

There are treatments for all patients with cancer of the pancreas. Three kinds of treatment are used:

- surgery (taking out the cancer or relieving symptoms caused by the cancer)
- radiation therapy (using high-dose x-rays or other high-energy rays to kill cancer cells)
- chemotherapy (using drugs to kill cancer cells)

The use of biological therapy (using the body's immune system to fight cancer) is being tested for pancreatic cancer.

Surgery may be used to take out the tumor. Your doctor may take out the cancer using one of the following operations:

- A Whipple procedure removes the head of the pancreas, part of the small intestine, and some of the tissues around it. Enough of the pancreas is left to continue making digestive juices and insulin.
- Total pancreatectomy takes out the whole pancreas, part of the small intestine, part of the stomach, the bile duct, the gallbladder, spleen, and most of the lymph nodes in the area.
- Distal pancreatectomy takes out only the tail of the pancreas.

If your cancer has spread and it cannot be removed, your doctor may do surgery to relieve symptoms. If the cancer is blocking the small intestine and bile builds up in the gallbladder, your doctor may do surgery to go around (bypass) all or part of the small intestine. During this operation, your doctor will cut the gallbladder or bile duct and sew it to the small intestine. This is called biliary bypass. Surgery or x-ray procedures may also be done to put in a tube (catheter) to drain bile that has built up in the area. During these procedures, your doctor may make the catheter drain through a tube to the outside of the body or the catheter may go around the blocked area and drain the bile to the small intestine. In addition, if the cancer is blocking the flow of food from the stomach, the stomach may be sewn directly to the small intestine so you can continue to eat normally.

Radiation therapy uses high-energy x-rays to kill cancer cells and shrink tumors. Radiation may come from a machine outside the body (external radiation therapy) or from putting materials that produce radiation (radioisotopes) through thin plastic tubes in the area where the cancer cells are found (internal radiation therapy).

Chemotherapy uses drugs to kill cancer cells. Chemotherapy may be taken by pill, or it may be put into the body by a needle in the vein or muscle. Chemotherapy is called a systemic treatment because the drug enters the bloodstream, travels through the body, and can kill cancer cells outside the pancreas.

Biological therapy tries to get your own body to fight cancer. It uses materials made by your own body or made in a laboratory to boost, direct, or restore your body's natural defenses against disease. Biological therapy is sometimes called biological response modifier (BRM) therapy or immunotherapy. Biological therapy is being tested in clinical trials.

Treatment by Stage

Treatment for cancer of the pancreas depends on the stage of your disease, your age, and your overall condition.

You may receive treatment that is considered standard based on its effectiveness in a number of patients in past studies, or you may choose to go into a clinical trial. Most patients with cancer of the pancreas are not cured with standard therapy and some standard treatments may have more side effects than are desired. For these reasons, clinical trials are designed to find better ways to treat cancer patients and are based on the most up-to-date information. Clinical trials are going on in most parts of the country for all stages of cancer of the pancreas. If you wish to know more about clinical trials, call the Cancer Information Service at 1-800-4-CANCER (1-800-422-6237).

Stage I Pancreatic Cancer

Your treatment may be one of the following:

1. Surgery to remove the head of the pancreas, part of the small intestine, and some of the surrounding tissues (Whipple procedure).
2. Surgery to remove the entire pancreas and the organs around it (total pancreatectomy).
3. Surgery to remove the tail of the pancreas (distal pancreatectomy) for tumors in the tail of the pancreas.
4. Surgery followed by chemotherapy and radiation therapy.
5. Clinical trials of radiation therapy with or without chemotherapy given before, during, or after surgery.

Stage II Pancreatic Cancer

Your treatment may be one of the following:

1. Surgery or other treatments to reduce symptoms.
2. External radiation therapy with or without chemotherapy.
3. Surgery to remove all or part of the pancreas with or without chemotherapy and radiation therapy.
4. Clinical trials of radiation therapy and chemotherapy given before surgery.
5. Clinical trials of radiation therapy plus drugs to make cancer cells more sensitive to radiation (radiosensitizers).
6. Clinical trials of chemotherapy.
7. Clinical trials of radiation therapy given during surgery with or without internal radiation therapy.

Stage III Pancreatic Cancer

Your treatment may be one of the following:

1. Surgery or other treatments to reduce symptoms.

2. External radiation therapy with or without chemotherapy.
3. Surgery to remove all or part of the pancreas with or without chemotherapy and radiation therapy.
4. Clinical trials of radiation therapy given before surgery.
5. Clinical trials of surgery plus radiation therapy plus drugs to make cancer cells more sensitive to radiation (radiosensitizers).
6. Clinical trials of chemotherapy.
7. Clinical trials of radiation therapy given during surgery, with or without internal radiation therapy.

Stage IV Pancreatic Cancer

Your treatment may be one of the following:

1. Surgery or other treatments to reduce symptoms.
2. Treatments for pain.
3. Clinical trials of chemotherapy or biological therapy.

Recurrent Pancreatic Cancer

Your treatment may be one of the following:

1. Chemotherapy.
2. Surgery or other treatments to reduce symptoms.
3. External radiation therapy to reduce symptoms.
4. Treatments for pain.
5. Other medical care to reduce symptoms.
6. Clinical trials of chemotherapy or biological therapy.

To Learn More

To learn more about cancer of the pancreas, call the National Cancer Institute's Cancer Information Service at 1-800-4-CANCER (1-800-422-6237). By dialing this toll-free number, you can speak with someone who can answer your questions.

The Cancer Information Service can also send you free booklets. The following booklets about cancer of the pancreas may be helpful to you:

- What You Need to Know About Cancer of the Pancreas
- Research Report: Cancer of the Pancreas

The following general booklets on questions related to cancer may also be helpful:

- What You Need to Know About Cancer
- Taking Time: Support for People with Cancer and the People Who Care About Them
- What Are Clinical Trials All About?
- Chemotherapy and You: A Guide to Self-Help During Treatment
- Radiation Therapy and You: A Guide to Self-Help During Treatment
- Eating Hints for Cancer Patients
- Advanced Cancer: Living Each Day
- When Cancer Recurs: Meeting the Challenge Again

There are many other places you can get material about cancer treatment and services to help you. You can check the social service office at your hospital for local and national agencies that help with your finances, getting to and from treatment, care at home, and dealing with your problems. The American Cancer Society, for example, has many free services. Their local offices are listed in the white pages of the telephone book.

You can also write to the National Cancer Institute at this address:

National Cancer Institute
Office of Cancer Communications
31 Center Dr, MSC 2580
Bethesda, MD 20892-2580

■ **Document Source:**
U.S. Department of Health and Human Services, Public Health Service
National Institutes of Health
National Cancer Institute

Medical Sciences Bulletin

STOMACH AND DUODENAL ULCERS

What is an ulcer?

During normal digestion, food moves from the mouth down the esophagus into the stomach. The stomach produces hydrochloric acid and an enzyme called pepsin to digest the food. From the stomach, food passes into the upper part of the small intestine, called the duodenum, where digestion and nutrient absorption continue.

An ulcer is a sore or lesion that forms in the lining of the stomach or duodenum where acid and pepsin are present. Ulcers in the stomach are called gastric or stomach ulcers. Those in the duodenum are called duodenal ulcers. In general, ulcers in the stomach and duodenum are referred to as peptic ulcers. Ulcers rarely occur in the esophagus or in the first portion of the duodenum, the duodenal bulb.

Who has ulcers?

About 20 million Americans develop at least one ulcer during their lifetime. Each year:

- Ulcers affect about four million people.
- More than 40,000 people have surgery because of persistent symptoms or problems from ulcers.
- About 6,000 people die of ulcer-related complications.

Ulcers can develop at any age, but they are rare among teenagers and even more uncommon in children. Duodenal ulcers occur for the first time usually between the ages of 30 and 50. Stomach ulcers are more likely to develop in people over age 60. Duodenal ulcers occur more frequently in men than women; stomach ulcers develop more often in women than men.

What causes ulcers?

For almost a century, doctors believed lifestyle factors such as stress and diet caused ulcers. Later, researchers discovered that an imbalance between digestive fluids (hydrochloric acid and pepsin) and the stomach's ability to defend itself against these powerful substances resulted in ulcers.

Today, research shows that most ulcers develop as a result of infection with bacteria called *Helicobacter pylori* (*H. pylori*). While all three of these factors—lifestyle, acid and pepsin, and *H. pylori*—play a role in ulcer development, *H. pylori* is now considered the primary cause.

Lifestyle

While scientific evidence refutes the old belief that stress and diet cause ulcers, several lifestyle factors continue to be suspected of playing a role. These factors include cigarettes, foods and beverages containing caffeine, alcohol, and physical stress.

Smoking

Studies show that cigarette smoking increases one's chances of getting an ulcer. Smoking slows the healing of existing ulcers and also contributes to ulcer recurrence.

Caffeine

Coffee, tea, colas, and foods that contain caffeine seem to stimulate acid secretion in the stomach, aggravating the pain of an existing ulcer. However, the amount of acid secretion that occurs after drinking decaffeinated coffee is the same as that produced after drinking regular coffee. Thus, the stimulation of stomach acid cannot be attributed solely to caffeine.

Alcohol

Research has not found a link between alcohol consumption and peptic ulcers. However, ulcers are more common in people who have cirrhosis of the liver, a disease often linked to heavy alcohol consumption.

Stress

Although emotional stress is no longer thought to be a cause of ulcers, people with ulcers often report that emotional stress increases ulcer pain. Physical stress, however, increases the risk of developing ulcers particularly in the stomach. For example, people with injuries such as severe burns and people undergoing major surgery often require rigorous treatment to prevent ulcers and ulcer complications.

Acid and Pepsin

Researchers believe that the stomach's inability to defend itself against the powerful digestive fluids, acid and pepsin, contributes to ulcer formation. The stomach defends itself from these fluids in several ways. One way is by producing mucus—a lubricant-like coating that shields stomach tissues. Another way is by producing a chemical called bicarbonate. This chemical neutralizes and breaks down digestive fluids into substances less harmful to stomach tissue. Finally, blood circulation to the stomach lining, cell renewal, and cell repair also help protect the stomach.

Nonsteroidal anti-inflammatory drugs (NSAIDs) make the stomach vulnerable to the harmful effects of acid and pepsin. NSAIDs such as aspirin, ibuprofen, and naproxen sodium are present in many non-prescription medications used to treat fever, headaches, and minor aches and pains. These, as well as prescription NSAIDs used to treat a variety of arthritic conditions, interfere with the stomach's ability to produce mucus and bicarbonate and affect blood flow to the stomach and cell repair. They can all cause the stomach's defense mechanisms to fail, resulting in an increased chance of developing stomach ulcers. In most cases, these ulcers disappear once the person stops taking NSAIDs.

Helicobacter pylori

H. pylori is a spiral-shaped bacterium found in the stomach. Research shows that the bacteria (along with acid secretion) damage stomach and duodenal tissue, causing inflammation and ulcers. Scientists believe this damage occurs because of *H. pylori's* shape and characteristics.

H. pylori survives in the stomach because it produces the enzyme urease. Urease generates substances that neutralize the stomach's acid—enabling the bacteria to survive. Because of their shape and the way they move, the bacteria can penetrate the stomach's protective mucous lining. Here, they can produce substances that weaken the stomach's protective mucus and make the stomach cells more susceptible to the damaging effects of acid and pepsin.

The bacteria can also attach to stomach cells, further weakening the stomach's defensive mechanisms and producing local inflammation. For reasons not completely understood, *H. pylori* can also stimulate the stomach to produce more acid.

Excess stomach acid and other irritating factors can cause inflammation of the upper end of the duodenum, the duodenal bulb. In some people, over long periods of time, this inflammation results in production of stomach-like cells called duodenal gastric metaplasia. *H. pylori* then attacks these cells causing further tissue damage and inflammation, which may result in an ulcer.

Within weeks of infection with *H. pylori*, most people develop gastritis—an inflammation of the stomach lining. However, most people will never have symptoms or problems related to the infection. Scientists do not yet know what is different in those people who develop *H. pylori*-related symptoms or ulcers. Perhaps, hereditary or environmental factors yet to be discovered cause some individuals to develop problems. Alternatively, symptoms and ulcers may result from infection with more virulent strains of bacteria. These unanswered questions are the subject of intensive scientific research.

Studies show that *H. pylori* infection in the United States varies with age, ethnic group, and socioeconomic class. The bacteria are more common in older adults, African Americans, Hispanics, and lower socioeconomic groups. The organism appears to spread through the fecal-oral route (when infected stool comes into contact with hands, food, or water). Most individuals seem to be infected during childhood, and their infection lasts a lifetime.

The History of *Helicobacter pylori*

In 1982, Australian researchers Barry Marshall and Robin Warren discovered spiral-shaped bacteria in the stomach, later named *Helicobacter pylori* (*H. pylori*). After closely studying *H. pylori's* effect on the stomach, they proposed that the bacteria were the underlying cause of gastritis and peptic ulcers.

Marshall and Warren came to this conclusion because in their studies all patients with duodenal ulcers and 80 percent of patients with stomach ulcers had the bacteria. The 20 percent of patients with stomach ulcers who did not have *H. pylori* were those who had taken NSAIDs such as aspirin and ibuprofen, which are a common cause of stomach ulcers.

Although their findings seem conclusive, Marshall and Warren's theory was hotly debated and remained in dispute. The debate continued even after Marshall and colleague performed an experiment in which they infected themselves with *H. pylori* and developed gastritis.

Evidence linking *H. pylori* to ulcers mounted over the next 10 years as numerous studies from around the world confirmed its presence in most people with ulcers. Moreover, researchers from the United States and Europe proved that using antibiotics to eliminate *H. pylori* healed ulcers and prevented recurrence in about 90 percent of cases.

To further investigate these findings, the National Institutes of Health (NIH) established a panel to closely review the link between *H. pylori* and peptic ulcer disease. At the February 1994 Consensus Development Conference, the panel concluded that *H. pylori* plays a significant role in the development of ulcers and that antibiotics with other medicines can cure peptic ulcer disease.

What are the symptoms of ulcers?

The most common ulcer symptom is a gnawing or burning pain in the abdomen between the breastbone and the naval. The pain often occurs between meals and in the early hours of the morning. It may last from a few minutes to a few hours and may be relieved by eating or by taking antacids.

Less common ulcer symptoms include nausea, vomiting, and loss of appetite and weight. Bleeding from ulcers may occur in the stomach and duodenum. Sometimes people are unaware that they have a bleeding ulcer, because blood loss is slow and blood may not be obvious in the stool. These people may feel tired and weak. If the bleeding is heavy, blood will appear in vomit or stool. Stool containing blood appears tarry or black.

How are ulcers diagnosed?

The NIH Consensus Panel emphasized the importance of adequately diagnosing ulcer disease and *H. pylori* before starting treatment. If the person has an NSAID-induced ulcer, treatment is quite different from the treatment for a person with an *H. pylori*-related ulcer. Also, a person's pain may be the result of nonulcer dyspepsia (persistent pain or discomfort in the upper abdomen including burning, nausea, and bloating), and not at all related to ulcer disease. Currently, doctors have a number of options available for diagnosing

ulcers, such as performing endoscopic and x-ray examinations, and for testing for *H. pylori*.

Locating and Monitoring Ulcers

Doctors may perform an upper GI series to diagnose ulcers. An upper GI series involves taking an x-ray of the esophagus, stomach, and duodenum to locate an ulcer. To make the ulcer visible on the x-ray image, the patient swallows a chalky liquid called barium.

An alternative diagnostic test is called an endoscopy. During this test, the patient is lightly sedated and the doctor inserts a small flexible instrument with a camera on the end through the mouth into the esophagus, stomach, and duodenum. With this procedure, the entire upper GI tract can be viewed. Ulcers or other conditions can be diagnosed and photographed, and tissue can be taken for biopsy, if necessary.

Once an ulcer is diagnosed and treatment begins, the doctor will usually monitor clinical progress. In the case of a stomach ulcer, the doctor may wish to document healing with repeat x-rays or endoscopy. Continued monitoring of a stomach ulcer is important because of the small chance that the ulcer may be cancerous.

Testing for H. pylori

Confirming the presence of *H. pylori* is important once the doctor has diagnosed an ulcer because elimination of the bacteria is likely to cure ulcer disease. Blood, breath, and stomach tissue tests may be performed to detect the presence of *H. pylori*. While some of the tests for *H. pylori* are not approved by the U.S. Food and Drug Administration (FDA), research shows these tests are highly accurate in detecting the bacteria. However, blood tests on occasion give false positive results, and the other tests may give false negative results in people who have recently taken antibiotics, omeprazole (Prilosec), or bismuth (Pepto-Bismol).

Blood Tests

Blood tests such as the enzyme-linked immunosorbent assay (ELISA) and quick office-based tests identify and measure *H. pylori* antibodies. The body produces anti bodies against *H. pylori* in an attempt to fight the bacteria. The advantages of blood tests are their low cost and availability to doctors. The disadvantage is the possibility of false positive results in patients previously treated for ulcers since the levels of *H. pylori* antibodies fall slowly. Several blood tests have FDA approval.

Breath Tests

Breath tests measure carbon dioxide in exhaled breath. Patients are given a substance called urea with carbon to drink. Bacteria break down this urea and the carbon is absorbed into the blood stream and lungs and exhaled in the breath. By collecting the breath, doctors can measure this carbon and determine whether *H. pylori* is present or absent. Urea breath tests are at least 90 percent accurate for diagnosing the bacteria and are particularly suitable to follow-up treatment to see if bacteria have been eradicated. These tests are awaiting FDA approval.

Tissue Tests

If the doctor performs an endoscopy to diagnose an ulcer, tissue samples of the stomach can be obtained. The doctor may then perform one of several tests on the tissue. A rapid urease test detects the bacteria's enzyme urease. Histology involves visualizing the bacteria under the microscope. Culture involves specially processing the tissue and watching it for growth of *H. pylori* organisms.

How are ulcers treated?

Lifestyle Changes

In the past, doctors advised people with ulcers to avoid spicy, fatty, or acidic foods. However, a bland diet is now known to be ineffective for treating or avoiding ulcers. No particular diet is helpful for most ulcer patients. People who find that certain foods cause irritation should discuss this problem with their doctor. Smoking has been shown to delay ulcer healing and has been linked to ulcer recurrence, therefore, persons with ulcers should not smoke.

Medicines

Doctors treat stomach and duodenal ulcers with several types of medicines including H2 blockers, acid pump inhibitors, and mucosal protective agents. When treating *H. pylori*, these medications are used in combination with antibiotics.

H2 Blockers

Currently, most doctors treat ulcers with acid-suppressing drugs known as H2 blockers. These drugs reduce the amount of acid the stomach produces by blocking histamine, a powerful stimulant of acid secretion.

H2 blockers reduce pain significantly after several weeks. For the first few days of treatment, doctors often recommend taking an antacid to relieve pain.

Initially, treatment with H2 blockers lasts six to eight weeks. However, because ulcers recur in 50 to 80 percent of cases, many people must continue maintenance therapy for years. This may no longer be the case if *H. pylori* infection is treated. Most ulcers do not recur following successful eradication. Nizatidine (Axid) is approved for treatment of duodenal ulcers but is not yet approved for treatment of stomach ulcers. H2 blockers that are approved to treat both stomach and duodenal ulcers are

- Cimetidine (Tagamet)
- Ranitidine (Zantac)
- Famotidine (Pepcid)

Acid Pump Inhibitors

Like H2 blockers, acid pump inhibitors modify the stomach's production of acid. However, acid pump inhibitors more completely block stomach acid production by stopping the stomach's acid pump—the final step of acid secretion. The

FDA has approved use of omeprazole for short-term treatment of ulcer disease. Similar drugs, including lansoprazole, are currently being studied.

Mucosal Protective Medications

Mucosal protective medications protect the stomach's mucous lining from acid. Unlike H2 blockers and acid pump inhibitors, protective agents do not inhibit the release of acid. These medications shield the stomach's mucous lining from the damage of acid. Two commonly prescribed protective agents are

- Sucralfate (Carafate). This medication adheres to the ulcer, providing a protective barrier that allows the ulcer to heal and inhibits further damage by stomach acid. Sucralfate is approved for short-term treatment of duodenal ulcers and for maintenance treatment.
- Misoprostol (Cytotec). This synthetic prostaglandin, a substance naturally produced by the body, protects the stomach lining by increasing mucus and bicarbonate production and by enhancing blood flow to the stomach. It is approved only for the prevention of NSAID-induced ulcers.

Two common nonprescription protective medications are

- Antacids. Antacids can offer temporary relief from ulcer pain by neutralizing stomach acid. They may also have a mucosal protective role. Many brands of antacids are available without prescription.
- Bismuth Subsalicylate. Bismuth subsalicylate has both a protective effect and an antibacterial effect against *H. pylori*.

Antibiotics

The discovery of the link between ulcers and *H. pylori* has resulted in a new treatment option. Now, in addition to treatment aimed at decreasing the production of stomach acid, doctors may prescribe antibiotics for patients with *H. pylori*. This treatment is a dramatic medical advance because eliminating *H. pylori* means the ulcer may now heal and most likely will not come back.

Typical Two-Week, Triple Therapy

- Metronidazole four times a day
- Tetracycline (or amoxicillin) four times a day
- Bismuth subsalicylate four times a day

Typical Two-Week, Dual Therapy

- Amoxicillin two to four times a day, or clarithromycin three times a day
- Omeprazole two times a day

The most effective therapy, according to the NIH Panel, is a two-week, triple therapy. This regimen eradicates the bacteria and reduces the risk of ulcer recurrence in 90 percent of people with duodenal ulcers. People with stomach ulcers that are not associated with NSAIDs also benefit from bacterial eradication. While triple therapy is effective, it is sometimes difficult to follow because the patient must take three different medications four times each day for two weeks.

In addition, the treatment commonly causes side effects such as yeast infection in women, stomach upset, nausea, vomiting, bad taste, loose or dark bowel movements, and dizziness. The two-week, triple therapy combines two antibiotics, tetracycline (e.g., Achromycin or Sumycin) and metronidazole (e.g., Flagyl) with bismuth subsalicylate (Pepto-Bismol). Some doctors may add an acid-suppressing drug to relieve ulcer pain and promote ulcer healing. In some cases, doctors may substitute amoxicillin (e.g., Amoxil or Trimox) for tetracycline or, if they expect bacterial resistance to metronidazole, other antibiotics such as clarithromycin (Biaxin).

As an alternative to triple therapy, several two-week, dual therapies are about 80 percent effective. Dual therapy is simpler for patients to follow and causes fewer side effects. A dual therapy might include an antibiotic, such as amoxicillin or clarithromycin, with omeprazole, a drug that stops the production of acid.

Again, an accurate diagnosis is important. Accurate diagnosis and appropriate treatment prevent people without ulcers from needless exposure to the side effects of antibiotics and should lessen the risk of bacteria developing resistance to antibiotics.

Although all of the above antibiotics are sold in the United States, the FDA has not yet approved the use of antibiotics for treatment of *H. pylori* or ulcers. Doctors may choose to prescribe antibiotics to their ulcer patients as "off label" prescriptions as they do for many conditions.

When is surgery needed?

In most cases, anti-ulcer medicines heal ulcers quickly and effectively. Eradication of *H. pylori* prevents most ulcers from recurring. However, people who do not respond to medication or who develop complications may require surgery. While surgery is usually successful in healing ulcers and preventing their recurrence and future complications, problems can sometimes result.

At present, standard open surgery is performed to treat ulcers. In the future, surgeons may use laparoscopic methods. A laparoscope is a long tube-like instrument with a camera that allows the surgeon to operate through small incisions while watching a video monitor.

The common types of surgery for ulcers—vagotomy, pyloroplasty, and antrectomy—are described below

Vagotomy

A vagotomy involves cutting the vagus nerve, a nerve that transmits messages from the brain to the stomach. Interrupting the messages sent through the vagus nerve reduces acid secretion. However, the surgery may also interfere with stomach emptying. The newest variation of the surgery involves cutting only parts of the nerve that control the acid-secreting cells of the stomach, thereby avoiding the parts that influence stomach emptying.

Antrectomy

Another surgical procedure is the antrectomy. This operation removes the lower part of the stomach (antrum), which produces a hormone that stimulates the stomach to secrete digestive juices. Sometimes a surgeon may also remove an adjacent part of the stomach that secretes pepsin and acid. A vagotomy is usually done in conjunction with an antrectomy.

Pyloroplasty

Pyloroplasty is another surgical procedure that may be performed along with a vagotomy. Pyloroplasty enlarges the opening into the duodenum and small intestine (pylorus), enabling contents to pass more freely from the stomach.

What are the complications of ulcers?

People with ulcers may experience serious complications if they do not get treatment. The most common problems include bleeding, perforation of the organ walls, and narrowing and obstruction of digestive tract passages.

Bleeding

As an ulcer eats into the muscles of the stomach or duodenal wall, blood vessels may also be damaged, which causes bleeding. If the affected blood vessels are small, the blood may slowly seep into the digestive tract. Over a long period of time, a person may become anemic and feel weak, dizzy, or tired.

If a damaged blood vessel is large, bleeding is dangerous and requires prompt medical attention. Symptoms include feeling weak and dizzy when standing, vomiting blood, or fainting. The stool may become a tarry black color from the blood.

Most bleeding ulcers can be treated endoscopically—the ulcer is located and the blood vessel is cauterized with a heating device or injected with material to stop bleeding. If endoscopic treatment is unsuccessful, surgery may be required.

Perforation

Sometimes an ulcer eats a hole in the wall of the stomach or duodenum. Bacteria and partially digested food can spill through the opening into the sterile abdominal cavity (peritoneum). This causes peritonitis, an inflammation of the abdominal cavity and wall. A perforated ulcer that can cause sudden, sharp, severe pain usually requires immediate hospitalization and surgery.

Narrowing and Obstruction

Ulcers located at the end of the stomach where the duodenum is attached can cause swelling and scarring, which can narrow or close the intestinal opening. This obstruction can prevent food from leaving the stomach and entering the small intestine. As a result, a person may vomit the contents of the stomach. Endoscopic balloon dilation, a procedure that uses a balloon to force open a narrow passage, may be performed.

If the dilation does not relieve the problem, then surgery may be necessary.

Points to Remember

- An ulcer is a sore or lesion that forms in the lining of the stomach or duodenum where the digestive fluids acid and pepsin are present.
- Recent research shows that most ulcers develop as a result of infection with bacteria called *Helicobacter pylori* (*H. pylori*). The bacteria produce substances that weaken the stomach's protective mucus and make the stomach more susceptible to damaging effects of acid and pepsin. *H. pylori* can also cause the stomach to produce more acid. Although acid and pepsin and lifestyle factors such as stress and smoking cigarettes play a role in ulcer formation, *H. pylori* is now considered the primary cause.
- Nonsteroidal anti-inflammatory drugs such as aspirin make the stomach vulnerable to the harmful effects of acid and pepsin, leading to an increased chance of stomach ulcers.
- Ulcers do not always cause symptoms. When they do, the most common symptom is a gnawing or burning pain in the abdomen between the breastbone and navel. Some people have nausea, vomiting, and loss of appetite and weight.
- Bleeding from an ulcer may occur in the stomach and duodenum. Symptoms may include weakness and stool that appears tarry or black. However, sometimes people are not aware they have a bleeding ulcer because blood may not be obvious in the stool.
- Ulcers are diagnosed with x-ray or endoscopy. The presence of *H. pylori* may be diagnosed with a blood test, breath test, or tissue test. Once an ulcer is diagnosed and treatment begins, the doctor will usually monitor progress.
- Doctors treat ulcers with several types of medicines aimed at reducing acid production, including H2 blockers, acid pump inhibitors, and mucosal protective drugs. When treating *H. pylori*, these medications are used in combination with antibiotics.
- According to an NIH panel, the most effective treatment for *H. pylori* is a two-week, triple therapy of metronidazole, tetracycline or amoxicillin, and bismuth subsalicylate.
- Surgery may be necessary if an ulcer recurs or fails to heal or if complications such as bleeding, perforation, or obstruction develop.

Conclusion

Although ulcers may cause discomfort, rarely are they life-threatening. With an understanding of the causes and proper treatment, most people find relief. Eradication of *H. pylori* infection is a major medical advance that can permanently cure most peptic ulcer disease.

Additional Reading

DeCross AJ, Peura DA. Role of *H. pylori* in peptic ulcer disease. *Contemporary Gastroenterology*, 1992; 5(4): 18-28.

Fedotin MS. *Helicobacter pylori* and peptic ulcer disease: Reexamining the therapeutic approach. *Postgraduate Medicine*, 1993; 94(3): 38-45.

Gilbert G, Chan CH, Thomas E. Peptic ulcer disease: How to treat it now. *Postgraduate Medicine*, 1991; 89(4): 91-98.

Larson DE, Editor-in-Chief. *Mayo Clinic Family Health Book*. New York: William Morrow and Company, Inc., 1990. General medical guide with sections on stomach problems and ulcers.

■ **Document Source:**
U.S. Department of Health and Human Services, Public Health Service
National Institutes of Health
National Institute of Diabetes and Digestive and Kidney Diseases
NIH Publication No. 95-38
January 1995

SURPRISE CAUSE OF GASTRITIS REVOLUTIONIZES ULCER TREATMENT

by Ricki Lewis, PhD

Mention "ulcer" and most people envision a stressed-out, workaholic, junk-food-gobbling worrywart. Since the turn of the century, ulcers have been equated with stress and poor diet. But that image may be substantially incorrect. Now, the medical community is beginning to look at painful ulcers in a new light—as an easily treatable bacterial infection. The name of the bug—*Helicobacter pylori*.

For many of the four million ulcer sufferers in the United States, the new view of ulcers may mean a course of antibiotics. This treatment may reduce recurrence to below the 10 to 15 percent a year for current, non-antibiotic drug therapies. In ulcer sufferers who receive no treatment, recurrence is up to 80 percent.

"Now there is the possibility of curing the condition, which was unthought-of before," says Hugo Gallo-Torres, MD, medical officer in the Food and Drug Administration's division of gastrointestinal and coagulation drug products.

The agency is considering particular combinations of drugs for ulcer treatment, following conclusions of a consensus development conference convened by the National Institutes of Health in February 1994. The conference gathered experts to review data accumulating since 1983 implicating bacteria in causing ulcers. The drugs under consideration aren't new, but their use to treat ulcers is.

Anatomy of an Ulcer

Sufferers describe an ulcer as a burning, cramping, gnawing, or aching in the abdomen that comes in waves, for three to four days at a time, but may subside completely for weeks or months. Pain is worst before meals and at bedtime, when the stomach is usually empty. The ulcer itself is an open sore in the lining of the stomach (gastric ulcer) or in the upper part of the small intestine, or duodenum (duodenal ulcer). Both types are also called peptic ulcers.

The stomach is the most acidic part of the body, setting the stage both for ulcer development and infection. Three types of cells pump out the ingredients of gastric juice;

mucous-secreting cells, chief cells that release digestive enzymes, and parietal cells that produce hydrochloric acid. The mucous-secreting cells also produce histamine, which stimulates the parietal cells to release acid. The stomach needs the acid environment for the digestive enzyme pepsin to break down proteins in foods.

Acidity is measured using the pH scale. A neutral pH is neither acid nor base—it has a value of 7; acids are less than 7, and bases (also called alkaline substances) are greater than 7. Many body fluids, including blood, tears, pancreatic juice, and bile, are in the 7 to 8 pH range. Gastric juice, in contrast, has a pH of 1.6 to 1.8. That's more acidic than lemon juice, cola drinks, and coffee. The environment in the small intestine is far less acidic than in the stomach, but because it receives the acidic mixture of semi-digested food from the stomach, it is prone to ulceration too.

The stomach's innermost lining, the mucosa, protects it from digesting itself. The mucosa consists of lining cells, connective tissue, and muscle. An ulcer hurts when it penetrates the mucosa into the underlying submucosa, which is rich in nerves and blood vessels.

A vat of churning acidic goop may not seem a hospitable place for a microbe, but the type that causes ulcers thrives in the low pH environment. "They have outgrowths called flagella that allow them to penetrate the mucous layers of the stomach, where the pH is more tolerable. Eradicating these bacteria is not simple," says Gallo-Torres. The antibiotic drug must be able to kill the bacteria, yet also resist breakdown in the acidic surroundings.

Researchers aren't certain how people acquire the bacteria. However, person-to-person transmission is believed to be the most likely route in developed countries. In developing countries, fecal-oral transmission may play a more important role, similar to the way a person contracts cholera and hepatitis B.

Early in the 20th century, the prescription for an ulcer was bed rest and a bland diet, in a hospital if the patient could afford it. Antacids were added to the treatment regimen when researchers learned that ulcer patients produce excess stomach acid. By 1971, the control site of acid secretion was identified—histamine (H_2) receptors on the parietal cells.

When histamine binds such receptors, acid output increases. Four approved ulcer drugs—Zantac (ranitidine), Tagemet (cimetidine), Pepcid (famotidine), and Axid (nizatidine)—block H_2 receptors, thwarting the signal to secrete acid. A second type of ulcer drug, called an acid or proton pump inhibitor, works at a different point in digestion, blocking parietal cells from releasing acid. Prilosec (omeprazole) is the only acid-pump inhibitor approved in the United States at this time.

The problem with existing drugs is that they only temporarily improve symptoms; the ulcer is likely to return. If bacteria causing some ulcers are eradicated, however, the likelihood of ulcer recurrence is much less because the problem is attacked at its source. But acceptance of the role of bacteria in the production of peptic ulcer disease has been slow.

Discovering the Infection Connection

In 1982, two young Australian physicians, Barry J. Marshall and Robin Warren, isolated bacteria from patients with ulcers or gastritis (stomach inflammation). In a paper published in the medical journal *Lancet* in early 1983, they proposed that a spiral-shaped bacterium, later named *Helicobacter pylori*, causes gastritis and possibly ulcers. But few physicians accepted their work, so entrenched was the idea that ulcers stem from stress. So Marshall and Warren took drastic measures to prove their point—they swallowed some of the bacteria. And their digestive tracts soon became inflamed.

But most of the medical community felt this was not sufficient proof to definitively implicate the bacteria in causing ulcers. A medical dictionary published in 1986, for example, lists the causes of ulcers in order of importance as high acid, irritation, decreased blood supply to the digestive tract, decreased mucus, and last, with question mark, infection.

"We had treated ulcers with antisecretory compounds for so many years, it was hard to accept that a germ, a bacterium, would produce a disease like that. It took a while. Even academicians were not convinced. Gradually other people found the same thing," says Gallo-Torres.

The accumulating evidence became the basis of the February 1994 consensus development conference, which concluded: "Ulcer patients with *Helicobacter pylori* infection require treatment with anti-microbial agents in addition to anti-secretory drugs."

In a nutshell, the evidence for the link between bacteria and ulcers is that

- All patients examined who are infected with the bacteria have evidence at the tissue level of gastritis (inflammation), but most are asymptomatic.
- Clearing up the infection cures the gastric inflammation.
- Giving the bacteria to laboratory animals (and Warren and Marshall) causes gastritis.

However, even though nearly all people who are infected develop gastritis, not all develop ulcers. This suggests that other factors—such as heredity, diet, stress, and other environmental influences—may be important for the development of peptic ulcers. According to the consensus development report, "the strongest evidence for the pathogenic role of *H. pylori* in peptic ulcer disease is the marked decrease in recurrence rate of ulcers following the eradication of infection."

How common are bacterial ulcers? The consensus report estimates that "almost all" duodenal ulcers are attributable to *H. pylori*, as are about 80 percent of gastric ulcers, making the microbes a very major cause. A very small percentage of ulcer sufferers develop ulcers from using aspirin or a nonsteroidal anti-inflammatory drug (NSAID) such as Voltaren (diclofenac), Feldene (piroxicam), or Ansaid (flurbiprofen). Ibuprofen, also an NSAID, is less likely to cause gastric inflammation.

Diagnosis

For ulcer patients, diagnosis and treatment are changing.

Several different tests detect *H. pylori*. "You can biopsy [take tissue samples of] gastric and duodenal mucosa, then culture bacteria and identify them. But this approach is not very sensitive because it depends upon where you biopsy," says Gallo-Torres.

To sample stomach or intestinal tissue, a physician snakes a lighted tube called an endoscope down through the throat. Less invasive techniques are available, too. Blood tests can detect IgG antibodies to *H. pylori* in a person's blood, representing the immune system's response to the microbe. These tests are cleared for marketing by FDA.

Other diagnosis tests in development, but not yet established by FDA, are based on the ability of *H. pylori* to break down urea, human metabolic waste, with an enzyme called urease, which humans do not produce. Elevated levels of breakdown products of urea, detected in a person's breath after drinking chemically labeled urea, indicate *H. pylori* infection.

Can the ulcer bacterium also cause cancer?

It's been known for several years that people with a form of stomach cancer called gastric carcinoma are very often infected with *H. pylori*, and there is evidence that the infection precedes the cancer. More recently, researchers linked the microbe to a second type of stomach cancer, called primarily gastric lymphoma.

This second type of malignancy affects lymphoid tissue—antibody-producing cells in the stomach. However, such cells are not normally present in the stomach unless there is an infection.

In the May 5, 1994, issue of *The New England Journal of Medicine*, a multi-center team led by Julie Parsonnet, MD, of Stanford University, reported that people with gastric lymphoma also have *H. pylori* infection and that the infection precedes the cancer. In an accompanying editorial, Peter G. Isaacson, DM, of University College of London Medical School, suggests that the bacterial infection initiates a chain reaction leading to cancer. He suggests that first infection causes chronic gastritis; then, the inflammation causes stomach lining tissue to overgrow; and, ultimately, excess growth may blossom into cancer, given some as-yet unidentified environmental trigger or genetic susceptibility.

But, so far, the link between *H. pylori* and cancer is far more tenuous than that between the bacteria and gastritis or ulcers. Fewer than 1 percent of people infected with the microbe develop cancer, and some populations in which many people are infected have very low stomach cancer rates. These facts, researchers say, suggest that several factors are at play. Still, it will be interesting to see if antibiotic/anti-secretory treatment can reduce incidence of these already rare cancers.

The consensus development conference convened to study *H. pylori* in February 1994 concluded, "if there is any causal relationship between *H. pylori* infection and gastric cancer, clearly other facts are also important." They recommend further study into whether eradicating the infection can prevent cancer.

Treatment

Quite a few helpful drugs are already on the market, though they are not approved for treating ulcers. FDA's role now is to wade through studies, old and new, to identify the best combinations of drugs, a process that was under way when this issue of *FDA Consumer* went to press. FDA is also considering new drugs to treat bacterial ulcers.

"We would really like to inform physicians quickly and also evaluate the data. There are many regimens proposed," says Gallo-Torres.

The consensus development conference examined several treatment plans. Its report said that there had been extensive studies of bismuth subsalicylate (better known as Pepto Bismol), an antiprotozoan drug, Flagyl (metronidazole), and either the antibiotic tetracycline (giving an overall 90 percent cure rate) or amoxicillin (with an overall 80 percent cure rate).

According to the consensus development report, there had been one study of another regimen, consisting of amoxicillin, metronidazole, and ranitidine, that showed a 90 percent effective rate. However, all of these approaches require a patient to take several different pills several times a day. The committee reported that a two-drug alternative, consisting of amoxicillin, taken four times a day, and Priolsec (omeprazole), taken twice a day, offers 80 percent effectiveness. However, at press time, FDA had not verified these regimens.

Clearly, doctors will have many choices. But at the time of the conference, only 1 to 2 percent of US physicians were treating an ulcer as they would a bacterial infection, according to the conference report.

Concluded conference member Daniel K. Podolsky, MD, of Massachusetts General Hospital, "These recommendations represent a sea change in how we approach this problem. From this time forward, I would consider use of these drugs to be essential."

As data confirming the bacteria-ulcer link continue to pour in, medical researchers are already asking questions that will form the basis of future studies: What factors cause bacterial gastritis to develop into an ulcer? Do children have bacterial ulcers? Can the new treatments prevent complications, such as bleeding ulcers? Does *H. pylori* cause stomach cancer, and, if so, can we prevent it?

Meanwhile, the future of current ulcer sufferers looks brighter than ever. Says consensus team member Ann L.B. Williams, MD, of George Washington University Medical College, "We now have an opportunity to cure a disease that previously we had only been able to suppress or control."

■ Document Source:
U.S. Department of Health and Human Service, Public Health Service
Food and Drug Administration
FDA Consumer
December 1994

GENETIC DISORDERS

■ ■ ■

FACTS ABOUT DOWN SYNDROME

Down syndrome, the most common genetic birth defect associated with mental retardation, occurs equally across all races and levels of society. The effects of the disorder on physical and mental development are severe and are expressed throughout the life span. The individual's family is also affected emotionally, economically, and socially.

This booklet, based primarily on knowledge gained from research studies and programs developed at Mental Retardation Research Centers throughout the United States, presents current information about Down syndrome for families of children with the disorder and those who care for them. The Research Centers are supported by the National Institute of Child Health and Human Development (NICHD), National Institutes of Health (NIH), which has primary responsibility for research on mental retardation.

Genetic and Physical Aspects

Down syndrome is a combination of physical abnormalities and mental retardation characterized by a genetic defect in chromosome pair 21. All normal cells in the human body, except ova and sperm cells, have 46 chromosomes—44 autosomes and two sex chromosomes. Normal reproductive cells contain 23 chromosomes—22 autosomes and one sex chromosome.

In all other (nonreproductive) body cells, chromosomes occur in pairs. The 22 pairs of autosomes are identified by number while the remaining pair of sex chromosomes is designated XX for females or XY for males. Each autosome appears identical to its partner, but each pair is different in its genetic content, and frequently in appearance, from all other pairs.

The genetic defect associated with Down syndrome is the presence of extra material on the chromosome pair designated 21. Although other genetic disorders may be associated with an extra chromosome, only Down syndrome is characterized by extra chromosome 21 material. The forms in which this extra material can appear are classified as:

Trisomy 21—the presence of three rather than the normal pair of chromosomes designated as 21. The genetic abnormality most frequently associated with Down syndrome (95 percent of all cases), trisomy 21, results from an error in cell division during the development of the egg or sperm, or during fertilization.

Translocation—an interchange of chromosomes or parts of chromosomes which may result in a mismatched pair. Children with translocation Down syndrome, which occurs in about four percent of the cases, have an extra number 21 chromosome which has broken and become attached to another chromosome. In certain cases, a person can carry a broken chromosome 21 without showing any symptoms of Down syndrome because the correct amount of genetic material is there, even though some of it is out of place.

Normally, children receive one chromosome of pair 21 from each parent. However, a parent with a translocation can pass on his or her normal chromosome 21 *plus* the translocated chromosome 21, giving the child too much genetic material for chromosome 21.

Mosaicism—a very rare form of Down syndrome, appearing in about one percent of individuals with the disorder. Affected persons have cells with different chromosome counts (for example, 46 in some cells and 47 in others). Mosaicism is not carried in the parents' chromosomes; it is accidental, resulting from an error in cell division of the fertilized egg. Since only some of their cells have an abnormal number of chromosomes, babies with mosaic Down syndrome may have only some of the features of the disorder.

The distinct physical characteristics of Down syndrome include slanting eyes; slightly protruding lips; small ears; slightly protruding tongue; short hands, feet and trunk; and sometimes, an unusual crease on the palm of the infant's hand. Congenital heart defects are common and nystagmus (involuntary movement of the eyes), enlarged liver and spleen also occur. In 99 percent of cases, there is mild to severe mental retardation.

Surveys show the average incidence of Down syndrome to be about one in 800 live births. However, the risk of bearing a child with the disorder increases dramatically with advancing maternal age. For example, the incidence is less than one in 1,000 live births to women under 30, increasing to one in 35 to mothers aged 44.

The sharp rise in the incidence of babies with Down syndrome born to older women may occur for several reasons.

Although males produce new sperm continually, women are born with all the oocytes (eggs) they will ever have. An oocyte remains in a state of incomplete development until the process begins that results in ovulation. Thus, a 35-year-old woman has 35-year-old oocytes.

Many body functions decline with age, and oocytes in the older woman simply may be past their prime. Or they may have been exposed over the years to damaging internal and external influences, including medications, radiation, or other harmful agents.

Until recently, the mother was believed to be the source of the extra genetic material. However, researchers, using new laboratory techniques, have demonstrated that in about 25 percent of cases studied, the father is the source of the extra chromosome. Because older fathers have been associated with increased incidence of other genetic disorders, researchers are looking more closely at the possible effect of the father's age on the incidence of Down syndrome. In one project, involving only a small number of cases, a paternal age effect for fathers over age 55 was reported.

Although individuals with Down syndrome are living longer than in the past, due in part to improved surgical treatment of congenital heart defects, the use of antibiotics for treating infection, and avoidance of early institutionalization, their life expectancy still remains much less than for the general population.

Of special concern is the much greater risk that children with Down syndrome have of developing leukemia—20 times greater than normal children. Not only is the risk greater, but the children die earlier—the peak age of leukemia deaths in normal children is age four, but for those with Down syndrome it is one year.

Relationship of Down Syndrome to Maternal Age

Mother's Age	Incidence of Down Syndrome
under 30	less than 1 in 1,000
30	1 in 900
35	1 in 400
36	1 in 300
37	1 in 230
38	1 in 180
39	1 in 135
40	1 in 105
42	1 in 60
44	1 in 35
46	1 in 20
48	1 in 12

The Outlook

The individual with Down syndrome presents unusual and demanding problems at virtually every stage of life, beginning at birth.

In most cases, the first medical exam identifies the newborn with Down syndrome. Expecting a normal infant, most parents are intensely disappointed when the physician explains their new baby's condition to them. Parents generally experience an initial period of shock, followed by denial, grief, anger, adjustment, and finally, acceptance. These events do not necessarily occur in this sequence, nor does everyone experience all of these stages.

Faced with an abrupt change in their hopes and plans for the new child, parents need early counseling and guidance to help them cope with the situation and plan for their child's future.

The presence of a retarded child in the home is not necessarily detrimental to the happiness and welfare of siblings or to the family as a whole. With professional guidance, an accepting community attitude, and the help of parent support organizations, a congenial home atmosphere can evolve. All children, but especially those with Down syndrome, benefit from loving and caring homes.

In addition to help in managing medical problems, professional guidance usually includes genetic counseling for parents and a discussion of the family's plans for the future.

Since stereotypes of Down syndrome persist, early and sound information for new parents and other family members is very important. In the past, most physicians recommended placing the infant in an institution immediately upon discharge from the hospital nursery. New developments in care and treatment now permit other courses, but, unfortunately, parents are not always made aware of these approaches or to alternatives to institutionalization.

To help keep professionals and parents informed about new developments, and to provide friendly support to new Down syndrome families, parent groups have formed in many communities, sometimes as chapters of national organizations. Often, a hospital social worker will help new parents contact such groups.

In the past 20 years, through the efforts of the comprehensive, multidisciplinary University Affiliated Programs and the NICHD-supported Mental Retardation Research Centers, a new generation of professionals, skilled and knowledgeable in meeting the needs of families affected by Down syndrome, has evolved.

Work at the centers ranges from training health professionals to investigating the causes of mental retardation, particularly Down syndrome. Because the syndrome results from a chromosomal error, most studies are concerned with genetic aspects. However, because of the complexity of the studies and the need for additional research, preventing Down syndrome through genetics research remains a distant goal.

Research has provided strategies for recognizing Down syndrome and other genetic defects through advances in prenatal diagnosis. For example, NICHD-supported studies have demonstrated the safety and efficiency of amniocentesis and related technologies.

Health and Development

Since significant health and developmental problems occur in the child with Down syndrome during the first few years of life, close monitoring is necessary throughout this period.

Medical management and surgical correction, when indicated, of the life-threatening congenital defects frequently associated with Down syndrome are essential to assure the child's optimal health and well-being. Today, most experts agree that surgical procedures to correct defects should not be withheld, as occasionally happens, simply because the child has Down syndrome. In a few cases, cosmetic surgery has been used to alter the distinct physical characteristics of the syndrome; however, the use of cosmetic surgery does not appeal to everyone.

Children with Down syndrome are more susceptible to infections than normal children and, as a result, often suffer chronic respiratory infection, recurrent pneumonia, and repeated bouts of tonsillitis. Researchers believe that children with the disorder have a deficient immune response. According to several studies, they not only have fewer of the cells needed for normal immunologic response to infection but the cells they have do not function well.

Hearing loss occurs more frequently among individuals with Down syndrome than in the normal population. Because affected persons are particularly vulnerable to deficiencies in speech and language development, careful screening and testing for hearing loss should be done and corrective procedures started as early as possible.

Development delays are evident from the early months of life. Infants are slow to turn over, sit, stand, speak, and respond, and parents or others caring for them may not interact with them—smiling and talking while feeding them or changing their diapers, for example—as readily as with normally developing babies.

Such early interaction is even more important for Down syndrome children, however, because their weak motor development reduces their own self-initiated activities, like rolling over or reaching for objects. Proponents of home care point out that children reared in a home atmosphere function better than those reared in institutions, because opportunities for early interaction in institutions are generally inadequate.

Compared with early delay in postural motor development (sitting, standing, walking), the delay in speech and language development encountered by the child with Down syndrome is more noticeable. In addition, beginning in the second year of life, there is an apparent decline in intelligence because language and speech become increasingly more important in intelligence tests.

The reasons for the special difficulty that Down syndrome children have in speech and language are not fully understood. Part of the difficulty stems from the characteristic overlarge and protruding tongue, and in some instances surgical correction of this condition has been helpful. The acquisition of speech and language also depends upon the patterns of vocal and verbal interactions between child and parents and upon cognitive processes.

At this time, there is no known medical regimen that can reverse the pattern of early developmental delay observed in children with the syndrome. Various forms of medication, including chemicals and vitamins, have been tested, without success. Most often, the gains observed are attributed to changes in the quality and quantity of parental care associated with the treatment being tested. This has led to increased interest by researchers and parents in early intervention programs.

Preliminary results from one early intervention program, operating at the Mental Retardation Research Center, University of Washington, Seattle, is encouraging. Children with Down syndrome who entered the project as infants are now in elementary school, or about to begin. Researchers are finding that in a variety of developmental tasks, children in the program exceed the development of other children with Down syndrome not in the program. In addition, the program appears to reduce the severity of retardation.

On the other hand, a six-month, less intensive intervention program at McGill University in Montreal did not produce beneficial gains—contrasting results that only point to the need for more information about early intervention efforts.

Not all families have easy access to specialized resources for their handicapped child. In these situations, efforts have focused on enhancing the ability of parents to teach their children speech and language and self-help and social skills through home-based programs.

If effective early intervention programs can be designed and used in the preschool years, the subsequent educational progress of a child with Down syndrome may be altered significantly. A child may then be classified as educable, rather than trainable, and therefore qualified for different educational opportunities and strategies.

An "educable" person is defined as one who is capable of learning such basic skills as reading and arithmetic and is quite capable of self-care and independent living (those with mild retardation are generally considered educable). Although trainable (moderately retarded) persons are very limited in educational attainments, they can profit from simple training for self-care and vocational tasks.

The Elementary School Years

Under Public Law 94-12, each state is required to have a goal that "all handicapped children have available to them . . . a free public education and related services designed to meet their unique needs."

School entry for children with Down syndrome brings with it the need to determine what is an *appropriate* education designed to meet their special situation. Because the physical characteristics associated with the syndrome easily identify and label the child, the old stereotype of a trainable but uneducable person is readily aroused and can affect early school placement.

As increasing numbers of children with Down syndrome are cared for in their home communities and receive school instruction, the demand for research on their unique learning problems is expected to increase. And as expectations rise for their academic achievement, increased research concern for special educational strategies can also be expected.

Adolescence

At adolescence, children with Down syndrome tend to be overweight. This may be due to general body type (short stature and decreased muscle tone), lack of physical activity associated with social isolation and reduced outlets for activity, and excessive eating of high-calorie foods. In addition to detracting from the adolescent's appearance, the weight gain has negative implications for later health and longevity. A supervised regimen of diet and exercise through the elementary school years, or even earlier, may have a beneficial effect.

Parental concern for the social and sexual life of their child with Down syndrome usually intensifies at adolescence. Unless earlier efforts have been highly successful, the child's social isolation increases outside of structured school and other group situations. Although persons with Down syndrome seldom reproduce, it is necessary to provide them with a healthy understanding and orientation toward sexuality. Pregnancy has been rare, probably as a result of sexual isolation in institutions, but sometimes does occur. About half the infants born of such pregnancies have Down syndrome. Males with trisomy 21 not associated with mosaicism or translocation have not been known to reproduce.

Generally, few services and programs exist for adolescents with the disorder and their families. In the past, both research and service efforts have concentrated on younger persons. The national trend toward "mainstreaming" is a fairly recent development, and the present generation of adolescents with Down syndrome is the first raised under conditions of greater educational and community opportunity. The long-range effects of these new opportunities on adolescents and upon community attitudes remain to be determined.

The Adult Years

For more than a century, researchers have observed that individuals born with Down syndrome tend to age prematurely. This phenomenon has become more apparent with the increased longevity of affected persons. Because intellectual deterioration—a striking symptom in the senile dementias—is more difficult to assess in retarded individuals, the judgment of premature aging in a person with Down syndrome is generally based on emotional deterioration as shown by changes in personality and behavior.

Neurological signs such as tremors, incoordination and changes in reflexes are often noted among older persons with Down syndrome. Brain tissue research has revealed the same type of degenerative changes in Down syndrome as in Alzheimer's disease, the most common form of the senile dementias, but the relationship between Alzheimer's disease and Down syndrome is not yet well understood. Studies underway at NIH and elsewhere are expected to yield more knowledge about both disorders.

Parents who elect to raise a child with Down syndrome at home face many problems and demands throughout the child's life. As the child grows older, and as the parents age, parents become more concerned about who will care for their child in case they become ill or die.

In some cases, families arrange for the older child or adult to move into a group home for mentally retarded persons in the community. In this way, family ties are maintained, yet the child is no longer totally dependent on the parents.

Still to be determined are the effects of deinstitutionalization on adults with Down syndrome and their families.

NICHD continues to support research into the causes of mental retardation. Through its Mental Retardation Research Centers, the Institute also funds research on better management, treatment, and programs for individuals and families affected by Down syndrome.

Voluntary agencies, like those listed below, comprised of interested persons and parents and families of individuals with Down syndrome, are excellent sources of information:

March of Dimes Birth Defects Foundation
1275 Mamaroneck Ave
White Plains, NY 10605

Down's Syndrome Congress
1640 West Roosevelt Rd, Rm 156-E
Chicago, IL 60608

National Association for Retarded Citizens
709 Avenue E East
Arlington, TX 76011

National Down Syndrome Society
146 East 57th St
New York, NY 10022

Mental Retardation Research Centers Supported by the NICHD

Child Development Research and Evaluation Center, Boston Children's Hospital Medical Center; 300 Longwood Avenue; Boston, Massachusetts 02115

Eunice Kennedy Shriver Center for Mental Retardation; 200 Trapelo Road; Waltham, Massachusetts 02154

Rose F. Kennedy Center for Research in Mental Retardation and Human Development, Albert Einstein College of Medicine, 1410 Pelham Parkway South, Bronx, New York 10461

Child Development Research Institute, Frank Porter Graham Child Development Center, University of North Carolina, Chapel Hill, North Carolina 27514

Mental Retardation Research Center, Neuropsychiatric Institute, Center for the Health Sciences, University of California at Los Angeles; 760 Westwood Plaza; Los Angeles, California 90024

The John F. Kennedy Child Development Center, University of Colorado Health Sciences Center, B.F. Stolinsky Research Laboratories, 4200 East Ninth Avenue, Denver, Colorado 80220

The Joseph P. Kennedy, Jr., Mental Retardation Research Center, School of Medicine, University of Chicago, Wyler's Children's Hospital, Chicago, Illinois 60637

Center for Research in Human Development, University of Kansas, New Haworth Hall, University of Kansas, Lawrence, Kansas 66045

The John F. Kennedy Center for Research on Education and Human Development, George Peabody College of Vanderbilt University, Nashville, Tennessee 37203

Child Development and Mental Retardation Research Center, University of Washington, WJ-10, Seattle, Washington 98195

Harry A. Waisman Center on Mental Retardation and Human Development, University of Wisconsin, 1500 Highland Avenue, University of Wisconsin, Madison, Wisconsin 53706

Cincinnati Mental Retardation Research Center, Children Hospital Research Foundation, Elland and Bethesda Avenues, Cincinnati, Ohio 45229

"Facts About Down Syndrome" was prepared by Drs. Theodore Tjossem and Felix De La Cruz of the Mental Retardation and Disabilities Branch, and Ms. Joan Z. Muller of the Office of Research Reporting, National Institute of Child Health and Human Development (NICHD), and is reprinted from the November/December 1983 issue of *Children Today* magazine.

The Institute, part of the federal government's National Institutes of Health, conducts and supports research on the various processes that determine the health of children, adults, families and populations. For more copies of this fact sheet or others in this series, write to the Office of Research Reporting, NICHD, NIH, Building 31, Room 2A32, 9000 Rockville Pike, Bethesda, MD 20205.

Other Publications in This Series:

- *Facts About Anorexia Nervosa*
- *Facts About Cesarean Childbirth*
- *Facts About Dysmenorrhea and Premenstrual Syndrome*
- *Facts About Oral Contraceptives*
- *Facts About Precocious Puberty*

- *Facts About Pregnancy and Smoking*
- *Facts About Premature Birth*

■ Document Source:
U.S. Department of Health and Human Services, Public Health Service
National Institutes of Health
National Institute of Child Health and Human Development

GENITOURINARY SYSTEM DISORDERS

■■■

END-STAGE RENAL DISEASE: CHOOSING A TREATMENT THAT'S RIGHT FOR YOU

When Your Kidneys Fail

Healthy kidneys clean the blood by filtering out extra water and wastes. They also make hormones that keep your bones strong and blood healthy. When both of your kidneys fail, your body holds fluid. Your blood pressure rises. Harmful wastes build up in your body. Your body doesn't make enough red blood cells. When this happens, you need treatment to replace the work of your failed kidneys.

Treatment Choice: Hemodialysis

Hemodialysis is a procedure that cleans and filters your blood. It rids your body of harmful wastes and extra salt and fluids. It also controls blood pressure and helps your body keep the proper balance of chemicals such as potassium, sodium, and chloride.

Hemodialysis uses a dialyzer, or special filter, to clean your blood. The dialyzer connects to a machine. During treatment, your blood travels through tubes into the dialyzer. The dialyzer filters out wastes and extra fluids. Then the newly cleaned blood flows through another set of tubes and back into your body.

Before your first treatment, an access to your bloodstream must be made. The access provides a way for blood to be carried from your body to the dialysis machine and then back into your body. The access can be internal (inside the body—usually under your skin) or external (outside the body).

Hemodialysis can be done at home or at a center. At a center, nurses or trained technicians perform the treatment. At home, you perform hemodialysis with the help of a partner, usually a family member or friend.

If you decide to do home dialysis, you and your partner will receive special training. Hemodialysis usually is done three times a week. Each treatment lasts from two to four hours. During treatment, you can read, write, sleep, talk, or watch TV.

Possible Complications

Side effects can be caused by rapid changes in your body's fluid and chemical balance during treatment. Muscle cramps and hypotension are two common side effects. Hypotension, a sudden drop in blood pressure, can make you feel weak, dizzy, or sick to your stomach.

It usually takes a few months to adjust to hemodialysis. You can avoid many of the side effects if you follow the proper diet and take your medicines as directed. You should always report side effects to your doctor. They often can be treated quickly and easily.

Your Diet

Hemodialysis and a proper diet help reduce the wastes that build up in your blood. A dietitian can help you plan meals according to your doctor's orders. When choosing foods, you should remember to

- Eat balanced amounts of foods high in protein such as meat and chicken. Animal protein is better used by your body than the protein found in vegetables and grains.
- Watch the amount of potassium you eat. Potassium is a mineral found in salt substitutes, some fruits, vegetables, milk, chocolate, and nuts. Too much or too little potassium can be harmful to your heart.
- Limit how much you drink. Fluids build up quickly in your body when your kidneys aren't working. Too much fluid makes your tissues swell. It also can cause high blood pressure and heart trouble.
- Avoid salt. Salty foods make you thirsty and cause your body to hold water.
- Limit foods such as milk, cheese, nuts, dried beans, and soft drinks. These foods contain the mineral phosphorus. Too much phosphorus in your blood causes calcium to be pulled from your bones. Calcium helps keep bones strong and healthy. To prevent bone problems, your doctor may give you special medicines. You must take these medicines every day as directed.

Pros and Cons

Each person responds differently to similar situations. What may be a negative factor for one person may be positive for another. However, in general, the following are pros and cons for each type of hemodialysis.

In-Center Hemodialysis

Pros

- You have trained professionals with you at all times.
- You can get to know other patients.

Cons

- Treatments are scheduled by the center.
- You must travel to the center for treatment.

Home Hemodialysis

Pros

- You can do it at the hours you choose. (But you still must do it as often as your doctor orders.)
- You don't have to travel to a center.
- You gain a sense of independence and control over your treatment.

Cons

- Helping with treatments may be stressful to your family.
- You need training.
- You need space for storing the machine and supplies at home.

Questions You May Want to Ask:

- Is hemodialysis the best treatment choice for me? Why or why not?
- If I am treated at a center, can I go to the center of my choice?
- What does hemodialysis feel like? Does it hurt?
- What is self-care dialysis?
- How long does it take to learn home hemodialysis? Who will train my partner and me?
- What kind of blood access is best for me?
- As a hemodialysis patient, will I be able to keep working? Can I have treatments at night if I plan to keep working?
- How much should I exercise?
- Who will be on my health care team? How can they help me?
- Who can I talk with about sexuality, family problems, or money concerns?
- How/where can I talk to other people who have faced this decision?

Treatment Choice: Peritoneal Dialysis

Peritoneal dialysis is another procedure that replaces the work of your kidneys. It removes extra water, wastes, and chemicals from your body. This type of dialysis uses the lining of your abdomen to filter your blood. This lining is called the peritoneal membrane.

A cleansing solution, called dialysate, travels through a special tube into your abdomen. Fluid, wastes, and chemicals pass from tiny blood vessels in the peritoneal membrane into the dialysate. After several hours, the dialysate gets drained from your abdomen, taking the wastes from your blood with it. Then you fill your abdomen with fresh dialysate and the cleaning process begins again.

Before your first treatment, a surgeon places a small, soft tube called a catheter into your abdomen. This catheter always stays there. It helps transport the dialysate to and from your peritoneal membrane. There are three types of peritoneal dialysis.

1. Continuous Ambulatory Peritoneal Dialysis (CAPD)—CAPD is the most common type of peritoneal dialysis. It needs no machine. It can be done in any clean, well-lit place. With CAPD, your blood is always being cleaned. The dialysate passes from a plastic bag through the catheter and into your abdomen. The dialysate stays in your abdomen with the catheter sealed. After several hours, you drain the solution back into the bag. Then you refill your abdomen with fresh solution through the same catheter. Now the cleaning process begins again. While the solution is in your body, you may fold the empty plastic bag and hide it under your clothes, around your waist, or in a pocket.
2. Continuous Cyclic Peritoneal Dialysis (CCPD)—CCPD is like CAPD except that a machine, which connects to your catheter, automatically fills and drains the dialysate from your abdomen. The machine does this at night while you sleep.
3. Intermittent Peritoneal Dialysis (IPD)—IPD uses the same type of machine as CCPD to add and drain the dialysate. IPD can be done at home, but it's usually done in the hospital. IPD treatments take longer than CCPD.

CAPD is a form of self-treatment. It needs no machine and no partner. However, with IPD and CCPD, you need a machine and the help of a partner (family member, friend, or health professional).

With CAPD, the dialysate stays in your abdomen for about four to six hours. The process of draining the dialysate and replacing fresh solution takes 30 to 40 minutes. Most people change the solution four times a day.

With CCPD, treatments last from 10 to 12 hours every night.

With IPD, treatments are done several times a week, for a total of 36 to 42 hours per week. Sessions may last up to 24 hours.

Possible Complications

Peritonitis, or infection of the peritoneum, can occur if the opening where the catheter enters your body gets infected. You can also get it if there is a problem connecting or disconnecting the catheter from the bags. Peritonitis can make you feel sick. It can cause a fever and stomach pain.

To avoid peritonitis, you must be careful to follow the procedure exactly. You must know the early signs of peritonitis. Look for reddening or swelling around the catheter. You should also note if your dialysate looks cloudy. It is important to report these signs to your doctor so that the peritonitis can be treated quickly to avoid serious problems.

Your Diet

Diet for peritoneal dialysis is slightly different than diet for hemodialysis.

- You may be able to have more salt and fluids.
- You may eat more protein.
- You may have different potassium restrictions.
- You may need to cut back on the number of calories you eat. This limitation is because the sugar in the dialysate may cause you to gain weight.

Pros and Cons

There are pros and cons to each type of peritoneal dialysis.

CAPD

Pros

- You can perform treatment alone.
- You can do it at times you choose.
- You can do it in many locations.
- You don't need a machine.

Cons

- It disrupts your daily schedule.

CCPD

Pros

- You can do it at night, mainly while you sleep.

Cons

- You need a machine and help from a partner.

IPD

Pros

- Health professionals usually perform treatments.

Cons

- You may need to go to a hospital.
- It takes a lot of time.
- You need a machine.

Dialysis Is Not a Cure

Hemodialysis and peritoneal dialysis are treatments that try to replace your failed kidneys. These treatments help you feel better and live longer, but they are not cures for ESRD. While patients with ESRD are now living longer than ever, ESRD

can cause problems over the years. Some problems are bone disease, high blood pressure, nerve damage, and anemia (having too few red blood cells). Although these problems won't go away with dialysis, doctors now have new and better ways to treat or prevent them. You should discuss these treatments with your doctor.

Questions You May Want to Ask

- Is peritoneal dialysis the best treatment choice for me? Why or why not? Which type?
- How long will it take me to learn peritoneal dialysis?
- What does peritoneal dialysis feel like? Does it hurt?
- How will peritoneal dialysis affect my blood pressure?
- How do I know if I have peritonitis? How is peritonitis treated?
- As a peritoneal dialysis patient, will I be able to continue working?
- How much should I exercise?
- Who will be on my health care team? How can they help me?
- Who can I talk with about sexuality, finances, or family concerns?
- How/where can I talk to other people who have faced this decision?

Kidney Transplantation

Kidney transplantation is a procedure that places a healthy kidney from another person into your body. This one new kidney does all the work that your two failed kidneys cannot do.

A surgeon places the new kidney inside your body between your upper thigh and abdomen. The surgeon connects the artery and vein of the new kidney to your artery and vein. Your blood flows through the new kidney and makes urine, just like your own kidneys did when they were healthy. The new kidney may start working right away or may take up to a few weeks to make urine. Your own kidneys are left where they are, unless they are causing infection or high blood pressure.

You may receive a kidney from a member of your family. This kind of donor is called a living-related donor. You may receive a kidney from a person who has recently died. This type of donor is called a cadaver donor. Sometimes a spouse or very close friend may donate a kidney. This kind of donor is called a living-unrelated donor.

It is very important for the donor's blood and tissues to closely match yours. This match will help prevent your body's immune system from fighting off, or rejecting, the new kidney. A lab will do special tests on blood cells to find out if your body will accept the new kidney.

The time it takes to get a kidney varies. There are not enough cadaver donors for every person who needs a transplant. Because of this, you must be placed on a waiting list to receive a cadaver donor kidney. However, if a relative gives you a kidney, the transplant operation can be done sooner.

The surgery takes from three to six hours. The usual hospital stay may last from 10 to 14 days. After you leave the hospital, you will go to the clinic for regular followup visits.

If a relative or close friend gives you a kidney, he or she will probably stay in the hospital for one week or less.

Possible Complications

Transplantation is not a cure. There is always a chance that your body will reject your new kidney, no matter how good the match. The chance of your body accepting the new kidney depends on your age, race, and medical condition.

Normally, 75 to 80 percent of transplants from cadaver donors are working one year after surgery. However, transplants from living relatives often work better than transplants from cadaver donors. This fact is because they are usually a closer match.

Your doctor will give you special drugs to help prevent rejection. These are called immunosuppressants. You will need to take these drugs every day for the rest of your life. Sometimes these drugs cannot stop your body from rejecting the new kidney. If this happens, you will go back to some form of dialysis and possibly wait for another transplant.

Treatment with these drugs may cause side effects. The most serious is that they weaken your immune system, making it easier for you to get infections. Some drugs also cause changes in how you look. Your face may get fuller. You may gain weight or develop acne or facial hair. Not all patients have these problems, and makeup and diet can help.

Some of these drugs may cause problems such as cataracts, extra stomach acid, and hip disease. In a smaller number of patients, these drugs also may cause liver or kidney damage when used for a long period of time.

Your Diet

Diet for transplant patients is less limiting than it is for dialysis patients. You may still have to cut back on some foods, though. Your diet probably will change as your medicines, blood values, weight, and blood pressure change.

- You may need to count calories. Your medicine may give you a bigger appetite and cause you to gain weight.
- You may have to limit eating salty foods. Your medications may cause salt to be held in your body, leading to high blood pressure.
- You may need to eat less protein. Some medications cause a higher level of wastes to build up in your bloodstream.

Pros and Cons

There are pros and cons to kidney transplantation.

Pros

- It works like a normal kidney.
- It helps you feel healthier.
- You have fewer diet restrictions.
- There's no need for dialysis.

Cons

- It requires major surgery.
- You may need to wait for a donor.
- One transplant may not last a lifetime. Your body may reject the new kidney.
- You will have to take drugs for the rest of your life.

Questions You May Want to Ask

- Is transplantation the best treatment choice for me? Why or why not?
- What are my chances of having a successful transplant?
- How do I find out if a family member or friend can donate?
- What are the risks to a family member or friend if he or she donates?
- If a family member or friend doesn't donate, how do I get placed on a waiting list for a kidney? How long will I have to wait?
- What are the symptoms of rejection?
- Who will be on my health care team? How can they help me?
- Who can I talk to about sexuality, finances, or family concerns?
- How/where can I talk to other people who have faced this decision?

Conclusion

It's not always easy to decide which type of treatment is best for you. Your decision depends on your medical condition, lifestyle, and personal likes and dislikes. Discuss the pros and cons of each with your health care team. If you start one form of treatment and decide you'd like to try another, talk it over with your doctor. The key is to learn as much as you can about your choices. With that knowledge, you and your doctor will choose a treatment that suits you best.

Paying for Treatment

Treatment for ESRD is expensive, but the federal government helps pay for much of the cost. Often, private insurance or state programs pay the rest.

Medicare

Medicare pays for 80 percent of the cost of your dialysis treatments or transplant, no matter how old you are. To qualify

- You must have worked long enough to be insured under Social Security (or be the child of someone who has) or
- You already must be receiving Social Security benefits.

You should apply for Medicare as soon as possible after beginning dialysis. Often, a social worker at your hospital or dialysis center will help you apply.

Private Insurance

Private insurance often pays for the entire cost of treatment. Or it may pay for the 20 percent that Medicare does not cover. Private insurance also may pay for your prescription drugs.

Medicaid

Medicaid is a state program. Your income must be below a certain level to receive Medicaid funds. Medicaid may pay for your treatments if you cannot receive Medicare. In some states, it also pays the 20 percent that Medicare does not cover. It also may pay for some of your medicines. To apply for Medicaid, talk with your social worker or contact your local health department.

Veterans Administration (VA) Benefits

If you are a veteran, the VA can help pay for treatment. Contact your local VA office for more information.

Social Security Income (SSI) and Social Security Disability Income (SSDI)

These benefits are available from the Social Security Administration. They assist you with the costs of daily living. To find out if you qualify, talk to your social worker or call your local Social Security office.

Organizations That Can Help

There are several groups that offer information and services to kidney patients. You may wish to contact the following:

American Kidney Fund
6110 Executive Blvd, Ste 1010
Rockville, MD 20852
(800) 638-8299

American Association of Kidney Patients
1 Davis Blvd, Ste LL1
Tampa, FL 33606
(813) 251-0725

National Kidney Foundation, Inc.
30 East 33rd St
New York, NY 10016
(800) 622-9010

National Kidney and Urologic Diseases Information Clearinghouse
Box NKUDIC
9000 Rockville Pike
Bethesda, MD 20892
(301) 654-4415

Additional Reading

If you would like to learn more about ESRD and its treatment, you may be interested in reading:

Your New Life With Dialysis: A Patient Guide for Physical and Psychological Adjustment.
Edith T. Oberley, MA, and Terry D. Oberley, MD, PhD
Fourth edition, 1991
Charles C. Thomas Publishers
2600 S First St
Springfield, IL 62794-9265

Understanding Kidney Transplantation
Edith T. Oberley, MA, and Neal R. Glass, MD, FACS
Charles C. Thomas Publishers, 1987

2600 S First St
Springfield, IL 62794-9265

Kidney Disease: A Guide for Patients and Their Families
American Kidney Fund
6110 Executive Blvd, Ste 1010
Rockville, MD 20852
(800) 638-8299

National Kidney Foundation Patient Education Brochures
Includes information on treatment, diet, work, and exercise.
National Kidney Foundation, Inc.
30 East 33rd St
New York, NY 10016
(800) 622-9010

Medicare Coverage of Kidney Dialysis and Kidney Transplant Services: A Supplement to Your Medicare Handbook
Publication Number HCFA-02183
U.S. Department of Health and Human Services Health Care Financing Administration
1331 H Street, NW, Suite 500
Washington, DC 20005
(301) 966-7843

Renalife Magazine
American Association of Kidney Patients (AAKP)
1 Davis Blvd, Ste LL1
Tampa, FL 33606
(813) 251-0725
Published quarterly.

Family Focus Newsletter
National Kidney Foundation, Inc.
30 East 33rd St
New York, NY 10016
(800) 622-9010

For Patients Only Magazine
20335 Ventura Blvd, Ste 400
Woodland Hills, CA 91364
(818) 704-5555
Published six times per year.

■ **Document Source:**
U.S. Department of Health and Human Services, Public Health Service
National Institutes of Health
National Institute of Diabetes, and Digestive and Kidney Diseases
NIH Publication No. 94-2412
June 1994

IMPOTENCE

Impotence is a consistent inability to sustain an erection sufficient for sexual intercourse. Medical professionals often use the term "erectile dysfunction" to describe this disorder and to differentiate it from other problems that interfere with sexual intercourse, such as lack of sexual desire and problems with ejaculation and orgasm. This fact sheet focuses on impotence defined as erectile dysfunction.

Impotence can be a total inability to achieve erection, an inconsistent ability to do so, or a tendency to sustain only brief erections. These variations make defining impotence and estimating its incidence difficult. Experts believe impotence affects between 10 and 15 million American men. In 1985, the National Ambulatory Medical Care Survey counted 525,000 doctor-office visits for erectile dysfunction.

Impotence usually has a physical cause, such as disease, injury, or drug side effects. Any disorder that impairs blood flow in the penis has the potential to cause impotence. Incidence rises with age: about five percent of men at the age of 40 and between 15 and 25 percent of men at the age of 65 experience impotence. Yet, it is not an inevitable part of aging.

Impotence is treatable in all age groups, and awareness of this fact has been growing. More men have been seeking help and returning to near-normal sexual activity because of improved, successful treatments for impotence. Urologists, who specialize in problems of the urinary tract, have traditionally treated impotence—especially complications of impotence.

How does an erection occur?

The penis contains two chambers, called the *corpora cavernosa*, which run the length of the organ. A spongy tissue fills the chambers. The *corpora cavernosa* are surrounded by a membrane, called the *tunica albuginea*. The spongy tissue contains smooth muscles, fibrous tissues, spaces, veins, and arteries. The urethra, which is the channel for urine and ejaculate, runs along the underside of the *corpora cavernosa*.

Erection begins with sensory and mental stimulation. Impulses from the brain and local nerves cause the muscles of the *corpora cavernosa* to relax, allowing blood to flow in and fill the open spaces. The blood creates pressure in the *corpora cavernosa*, making the penis expand. The *tunica albuginea* helps to trap the blood in the *corpora cavernosa*, thereby sustaining erection. Erection is reversed when muscles in the penis contract, stopping the inflow of blood and opening outflow channels.

What causes impotence?

Since an erection requires a sequence of events, impotence can occur when any of the events is disrupted. The sequence includes nerve impulses in the brain, spinal column, and area of the penis, and response in muscles, fibrous tissues, veins, and arteries in and near the *corpora cavernosa*.

Damage to arteries, smooth muscles, and fibrous tissues, often as a result of disease, is the most common cause of impotence. Diseases—including diabetes, kidney disease, chronic alcoholism, multiple sclerosis, atherosclerosis, and vascular disease—account for about 70 percent of cases of impotence. Between 35 and 50 percent of men with diabetes experience impotence.

Surgery (for example, prostate surgery) can injure nerves and arteries near the penis, causing impotence. Injury to the penis, spinal cord, prostate, bladder, and pelvis can lead to impotence by harming nerves, smooth muscles, arteries, and fibrous tissues of the *corpora cavernosa*.

Also, many common medicines produce impotence as a side effect. These include high blood pressure drugs, antihistamines, antidepressants, tranquilizers, appetite suppressants, and cimetidine (an ulcer drug).

Experts believe that psychological factors cause 10 to 20 percent of cases of impotence. These factors include stress, anxiety, guilt, depression, low self-esteem, and fear of sexual failure. Such factors are broadly associated with more than 80 percent of cases of impotence, usually as secondary reactions to underlying physical causes.

Other possible causes of impotence are smoking, which affects blood flow in veins and arteries, and hormonal abnormalities, such as insufficient testosterone.

How is impotence diagnosed?

Patient History

Medical and sexual histories help define the degree and nature of impotence. A medical history can disclose diseases that lead to impotence. A simple recounting of sexual activity might distinguish between problems with erection, ejaculation, orgasm, or sexual desire.

A history of using certain prescription drugs or illegal drugs can suggest a chemical cause. Drug effects account for 25 percent of cases of impotence. Cutting back on or substituting certain medications often can alleviate the problem.

Physical Examination

A physical examination can give clues for systemic problems. For example, if the penis does not respond as expected to certain touching, a problem in the nervous system may be a cause. Abnormal secondary sex characteristics, such as hair pattern, can point to hormonal problems, which would mean the endocrine system is involved. A circulatory problem might be indicated by, for example, an aneurysm in the abdomen. And unusual characteristics of the penis itself could suggest the root of the impotence—for example, bending of the penis during erection could be the result of Peyronie's disease.

Laboratory Tests

Several laboratory tests can help diagnose impotence. Tests for systemic diseases include blood counts, urinalysis, lipid profile, and measurements of creatinine and liver enzymes. For cases of low sexual desire, measurement of testosterone in the blood can yield information about problems with the endocrine system.

Other Tests

Monitoring erections that occur during sleep (nocturnal penile tumescence) can help rule out certain psychological causes of impotence. Healthy men have involuntary erections during sleep. If nocturnal erections do not occur, then the cause of impotence is likely to be physical rather than psychological. Tests of nocturnal erections are not completely reliable, however. Scientists have not standardized such tests and have not determined when they should be applied for best results.

Psychosocial Examination

A psychosocial examination, using an interview and questionnaire, reveals psychological factors. The man's sexual partner also may be interviewed to determine expectations and perceptions encountered during sexual intercourse.

How is impotence treated?

Most physicians suggest that treatments for impotence proceed along a path moving from least invasive to most invasive. This means cutting back on any harmful drugs is considered first. Psychotherapy and behavior modifications are considered next, followed by vacuum devices, oral drugs, locally injected drugs, and surgically implanted devices (and, in rare cases, surgery involving veins or arteries).

Psychotherapy

Experts often treat psychologically based impotence using techniques that decrease anxiety associated with intercourse. The patient's partner can help apply the techniques, which include gradual development of intimacy and stimulation. Such techniques also can help relieve anxiety when physical impotence is being treated.

Drug Therapy

Drugs for treating impotence can be taken orally or injected directly into the penis. Oral testosterone can reduce impotence in some men with low levels of natural testosterone. Patients also have claimed effectiveness of other oral drugs, including yohimbine hydrochloride, dopamine and serotonin agonists, and trazodone—but no scientific studies have proved the effectiveness of these drugs in relieving impotence. Some observed improvements following their use may be examples of the placebo effect, that is, a change that results simply from the patient's believing that an improvement will occur.

Many men gain potency by injecting drugs into the penis, causing it to become engorged with blood. Drugs such as papaverine hydrochloride, phentolamine, and prostaglandin E1 widen blood vessels. These drugs may create unwanted side effects, however, including persistent erection (known as priapism) and scarring. Nitroglycerin, a muscle relaxant, sometimes can enhance erection when rubbed on the surface of the penis.

Research on drugs for treating impotence is expanding rapidly. Patients should ask their doctors about the latest advances.

Vacuum Devices

Mechanical vacuum devices cause erection by creating a partial vacuum around the penis, which draws blood into the penis, engorging it and expanding it. The devices have three components: a plastic cylinder, in which the penis is placed; a pump, which draws air out of the cylinder; and an elastic band, which is placed around the base of the penis, to maintain the erection after the cylinder is removed and during intercourse by preventing blood from flowing back into the body.

One variation of the vacuum device involves a semirigid rubber sheath that is placed on the penis and remains there after attaining erection and during intercourse.

Surgery

Surgery usually has one of three goals:

1. To implant a device that can cause the penis to become erect;
2. To reconstruct arteries to increase flow of blood to the penis;
3. To block off veins that allow blood to leak from the penile tissues.

Implanted devices, known as prostheses, can restore erection in many men with impotence. Possible problems with implants include mechanical breakdown and infection. Mechanical problems have diminished in recent years because of technological advances.

Malleable implants usually consist of paired rods, which are inserted surgically into the *corpora cavernosa*, the twin chambers running the length of the penis. The user manually adjusts the position of the penis and, therefore, the rods. Adjustment does not affect the width or length of the penis.

Inflatable implants consist of paired cylinders, which are surgically inserted inside the penis and can be expanded using pressurized fluid. Tubes connect the cylinders to a fluid reservoir and pump, which also are surgically implanted. The patient inflates the cylinders by pressing on the small pump, located under the skin in the scrotum. Inflatable implants can expand the length and width of the penis somewhat. They also leave the penis in a more natural state when not inflated.

Surgery to repair arteries can reduce impotence caused by obstructions that block the flow of blood to the penis. The best candidates for such surgery are young men with discrete blockage of an artery because of an injury to the crotch area or fracture of the pelvis. The procedure is less successful in older men with widespread blockage.

Surgery to veins that allow blood to leave the penis usually involves an opposite procedure—intentional blockage. Blocking off veins (ligation) can reduce the leakage of blood that diminishes rigidity of the penis during erection. However, experts have raised questions about this procedure's long-term effectiveness.

What will the future bring?

Advances in injectable medications, implants, and vacuum devices have expanded the options for men seeking treatment for impotence. These advances also have helped increase the number of men seeking treatment.

One possible new treatment, currently in experimental stages, is a small pellet that a man can insert in the end of his penis. The pellet releases a drug that migrates into the erectile tissue and causes a temporary erection. There is no need for a needle. Whether or not this method proves to be safe and effective, ongoing improvements in traditional methods should continue to create more successful and widespread treatment of impotence.

Resources for More Information

Impotence Information Center
PO Box 9
Minneapolis, MN 55440
(800) 843-4315

Impotence Institute of America
8201 Corporate Drive, Suite 320
Landover, MD 20785
(301) 577-0650

Sexual Function Health Council American Foundation for Urologic Disease
300 West Pratt Street, Suite 401
Baltimore, MD 21201
(800) 242-2383

The Geddings Osbon, Sr. Foundation
PO Drawer 1593
Augusta, GA 30903-1593
(800) 433-4215

National Kidney and Urologic Diseases Information Clearinghouse
3 Information Way
Bethesda, MD 20892-3580
Fax: (301) 907-8906

The National Kidney and Urologic Diseases Information Clearinghouse is a service of the National Institute of Diabetes and Digestive and Kidney Diseases, part of the National Institutes of Health, under the U.S. Public Health Service. Authorized in 1987, the clearinghouse provides information about diseases of the kidneys and urologic system to people with such afflictions and to their families, health care professionals, and the public. The clearinghouse answers inquiries; develops, reviews, and distributes publications; and works closely with professional and patient organizations and government agencies to coordinate resources about kidney and urologic diseases.

Publications produced by the clearinghouse are reviewed carefully for scientific accuracy, content, and readability. Publications produced by outside sources are also reviewed carefully before being used to supplement clearinghouse materials when responding to inquiries.

■ **Document Source:**
   U.S. Department of Health and Human Services, Public Health Service
   National Institutes of Health
   National Institute of Diabetes and Digestive and Kidney Diseases
   NIH Publication No. 95-3923
   September 1995

INTERSTITIAL CYSTITIS: PROGRESS AGAINST DISABLING BLADDER CONDITION

by Evelyn Zamula

The woman knew she was going to be fired from her job. Since her 20s, this insurance firm middle manager has suffered from interstitial cystitis (IC), an inflammatory disease of the bladder wall.

The chief symptoms Marsha (not her real name) has are a smaller than normal bladder capacity, urgent and frequent urination, feelings of pressure and pain around the bladder and in the pelvic area, and painful sexual intercourse. Now 46 years old, she has coped with these symptoms fairly well until recently, when they have worsened. On some days, Marsha is in such agony that she can barely walk.

Though sympathetic at first, Marsha's supervisor become impatient with her frequent bouts of pain and trips to the bathroom, as well as time lost from sick days and doctor's appointments, even though she's made up every minute. When she started to miss policy meetings, Marsha began to get indications that she would be fired. Her boss would comment that she couldn't know what was going on because, "You aren't always here."

Finally, when Marsha needed to urinate every 20 minutes at work and 10 times during the night, leaving her exhausted and depressed in the morning, she became so fearful of being asked to leave that she decided to retire on disability instead. She hopes to return to her job when she feels better, but so far it hasn't been possible.

Marsha counts herself among the more fortunate of IC sufferers because she receives long-term disability benefits and has both Medicare and private medical insurance. Also, unlike many other women, whose marriages and relationships are put under severe stress by IC, Marsha is lucky to have a supportive husband.

Cause Elusive

No one knows what causes IC. It wasn't recognized as a disorder until about 20 years ago. In 1978, the Food and Drug Administration approved Rimso-50, a purified form of the industrial solvent dimethyl sulfoxide (DMSO), for symptomatic relief of IC. Before that, many patients were neither diagnosed nor treated.

Because physicians could find no organic cause, the prevailing medical opinion was that IC was a "hysterical female condition," even though at least 10 percent of cases are in men. Even Campbell's *Urology*, the definitive text of urologic diseases, stated as late as 1986 that IC was "daunting in its evasion of being understood. [It] may represent the end stage of a bladder that has been made irritable by emotional disturbance." The book further states that interstitial cystitis may be a pathway for the discharge of unconscious hatreds.

People with IC have had to put up with this type of disbelief for a long time. Kristene E. Whitmore, MD, chairwoman of the Department of Urology, Philadelphia Graduate Hospital, Philadelphia, PA, says, "The average number of doctors seen before diagnosis is five, and it takes three to five years to get that diagnosis."

When the columnist Ann Landers wrote about IC in 1987, she received 10,000 letters from patients or their families, relieved that the condition was finally being recognized. A 1987 study conducted by the Urban Institute in Washington, DC, found that IC makes people so miserable that they contemplate suicide four times more often than the general population and that they rate their quality of life lower than those who undergo kidney dialysis. Nearly 30 percent of IC patients can't work full-time, according to the study.

Although no bacteria or fungi or viruses are found in patients' urine, many researchers believe it's possible that IC is caused by an infectious agent that hasn't yet been identified.

Researchers have also suggested it may be an autoimmune disorder of the bladder's connective tissue, in which the body's defense mechanisms against invading bacteria turn suddenly against healthy tissue. In some patients, special white blood cells called mast cells, which are associated with inflammation, are found within the bladder's mucous lining. Or, some scientists theorize that the disorder may be an allergic reaction, because many patients have a history of allergies.

Some women go into remission during pregnancy, while others get worse, suggesting that in some patients hormones may be involved. Complicating the picture, many women with IC also suffer from a variety of other conditions, such as irritable bowel syndrome, migraine headaches, fibromyalgia (chronic aching of the muscles, joints, and connective tissues), low back pain, and similar disorders.

One theory in favor at present holds that the inner lining of the bladder (the glycosaminoglycan or GAG layer) that protects the bladder wall from toxic effects of urine may be "leaky," allowing substances in the urine to penetrate the bladder wall and trigger IC symptoms. A California study found that 70 percent of IC patients they examined had a "leaky" bladder lining.

More likely, any or all of these factors may exist, leading many researchers to conclude that IC is a syndrome, or a collection of signs and symptoms, rather than a specific disease. Others, such as Witmore, believe it's more than one disease and is different in every person.

Making a Diagnosis

Although there is no test that identifies IC, urologists rely on several criteria to make a diagnosis:

- Frequent and urgent urination, and pelvic or bladder pain, especially as the bladder is filling.
- Pinpoint hemorrhages that can often be seen on the bladder wall during cystoscopy (an examination of the bladder's interior with a long, lighted tube, performed under anesthesia). This is called nonulcerative IC, seen in about 95 percent of patients.

- Cracks, scars, and star-shaped sores called Hunner's ulcers that are found in the bladder wall in ulcerative IC. Bladder capacity is decreased because the usually elastic bladder walls become stiff and don't expand normally.

Because it's easier to define IC by what it isn't than by what it is, a diagnosis must rule out bacterial cystitis—the most common urinary tract infection—whose symptoms it most closely resembles. Bladder cancer, kidney stones, vaginitis, endometriosis, sexually transmitted diseases, and tuberculous and radiation cystitis, as well as prostate infections in men, are some other conditions that must be considered. Thus, interstitial cystitis becomes a diagnosis of exclusion.

Although about 10 times more women than men get IC, it's possible that men have been underdiagnosed. "We haven't been real sensitive in screening our prostatitis patients, so maybe more men have IC than we think," says Whitmore.

Symptoms usually begin between 20 and 50 years of age, but the average age of onset is 40. Some cases have been diagnosed in children. About 450,000 people in the United States are believed to have IC, but true numbers are hard to come by, because many cases are either undiagnosed or misdiagnosed. Although occasionally more than one member of a family has IC, the disorder is not believed to have a genetic component.

IC Symptoms

The symptoms of interstitial cystitis are similar to those of a urinary tract infection. Most people have some of the following symptoms:

- urgent need for frequent urination both day and night
- reduced bladder capacity
- feelings of pressure, pain, and tenderness around the bladder, pelvis, and genital area, which may increase is the bladder fills and decrease as it empties
- painful sexual intercourse
- in men, discomfort or pain in the prostatic area

Treating the Condition

There is no cure for IC. All doctors can do is try to relieve the symptoms, a challenging task, because they vary from person to person. People may have flareups and remissions, and different patients respond to different treatments. A particular type of therapy may work for a while and then lose its effectiveness. Sometimes, stress or a change of diet triggers symptoms. Occasionally, IC goes into remission spontaneously.

Paradoxically, the cytoscopy used to diagnose IC also seems to make some people feel better. To enable the doctor to look inside the bladder with the cystoscope, the bladder is filled with water. This bladder distention helps about 30 percent of patients, at least for the short term, probably because the bladder is stretched and capacity is increased. It's also possible that the procedure may interfere with the transmission of pain signals by nerves in the bladder. The fact that IC can only be diagnosed by cystoscopy under anesthesia explains why many cases are overlooked even by urologists.

In a similar procedure, Rimso-50 is instilled directly into the bladder by a catheter. The solution is retained in the bladder for about 15 minutes before being expelled by spontaneous voiding. This treatment is given every two weeks until maximum symptomatic relief is obtained, then repeated as needed.

For some patients, Rimso-50 treatments become less effective over time. About 50 percent of patients experience significant pain relief for an average of about 10 months. The drug works by penetrating the bladder wall to reduce inflammation and acts as a muscle relaxant by preventing muscle contractions that cause pain, frequency, and urgency.

Disadvantages of Rimso-50 include a garlic-like odor on the skin and breath that may last up to 72 hours. Some patients may develop a chemical cystitis after use of the drug that goes away within one or two days. patients taking Rimso-50 also require a blood test every six months to make sure the blood count and liver and kidney function are normal. Periodic ophthalmologic examinations are also recommended.

For More Info

More information about interstitial cystitis is available from

Interstitial Cystitis Association
PO Box 1553
Madison Square Station
New York, NY 10159
1-800-422-1626

American Foundation for Urologic Disease, Inc.
300 West Pratt St, Suite 401
Baltimore, MD 21201
1-800-242-2383

"You have to customize therapy for the person," says Whitmore, who advocates a number of untraditional therapies, many of which have not been reviewed by FDA for this purpose. They include acid-restricted diets, alkalization or urine, bladder holding and retraining (delaying voiding for increasingly long intervals), biofeedback and electric stimulation, acupuncture, muscle relaxants, antidepressants, anti-inflamatories, antihistamines and analgesics, and an experimental bladder "wash" consisting of an anesthetic, an antibiotic, an anticoagulant, and hydrocortisone.

From 40 to 60 percent of IC patients may benefit from low doses of the tricyclic antidepressant amitriptyline (Elavil and others), according to Vicki Ratner, MD, and colleagues in the *Journal of Women's Health,*, Vol. 1, No. 1, 1992. Physicians prescribe it not only to treat the depression that is common in IC patients, but to take advantage of its bladder-relaxing, allergy-fighting, pain-blocking, and sedating properties.

When pain is severe, some people may benefit from transcutaneous electrical nerve stimulation (TENS). Mild electrical impulses delivered to the body through wires placed on the lower back or abdomen or through devices implanted in the body may alter nerve transmissions to the bladder and help trigger release of pain-blocking hormones.

A bland diet helps some IC people. Doctors recommend avoiding high-acid foods, such as citrus fruits, that may irritate the bladder, or spicy foods that may cause the release of histamine. Restricting alcoholic beverages, carbonated sodas, coffee and other caffeinated products, and beverages and foods with artificial sweeteners appears to reduce symptoms in some people.

Surgery is an option when all else fails. Some urologists may remove the diseased portion of the bladder and attach a piece of the patient's bowel to the remaining healthy tissue to make a larger bladder. In other cases, the bladder is completely removed and urine is rerouted to a bag outside the body or a pouch inside the lower abdomen. However, about half of patients don't get pain relief from this procedure.

"I don't take the bladder out unless I've used all the tricks up my sleeve," says Whitmore. "When patients have bladders the size of a walnut or smaller, or when they have intractable pain, then they're candidates for cystectomy [bladder removal]. The operation has allowed some people to get out of the house and have a life."

Whitmore tells her patients that, as will all disorders of chronic pain, there is going to be a certain amount of anger, anxiety and depression. "I say to them, 'I have an 85 percent chance or greater to make you better, but I can't teach you how to cope with your illness, so you've got to get some help.' I encourage them to go for self-hypnosis, self-relaxation, and other coping techniques, or to seek therapy with psychologists or psychiatrists. I tell them, 'if you can't cope, you're not going to get better.'"

Researchers funded by the federal government, drug companies, and the Interstitial Cystitis Association have stepped up their efforts to find out more about the disorder. Philip Hanno, MD, chairman, Department of Urology, Temple University School of Medicine, Philadelphia, PA, expects that in the next decade, treatment for IC will be more beneficial than the therapy available now. He believes that ultimately there will be a cure for most cases of this painful and disabling condition.

■ **Document Source:**
U.S. Department of Health and Human Services, Public Health Service
Food and Drug Administration
FDA Consumer
September 1995

KIDNEY STONES IN ADULTS

Overview

Kidney stones are one of the most painful disorders to afflict humans. This ancient health problem has tormented people throughout history. Scientists have even found evidence of kidney stones in an Egyptian mummy estimated to be more than 7,000 years old.

Kidney stones are one of the most common disorders of the urinary tract. More than one million cases of kidney stones were diagnosed in 1985. It is estimated that 10 percent of all people in the United States will have a kidney stone at some point in time. Men tend to be affected more frequently than women.

Most kidney stones pass out of the body without any intervention by a physician. Cases that cause lasting symptoms or other complications may be treated by various techniques, most of which do not involve major surgery. Research advances also have led to a better understanding of the many factors that promote stone formation.

An Introduction to the Urinary Tract

The urinary tract, or system, consists of the kidneys, ureters, bladder, and urethra. The kidneys are two bean-shaped organs located below the ribs toward the middle of the back. The kidneys remove extra water and wastes from the blood, converting it to urine. They also keep a stable balance of salts and other substances in the blood. The kidneys produce hormones that help build strong bones and help form red blood cells.

Narrow tubes called ureters carry urine from the kidneys to the bladder, a triangle-shaped chamber in the lower abdomen. Like a balloon, the bladder's elastic walls stretch and expand to store urine. They flatten together when urine is emptied through the urethra to outside the body.

What is a kidney stone?

A kidney stone develops from crystals that separate from urine and build up on the inner surfaces of the kidney. Normally, urine contains chemicals that prevent or inhibit the crystals from forming. These inhibitors do not seem to work for everyone, however, and some people form stones. If the crystals remain tiny enough, they will travel through the urinary tract and pass out of the body in the urine without even being noticed.

Kidney stones may contain various combinations of chemicals. The most common type of stone contains **calcium** in combination with either **oxalate** or **phosphate.** These chemicals are part of a person's normal diet and make up important parts of the body, such as bones and muscles.

A less common type of stone is caused by infection in the urinary tract. This type of stone is called a **struvite** or infection stone. Much less common are the **uric acid** stone and the rare **cystine** stone.

Urolithiasis is the medical term used to describe stones occurring in the urinary tract. Other frequently used terms are **urinary tract stone disease** and **nephrolithiasis.** Doctors also use terms that describe the location of the stone in the urinary tract. For example, a **ureteral stone** (or ureterolithiasis) is a kidney stone found in the ureter. To keep things simple, the term "kidney stones" is used throughout this document.

Gallstones and kidney stones are not related. They form in different areas of the body. If a person has a gallstone, he or she is not necessarily more likely to develop kidney stones.

Who gets kidney stones?

For some unknown reason, the number of persons in the United States with kidney stones has been increasing over the past 20 years. White people are more prone to kidney stones than are black people. Although stones occur more frequently in men, the number of women who get kidney stones has been increasing over the past 10 years, causing the ratio to change. Kidney stones strike most people between the ages of 20 and 40. Once a person gets more than one stone, he or she is more likely to develop others.

What causes kidney stones?

Doctors do not always know what causes a stone to form. While certain foods may promote stone formation in people who are susceptible, scientists do not believe that eating any specific food causes stones to form in people who are not susceptible.

A person with a family history of kidney stones may be more likely to develop stones. Urinary tract infections, kidney disorders such as cystic kidney diseases, and metabolic disorders such as hyperparathyroidism are also linked to stone formation.

In addition, more than 70 percent of patients with adequate hereditary disease called renal tubular acidosis develop kidney stones.

Cystinuria and hyperoxaluria are two other rare inherited metabolic disorders that often cause kidney stones. In cystinuria, the kidneys produce too much of the amino acid cystine. Cystine does not dissolve in urine and can build up to form stones. With hyperoxaluria, the body produces too much of the salt oxalate. When there is more oxalate than can be dissolved in the urine, the crystals settle out and form stones.

Absorptive hypercalciuria occurs when the body absorbs too much calcium from food and empties the extra calcium into the urine. This high level of calcium in the urine causes crystals of calcium oxalate or calcium phosphate to form in the kidneys or urinary tract.

Other causes of kidney stones are hyperuricosuria (a disorder of uric acid metabolism), gout, excess intake of vitamin D, and blockage of the urinary tact. Certain diuretics (water pills) or calcium-based antacids may increase the risk of forming kidney stones by increasing the amount of calcium in the urine.

Calcium oxalate stones may also form in people who have a chronic inflammation of the bowel or who have had an intestinal bypass operation, or ostomy surgery. As mentioned above, struvite stones can form in people who have had a urinary tract infection.

What are the symptoms?

Usually, the first symptom of a kidney stone is extreme pain. The pain often begins suddenly when a stone moves in the urinary tract, causing irritation or blockage. Typically, a person feels a sharp, cramping pain the back and side in the area of the kidney or in the lower abdomen. Sometimes nausea and vomiting occur with this pain. Later, the pain may spread to the groin.

If the stone is too large to pass easily, the pain continues as the muscles in the wall of the tiny ureter try to squeeze the stone along into the bladder. As a stone grows or moves, blood may be found in the urine. As the stone moves down the ureter closer to the bladder, a person may feel the need to urinate more often or feel a burning sensation during urination.

If fever and chills accompany any of these symptoms, an infection may be present. In this case, a doctor should be contacted immediately.

How are kidney stones diagnosed?

Sometimes "silent" stones—those that do not cause symptoms—are found on x-rays taken during a general health exam. These stones would likely pass unnoticed.

More often, kidney stones are found on an x-ray or sonogram taken on someone who complains of blood in the urine or sudden pain. These diagnostic images give the doctor valuable information about the stone's size and location. Blood and urine tests help detect any abnormal substance that might promote stone formation.

The doctor may decide to scan the urinary system using a special x-ray test called an IVP (intravenous pyelogram). Together, the results from these tests help determine the proper treatment.

How are kidney stones treated?

Fortunately, most stones can be treated without surgery. Most kidney stones can pass through the urinary system with plenty of water (two to three quarts a day) to help move the stone along. In most cases, a person can stay home during this process, taking pain medicine as needed. The doctor usually asks the patient to save the passed stone(s) for testing.

The First Step: Prevention

People who have had more than one kidney stone are likely to form another. Therefore, prevention is very important. To prevent stones from forming, their cause must be determined. The urologist will order laboratory tests, including urine and blood tests. He or she will also ask about the patient's medical history, occupation, and dietary habits. If a stone has been removed, or if the patient has passed a stone and saved it, the lab can analyze the stone to determine its composition.

A patient may be asked to collect his or her urine for 24 hours after a stone has passed or been removed. The sample is used to measure urine volume and levels of acidity, calcium, sodium, uric acid, oxalate, citrate, and creatinine (a byproduct of protein metabolism). The doctor will use this information to determine the cause of the stone. A second 24-hour urine collection may be needed to determine if the prescribed treatment is working.

Lifestyle Changes

A simple and most important lifestyle change to prevent stones is to drink more liquids—water is best. A recurrent stone former should try to drink enough liquids throughout the day to produce at least two quarts of urine in every 24-hour period.

Patients with too much calcium or oxalate in the urine may need to eat fewer foods containing calcium and oxalate.

Not everyone will benefit from a low-calcium diet, however. Some patients who have high levels of oxalate in their urine may benefit from extra calcium in their diet. patients may be told to avoid food with added vitamin D and certain types of antacids that have a calcium base.

Patients who have a very acid urine may need to eat less meat, fish, and poultry. These foods increase the amount of acid in the urine.

To prevent cystine stones, patients should drink enough water each day to reduce the amount of cystine that escapes into the urine. This is difficult because more than a gallon of water may be needed every 24 hours, a third of which must be drunk during the night.

Medical Therapy

The doctor may prescribe certain medications to prevent calcium and uric acid stones. These drugs control the amount of acid or alkali in the urine, key factors in crystal formation. The drug allopurinol may also be useful in some cases of hypercalciuria and hyperuricosuria.

Another way a doctor may try to control hypercalciuria, and thus prevent calcium stones, is by prescribing certain diuretics, such as hydrochlorothiazide. These drugs decrease the amount of calcium released by the kidneys into the urine.

Some patients with absorptive hypercalciuria may be given the drug sodium cellulose phosphate. This drug binds calcium in the intestine and prevents it from leaking into the urine.

If cystine stones cannot be controlled by drinking more fluids, the doctor may prescribe the drug Thiola. This medication helps reduce the amount of cystine in the urine.

For struvite stones that have been totally removed, the first line of prevention is to keep the urine free of bacteria that can cause infection. The patient's urine will be tested on a regular basis to be sure that bacteria are not present.

If struvite stones cannot be removed the doctor may prescribe a new drug called aetohydroamic acid (AHA). AHA is used along with long-term antibiotic drugs to prevent the infection that leads to stone growth.

To prevent calcium stones that form in hyperparathyroid patients, a surgeon may remove all of the parathyroid glands (located in the neck). This is usually the treatment for hyperparathyroidism as well. In most cases, only one of the glands is enlarged. Removing the gland ends the patient's problem with kidney stones.

Surgical Treatment

Some type of surgery may be needed to remove a kidney stone if the stone

- does not pass after a reasonable period of time and causes constant pain,
- is too large to pass on its own,
- blocks the urine flow,
- causes ongoing urinary tract infection,
- damages the kidney tissue or causes constant bleeding, or
- has grown larger (as seen on follow up x-ray studies).

Until recently, surgery to remove a stone was very painful and required a lengthy recovery time (four to six weeks). Today, treatment for these stones is greatly improved. Many options exist that do not require major surgery.

Extracorporeal Shockwave Lithotripsy (ESWL)

Extracorporeal shockwave lithotripsy (ESWL) is the most frequently used surgical procedure for the treatment of kidney stones. ESWL uses shockwaves that are created outside of the body to travel through the skin and body tissues until the waves hit the dense stones. The stones become sand-like and are easily passed through the urinary tract in the urine.

There are several types of ESWL devices. One device positions the patient in the water bath while the shock waves are transmitted. Other devices have a soft cushion or membrane on which the patient lies. Most devices use either x-rays or ultrasound to help the surgeon pinpoint the stone during treatment. For most types of ESWL procedures, some type of anesthesia is needed.

In some cases, ESWL may be done on an outpatient basis. Recovery time is short, and most people can resume normal activities in a few days.

Complications may occur with ESWL. Most patients have blood in the urine for a few days after treatment. Bruising and minor discomfort on the back or abdomen due to the shockwaves are also common. To reduce the chances of complications, doctors usually tell patients to avoid taking aspirin and other drugs that affect blood clotting for several weeks before treatment.

In addition, the shattered stone fragments may cause discomfort as they pass through the urinary tract in the urine. In some cases, the doctor will insert a small tube called a stent through the bladder into the ureter to help the fragments pass. Sometimes the stone is not completely shattered with one treatment and additional treatments may be required.

Percutaneous Nephrolithotomy

Sometimes a procedure called percutaneous nephrolithotomy is recommended to remove a stone. This treatment is often used when the stone is quite large or in a location that does not allow effective use of EWSL.

In this procedure, the surgeon makes a tiny incision in the back and creates a tunnel directly into the kidney. Using an instrument called a nephroscope, the stone is located and removed. For large stones, some type of energy probe (ultrasonic or electrohydraulic) may be needed to break the stone into small pieces. Generally, patients stay in the hospital for several days and may have a small tube called a nephrostomy tube left in the kidney during the healing process

One advantage of percutaneous nephrolithotomy over ESWL is that the surgeon removes the stone fragments instead of relying on their natural passage from the kidney.

Uteroscopic Stone Removal

Although some ureteral stones can be treated with ESWL, urethroscopy may be needed for mid- and lower ureter stones. No incision is made in this procedure. Instead, the surgeon passes a small fiberoptic instrument called a ureteroscope through the urethra and bladder into the ureter. The surgeon then locates the stone and either removes it with a cage-like device or shatters it with a special instrument that produces a form of shockwave. A small tube or stent may be left in the ureter for a few days after treatment to help the lining of the ureter heal.

Is there any current research on kidney stones?

The Division of Kidney, Urologic, and Hematologic Diseases of the National Institutes of Diabetes and Digestive and Kidney Diseases (NIDDK) funds research on the causes, treatments, and prevention of kidney stones. The NIDDK is part of the federal government's National Institutes of Health in Bethesda, Maryland.

New drugs and the growing field of lithotripsy have greatly improved the treatment of kidney stones. Still, NIDDK researchers and grantees seek to answer questions such as

- Why do some people continue to have painful stones?
- How can doctors predict, or screen, who is as risk for getting stones?
- What are the long-term effects of lithotripsy?
- Do genes play a role in stone formation?
- What is the natural substance(s) found in urine that blocks stone formation?

Researchers are also working to develop new drugs with fewer side effects.

Prevention Points to Remember

- People who have a family history of stones or who have had more than one stone are likely to develop another.
- A good first step to prevent any type of stone is to drink plenty of liquids—water is best.
- If a person is at risk for developing stones, the doctor may perform certain blood and urine tests. These tests will determine which factors can be best altered to reduce that risk.
- Some patients will need medicines to prevent stones from forming.
- People with chronic urinary tract infections and stones will often need the stone removed if the doctor determines that the infection results from the stone's presence. Patients must receive careful followup to be sure that the infection has cleared.

Foods and Drinks Containing Calcium and Oxalate

Persons prone to forming calcium oxalate stones may be asked by their doctor to cut back on certain foods on this list.

- apples
- asparagus
- beer

- beets
- berries, various (e.g., cranberries, strawberries)
- black pepper
- broccoli
- cheese
- chocolate
- cocoa
- coffee
- cola drinks
- collards
- figs
- grapes
- ice cream
- milk
- oranges
- parsley
- peanut butter
- pineapples
- spinach
- Swiss chard
- rhubarb
- tea
- turnips
- vitamin C
- yogurt

Persons should not give up or avoid eating these types of foods without talking to their doctor first. In most cases, these foods can be eaten in limited amounts.

Additional Reading

Prevention and Treatment of Kidney Stones. National Institutes of Health Consensus Development Conference Statement. Available from the National Institutes of Health Consensus Program Clearinghouse PO Box 2577, Kensington, Maryland, 20891. (800) 644-6627.

Understanding Kidney Stones...Management for a Lifetime. Krames Communication, 110 Grundy Lane, San Bruno, CA 94066. (800) 333-3032.

Coe, F.L., et al., "The Pathogenesis and Treatment of Kidney Stones," *New England Journal of Medicine,* Vol. 327, No. 16, pp. 1141-1152, 1992.

Curhan, G.C., et al., A Prospective Study of Dietary Calcium and Other Nutrients and the Risk of Symptomatic Kidney Stones," *New England Journal of Medicine,* Vol. 328, No. 12, pp. 833-838, 1993.

Jenkins, A.D., "Upgrading Extracorporeal Shock Wave Lithotripsy," *Contemporary Urology,* October 1991, pp. 11-12.

Lawson, R.K. "Smaller Means Safer Intraureternal Eletrohydraulic Lithotripsy," *Comtemporary Urology,* October 1991, pp.51-58.

Lingeman, J.E., et al., "Kidney Stones: Acute Management," *Patient Care,* August 15, 1990, pp. 20-42.

Lingeman, J.E., et al., "Kidney Stones: Identifying the Causes," *Patient Care,* September 30, 1990, pp. 31-46.

O'Brien, W.M., Rotolo, J.E., Pahira, J.J., "New Approaches in the Treatment of Renal Calculi," *American Family Physician,* November 1987, pp. 181-94.

Other Resources

American Foundation for Urologic Disease
300 W Pratt St

Baltimore, MD 21201-2463
(800) 242-2383
(410) 727-2908

National Kidney Foundation
30 E 33rd St
New York, NY 10016
(800) 622-9010
(212) 889-2210

National Kidney and Urologic Diseases Information Clearinghouse
3 Information Way
Bethesda, MD 20892-3580

Oxalosis and Hyperoxaluria Foundation
PO Box 1632
Kent, WA 98035
(800) 484-9698 ext: 5100
(206) 631-0386

For information about hyperparathyroidism:

National Institute of Diabetes and Digestive and Kidney Diseases
Building 31, Room 9A04
9000 Rockville Pike
Bethesda, MD 20892
(301) 496-3583

For information about gout:

National Arthritis and Musculoskeletal and Skin Diseases Information Clearinghouse
Box AMS
9000 Rockville Pike
Bethesda, MD 20892
(301) 495-4484

■ **Document Source:**
U.S. Department of Health and Human Services, Public Health Service
National Institutes of Health
National Institute of Diabetes and Digestive and Kidney Diseases
NIH Publication No. 94-2495
April 1994

PEYRONIE'S DISEASE

Peyronie's disease, a condition of uncertain cause, is characterized by a plaque, or hard lump, that forms on the penis. The plaque develops on the upper or lower side of the penis in layers containing erectile tissue. It begins as a localized inflammation and can develop into a hardened scar.

Peyronie's disease often occurs in a mild form that heals without treatment in six to 15 months. But in severe cases, the hardened plaque reduces flexibility, causing pain and forcing the penis to bend or arc during erection.

The plaque itself is benign, or noncancerous. A plaque on the top of the shaft (most common) causes the penis to bend upward; a plaque on the underside causes it to bend downward. In some cases, the plaque develops on both top and bottom, leading to indentation and shortening of the penis. At times, pain, bending, and emotional distress prohibit sexual intercourse.

One study found Peyronie's disease occurring in 1 percent of men. Although the disease occurs mostly in middle-aged men, younger and older men can acquire it. About 30 percent of people with Peyronie's disease develop fibrosis (hardened cells) in other elastic tissues of the body, such as on the hand or foot. A common example is a condition known as Dupuytren's contracture of the hand. In some cases, men who are related by blood tend to develop Peyronie's disease, which suggests that familial factors might make a man vulnerable to the disease.

Men with Peyronie's disease usually seek medical attention because of painful erections and difficulty with intercourse. Since the cause of the disease and its development are not well understood, doctors treat the disease empirically; that is, they prescribe and continue methods that seem to help. The goal of therapy is to keep the Peyronie's patient sexually active. Providing education about the disease and its course often is all that is required. No strong evidence shows that any treatment other than surgery is effective. Experts usually recommend surgery only in long-term cases in which the disease is stabilized and the deformity prevents intercourse.

A French surgeon, Francois de la Peyronie, first described Peyronie's disease in 1743. The problem was noted in print as early as 1687. Early writers classified it as a form of impotence. Peyronie's disease can be associated with impotence; however, experts now recognize impotence as one factor associated with the disease—a factor that is not always present.

Course of the Disease

Many researchers believe the plaque of Peyronie's disease develops following trauma (hitting or bending) that causes localized bleeding inside the penis. A chamber (actually two chambers known as the *corpora cavernosa*) runs the length of the penis. The inner-surface membrane of the chamber is a sheath of elastic fibers. A connecting tissue, called a septum, runs along the center of the chamber and attaches at the top and bottom.

If the penis is abnormally bumped or bent, an area where the septum attaches to the elastic fibers may stretch beyond a limit, injuring the lining of the erectile chamber and, for example, rupturing small blood vessels. As a result of aging, diminished elasticity near the point of attachment of the septum might increase the chances of injury.

The damaged area might heal slowly or abnormally for two reasons: repeated trauma and a minimal amount of bloodflow in the sheath-like fibers. In cases that heal within about a year, the plaque does not advance beyond an initial inflammatory phase. In cases that persist for years, the plaque undergoes fibrosis, or formation of tough fibrous tissue, and even calcification, or formation of calcium deposits.

While trauma might explain acute cases of Peyronie's disease, it does not explain why most cases develop slowly and with no apparent traumatic event. It also does not explain why some cases disappear quickly, and why similar conditions such as Dupuytren's contracture do not seem to result from severe trauma.

Treatment

Because the plaque of Peyronie's disease often shrinks or disappears without treatment, medical experts suggest waiting one to two years or longer before attempting to correct it surgically. During that wait, patients often are willing to undergo treatments that have unproven effectiveness.

Some researchers have given men with Peyronie's disease vitamin E orally in small-scale studies and have reported improvements. Yet, no controlled studies have established the effectiveness of vitamin E therapy. Similar inconclusive success has been attributed to oral application of para-aminobenzoate, a substance belonging to the family of B-complex molecules.

Researchers have injected chemical agents such as collagenase, dimethyl sulfoxide, steroids, and calcium channel blockers directly into the plaques. None of these has produced convincing results. Steroids, such as cortisone, have produced unwanted side effects, such as atrophy, or death of healthy tissues. Perhaps the most promising directly injected agent is collagenase, an enzyme that attacks collagen, the major component of Peyronie's plaques.

Radiation therapy, in which high-energy rays are aimed at the plaque, also has been used. Like some of the chemical treatments, radiation appears to reduce pain, yet it has no effect on the plaque itself and can cause unwelcome side effects. Currently, none of the treatments mentioned here has equalled the body's natural ability to eliminate Peyronie's disease. The variety of agents and methods used points to the lack of a proven, effective treatment.

Peyronie's disease has been treated with some success by surgery. The two most common surgical methods are: removal or expansion of the plaque followed by placement of a patch of skin or artificial material, and removal or pinching of tissue from the side of the penis opposite the plaque, which cancels out the bending effect. The first method can involve partial loss of erectile function, especially rigidity. The second method, known as the Nesbit procedure, causes a shortening of the erect penis.

Some men choose to receive an implanted device that increases rigidity of the penis. In some cases, an implant alone will straighten the penis adequately. In other cases, implantation is combined with a technique of incisions and grafting or plication (pinching or folding the skin) if the implant alone does not straighten the penis.

Most types of surgery produce positive results. But because complications can occur, and because many of the phenomena associated with Peyronie's disease (for example, shortening of the penis) are not corrected by surgery, most doctors prefer to perform surgery only on the small number of men with curvature so severe that it prevents sexual intercourse.

Sources of More Information

American Foundation for Urologic Disease
300 W Pratt St
Suite 401
Baltimore, MD 21201

National Organization for Rare Disorders
PO Box 8923
New Fairfield, CT 06812-1783
(800) 999-6673

National Kidney and Urologic Diseases Information Clearinghouse
3 Information Way

Bethesda, MD 20892-3580

The National Kidney and Urologic Diseases Information Clearinghouse is a service of the National Institute of Diabetes and Digestive and Kidney Diseases, part of the National Institutes of Health, under the U.S. Public Health Service. Authorized in 1987, the clearinghouse provides information about diseases of the kidneys and urologic system to people with such afflictions and to their families, health care professionals, and the public. The clearinghouse answers inquiries; develops, reviews, and distributes publications; and works closely with professional and patient organizations and government agencies to coordinate resources about kidney and urologic diseases.

Publications produced by the clearinghouse are reviewed carefully for scientific accuracy, content, and readability. Publications produced by outside sources are also reviewed carefully before being used to supplement clearinghouse materials when responding to inquiries.

■ Document Source:
U.S. Department of Health and Human Services, Public Health Service
National Institutes of Health
National Institute of Diabetes and Digestive and Kidney Diseases
NIH Publication No. 95-3902
May 1995

PROSTATE PROBLEMS

The prostate is a small organ about the size of a walnut. It lies below the bladder (where urine is stored) and surrounds the urethra (the tube that carries urine from the bladder). The prostate makes a fluid that becomes part of semen. Semen is the white fluid that contains sperm.

Prostate problems are common in men 50 and older. Most can be treated successfully without harming sexual function. A urologist (a specialist in diseases of the urinary system) is the kind of doctor most qualified to diagnose and treat many prostate problems.

Noncancerous Prostate Problems

Acute prostatitis is a bacterial infection of the prostate. It can occur in men at any age. Symptoms include fever, chills, and pain in the lower back and between the legs. This problem also can make it hard or painful to urinate. Doctors prescribe antibiotics for acute prostatitis and recommend that the patient drink more liquids. Treatment is usually successful.

Chronic prostatitis is a prostate infection that comes back again and again. The symptoms are similar to those of acute prostatitis except that there is usually no fever. Also, the symptoms are usually milder in chronic prostatitis. However, they can last a long time.

Chronic prostatitis is hard to treat. Antibiotics often work when the infection is caused by bacteria. But sometimes no disease causing bacteria can be found. In some cases, it helps to massage the prostate to release fluids. Warm baths also may bring relief. Chronic prostatitis clears up by itself in many cases.

Benign prostatic hypertrophy (BPH) is enlargement of the prostate. This condition is common in older men. More than half of men in their 60s have BPH. Among men in their 70s and 80s, the figure may go as high as 90 percent.

An enlarged prostate may eventually block the urethra and make it hard to urinate. Other common symptoms are dribbling after urination and the urge to urinate often, especially at night. In rare cases, the patient is unable to urinate.

A doctor usually can detect an enlarged prostate by rectal exam. The doctor also may examine the urethra, prostate, and bladder using a cytoscope, an instrument that is inserted through the penis.

BPH Treatment Choices

There are several different ways to treat BPH:

- *Watchful waiting* is often chosen by men who are not bothered by symptoms of BPH. They have no treatment but get regular checkups and wait to see whether or not the condition gets worse.
- *Alpha blockers* are drugs that help relax muscles near the prostate and may relieve symptoms. Side effects can include headaches. Also, these medicines sometimes make people feel dizzy, lightheaded, or tired. Alpha blockers are new drugs, so doctors do not know their long-term effects. Some common alpha blockers are doxazosin (Cardura), prazosin (Minipress), and terazosin (Hytrin).
- *Finasteride* (Proscar) is a drug that inhibits the action of the male hormone testosterone. It can shrink the prostate. Side effects of finasteride include declining interest in sex, problems getting an erection, and problems with ejaculation. Again, because it is new, doctors do not know its long-term effects.
- *Surgery* is the treatment most likely to relieve BPH symptoms. However, it also has the most complications. Doctors use three kinds of surgery for BPH:
  - Transurethral resection of the prostate (TURP) is the most common. After the patient is given anesthesia, the doctor inserts a special instrument into the urethra through the penis. With the instrument, the doctor then removes part of the prostate to lessen its obstruction.
  - Transurethral incision of the prostate (TUIP) may be used when the prostate is not too enlarged. In this procedure, the doctor passes an instrument through the urethra to make one or two small cuts in the prostate.
  - Open surgery is used when the prostate is very enlarged. In open surgery, the surgeon makes an incision in the abdomen or between the scrotum and the anus to remove prostate tissue.

Men should carefully weigh the risks and benefits of each of these options. The Agency for Health Care Policy and Research has designed a booklet to help in choosing a treatment; call 800-358-9295 and ask for their free patient guide on prostate enlargement.

Prostate Cancer

Prostate cancer is one of the most common forms of cancer among American men. About 80 percent of all cases occur in men over 65. For unknown reasons, prostate cancer is more common among African American men than white men.

In the early stages of prostate cancer, the disease stays in the prostate and is not life-threatening. But without treatment, cancer can spread to other parts of the body and eventually cause death. Some 40,000 men die every year from prostate cancer that has spread.

Diagnosis. To find the cause of prostate symptoms, the doctor takes a careful medical history and performs a physical exam. The physical includes a digital rectal exam, in which the doctor feels the prostate through the rectum. Hard or lumpy areas may mean that cancer is present.

Some doctors also recommend a blood test for a substance called prostate specific antigen (PSA). PSA levels may be high in men who have prostate cancer or BPH. However, the test is not always accurate. Researchers are studying changes in PSA levels over time to learn whether the test may someday be useful for early diagnosis of prostate cancer.

If a doctor suspects prostate cancer, he or she may recommend a biopsy. This is a simple surgical procedure in which a small piece of prostate tissue is removed with a needle and examined under a microscope. If the biopsy shows prostate cancer, other tests are done to determine the type of treatment needed.

Prostate Cancer Treatment. Doctors have several ways to treat prostate cancer. The choice depends on many factors, such as whether or not the cancer has spread beyond the prostate, the patient's age and general health, and how the patient feels about the treatment options and their side effects. Approaches to treatment include:

- *Watchful waiting.* Some men decide not to have treatment immediately if the cancer is growing slowly and not causing symptoms. Instead, they have regular checkups so they can be closely monitored by their doctor. Men who are older or have another serious illness may choose this option.
- *Surgery* usually removes the entire prostate and surrounding tissues. This operation is called a radical prostatectomy. In the past, impotence was a side effect for nearly all men undergoing radical prostatectomy. But now, doctors can preserve the nerves going to the penis so that men can have erections after prostate removal.

  Incontinence, the inability to hold urine, is common for a time after radical surgery for cancer. Most men regain urinary control within several weeks. A few continue to have problems that require them to wear a device to collect urine.
- Another kind of surgery is a *transurethral resection,* which cuts cancer from the prostate but does not take out the entire prostate. This operation is sometimes done to relieve symptoms caused by the tumor before other treatment or in men who cannot have a radical prostatectomy.
- *Radiation therapy* uses high energy rays to kill cancer cells and shrink tumors. It is often used when cancer cells are found in more than one area. Impotence may occur in men treated with radiation therapy.

- *Hormone therapy* uses various hormones to stop cancer cells from growing. It is used for prostate cancer that has spread to distant parts of the body. Growth of breast tissue is a common side effect of hormone therapy.

More detailed information on the pros and cons of these treatment options is available from the Cancer Information Service at 800-422-6237; ask for the prostate cancer "PDQ for Patients."

Protecting Yourself

The best protection against prostate problems is to have regular medical checkups that include a careful prostate exam. See a doctor promptly if symptoms occur such as:

- a frequent urge to urinate,
- difficulty in urinating, or
- dribbling of urine.

Regular checkups are important even for men who have had surgery for BPH. BPH surgery does not protect against prostate cancer because only part of the prostate is removed. In all cases, the sooner a doctor finds a problem, the better the chances that treatment will work.

Resources

Agency for Health Care Policy and Research (AHCPR) Publications Clearinghouse
PO Box 8547
Silver Spring, MD 20907
800-358-9295

Ask for the free booklet called *Treating Your Enlarged Prostate*. It contains detailed information on the pros and cons of different treatments for BPH.

Cancer Information Service (CIS)
National Cancer Institute
Building 31, Room 10A24
Bethesda, MD 20892
800-4-CANCER

CIS staff can answer questions and mail free booklets about prostate cancer. The prostate cancer "PDQ for Patients" contains detailed information on diagnosis and treatment. Spanish-speaking CIS staff are available during daytime hours.

National Kidney and Urologic Diseases Information Clearinghouse
Box NKUDIC
Bethesda, MD 20892
301-468-6345

Ask for free materials on BPH.

American Cancer Society
1599 Clifton Rd NE
Atlanta, GA 30329
800-227-2345

Ask about their materials on prostate cancer.

Prostate Health Council
The American Foundation for Urologic Disease, Inc.
300 W Pratt St, Ste 401
Baltimore, MD 21201
800-242-2383

Ask for free brochures in English and Spanish on prostate disease and prostate cancer.

The National Institute on Aging Information Center
PO Box 8057

Gaithersburg, MD 20898-8057
1-800-222-2225
1-800-222-4225 (TTY)

■ Document Source:
U.S. Department of Health and Human Services, Public Health Service
National Institutes of Health
National Institute on Aging
1994

Information from PDQ for Patients

TESTICULAR CANCER

Description

What is cancer of the testicle?

Cancer of the testicle (also called the testis), a rare kind of cancer in men, is a disease in which cancer (malignant) cells are found in the tissues of one or both testicles. The testicles are round and a little smaller than golf balls. Sperm (the male germ cells that can join with a female egg to develop into a baby) and male hormones are made in the testicles. There are two testicles located inside of the scrotum (a sac of loose skin that lies directly under the penis). The testicles are similar to the ovaries in women (the small sacs that hold the female egg cells).

Cancer of the testicle is the most common cancer in men 15 to 35 years old. Men who have an undescended testicle (a testicle that has never moved down into the scrotum) are at higher risk of developing cancer of the testicle than other men whose testicles have moved down into the scrotum. This is true even if surgery has been done to place the testicle in the appropriate place in the scrotum.

Like most cancers, cancer of the testicle is best treated when it is found (diagnosed) early. You should see a doctor if you have any swelling in your scrotum. Your doctor will examine the testicles and feel for any lumps. If the scrotum doesn't feel normal, your doctor may need to do an ultrasound exam, which uses sound waves to make a picture of the inside of the testes. Your doctor may need to cut out the testicle and look at it under a microscope to see if there are any cancer cells. It is very important that this be done correctly.

Your chance of recovery (prognosis) and choice of treatment depend on the stage of your cancer (whether it is just in the testicle or has spread to other places) and your general state of health.

Stage Explanation

Stages of Cancer of the Testicle

Once cancer of the testicle has been found, more tests will be done to find out if the cancer has spread from the testicle to other parts of the body (staging). Your doctor needs to know the stage of your disease to plan treatment. The following stages are used for cancer of the testicle:

Stage I

Cancer is found only in the testicle.

Stage II

Cancer has spread to the lymph nodes in the abdomen (lymph nodes are small, bean-shaped structures that are found throughout the body; they produce and store infection-fighting cells).

Stage III

Cancer has spread beyond the lymph nodes in the abdomen. There may be cancer in parts of the body far away from the testicles, such as the lungs and liver.

Recurrent

Recurrent disease means that the cancer has come back (recurred) after it has been treated. It may come back in the same place or in another part of the body. You should regularly examine your opposite testicle for possible recurrence for many years after your treatment.

Treatment Option Overview

How Cancer of the Testicle is Treated

There are treatments for all patients with cancer of the testicle, and most patients can be cured with available treatments. Four kinds of treatment are used:

- surgery (taking out the cancer in an operation)
- radiation therapy (using high-dose x-rays or other high-energy rays to kill cancer cells)
- chemotherapy (using drugs to kill cancer cells)
- bone marrow transplantation

Surgery is a common treatment for most stages of cancer of the testicle. Your doctor may take out the cancer by removing one or both testicles through an incision (cut) in the groin. This is called a radical inguinal orchiectomy. Some of the lymph nodes in the abdomen may also be removed (lymph node dissection).

Radiation therapy uses x-rays or other high-energy rays to kill cancer cells and shrink tumors. Radiation therapy for testicular cancer usually comes from a machine outside the body (external beam radiation).

Chemotherapy uses drugs to kill cancer cells. Chemotherapy may be taken by pill, or it may be put into the body by a needle in a vein. Chemotherapy is called a systemic treatment because the drugs enter the bloodstream, travel through the body, and can kill cancer cells outside the testicle.

Bone marrow transplantation is a newer type of treatment. For autologous bone marrow transplant, bone marrow is taken from you and treated with drugs to kill any cancer cells. The marrow is then frozen and you are given high-dose chemotherapy with or without radiation therapy to destroy all of your remaining marrow. The marrow you had taken out is then thawed and given to you through a needle in a vein to replace the marrow that was destroyed.

Treatment by Stage

Treatment for cancer of the testicle depends on the stage and cell type of your disease, your age, and your overall condition.

You may receive treatment that is considered standard based on its effectiveness in a number of patients in past studies, or you may choose to go into a clinical trial. Not all patients are cured with standard therapy and some standard treatments may have more side effects than are desired. For these reasons, clinical trials are designed to find better ways to treat cancer patients and are based on the most up-to-date information. Clinical trials are going on in many parts of the country for all stages of cancer of the testicle. If you want more information, call the Cancer Information Service at 1-800-4-CANCER (1-800-422-6237).

Stage I Testicular Cancer

Your treatment depends on what the cancer cells look like under a microscope (cell type). If you have a tumor called seminoma, your treatment will probably be surgery to remove the testis (radical inguinal orchiectomy), followed by external beam radiation to the lymph nodes in the abdomen.

If you have a tumor called a nonseminoma, your treatment may be one of the following:

1. Radical inguinal orchiectomy and removal of some of the lymph nodes in the abdomen (lymph node dissection). You may receive surgery that will preserve your fertility. Blood tests and chest x-rays must be done once each month for the first year following the operation and at least every two months during the second year. A CT scan, a special kind of x-ray, may also be done. If results of the tests don't look normal and your cancer has recurred (come back), your doctor will give you systemic chemotherapy as soon as possible.
2. Clinical trials of radical inguinal orchiectomy alone followed by careful testing to see if the cancer comes back. Your doctor must check you and do blood test and x-rays every month for two years. This option is chosen only if the tumor has certain special features.

Stage II Testicular Cancer

Your treatment depends on what the cancer cells look like under a microscope (cell type). If you have a tumor called a seminoma and your tumor is nonbulky (no lymph nodes can be felt in your abdomen, and no lymph nodes block the ureters [the tubes that carry urine from the kidney to the bladder]), your treatment will probably be surgery to remove the testis (radical inguinal orchiectomy). External beam radiation is then given to the lymph nodes in the abdomen.

If you have a tumor called a seminoma and your tumor is bulky (lymph nodes can be felt in your abdomen and/or the lymph nodes block the ureters, or if a CT scan shows them to be large), your treatment will probably be one of the following:

1. Radical inguinal orchiectomy followed by external beam radiation to the lymph nodes in the abdomen and the pelvis.

2. Radical inguinal orchiectomy followed by systemic chemotherapy.

If you have a tumor called a nonseminoma, your treatment will probably be one of the following:

1. Radical inguinal orchiectomy and removal of the lymph nodes in the abdomen (lymph node dissection). Your doctor will check you each month and do blood tests, chest x-rays, and CT scans. If the test results are not normal, you will probably receive systemic chemotherapy.
2. Radical inguinal orchiectomy and lymph node dissection, followed by systemic chemotherapy. Blood tests and chest x-rays must be done once each month for the first year after the operation. CT scans are also done regularly.
3. Radical inguinal orchiectomy followed by systemic chemotherapy. If x-rays following chemotherapy show that cancer remains, surgery may be done to remove the cancer. After the operation, your doctor will check you each month and do blood tests, chest x-rays, and CT scans.
4. Clinical trials of systemic chemotherapy instead of lymph node dissection (in selected patients).
5. Clinical trials of high-dose systemic chemotherapy with autologous bone marrow transplantation.

Stage III Testicular Cancer

Your treatment depends on what the cancer cells look like under a microscope (cell type). If you have a tumor called a seminoma, your treatment will probably be one of the following:

1. Surgery to remove the testis (radical inguinal orchiectomy), followed by systemic chemotherapy.
2. Clinical trials of radical inguinal orchiectomy followed by systemic chemotherapy and external beam radiation therapy.

If you have a tumor called a nonseminoma, your treatment will probably be one of the following:

1. Systemic chemotherapy. Clinical trials are testing new chemotherapy drugs.
2. Systemic chemotherapy, followed by surgery to take out any masses that remain to see if there are any cancer cells left. If cancer cells remain, you will probably receive more systemic chemotherapy.
3. Clinical trials of systemic chemotherapy.
4. Clinical trials of high-dose systemic chemotherapy with autologous bone marrow transplantation.

Recurrent Testicular Cancer

Your treatment will probably be one of the following:

1. Systemic chemotherapy.
2. High-dose systemic chemotherapy with autologous bone marrow transplantation.
3. Surgery.
4. Clinical trials testing new chemotherapy drugs.

To Learn More

To learn more about cancer of the testicle, call the National Cancer Institute's Cancer Information Service at 1-800-4-CANCER (1-800-422-6237). By dialing this toll-free number, you can speak with someone who can answer your questions.

The Cancer Information Service can also send you free booklets. The following booklets about cancer of the testicle may be helpful to you:

- What You Need to Know about Testicular Cancer
- Testicular Self-Examination

The following general booklets on questions related to cancer may also be helpful:

- What You Need to Know About Cancer
- Taking Time: Support for People with Cancer and the People Who Care About Them
- What Are Clinical Trials All About?
- Chemotherapy and You: A Guide to Self-Help During Treatment
- Radiation Therapy and You: A Guide to Self-Help During Treatment
- Eating Hints for Cancer Patients
- Advanced Cancer: Living Each Day
- When Cancer Recurs: Meeting the Challenge Again

There are many other places you can get material about cancer treatment and services to help you. You can check the social service office at your hospital for local and national agencies that help with your finances, getting to and from treatment, care at home, and dealing with your problems. The American Cancer Society, for example, has many free services. Their local offices are listed in the white pages of the telephone book.

You can also write to the National Cancer Institute at this address:

National Cancer Institute
Office of Cancer Communications
31 Center Dr, MSC 2580
Bethesda, MD 20892-2580

■ **Document Source:**
U.S. Department of Health and Human Services, Public Health Service
National Institutes of Health
National Cancer Institute
February 1996

UNDERSTANDING INCONTINENCE

How Your Body Makes, Stores, and Releases Urine

When you eat and drink, your body absorbs the liquid. The kidneys filter out waste products from the body fluids and make urine.

Urine travels down tubes called ureters into a muscular sac called the urinary bladder, which stores the urine.

When you are ready to go to the bathroom, your brain tells your system to relax.

Urine travels out of your bladder through a tube called the urethra. You release urine by relaxing the urethral sphincter and contracting the bladder muscles. The urethral sphincter is a group of muscles that tightens to hold urine in and loosens to let it out.

Purpose of this Booklet

Many people lose urine when they don't want to. When this happens enough to be a problem, it is called urinary incontinence.

Urinary incontinence is very common. But some people are too embarrassed to get help. The good news is that millions of men and women are being successfully treated and cured.

Reading this booklet will help you. But it is important to tell your health care provider (such as a doctor or nurse) about the problem. You may even want to bring this booklet with you to help you talk about your incontinence.

Causes of Urinary Incontinence

Urinary incontinence is not a natural part of aging. It can happen at any age and can be caused by many physical conditions. Many causes of incontinence are temporary and can be managed with simple treatment. Some causes of temporary incontinence are

- Urinary tract infection
- Vaginal infection or irritation
- Constipation
- Effects of medicine

Incontinence can be caused by other conditions that are not temporary. Other causes of incontinence are

- Weakness of muscles that hold the bladder in place
- Weakness of the bladder itself
- Weakness of the urethral sphincter muscles
- Overactive bladder muscles
- Blocked urethra (can be from prostate enlargement)
- Hormone imbalance in women
- Neurologic disorders
- Immobility (not being able to move around)

In almost every case, these conditions can be treated. Your health care provider will help to find the exact cause of your incontinence.

Types of Incontinence

There are also many different types of incontinence. Some people have more than one type of incontinence. You should be able to identify the type of incontinence you have by comparing it to the list below.

Urge Incontinence

People with urge incontinence lose urine as soon as they feel a strong need to go to the bathroom. If you have urge incontinence you may leak urine

- When you can't get to the bathroom quickly enough
- When you drink even a small amount of liquid, or when you hear or touch running water

You may also

- Go to the bathroom very often; for example, every two hours during the day and night. You may even wet the bed

Stress Incontinence

People with stress incontinence lose urine when they exercise or move in a certain way. If you have stress incontinence, you may leak urine

- When you sneeze, cough, or laugh
- When you get up from a chair or get out of bed
- When you walk or do other exercise

You may also
- Go to the bathroom often during the day to avoid accidents

Overflow Incontinence

People with overflow incontinence may feel that they never completely empty their bladder. If you have overflow incontinence, you may

- Often lose small amounts of urine during the day and night
- Get up often during the night to go to the bathroom
- Often feel as if you have to empty your bladder but can't
- Pass only a small amount of urine but feel as if your bladder is still partly full
- Spend a long time at the toilet, but produce only a weak, dribbling stream of urine

Some people with overflow incontinence do not have the feeling of fullness, but they lose urine day and night.

Finding the Cause of Urinary Incontinence

Once you tell your health care provider about the problem, finding the cause of your urinary incontinence is the next step.

Your health care provider will talk with you about your medical history and urinary habits. You may be asked to keep a record of your usual habits in a bladder record. You probably will have a physical examination and urine tests. You may have other tests, as well. These tests will help find the exact cause of your incontinence and the best treatment for you. The table at the end of this booklet lists some of the tests you may be asked to take.

Treating Urinary Incontinence

Once the type and cause of your urinary incontinence are known, treatment can begin. Urinary incontinence is treated in one or more of three ways: behavioral techniques, medication, and surgery.

Behavioral Techniques

Behavioral techniques teach you ways to control your own bladder and sphincter muscles. They are very simple and work well for certain types of urinary incontinence. Two types of behavioral techniques are commonly used—bladder training and pelvic muscle exercises. You may also be asked to change the amount of liquid that you drink. You may be asked to drink more or less water depending on your bladder problem.

Bladder training is used for urge incontinence and may also be used for stress incontinence. Both men and women can benefit from bladder training. People learn different ways to control the urge to urinate. Distraction (thinking about other things) is just one example. A technique called prompted voiding—urinating on a schedule—is also used. This technique has been quite successful in controlling incontinence in nursing home patients.

Pelvic muscle exercises called Kegel exercises are used for stress incontinence. The Kegel exercises help to strengthen weak muscles around the bladder.

Medication

Some people need to take medicine to treat conditions that cause urinary incontinence. The most common types of medicine treat infection, replace hormones, stop abnormal bladder muscle contractions, or tighten sphincter muscles. Your health care provider may recommend medication for your condition. You will be taught how and when to take it.

Surgery

Surgery is sometimes needed to help treat the cause of incontinence. Surgery can be used to

- Return the bladder neck to its proper position in women with stress incontinence
- Remove tissue that is causing a blockage
- Correct severely weakened pelvic muscles
- Enlarge a small bladder to hold more urine

There are many different surgical procedures that may be used to treat incontinence. The type of operation you may need depends on the type and cause of your incontinence. Your doctor will discuss the specific procedure you might need.

> Be sure to ask questions so that you fully understand the procedure.

Other Measures and Supportive Devices

Some other products can be used to help manage incontinence. These include pads and catheters. Catheters are used when a person cannot urinate. A catheter is a tube that is placed in the bladder to drain urine into a bag outside the body. The catheter usually is left inside the bladder, but some catheters are not left in. They are put in and taken out of the bladder as needed to empty it every few hours. Condom catheters (mostly used in men) attach to the outside of the body and are not placed directly in the bladder. Specially designed pads are available to help men and women with incontinence.

> Catheters and pads are not the first and only treatment for incontinence. They should only be used to make other treatments more effective or when other treatments have failed.

What to Do Next

Your health care provider will tell you about the type of incontinence you have and will recommend a treatment. While you are being treated, be sure to

- Ask questions
- Follow instructions
- Take all of your medicine
- Report side effects of your medicine, if any
- Report any changes, good and bad, to your health care provider

> . . .and remember, incontinence is not a natural part of aging. In most cases, it can be successfully treated and reversed.

Risks and Benefits of Treatment

Three types of treatment are recommended for urinary incontinence:

- Behavioral techniques
- Medicine
- Surgery

How well each of these treatments works depends on the cause of the incontinence and, in some cases, patient effort. The risks and benefits described below are based on current medical knowledge and expert opinion. How well a treatment works may also depend on the individual patient. A treatment that works for one patient may not be as effective for another patient. Therefore, it is important to talk with a health care provider about treatment choices.

Behavioral techniques. There are no risks for this type of treatment.

Medicine. As with most drugs, there is a risk of having a side effect. If you are taking medicine for other conditions, the drugs could react with each other. Therefore, it is impor-

tant to work with the health care provider and report all of your medicines and any side effects as soon as they happen.

Surgery. With any surgery there is a possibility of a risk or complication. It is important to discuss these risks with your surgeon.

Coping with Incontinence

Several national organizations help people with urinary incontinence. They may be able to put you in touch with local groups that can give you more information, ideas, and emotional support in coping with urinary incontinence.

Alliance for Aging Research (information on bladder training program)
2021 K Street, NW, Suite 305
Washington, DC 20006
(202) 293-2856

Bladder Health Council
c/o American Foundation for Urologic Disease
300 West Pratt Street, Suite 401
Baltimore, MD 21201
(800) 242-2383
(410) 727-2908

National Association for Continence (formerly Help for Incontinent People)
PO Box 8310
Spartanburg, SC 29305
(864) 579-7900
(800) BLADDER or (800) 252-3337

International Continence Society
The Continence Foundation
2 Doughty Street
London WC1N 2PH
4471-404 6875

Simon Foundation for Continence
Box 835
Wilmette, IL 60091
(800) 23-SIMON
(708) 864-3913

For Further Information

The information in this booklet was taken from the *Clinical Practice Guideline Update on Urinary Incontinence in Adults: Acute and Chronic Management.* The guideline was developed by an expert panel of doctors, nurses, other health care providers, and consumers sponsored by the Agency for Health Care Policy and Research. Other guidelines on common health problems are being developed and will be released in the near future. For more information about the guidelines or to receive additional copies of this booklet, contact: Agency for Health Care Policy and Research, Publications Clearinghouse, Post Office Box 8547, Silver Spring, MD 20907, (800) 358-9295.

■ **Document Source:**
U.S. Department of Health and Human Services, Public Health Service
Agency for Health Care Policy and Research
AHCPR Publication No. 0685
1996

HEART DISEASE AND BLOOD VESSEL DISORDERS

■ ■ ■

ABOUT CAROTID ENDARTERECTOMY

Carotid endarterectomy (care-rot'tid end-art-ter-rec'toe-me) is a surgical procedure that removes blockage from the carotid arteries, which are blood vessels located in the neck that supply blood to the brain. This procedure allows blood to flow more freely to the brain. When blood is prevented from traveling to the brain, a medical emergency called a *stroke* can occur.

This booklet will explain

- Why you may need to have a carotid endarterectomy
- How the blockage is removed from the carotid arteries
- What to expect before and after the operation

Remember, although this procedure has a high success rate, it does have some risks. No two people undergoing a carotid endarterectomy are alike. The reasons for and the outcome of any operation depend on your overall health, your age, and the severity and degree of arterial blockage, as well as any accompanying cardiovascular disease.

This booklet is not intended to take the place of your surgeon's professional opinion. Rather, it can help you begin to understand the basics of this surgical procedure. Read this material carefully. If you have additional questions, you should discuss them openly with your surgeon.

About Arterial Blockage

Cerebrovascular disease is a condition that affects the blood vessels leading to and passing through the brain. If you are being treated by a doctor for cerebrovascular disease, you should know that the objective of such treatment is to prevent stroke and *transient ischemic attacks (TIAs),* or ministrokes. Strokes and ministrokes occur when there is a marked reduction in blood flow and oxygen to the brain. A decrease in oxygen-rich blood can result in the destruction of brain tissue. All human beings' brains must be nourished with oxygenated blood if people are to function normally.

A reduction of blood flow to the brain can be caused by a narrowing of the arteries leading to the brain. This narrowing can be caused by a blood clot or piece of fatty plaque that interferes with the passage of blood to the brain, thus causing a stroke. Strokes can also occur because of uncontrolled high blood pressure or the bursting of a weakened blood vessel in the brain.

Often, preventive measures are used to decrease the chances of having a stroke. Low doses of aspirin and similar "blood thinning" drugs such as warfarin (Coumadin) that prevent the formation of clots and drugs that lower blood pressure are used to reduce the chances of having a stroke. Increasingly, a surgical procedure is used to repair seriously blocked arteries or to reposition blood vessels that supply the brain with oxygenated blood.

Strokes occur most frequently in people who have high blood pressure, smoke, have diabetes (high blood sugar), are overweight, or have high cholesterol levels. Strokes can be mild or can inflict lasting damage to the brain. This damage results in a wide range of disabilities—from speech impairment to complete paralysis.

Strokes sometimes can be caused by a narrowing in one of the carotid arteries of the neck, the major vessels that supply blood to the brain. Carotid arterial blockage can now be pinpointed precisely through the use of ultrasound scans that work like sonar or through a special x-ray test called *arteriography,* or magnetic scan angiography.

Where are the carotid arteries?

The carotid arteries, which lie on either side of the neck, are the two major arteries that supply blood to the head. The carotid artery forks into two smaller arteries. Clots and plaque can form at this fork in the artery, thus interfering with or completely cutting off blood flow.

What are the symptoms of carotid arterial blockage?

Patients with carotid arterial blockage may have disturbances in one or more of the five "S's": *strength, sensation, sight, speech,* and *steadiness.* Two other "S's"—*sleepiness* and *severe headache*—may also signal brain hemorrhage. Patients may have mental deterioration and loss of memory. There may be temporary blindness in one eye or other visual defects. Numbness, weakness, or paralysis of an extremity or of one entire side of the body may exist. Difficulty in speech or the ability to swallow may occur. Coma and, rarely, convulsions may also be experienced. Obviously, these are severe symptoms that need immediate medical attention. But you should also understand that some people can have significant blockage of a carotid artery and have no symptoms at all. Strokes left untreated, as well as arterial blockage, are life-threatening conditions.

How is a carotid endarterectomy performed?

In this procedure, the surgeon makes an incision into the carotid artery. The surgeon uses a dissecting tool to remove the plaque that is clogging the inside of the artery. Removing the plaque is done through a process that is much like the way in which a roto-rooter removes a clog in a drain. The passageway is made broader, thus permitting increased blood flow. The artery is then closed; the surgeon may employ a technique that uses a patch of vein or plastic to enlarge the artery.

Is the operation better than drug therapy?

Strong evidence now exists that a surgical procedure provides better protection against stroke than aspirin does in patients with severe (greater than 70 percent) obstruction of the carotid artery and symptoms of stroke or TIAs. Research also indicates that an operation may be more beneficial than aspirin alone for carotid blockage in patients who do not have symptoms, but have severe narrowing of the arteries. Oral anticoagulant drugs, or "blood thinners," only variably reduce the incidence of TIAs. They do not reduce the risk of completed strokes and may cause bleeding complications. A successful carotid endarterectomy can abolish disabling TIAs.

Who can have this procedure?

Generally, carotid endarterectomy is performed on patients who have an increased risk of stroke with at least 70 percent blockage of one or both carotid arteries.

Through a series of tests, your surgeon will locate and evaluate the blockage in the carotid arteries. Other factors will also be assessed before this procedure is recommended. For instance, active coronary heart disease may make this operation too risky to perform. Similarly, if a patient has other diseases, such as cancer, this operation may not be recommended. Furthermore, uncontrolled high blood pressure must be reduced before this operation is performed. If symptoms of impending stroke prevail, the doctor may opt to treat the blockage another way. The procedure is not performed to fix existing brain damage.

A patient must be physically strong enough to endure the operation and the tests leading to the operation. Age can be,

but is not necessarily, a barrier in performing this procedure. Patients who are 80 years old and over have been successfully treated with carotid endarterectomy.

Preparing for the Operation

If your surgeon decides that you are a candidate for carotid endarterectomy, you will undergo a series of tests prior to admission to the hospital to determine the overall health of your cardiovascular system (that is, your blood vessels and heart). You may be given standard tests to measure your complete blood count and electrolyte levels, as well as an analysis of your urine. Your surgeon may require additional studies, depending on your age and condition. Prior to the operation, you will dress in a surgical cap and gown, receive a sedative by injection, and have a needle placed in the back of your hand or in your forearm for connection to an intravenous line in the operating room. You may be given a general, local, or regional anesthetic. The procedure generally takes two hours.

Immediately Following the Operation

Regardless of the type of anesthesia you received, you will remain overnight in the intensive care nursing area following the operation. Here, complications such as wound bleeding, low blood pressure, and mental status can be assessed and treated swiftly. Because you may have received intravenous fluids during the procedure, blood and electrolyte tests will be done. You may have your heart monitored by a continuous electrocardiogram to confirm that your heart is beating normally.

You will also undergo a series of neurological examinations to evaluate the strength of your arms and legs, your fine hand movements, and your ability to speak, see, and think clearly. These examinations will be done repeatedly, particularly in the first hours after the operation, until you are deemed to be in stable condition.

As with most operations, no drugs, food, or water will be administered orally for several hours or until the day following your procedure, to allow the neck area to begin its healing process. (However, if you're thirsty, you will probably be given ice chips to suck on.) You may be given aspirin in the recovery room. This aspirin therapy may be continued indefinitely—perhaps for the remainder of your life.

Once stabilized, you will be moved to a regular nursing unit where full activity will be encouraged during your two-to-five day convalescence.

Recovery

About one month after your operation, an outpatient examination will be done to assess brain function and wound healing. Your surgeon will check your wound and will determine whether your blood pressure is normal. After that, a yearly exam will be scheduled. At your yearly exam, you may undergo a series of noninvasive tests, such as ultrasound imaging and a test for blood flow detection, on the carotid artery that was cleared to ensure that narrowing has not recurred. Your blood pressure and cholesterol level will also be checked. More importantly, you will be instructed to report any unexpected symptoms associated with a deterioration in your condition, such as speech or visual impairment and weakness or numbness, *as soon as they occur.*

Long-Term Results

As a surgical procedure, carotid endarterectomy does have serious complications of death or disabling stroke, but the risk is no greater than that of leaving the disease untreated for one year. According to the experts, it is currently estimated that a 95 percent chance exists that patients will come through the procedure successfully.

Patients who have undergone carotid endarterectomy have been found to reduce their risk of stroke by as much as 71 percent. If you control or eliminate additional risk factors, such as smoking, high cholesterol, high blood pressure, and obesity, you can increase your chances of good health in the years following your operation.

Surgery by Surgeons

A fully trained surgeon is a physician who, after medical school, has gone through years of training in an accredited residency program to learn the specialized skills of a surgeon. One good sign of a surgeon's competence is certification by a national surgical board approved by the American Board of Medical Specialties. All board-certified surgeons have satisfactorily completed an approved residency training program and have passed a rigorous specialty examination.

The letters FACS (Fellow of the American College of Surgeons) after a surgeon's name are a further indication of a physician's qualifications. Surgeons who become Fellows of the College have passed a comprehensive evaluation of their surgical training and skills; they also have demonstrated their commitment to high standards of ethical conduct. This evaluation is conducted according to national standards that were established to ensure that patients receive the best possible surgical care.

Reviewed by Robert W. Barnes, MD, FACS, Professor and Chairman, Department of Surgery, The University of Arkansas for Medical Sciences, Little Rock, AR, and James T. Robertson, MD, FACS, Professor and Chairman, Department of Neurosurgery, University of Tennessee, Memphis, TN.

■ **Document Source:**
American College of Surgeons
55 East Erie Street
Chicago, IL 60611
January 1995

See also: Stroke Prevention: Atrial Fibrillation and Stroke (page 478); Stroke Prevention: Reducing Risks and Recognizing Symptoms (page 479); Stroke Treatment and Recovery (page 480)

FACTS ABOUT ANGINA

What is angina?

Angina pectoris ("angina") is a recurring pain or discomfort in the chest that happens when some part of the heart does not receive enough blood. It is a common symptom of coronary heart disease (CHD), which occurs when vessels that carry blood to the heart become narrowed and blocked due to atherosclerosis.

Angina feels like a pressing or squeezing pain, usually in the chest under the breast bone, but sometimes in the shoulders, arms, neck, jaws, or back. Angina is usually precipitated by exertion. It is usually relieved within a few minutes by resting or by taking prescribed angina medicine.

What brings on angina?

Episodes of angina occur when the heart's need for oxygen increases beyond the oxygen available from the blood nourishing the heart. Physical exertion is the most common trigger for angina. Other triggers can be emotional stress, extreme cold or heat, heavy meals, alcohol, and cigarette smoking.

Does angina mean a heart attack is about to happen?

An episode of angina is not a heart attack. Angina pain means that some of the heart muscle is not getting enough blood temporarily—for example, during exercise, when the heart has to work harder. The pain does **NOT** mean that the heart muscle is suffering irreversible, permanent damage. Episodes of angina seldom cause permanent damage to heart muscle.

In contrast, a heart attack occurs when the blood flow to a part of the heart is suddenly and permanently cut off. This causes permanent damage to the heart muscle. Typically, the chest pain is more severe, lasts longer, and does not go away with rest or with medicine that was previously effective. It may be accompanied by indigestion, nausea, weakness, and sweating. However, the symptoms of a heart attack are varied and may be considerably milder.

When someone has a repeating but stable pattern of angina, an episode of angina does not mean that a heart attack is about to happen. Angina means that there is underlying coronary heart disease. Patients with angina are at an increased risk of heart attack compared with those who have no symptoms of cardiovascular disease, but the episode of angina is not a signal that a heart attack is about to happen. In contrast, when the pattern of angina changes—if episodes become more frequent, last longer, or occur without exercise—the risk of heart attack in subsequent days or weeks is much higher.

People with angina should talk with their physician to learn the pattern of their angina—what causes an angina attack, what it feels like, how long episodes usually last, and whether medication relieves the attack. If the pattern changes sharply or if the symptoms are those of a heart attack, the patient should get medical help immediately, perhaps best done by seeking an evaluation at a nearby hospital emergency room.

Is all chest pain angina?

No, not at all. Not all chest pain is from the heart, and not all pain from the heart is angina. For example, if the pain lasts for less than 30 seconds or if it goes away during a deep breath, after drinking a glass of water, or by changing position, it almost certainly is **NOT** angina and should not cause concern. But prolonged pain, unrelieved by rest and accompanied by other symptoms, may signal a heart attack.

How is angina diagnosed?

Usually the doctor can diagnose angina by noting the symptoms and how they arise. However, one or more diagnostic tests may be needed to exclude angina or to establish the severity of the underlying coronary disease. These include the electrocardiogram (ECG) at rest, the stress test, and x-rays of the coronary arteries (coronary "arteriogram" or "angiogram").

The ECG records electrical impulses of the heart. These may indicate that the heart muscle is not getting as much oxygen as it needs ("ischemia"); they may also indicate abnormalities in heart rhythm or some of the other possible abnormal features of the heart. To record the ECG, a technician positions a number of small contacts on the patient's arms, legs, and across the chest to connect them to an ECG machine.

For many patients with angina, the ECG at rest is normal. This is not surprising because the symptoms of angina occur during stress. Therefore, the functioning of the heart may be tested under stress, typically exercise. In the simplest stress test, the ECG is taken before, during, and after exercise to look for stress-related abnormalities. Blood pressure is also measured during the stress test, and symptoms are noted.

A more complex stress test involves picturing the blood flow pattern in the heart muscle during peak exercise and after rest. A tiny amount of a radioisotope, usually thallium, is injected into a vein at peak exercise and is taken up by normal heart muscle. A radioactivity detector and computer record the pattern of radioactivity distribution to various parts of the heart muscle. Regional differences in radioisotope concentration and in the rates at which the radioisotopes disappear are measures of unequal blood flow due to coronary artery narrowing, or due to failure of uptake in scarred heart muscle.

The most accurate way to assess the presence and severity of coronary disease is a coronary angiogram, an x-ray of the coronary artery. A long thin flexible tube (a "catheter") is threaded into an artery in the groin or forearm and advanced through the arterial system into one of the two major coronary arteries. A fluid that blocks x-rays (a "contrast medium" or "dye") is injected. X-rays of its distribution show the coronary arteries and their narrowing.

How is angina treated?

The underlying coronary artery disease that causes angina should be treated by controlling existing "risk factors." These include high blood pressure, cigarette smoking, high blood cholesterol levels, and excess weight. If the doctor has prescribed a drug to lower blood pressure, it should be taken as directed. Advice is available on how to eat to control weight, blood cholesterol levels, and blood pressure. A physician can also help patients to stop smoking. Taking these steps reduces the likelihood that coronary artery disease will lead to a heart attack.

Most people with angina learn to adjust their lives to minimize episodes of angina by taking sensible precautions and using medications if necessary.

Usually the first line of defense involves changing one's living habits to avoid bringing on attacks of angina. Controlling physical activity, adopting good eating habits, moderating alcohol consumption, and not smoking are some of the precautions that can help patients live more comfortably and with less angina. For example, if angina comes on with strenuous exercise, exercise a little less strenuously, but do exercise. If angina occurs after heavy meals, avoid large meals and rich foods that leave one feeling stuffed. Controlling weight, reducing the amount of fat in the diet, and avoiding emotional upsets may also help.

Angina is often controlled by drugs. The most commonly prescribed drug for angina is nitroglycerin, which relieves pain by widening blood vessels. This allows more blood to flow to the heart muscle and also decreases the work load of the heart. Nitroglycerin is taken when discomfort occurs or is expected. Doctors frequently prescribe other drugs, to be taken regularly, that reduce the heart's workload. Beta blockers slow the heart rate and lessen the force of the heart muscle contraction. Calcium channel blockers are also effective in reducing the frequency and severity of angina attacks.

What if medications fail to control angina?

Doctors may recommend surgery or angioplasty if drugs fail to ease angina or if the risk of heart attack is high. Coronary artery bypass surgery is an operation in which a blood vessel is grafted onto the blocked artery to bypass the blocked or diseased section so that blood can get to the heart muscle. An artery from inside the chest (an "internal mammary" graft) or a long vein from the leg (a "saphenous vein" graft) may be used.

Balloon angioplasty involves inserting a catheter with a tiny balloon at the end into a forearm or groin artery and threading its tip into the narrowed coronary artery. The balloon is inflated briefly to open the vessel in places where the artery is narrowed. Other catheter techniques are also being developed for opening narrowed coronary arteries, including laser and mechanical devices applied by means of catheters.

Can a person with angina exercise?

Yes. It is important to work with the doctor to develop an exercise plan. Exercise may increase the level of pain-free activity, relieve stress, improve the heart's blood supply, and help control weight. A person with angina should start an exercise program only with the doctor's advice. Many doctors tell angina patients to gradually build up their fitness level—for example, start with a five-minute walk and increase over weeks or months to 30 minutes or hour hour. The idea is to gradually increase stamina by working at a steady pace, but avoiding sudden bursts of effort.

What is the difference between "stable" and "unstable" angina?

It is important to distinguish between the typical, stable pattern of angina and "unstable" angina.

Angina pectoris often recurs in a regular or characteristic pattern. Commonly, a person recognizes that he or she is having angina only after several episodes have occurred, and a pattern has evolved. The level of activity or stress that provokes the angina is somewhat predictable, and the pattern changes only slowly. This is "stable" angina, the most common variety.

Instead of appearing gradually, angina may first appear as a very severe episode or as frequently recurring bouts of angina. Or, an established stable pattern of angina may change sharply; it may be provoked by far less exercise than in the past, or it may appear at rest. Angina in these forms is referred to as "unstable angina" and needs prompt medical attention.

The term "unstable angina" is also used when symptoms suggest a heart attack, but hospital tests do not support that diagnosis. For example, a patient may have typical but prolonged chest pain and poor response to rest and medication, but there is no evidence of heart muscle damage either on the electrocardiogram or in blood enzyme tests.

Are there other types of angina?

There are two other forms of angina pectoris. One, long recognized but quite rare, is called Prinzmetal's, or variant, angina. This type is caused by vasospasm, a spasm that narrows the coronary artery and lessens the flow of blood to the heart. The other is a recently discovered type of angina called microvascular angina. Patients with this condition experience chest pain but have no apparent coronary artery blockages. Doctors have found that the pain results from poor function of tiny blood vessels nourishing the heart as well as the arms and legs. Microvascular angina can be treated with some of the same medications used for angina pectoris.

Additional Resources

Facts About Blood Cholesterol (revised 1994), NIH Publication No. 94-2696

Facts About Coronary Heart Disease (reprinted 1993), NIH Publication No. 93-2265

Facts About Heart Failure (reprinted 1995), NIH Publication No. 95-923

Facts About Heart Disease and Women: So You Have Heart Disease, NIH Publication No. 95-2645

High Blood Presure and What You Can Do About It, No. 55-222A

So You Have High Blood Cholesterol (revised 1993), NIH Publication No. 93-2922

Step by Step: Eating to Lower Your High Blood Cholesterol (revised 1994), NIH Publication No. 94-2920

For Further Information

Call or Write:

National Heart, Lung, and Blood Institute Information Office
PO Box 30105
Bethesda, MD 20892-0105
Telephone: (301) 251-1222

■ Document Source:
U.S. Department of Health and Human Services, Public Health Service
National Institutes of Health
National Heart, Lung, and Blood Institute
NIH Publication No. 95-2890
Reprinted September 1995

FACTS ABOUT ARRHYTHMIAS/RHYTHM DISORDERS

What is an arrhythmia?

An arrhythmia is a change in the regular beat of the heart. The heart may seem to skip a beat or beat irregularly or very fast or very slowly.

Does having an arrhythmia mean that a person has heart disease?

No, not necessarily. Many arrhythmias occur in people who do not have underlying heart disease.

What causes arrhythmias?

Many times, there is no recognizable cause of an arrhythmia. Heart disease may cause arrhythmias. Other causes include: stress, caffeine, tobacco, alcohol, diet pills, and cough and cold medicines.

Are arrhythmias serious?

The vast majority of people with arrhythmias have nothing to fear. They do not need extensive exams or special treatments for their condition.

In some people, arrhythmias are associated with heart disease. In these cases, heart disease, not the arrhythmia, poses the greatest risk to the patient.

In a very small number of people with serious symptoms, arrhythmias themselves are dangerous. These arrhythmias require medical treatment to keep the heartbeat regular. For example, a few people have a very slow heartbeat (brady-cardia), causing them to feel lightheaded or faint. If left untreated, the heart may stop beating and these people could die.

How common are arrhythmias?

Arrhythmias occur commonly in middle-age adults. As people get older, they are more likely to experience an arrhythmia.

What Makes a Heart Beat

The heartbeat usually starts in the sinus node located in the right atrium.

The sinus node sends an electrical signal throughout the atria and to the atrioventricular (AV) node.

The signal then travels down special pathways that conduct it to the ventricles.

As the signal travels through the heart, the heart contracts or beats.

What are the symptoms of an arrhythmia?

Most people have felt their heart beat very fast, experienced a fluttering in their chest, or noticed that their heart skipped a beat. Almost everyone has also felt dizzy, faint, or out of breath or had chest pains at one time or another. One of the most common arrhythmias is sinus arrhythmia, the change in heart rate that can occur normally when we take a breath. These experiences may cause anxiety, but for the majority of people, they are completely harmless.

You should not panic if you experience a few flutters or your heart races occasionally. But if you have questions about your heart rhythm or symptoms, check with your doctor.

What happens in the heart during an arrhythmia?

Describing how the heart beats normally helps to explain what happens during an arrhythmia.

The heart is a muscular pump divided into four chambers—two atria located on the top and two ventricles located on the bottom.

Normally, each heartbeat starts in the right atrium. Here, a specialized group of cells called the sinus node, or natural pacemaker, sends an electrical signal. The signal spreads throughout the atria to the area between the atria called the atrioventricular (AV) node.

The AV node connects to a group of special pathways that conduct the signal to the ventricles below. As the signal travels through the heart, the heart contracts. First, the atria contract, pumping blood into the ventricles. A fraction of a second later, the ventricles contract, sending blood throughout the body.

Usually the whole heart contracts between 60 and 100 times per minute. Each contraction equals one heartbeat.

An arrhythmia may occur for one of several reasons:

- Instead of beginning in the sinus node, the heartbeat begins in another part of the heart.
- The sinus node develops an abnormal rate or rhythm.
- A patient has a heart block.

Arrhythmia Types

Originating in the Atria

Sinus arrhythmia. Cyclic changes in the heart rate during breathing. Common in children and often found in adults.

Sinus tachycardia. The sinus node sends out electrical signals faster than usual, speeding up the heart rate.

Sick sinus syndrome. The sinus node does not fire its signals properly, so that the heart rate slows down. Sometimes, the rate changes back and forth between a slow (bradycardia) and fast (tachycardia) rate.

Premature supraventricular contractions or premature atrial contractions (PAC). A beat occurs early in the atria, causing the heart to beat before the next regular heartbeat.

Supraventricular tachycardia (SVT), paroxysmal atrial tachycardia (PAT). A series of early beats in the atria speed up the heart rate (the number of times a heart beats per minute). In paroxysmal tachycardia, repeated periods of very fast heartbeats begin and end suddenly.

Atrial flutter. Rapidly fired signals cause the muscles in the atria to contract quickly, leading to a very fast, steady heartbeat.

Atrial fibrillation. Electrical signals in the atria are fired in a very fast and uncontrolled manner. Electrical signals arrive in the ventricles in a completely irregular fashion, so the heart beat is completely irregular.

Wolff-Parkinson-White syndrome. Abnormal pathways between the atria and ventricles cause the electrical signal to arrive at the ventricles too soon and to be transmitted back into the atria. Very fast heart rates may develop as the electrical signal ricochets between the atria and ventricles.

Originating in the Ventricles

Premature ventricular complexes (PVC). An electrical signal from the ventricles causes an early heart beat that generally goes unnoticed. The heart then seems to pause until the next beat of the ventricle occurs in a regular fashion.

Ventricular tachycardia. The heart beats fast due to electrical signals arising from the ventricles (rather than from the atria).

Ventricular fibrillation. Electrical signals in the ventricles are fired in a very fast and uncontrolled manner, causing the heart to quiver rather than beat and pump blood.

What is a heart block?

Heart block is a condition in which the electrical signal cannot travel normally down the special pathways to the ventricles. For example, the signal from the atria to the ventricles may be (1) delayed, but each one conducted; (2) delayed with only some getting through; or (3) completely interrupted. If there is no conduction, the beat generally originates from the ventricles and is very slow.

What are the different types of arrhythmias?

There are many types of arrhythmias. Arrhythmias are identified by where they occur in the heart (atria or ventricles) and by what happens to the heart's rhythm when they occur.

Arrhythmias arising in the atria are called atrial or supraventricular (above the ventricles) arrhythmias. Ventricular arrhythmias begin in the ventricles. In general, ventricular arrhythmias caused by heart disease are the most serious.

How does the doctor know that I have an arrhythmia?

Sometimes an arrhythmia can be detected by listening to the heart with a stethoscope. However, the electrocardiogram is the most precise method for diagnosing the arrhythmia.

An arrhythmia may not occur at the time of the exam even though symptoms are present at other times. In such cases, tests will be done, if necessary, to find out whether an arrhythmia is causing the symptoms.

What tests can be done?

First, the doctor will take a medical history and do a thorough physical exam. Then, one or more tests may be used to check for an arrhythmia and to decide whether it is caused by heart disease.

How are arrhythmias treated?

Many arrhythmias require no treatment whatsoever.

Serious arrhythmias are treated in several ways depending on what is causing the arrhythmia. Sometimes the heart disease is treated to control the arrhythmia. Or, the arrhythmia itself may be treated using one or more of the following treatments.

- **Drugs**

    There are several kinds of drugs used to treat arrhythmias. One or more drugs may be used.

    Drugs are carefully chosen because they can cause side effects. In some cases, they can cause arrhythmias or make arrhythmias worse. For this reason, the benefits of the drug are carefully weighed against any risks associated with taking it. It is important not to change the dose or type of your medication unless you check with your doctor first.

    If you are taking drugs for an arrhythmia, one of the following tests will probably be used to see whether treatment is working: a 24-hour electrocardiogram (ECG) while you are on drug therapy, an exercise ECG, or a special technique to see how easily the arrhythmia can be caused. Blood levels of anti-arrhythmic drugs may also be checked.

- **Cardioversion**

    To quickly restore a heart to its normal rhythm, the doctor may apply an electrical shock to the chest wall. Called cardioversion, this treatment is most often used in emer-

gency situations. After cardioversion, drugs are usually prescribed to prevent the arrhythmia from recurring.

Tests for Detecting Arrhythmias

Electrocardiogram (ECG or EKG). A record of the electrical activity of the heart. Disks are placed on the chest and connected by wires to a recording machine. The heart's electrical signals cause a pen to draw lines across a strip of graph paper in the ECG machine. The doctor studies the shapes of these lines to check for any changes in the normal rhythm. The types of ECGs are:

- **Resting ECG.** The patient lies down for a few minutes while a record is made. In this type of ECG, disks are attached to the patient's arms and legs as well as to the chest.
- **Exercise ECG (stress test).** The patient exercises either on a treadmill machine or bicycle while connected to the ECG machine. This test tells whether exercise causes arrhythmias or makes them worse or whether there is evidence of inadequate blood flow to the heart muscle ("ischemia").
- **24-hour ECG (Holter) monitoring.** The patient goes about his or her usual daily activities while wearing a small, portable tape recorder that connects to the disks on the patient's chest. Over time, this test shows changes in rhythm (or "ischemia") that may not be detected during a resting or exercise ECG.
- **Transtelephonic monitoring.** The patient wears the tape recorder and disks over a period of a few days to several weeks. When the patient feels an arrhythmia, he or she telephones a monitoring station where the record is made. If access to a telephone is not possible, the patient has the option of activating the monitor's memory function. Later, when a telephone is accessible, the patient can transmit the recorded information from the memory to the monitoring station. Transtelephonic monitoring can reveal arrhythmias that occur only once every few days or weeks.
- **Electrophysiologic study (EPS).** A test for arrhythmias that involves cardiac catheterization. Very thin, flexible tubes (catheters) are placed in a vein of an arm or leg and advanced to the right atrium and ventricle. This procedure allows doctors to find the site and type of arrhythmia and how it responds to treatment.

- **Automatic implantable defibrillators**

    These devices are used to correct serious ventricular arrhythmias that can lead to sudden death. The defibrillator is surgically placed inside the patient's chest. There, it monitors the heart's rhythm and quickly identifies serious arrhythmias. With an electrical shock, it immediately disrupts a deadly arrhythmia.
- **Artificial pacemaker**

    An artificial pacemaker can take charge of sending electrical signals to make the heart beat if the heart's natural pacemaker is not working properly or its electrical pathway is blocked. During a simple operation, this electrical device is placed under the skin. A lead extends from the device to the right side of the heart, where it is permanently anchored.

- **Surgery**

    When an arrhythmia cannot be controlled by other treatments, doctors may perform surgery. After locating the heart tissue that is causing the arrhythmia, the tissue is altered or removed so that it will not produce the arrhythmia.

How can arrhythmias be prevented?

If heart disease is not causing the arrhythmia, the doctor may suggest that you avoid what is causing it. For example, if caffeine or alcohol is the cause, the doctor may ask you not to drink coffee, tea, colas, or alcoholic beverages.

Is research on arrhythmias being done?

The National Heart, Lung, and Blood Institute (NHLBI) supports basic research on normal and abnormal electrical activity in the heart to understand how arrhythmias develop. Clinical studies with patients aim to improve the diagnosis and management of different arrhythmias. These studies will someday lead to better diagnostic and treatment strategies.

Where can I find publications about heart disease?

To obtain publications about heart disease, you may want to contact your

- local American Heart Association chapter
- local or state health department

The National Heart, Lung, and Blood Institute also has publications about heart disease. For more information, contact:

NHLBI Information Center
PO Box 30105
Bethesda, MD 20892-0105
Telephone: (301) 251-1222

■ **Document Source:**
   U.S. Department of Health and Human Services, Public Health Service
   National Institutes of Health
   National Heart, Lung, and Blood Institute
   NIH Publication No. 95-2264
   Reprinted September 1995

FACTS ABOUT HEART FAILURE

What is heart failure?

Heart failure occurs when the heart loses its ability to pump enough blood through the body. Usually, the loss in pumping action is a symptom of an underlying heart problem, such as coronary artery disease.

The term *heart failure* suggests a sudden and complete stop of heart activity. But, actually, the heart does not suddenly stop. Rather, heart failure usually develops slowly, often over years, as the heart gradually loses its pumping ability and works less efficiently. Some people may not become aware of their condition until symptoms appear years after their heart began its decline.

How serious the condition is depends on how much pumping capacity the heart has lost. Nearly everyone loses some pumping capacity as he or she ages. But the loss is significantly more in heart failure and often results from a heart attack or other disease that damages the heart.

The severity of the condition determines the impact it has on a person's life. At one end of the spectrum, the mild form of heart failure may have little effect on a person's life; at the other end, severe heart failure can interfere with even simple activities and prove fatal. Between those extremes, treatment often helps people lead full lives.

But all forms of heart failure, even the mildest, are a serious health problem, which must be treated. To improve their chance of living longer, patients must take care of themselves, see their physician regularly, and closely follow treatments.

Is there only one type of heart failure?

The term congestive heart failure is often used to describe all patients with heart failure. In reality, congestion (the buildup of fluid) is just one feature of the condition and does not occur in all patients. There are two main categories of heart failure although, within each category, symptoms and effects may differ from patient to patient. The two categories are:

- Systolic heart failure—This occurs when the heart's ability to contract decreases. The heart cannot pump with enough force to push a sufficient amount of blood into the circulation. Blood coming into the heart from the lungs may back up and cause fluid to leak into the lungs, a condition known as pulmonary congestion.
- Diastolic heart failure—This occurs when the heart has a problem relaxing. The heart cannot properly fill with blood because the muscle has become stiff, losing its ability to relax. This form may lead to fluid accumulation, especially in the feet, ankles, and legs. Some patients may have lung congestion.

How common is heart failure?

Between two and three million Americans have heart failure, and 400,000 new cases are diagnosed each year. The condition is slightly more common among men than women and is twice as common among African Americans as whites.

Heart failure causes 39,000 deaths a year and is a contributing factor in another 225,000 deaths. The death rate attributed to heart failure rose by 64 percent from 1970 to 1990, while the death rate from coronary heart disease dropped by 49 percent during the same period. Heart failure mortality is about twice as high for African Americans as for whites for all age groups.

In a sense, heart failure's growing presence as a health problem reflects the nation's changing population: More people are living longer. People age 65 and older represent the fastest growing segment of the population, and the risk of heart failure increases with age. The condition affects one percent of people age 50, but about five percent of people age 75.

What causes heart failure?

As stated, the heart loses some of its blood-pumping ability as a natural consequence of aging. However, a number of other factors can lead to a potentially life-threatening loss of pumping activity.

As a symptom of underlying heart disease, heart failure is closely associated with the major risk factors for coronary heart disease: smoking, high cholesterol levels, hypertension (persistent high blood pressure), diabetes and abnormal blood sugar levels, and obesity. A person can change or eliminate those risk factors and thus lower their risk of developing or aggravating their heart disease and heart failure.

Among prominent risk factors, hypertension (high blood pressure) and diabetes are particularly important. Uncontrolled high blood pressure increases the risk of heart failure by about 200 percent, compared with those who do not have hypertension. Moreover, the degree of risk appears directly related to the severity of the high blood pressure.

Persons with diabetes have about a two- to eightfold greater risk of heart failure than those without diabetes. Women with diabetes have a greater risk of heart failure than men with diabetes. Part of the risk comes from diabetes' association with other heart failure risk factors, such as high blood pressure, obesity, and high cholesterol levels. However, the disease process in diabetes also damages the heart muscle.

The presence of coronary disease is among the greatest risks for heart failure. Muscle damage and scarring caused by a heart attack greatly increase the risk of heart failure. Cardiac arrhythmias, or irregular heartbeats, also raise heart failure risk. Any disorder that causes abnormal swelling or thickening of the heart sets the stage for heart failure.

In some people, heart failure arises from problems with heart valves, the flap-like structures that help regulate blood flow through the heart. Infections in the heart are another source of increased risk for heart failure.

A single risk factor may be sufficient to cause heart failure, but a combination of factors dramatically increases the risk. Advanced age adds to the potential impact of any heart failure risk.

Finally, genetic abnormalities contribute to the risk for certain types of heart disease, which in turn may lead to heart failure. However, in most instances, a specific genetic link to heart failure has not been identified.

What are the symptoms?

A number of symptoms are associated with heart failure, but none is specific for the condition. Perhaps the best known symptom is shortness of breath ("dyspnea"). In heart failure, this may result from excess fluid in the lungs. The breathing difficulties may occur at rest or during exercise. In some cases, congestion may be severe enough to prevent or interrupt sleep.

Fatigue or easy tiring is another common symptom. As the heart's pumping capacity decreases, muscles and other tissues receive less oxygen and nutrition, which are carried in the blood. Without proper "fuel," the body cannot perform as much work, which translates into fatigue.

Fluid accumulation, or edema, may cause swelling of the feet, ankles, legs, and, occasionally, the abdomen. Excess fluid retained by the body may result in weight gain, which sometimes occurs fairly quickly.

Persistent coughing is another common sign, especially coughing that regularly produces mucus or pink, blood-tinged sputum. Some people develop raspy breathing or wheezing.

Because heart failure usually develops slowly, the symptoms may not appear until the condition has progressed over years. The heart hides the underlying problem by making adjustments that delay—but do not prevent—the eventual loss in pumping capacity. The heart adjusts, or compensates, in three ways to cope with and hide the effects of heart failure:

- Enlargement ("dilatation"), which allows more blood into the heart;
- Thickening of muscle fibers ("hypertrophy") to strengthen the heart muscle, which allows the heart to contract more forcefully and pump more blood; and
- More frequent contraction, which increases circulation.

By making these adjustments, or compensating, the heart can temporarily make up for losses in pumping ability, sometimes for years. However, compensation has its limits. Eventually, the heart cannot offset the lost ability to pump blood, and the signs of heart failure appear.

How do doctors diagnose heart failure?

In many cases, physicians diagnose heart failure during a physical examination. Readily identifiable signs are shortness of breath, fatigue, and swollen ankles and feet. The physician also will check for the presence of risk factors, such as hypertension, obesity, and a history of heart problems. Using a stethoscope, the physician can listen to a patient breathe and identify the sounds of lung congestion. The stethoscope also picks up the abnormal heart sounds indicative of heart failure.

Facts About Heart Failure

If neither the symptoms nor the patient's history point to a clear-cut diagnosis, the physician may recommend any of a variety of laboratory tests, including, initially, an electrocardiogram, which uses recording devices placed on the chest to evaluate the electrical activity of a patient's heartbeat.

Echocardiography is another means of evaluating heart function from outside the body. Sound waves bounced off the heart are recorded and translated into images. The pictures can reveal abnormal heart size, shape, and movement. Echocardiography also can be used to calculate a patient's ejection fraction, a measure of the amount of blood pumped out when the heart contracts.

Another possible test is the chest x-ray, which also determines the heart's size and shape, as well as the presence of congestion in the lungs.

Tests help rule out other possible causes of symptoms. The symptoms of heart failure can result when the heart is made to work too hard, instead of from damaged muscle. Conditions that overload the heart occur rarely and include severe anemia and thyrotoxicosis (a disease resulting from an overactive thyroid gland).

What treatments are available?

Heart failure caused by an excessive workload is curable by treating the primary disease, such as anemia or thyrotoxicosis. Also curable are forms caused by anatomical problems, such as a heart valve defect. These defects can be surgically corrected.

However, for the common forms of heart failure—those due to damaged heart muscle—no known cure exists. But treatment for these forms may be quite successful. The treatment seeks to improve patients' quality of life and length of survival through lifestyle change and drug therapy.

Patients can minimize the effects of heart failure by controlling the risk factors for heart disease. Obvious steps include quitting smoking, losing weight if necessary, abstaining from alcohol, and making dietary changes to reduce the amount of salt and fat consumed. Regular, modest exercise is also helpful for many patients, though the amount and intensity should be carefully monitored by a physician.

But, even with lifestyle changes, most heart failure patients must take medication. Many patients receive two or more drugs.

Several types of drugs have proven useful in the treatment of heart failure:

- Diuretics help reduce the amount of fluid in the body and are useful for patients with fluid retention and hypertension.
- Digitalis increases the force of the heart's contractions, helping to improve circulation.
- Results of recent studies have placed more emphasis on the use of drugs known as angiotensin converting enzyme (ACE) inhibitors. Several large studies have indicated that ACE inhibitors improve survival among heart failure patients and may slow, or perhaps even prevent, the loss of heart pumping activity.

Originally developed as a treatment for hypertension, ACE inhibitors help heart failure patients by, among other things, decreasing the pressure inside blood vessels. As a result, the heart does not have to work as hard to pump blood through the vessels.

Patients who cannot take ACE inhibitors may get a nitrate and/or a drug called hydralazine, each of which helps relax tension in blood vessels to improve blood flow.

Sometimes, heart failure is life-threatening. Usually, this happens when drug therapy and lifestyle changes fail to control its symptoms. In such cases, a heart transplant may be the only treatment option. However, candidates for transplantation often have to wait months or even years before a suitable donor heart is found. Recent studies indicate that some transplant candidates improve during this waiting period through drug treatment and other therapy, and can be removed from the transplant list.

Transplant candidates who do not improve sometimes need mechanical pumps, which are attached to the heart. Called left ventricular assist devices (LVADs), the machines take over part or virtually all of the heart's blood-pumping activity. However, current LVADs are not permanent solutions for heart failure but are considered bridges to transplantation.

An experimental surgical procedure for severe heart failure is available at a few U.S. medical centers. The procedure, called cardiomyoplasty, involves detaching one end of a muscle in the back, wrapping it around the heart, and then suturing the muscle to the heart. An implanted electric stimulator causes the back muscle to contract, pumping blood from the heart.

Common Heart Failure Medications

Listed below are some of the medications prescribed for heart failure. Not all medications are suitable for all patients, and more than one drug may be needed.

Also, the list provides the full range of possible side effects for these drugs. Not all patients will develop these side effects. If you suspect that you are having a side effect, alert your physician.

- **ACE Inhibitors**
  These prevent the production of a chemical that causes blood vessels to narrow. As a result, blood pressure drops, and the heart does not have to work as hard to pump blood.
  - *Side effects* may include coughing, skin rashes, fluid retention, excess potassium in the bloodstream, kidney problems, and an altered or lost sense of taste.

- **Digitalis**
  Increases the force of the heart's contractions. It also slows certain fast heart rhythms. As a result, the heart beats less frequently but more effectively, and more blood is pumped into the arteries.
  - *Side effects* may include nausea, vomiting, loss of appetite, diarrhea, confusion, and new heartbeat irregularities.

- **Diuretics**
  These decrease the body's retention of salt and so of water. Diuretics are commonly prescribed to reduce high blood pressure. Diuretics come in many types, with different periods of effectiveness.
  - *Side effects* may include loss of too much potassium, weakness, muscle cramps, joint pains, and impotence.

- **Hydralazine**
  This drug widens blood vessels, easing blood flow.
  - *Side effects* may include headaches, rapid heartbeat, and joint pain.

- **Nitrates**
  These drugs are used mostly for chest pain, but may also help diminish heart failure symptoms. They relax smooth muscle and widen blood vessels. They act to lower primarily systolic blood pressure.
  - *Side effects* may include headaches.

Making the Most of Your Doctor Visit

Here are some points you may want to discuss with your doctor. Don't hesitate to ask questions to clarify points. Also, ask your doctor to rephrase a reply you cannot understand. You may want to take a family member or friend to the appointment with you to help you better understand and remember what's said.

- Briefly describe your symptoms, even those you feel may not be important. You may want to keep a list so you will remember them.
- Tell the doctor all of the medications you take—including over-the-counter drugs—and any problems you may be having with them.
- Be sure you understand all of the doctor's instructions—especially for medications. Know what drug to take, when, how often, and in what amount.
- Find out what side effects are possible from any drug the doctor prescribes for you.
- Ask the meaning of any medical term you don't understand.
- If, after your appointment, you still have questions or are uncertain about your treatment, call the doctor's office to get the information you need.

Can a person live with heart failure?

Heart failure is one of the most serious symptoms of heart disease. About two-thirds of all patients die within five years of diagnosis. However, some live beyond five years, even into old age. The outlook for an individual patient depends on the patient's age, severity of heart failure, overall health, and a number of other factors.

As heart failure progresses, the effects can become quite severe, and patients often lose the ability to perform even modest physical activity. Eventually, the heart's reduced pumping capacity may interfere with routine functions, and patients may become unable to care for themselves. The loss in functional ability can occur quickly if the heart is further weakened by heart attacks or the worsening of other conditions that affect heart failure, such as diabetes and coronary heart disease.

Heart failure patients also have an increased risk of sudden death, or cardiac arrest, caused by an irregular heartbeat.

To improve the chances of surviving with heart failure, patients must take care of themselves.

Patients must

- See their physician regularly;
- Closely follow all of their physician's instructions;
- Take any medication according to instructions; and
- Immediately inform their physician of any significant change in their condition, such as an intensified shortness of breath or swollen feet.

Patients with heart failure also should

- Control their weight;
- Watch what they eat;

- Not smoke cigarettes or use other tobacco products; and
- Abstain from or strictly limit alcohol consumption.

Even with the best care, heart failure can worsen, but patients who don't take care of themselves are almost writing themselves a prescription for poor health.

The best defense against heart failure is the prevention of heart disease. Almost all of the major coronary risk factors can be controlled or eliminated: smoking, high cholesterol, high blood pressure, diabetes, and obesity.

A Question for Your Pharmacist

Your pharmacist is a good resource for information about medications. Ask if any drug you're taking interacts badly with certain foods or with other drugs, including nonprescription ones. Your pharmacist also can help you understand product package inserts and label instructions.

What is the outlook for heart failure?

Within the past decade, knowledge of heart failure has improved dramatically but, clearly, much more remains to be learned. The National Heart, Lung, and Blood Institute (NHLBI) supports numerous research projects aimed at building on what is already known about heart failure and at uncovering new knowledge about its process, diagnosis, and treatment. NHLBI research priorities for heart failure include

- Learning more about basic cellular changes that lead to heart failure;
- Developing tests to detect the earliest signs of heart failure;
- Identifying factors that cause heart failure to worsen;
- Determining how heart failure can be reversed once it starts;
- Understanding better the heart's ability to compensate for lost pumping ability; and
- Developing new therapies, especially those based on early signs of heart failure.

Glossary

Angiotensin converting enzyme (ACE) inhibitor: A drug used to decrease pressure inside blood vessels.

Arrhythmia: An irregular heartbeat.

Cardiomyoplasty: A surgical procedure that involves detaching one end of a back muscle and attaching it to the heart. An electric stimulator causes the muscle to contract to pump blood from the heart.

Congestive heart failure: A heart disease condition that involves loss of pumping ability by the heart, generally accompanied by fluid accumulation in body tissues, especially the lungs.

Diastolic heart failure: Inability of the heart to relax properly and fill with blood as a result of stiffening of the heart muscle.

Dyspnea: Shortness of breath.

Echocardiography: Recording sound waves bounced off the heart to produce images of the heart.

Edema: Abnormal fluid accumulation in body tissues.

Electrocardiogram (EKG or ECG): Measurement of electrical activity associated with heartbeats.

Heart failure: Loss of blood-pumping ability by the heart.

Left ventricular assist device: A mechanical device used to increase the heart's pumping ability.

Pulmonary congestion (or edema): Fluid accumulation in the lungs.

Sudden cardiac death: Cardiac arrest caused by an irregular heartbeat.

Systolic heart failure: Inability of the heart to contract with enough force to pump adequate amounts of blood through the body.

Valves: Flap-like structures that control the direction of blood flow through the heart.

■ Document Source:
  U.S. Department of Health and Human Services, Public Health Service
  National Institutes of Health
  National Heart, Lung, and Blood Institute
  NIH Publication No. 95-923
  Reprinted September 1995

See also: Living with Heart Disease: Is it Heart Failure? (page 238)

LIVING WITH HEART DISEASE: IS IT HEART FAILURE?

Your Heart

The human heart is a remarkable organ that continuously pumps blood to nourish and provide energy to the body. As big as a fist, this powerful muscle uses its own electrical system to pump blood. It pumps five to six quarts of blood a minute during rest, but more than 20 quarts a minute during exercise.

Normally, the heart automatically adjusts to changing demands. As the body needs more nourishment and energy (for example, when climbing stairs), the heart responds. It should beat faster and more forcefully, causing more blood to circulate through the body. The blood will carry more oxygen and nourishment to muscles and organs and then return to the heart to begin the process again.

If you have heart failure, your heart is weak and its pumping power is reduced. Although it still beats normally, your heart cannot pump as much blood with each beat. Your symptoms will depend on how severe your heart failure is.

Purpose of this Booklet

If you have heart failure due to reduced pumping power of your heart (left-ventricular systolic dysfunction), this booklet is for you. Understanding your condition and following a few simple guidelines can improve the quality of your life.

This booklet is designed to help you and your family be active partners with your health care team—doctors, nurses, and other professionals. It is your guide to living with heart failure. Share it with your family and other caregivers.

This booklet will tell you how and why heart failure affects your body. It also tells how to respond to symptoms and what to expect from treatment. You need to know as much as you can to improve the quality of your life. Be involved in managing your condition.

What is heart failure?

"Heart failure" simply means that your heart's pumping power is weaker than normal. Although it still beats, a weakened heart pumps too little blood rich with oxygen and nutrients to meet the body's needs. Walking, carrying groceries, or climbing stairs can be difficult. You may feel short of breath; the body is not getting all the oxygen it needs.

For most patients, heart failure is a chronic condition, which means it can be treated and managed, but not cured. If it is a complication of other medical conditions such as blocked coronary arteries or heart valve disease, surgery may help.

Causes of Heart Failure

The most common causes are

- Coronary artery disease, usually with previous heart attack (myocardial infarction [MI]).
- Heart muscle disorder (cardiomyopathy).
- High blood pressure (hypertension).
- Heart valve disease.

Sometimes the exact cause of heart failure is not found. However, the actual cause is not as important as your heart's reduced pumping power and what can be done about it.

Symptoms

Check your symptoms:

1. Difficulty breathing, especially with exertion or when lying flat in bed.
2. Waking up breathless at night.
3. Frequent dry, hacking cough, especially when lying down.
4. Fatigue, weakness.
5. Dizziness or fainting.
6. Swollen feet, ankles, and legs (edema).
7. Nausea, with abdominal swelling, pain, and tenderness.

Other medical problems can cause the same symptoms. A thorough physical exam and a complete health history, plus certain tests, are needed to diagnose heart failure and find its possible causes.

Causes of Symptoms

A healthy heart can increase how much oxygen-rich blood is pumped to vital organs and muscles as it is needed.

When a heart pumps with less power and force than normal, it cannot pump enough blood to organs and muscles. As a result, your body cannot do as much. Blood and fluids may collect or "pool" in the lungs. This can cause breathing problems when you lie down. Fluids can also collect in other parts of the body, swelling the feet, ankles, legs, and abdomen.

Your Health Care Team

Because heart failure is complex, a team of health care professionals is needed for special skills and expertise.

By working with your health care team in learning how to treat your condition, you may live longer and also improve the quality of your life.

Health care providers on the team may include

- Your primary care doctor—the doctor you normally see for health problems. General internists or family physicians normally provide primary care.
- A cardiologist, if your primary care doctor believes a heart specialist is needed.
- Other doctors, such as surgeons and other specialists, if needed and recommended by your primary care doctor or cardiologist.
- Clinical nurse specialists and nurse practitioners, who care for you and are sources of information, education, and counsel.
- Other health care professionals, including physician's assistants, nurses, dietitians, physical and occupational therapists, pharmacists, case managers, social workers, and other mental health professionals.

You and your family are important parts of this health care team. Before seeing other members of the health care team, write down your questions. Mark anything in this booklet you don't understand or would like to know more about. Using the list and this booklet, ask your health care provider questions. Tell him or her how you feel about your care.

Be involved in management of your condition.

How Your Heart's Chambers and Valves Work

Understanding how your heart works will help you understand the reasons behind the treatment plan your health care team designs for you. The more you know, the more you can be involved.

Blood moves through four chambers (two atriums and two ventricles) in the heart before circulating through the body. With each heartbeat, blood returns from the body through the veins, enters one of the chambers—the right atrium—and moves through the valve into the right ventricle below it. At the same time, blood from the lungs that is rich in oxygen enters the left atrium on the other side of the heart. From the left atrium, the blood passes through a valve into the left ventricle.

Next, the right ventricle contracts after getting blood from the right atrium, sending blood to the lungs to get oxygen. At the same time, the left ventricle contracts after getting blood from the left atrium. When the left ventricle contracts, it pumps blood through the aorta to arteries in all parts of the body.

The heart has four valves. Two prevent blood from flowing back between the atriums and ventricles. The other two valves prevent blood from flowing backward from the arteries and into the ventricles.

Normally, the left ventricle pumps one-half or more of the blood in it with each beat. With heart failure, the left ventricle cannot contract strongly enough, pumping two-fifths or less of the blood in it with each beat.

Diagnosis and Evaluation

Your health care team will want to know

- About your symptoms and how long you've had them.
- If you have ever had a heart attack, a heart murmur, or other heart problems. If so, how are these problems being treated?
- About your general health history and status. What other health problems do you have, and how are they being treated? Are your diet, activities, or exercise restricted? Have family members had heart problems?
- About your lifestyle and health habits. What is your daily life like? What do you do to prevent health problems?
- If you use tobacco, alcohol, or illegal drugs.

Be honest and candid. Information you share with health care providers is confidential. Evaluating, treating, and managing heart failure depends on accurate information, including facts that only you and your family can provide.

A health history, physical exam, chest x-ray, and electrocardiogram (called ECG or EKG) help diagnose heart failure.

Based on your symptoms and first test results, a test is needed to measure the amount of blood pumped from the heart with each beat (the ejection fraction). Patients with suspected heart failure should undergo echocardiography or radionuclide ventriculography to measure the ejection fraction.

Echocardiography uses sound waves to make images of the heart and its chambers. The procedure is safe and does not require entering the body with any instruments or devices.

Radionuclide ventriculography is a special test that tracks very low doses of a radioactive substance as it travels through the heart. The radioactive substance is safe and completely leaves the body.

A normal heart pumps one-half (50 percent) or more of the blood in the left ventricle with each heartbeat. With heart failure, the weakened heart may pump two-fifths (40 percent) or less, and less blood is pumped with less force to all parts of your body.

Managing Heart Failure

To manage heart failure, follow the instructions of your health care team. You may reduce symptoms and improve how you feel if you take medicines as prescribed and change how you live.

Work with your health care team to make the best choices and set goals to keep life interesting and enjoyable.

Your management plan consists of

- Medicines
- Diet
- Daily activities
- Exercise
- Lifestyle and health habits
- Family support

If you do not want to change how you live or take medicines as prescribed, tell your health care provider. Explain your reasons to your health care provider.

Work with your health care team to learn how to treat your condition.

Medicines

Importance

Taking medicine every day is vital to treating heart failure. Depending on your symptoms and diagnosis, your doctor may start treatment by prescribing one medicine and then adding others later. Sometimes, treatment will begin with two or more medicines.

It may take several days or weeks to find the right doses of prescribed medicines. Be patient as you and your health care provider work together to find

- The right medicines for you
- The right amount of each one
- The best time of day to take each medicine

The benefits of these medicines will be lost or reduced if you do not take your medicines as prescribed. Skipping doses or not refilling a medicine's prescription can cause serious problems. Do not take more than the prescribed dose of any medicine.

Be sure to tell your health care provider about other health conditions you have and other medicines you take. These medicines include nonprescription medicines such as aspirin, antacids, and cold remedies.

Side Effects

Any medicine can have unplanned results. If you have any side effects, tell your health care provider right away. He or she can work with you to lessen bothersome effects. If the first medicines prescribed do not work as expected, others are available.

Ask your health care team about side effects caused by taking prescribed medicines with

- Other prescribed medicines
- Medicines you can buy without a doctor's prescription (such as aspirin, antacids, and cold remedies)
- Certain foods

Always report side effects to your health care provider. He or she will know what to do about side effects.

Common Kinds of Medicines

Medicines commonly prescribed for treating heart failure include

- ACE inhibitors (angiotensin-converting enzyme inhibitors) to make it easier for the heart to pump
- Diuretics, or "water pills," to help remove excess fluid and salt from the body
- Digitalis to strengthen each heartbeat, allowing more blood to be pumped

When other heart or health problems exist with heart failure, your doctor may prescribe additional medicines, such as drugs to lower blood pressure.

ACE Inhibitors

ACE inhibitors have been shown to help heart failure patients live longer and feel better. The drugs relax blood vessels and make it easier for the heart to pump. For some people, it may take weeks before they feel better from taking the medicine.

Depending on your initial diagnosis and evaluation, an ACE inhibitor may be the first medicine prescribed. Based on your symptoms, a diuretic and digitalis may be prescribed with the ACE inhibitor or added later.

Captopril, enalapril, lisinopril, and quinapril are generic names for ACE inhibitors now being used for heart failure. Others may be used in the future.

Although most patients take an ACE inhibitor without problems, some patients have side effects. They include

- Cough
- Dizziness
- Skin rash

Tell your health care provider if any of these symptoms occur.

ACE inhibitors may also produce high potassium levels and affect kidney function. Blood tests are needed to monitor these actions.

If you have any side effects, tell your health care provider right away.

Diuretics

By making you urinate more often, diuretics keep fluid from collecting in your feet, ankles, legs, and abdomen. Skipping doses can cause swelling in these parts of the body and shortness of breath when lying down or during physical activity.

The most commonly used diuretics are hydrochlorothiazide and furosemide (Lasix).

Regular use of some diuretics can lead to the body losing too much potassium and to other imbalances. Blood tests are needed to monitor these levels.

To replace lost potassium, you may have to

- Eat more foods rich in potassium, including bananas and raisins, and drink orange juice and other citrus juices.
- Take a prescribed potassium supplement.

Diuretics may also cause

- Leg cramps
- Dizziness or lightheadedness
- Incontinence (accidental urine leakage)

- Gout (a type of arthritis)
- Skin rash

Tell your health care provider if you have any of these symptoms. (Urinating more often is not a side effect. It is caused by the diuretic.)

Digitalis

Digitalis helps the heart pump more effectively and may improve your ability to exercise. Prescribed as digoxin or Lanoxin, digitalis is taken daily by many heart patients.

Digitalis has been proven safe for most patients. If too much digitalis is in your body, you may have

- Nausea, loss of appetite
- Mental confusion
- Blurred or yellow-colored vision
- Rapid, forceful heartbeat (palpitations)

Tell your health care provider right away if you have these side effects. Do not stop taking digitalis unless told to do so by your health care provider.

Keeping Track of Your Medicines

Having a system can help tell you when to take medicines, especially if you take several each day. Use the form in the back of this booklet each day to remind you

- Which medicines to take each day
- What each pill looks like
- When to take them
- When each medicine was taken

Make copies of the blank form in the back for future use. **Always carry with you a list giving the doses of each medicine you take.** In an emergency, this information can help medical workers help you.

Cost of Medicines

The retail cost of medicines varies greatly among different pharmacies. If cost is a problem, ask your health care provider or pharmacist if there is a lower cost and acceptable generic form of your medicine. You can also compare prices of different pharmacies and mail-order prescription services.

If needed, financial assistance may be available through social service agencies where you live. You also may qualify for help through programs established by drug companies.

Let your health care provider know if the cost of medicines is a problem. Your health care team can help you apply for assistance.

Diet

In addition to taking medicines, you must change and then monitor your diet. Because salt (sodium) causes fluid to build up in the body, you must restrict salt intake. If you do not, your feet, ankles, legs, and abdomen may swell, and you may find it hard to breathe. If severe, these symptoms may require hospital treatment.

Your health care provider will tell you how much salt, if any, can be in your diet. You and your family may be asked to see a dietitian, nurse specialist, or other health educator for special diet instructions and counseling. They may also suggest new ways to prepare foods and how to modify family recipes. For example, lemon juice and many spices and herbs can add flavor to unsalted foods.

Be especially aware of foods with "hidden" salt such as frozen or canned foods, cheeses, and processed meats. Foods such as hot dogs, salami, and canned soups often contain a lot of salt. Check the nutrition labels for salt content.

If you drink alcoholic beverages, you may have to stop or have only one drink per day. One drink means a glass of beer or wine, or a mixed drink or cocktail containing no more than one ounce of alcohol.

Changing your diet can be complicated and confusing. The goal is to reduce salt, and possibly fat, in your food, without sacrificing the pleasure of eating. If you have trouble changing your diet, ask your health care team for help.

Watch your weight. Obtain an accurate scale and weigh yourself each morning after urinating, but before eating breakfast or dressing.

If you gain three to five pounds since last visiting your health care provider, tell him or her promptly. The weight gain may mean your body is retaining fluid.

Daily Activities

How heart failure affects you depends on how severe it is. Mild heart failure may have little effect on work or recreation. Severe heart failure may restrict what used to be easy. Talk to your health care team about

- Work. Can you still work? Full time or part time?
- Recreation. Can you go hiking, play golf, swim, and attend sporting events?
- Leisure. Can you travel, work in the garden, and do volunteer work?
- Sex. Can you have sexual intercourse?

Involve your family members in discussions about activities. They need to know how to support and help you. This is especially true when what you can do changes over time. Some activities (such as work or recreation) may become more difficult while others do not change.

Do not be afraid of discussing private aspects of your life. Your health care team must rely on what you say to help reduce symptoms and improve the quality of your life.

> Heart failure means you may have to change your lifestyle and health habits.

As you learn to live with heart failure, you may discover new satisfactions and pleasures. Changes to daily life can be positive and rewarding. Work restrictions may lead to interesting and enjoyable leisure activities. Recreation may become a valuable part of daily life. Sexual relations can be very enjoyable as you and your partner discover less demanding ways to express and share affection.

Exercise

Exercise regularly within your doctor's guidelines. Many people with heart failure say they feel better when they exercise regularly. Usually, you can exercise safely at home or in a supervised rehabilitation setting such as a hospital, health club, recreation center, YMCA, or YWCA.

Exercise includes

- Walking
- Cycling
- Swimming
- Low-impact aerobic routines

Your health care provider will advise you about the right kind and amount of exercise. Find out before starting. You may be asked to see a cardiac rehabilitation specialist to help plan and monitor an exercise program. Also, you may need an exercise stress test to see how much you can do safely.

Lifestyle and Health Habits

Your lifestyle reflects attitudes and values. Health habits involve what you do to reduce chances of illness or injury. Heart failure means you may have to change your lifestyle and health habits.

Examine your lifestyle and health habits. The following changes can reduce the symptoms of heart failure and improve the quality of your life:

- Lose weight if you are overweight
- Do not smoke or chew tobacco
- Eliminate or reduce alcohol
- Do not use illegal drugs

You should also

- Avoid exercise that exceeds your exercise guidelines
- Avoid coming in contact with people who have colds
- Get a flu and pneumonia shot

You may want to make other changes too, such as learning how to reduce stress. Work with your health care team to decide which choices are best.

Family Support

Your family can be a great source of support and encouragement. As much as possible, include family members in all decisions that affect you. These decisions involve your lifestyle and your ability to work and earn a living. Support by family members can be especially important as you adjust to lifestyle changes and if you face emotional difficulties. Let family members know how they can help.

Family members can help you

- Keep track of medicines
- Prepare special meals
- Exercise
- Find more information on treating heart failure
- Join a support group

The diagnosis of heart failure may affect your family as much as you. Family support can help you change your lifestyle and health habits.

Chest Pain (Angina)

Some people have chest pain (angina) in addition to heart failure symptoms. Angina is caused by blockage in the coronary arteries. When angina is a symptom, a test called cardiac angiography (heart catheterization with angiography) may be needed.

In this diagnostic procedure, fluid is injected into the coronary arteries through a long, thin tube called a catheter. Special x-rays show where and how much arteries are blocked. Ask your health care provider about expected benefits and risks of the procedure before agreeing to it.

The results of cardiac angiography are usually used to help health care providers plan your care. Treatment may include surgery. Cardiac angiography may not be needed if you do not want heart surgery. Ask your health care provider how information from the procedure will affect your care.

Heart Surgery

If a heart valve problem or coronary artery disease is suspected as the cause of your heart failure, you may be asked to consider heart surgery. Detailed information should be provided. You should know what may result from heart surgery. You should know its

- Benefits
- Risks, including the risks of doing nothing
- Alternatives, including their benefits and risks
- Total cost and how much is paid by insurance

Before deciding to have surgery, ask for a second opinion from another health care provider. Health insurance often requires a second opinion before surgery.

If heart surgery is a realistic choice for you, seek an experienced surgeon and hospital for the surgery. Ask for information about their success rates and costs before selecting a surgeon and hospital.

Heart Valve Surgery

Repairing or replacing one or more heart valves may be needed if heart failure is caused by heart valve problems. This surgery is common and has proven to be successful in many cases.

Coronary Artery Bypass Graft Surgery and Angioplasty

Coronary artery bypass graft (CABG) surgery is major surgery. In it, veins or arteries from other parts of the body are used to bypass blocked coronary arteries on the heart to restore more normal blood flow to the heart. As a muscle, the heart needs its own blood supply for nourishment so it can pump blood throughout the body.

An alternative to CABG surgery is angioplasty (or PTCA, percutaneous transluminal coronary angioplasty). In this major procedure, a catheter (long, thin tube) is inserted into the arteries on the heart. Inflating the small balloon on the catheter's tip expands the coronary artery and crushes the blockage, restoring blood flow.

Current research indicates that CABG surgery may benefit many people with angina (chest pain) and worsening heart failure resulting from coronary artery disease. The long-term benefits of angioplasty for such patients have not been established by research.

After heart surgery, you must follow a plan for managing and monitoring your heart health.

Heart Transplant Surgery

Heart transplantation is considered only in cases of very severe heart failure. Heart transplants are only performed in specialized centers.

Monitoring Your Progress

Managing heart failure requires keeping track of symptoms and monitoring how well you follow instructions of your health care team. Report changes in your health to your health care provider.

Your Responsibilities

As part of your health care team, you should

- Monitor your general health and report any changes in how you feel.
- Report changes in your symptoms.
- Take medicines as prescribed and report any side effects.
- Follow your guidelines for activities and exercise, and report when you are not able to do an activity or exercise easily.
- Follow a prescribed diet.
- Report any sudden weight changes.

Family Responsibilities

Your family is part of your health care team. Ask family members for help in monitoring your condition. They should know when to report new symptoms, or a change in symptoms, to your health care provider if you do not.

When calling the health care provider's office, your family should

- Say you are being treated for heart failure.
- Describe your symptoms.
- Describe what has already been done to bring relief or comfort.
- Give the names and amounts of medicines you take.

The Future

Ask your primary care doctor to explain how heart failure is likely to affect your life. Many people adjust to limits imposed by heart failure and still lead active lives.

Although a sudden change in symptoms is not expected, certain activities may become harder because you are tired and short of breath. If your symptoms do change suddenly, call your health care provider right away.

Emergencies

In an emergency, such as if your heart or breathing stops, acceptance of medical care and treatment is assumed. However, you have a right to accept or refuse any medical care and treatment in advance. You can direct that you do not want emergency medical workers to restore the heartbeat or use special equipment to breathe for you.

Specific instructions for family members and others may be needed so they will know how to react in a medical emergency. A legal document called an advance directive lets others know what to do in a medical emergency. This document states what life-saving measures you want taken if you cannot think clearly or speak for yourself.

Advance directives include these legal documents:

- Living wills
- Medical durable power of attorney
- "No cardiopulmonary resuscitation (CPR)" instructions
- Substitute decision makers (medical proxies)

If you do not have an advance directive, discuss your medical care and treatment wishes with your family and health care team before preparing one. Ask your health care team or attorney for more information about advance directives. These decisions may be difficult. Your health care team will help you understand how these decisions may affect you. Individual state laws govern the content and use of advance directives.

Support Groups and Counseling

Diagnosis of heart failure can generate a wide range of feelings. You and your family should express these feelings to your health care team. Seek help in dealing with feelings that cause problems.

In addition to professional counseling, local support groups can be a source of help. These groups offer the chance for you to talk about your feelings with other heart patients and families during regular meetings. Support groups may also offer educational programs about heart problems.

Ask your health care team about support groups where you live. If no support group exists, your health care team may help you start one.

Many people adjust to limits imposed by heart failure and still lead active lives.

For more information about support groups for heart patients and their families, contact

The Mended Hearts, Inc.
7272 Greenville Avenue
Dallas, TX 75231
(214) 706-1442

The Coronary Club, Inc.
9500 Euclid Avenue, E-37
Cleveland, OH 44195
(216) 444-3690

Additional Resources

If you want more information about heart failure and its treatment, bookstores and your local public library have helpful books and articles about the subject. Hospitals and health care providers may also have booklets, brochures, videotapes, and audiotapes about heart failure for patients. You may also contact

The American Heart Association
7272 Greenville Ave
Dallas, TX 75231-4596
(800) AHA-USA1 (242-8721)

National Heart, Lung, and Blood Institute Information Center Public Health Service
PO Box 30105
Bethesda, MD 20824
(301) 251-1222

For More Information

Information in this booklet was taken from *Heart Failure: Evaluation and Care of Patients With Left-Ventricular Systolic Dysfunction: Clinical Practice Guideline.* The guideline was developed by a private, non-federal expert panel of physicians, nurses, pharmacists, and consumers. Development of the guideline was sponsored by the Agency for Health Care Policy and Research (AHCPR), an agency of the U.S. Public Health Service. Other guidelines on common health problems have been issued and are under development for release in the future.

For more information on guidelines and to receive more copies of this booklet, call toll free (800) 358-9295 or write to

AHCPR Publications Clearinghouse
PO Box 8547
Silver Spring, MD 20907

■ **Document Source:**
U.S. Department of Health and Human Services, Public Health Service
Agency for Health Care Policy and Research
Executive Office Center, Ste 501
2101 E Jefferson St
Rockville, MD 20852
AHCPR Publication No. 94-0614
June 1994

See also: Facts about Heart Failure (page 234)

RECOVERING FROM HEART PROBLEMS THROUGH CARDIAC REHABILITATION

The Keys to Heart Health

- **Exercise:** Regular physical activity that is tailored to your abilities, needs, and interests.
- **Education:** Learning about your heart problem, its causes and treatments, and how you can manage it.

- **Counseling:** Advice on why and how to change your lifestyle to lower your risk of further heart problems.
- **Behavior change:** Learning specific skills to enable you to stop unhealthy behaviors such as smoking or to begin healthy behaviors such as eating a heart-healthy diet.

Purpose of this Booklet

Cardiac rehabilitation (rehab) services are designed to help patients with heart disease recover faster and return to full and productive lives. Cardiac rehab includes exercise, education, counseling, and learning ways to live a healthier life. Together with medical and surgical treatments, cardiac rehab can help you feel better and live a healthier life. You can benefit from cardiac rehab if you

- Have heart disease, such as angina or heart failure, or have had a heart attack
- Have had coronary bypass surgery or a balloon catheter (PTCA) procedure on your heart
- Have had a heart transplant

Cardiac rehab can make a difference. It is a safe and effective way to help you

- Feel better faster
- Get stronger
- Reduce stress
- Reduce the risks of future heart problems
- Live longer

Almost everyone with heart disease can benefit from some type of cardiac rehab. No one is too old or too young. Women benefit from cardiac rehab as much as men.

This booklet can help you learn how to lower your risk for future heart problems. You will also learn tips for finding a cardiac rehab plan that is right for you.

Most important, you will learn what you can do to be healthier.

When you have heart disease, breaking old habits and learning new ones can be stressful. Wondering about your future health can be stressful, too. But the support of family and friends, as well as health care providers, can make a big difference in how well you adjust to these changes. Share this booklet with others so they will learn about cardiac rehab and how they can help you.

Risk Factors for Coronary Disease

The controllable risk factors for coronary disease are shown below. There are some risk factors that you cannot change, such as older age or a family history of heart disease. But you *can* change or control the ones shown below. Cardiac rehab can help you do this.

Coronary Disease Risk Factors You Can Control

- Smoking
- High blood pressure
- High blood cholesterol
- Sedentary lifestyle
- Overweight
- Diabetes
- Stress

The Cardiac Rehab Team

Cardiac rehab services can involve many health care providers. Your team may include

- Doctors (your family doctor, a heart specialist, perhaps a surgeon)
- Nurses
- Exercise specialists
- Physical and occupational therapists
- Dietitians
- Psychologists or other behavior therapists

Sometimes a primary care provider, such as your family doctor or nurse practitioner, works alone, playing many roles, or refers patients to other health care specialists as needed.

But the most important member of your cardiac rehab team is you. No one else can make you exercise. Or quit smoking. Or eat a more healthful diet.

To be an active member of the cardiac rehab team:

- Learn about your heart condition.
- Learn what you can do to help your heart.
- Follow the treatment plan.
- Feel free to ask questions.
- Report symptoms or problems.

A support network can help you. Your support network may be family, friends, or a group of other people with heart problems.

Family members and friends can make a difference. They may want to learn more about heart problems so their help can be even more valuable. For example, family members may have to learn to let you do things for yourself. Or they may want to learn about preparing heart-healthy meals. Your family and friends can give you emotional support as you adjust to a new, healthier lifestyle.

You may also want the support of other people who have heart disease. Ask your cardiac rehab team if they know of a support group you can join, or get in touch with one of the organizations listed in the back of this booklet.

How do I get started?

Cardiac rehab often begins in the hospital after a heart attack, heart surgery, or other heart treatment. It continues in an outpatient setting after you leave the hospital. Once you learn the habits of heart-healthy living, stick with them for life.

- **In an outpatient setting.** Outpatient rehab may be located at the hospital, in a medical or professional center, in a community facility such as the YMCA, or at your place of work. You may even have cardiac rehab at home. You will be advised to increase the amount of exercise you do. You will also receive education and encouragement to control your risk factors.
- **For life.** After you have learned the skills of heart-healthy living, you should continue to use them for life.

You need your doctor's approval to get started in cardiac rehab. Tell your doctor or nurse that you're interested in cardiac rehab and ask which rehab services or plans are best for you.

How does cardiac rehab work?

Cardiac rehab has two major parts:

1. Exercise training to help you learn how to exercise safely, strengthen your muscles, and improve your stamina. Your exercise plan will be based on your individual ability, needs, and interests.
2. Education, counseling, and training to help you understand your heart condition and find ways to reduce your risk of future heart problems. The cardiac rehab team will help you learn how to cope with the stress of adjusting to a new lifestyle and to deal with your fears about the future.

Cardiac rehab often takes place in groups. However, each patient's plan is based on his or her specific risk factors and special needs.

Cardiac rehab helps you recognize and change unhealthy habits you may have and establish new, more healthy ones. Your rehab may last six weeks, six months, or even longer. It is important that you complete the recommended rehab plan.

No matter how difficult it seems, your hard work in cardiac rehab will have lifetime benefits.

Is it safe for me?

Cardiac rehab is safe. Studies show that serious health problems caused by cardiac rehab exercise are rare. The cardiac rehab team is trained to handle emergencies. Your health care provider can help you choose a plan that is safe for you. Many patients can safely exercise without supervision once they learn their own exercise plan.

Checking how your heart reacts and adapts to exercise is an important part of cardiac rehab. You may be connected to an EKG transmitter while you exercise. If your cardiac rehab is done at home, you may be connected to an EKG machine by telephone, or you may phone the cardiac rehab team to let them know how you are doing. In some settings, you check your own pulse rate or estimate how hard you are exercising.

What's in it for me?

The goals of cardiac rehab are different for each patient. In helping set your personal goals, your health care team will look at your general health, your personal heart problem, your risks for future heart problems, your doctor's recommendations, and, of course, your own preferences.

Cardiac rehab can reduce your symptoms and your chances of having more heart problems. And it has many other benefits:

- Exercise tones your muscles and improves your energy level and spirits. It helps both your heart and your body get stronger and work better. Exercise also can get you back to work and other activities faster.
- A healthy diet can lower blood cholesterol, control weight, and help prevent or control high blood pressure and other problems such as diabetes. Plus, you will feel better and have more energy.
- Cardiac rehab can help you quit smoking. Kicking the habit means less risk of lung cancer, emphysema, and bronchitis, as well as less risk of heart attack, stroke, and other heart and blood vessel problems. It means more energy, and it means better health for your loved ones.
- You can learn to manage stress instead of letting it manage you. You will feel better and improve your heart health.

Aerobic exercise raises your pulse rate and makes you perspire. It helps improve the flow of oxygen-rich blood throughout your body.

Strength training, such as using weights, improves your muscle strength and your stamina.

Both types of exercise in the right amount are safe and important for your heart health.

Make a habit of the heart-healthy lifestyle you learn in cardiac rehab. Your life depends on it!

How do I find a plan that's right for me?

Your doctor or nurse may recommend a cardiac rehab plan or help you to arrange for exercise training, education, counseling, and other services. Many hospitals and outpatient health care centers offer cardiac rehab so do some local schools and community centers. You can also check the Yellow Pages of your telephone book.

When choosing a cardiac rehab plan, ask about

- **Time.** Is it offered when you can get there without causing added stress? Cardiac rehab services offered at the workplace are sometimes an option.
- **Place.** Is it easy to get to? Keep in mind that traffic problems can add to your stress. Is there parking? Public transportation?
- **Setting.** Is it an individual or group plan? Is it home-based or in a facility? Think about whether you want to be in a group with professional supervision.
- **Services.** Does it offer a wide range of services? More importantly, does it include the areas you need help with, such as quitting smoking?
- **Cost.** Is it affordable? Is it covered by insurance? Your insurance may cover all or part of the cost of some

cardiac rehab services but not others. Find out what will be covered and for how long. Consider what you can afford and for how long.

Cardiac rehab has life-long favorable effects, so choose a plan that will serve your needs. For example, if you smoke, look for a plan that will help you quit. Choose a plan that includes activities you enjoy, such as regular walking in a shopping mall or park. Before you sign up, visit and ask any questions you may have.

How can I get the most out of cardiac rehab?

Studies show that controlling your risk factors for heart disease can help you lead a healthier life. So make sure your cardiac rehab plan works for you. Here's how:

- **Plan.** Work with your health care team to design or change your services to meet your needs.
- **Communicate.** Ask questions. If you don't understand the answers, keep asking until you do. Report changes in your feelings or symptoms.
- **Take charge of your recovery.** No one else can do it for you. Your new lifestyle is healthy for your heart, so stick with it for life.

To gain more control over your cardiac rehab, remember your goals and keep important information where you can find it. You may want to have a special calendar just for your rehab activities or keep a notebook.

Sometimes people who have big changes in their lives feel depressed. Some people with heart problems feel depressed when they find out about their disease or after surgery. Cardiac rehab may help you feel better, but if you are seriously depressed, you will need additional help. When you are depressed, it is hard to do things to help yourself get better, such as going to cardiac rehab or getting back to your usual activities. If you are depressed, tell your doctor. Depression can be treated. Information on a patient guide about depression is given at the end of this document.

Where can I get more information and support?

For additional information about heart disease and ways you can help yourself through cardiac rehab, contact:

American Association of Cardiovascular and Pulmonary Rehabilitation (national program directory)
(608) 831-7561

American Heart Association (patient education materials)
800-AHA-USA1 (800-242-8721)

Mended Hearts, Inc. (patient support group)
(214) 706-1442

National Heart, Lung, and Blood Institute (patient education materials)
(301) 251-1222

For Further Information

The information in this booklet is based on the *Clinical Practice Guideline on Cardiac Rehabilitation*. The guideline was developed by a non-federal panel of experts sponsored by the Agency for Health Care Policy and Research (AHCPR), a U.S. Government agency. Additional support came from the National Heart, Lung, and Blood Institute. Other guidelines on common health problems are available from AHCPR, and more are being developed.

Three other patient guides available from AHCPR may be of interest to people participating in cardiac rehab:

- *Managing Unstable Angina* (AHCPR Publication No. 94-0604).
- *Living With Heart Disease: Is It Heart Failure?* (AHCPR Publication No. 94-0614).
- *Depression Is a Treatable Illness* (AHCPR Publication No. 93-0553).

For more information about these and other guidelines, or to get more copies of this booklet, call toll free: 800-358-9295 or write to:

Agency for Health Care Policy and Research Publications Clearinghouse
PO Box 8547
Silver Spring, MD 20907

These and other guidelines are available online through a free electronic service from the National Library of Medicine called HSTAT.

Copies of this brochure and other consumer brochures are free through InstantFAX, which operates all day every day. If you have a fax machine equipped with a touchtone telephone, dial (301) 594-2800, push 1, and then press the start button for instructions and a list of publications.

■ **Document Source:**
U.S. Department of Health and Human Services, Public Health Service
Agency for Health Care Policy and Research
Executive Office Center, Ste 501
2101 E Jefferson St
Rockville, MD 20852
AHCPR Publication No. 96-0674
October 1995

INFECTIOUS DISEASES

■ ■ ■

CHRONIC FATIGUE SYNDROME

The Centers for Disease Control and Prevention (CDC) is actively engaged in Chronic Fatigue Syndrome research. This document reflects current and reliable information. At this time, CDC is not equipped to handle counseling but suggests that you call your nearest support group.

General Description

Chronic Fatigue Syndrome, or CFS, is characterized by persistent and debilitating fatigue and additional nonspecific symptoms such as sore throat, headache, tender muscles, joint pains, difficulty thinking, and loss of short-term memory. On physical examination, patients may have nonspecific findings such as low-grade fever and redness in the throat, but frequently no abnormalities are found. No laboratory test or panel of tests is available to diagnose CFS, so the diagnosis is made solely on clinical grounds. The cause of CFS is unknown.

In some individuals, CFS appears to develop after an acute illness like influenza or infectious mononucleosis, both of which usually resolve within a few months, or after periods of unusual stress. In other persons, however, CFS appears to develop gradually with no precipitating event. Symptoms are usually most severe early in the course of illness. Later in the illness, periods of partial improvement may be followed by relapses or recovery. While some patients have recovered after several months of illness, others have remained ill for many years. The average duration and full clinical picture of CFS over time is unknown. The degree to which CFS patients are disabled varies widely. Some patients continue to function at home and at work, although at a reduced level of activity, while others become severely disabled and cannot perform many of the routine activities of daily living.

CFS affects females and males, and adolescents as well as adults. Most reported cases, however, have occurred in young to middle-aged adults with females diagnosed more frequently than males. It is unclear to what extent these demographic characteristics reflect biases among reported cases. CFS does not appear to be directly transmissible from person to person, and there is no justification for CFS patients to be isolated. No deaths from CFS have been reported.

Epidemiologic studies of CFS have not documented clear and consistent risk factors.

The total number of persons with CFS in the United States is unknown. CDC has conducted surveillance for CFS in four cities across the United States since 1989. Preliminary analysis of the first three years of data indicates that, in these sites, two to seven adults out of 100,000 have CFS. These figures, or prevalence rates, are based upon persons who meet all of the criteria in the CFS research case definition, which was published in the Annals of Internal Medicine in 1988. Because this case definition was deliberately designed to be restrictive for purposes of research, these prevalence rates probably represent low estimates. They should not be used to estimate the overall number of CFS patients in the rest of the United States because the cities chosen for CFS surveillance were not selected randomly.

Case Definition of CFS

In 1987, a panel of experts met at CDC in order to define chronic fatigue syndrome for research purposes. The criteria chosen to define CFS cases were deliberately selected to be restrictive in order to facilitate research. The goal of the case definition was to identify CFS patients who were relatively similar in terms of their illness. The case definition was not designed to diagnose all persons with CFS or to process CFS-associated disability claims. This research case definition, which was published in March 1988 in the Annals of Internal Medicine, essentially requires

1. the presence of new and debilitating persistent or relapsing fatigue for at least six months, and
2. the exclusion, by medical examination and laboratory testing, of other clinical conditions (including psychiatric disorders) that may also cause prolonged fatigue, and
3. the presence of a combination of eight or more symptom and physical sign criteria during six or more months of illness. The symptom criteria are mild fever, sore throat, painful lymph nodes, generalized muscle weakness, muscle aches, prolonged fatigue following exercise, generalized headaches, joint pains, various nervous system complaints, sleep alterations, and development of the symptom com-

plex over a few hours to a few days. The physical examination criteria are low-grade fever, an inflamed pharynx without pus, and enlarged lymph nodes.

Diagnostic Evaluation

Severe persistent fatigue and other CFS symptoms can be associated with many other illnesses. These illnesses include underlying major depression and anxiety disorders, autoimmune diseases such as systemic lupus erythematosus, malignancies such as ovarian cancer, lymphoma or leukemia, infectious diseases such as endocarditis, hepatitis, syphilis, or AIDS, and a variety of other diseases such as anemia, diabetes, and diseases of the thyroid, heart, lungs, liver, kidneys, gastrointestinal tract, and endocrine system.

The exclusion of other possible diseases as a cause of CFS symptoms is the most important part of the diagnostic evaluation. Since many of these diseases can be treated or managed appropriately following diagnosis, and since some of these conditions can be progressive or even fatal if untreated, it is absolutely imperative that a thorough medical evaluation be done before a diagnosis of CFS is made.

The role of laboratory and radiologic testing in the diagnostic workup of CFS is to exclude other possible diseases. There are no laboratory tests currently available, including tests for infections, tests for activation of the body's natural defenses against infection, or tests for immune function, that can identify CFS. In particular, tests for Epstein-Barr virus, or EBV, human T-cell lymphotropic virus type-II, or HTLV-II, human spumavirus, and immunologic abnormalities should not be used to diagnose CFS. Such tests do not distinguish people with CFS from healthy people and are expensive. Some physicians have reported finding brain abnormalities in CFS patients using radiologic tests such as magnetic resonance imaging, known as MRI scans, or nuclear medicine brain scans such as PET or SPECT scans. The meaning of these findings is unknown. They are not unique to CFS and are not found in all CFS patients. Therefore, MRI and nuclear medicine scans, which are very expensive, should not be routinely used to diagnose CFS. These radiologic scans should only be used, when clinically warranted, to exclude the possibility of another brain disease.

CDC cannot recommend specific physicians for referral. Our general recommendation is to contact the county medical society, closest university, or a local CFS patient support group for a referral to an internist, infectious disease specialist, or other physician who is knowledgeable about CFS.

Possible Causes of CFS

The cause of CFS is unknown. It is also unknown whether or not CFS is a single illness or a group of different illnesses that share common symptoms. A number of theories about the underlying cause or causes of CFS have been proposed. Some theories have focused on possible underlying viral infections, while others have focused on possible underlying immunologic, hormonal, neurologic, and psychological dysfunc-

tion. Some of the more prominent theories are discussed in more detail.

Possible Viral Causes

Epstein-Barr virus, or EBV, which is the virus that causes mononucleosis, was widely thought to be responsible for CFS in the 1980s. Later studies, however, indicated that EBV was not the cause of CFS. Most adults have antibody to EBV, and a positive test for EBV, even at a high level of antibody, does not diagnose CFS. In addition to EBV, several other viruses have been proposed as possible causes of CFS, including cytomegalovirus, Coxsackie B virus, adenovirus type 1, and human herpesvirus 6 or HHV-6. Although it is possible that viral infections play a role in causing CFS in some patients, none of these viruses has been consistently associated with CFS. More recently, there have been reports suggesting associations between CFS and human retroviruses. These reports, which suggested that CFS may be associated with human spumavirus and viruses like human T-cell lymphotropic virus type-II, received a great deal of attention and generated a great deal of excitement. Since then, however, three published studies have failed to verify an association between CFS and any known human retroviruses. At present, there does not appear to be an association between human retroviruses and CFS. The only role for retroviral testing in the diagnosis of CFS should be to exclude the possibility of infection with human immunodeficiency virus, or HIV.

Possible Immunologic Causes

Several subtle immunologic abnormalities have been described in some patients with CFS. Results of immunologic studies as a whole have been confusing, and the results of some published findings are in conflict. Recently, a panel of distinguished immunologists and virologists from the National Chronic Fatigue Syndrome Advisory Council issued an official statement regarding immunologic and virologic aspects of chronic fatigue syndrome. In their statement, the following points were made:

1. No test is diagnostic for CFS.
2. There is evidence of immune abnormalities in CFS studies, which suggests a pattern of chronic immune activation. However, similar findings can be found in other chronic disorders such as chronic infections, autoimmune disorders, and allergies.
3. Among the most frequently identified abnormalities are the following: chronic activation of T-cells, decreased function of natural killer cells, reduction of subsets of CD8 positive suppressor cells, and increased levels of antibody to Epstein-Barr virus early antigen.
4. Other immune abnormalities have been inconsistently reported. These include: failure to respond to skin tests, deficiencies of immunoglobulin subclasses, and abnormal CD4 and CD8 numbers and ratios.

Recently, researchers at the National Institutes of Health reported finding slightly lower percentages of naive CD4

T-cells circulating in the blood of CFS patients than in controls.

The significance of these reported immunologic abnormalities is uncertain, but to keep these reports in perspective, the following points should be kept in mind. While it is possible that immunologic abnormalities may be part of the process that causes CFS, these abnormalities may also represent nonspecific immune changes that occur as part of many chronic diseases. It is clear, however, that severe suppression of the immune system, such as that seen in AIDS, does not occur in CFS. The opportunistic infections common to AIDS are not seen in CFS.

Possible Psychological Causes

The role of psychological factors and psychiatric diseases in causing CFS is highly controversial and particularly difficult to study. It is clear that psychiatric disease, and especially depression, is frequently found in individuals with persistent fatigue and among patients referred for evaluation for CFS. Approximately half of the individuals referred to the CDC's CFS surveillance system have evidence of psychiatric illness, which was present before the start of their CFS symptoms. It is also clear that CFS patients commonly experience depression or anxiety sometime during the course of their illness.

These kinds of findings have led some researchers to conclude that CFS is one specific manifestation of underlying psychiatric illness. Other researchers, however, point out that many patients who develop CFS do not have evidence of prior psychiatric disease and that the depression or anxiety that develops after the start of CFS symptoms may be a part of the CFS disease process or simply a natural reaction to any chronic illness.

Treatment

Treatment for CFS should be initiated only after the possibility of another disease has been excluded as thoroughly as possible. No medication has been shown to be effective for curing CFS in well conducted clinical trials. The current standard of treatment is to treat the symptoms of CFS.

Most experts begin by recommending a regimen of adequate rest, balanced diet, and physical conditioning. Moderate exercise is generally helpful to minimize loss of physical conditioning, but patients should take care to avoid over-exertion since this can lead to relapses of severe fatigue and other symptoms. Nonsteroidal anti-inflammatory medications can be useful for treating headaches and muscle and joint pains. Since all medications can have side effects, a physician should be consulted for specific recommendations regarding drugs.

Among the numerous medications claimed to be effective for treating CFS are a variety of antiviral and immune system modulating drugs, vitamins, and holistic remedies. While some of these treatments may be of benefit to some patients, other treatments are expensive, are of no proven use, and are potentially harmful to the patient. If you are in doubt about a specific therapy, one or more reputable physicians in your area should be consulted.

Acyclovir and gamma globulin are two medications that have undergone rigorous clinical testing in CFS patients. Acyclovir, which is usually used to treat herpes infections, was shown to be no more effective than a placebo in treating CFS patients. Gamma globulin, which is composed of antibodies pooled from many individuals, was tested in two trials. One trial conducted in the United States showed no benefit. The other trial, conducted in Australia, showed minimal benefit, but this benefit was lost after the trial ended. Currently, two other medications, cortisol and ampligen, are undergoing controlled trials.

For Further Information

There are several national and local nonprofit support groups for persons with chronic fatigue syndrome. These groups publish periodic newsletters, provide lists of interested physicians, and facilitate contact between affected persons. The CDC does not endorse these organizations or their published information but provides the names and addresses of the two largest national organizations for further information. These are

1. The National CFS Association, 919 Scott Avenue, Kansas City, KS 66105. Tel. (913) 321-2278.
2. The CFIDS Association, Community Health Services, PO Box 220398, Charlotte, NC 28222-0398. Tel. (704) 362-2343

■ Document Source:
U.S. Department of Health and Human Services, Public Health Service
Centers for Disease Control and Prevention
Date last revised: March 9, 1995

DIPHTHERIA, TETANUS, AND PERTUSSIS VACCINE (DTP)

About the Diseases

Diphtheria, tetanus (lockjaw), and pertussis (whooping cough) are serious diseases. Diphtheria and pertussis spread when germs pass from an infected person to the nose or throat of others. Tetanus is caused by a germ that enters the body through a cut or wound.

Diphtheria causes

- a thick coating in the nose, throat, or airway

It can lead to

- breathing problems
- heart failure
- paralysis
- death

Tetanus causes

- serious, painful spasms of all muscles

It can lead to

- "locking" of the jaw so the patient cannot open his or her mouth or swallow
- death

Pertussis causes

- coughing and choking for several weeks (makes it hard for infants to eat, drink, or breathe)

It can lead to

- pneumonia
- seizures (jerking and staring spells)
- brain damage
- death

About the Vaccines

Benefits of the Vaccines

Vaccination is the best way to protect against diphtheria, tetanus, and pertussis. Because most children get the vaccines, there are now many fewer cases of these diseases. There would be many more cases if we stopped vaccinating children.

DTP

Most children should have a total of five DTP vaccines. They should have DTP at:

- two months of age
- four months of age
- six months of age
- 12 to 18 months of age
- four to six years of age

Other vaccines may be given at the same time as DTP.

Related Vaccines

DTaP (Diphtheria Tetanus acellular Pertussis)

- Like DTP, it prevents diphtheria, tetanus, and pertussis.
- It is only given for the fourth and fifth doses.
- It is less likely to cause the mild problems we see after DTP and is probably less likely to cause some of the moderate problems.

DT (Diphtheria Tetanus)

- Unlike DTP, it does not prevent pertussis. For this reason, it is usually not recommended.

Who should get DTP vaccine?

Most doctors recommend that almost all young children get DTP or DTaP vaccine. Some children should get DT. With all vaccines, there are some cautions.

Tell your doctor or nurse if the child getting the vaccine

- ever had a serious allergic reaction or other problem after getting DTP, DTaP, or DT
- now has moderate or severe illness
- has ever had a seizure
- has a parent, brother, or sister who has had seizures
- has a brain problem that is getting worse

If you are not sure, ask your doctor or nurse.

What are the risks from these vaccines?

As with any medicine, there are very small risks that serious problems, even death, could occur after getting a vaccine.

The risks from the vaccine are **much smaller** than the risks from the diseases if people stopped using vaccine.

Below is a list of problems that may occur after getting the vaccine. *If your child ever had one of the moderate or severe problems listed below or any other serious problem after DTP, DTaP, or DT, discuss it with your doctor or nurse before this vaccination.*

Mild Problems

If these problems occur, they usually start within hours to a day or two after vaccination. They usually last up to one to two days:

- soreness, redness, or swelling where the shot was given
- fever
- fussiness, drowsiness, less appetite

Acetaminophen or ibuprofen (nonaspirin) may be used to prevent or reduce fever and soreness. This is especially important for children who have had seizures or have a parent, brother, or sister who has had seizures.

Moderate Problems

Once for every 100 to 1,000 doses:

- on-going crying for three hours or more
- fever of 105 or higher
- an unusual, high-pitched cry

Once for every 1,750 doses:

- a seizure (jerking and staring spell) usually caused by fever
- "shock-collapse" (becomes pale, limp, and less alert)

Severe Problems

These problems happen **very rarely**:

- serious allergic reaction after DT or DTP
- a long seizure
- decreased consciousness or coma. Some of these children may have lasting brain damage. There is disagree-

ment about whether or not DTP causes the lasting brain damage. If it does, it is very rare.

What to Do If There Is a Serious Reaction

- Call a doctor or get the person to a doctor right away.
- Write down what happened and the date and time it happened.
- Ask your doctor, nurse, or health department to file a Vaccine Adverse Event Report form or call (800) 822-7967 (toll-free).

The National Vaccine Injury Compensation Program gives compensation (payment) for persons thought to be injured by vaccines. For details, call (800) 338-2382 (toll-free).

If you want to learn more, ask your doctor or nurse. She/he can give you the vaccine package insert or suggest other sources of information.

■ **Document Source:**
U.S. Department of Health and Human Services, Public Health Service
Centers for Disease Control and Prevention

FIRST VACCINE FOR CHICKENPOX

by Isadora B. Stehlin

The days when nearly everyone spent a week of their childhood with the itchy, miserable rash of chickenpox may be on the wane. Last March 17, the Food and Drug Administration licensed a new vaccine, Varivax (varicella virus vaccine live). Commonly known as the chickenpox vaccine, it will prevent the typical cases of itchy, uncomfortable, week-long rashes and mild fevers, and the rarer cases of serious illness caused by the virus.

Although chickenpox is generally mild and not normally life-threatening, the Centers for Disease Control and Prevention estimates that there are 9,300 chickenpox-related hospitalizations and 50 to 100 deaths annually, mainly among young children.

Before receiving approval from FDA, researchers tested Varivax in about 11,000 children and adults. Scientists predict that it will be 70 to 90 percent effective in preventing the disease. Of those who did get chickenpox after vaccination, almost all had a mild form of the disease.

Adverse reactions to the vaccine were generally mild and included pain, rash, hardness, and swelling at the injection site, fever, and generalized rashes.

Mary L. Kumar, MD, chief of pediatric infectious diseases at MetroHealth Clinic in Cleveland, tested the vaccine on about 500 children and 200 adults in the Cleveland area. She says the vaccine trials were very easy to recruit for. "We actually had people calling us," Kumar explains, adding that there was not only great interest from parents who wanted to spare their children from the disease but also from adults in health-care professions who were concerned about getting chickenpox themselves and about infecting susceptible patients.

Will it last?

Throughout the development of the chickenpox vaccine, there has been concern about whether the vaccine would confer lifetime immunity or simply delay infection until adulthood. When adults get chickenpox, the cases are usually more severe and the risk of complications such as pneumonia greater.

"Over the period of time it's been looked at carefully, which is about five years, we're not able to find evidence for substantial waning in immunity," says Philip Krause, MD, senior research investigator in FDA's Center for Biologics Evaluation and Research. "It's complicated to determine how long immunity lasts, because right now people who are vaccinated are exposed to children who have [naturally acquired] chickenpox and they presumably are getting a booster effect from those repeated exposures."

"Longer is more difficult to tell," says Krause. "The only way to sort that out is going to be to see what happens after the vaccine is introduced." At FDA's request, Merck will follow several thousand vaccinated children for 15 years to determine the long-term effects of the vaccine and possible need for a booster immunization.

Shingles

As with the question of immunity, more time is needed to answer another question about the vaccine—will it cause shingles in adulthood?

Shingles is the second act of chickenpox. Once someone has had chickenpox, the virus doesn't die, it simply becomes dormant. It lingers in the body's nerve cells next to the spinal cord. Then, for reasons still not definitely known, but possibly related to a weakened immune system, the virus reactivates and infects nerve fibers, causing severe pain, burning, or itching. Because weakened immunity often accompanies aging, shingles usually occurs after age 50.

Can the chickenpox vaccine, which is a weakened form of the live virus, cause shingles?

"Nobody's sure what the effect will be," says Krause. "We really don't have the data to say what's going to happen in 20 to 30 years. Based on our knowledge of how the virus works and the data available so far, it doesn't appear that the rate of shingles cases in vaccinated individuals will be any greater than in the naturally infected population. There's some data in children who were immunocompromised that suggests that the vaccine may reduce the likelihood of shingles over the short term. But more data are required to determine the effect of the vaccine on shingles in healthy individuals over a lifetime."

Just One or Two Shots

A single injection of the vaccine is recommended for children ages 12 months to 12 years, while two injections four to eight weeks apart are recommended for adolescents and adults who have never had chickenpox.

"We're not really sure why teens and adults don't get immunity with one shot," says Krause. "The immune response to a single shot if you're 13 or older is not nearly as good as it is if you're younger. But two shots provide immune responses comparable to what younger people get."

For children, the vaccine has been shown to be safe and effective and can be administered at the same time as the measles, mumps, and rubella vaccine. (The MMR vaccine is given at 15 months and again between four and six years or before junior high or middle school. See "Kids' Vaccinations Get a Little Easier," in the March 1994 *FDA Consumer.*) Public health officials hope that being able to give the chickenpox vaccine along with an already scheduled vaccine will encourage vaccination.

Vaccine Development

Varivax's development began with a sample of varicella (chickenpox) virus isolated from the blood of a three-year-old Japanese boy in 1972. Japanese researcher Michiaki Takahashi, MD, attenuated (weakened) the virus by growing it in different human and animal host cells. He then tested the weakened virus in children as a vaccine against chickenpox.

His tests were successful, and in 1981, Merck obtained the rights to use the "Oka" strain (named after the three-year-old boy) to develop its own vaccine.

Merck began clinical trials of the vaccine for safety and effectiveness. But obtaining successful test results was only half the battle for Merck to bring the vaccine to market. Making enough vaccine to meet demand was the other.

Unlike other weakened live viruses used for vaccines that spontaneously emerge from cultivated cells, varicella stays in the cell.

"In the case of varicella, we have to collect the infected cells and then break them open," explains Barry D. Garfinkle, PhD, Merck's vice president for vaccine quality operations. "We do this using an ultrasonic device."

The ultrasound creates heat and, in this case, creates problems. Although the varicella virus is extremely virulent in its natural environment inside the human host, once it's removed from the infected cells in the lab, "varicella is very, very sensitive to elevated temperatures," says Garfinkle.

"We have to use the right amount of [ultrasound] to get the virus freed but not so much that we damage the virus," says Garfinkle. "Getting those parameters correct took us a while."

To this end, Merck built a new facility in West Point, PA, where robots handle most of the vaccine production. Garfinkle explains that using robots allows for better control of the exacting ultrasound procedure.

Merck submitted data on Varivax's safety and effectiveness to FDA in May 1993.

In January 1994, FDA's Vaccines and Related Biological Products Advisory Committee concluded that the vaccine was safe and effective. But the committee advised FDA to address several questions before making a final decision, including how to address whether vaccinating children would shift the disease to adults and whether doctors could give Varivax at the same time as other vaccines.

In January 1995, FDA presented to the committee clinical data from the manufacturer resolving those issues.

Easy to Catch

An estimated 3.7 million Americans get chickenpox each year, with more than 90 percent of cases in people younger than 15.

Chickenpox is transmitted through fluid from broken blisters and through coughing or sneezing. A person is contagious for one or two days before the rash appears until all the lesions are dried, which usually takes four to five days. The average incubation period (the time between exposure to the virus and the onset of illness) is 10 to 21 days.

Those at greatest risk for a serious case of chickenpox are people age 13 and older, and anyone with impaired immunity. Chickenpox can also be serious for fetuses and newborn babies. When a woman breaks out in chickenpox just before or after delivery, her baby may develop a severe form of the disease; as many as five percent of these babies die. Infection early in pregnancy may cause the fetus to develop limb abnormalities, scarring of internal organs, or damage to the central nervous system.

In addition, "there are a fair number of complications that require hospitalization of otherwise healthy children," says Kumar.

That was the case for Brittany Evans (not her real name). The only risk factor for the healthy two-and-half-year-old was her five-year-old sister's routine bout with chickenpox two weeks before.

"Frequently in a family, the second and third cases can be more severe," explains Kumar. Siblings generally spend more time with each other than with friends and schoolmates, and this gives the virus the opportunity to infect siblings when it's most virulent.

Brittany's chickenpox broke out on Friday, March 10. By the next Wednesday, she was covered with blisters and running a fever of almost 105 degrees Fahrenheit.

"She had [blisters] between her fingers so bad she couldn't get her fingers side by side," says her mother. "I couldn't rub my hand along her tummy and find a spot that didn't have a blister."

Brittany was admitted to Shady Grove Hospital in Gaithersburg, MD, on March 17 (ironically, the same day the vaccine was licensed). She spent three days there to make sure she didn't become dangerously dehydrated from the high fever. Her body's own defenses finally overcame the virus, and she recovered.

On April 10, the American Academy of Pediatrics recommended the vaccine for all healthy children between the ages of 12 months and 13 years who have not had chickenpox. For children between 12 and 18 months, the academy recommends giving the chickenpox vaccine at the same time as the first measles, mumps, and rubella shot. Older children should be vaccinated at the earliest convenient time.

While some doctors still question the need for vaccinating against a generally mild disease, Kumar agrees with the academy's recommendations because of the need to prevent unforeseen complications and hospitalizations.

Brittany's mom isn't a medical expert, but she says, "I never want to go through this again. My husband and I are thinking about having another child, and I'll get the next one the vaccine, without a doubt."

Treating Chickenpox

Public health officials don't know yet how many children will be vaccinated, since the chickenpox vaccine isn't required for school admission at this time.

In otherwise healthy children and adults, the disease should be allowed to run its course. But that doesn't mean the symptoms should be ignored. Calamine lotion applied to the lesions may offer some relief from the infamous itch of the chickenpox rash. Soaking in a cornstarch, baking soda, or oatmeal bath may also do the trick. However, because any relief is at best temporary, doctors advise parents to cut children's nails very short, since scratching can lead to secondary skin infection by bacteria on the skin, such as staphylococcus ("staph") and permanent scarring. A daily bath with soap is also recommended to clean as much bacteria off the skin as possible.

A nonaspirin pain reliever and fever reducer such as acetaminophen (Datril, Tempra, Tylenol, and others) can ease headaches, fever, or general malaise. Aspirin or any medication that contains aspirin or salicylates should never be used because of the risk of Reye syndrome, a rare but serious illness that typically strikes children and teenagers just as they appear to be recovering from the flu or chickenpox.

If a doctor visit is necessary, pediatricians usually make special arrangements to see children who might have chickenpox to avoid exposing others.

"They might see [those children] after hours or when the office isn't busy," says Mary L. Kumar, MD, a pediatrician in Cleveland. Although diagnosis may be possible over the phone, "I like to take a look myself," she says. "Over the phone can be pretty accurate if other children in the family just had chickenpox. But there are many other rashes that can look somewhat like the varicella [chickenpox] rash, so I don't think it's easy over the phone to be certain."

During the course of the infection, the doctor should be called if the patient's temperature goes above 102 degrees Fahrenheit (39 degrees Celsius) or any fever lasts longer than four days, or if areas of the rash become very red, warm, or tender, which may signal a bacterial infection requiring antibiotics.

In February 1992, FDA approved the use of oral Zovirax (acyclovir) to treat chickenpox in otherwise healthy children. (FDA had already approved the drug to treat genital herpes and shingles.) When a patient receives oral Zovirax within 24 hours after the rash appears, the number of lesions are reduced, and average recovery time is shortened approximately one day.

However, the American Academy of Pediatrics does not recommend the use of oral Zovirax in otherwise healthy children. The academy says the medication's relief of chickenpox symptoms is minimal; it's extremely difficult to start it during the first 24 hours; and there is a potential for unforeseen dangers when treating large numbers of children who are at low risk of developing complications. The academy recommends use of oral Zovirax only in people at high risk for severe chickenpox or complications, including

- healthy nonpregnant teenagers and adults
- children over one year who have chronic skin or lung disorders, or who must take aspirin daily for conditions such as arthritis
- children taking corticosteroids for conditions such as asthma.

A biological product that actually prevents infection is available for people at high risk. But the product, varicella-zoster immune globulin, or VZIG (doctors pronounce it "vee-zig"), must be administered within 96 hours of exposure, long before symptoms appear. And it serves little purpose to the otherwise healthy population because VZIG gives only temporary protection.

VZIG is prepared from the plasma of normal blood donors who have high levels of antibodies to the varicella virus, which causes chickenpox. It confers a "passive" immunization that lasts only about three months.

The Centers for Disease Control and Prevention recommend VZIG for the following:

- high-risk individuals who have no immunity to chickenpox
- immunocompromised children and adults
- newborns whose mothers came down with chickenpox five days before to two days after delivery
- premature infants exposed after birth.

VZIG may be recommended for mothers who are exposed during the first trimester. However, taking VZIG at this time only benefits the mother's health. There is no indication that VZIG can prevent the birth defects associated with the chickenpox virus.

Those at highest risk for complications are not candidates for the chickenpox vaccine. (Healthy teenagers and adults, who are considered at high risk for chickenpox complications simply because of their age, can get the vaccine.)

"People who have compromised immune systems are more likely to get worse reactions to the vaccine because it is a live virus," says FDA's Philip R. Krause, MD. "The hope is that if enough healthy children get the vaccine, there will be less natural chickenpox floating around, and [high-risk] people will not be exposed."

■ **Document Source:**
U.S. Department of Health and Human Services, Public Health Service
Food and Drug Administration
FDA Consumer
September 1995

HOW TO AVOID THE FLU

by Evelyn Zamula

Though flu is expected to make its usual rounds this winter, many Americans won't have to suffer its high fever, characteristic cough, and possibly serious complications. A safe, effective vaccine is available.

It was not always so.

In 1918-1919—during the worst flu epidemic of all time—doctors had meager resources to fight the disease. To relieve symptoms, they relied on aspirin and other simple remedies. An influenza vaccine and antibiotics to combat pneumonia and other flu complications were years away from development. It has been estimated that over 20 million people died, and possibly half the world's population came down with the flu in this global epidemic, or pandemic.

Influenza epidemics spread quickly through large populations because flu viruses are highly contagious. During flu's acute phase, respiratory tract secretions are rich in infectious virus and the disease is transmitted easily by sneezing and coughing. The incubation period lasts one to three days. Then symptoms—such as chills and fever that develop within 24 hours, headache often accompanied by sensitivity to light, sore muscles, backache, weakness, and fatigue—appear suddenly. Respiratory tract symptoms may be mild at first, with a dry, unproductive cough, scratchy sore throat, and runny nose. As the person's temperature rises—sometimes to as high as 104 degrees Fahrenheit—the muscle aches and headache get worse, and secondary bacterial infections, such as bronchitis and pneumonia, may move in. Ear infections are a common complication in children.

With no complications, acute symptoms usually subside after two or three days and the fever ends, although it may last as long as five days. Weakness and fatigue may persist for several weeks.

Vaccine Most Important Defense

Today, we have several ways to defend people from influenza. The most important tool is immunization by a killed virus vaccine. Flu vaccines are licensed by FDA, and the exact composition of the vaccine varies each year, depending on the flu strains scientists expect to be most common.

Influenza viruses have the ability to change themselves, or mutate, thereby becoming different viruses. Having the flu once does not confer lasting immunity, as is the case with some childhood viral diseases. The antibodies people produce in response to the one flu virus don't recognize and, therefore, don't provide immunity to a different flu virus. Because the immunity conferred by a flu shot lasts for only about a year—and because different flu strains may circulate each season—individuals who want to be protected from flu should be vaccinated annually.

It takes two to four weeks for antibodies to develop after the vaccine is given. Therefore, the ideal time to get the flu vaccine is mid-October to mid-November, before the start of the flu season, which lasts from about December to March in the Northern Hemisphere. (Travelers should be aware that flu season lasts all year in some tropical climates and in the Southern Hemisphere occurs from April to September.)

Who should get vaccine?

Vaccination is available to anyone who wants it and whose doctor agrees it would be beneficial. The Public Health Service's Advisory Committee on Immunization Practices (ACIP) strongly recommends vaccination for

- People age 65 or older. (Effective May 1993, Medicare Part B pays for flu shots.)
- People over six months who have underlying medical conditions that put them at increased risk for flu complications. These include
  - chronic cardiovascular disorders or lung disease, including asthma in children.
  - chronic metabolic diseases requiring hospitalization during the preceding year or regular checkups. These diseases include diabetes, kidney disorders, blood disorders, and impaired immune systems due to HIV infection or chemotherapy.
- Residents of nursing homes and other facilities that provide care for chronically ill persons of any age.
- Children and teenagers (six months to 18 years of age) who have to take aspirin regularly and therefore may be at risk of developing Reye syndrome after influenza. (Children who have symptoms of flu or chickenpox should not be given products containing aspirin or other salicylates without consulting a doctor.)

To reduce the risk of transmitting flu to high-risk persons, such as the elderly, transplant patients, and people with AIDS (who may have low antibody response to the flu vaccine)—and also to protect themselves from infection—ACIP recommends vaccination for doctors, nurses, hospital employees, employees of nursing homes and chronic-care facilities, visiting nurses, and home-care providers. Students, police, firefighters, and other essential workers and community service providers may also find vaccination useful.

In most cases, children at high risk for influenza complications may receive the flu vaccine when they receive other routine vaccinations, including DTP (diphtheria, tetanus, and pertussis) and pneumococcal vaccines. Pregnant women who have a high-risk condition should be immunized regardless of the stage of pregnancy; healthy pregnant women may also want to consult their health care providers about being vaccinated.

Side Effects

The flu vaccine cannot cause flu because it contains only inactivated viruses. Any respiratory disease that appears immediately after vaccination is coincidental. However, the vaccine may have some side effects, especially in children who have not been exposed to the flu virus in the past.

The most commonly reported side effect in children and adults is soreness at the vaccination site that lasts up to two days. Fever, malaise, sore muscles, and other symptoms may begin six to 12 hours after vaccination and may last as long as two days.

People should be aware that they may test HIV-positive with the ELISA test after a recent flu shot, says the national Centers for Disease Control and Prevention. CDC recommends retesting with the more accurate Western Blot test to rule out false positives.

The vaccine is not for everyone. People allergic to eggs—the vaccine is made from highly purified, egg-grown viruses that have been made noninfectious—or other vaccine components should consult a doctor before getting a flu shot because they may develop hives, allergic asthma, difficulty breathing, and other allergic symptoms. The vaccine should not be given to any person ill with a high fever until the fever and other symptoms have abated.

Drugs Help Some People

For these individuals, and persons expected to develop low levels of antibodies in response to the influenza vaccine because they have impaired immune systems, influenza-specific antiviral drugs can be used for prevention during the flu season or after infection to relieve influenza symptoms.

The antiviral agents Symmetrel (amantadine), approved by FDA in 1976, and Flumadine (rimantadine), a chemically similar drug approved by FDA in September 1993, are safe and effective in preventing signs and symptoms of infection caused by various strains of the influenza A virus in children over one, healthy adults, and elderly patients. These drugs may also be used for family members or close contacts of influenza A patients and for elderly nursing home patients who have been vaccinated but may need added protection. When a vaccine is expected to be ineffective because an epidemic is caused by strains other than those covered by the vaccine, antiviral drugs may be used to provide protection.

Either drug may be used following vaccination during a flu epidemic to provide protection during the two- to four-week period before antibodies develop. If an adult has already come down with the flu, treatment with Symmetrel or Flumadine has been shown to reduce symptoms and shorten the illness if administered within 48 hours after symptoms appear. Children with the flu can be treated with Symmetrel.

About 5 to 10 percent of people who take Symmetrel experience nausea, dizziness, and insomnia. There have been reports of more serious neurological adverse events, including seizures and aggravations of psychiatric illnesses. Flumadine has similar side effects, but at a lower rate.

Though many flu victims use over-the-counter preparations, such as decongestants and fever reducers, to make them feel more comfortable, none of these products affects the course of the disease.

Prevention Worthwhile

Every year, about 20 percent of the U.S. population may become infected with flu, although each flu season is different. About 1 percent of those infected will require hospitalization because of complications, mostly bacterial pneumonia. Among those hospitalized, as many as 8 percent may die—about 20,000 people in an average year. But the 1957-1958 "Asian flu" caused 70,000 deaths and the 1968-1969 "Hong Kong flu" carried off 34,000. The toll is usually greatest among the elderly.

The economic costs run high, too. From 15 million to 111 million workdays are lost each year, depending on the severity of the epidemic. Added to that are the costs of over-the-counter and prescription medicines, physician visits, hospitalization, and lost productivity.

It's no contest between the cost of a flu shot and the physical and other costs exacted by a bad case of the flu. A yearly vaccination early in the flu season is the best way to avoid this miserable disease.

■ **Document Source:**
U.S. Department of Health and Human Services, Public Health Service
Food and Drug Administration
FDA Consumer Magazine
November 1994

MEASLES, MUMPS, AND RUBELLA VACCINE (MMR)

About the Diseases

Measles, mumps, and rubella (German measles) are serious diseases. They spread when germs pass from an infected person to the nose or throat of others.

Measles causes

- rash
- cough
- fever

It can lead to

- ear infection
- pneumonia
- diarrhea
- seizures (jerking and staring spells)
- brain damage
- death

Mumps causes

- fever
- headache
- swollen glands under the jaw

It can lead to

- hearing loss
- meningitis (infection of brain and spinal cord coverings)
- Males can have painful, swollen testicles.

Rubella causes

- rash
- mild fever
- swollen glands arthritis (mostly in women)
- Pregnant women can lose their babies.

Babies can be born with birth defects such as

- deafness
- blindness
- heart disease
- brain damage
- other serious problems

About the Vaccines

Benefits of the Vaccines

Vaccination is the best way to protect against measles, mumps, and rubella. Because most children get the MMR vaccines, there are now many fewer cases of these diseases. There would be many more cases if we stopped vaccinating children.

MMR Schedule

Most children should have a total of two MMR vaccines. They should have MMR at

- 12 to 15 months of age
- four to six years of age or before middle school or junior high school

Other vaccines may be given at the same time as MMR.

Who should get MMR vaccine?

Most doctors recommend that almost all young children get MMR vaccine. But there are some cautions. Tell your doctor or nurse if the person getting the vaccine is less able to fight serious infections because of

- a disease she/he was born with
- treatment with drugs such as long-term steroids
- any kind of cancer
- cancer treatment with x-rays or drugs

Also:

- People with AIDS or HIV infection usually *should get* MMR vaccine.
- Pregnant women should wait until after pregnancy for MMR vaccine.
- People with a serious allergy to eggs or the drug neomycin should tell the doctor or nurse. If you are not sure, ask the doctor or nurse.

Tell your doctor or nurse if the person getting the vaccine

- ever had a serious allergic reaction or other problem after getting MMR
- now has moderate or severe illness
- has ever had a seizure

- has a parent, brother, or sister who has had seizures
- has gotten immune globulin or other blood products (such as a transfusion) during the past several months

If you are not sure, ask your doctor or nurse.

What are the risks from MMR vaccine?

As with any medicine, there are very small risks that serious problems, even death, could occur after taking a vaccine.

The risks from the vaccine are much smaller than the risks from the diseases if people stopped using vaccine.

Almost all people who get MMR have no problems from it.

Mild or Moderate Problems

- Soon after the vaccination, there may be soreness, redness, or swelling where the shot was given.
- one to two weeks after the **first** dose, there may be
  - rash (five-15 out of every 100 doses)
  - fever of 103 or higher (five-15 out of every 100 doses). This usually lasts one to two days.
  - swelling of the glands in the cheeks, neck, or under the jaw.
  - a seizure (jerking and staring spell) usually caused by fever. This is rare.
- one to three weeks after the **first** dose, there may be
  - pain, stiffness, or swelling in one or more joints lasting up to three days (one out of every 100 doses in children; up to 40 out of every 100 doses in young women). Rarely, pain or stiffness lasts a month or longer, or may come and go; this is most common in young and adult women. Acetaminophen or ibuprofen (non-aspirin) may be used to reduce fever and soreness.

Severe Problems

These problems happen **very rarely:**

- serious allergic reaction
- low number of platelets (a type of blood cell) that can lead to bleeding problems. This is almost always temporary.
- long seizures, decreased consciousness, or coma

Problems following MMR are much less common after the **second** dose.

What to Do if There Is a Serious Reaction

- Call a doctor or get the person to a doctor right away.
- Write down what happened and the date and time it happened.
- Ask your doctor, nurse, or health department to file a Vaccine Adverse Event Report form or call (800) 822-7967 (toll-free).

The **National Vaccine Injury Compensation Program** gives compensation (payment) for persons thought to be injured by vaccines. For details call (800) 338-2382 (toll-free).

If you want to learn more, ask your doctor or nurse. She/he can give you the vaccine package insert or suggest other sources of information.

■ **Document Source:**
U.S. Department of Health and Human Services, Public Health Service
Centers for Disease Control and Prevention

POLIO VACCINE

About the Disease

Polio is a serious disease. It spreads when germs pass from an infected person to the mouths of others. Polio can

- Paralyze a person (make arms and legs unable to move)
- Cause death

About the Vaccines

Benefits of the Vaccines

Vaccination is the best way to protect against polio. Because most children get the polio vaccines, there are now very few cases of this disease. Before most children were vaccinated, there were thousands of cases of polio.

There are two kinds of polio vaccine.

OPV, or Oral Polio Vaccine, is the one most often given to children. It is given by mouth as drops. It is easy to give and works well to stop the spread of polio.

IPV or Inactivated Polio Vaccine is given as a shot in the leg or arm.

OPV Schedule

Most children should have a total of four OPV vaccines. They should have OPV at

- two months of age
- four months of age
- six to 18 months of age
- four to six years of age

Other vaccines may be given at the same time as OPV.

Who should get OPV?

Most doctors recommend that almost all young children get OPV. But there are some cautions. Tell your doctor or nurse if the person getting the vaccine or anyone else in close contact with the person getting the vaccine is less able to fight serious infections because of

- a disease she/he was born with
- treatment with drugs such as long-term steroids
- any kind of cancer

- cancer treatment with x-rays or drugs
- AIDS or HIV infection

If so, your doctor or nurse will probably give IPV instead of OPV.

If you are older than age 18 years, you usually do not need polio vaccine.

Travel

If you are traveling to a country where there is polio, you should get either OPV or IPV.

Pregnancy

If protection is needed during pregnancy, OPV or IPV can be used.

Allergy to Neomycin or Streptomycin

Does the person getting the vaccine have an allergy to the drugs neomycin or streptomycin? If so, she/he should get OPV, but not IPV. Ask your doctor or nurse if you are not sure.

Tell your doctor or nurse if the person getting the vaccine

- ever had a serious allergic reaction or other problem after getting polio vaccine
- now has moderate or severe illness

If you are not sure, ask your doctor or nurse.

What are the risks from polio vaccine?

As with any medicine, there are very small risks that serious problems, even death, could occur after getting a vaccine.

The risks from the vaccine are **much smaller** than the risks from the disease if people stopped using vaccine.

Almost all people who get polio vaccine have no problems from it.

Risks from OPV

Risks to the person taking OPV:

There is a very small chance of getting polio disease from the vaccine.

- about one case occurs for every one and a half million first doses
- about one case occurs for every 30 million later doses

Risks to people who never took polio vaccine who have close contact with the person taking OPV:

After a person gets OPV, it can be found in his or her mouth and stool. If you never took polio vaccine, there is a very small chance of getting polio disease from close contact with a child who got OPV in the past 30 days. (Examples of close contact include changing diapers or kissing.)

- about one case occurs for every two million first doses
- about one case occurs for every 15 million later doses

Talk to your doctor or nurse about getting IPV.

Risks from IPV

This vaccine is not known to cause problems except mild soreness where the shot is given.

What to Do If There Is a Serious Reaction

- Call a doctor or get the person to a doctor right away.
- Write down what happened and the date and time it happened.
- Ask your doctor, nurse, or health department to file a Vaccine Adverse Event Report form or call (800) 822-7967 (toll-free).

The National Vaccine Injury Compensation Program gives compensation (payment) to persons thought to be injured by vaccines. For details, call (800) 338-2382 (toll-free).

If you want to learn more, ask your doctor or nurse. She/he can give you the vaccine package insert or suggest other sources of information.

■ **Document Source:**
   U.S. Department of Health and Human Services, Public Health Service
   Centers for Disease Control and Prevention

THE RISE OF ANTIBIOTIC-RESISTANT INFECTIONS

by Ricki Lewis, PhD

When penicillin became widely available during the Second World War, it was a medical miracle, rapidly vanquishing the biggest wartime killer—infected wounds. Discovered initially by a French medical student, Ernest Duchesne, in 1896, and then rediscovered by Scottish physician Alexander Fleming in 1928, the product of the soil mold *Penicillium* crippled many types of disease-causing bacteria. But just four years after drug companies began mass-producing penicillin in 1943, microbes began appearing that could resist it.

The first bug to battle penicillin was *Staphylococcus aureus*. This bacterium is often a harmless passenger in the human body, but it can cause illness, such as pneumonia or toxic shock syndrome, when it overgrows or produces a toxin.

In 1967, another type of penicillin-resistant pneumonia, caused by *Streptococcus pneumoniae* and called pneumococcus, surfaced in a remote village in Papua New Guinea. At about the same time, American military personnel in southeast Asia were acquiring penicillin-resistant gonorrhea from prostitutes. By 1976, when the soldiers had come home, they brought the new strain of gonorrhea with them, and physicians had to find new drugs to treat it. In 1983, a hospital-acquired intestinal infection caused by the bacterium *Enterococcus faecium* joined the list of bugs that outwit penicillin.

Antibiotic resistance spreads fast. Between 1979 and 1987, for example, only 0.02 percent of pneumococcus strains infecting a large number of patients surveyed by the national Centers for Disease Control and Prevention (CDC) were penicillin-resistant. CDC's survey included 13 hospitals in 12 states. Today, 6.6 percent of pneumococcus strains are resistant, according to a report in the June 15, 1994, *Journal of the American Medical Association* by Robert F. Breiman, M D, and colleagues at CDC. The agency also reports that in 1992, 13,300 hospital patients died of bacterial infections that were resistant to antibiotic treatment.

Why has this happened?

"There was complacency in the 1980s. The perception was that we had licked the bacterial infection problems. Drug companies weren't working on new agents. They were concentrating on other areas, such as viral infections," says Michael Blum, MD, medical officer in the Food and Drug Administration's division of anti-infective drug products. "In the meantime, resistance increased to a number of commonly used antibiotics, possibly related to overuse of antibiotics. In the 1990s, we've come to a point for certain infections that we don't have agents available."

According to a report in the April 28, 1994, *New England Journal of Medicine*, researchers have identified bacteria in patient samples that resist all currently available antibiotic drugs.

Survival of the Fittest

The increased prevalence of antibiotic resistance is an outcome of evolution. Any population of organisms, bacteria included, naturally includes variants with unusual traits—in this case, the ability to withstand an antibiotic's attack on a microbe. When a person takes an antibiotic, the drug kills the defenseless bacteria, leaving behind—or "selecting," in biological terms—those that can resist it. These renegade bacteria then multiply, increasing their numbers a millionfold in a day, becoming the predominant microorganism.

The antibiotic does not technically cause the resistance, but allows it to happen by creating a situation where an already existing variant can flourish. "Whenever antibiotics are used, there is selective pressure for resistance to occur. It builds upon itself. More and more organisms develop resistance to more and more drugs," says Joe Cranston, PhD, director of the department of drug policy and standards at the American Medical Association in Chicago.

A patient can develop a drug-resistant infection either by contracting a resistant bug to begin with, or by having a resistant microbe emerge in the body once antibiotic treatment begins. Drug-resistant infections increase risk of death and are often associated with prolonged hospital stays, and sometimes complications. These might necessitate removing part of a ravaged lung or replacing a damaged heart valve.

Bacterial Weaponry

Disease-causing microbes thwart antibiotics by interfering with their mechanism of action. For example, penicillin kills bacteria by attaching to their cell walls, then destroying a key part of the wall. The wall falls apart, and the bacterium dies. Resistant microbes, however, either alter their cell walls so penicillin can't bind or produce enzymes that dismantle the antibiotic.

In another scenario, erythromycin attacks ribosomes, structures within a cell that enable it to make proteins. Resistant bacteria have slightly altered ribosomes to which the drug cannot bind. The ribosomal route is also how bacteria become resistant to the antibiotics tetracycline, streptomycin, and gentamicin.

Antibiotic resistance can occur in three different ways:" spontaneous mutation of a bacterium's own genetic material (DNA), acquisition of DNA from another bacterium through transformation, and acquisition via plasmid transmission.

A Vicious Cycle

Though bacterial antibiotic resistance is a natural phenomenon, societal factors also contribute to the problem. These factors include increased infection transmission, coupled with inappropriate antibiotic use.

More people are contracting infections. Sinusitis among adults is on the rise, as are ear infections in children. A report by CDC's Linda F. McCaig and James M. Hughes, MD, in the Jan. 18, 1995, *Journal of the American Medical Association*, tracks antibiotic use in treating common illnesses. The report cites nearly six million antibiotic prescriptions for sinusitis in 1985 and nearly 13 million in 1992. Similarly, for middle ear infections, the numbers are 15 million prescriptions in 1985 and 23.6 million in 1992.

Causes for the increase in reported infections are diverse. Some studies correlate the doubling in doctor's office visits for ear infections for preschoolers between 1975 and 1990 to increased use of daycare facilities. Homelessness contributes to the spread of infection. Ironically, advances in modern medicine have made more people predisposed to infection. People on chemotherapy and transplant recipients taking drugs to suppress their immune function are at greater risk of infection.

"There are the number of immunocompromised patients, who wouldn't have survived in earlier times," says Cranston. "Radical procedures produce patients who are in difficult shape in the hospital, and are prone to nosocomial [hospital-acquired] infections. Also, the general aging of patients who live longer, get sicker, and die slower contributes to the problem," he adds.

Though some people clearly need to be treated with antibiotics, many experts are concerned about the inappropriate use of these powerful drugs. "Many consumers have an expectation that when they're ill, antibiotics are the answer. They put pressure on the physician to prescribe them. Most of the time the illness is viral, and antibiotics are not the answer. This larger burden of antibiotics is certainly selecting resistant bacteria," says Blum.

Another much-publicized concern is use of antibiotics in livestock, where the drugs are used in well animals to prevent disease, and the animals are later slaughtered for food. "If an animal gets a bacterial infection, growth is slowed and it doesn't put on weight as fast," says Joe Madden, PhD, strategic manager of microbiology at FDA's Center for Food Safety and Applied Nutrition. In addition, antibiotics are sometimes administered at low levels in feed for long durations to increase the rate of weight gain and improve the efficiency of converting animal feed to units of animal production.

FDA's Center for Veterinary Medicine limits the amount of antibiotic residue in poultry and other meats, and the U.S. Department of Agriculture monitors meats for drug residues. According to Margaret Miller, PhD, deputy division director at the Center for Veterinary Medicine, the residue limits for antimicrobial animal drugs are set low enough to ensure that the residues themselves do not select resistant bacteria in (human) gut flora.

FDA is investigating whether bacteria resistant to quinolone antibiotics can emerge in food animals and cause disease in humans. Although thorough cooking sharply reduces the likelihood of antibiotic-resistant bacteria surviving in a meat meal to infect a human, it could happen. Pathogens resistant to drugs other than fluoroquinolones have sporadically been reported to survive in a meat meal to infect a human. In 1983, for example, 18 people in four midwestern states developed multi-drug-resistant *Salmonella* food poisoning after eating beef from cows fed antibiotics. Eleven of the people were hospitalized, and one died.

A study conducted by Alain Cometta, MD, and his colleagues at the Centre Hospitalier Universitaire Vaudois in Lausanne, Switzerland, and reported in the April 28, 1994, *New England Journal of Medicine*, showed that increase in antibiotic resistance parallels increase in antibiotic use in humans. They examined a large group of cancer patients given antibiotics called fluoroquinolones to prevent infection. The patients' white blood cell counts were very low as a result of their cancer treatment, leaving them open to infection.

Between 1983 and 1993, the percentage of such patients receiving antibiotics rose from 1.4 to 45. During those years, the researchers isolated *Escherichia coli* bacteria annually from the patients and tested the microbes for resistance to five types of fluoroquinolones. Between 1983 and 1990, all 92 *E. coli* strains tested were easily killed by the antibiotics. But from 1991 to 1993, 11 of 40 tested strains (28 percent) were resistant to all five drugs.

Towards Solving the Problem

Antibiotic resistance is inevitable, say scientists, but there are measures we can take to slow it. Efforts are underway on several fronts—improving infection control, developing new antibiotics, and using drugs more appropriately.

Barbara E. Murray, MD, of the University of Texas Medical School at Houston writes in the April 28, 1994, *New England Journal of Medicine* that simple improvements in public health measures can go a long way towards preventing infection. Such approaches include more frequent hand washing by health care workers, quick identification and isolation of patients with drug-resistant infections, and improving sewage systems and water purity in developing nations.

Drug manufacturers are once again becoming interested in developing new antibiotics. These efforts have been spurred both by the appearance of new bacterial illnesses, such as Lyme disease and Legionnaire's disease, and resurgences of old foes, such as tuberculosis, due to drug resistance.

FDA is doing all it can to speed development and availability of new antibiotic drugs. "We can't identify new agents—that's the job of the pharmaceutical industry. But once they have identified a promising new drug for resistant infections, what we can do is to meet with the company very early and help design the development plan and clinical trials," says Blum.

In addition, drugs in development can be used for patients with multi-drug-resistant infections on an "emergency IND (compassionate us)" basis, if the physician requests this of FDA, Blum adds. This is done for people with AIDS or cancer, for example.

No one really has a good idea of the extent of antibiotic resistance, because it hasn't been monitored in a coordinated fashion. "Each hospital monitors its own resistance, but there is no good national system to test for antibiotic resistance," says Blum.

This may soon change. CDC is encouraging local health officials to track resistance data, and the World Health Organization has initiated a global computer database for physicians to report outbreaks of drug-resistant bacterial infections.

Experts agree that antibiotics should be restricted to patients who can truly benefit from them—that is, people with bacterial infections. Already this is being done in the hospital setting, where the routine use of antibiotics to prevent infection in certain surgical patients is being reexamined.

"We have known since way back in the antibiotic era that these drugs have been used inappropriately in surgical prophylaxis [preventing infections in surgical patients]. But there is more success [in limiting antibiotic use] in hospital settings, where guidelines are established, than in the more typical outpatient settings," says Cranston.

Murray points out an example of antibiotic prophylaxis in the outpatient setting—children with recurrent ear infections given extended antibiotic prescriptions to prevent future infections.

Another problem with antibiotic use is that patients often stop taking the drug too soon, because symptoms improve. However, this merely encourages resistant microbes to proliferate. The infection returns a few weeks later, and this time a different drug must be used to treat it.

Targeting TB

Stephen Weis and colleagues at the University of North Texas Health Science Center in Fort Worth reported in the April 28, 1994, *New England Journal of Medicine* on research they conducted in Tarrant County, Texas, that vividly illustrates how helping patients to take the full course of their medication can actually lower resistance rates. The subject—tuberculosis.

TB is an infection that has experienced spectacular ups and downs. Drugs were developed to treat it, complacency set in that it was beaten, and the disease resurged because patients stopped their medication too soon and infected others. Today, one in seven new TB cases is resistant to the two drugs most commonly used to treat it (isoniazid and rifampin), and 5 percent of these patients die.

In the Texas study, 407 patients from 1980 to 1986 were allowed to take their medication on their own. From 1986 until the end of 1992, 581 patients were closely followed, with nurses observing them take their pills. By the end of the study, the relapse rate—which reflects antibiotic resistance—fell from 20.9 to 5.5 percent. This trend is especially significant, the researchers note, because it occurred as risk factors for spreading TB—including AIDS, intravenous drug use, and homelessness—were increasing. The conclusion: Resistance can be slowed if patients take medications correctly.

The Greatest Fear—Vancomycin Resistance

When microbes began resisting penicillin, medical researchers, fought back with chemical cousins, such as methicillin and oxacillin. By 1953, the antibiotic armamentarium included chloramphenicol, neomycin, terramycin, tetracycline, and cephalosporins. But today, researchers fear that we may be nearing an end to the seemingly endless flow of antimicrobial drugs.

At the center of current concern is the antibiotic vancomycin, which for many infections is literally the drug of "last resort," says Michael Blum, MD, medical officer in FDA's division of anti-infective drug products. Some hospital-acquired staph infections are resistant to all antibiotics except vancomycin.

Now vancomycin resistance has turned up in another common hospital bug, enterococcus. And since bacteria swap resistance genes like teenagers swap T-shirts, it is only a matter of time, many microbiologists believe, until vancomycin-resistant staph infections appear. *"Staph aureus* may pick up vancomycin resistance from enterococci, which are found in the normal human gut," says Madden. And the speed with which vancomycin resistance has spread through enterococci has prompted researchers to use the word "crisis" when discussing the possibility of vancomycin-resistant staph.

Vancomycin-resistant enterococci were first reported in England and France in 1987 and appeared in one New York City hospital in 1989. By 1991, 38 hospitals in the United States reported the bug. By 1993, 14 percent of patients with enterococcus in intensive-care units in some hospitals had vancomycin-resistant strains, a 20-fold increase from 1987. A frightening report came in 1992, when a British researcher observed a transfer of a vancomycin-resistant gene from enterococcus to *Staph aureus* in the laboratory. Alarmed, the researcher immediately destroyed the bacteria.

Narrowing the Spectrum

Appropriate prescribing also means that physicians use "narrow spectrum" antibiotics—those that target only a few bacterial types—whenever possible, so that resistances can be restricted. The only national survey of antibiotic prescribing practices of office physicians, conducted by the National Center for Health Statistics, finds that the number of prescriptions has not risen appreciably from 1980 to 1992, but there has been a shift to using costlier, broader spectrum agents. This prescribing trend heightens the resistance problem, write McCaig and Hughes, because more diverse bacteria are being exposed to antibiotics.

One way FDA can help physicians choose narrower spectrum antibiotics is to ensure that labeling keeps up with evolving bacterial resistances. Blum hopes that the surveillance information on emerging antibiotic resistance from CDC will enable FDA to require that product labels be updated with the most current surveillance information.

Many of us have come to take antibiotics for granted. A child develops strep throat or an ear infection, and soon a bottle of "pink medicine" makes everything better. An adult suffers a sinus headache, and antibiotic pills quickly control it. But infections can and do still kill. Because of a complex combination of factors, serious infections may be on the rise. While awaiting the next "wonder drug," we must appreciate, and use correctly, the ones that we already have.

■ Document Source:
U.S. Department of Health and Human Services, Public Health Service
Food and Drug Administration
FDA Consumer
September 1995

TETANUS AND DIPHTHERIA VACCINE (Td)

About the Diseases

Tetanus (lockjaw) and diphtheria are serious diseases. Tetanus is caused by a germ that enters the body through a cut or wound. Diphtheria spreads when germs pass from an infected person to the nose or throat of others.

Tetanus causes

- serious, painful spasms of all muscles

It can lead to

- "locking" of the jaw so the patient cannot open his or her mouth or swallow

Diphtheria causes

- a thick coating in the nose, throat, or airway

It can lead to

- breathing problems
- heart failure
- paralysis
- death

About the Vaccines

Benefits of the Vaccines

Vaccination is the best way to protect against tetanus and diphtheria. Because of vaccination, there are many fewer cases of these diseases. Cases are rare in children because most get DTP (Diphtheria, Tetanus, and Pertussis), DTaP (Diphtheria, Tetanus, and acellular Pertussis), or DT (Diphtheria and Tetanus) vaccines. There would be many more cases if we stopped vaccinating people.

When should you get Td vaccine?

Td is made for people seven years of age and older.

People who have not gotten at least three doses of any tetanus and diphtheria vaccine (DTP, DTaP, or DT) during their lifetime should do so using Td. After a person gets the third dose, a Td dose is needed every 10 years all through life.

Other vaccines may be given at the same time as Td.

Tell your doctor or nurse if the person getting the vaccine:

- ever had a serious allergic reaction or other problem with Td, or any other tetanus and diphtheria vaccine (DTP, DTaP, or DT)
- now has a moderate or severe illness
- is pregnant

If you are not sure, ask your doctor or nurse.

What are the risks from Td vaccine?

As with any medicine, there are very small risks that serious problems, even death, could occur after getting a vaccine.

The risks from the vaccine are much smaller than the risks from the diseases if people stopped using vaccine.

Almost all people who get Td have no problems from it.

Mild Problems

If these problems occur, they usually start within hours to a day or two after vaccination. They may last one to two days:

- soreness, redness, or swelling where the shot was given

These problems can be worse in adults who get Td vaccine very often.

Acetaminophen or ibuprofen (non-aspirin) may be used to reduce soreness.

Severe Problems

These problems happen very rarely:

- serious allergic reaction.
- deep, aching pain and muscle wasting in upper arm(s). This starts two days to four weeks after the shot, and may last many months.

What to Do If There Is a Serious Reaction

- Call a doctor or get the person to a doctor right away.
- Write down what happened and the date and time it happened.

- Ask your doctor, nurse, or health department to file a Vaccine Adverse Event Report form or call (800) 822-7967 (toll-free)

The National Vaccine Injury Compensation Program gives compensation (payment) for persons thought to be injured by vaccines. For details call (800) 338-2382 (toll-free)

■ **Document Source:**
U.S. Department of Health and Human Services, Public Health Service
Centers for Disease Control and Prevention

See also: First Vaccine for Chicken Pox (page 252)

TUBERCULOSIS: GENERAL INFORMATION

Tuberculosis (TB) is a disease that is spread from person to person through the air. TB usually affects the lungs, but it can also affect other parts of the body, such as the brain, the kidneys, or the spine. TB germs are put into the air when a person with TB disease of the lungs or throat coughs or sneezes. When a person inhales air that contains TB germs, he or she may become infected. People with TB infection do not feel sick and do not have any symptoms. However, they may develop TB disease at some time in the future.

The general symptoms of TB disease include feeling sick or weak, weight loss, fever, and night sweats. The symptoms of TB of the lungs include coughing, chest pain, and coughing up blood. Other symptoms depend on the part of the body that is affected.

The Difference between TB Infection and TB Disease

People with TB infection but not TB disease have the germ that causes TB in their bodies. They are not sick because the germs are inactive in their bodies. They cannot spread the germs to others. However, these people may develop TB disease in the future. They are often prescribed treatment to prevent them from developing the disease.

People with TB disease are sick from germs that are active in their body. They usually have symptoms of TB, such as feeling sick, coughing, weight loss, fever, or night sweats. Usually, people with TB disease of the lungs or throat are capable of spreading the disease to others. They are prescribed drugs that can cure TB.

How is TB spread?

TB is spread from person to person through the air. When people with TB disease of the lungs or throat cough or sneeze, they can put TB germs into the air. Then other people who breathe in the air containing these germs can become infected.

People with TB disease are most likely to spread it to people they spend time with every day, such as family members or coworkers. If you think you have been around someone who has TB disease, you should go to your doctor or the local health department for tests. It is important to remember that people who have TB infection but not TB disease cannot spread the germ to others.

What is a tuberculin skin test?

The tuberculin skin test is used for finding out whether a person is infected with the TB germ. It does not tell whether a person has TB disease. For the skin test, a small amount of fluid called tuberculin is injected under the skin in the lower part of the arm. Two or three days later, a health care worker looks for a reaction on the arm.

What does a positive reaction mean?

A positive reaction to the tuberculin skin test usually means that the person has been infected with the TB germ. It does not necessarily mean that the person has TB disease. Other tests, such as a chest x-ray and a sample of phlegm, are needed to see whether the person has TB disease. People who have a positive reaction to the skin test but who do not have TB disease cannot spread the germs to others. They may be given a drug to prevent them from developing TB disease. People who have TB disease must take several drugs to cure the disease.

Skin Testing for Persons Who Have Been Vaccinated with BCG

BCG, or bacille Calmette-Guérin, is a vaccine for TB disease. BCG is used in many countries, but it is not used widely in the United States.

BCG vaccination does not completely prevent people from getting TB. People who have been vaccinated with BCG can be given a tuberculin skin test. Although BCG can cause a positive reaction to the skin test, it is more likely that a positive reaction is caused by TB infection if

1. the reaction is large,
2. the person was vaccinated a long time ago,
3. the person has been around someone with TB disease,
4. other family members have had TB disease, or
5. the person is from a country where TB is very common.

Preventive Therapy

If you have TB infection but not TB disease, your doctor may want you to take a drug to prevent you from developing the disease. The decision about taking preventive therapy will be based on your age and on the chances that you will develop the disease. Some people are more likely than others to develop TB disease once they have TB infection: people with HIV infection, people who were recently exposed to someone with TB disease, and people with certain medical conditions.

The drug used to prevent TB is isoniazid. It is taken for six to 12 months. Isoniazid may cause liver problems in certain people, especially older people and people with liver disease. Therefore, people who are taking isoniazid should be monitored carefully for signs of adverse reactions.

Treatment for TB Disease

TB disease can be cured by taking several drugs for six to nine months. It is very important that people who have TB disease take the drugs exactly as prescribed. If they stop taking the drugs too soon or if they do not take the drugs correctly, the germs that are still alive may become resistant to those drugs. TB that is resistant to drugs is harder to treat.

In some situations, staff of the local health department meet regularly with patients who have TB to help them remember to take their medications. This is called directly observed therapy.

Trends in TB

About eight million new cases of TB occur each year in the world. The number of TB cases reported in the United States has increased every year since 1985. In 1993, 25,313 cases of TB disease were reported in the United States. Also, about 10 to 15 million people in the United States are infected with the TB germ; these people may develop TB disease in the future.

■ **Document Source:**
U.S. Department of Health and Human Services, Public Health Service
Centers for Disease Control and Prevention

LIVER AND GALLBLADDER DISORDERS

■ ■ ■

ADULT PRIMARY LIVER CANCER

Description

What is adult primary liver cancer?

Adult primary liver cancer is a disease in which cancer (malignant) cells start to grow in the tissues of the liver. The liver is one of the largest organs in the body, filling the upper right side of the abdomen and protected by the rib cage. The liver has many functions. It has an important role in making your food into energy. The liver also filters and stores blood.

Primary liver cancer is different from cancer that has spread from another place in the body to the liver (liver metastases).

A separate PDQ statement is available for childhood liver cancer. Adult primary liver cancer is very rare in the United States. People who have hepatitis B or C (viral infections of the liver) or a disease of the liver called cirrhosis are more likely than other people to get adult primary liver cancer.

Like most cancers, liver cancer is best treated when it is found (diagnosed) early. You should see your doctor if you have a hard lump just below the rib cage on the right side where the liver has swollen, you feel discomfort in your upper abdomen on the right side, you have pain around your right shoulder blade, or your skin turns yellow (jaundice).

If you have symptoms, your doctor may order special x-rays, such as a computed tomographic scan or a liver scan. If a lump is seen on an x-ray, your doctor may use a needle inserted into your abdomen to remove a small amount of tissue from your liver. This procedure is called a needle biopsy, and your doctor usually will use an x-ray for guidance. Your doctor will have the tissue looked at under a microscope to see if there are any cancer cells. Before the test, you will be given a local anesthetic (a drug that causes loss of feeling for a short period of time) in the area so that you do not feel pain.

Your doctor may also want to look at the liver with an instrument called a laparoscope, which is a small tube-shaped instrument with a light on the end. For this test, a small cut is made in the abdomen so that the laparoscope can be inserted. Your doctor may also take a small piece of tissue (biopsy specimen) during the laparoscopy and look at it under the microscope to see if there are any cancer cells. You will be given an anesthetic so you do not feel pain.

Your doctor may also order an examination called an angiography. During this examination, a tube (catheter) is inserted into the main blood vessel that takes blood to the liver. Dye is then injected through the tube so that the blood vessels in the liver can be seen on an x-ray. Angiography can help your doctor tell whether the cancer is primary liver cancer or cancer that has spread from another part of the body. This test is usually done in the hospital.

Certain blood tests (such as alpha-fetoprotein, or AFP) may also help your doctor diagnose primary liver cancer.

Your chance of recovery (prognosis) and choice of treatment depend on the stage of your cancer (whether it is just in the liver or has spread to other places) and your general state of health.

Stage Explanation

Stages of Adult Primary Liver Cancer

Once adult primary liver cancer is found, more tests will be done to find out if the cancer cells have spread to other parts of the body (staging). The following stages are used for adult primary liver cancer:

Localized Resectable

Cancer is found in one place in the liver and can be totally removed in an operation.

Localized Unresectable

Cancer is found only in one part of the liver, but the cancer cannot be totally removed.

Advanced

Cancer has spread through much of the liver or to other parts of the body.

Recurrent

Recurrent disease means that the cancer has come back (recurred) after it has been treated. It may come back in the liver or in another part of the body.

Treatment Option Overview

How adult primary liver cancer is treated

There are treatments for all patients with adult primary liver cancer. Three kinds of treatment are used:

- surgery (taking out the cancer in an operation)
- radiation therapy (using high-dose x-rays to kill cancer cells)
- chemotherapy (using drugs to kill cancer cells)

Hyperthermia (warming the body to kill cancer cells) and biological therapy (using the body's immune system to fight cancer) are being tested in clinical trials.

Surgery may be used to take out the cancer or to replace the liver.

- Resection of the liver takes out the part of the liver where the cancer is found.
- A liver transplant is the removal of the entire liver and replacement with a healthy liver donated from someone else. Only a very few patients with liver cancer are eligible for this procedure.
- Cryosurgery is a type of surgery that kills cancer by freezing it.

Chemotherapy is the use of drugs to kill cancer cells. Chemotherapy for liver cancer is usually put into the body by inserting a needle into a vein or artery. This type of chemotherapy is called a systemic treatment because the drug enters the bloodstream, travels through the body, and can kill cancer cells outside the liver. In another type of chemotherapy called regional chemotherapy, a small pump containing drugs is placed in the body. The pump puts drugs directly into the blood vessels that go to the tumor.

If your doctor removes all the cancer that can be seen at the time of the operation, you may be given chemotherapy after surgery to kill any remaining cells. Chemotherapy that is given after surgery to remove the cancer is called adjuvant chemotherapy.

Radiation therapy is the use of x-rays or other high-energy rays to kill cancer cells and shrink tumors. Radiation may come from a machine outside the body (external-beam radiation therapy) or from putting materials that contain radiation through thin plastic tubes (internal radiation therapy) in the area where the cancer cells are found. Drugs may be given with the radiation therapy to make the cancer cells more sensitive to radiation (radiosensitization).

Radiation may also be given by attaching radioactive substances to antibodies (radiolabeled antibodies) that search out certain cells in the liver. Antibodies are made by your body to fight germs and other harmful things; each antibody fights specific cells.

Hyperthermia therapy is the use of a special machine to heat your body for a certain period of time to kill cancer cells. Because cancer cells are often more sensitive to heat than normal cells, the cancer cells die and the tumor shrinks.

Biological therapy is the use of methods to get your body to fight cancer. Materials made by your body or made in a laboratory are used to boost, direct, or restore your body's natural defenses against disease. Biological therapy is some-times called biological response modifier therapy or immunotherapy.

Treatment by stage

Treatments for adult primary liver cancer depend on the stage of your disease, the condition of your liver, your age, and your general health. You may receive treatment that is considered standard based on its effectiveness in a number of patients in past studies, or you may choose to go into a clinical trial. Many patients are not cured with standard therapy, and some standard treatments may have more side effects than are desired. For these reasons, clinical trials are designed to find better ways to treat cancer patients and are based on the most up-to-date information. Clinical trials are going on in most parts of the country for most stages of adult liver cancer. If you want more information, call the Cancer Information Service at 1-800-4-CANCER (1-800-422-6237); TTY at 1-800-332-8615.

Localized Resectable Adult Primary Liver Cancer

Treatment is usually surgery (resection). Liver transplantation may be done in certain patients. Clinical trials are testing adjuvant systemic or regional chemotherapy following surgery.

Localized Unresectable Adult Primary Liver Cancer

Your treatment may be one of the following:

1. A clinical trial of liver transplantation (in certain patients).
2. A clinical trial of regional chemotherapy, including local infusion of chemotherapy.
3. A clinical trial of systemic chemotherapy.
4. A clinical trial of surgery followed by chemotherapy. Hyperthermia or radiation therapy with or without drugs to make the cancer cells more sensitive to radiation may be given in addition to chemotherapy.
5. A clinical trial of local injection of pure alcohol, or cryosurgery.
6. A clinical trial of radiation therapy.

Advanced Adult Primary Liver Cancer

Your treatment may be one of the following:

1. A clinical trial of biological therapy.
2. A clinical trial of chemotherapy.
3. A clinical trial of chemotherapy, radiation therapy, and drugs to make the cancer cells more sensitive to radiation (radiosensitizers).
4. A clinical trial of external radiation therapy plus chemotherapy followed by radiolabeled antibodies.

Recurrent Adult Primary Liver Cancer

Treatment for recurrent adult primary liver cancer depends on what treatment you have already received, the part of the body where the cancer has come back, whether the liver has cirrhosis, and other factors. You may wish to consider taking part in a clinical trial.

To Learn More

To learn more about adult primary liver cancer, call the National Cancer Institute's Cancer Information Service at 1-800-4-CANCER (1-800-422-6237); TTY at 1-800-332-8615. By dialing this toll-free number, you can speak with someone who can answer your questions.

The Cancer Information Service can also send you booklets. The following booklet about liver cancer may also be helpful to you:

- In Answer to Your Questions About Liver Cancer

The following general booklets on questions related to cancer may also be helpful:

- What You Need To Know About Cancer
- Taking Time: Support for People with Cancer and the People Who Care About Them
- What Are Clinical Trials All About?
- Chemotherapy and You: A Guide to Self-Help During Treatment
- Radiation Therapy and You: A Guide to Self-Help During Treatment
- Eating Hints for Cancer Patients
- Advanced Cancer: Living Each Day
- When Cancer Recurs: Meeting the Challenge Again

There are many other places you can get information about cancer treatment and services to help you. You can check the social service office at your hospital for local and national agencies that help with your finances, getting to and from treatment, care at home, and dealing with your problems. The American Cancer Society, for example, has many free services. Their local offices are listed in the white pages of the telephone book.

You can also write to the National Cancer Institute at this address:

National Cancer Institute
Office of Cancer Communications
31 Center Drive, MSC 2580
Bethesda, MD 20892-2580

■ Document Source:
  U.S. Department of Health and Human Services, Public Health Service
  National Institutes of Health
  National Cancer Institute
  June 1996

CHILDHOOD LIVER CANCER

Description

What is childhood liver cancer?

Childhood liver cancer, also called hepatoma, is a rare disease in which cancer (malignant) cells are found in the tissues of your child's liver. The liver is one of the largest organs in the body, filling the upper right side of the abdomen and protected by the rib cage. The liver has many functions. It plays an important role in making your food into energy and also filters and stores blood.

Primary liver cancer is different from cancer that has spread from another place in the body to the liver (liver metastases). For information on the treatment of adult liver cancer, see the PDQ patient information statement on adult primary liver cancer.

There are two types of cancer that start in the liver (hepatoblastoma and hepatocellular cancer), based on how the cancer cells look under a microscope. Hepatoblastoma is more common in young children before age 3 and may be caused by an abnormal gene. Children of families whose members carry a gene related to a certain kind of colon cancer may be more likely to develop hepatoblastoma (genes carry the hereditary information that you get from your parents). Children infected with hepatitis B or C (viral infections of the liver) are more likely than other children to get hepatocellular cancer. Hepatocellular cancer is found in children from birth to age 4 or in children ages 12 to 15.

Like most cancers, childhood liver cancer is best treated when it is found (diagnosed) early. If your child has symptoms, your child's doctor may order special x-rays, such as a CT scan or a liver scan. If a lump is seen on an x-ray, your child's doctor may remove a small amount of tissue from the liver using a needle inserted into the abdomen. This is called a needle biopsy and is usually done using an x-ray to guide the doctor. Your child's doctor will have the tissue looked at under the microscope to see if there are any cancer cells.

Your child's chance of recovery (prognosis) and choice of treatment depend on the stage of your child's cancer (whether it is just in the liver or has spread to other places), how the cancer cells look under a microscope (the histology), and your child's general state of health.

Stage Explanation

Stages of Childhood Liver Cancer

Once liver cancer is found, more tests will be done to find out if the cancer cells have spread to other parts of the body. This is called staging. Your child's doctor needs to know the stage of disease in order to plan treatment. The following stages are used for childhood liver cancer:

Stage I

Stage I childhood liver cancer means the cancer can be removed with surgery.

Stage II

Stage II childhood liver cancer means that most of the cancer may be removed in an operation but very small (microscopic) amounts of cancer are left in the liver following surgery.

Stage III

Stage III childhood liver cancer means that some of the cancer may be removed in an operation, but some of the tumor cannot be removed and remains either in the abdomen or in the lymph nodes.

Stage IV

Stage IV childhood liver cancer means the cancer has spread to other parts of the body.

Recurrent

Recurrent disease means that the cancer has come back (recurred) after it has been treated. It may come back in the liver or in another part of the body.

Treatment Option Overview

How Childhood Liver Cancer Is Treated

There are treatments for all children with liver cancer. Three kinds of treatment are used:

- surgery (taking out the cancer in an operation)
- chemotherapy (using drugs to kill cancer cells)
- radiation therapy (using high-dose x-rays to kill cancer cells)

Surgery may be used to take out the cancer and part of the liver where the cancer is found. Sometimes the entire liver may be surgically removed and replaced by a liver transplant from a donor.

Chemotherapy uses drugs to kill cancer cells. Chemotherapy may be given to your child before surgery to help reduce the size of the liver cancer. Your child may be given chemotherapy after surgery to kill any remaining cells. Chemotherapy given after surgery when the doctor has removed the cancer is called adjuvant chemotherapy. Chemotherapy for childhood liver cancer is usually put into the body through a needle in a vein or artery. This type of chemotherapy is called a systemic treatment because the drug enters the bloodstream, travels through the body, and can kill cancer cells outside the liver. In another type of chemotherapy, called direct infusion chemotherapy, drugs are injected directly into the blood vessels that go into the liver.

Sometimes a special treatment called chemo-embolization is used to treat childhood liver cancer. Chemotherapy drugs are injected into the main artery of the liver with substances that block or slow the flow of blood into the cancer. This lengthens the time the drugs have to kill the cancer cells and it also prevents the cancer cells from getting oxygen or other materials that they need to grow.

Radiation therapy uses x-rays or other high-energy rays to kill cancer cells and shrink tumors. Radiation may come from a machine outside the body (external radiation therapy) or from putting materials that produce radiation (radioisotopes) through thin plastic tubes in the area where the cancer cells are found (internal radiation therapy).

Treatment by Stage

Treatments for childhood liver cancer depend on the type (hepatoblastoma or hepatocellular carcinoma) and stage of your child's disease and your child's age and general health.

Your child may receive treatment that is considered standard based on its effectiveness in a number of patients in past studies, or you may choose to have your child take part in a clinical trial. Not all patients are cured with standard therapy and some standard treatments may have more side effects than are desired. For these reasons, clinical trials are designed to test new treatments and to find better ways to treat cancer patients. Clinical trials are going on in many parts of the country for most stages of childhood liver cancer. If you want more information, call the Cancer Information Service at 1-800-4-CANCER (1-800-422-6237); TTY at 1-800-332-8615.

Stage I Childhood Liver Cancer

Stage I Hepatoblastoma

Your child's treatment will probably be complete removal of the liver cancer by surgery followed by adjuvant chemotherapy.

Stage I Hepatocellular Carcinoma

Your child's treatment will probably be complete removal of the liver cancer by surgery followed by adjuvant chemotherapy.

Stage II Childhood Liver Cancer

Stage II Hepatoblastoma

Your child's treatment will probably be removal of the liver cancer by surgery followed by chemotherapy.

Stage II Hepatocellular Carcinoma

Your child's treatment will probably be removal of the liver cancer by surgery followed by chemotherapy. For more information, please see the PDQ patient information statement on adult primary liver cancer.

Stage III Childhood Liver Cancer

Stage III Hepatoblastoma

Your child's treatment may be one or more of the following:

1. Chemotherapy to reduce the size of the tumor followed by surgery to remove as much of the cancer as possible.
2. Chemotherapy.
3. Radiation therapy.
4. Direct infusion of drugs into blood vessels going into the liver.
5. Liver transplant: Surgical removal of the liver followed by replacement with a donor's liver.

Stage III Hepatocellular Carcinoma

Your child's treatment will probably be chemotherapy to reduce the size of the tumor followed by surgery to remove as much of the cancer as possible. For more information, please see the PDQ patient information statement on adult primary liver cancer.

Stage IV Childhood Liver Cancer

Stage IV Hepatoblastoma

Your child's treatment may be one or more of the following:

1. Chemotherapy to reduce the size of the tumor followed by surgery to remove as much of the cancer as possible followed by chemotherapy.
2. Surgical removal of cancer that has spread to the lungs.
3. Chemotherapy.
4. Radiation therapy followed by additional surgery.
5. Direct infusion of chemotherapy drugs into blood vessels going into the liver.
6. Chemotherapy drugs injected into the main liver artery with substances that block or slow the flow of blood (chemo-embolization chemotherapy).
7. Liver transplant: Surgical removal of the liver followed by replacement with a donor's liver.
8. Clinical trials are testing new therapies and should be considered for your child.

Stage IV Hepatocellular Carcinoma

Your child's treatment will probably be chemotherapy to reduce the size of the tumor followed by surgery to remove as much of the cancer as possible. For more information, please see the PDQ patient information statement on adult primary liver cancer.

Recurrent Childhood Liver Cancer

Recurrent Hepatoblastoma

Treatment depends on where the cancer recurred and how the cancer was treated before. Treatment may include additional surgery. Clinical trials are testing new therapies and should be considered for your child.

Recurrent Hepatocellular Carcinoma

Clinical trials are testing new therapies and should be considered for your child.

To Learn More

To learn more about childhood liver cancer, call the National Cancer Institute's Cancer Information Service at 1-800-4-CANCER (1-800-422-6237); TTY at 1-800-332-8615. By dialing this toll-free number, you can speak with someone who can answer your questions.

The Cancer Information Service can also send you booklets. The following booklet about liver cancer may be helpful to you:

- In Answer to Your Questions About Liver Cancer

The following booklets on childhood cancer may be helpful to you:

- Young People with Cancer: A Handbook for Parents
- Talking with Your Child About Cancer

- Managing Your Child's Eating Problems During Cancer Treatment
- When Someone in Your Family Has Cancer

The following general booklets on questions related to cancer may also be helpful:

- Taking Time: Support for People with Cancer and the People Who Care About Them
- What Are Clinical Trials All About?
- Chemotherapy and You: A Guide to Self-Help During Treatment
- Radiation Therapy and You: A Guide to Self-Help During Treatment
- What You Need To Know About Cancer

There are many other places you can get material about cancer treatment and services to help you. You can check the social service office at your hospital for local and national agencies that help with your finances, getting to and from treatment, care at home, and dealing with your problems. The American Cancer Society, for example, has many free services. Candlelighters Childhood Cancer Foundation (1-800-366-2223) has free services and publications including newsletters, bibliographies, and information for parents and brothers and sisters of children with cancer. It can also refer you to a local parent peer support group in the United States or abroad. Local offices for these organizations are listed in the white pages of the telephone book.

You can also write to the National Cancer Institute at this address:

National Cancer Institute
Office of Cancer Communications
31 Center Dr, MSC 2580
Bethesda, MD 20892-2580

■ **Document Source:**
U.S. Department of Health and Human Services, Public Health Service
National Institutes of Health
National Cancer Institute
June 1996

CHRONIC HEPATITIS

Definition

Chronic Hepatitis (CAH) is ongoing injury to the cells of the liver with inflammation which lasts for longer than six months. The causes of chronic hepatitis are several: viruses, metabolic or immunologic abnormalities and medications.

Symptoms

Symptoms result from the liver cell injury, the inflammation or from the resulting scarring which is called cirrhosis. Chronic hepatitis may follow acute hepatitis B or C (formerly called non-A, non-B) or may develop quietly without an acute illness.

Liver biopsy is helpful in that it confirms the diagnosis, aids in establishing the cause (etiology) and can demonstrate the presence of cirrhosis. It is less helpful in judging the response to treatment.

Causes

Hepatitis B and C are the most common causes of chronic hepatitis. Together they account for more than 75 percent of the cases in the world. Hepatitis B is far more common in China and sub-Saharan Africa and among male homosexuals and IV drug users.

Chronic hepatitis C behaves differently from hepatitis B. The disease is generally mild, with fatigue being the main symptom. However, ten or more years later, the complications of cirrhosis appear in some patients, sometimes unexpectedly. By contrast with hepatitis B, the percentage of patients infected who develop cirrhosis is much greater. While primary liver cancer can also develop from hepatitis C, it appears to be much less common than after hepatitis B.

Autoimmune Chronic Hepatitis varies from a mild to serious disease. The percentage of patients who develop cirrhosis is high and it may appear early. Most of the patients are young women but postmenopausal women and males may get the disease. Only a few cases of primary liver cancer have been reported with this disease. Twenty-five percent of the cases of chronic hepatitis result from damage to the liver by the immune system. The trigger for autoimmune chronic hepatitis is unknown, but the damage to the liver is caused by the individual's lymphocytes and by antibodies produced in the individual's own tissue. Autoimmune chronic hepatitis is usually a progressive disease ending in cirrhosis.

Hepatitis A and E (formerly called epidemic or enteric non-A, non-B) are rarely, if ever, responsible for causes of chronic hepatitis.

Hepatitis D infection needs the hepatitis B virus to multiply. Hepatitis D can cause acute hepatitis in someone who is a carrier of the hepatitis B virus and can cause acute hepatitis at the same time that the hepatitis B virus does. In any event, the combination of hepatitis B and D is worse then hepatitis B alone and is more likely to cause serious chronic hepatitis and cirrhosis. IV drug users have a high incidence of hepatitis D.

Other Causes

Viruses of the herpes family, which cause cold sores, genital herpes, chicken pox, shingles and infectious mononucleosis, can cause acute hepatitis, especially when the immune system is not functioning properly. It is unlikely that they will produce chronic hepatitis. Other viruses, as yet undiscovered, may be responsible for some cases of chronic hepatitis.

Drug-Induced Hepatitis

Few medications still in use and several that have been withdrawn from the market can also cause chronic hepatitis. These include: isoniazid, used for tuberculosis; methyldopa,

used for hypertension; nitrofurantoin, used for urinary tract infections; phenytoin, used for seizure disorders and selected other prescription medications. These medications must be taken for long periods of time and the number of cases of chronic hepatitis produced by these medications is small.

Chronic hepatitis caused by drugs is usually recognized early. Stopping the medicine before cirrhosis has developed usually reverses the disease.

Inherited Disorders

Some inherited disorders of metabolism also can appear as chronic hepatitis. The most frequent of these conditions is Wilson's disease, a familial disorder of copper metabolism. Alpha-1-antitrypsin deficiency and tyrosinemia may appear as chronic hepatitis although other features help in distinguishing these rare conditions from those caused by viruses.

Signs and Symptoms

Fatigue, mild discomfort in the upper abdomen, loss of appetite and aching joints are the common symptoms of chronic hepatitis. Fatigue is by far the most common symptom and it might be quite disabling. Often it gets worse as the day wears on. Some patients, however, may have no symptoms. Others may have signs of liver failure, inducing jaundice, abdominal swelling (due to fluid retention called ascites), or coma, depending on the severity of the liver disease and whether or not cirrhosis has developed. Most complications are vague and may be mistaken for other diseases or simply a consequence of aging. Disorders of other organs like the thyroid, intestine, eyes, joints, blood, spleen, kidneys and skin may occur in about 20 percent of patients depending on the cause of the chronic hepatitis.

When the hepatitis is mild and limited in extent, it is called chronic persistent hepatitis (CPH). When it is more extensive and seems to be destroying the cells of the liver, it is called chronic active hepatitis (CAH).

Treatment

Interferon has been approved for the treatment of hepatitis B and C. The treatment has been shown to reduce the inflammation and liver damage caused by the virus in 25-30 percent of cases by eliminating the virus, thus reducing the development of scar tissue and avoiding the development of cirrhosis.

In people treated with interferon studies show that 50 percent will respond to treatment and 50 percent of those patients will relapse when interferon is stopped. Research is going on to address the relapse rate.

Additional clinical trials are being conducted to identify the most effective dose and duration of therapy with interferon. Studies are continuing in an attempt to reduce the side effects of the medication that exists. These include "flu-like" symptoms, and less often, fever, depression, hair loss, nausea and vomiting. Currently, the treatment consists of an injection three times a week over a period of six months.

Blood tests are needed to monitor progress during treatment and a liver biopsy (retrieving a small specimen of the liver through a needle inserted into the liver) is an accepted procedure prior to and following treatment.

Fifty percent of the patients treated will experience remission of the disease. When the treatment is stopped 50 percent will relapse. However, only about 20 percent of untreated patients will go on to develop cirrhosis over a period of years. Research into the management of those who relapse is ongoing.

Interferon does not seem to work well in patients

- with substance abuse (alcohol or illegal drugs)
- who are not very sick
- whose test results are not very abnormal
- whose immune system is not functioning well because of AIDS
- with hepatitis B who were infected from their mothers at birth
- carriers who are no longer contagious or infectious
- with significant heart, lung or kidney diseases
- or couples who are trying to conceive

Knowing the cause of the disease is helpful in estimating the prognosis.

Only a small percentage of patients with chronic hepatitis B develop cirrhosis. In those patients, cirrhosis develops early in the course of the disease with complications appearing in the first few years. Chronic hepatitis often causes acute hepatitis or flare-ups and periods with no signs. Scarring becomes more extensive with each flare-up. Patients in the Orient have about a 15 percent chance of developing primary liver cancer, usually after the age of 50, with men more likely candidates than women. This complication is much less common in the Western World.

The disease becomes life-threatening only after cirrhosis has developed. More than half of all patients live at least 15 years from the time of the first diagnosis and this number is continuously improving. Previously, prognosis was thought to depend on what was found on liver biopsy. This is now only partly true. Prognosis is worse and complications more numerous and severe if cirrhosis has already developed. Much attention has been paid to the location and extent of the inflammation of the liver.

Steroid therapy remains the only useful treatment for autoimmune disease, but it may have to be given for a lifetime and may also not prevent the ultimate development of cirrhosis.

Liver transplantation has become an accepted form of therapy when chronic hepatitis becomes life-threatening, usually as a result of complications of cirrhosis. Recurrence of hepatitis C or autoimmune hepatitis does not seem to occur, but hepatitis B, if virus is still present and the patient is contagious, will recur in the new liver and often be acute. Attempts are being made to prevent this recurrence.

The most important treatment for hepatitis B is prevention. Hepatitis B vaccines should be given to all who are exposed to this disease on a regular basis. All pregnant women should be tested for hepatitis B. Carriers of hepatitis B, many of them unaware that they are infected, can pass it on to their babies as well as their sexual contacts. All newborns should be vaccinated against hepatitis B. Three injections are needed to provide adequate immunity.

An important aspect of treatment is supportive care. Diet should be well balanced. The use of high carbohydrate, high protein or low fat diets have no scientific basis, and in some instances, such diets may be harmful. Vitamin and mineral supplementation also has no place in the management of chronic hepatitis unless some deficiency is present. No substance is known that will help the main symptom, fatigue. However, a good physical fitness program may lessen this distressing symptom. Patients should be advised to limit the amount of salt that they use in an attempt to forestall the accumulation of fluids as ascites or ankle swelling. Since almost all drugs must be detoxified by the liver, and since the injured liver does not perform this task well, limiting the amount of drugs that a patient uses to only essential ones is important. This includes discouraging the use of sedatives and tranquilizers.

Looking to the Future

Learning more about the viruses responsible for chronic hepatitis and how to control them will occur in the next decade. Similarly, learning about the body's immune system and how to control it has already begun. Preventive efforts will be enhanced so that fewer cases of chronic hepatitis will develop. The goal of eliminating this group of diseases seems to be just over the horizon, and while our skills at transplantation are rapidly increasing, the form of therapy for chronic hepatitis, like the disease itself, will disappear.

■ Document Source:
The American Liver Foundation
1425 Pompton Ave
Cedar Grove, NJ 07009
1-800-223-0179
Copyright, The American Liver Foundation
April 1993

CIRRHOSIS: MANY CAUSES

Basic Facts About the Liver

Your liver, the largest organ in your body, weights about three pounds and is roughly the size of a football. It lies in the upper right side of your abdomen situated mostly under the lower ribs. The normal liver is soft and smooth and is connected to the small intestine by the bile duct which carries bile formed in the liver to the intestines.

Nearly all of the blood that leaves the stomach and intestines must pass through the liver. Acting as the body's largest chemical factory, it has thousands of functions including

- the production of clotting factors, blood proteins, bile and more than a thousand different enzymes
- the metabolism of cholesterol
- the storage of energy (glycogen) to fuel muscles
- maintenance of normal blood sugar concentration

- the regulation of several hormones
- and the detoxification of drugs and poisons including alcohol. It is no wonder that liver disease can cause widespread disruption of body function. While many liver diseases can occur, one of the most important is cirrhosis.

What is cirrhosis?

Cirrhosis is a term that refers to a group of chronic liver diseases in which normal liver cells are damaged and replaced by scar tissue, decreasing the amount of normal liver tissue. The distortion of the normal liver structure by the scar tissue interferes with the flow of blood through the liver. It also handicaps the function of the liver which, with the loss of normal liver tissue, leads to failure of the liver tissue to perform some of its critically important functions. Cirrhosis and other liver diseases take the lives of over 25,000 Americans each year and rank eighth as a cause of death.

What causes cirrhosis?

There are a number of conditions that can lead to cirrhosis:

- excessive intake of alcohol (most common)
- types B, C and D of chronic viral hepatitis,
- inherited or congenital disease
    hemochromatosis: abnormal accumulation of iron in the liver and other organs because of the increased absorption of iron from the intestine.
    Wilson's disease: abnormal accumulation of copper in the liver and other organs due to the decreased excretion of copper from the liver.
    alpha 1 -antitrypsin deficiency: inherited absence of a specific enzyme in the liver.
    glycogen storage diseases: inability to properly utilize sugars.
    autoimmune hepatitis
- prolonged obstruction or other diseases of the bile ducts (biliary cirrhosis, sclerosing cholangitis)
- prolonged exposure to environmental toxins
- some forms of heart disease (cardiac cirrhosis)
- severe reaction to drugs
- schistosomiasis (parasitic infection)

Can the condition responsible for cirrhosis be identified?

Causes of the cirrhosis can be identified by certain factors:

In alcoholic cirrhosis
- history of regular and excessive alcoholic intake
- physical and behavioral changes
- examination of liver tissue obtained by needle biopsy under local anesthesia

In active viral hepatitis infection
- blood tests
- liver biopsy

Does heavy drinking always lead to cirrhosis?

While almost everyone who drinks excessive amounts of alcohol sustains some liver damage, it does not necessarily develop into cirrhosis. In those individuals who drink one-half to one pint (8 to 16 ounces) of hard liquor per day (or the equivalent in other alcoholic drinks), for 15 years or more, about one-third develop cirrhosis. Another third develop fatty livers, while the remainder have only minor liver problems.

In general, the more you drink, the greater the frequency and regularity of excessive intake, the more likely that cirrhosis is to result. A poor diet, long considered to be the main factor in the development of cirrhosis in the alcoholic, is probably only a contributing factor.

Alcohol by itself, in large amounts, is a poison which can cause cirrhosis.

Can social drinkers get cirrhosis?

Some individuals who are "social drinkers," not alcoholics, can develop cirrhosis. Factors affecting the development of cirrhosis include

- the amount of alcohol consumed
- the regularity of intake
- natural tendency
- perhaps the state of nutrition

It is not known why some individuals are more prone to adverse reactions to alcohol than others. Women are less tolerant of alcohol than men. Researchers believe that this is because men have a greater ability than women to break down the alcohol for elimination. Studies show that a much higher percentage of women, consuming less alcohol than men, go on to cirrhosis.

Does hepatitis always result in cirrhosis?

Some patients with chronic viral hepatitis develop cirrhosis. There are five known types of viral hepatitis, each caused by a different virus.

- Acute hepatitis A and acute hepatitis E do not lead to chronic hepatitis.
- Acute hepatitis B leads to chronic infection in approximately 5 percent of adult patients. In a few of these patients, the chronic hepatitis B progresses to cirrhosis.
- Acute hepatitis D infects individuals already infected by hepatitis B.
- Acute hepatitis C becomes chronic in approximately 80 percent of adults. A minority of these patients (20-30 percent) will progress to cirrhosis, typically over many years.

What are the signs and symptoms of cirrhosis?

The onset of cirrhosis is often "silent" with few specific symptoms to identify what is happening in the liver. As continued scarring and destruction occur, the following signs and symptoms may appear:

- loss of appetite
- nausea and vomiting
- weight loss
- enlargement of the liver
- jaundice—yellow discoloration of the whites of the eyes and skin occurs because bile pigment can no longer be removed by the liver
- itching—due to the retention of bile products in the skin
- ascites—abdominal swelling due to an accumulation of fluid caused by the obstruction of blood flow through the liver
- vomiting of blood—frequently occurs from swollen, ruptured varies (veins that burst) in the lower end of the esophagus due to the increased pressure in these vessels caused by scar tissue formation
- increased sensitivity to drugs—due to inability of the liver to inactivate them
- encephalopathy (impending coma)—subtle mental changes advancing to profound confusion and coma.

Many patients may have no symptoms and are found to have cirrhosis by physical examination and laboratory tests, which may have been performed in the course of treatment for unrelated illnesses.

How is cirrhosis treated?

Treatment depends on the type and stage of the cirrhosis. It aims at stopping the progress of the cirrhosis, reversing (to whatever extent possible) the damage which has already occurred, and treating complications that are disabling or life-threatening. Stopping or reversing the process requires removal of the cause.

In alcoholic cirrhosis:
- abstinence from alcohol
- an adequate, wholesome diet

In cirrhosis caused by viral hepatitis:
- an approved approach is the use of interferon to improve immune responses to viral infection

In certain types of cirrhosis caused by autoimmune hepatitis:
- corticosteroids alone or with azathioprine may be an effective treatment

In cirrhotic patients with jaundice:
- supplemental fat soluble vitamins may be helpful

Wilson's disease:
- removal of excessive copper by drugs that deplete the body's copper

Hemochromatosis:
- removal of excess iron by phlebotomy (removal of one pint of blood per week)

Most types of cirrhosis:
- liver transplantation with replacement of the diseased organ when advanced liver failure occurs

What are the complications of cirrhosis?

Complications of cirrhosis include ascites, coma and hemorrhage from esophageal varices.

- Ascites is treated by reducing the intake of salt and the administration of drugs to improve excretion of salt and water (diuretics). In some instances, large amounts of fluid are removed by direct catheter drainage through the abdominal wall (large volume paracentesis).
- Treatment of coma, or impending coma (encephalopathy), includes specific medications, reducing the intake of protein foods, and control of intestinal hemorrhage.
- Treatment of hemorrhage from varices (internal varicose veins) includes sclerotherapy (injection of the enlarged vein with a chemical that causes scarring). Other treatments include: drugs to reduce the likelihood of bleeding or rebleeding, compression of the bleeding varices with a specially constructed balloon, and a new radiological procedure called transjugular intrahepatic portosystemic shunt (TIPS).

How can I avoid cirrhosis?

1. **Do not drink to excess.**
   Avoid the use of alcoholic beverages. Alcohol destroys liver cells. How well damaged cells regenerate varies with each individual. Prior injury to the liver by unknown and unrecognized viruses or chemicals can also affect the regeneration process.

2. **Take precautions when using man-made chemicals.**
   The liver must process many chemicals which were not present in the past. More research is needed to determine the effects on the liver of many of these compounds. When using chemicals at work, in cleaning your home or working in your garden

   - be sure there is good ventilation
   - follow directions for use of all products
   - never mix chemical products
   - avoid getting chemicals on the skin, where they can be absorbed, and wash promptly if you do
   - avoid inhaling chemicals
   - wear protective clothing

3. **Seek medical advice.**
   Remain under supervision of a physician if you develop viral hepatitis until your recovery is assured.

How might cirrhosis affect other diseases I might have or treatment of them?

The responsibility of the liver for the proper functioning of the whole body is so great that the chronic disease of the liver may modify the body's responses to a variety of illnesses. Abnormal function of the liver in cirrhosis may

- affect the dose of medicine required in the treatment of other conditions
- affect the treatment of diabetes
- alter response of the body to infection
- alter tolerance for surgical procedures

Patients with cirrhosis are particularly prone to develop fatal bacterial infections, kidney malfunctions, stomach ulcers, gallstones, a type of diabetes and cancer of the liver.

What are my prospects for reasonable health and survival with treatment?

Treatment at this stage, with proper adherence to the physician's recommendations, leads to improvement in the majority of cases and the patient is able to pursue a normal life and activities.

When cirrhosis is not discovered until extensive damage has resulted, the outlook may be less favorable for improvement, and complications such as ascites and hemorrhage are more likely to be encountered.

> Experts estimate that more than half of all liver diseases could be prevented if people acted upon the knowledge we already have.

Each year more than 25 million Americans are afflicted with liver and gallbladder diseases and more than 25,000 die of chronic liver disease and cirrhosis. There are few effective treatments for most life-threatening liver diseases, except for liver transplants. Meanwhile, patients and their families must cope with medical, financial and emotional problems.

Research has recently opened up exciting new paths for investigation, **but much more remains to be done** to find cures for more than 100 different liver diseases and help millions of Americans who are suffering. To increase the number of liver researchers, the American Liver Foundation encourages young scientific investigators to pursue careers in liver research by supporting bright, highly-trained men and women in their quest for answers.

Research and education have made a difference. When the Foundation first became operational in 1979, reported deaths due to chronic liver diseases and cirrhosis exceeded 50,000 each year. By 1992, that figure was reduced to 26,000.

Concerned contributors like you have enabled us to increase Foundation-supported research tenfold since 1980.

In the past year the foundation has counselled, encouraged, and informed over 35,000 anxious victims of liver disease. We distributed two million brochures to patients and referred hundreds to medical specialists. We thank you for your thoughtful support and confidence in our efforts. You have enabled us to touch the lives of millions of Americans who look to the American Liver Foundation for guidance, support and encouragement.

The liver is a large organ and is able to perform its vital functions despite some damage. It also has the ability to repair itself to a limited degree. Cells that die are replaced by new cells. If the cause of cirrhosis can be removed, these factors provide hope for both improvement and carrying on a normal life.

An increasing number of scientific investigators conducting liver research give hope for new breakthroughs in treatment, management and cures for liver diseases in the foreseeable future.

The American Liver Foundation is the only national non-profit voluntary health organization dedicated to preventing, treating, and curing liver diseases through research and education.

For further information contact

American Liver Foundation
1425 Pompton Ave
Cedar Grove, NJ 07009
1-800-223-0179

■ Document Source:
**The American Liver Foundation
1425 Pompton Ave
Cedar Grove, NJ 07009
Copyright, The American Liver Foundation
Rev January 1995**

FACTS ON LIVER TRANSPLANTATION

Although the first human liver transplant was done in 1963, the procedure did not gain widespread acceptance in medical practice until the 1980's. With this acceptance, questions from patients, relatives, healthcare workers and the public have increased. This pamphlet is designed to answer some of the most common questions.

1. What diseases are treated by liver transplantation?

A large number of diseases are capable of interfering with the liver's function sufficiently to threaten the life of the patient and most are potentially treatable by liver transplantation.

2. Which liver diseases are the most common?

In adults, cirrhosis, the death of liver cells due to a variety of causes, is one of the most common reasons for which liver transplantation is done. In children, the disease most often treated by liver transplantation is biliary atresia, a failure of the bile ducts to develop normally to drain bile from the liver.

3. What about alcohol-related liver disease?

Most people who develop cirrhosis of the liver due to excessive use of alcohol do not need a liver transplant. Abstinence from alcohol and treatment of complications will usually allow them to live for prolonged periods without a transplant. For patients with advanced liver disease, where prolonged abstinence and medical treatment fails to restore health, transplantation is a consideration.

4. And cancer of the liver?

Most cancers of the liver begin somewhere else in the body and spread to the liver. These are not curable with a liver transplant. Likewise the tumors which start in the liver have usually spread to other organs by the time they are detected and are rarely cured by liver transplantation. Transplantation at an early stage of liver cancer may result in long-term survival for some patients.

5. Are there alternative treatments for liver disease?

There are effective medicines for some liver diseases, while for others only treatment for complications is available. Treatment of complications may be all that is required if the liver is not failing. Frequently medical treatment delays, but does not eliminate, the need for transplantation.

6. Is liver transplantation a treatment of last resort, when everything else has failed?

Yes and no. If medical treatment is likely to allow prolonged survival with good quality of life, transplantation would be reserved for the future. However, ideally the surgery is undertaken before the terminal stage of the disease when the person is too ill to withstand major surgery and will not survive until a suitable donor is available.

7. How is the decision made to transplant?

This is a decision made in consultation with all individuals involved in the patient's care, including the patient and/or family. The patient and family's input is vital and they must clearly understand the risks involved with proceeding to transplantation.

8. What are the major risks?

Before surgery, the risks are mainly the development of some acute complication of the disease which might render the patient unacceptable for surgery. With transplantation there are risks common to all forms of major surgery, as well as technical difficulties in removing the diseased liver and implanting the donor liver. One of the major risks for the patient is not having any liver function for a brief period. Immediately after surgery, bleeding, poor function of the grafted liver, and infections are major risks. The patient is carefully monitored for several weeks for signs of rejection of the liver.

9. What are the overall chances of surviving a liver transplant?

This depends on many factors but overall 60–75 percent of adult patients and 80–90 percent of children survive and are discharged from the hospital.

10. How long does it take to recover?

In part this depends on how ill the individual was prior to the surgery. Most patients should count on spending a few days in an intensive care unit and about four weeks in the hospital, as a minimum.

11. What happens during this recovery period?

Initially, in the intensive care unit there is very careful monitoring of all body functions including the liver. Once the patient is transferred to the ward, the frequency of blood testing, etc. is decreased, eating is allowed and physiotherapy is used to regain muscle strength. The drug or drugs to prevent rejection are initially given by vein, but later by mouth. During the transplantation, frequent tests are done to monitor liver function and detect any evidence of rejection.

12. If a transplanted liver fails to function, or is rejected, what can be done?

There are varying degrees of failure of the liver, however, and even with imperfect function, the patient will remain quite well. Occasionally, when circumstances and time permit, a failing transplanted liver can be replaced by a second (or even third) transplant. Unfortunately, there is no dialysis treatment for livers as is possible with kidneys. Researchers are experimenting with devices to keep patients with failing livers alive while waiting for a new liver.

13. What side-effects do patients commonly experience from the drugs used to treat or prevent rejection?

All the drugs used for rejection increase the person's susceptibility to infections (and possibly to the development of tumors). Various medicines are used, and each has its own effects. Cortisone-like drugs produce some fluid retention and puffiness of the face, risk of worsening diabetes and osteoporosis (a loss of mineral from bone). Cyclosporine produces some tendency to develop high blood pressure and the growth of body hair. The dose of this medication must be very carefully regulated. Kidney damage can occur from cyclosporine but this can usually be avoided by monitoring the drug levels in the blood. Common side effects for FK-506 include headaches, tremor, diarrhea, increased tension, nausea, increased levels of potassium and glucose and kidney dysfunction.

14. Do recipients of liver transplant have to take these medicines for the rest of their lives?

Usually. However, as the body adjusts to the transplanted liver, the amount of medicine needed to control rejection is reduced. There are patients who have been successfully taken off these drugs. Researchers are attempting to determine why this has been successful in these cases.

15. How frequent is medical follow-up?

Routine follow-up consists of monthly blood tests, measuring of blood pressure by a local physician, with annual or semi-annual checkups at the transplant center.

16. Are patients more susceptible to other infections?

Recipients should avoid exposure to infections as the immune system is depressed. Illness should be reported to the doctor immediately and medicines taken only under medical supervision.

17. What about physical activity after a liver transplant?

Most patients are able to return to a normal or near-normal existence and can participate in fairly vigorous physical exercise six to twelve months after a successful liver transplant.

18. What about sexual activity?

As with other physical activities, sexual activity may be resumed.

19. Is it safe for women to become pregnant after transplantation?

Studies have shown that women who undergo liver transplantation can conceive and give birth normally, although they have to be monitored carefully because of a higher incidence of premature births.

Mothers are advised against nursing babies because of the possibility of immunosuppressive drugs being ingested by the infants through breast milk.

20. What about diet?

Transplant patients have a tendency to gain weight because of their retention of water. They are advised to lower their intake of salt to reduce or eliminate this water retention. Otherwise patients should maintain a balanced diet.

21. Can there be a recurrence of the original disease in the transplanted liver?

If the disease was caused by hepatitis B or C viruses then recurrence is likely. Other types of liver disease do not recur.

22. From the description, patients with successful liver transplants seem very healthy. How long can this good health last?

The newness of this procedure makes this question difficult to answer. There is every indication that those who are well after one year remain so indefinitely.

23. Where do the donor livers come from?

Livers are donated, with the consent of the next of kin, from individuals who have brain death, usually as a result of a head injury or brain hemorrhage. When such a donor is identified, transplant centers are contacted by a computer network and arrangements are made to retrieve whatever organs may be donated. Frequently this involves a team from a transplant center flying to the donor hospital to remove the organs, and returning with them for the transplant operation.

24. Do the donor and the recipient have to be matched by tissue type, sex, age, etc.?

No. For liver transplants, the only requirements are that the donor and recipient need to be approximately the same size, and of compatible blood types. No other matching is necessary.

25. What happens if there are two suitable recipients for a donated liver?

This is unusual in practice but the decision would be to transplant the patient with the more urgent need.

26. How can I donate my organs?

If you wish to be an organ donor, carry an organ donor card and place an organ donor sticker on your medical identification card. It is important to discuss organ donation with family members since they will have to give consent. An organ donor card is available from the American Liver Foundation.

27. Is there financial help?

The cost of a liver transplant, including presurgery expenses and immunosuppressive drugs following the operation, is about $280,000 for the first year. Many patients pay for all or a good portion of this expense through private insurance or Medicare. Other expenses are covered through donations. The American Liver Foundation will act as a trustee, at no cost, for funds raised through private donations. In addition, The Transplant Foundation, a non-profit organization at 8002 Discovery Drive, Suite 310, Richmond, VA 23229, 804-285-5115 provides grants for immunosuppressive drugs to patients who can demonstrate a financial need.

The American Liver Foundation is the only national non-profit voluntary health organization dedicated to preventing, treating, and curing liver disease through research and education.

Experts estimate that more than half of all liver diseases could be prevented if people acted upon the knowledge we already have.

Each year more than 25 million Americans are afflicted with liver and gallbladder diseases and more than 27,000 die of chronic liver disease and cirrhosis. There are few effective treatments for most life-threatening chronic liver diseases, except for liver transplants. Research has recently opened up exciting new paths for investigation, but much more remains to be done to find cures for more than 100 different liver diseases.

Meanwhile, patients and their families must cope with medical, financial and emotional problems.

For more information on the Foundation's programs:

The American Liver Foundation
1425 Pompton Ave
Cedar Grove, NJ 07009
1-201-256-2550
1-800-223-0179

■ **Document Source:**
   The American Liver Foundation
   1425 Pompton Ave
   Cedar Grove, NJ 07009
   Copyright, The American Liver Foundation
   Rev February 1995

FATTY LIVER

What Is fatty liver?

Fatty liver is the accumulation of fat in liver cells. *Simple fatty liver* is not a disease, since it does not damage the liver, but is a condition that can be identified by taking a sample of liver tissue (liver biopsy) and examining it under a microscope. Another term often used to describe this condition is *fatty infiltration of the liver.*

What causes fatty liver?

Fat accumulates in the liver usually in connection with heavy use of alcohol, extreme weight gain or diabetes mellitus. Fatty liver can also occur with poor diet and certain illnesses, such as tuberculosis, intestinal bypass surgery for obesity, and certain drugs such as corticosteroids.

How is fatty liver identified?

Fatty liver is usually suspected in a patient with the diseases or conditions described above. The patient may have an enlarged liver or minor elevation of liver enzyme tests. Several studies show that fatty liver is one of the most common causes of isolated minor elevation of liver enzymes found in routine blood screening.

To find out for certain whether a patient has fatty liver requires that a sample of liver tissue be obtained (biopsy). Images of the liver obtained by an ultrasound test or by a computed tomography (CT) scan can suggest the presence of a fatty liver. In the ultrasound test, a fatty liver will produce a bright image in a ripple pattern. A CT scan will show a liver that is less dense than normal.

How does fat get into the liver?

It is not certain how fatty liver occurs. A patient has fatty liver when the fat increases the weight of the liver by 5 percent. Possible explanations for fatty liver include the transfer of fat from other parts of the body, or an increase in the extraction of fat presented to the liver from the intestine. Other explanations are that the liver reduces the rate it breaks down and removes fat. Eating fatty food by itself does not produce a fatty liver.

Can fatty liver lead to other liver diseases?

Simple fatty liver is not associated with any other liver abnormalities such as scarring or inflammation. It is a common finding in patients who are very overweight or have diabetes mellitus.

Patients who drink too much alcohol for many years may develop alcoholic liver damage that includes fatty liver. Alcoholism could also result in inflammation of the liver (alcoholic hepatitis) and/or scarring (alcoholic cirrhosis). Evidence suggests that while fatty liver is usually present in patients with excessive intake of alcohol, fatty liver does not by itself lead up to the development of alcoholic hepatitis or alcoholic cirrhosis.

An inflammation of the liver associated with an increase of fat deposits may occur in middle-aged, overweight, and often diabetic patients who do not drink alcohol. This disease, which resembles alcoholic hepatitis, is called nonalcoholic steatohepatitis (NASH). This fatty tissue in the liver may break up (steatonecrosis) and the patient may develop cirrhosis (scarring of the liver). Some studies have shown that 20 percent to 40 percent of people who are grossly overweight will develop NASH. However, just because a patient is grossly overweight does not mean they will develop NASH. Some researchers have connected the development of NASH with poor control of diabetes mellitus, rapid weight loss, or in women, the taking of hormones (estrogen).

Can fatty liver be treated?

The treatment of fatty liver is related to the cause. It is important to remember that simple fatty liver does not require treatment, since it does not result in damage to liver cells or clinical disease. Obese patients with fatty liver will have reduction or loss of excess fat in liver cells, as well as in other cells in the body, if substantial weight loss can be achieved. Patients who drink alcohol to excess will also have a loss of fat in the liver when alcohol is discontinued. Good control of diabetes mellitus with diet, drugs, or insulin also decreases the fat content in the liver.

The American Liver Foundation is the only national, non-profit voluntary health organization dedicated to preventing, treating, and curing liver disease through research and education.

■ Document Source:
  The American Liver Foundation
  1425 Pompton Ave
  Cedar Grove, NJ 07009
  1-800-223-0179
  Copyright, The American Liver Foundation
  1995

GALLSTONES: A NATIONAL HEALTH PROBLEM

This year, over one million people in the United States will discover that they have gallstones. They will join an estimated 20 million Americans, approximately 10 percent of the population, who have gallstones. Gallstones form within the gallbladder. Cholecystectomy, the surgical removal of the gallbladder, is the most common surgical procedure performed in the United States. Approximately 500,000 persons will undergo surgery to remove their gallbladder this year simply because of gallstones.

Who is at risk to develop gallstones?

People with certain characteristics have been associated with the development of gallstone disease. These include:

- People who are overweight
- Older people
- Pregnant women
- Women who use hormone contraceptives and post-menopausal hormones
- People with a family history of gallstones
- People of American Indian ancestry
- People with diseases of the small intestine
- People who have recently lost weight

The three most important risk factors for developing gallstone disease are body weight, increasing age and being female. The risk of developing gallstones in obese persons is three to sevenfold greater than for persons of normal weight. Women are more likely to develop gallstones than men.

Approximately 12 percent of all women, but only 8 percent of men, have gallstones. The risk of gallstones increases with age for men and women. By age 60, nearly 10 percent of men and over 20 percent of women have gallstones.

Rapid weight reduction has also been associated with the development of gallstones. However, several studies now demonstrate that it is not the actual weight loss which causes gallstones to form. Why gallstones form during weight loss is unclear.

We are just beginning to understand answers to questions, such as what causes gallstones to form and the relative roles of the liver and gallbladder in gallstone formation. Although many risk factors for developing gallstones have been identified, we still do not understand why some persons with many of these risk factors do not develop gallstones while others do. Researchers are working on answers to these questions.

What is the gallbladder and what does it do?

The gallbladder is a small pear-shaped organ that averages three to six inches in length. It lies underneath the liver in the upper right side of the abdomen. It is connected to the liver and small intestine by small tubes called bile ducts. Bile, a greenish-brown fluid, is utilized by the body to digest fatty foods and assists in the absorption of certain vitamins and minerals. The gallbladder serves as a reservoir for bile. Between meals, bile accumulates and is concentrated within this organ. During meals, the gallbladder contracts and empties bile into the intestine to assist in digestion.

What are gallstones and how are they formed?

Gallstones are lumps of solid material that form within the gallbladder. There are two major types of gallstones:

- **Cholesterol gallstones** are composed mainly of cholesterol which is made in the liver. These account for nearly 80 percent of all cases of gallstones in the United States.
- **Pigment gallstones** are composed of calcium salts, bilirubin and other material. They account for the remaining 20 percent of gallstones in this country.

Excess cholesterol is removed from the blood by the liver and is then secreted into bile. When bile contains too much cholesterol, small crystals form in bile and they fall to the bottom of the gallbladder. This is like adding too much sugar to coffee and finding sugar at the bottom of the cup. Cholesterol crystals fuse together in the gallbladder to form stones of varying sizes.

Pigment gallstones are formed by the secretion of excess bile pigments and bilirubin into bile. The excess pigments and bilirubin form crystals in the gallbladder.

Gallstones vary in size. They may be as small as tiny specks, or as large as a small ball. The vast majority measure less than 20 mm, about 1 inch, across. Over time, gallstones may grow in size and/or numbers. However, many gallstones remain the same size for years.

Gallbladder sludge occurs when multiple crystals of cholesterol and bilirubin pigments accumulate within the gallbladder but do not fuse together to form a gallstone. Gallbladder sludge typically occurs with fasting and resolves spontaneously. In some, but not all persons, gallbladder sludge can develop into gallstones. In the majority of cases, gallbladder sludge is asymptomatic. However, sludge may cause symptoms identical to those attributed to gallstones.

How often do gallstones cause problems?

Approximately 80 percent of all gallstones are completely asymptomatic and "silent." These stones cause no problems and there is no need for treatment. Once symptoms arise, they not only persist but they increase in frequency. The chance that a "silent" gallstone will become symptomatic is 2 percent for each year. The longer gallstones are present, the more likely it is that they could cause symptoms. However, it will take approximately 25 years for the majority of persons with asymptomatic gallstones to develop symptoms. When symptoms occur in the elderly they can be more difficult to treat, especially if the person has other medical problems.

What are the signs and symptoms of gallstone disease?

Symptoms of gallbladder disease occur when gallstones irritate the gallbladder. The most common symptoms associated with gallstone disease include

- Severe and intermittent pain in the right upper abdomen. This pain can also spread to the chest, shoulders or back. Sometimes this pain may be mistaken for a heart attack.
- Chronic indigestion and nausea

In addition to these symptoms, gallstones can also cause more serious complications. These occur when stones are expelled from the gallbladder during contraction and become lodged within bile ducts. This can lead to infection and obstruction of these ducts. When this occurs it is called acute cholecystitis (if the infection is within the gallbladder) or cholangitis (if the infection is within the bile ducts). Occasionally gallstones may block the bile duct at the entrance to the pancreas and intestine causing pancreatitis (inflammation of the pancreas). Gallstones are the most common cause of acute pancreatitis. If gallstones block the bile ducts for many years then liver damage occurs, leading to liver failure. In rare cases large gallstones may move into the small intestine and cause obstruction near the junction of the small and large intestine. The most common symptoms associated with these complications include the following:

- Severe and steady pain in the right upper abdomen that does not resolve on its own
- Fever and chills
- Severe nausea with vomiting
- Severe pain in the middle of the abdomen and back
- Jaundice, a yellow discoloration of the skin and eyes

How are gallstones identified?

Nearly all gallstones can be easily identified by an ultrasound examination. This is a simple and painless procedure in which sound waves are utilized to create pictures of the gallbladder, bile ducts and its contents. This test is highly sensitive for identifying either gallstones or sludge within the gallbladder.

Cholecystography is a test in which pills containing dyes are taken. These dyes are absorbed and excreted by the liver into the bile. Dye accumulates within the gallbladder and an X-ray is taken.

If gallstones are suspected within the bile ducts, then more specific and complicated testing may need to be performed. The most common test to evaluate bile ducts is called **ERCP** (endoscopic retrograde cholangio-pancreatography). This involves swallowing a small flexible tube through which a physician looks. The tube is then passed through the stomach and into the small intestine where the bile duct enters. Dye is then injected into the bile ducts and X-rays are taken.

If it is impossible to perform the **ERCP**, then a **PTC** (percutaneous transhepatic cholangiogram) can be done. In this test, a very thin needle is passed through the abdomen into the bile ducts, dye is injected and an X-ray is taken.

How can gallstones be treated?

Surgery

The gallbladder is an important organ, but is not essential for life. Many patients with gallstones or its complications have their gallbladders surgically removed safely. Until recently this was performed by "open" surgery, where the surgeon makes a large abdominal incision. Now the preferred surgical technique is to remove the gallbladder through a half-inch incision using a pencil-thin scope, a tiny video camera and long, thin instruments that are inserted through other tiny incisions.

This procedure is called laparoscopic cholecystectomy. It is used in 80 percent of the gallbladder removals because it is relatively safe, reduces the hospital stay to a day or two, is less painful and allows the patient to return to work or normal activity in a short time. An expert medical committee of the National Institutes of Health said the laparoscopic technique is used in 400,000 of the 500,000 gallbladder removals performed annually.

The risk of surgically removing the gallbladder increases with the patient's age and when the patient has other medical illnesses. When the gallbladder is removed bile flows directly from the liver into the small intestine. For most patients this has little to no effect on digestion. However, some patients may continue to have symptoms of gas, intermittent pain, bloating and nausea.

Medication

An oral medication, ursodiol, dissolves cholesterol gallstones and is a safe and effective alternative to gallbladder surgery for many patients. Ursodiol is a natural bile salt which alters the composition of the bile excreted by the liver. The time required to dissolve is directly related to the size of the stone. Multiple small stones dissolve more easily than a single large stone. On average, the time required to dissolve gallstones is approximately six months. Symptoms, however, resolve in the majority of patients soon after starting this medication. Gallstones frequently recur after medication is stopped.

Other Treatments

The following techniques are only used in special circumstances and are available only on a limited basis.

Shock wave lithotripsy is a technique which utilizes sound waves to crush and fragment stones into small pieces. The pieces are then dissolved by the oral medication ursodiol. This technique is best utilized for persons with a single large gallstone.

Contact dissolution involves inserting a needle through the abdomen into the gallbladder and instilling an agent which rapidly dissolves the stones. Utilizing this technique, most gallstones can be dissolved in hours. The needle is then removed.

Can gallstones be prevented?

Recent studies have suggested that persons at highest risk for gallstone formation, obese persons undergoing weight reduction, can virtually eliminate their risk for developing gallstones by taking the oral medication ursodiol. Prevention of gallstone formation with ursodiol in persons with other risk factors has not been investigated.

Each year more than 25 million Americans are afficted with liver and gallbladder diseases and more than 25,000 die of cirrhosis. There are few effective treatments for most life-threatening liver diseases, except for liver transplants. Research has recently opened up exciting new paths for investigation, but much more remains to be done to find cures for more than 100 different liver diseases.

The American Liver Foundation is a national, non-profit voluntary health organization dedicated to preventing, treating and curing hepatitis and all other liver and gallbladder diseases through research and education.

For further information contact

The American Liver Foundation
1425 Pompton Ave
Cedar Grove, NJ 07009
800-223-0179
800-GO-LIVER (465-4837)
888-4-HEP-ABC (443-7222)

■ **Document Source:**
 American Liver Foundation
 1425 Pompton Ave
 Cedar Grove, NJ 07009
 Copyright, The American Liver Foundation
 1996

LIVER FUNCTION TESTS

The term "liver function tests" and its abbreviated form "LFTs" is a commonly used term that is applied to a variety of blood tests that assess the general state of the liver and biliary system. Routine blood tests can be divided into those tests that are true LFTs, such as serum albumin or prothrombin time, and those tests that are simply markers of liver or biliary tract disease, such as the various liver enzymes. In addition to the usual liver tests obtained on routine automated chemistry panels, physicians may order more specific liver tests such as viral serologic tests or autoimmune tests that, if positive, can determine the specific cause of a liver disease.

There are two general categories of "liver enzymes." The first group includes the alanine aminotransferase (ALT) and the aspartate aminotransferase (AST), formerly referred to as the SGPT and SGOT. These are enzymes that are indicators of liver cell damage. The other frequently used liver enzymes are the alkaline phosphatase (alk. phos.) and gamma-glutamyltranspeptidase (GGT) that indicate obstruction to the biliary system, either within the liver or in the larger bile channels outside the liver.

The ALT and AST are enzymes that are located in liver cells and leak out and make their way into the general circulation when liver cells are injured. The ALT is thought to be a more specific indicator of liver inflammation, since the AST may be elevated in diseases of other organs such as the heart or muscle. In acute liver injury, such as acute viral hepatitis, the ALT and AST may be elevated to the high 100s or over 1,000 U/L. In chronic hepatitis or cirrhosis, the elevation of these enzymes may be minimal (less than 2-3 times normal) or moderate (100-300 U/L). Mild or moderate elevations of ALT or AST are nonspecific and may be caused by a wide range of liver diseases. ALT and AST are often used to monitor the course of chronic hepatitis and the response to treatments, such as prednisone and interferon.

The alkaline phosphatase and the GGT are elevated in a large number of disorders that affect the drainage of bile, such as a gallstone or tumor blocking the common bile duct, or alcoholic liver disease or drug-induced hepatitis, blocking the flow of bile in smaller bile channels within the liver. The alkaline phosphatase is also found in other organs, such as bone, placenta, and intestine. For this reason, the GGT is utilized as a supplementary test to be sure that the elevation of alkaline phosphatase is indeed coming from the liver or the biliary tract. In contrast to the alkaline phosphatase, the GGT is not elevated in diseases of bone, placenta, or intestine. Mild or moderate elevation of GGT in the presence of a normal alkaline phosphatase is difficult to interpret and is often caused by changes in the liver cell enzymes induced by alcohol or medications, but without causing injury to the liver.

Bilirubin is the main bile pigment in humans which, when elevated, causes the yellow discoloration of the skin and eyes called jaundice. Bilirubin is formed primarily from the breakdown of a substance in red blood cells called "heme." It is taken up from blood processed through the liver, and then secreted into the bile by the liver. Normal individuals have only a small amount of bilirubin circulating in blood (less than 1.2 mg/dL). Conditions which cause increased formation of bilirubin, such as destruction of red blood cells, or decrease its removal from the blood stream, such as liver disease may result in an increase in the level of serum bilirubin. Levels greater than 3 mg/dL are usually noticeable as jaundice. The bilirubin may be elevated in many forms of liver or biliary tract disease, and thus it is also relatively nonspecific. However, serum bilirubin is generally considered a true test of liver function (LFT), since it reflects the liver's ability to take up, process, and secrete bilirubin into the bile.

Two other commonly used indicators of liver function are the serum albumin and prothrombin time. Albumin is a major protein which is formed by the liver, and chronic liver disease causes a decrease in the amount of albumin produced. Therefore, in more advanced liver disease, the level of the serum albumin is reduced (less than 3.5 mg/dL). The prothrombin time, which is also called protime or PT, is a test that is used to assess blood clotting. Blood clotting factors are proteins made by the liver. When the liver is significantly injured, these proteins are not normally produced. The prothrombin time is also a useful test of liver function, since there is a good correlation between abnormalities in coagulation measured by the prothrombin time and the degree of liver dysfunction. Prothrombin time is usually expressed in seconds and compared to a normal control patient's blood.

Finally, specific and specialized tests may be used to make a precise diagnosis of the cause of liver disease. Elevations in serum iron, the percent of iron saturated in blood, or the iron storage protein ferritin may indicate the presence of hemochromatosis, a liver disease associated with excess iron storage. In another disease involving abnormal metabolism of metals, Wilson's disease, there is an accumulation of copper in the liver, a deficiency of serum ceruloplasmin and excessive excretion of copper into the urine. Low levels of serum alpha 1-antitrypsin may indicate the presence of lung and/or liver disease in children or adults with alpha 1-antitrypsin deficiency. A positive antimitochondrial antibody indicates the underlying condition of primary biliary cirrhosis. Striking elevations of serum globulin, another protein in blood, and the presence of antinuclear antibodies or antismooth muscle antibodies are clues to the diagnosis of autoimmune hepatitis. Finally, there are specific blood tests that allow the precise diagnosis of hepatitis A, hepatitis B, hepatitis C, and hepatitis D.

In summary, blood tests are used to diagnose or monitor liver disease. They may be simply markers of disease (e.g., ALT, AST, alkaline phosphatase, and GGT), more true indicators of overall liver function (serum bilirubin, serum albumin, and prothrombin time) or specific tests that allow the diagnosis of an underlying cause of liver disease. Interpretation of these liver tests is a sophisticated process that your physician will utilize in the context of your medical history, physical examination, and other tests such as X-rays or imaging studies of the liver.

The American Liver Foundation is the only national voluntary nonprofit health organization dedicated to treating, curing and preventing hepatitis and other liver and gallbladder diseases through research and education.

■ **Document Source:**
The American Liver Foundation
1425 Pompton Ave
Cedar Grove, NJ 07009
1-800-223-0179
Copyright, The American Liver Foundation
1995

LUNG AND RESPIRATORY SYSTEM DISORDERS

■■■

CHRONIC OBSTRUCTIVE PULMONARY DISEASE

What is chronic obstructive pulmonary disease?

Chronic obstructive pulmonary disease (COPD), also called chronic obstructive lung disease, is a term that is used for two closely related diseases of the respiratory system: *chronic bronchitis* and *emphysema*. In many patients these diseases occur together, although there may be more symptoms of one than the other. Most patients with these diseases have a long history of heavy cigarette smoking.

COPD gets gradually worse over time. At first there may be only a mild shortness of breath and occasional coughing. Then a chronic cough develops with clear, colorless sputum. As the disease progresses, the cough becomes more frequent and more and more effort is needed to get air into and out of the lungs. In later stages of the disease, the heart may be affected. Eventually death occurs when the function of the lungs and heart is no longer adequate to deliver oxygen to the body's organs and tissues.

Cigarette smoking is the most important risk factor for COPD; it would probably be a minor health problem if people did not smoke. Other risk factors include age, heredity, exposure to air pollution at work and in the environment, and a history of childhood respiratory infections. Living in low socioeconomic conditions also seems to be a contributing factor.

More than 13.5 million Americans are thought to have COPD. It is the fifth leading cause of death in the United States. Between 1980 and 1990, the total death rate from COPD increased by 22 percent. In 1990, it was estimated that there were 84,000 deaths due to COPD, approximately 34 per 100,000 people. Although COPD is still much more common in men than women, the greatest increase in the COPD death rate between 1979 and 1989 occurred in females, particularly in black females (117.6 percent for black females vs. 93 percent for white females). These increases reflect the increased number of women who smoke cigarettes.

COPD attacks people at the height of their productive years, disabling them with constant shortness of breath. It destroys their ability to earn a living, causes frequent use of the health care system, and disrupts the lives of the victims' family members for as long as 20 years before death occurs.

In 1990, COPD was the cause of approximately 16.2 million office visits to doctors and 1.9 million hospital days. The economic costs of this disease are enormous. In 1989, an estimated $7 billion was spent for care of persons with COPD and another $8 billion was lost to the economy by lost productivity due to morbidity and mortality from COPD.

What are chronic bronchitis and emphysema?

Chronic bronchitis, one of the two major diseases of the lungs grouped under COPD, is diagnosed when a patient has excessive airway mucus secretion leading to a persistent, productive cough. An individual is considered to have chronic bronchitis if cough and sputum are present on most days for a minimum of three- months for at least two successive years or for six months during one year. In chronic bronchitis, there also may be narrowing of the large and small airways making it more difficult to move air in and out of the lungs. An estimated 12.1 million Americans have chronic bronchitis.

In *emphysema* there is permanent destruction of the alveoli, the tiny elastic air sacs of the lung, because of irreversible destruction of a protein in the lung called *elastin* that is important for maintaining the strength of the alveolar walls. The loss of elastin also causes collapse or narrowing of the smallest air passages, called bronchioles, which in turn limits airflow out of the lung. The number of individuals with emphysema in the U.S. is estimated to be two million.

In the general population, emphysema usually develops in older individuals with a long smoking history. However, there is also a form of emphysema that runs in families. People with familial emphysema have a hereditary deficiency of a blood component, alpha-l-protease inhibitor, also called alpha-l-antitrypsin (AAT). The number of Americans with this genetic deficiency is quite small, probably no more than 70,000. It is estimated that one in 3,000 newborns have a genetic deficiency of AAT, and 1 to 3 percent of all cases of emphysema are due to AAT deficiency.

The destruction of elastin that occurs in emphysema is believed to result from an imbalance between two proteins in the lung—an enzyme called elastase which breaks down elastin, and AAT which inhibits elastase. In the normal individual, there is enough AAT to protect elastin so that abnormal elastin destruction does not occur. However, when there is a genetic deficiency of AAT, the activity of the elastase is not inhibited and elastin degradation occurs unchecked. If individuals with a severe genetic deficiency of alpha-l-protease inhibitor smoke, they usually have symptoms of COPD by the time they reach early middle age. Deficiency of alpha-l-protease inhibitor can be detected by blood tests available through hospital laboratories. People from families in which relatives have developed emphysema in their thirties and forties should be tested for AAT deficiency. If a deficiency is found, it is critical for these people not to smoke.

Some scientists believe that nonfamilial emphysema, usually called "smoker's emphysema," also results from an imbalance between elastin-degrading enzymes and their inhibitors. The elastase-AAT imbalance is thought to be a result of the effects of smoking, rather than inherited as in familial emphysema. Some evidence for this theory comes from studies on the effect of tobacco smoke on lung cells. These studies showed that tobacco smoke stimulates excess release of elastase from cells normally found in the lung. The inhaled smoke also stimulates more elastase-producing cells to migrate to the lung which in turn causes the release of even more elastase. To make matters worse, oxidants found in cigarette smoke inactivate a significant portion of the elastase inhibitors that are present, thereby decreasing the amount of active antielastase available for protecting the lung and further upsetting the elastase-antielastase balance.

Scientists believe that, in addition to smoking-related processes, there must be other factors that cause emphysema in the general population since only 15 to 20 percent of smokers develop emphysema. The nature and role of these other factors in smokers' emphysema are not yet clear.

What goes wrong with the lungs and other organs in chronic obstructive pulmonary disease?

The most important job that the lungs perform is to provide the body with oxygen and to remove carbon dioxide. This process is called *gas exchange,* and the normal anatomy of the lungs serves this purpose well. The lungs contain 300 million alveoli whose ultrathin walls form the gas exchange surface. Enmeshed in the wall of each of these air sacs is a network of tiny blood vessels, the capillaries, which bring blood to the gas exchange surface. When a person inhales, air flows from the nose and mouth through large and small airways into the alveoli. Oxygen from this air then passes through the thin walls of the inflated alveoli and is taken up by the red blood cells for delivery to the rest of the body. At the same time, carbon dioxide leaves the blood and passes through the alveolar walls into the alveoli. During exhalation, the lung pushes the used air out of the alveoli and through the air passages until it escapes from the nose or mouth. When COPD develops, the walls of the small airways and alveoli lose their elasticity. The airway walls thicken, closing off some of the smaller air passages and narrowing larger ones. The passageways also become plugged with mucus. Air continues to get into alveoli when the lung expands during inhalation, but it is often unable to escape during exhalation because the air passages tend to collapse during exhalation, trapping the "stale" air in the lungs. These abnormalities create two serious problems which affect gas exchange:

- Blood flow and air flow to the walls of the alveoli where gas exchange takes place are uneven or mismatched. In some alveoli there is adequate blood flow but little air, while in others there is a good supply of fresh air but not enough blood flow. When this occurs, fresh air cannot reach areas where there is good blood flow and oxygen cannot enter the bloodstream in normal quantities.

- Pushing the air through narrowed obstructed airways becomes harder and harder. This tires the respiratory muscles so that they are unable to get enough air to the alveoli. The critical step for removing carbon dioxide from the blood is adequate alveolar airflow. If airflow to the alveoli is insufficient, carbon dioxide builds up in the blood and blood oxygen diminishes. Inadequate supply of fresh air to the alveoli is called *hypoventilation.* Breathing oxygen can often correct the blood oxygen levels, but this does not help remove carbon dioxide. When carbon dioxide accumulation becomes a severe problem, mechanical breathing machines called respirators, or ventilators, must be used.

Pulmonary function studies of large groups of people show that lung function—the ability to move air into and out of the lungs—declines slowly with age even in healthy nonsmokers. Because healthy nonsmokers have excess lung capacity, this gradual loss of function does not lead to any symptoms. In smokers, however, lung function tends to worsen much more rapidly. If a smoker stops smoking before serious COPD develops, the rate at which lung function declines returns to almost normal. Unfortunately, because some lung damage cannot be reversed, pulmonary function is unlikely to return completely to normal.

COPD also makes the heart work much harder, especially the main chamber on the right side (right ventricle) which is responsible for pumping blood into the lungs. As COPD progresses, the amount of oxygen in the blood decreases which causes blood vessels in the lung to constrict. At the same time many of the small blood vessels in the lung have been damaged or destroyed as a result of the disease process. More and more work is required from the right ventricle to force blood through the remaining narrowed vessels. To perform this task, the right ventricle enlarges and thickens. When this occurs the normal rhythm of the heart may be disturbed by abnormal beats. This condition, in which the heart is enlarged because of lung problems, is called *cor pulmonale.* Patients with cor pulmonale tire easily and have chest pains and palpitations. If an additional strain is placed on the lungs and heart by a normally minor illness such as a cold, the heart may be unable to pump enough blood to meet the needs of other organs. This results in the inability of the liver and kidneys to carry out their normal functions which leads to swelling of the abdomen, legs, and ankles.

Another adjustment the body makes to inadequate blood oxygen is called *secondary polycythemia,* an increased production of oxygen-carrying red blood cells. The larger than normal number of red blood cells is helpful up to a point; however, a large overpopulation of red cells thickens the blood so much that it clogs small blood vessels causing a new set of problems. People who have a poor supply of oxygen usually have a bluish tinge to their skin, lips, and nailbeds, a condition called *cyanosis.*

Too little oxygen and too much carbon dioxide in the blood also affect the nervous system, especially the brain, and can cause a variety of problems including headache, inability to sleep, impaired mental ability, and irritability.

What is the course of chronic obstructive pulmonary disease?

Daily morning cough with clear sputum is the earliest symptom of COPD. During a cold or other acute respiratory tract infection, the coughing may be much more noticeable and the sputum often turns yellow or greenish. Periods of wheezing are likely to occur especially during or after colds or other respiratory tract infections. Shortness of breath on exertion develops later and progressively becomes more pronounced with severe episodes of breathlessness (*dyspnea*) occurring after even modest activity.

A typical course of COPD might proceed as follows. For a period of about 10 years after cigarette smoking begins, symptoms are usually not very noticeable. After this, the patient generally starts developing a chronic cough with the production of a small amount of sputum. It is unusual to develop shortness of breath during exertion below the age of 40, after which it becomes more common and may be well developed by the age of 50. However, although all COPD patients have these symptoms, not all cigarette smokers develop a notable cough and sputum production, or shortness of breath.

Most patients with COPD have some degree of reversible airways obstruction. It is therefore likely that, at first, treatment will lead to some improvement or stability in lung function. But as COPD progresses, almost all signs and symptoms except cough and sputum production tend to show a gradual worsening. This trend can show fluctuations, but over the course of four or five years, a slow deterioration becomes evident.

Repeated bouts of increased cough and sputum production disable most patients and recovery from coughing attacks may take a long time. Patients with severe lung damage sleep in a semi-sitting position because they are unable to breathe when they lie down. They often complain that they awaken during the night feeling "choked-up," and they need to sit up to cough.

Survival of patients with COPD is closely related to the level of their lung function when they are diagnosed and the rate at which they lose this function. Overall, the median survival is about 10 years for patients with COPD who have lost approximately two-thirds of their normally expected lung function at diagnosis.

How is chronic obstructive pulmonary disease detected?

Researchers are still looking for accurate methods to predict a person's chances of developing airway obstruction. None of the current ways used to diagnose COPD detects the disease before irreversible lung damage occurs. While many measures of lung function have been developed, those most commonly used determine: 1) air-containing volume of the lung (lung volume), 2) the ability to move air into and out of the lung, 3) the rate at which gases diffuse between the lung and blood, and 4) blood levels of oxygen and carbon dioxide.

Lung volumes are measured by breathing into and out of a device called a *spirometer.* Some types of spirometers are very simple mechanical devices which record volume changes as air is added to or removed from them. Other kinds are more sophisticated and use various types of electronic equipment to determine and record the volume of air moved into and out of the lungs. The three volume measures most relevant to COPD are forced vital capacity (FVC), residual volume (RV), and total lung capacity (TLC). The *forced vital capacity* is the maximum volume of air which can be forcibly expelled after inhaling as deeply as possible.

Not all of the air in the lungs is removed when measuring the vital capacity. The amount remaining is called the *residual volume.* The *total lung capacity* is the combination of the forced vital capacity and residual volume. While most of the measured lung volumes or capacities change to some degree with COPD, residual volume usually increases quite markedly. This increase is the result of the weakened airways collapsing before all the normally expired air can leave the lungs. The increased residual volume makes breathing even more difficult and labored.

Because COPD results in narrowed air passages, a measure of the rate at which air can be expelled from the lungs can also be used to determine how severe the narrowing has become. In this test, the *forced vital capacity maneuver,* the patient is asked to inhale as deeply as possible, and on signal, exhale as completely and as rapidly as possible. The volume of air exhaled within one second is then measured. This value is referred to as the *forced expiratory volume in one second* (FEV 1). When FEV 1 is used as an indicator of lung function, the average rate of decline in patients with chronic obstructive lung disease is observed to be two to three times the normal rate of 20-30 milliliters per year. This volume may also be expressed in terms of the percent of the vital capacity which can be expelled in one second. As COPD progresses, less air can be expelled in one second. A greater than expected annual fall in FEV 1 is the most sensitive test for COPD and a fairly good predictor of disability and early death.

Another measure of lung function is called *diffusing capacity.* For this, a more complicated test determines the amount of gas which can move in a given period of time from the alveolar side of the lung into the blood. A number of conditions can cause the diffusing capacity to decrease. However, in COPD the decrease is the result of the destruction of alveolar walls which leads to a significant decrease in surface area for diffusion of oxygen into the blood.

Because the primary function of the lung is to remove carbon dioxide from the blood and add oxygen, another indicator of pulmonary function is the blood levels of oxygen and carbon dioxide. As chronic obstructive pulmonary disease progresses, the amount of oxygen in the blood decreases and carbon dioxide increases.

In most cases, it is necessary to compare the results of several different tests in order to make the correct diagnosis, and to repeat some tests at intervals to determine the rate of disease progression or improvement. Measurement of FEV 1 and FEV 1/FVC ratio should be a routine part of the physical examination of every COPD patient. It is hoped that current research will result in more accurate and earlier measures for detecting lung destruction and diminished function.

How is chronic obstructive pulmonary disease treated?

Although there is no cure for COPD, the disease can be prevented in many cases. And, in almost all cases the disabling symptoms can be reduced. Because cigarette smoking is the most important cause of COPD, not smoking almost always prevents COPD from developing, and quitting smoking slows the disease process.

If the patient and medical team develop and adhere to a program of complete respiratory care, disability can be minimized, acute episodes prevented, hospitalizations reduced, and some early deaths avoided. On the other hand, none of the therapies has been shown to slow the progression of the disease, and only oxygen therapy has been shown to increase the survival rate.

Home oxygen therapy can improve survival in patients with advanced COPD who have *hypoxemia,* low blood oxygen levels. This treatment can improve a patient's exercise tolerance and ability to perform on psychological tests which reflect different aspects of brain function and muscle coordination. Increasing the concentration of oxygen in blood also improves the function of the heart and prevents the development of cor pulmonale. Oxygen can also lessen sleeplessness, irritability, headaches, and the overproduction of red blood cells. Continuous oxygen therapy is recommended for patients with low oxygen levels at rest, during exercise, or while sleeping. Many oxygen sources are available for home use; these include tanks of compressed gaseous oxygen or liquid oxygen and devices that concentrate oxygen from room air. However, oxygen is expensive with the cost per patient running into several hundred dollars per month, depending on the type of system and on the locale.

Medications frequently prescribed for COPD patients:

- *Bronchodilators* help open narrowed airways. There are three main categories: *sympathomimetics* (isoproterenol, metaproterenol, terbutaline, albuterol) which can be inhaled, injected, or taken by mouth; *parasympathomimetics* (atropine, ipratropium bromide); and *methylxanthines* (theophylline and its derivatives) which can be given intravenously, orally, or rectally.
- *Corticosteroids or steroids* (beclomethasone, dexamethasone, triamcinolone, flunisolide) lessen inflammation of the airway walls. They are sometimes used if airway obstruction cannot be kept under control with bronchodilators, and lung function is shown to improve on this therapy. Inhaled steroids given regularly may be of benefit in some patients and have few side effects.
- *Antibiotics* (tetracycline, ampicillin, erythromycin, and trimethoprim-sulfamethoxazole combinations) fight infection. They are frequently given at the first sign of a respiratory infection such as increased sputum production with a change in color of sputum from clear to yellow or green.
- *Expectorants* help loosen and expel mucus secretions from the airways.
- *Diuretics* help the body excrete excess fluid. They are given as therapy to avoid excess water retention associated with right-heart failure. Patients taking diuretics are monitored carefully because dehydration must be avoided. These drugs also may cause potassium imbalances which can lead to abnormal heart rhythms.
- *Digitalis* (usually in the form of digoxin) strengthens the force of the heartbeat. It is used very cautiously in patients who have COPD, especially if their blood oxygen tensions are low, because they are vulnerable to abnormal heart rhythms when taking this drug.
- *Other drugs* sometimes taken by patients with COPD are tranquilizers, pain killers (meperidine, morphine, propoxyphene, etc.), cough suppressants (codeine, etc.), and sleeping pills (barbiturates, etc.). All these drugs depress breathing to some extent; they are avoided whenever possible and used only with great caution.

A number of combination drugs containing various assortments of sympathomimetics, methylxanthines, expectorants, and sedatives are marketed and widely advertised. These drugs are undesirable for COPD patients for several reasons. It is difficult to adjust the dose of methylxanthines without getting interfering side effects from the other ingredients. The sympathomimetic drug used in these preparations is ephedrine, a drug with many side effects and less bronchodilating effect than other drugs now available. The combination drugs often contain sedatives to combat the unpleasant side effects of ephedrine. They also contain expectorants which have not been proven to be effective for all patients and may have some side effects.

Bullectomy, or surgical removal of large air spaces called *bullae* that are filled with stagnant air, may be beneficial in selected patients. Recently, use of lasers to remove bullae has been suggested.

Lung transplantation has been successfully employed in some patients with end-stage COPD. In the hands of an experienced team, the one-year survival in patients with transplanted lungs is over 70 percent.

Pulmonary rehabilitation programs, along with medical treatment, are useful in certain patients with COPD. The goals are to improve overall physical endurance and generally help to overcome the conditions which cause dyspnea and limit capacity for physical exercise and activities of daily living. General exercise training increases performance, maximum oxygen consumption, and overall sense of well-being. Administration of oxygen and nutritional supplements when necessary can improve respiratory muscle strength. Intermittent mechanical ventilatory support relieves dyspnea and rests respiratory muscles in selected patients. Continuous positive airway pressure (CPAP) is used as an adjunct to weaning from mechanical ventilation to minimize dyspnea during exercise. Relaxation techniques may also reduce the perception of ventilatory effort and dyspnea. Breathing exercises and breathing techniques, such as pursed lips breathing and relaxation, improve functional status.

Keeping air passages reasonably clear of secretions is difficult for patients with advanced COPD. Some commonly used methods for mobilizing and removing secretions are the following:

- *Postural bronchial drainage* helps to remove secretions from the airways. The patient lies in prescribed positions that allow gravity to drain different parts of the lung. This is usually done after inhaling an aerosol. In the basic position, the patient lies on a bed with his chest and head over the side and his forearms resting on the floor.
- *Chest percussion* or lightly clapping the chest and back, may help dislodge tenacious or copious secretions.
- *Controlled coughing* techniques are taught to help the patient bring up secretions.
- *Bland aerosols,* often made from solutions of salt or bicarbonate of soda, are inhaled. These aerosols thin and loosen secretions. Treatments usually last 10 to 15 minutes and are taken three or four times a day. Bronchodilators are sometimes added to the aerosols.

How can patients with chronic obstructive pulmonary disease cope best with their illness?

In most instances of COPD, some irreversible damage has already occurred by the time the doctor diagnoses the disease. At this point, the patient and the family should learn as much as possible about the disease and how to live with it. The goals, limitations, and techniques of treatment must be understood by the patient so that symptoms can be kept under control, and daily living can proceed as normally as possible. The doctor and other health care providers are good sources of information about COPD education programs. Patients and family members can usually take part in educational programs offered at a hospital or by a local branch of the American Lung Association.

Patients with COPD can help themselves in many ways. They can

- Stop smoking. Many programs are available to help smokers quit smoking and to stay off tobacco. Some

programs are based on behavior modification techniques; others combine these methods with nicotine gum or nicotine patches as aids to help smokers gradually overcome their dependence on nicotine.
- Avoid work-related exposures to dusts and fumes.
- Avoid air pollution, including cigarette smoke, and curtail physical activities during air pollution alerts.
- Refrain from intimate contact with people who have respiratory infections such as colds or the flu and get a one-time pneumonia vaccination (polyvalent pneumococcal vaccination) and yearly influenza shots.
- Avoid excessive heat, cold, and very high altitudes. (Note: Commercial aircraft cruise at high altitudes and maintain a cabin pressure equal to that of an elevation of 5,000 to 10,000 feet. This can result in hypoxemia for some COPD patients. However, with supplemental oxygen, most COPD patients can travel on commercial airlines.)
- Drink a lot of fluids. This is a good way to keep sputum loose so that it can be brought up by coughing.
- Maintain good nutrition. Usually a high protein diet, taken as many small feedings, is recommended.
- Consider "allergy shots." COPD patients often also have allergies or asthma which complicate COPD.

Of all the avoidable risk factors for COPD, smoking is by far the most significant. Cessation of smoking is the best way to decrease one's risk of developing COPD.

What types of research on chronic obstructive pulmonary disease is the national heart, lung, and blood institute supporting?

The National Heart, Lung, and Blood Institute (NHLBI) is supporting a number of research programs on COPD with the following objectives: 1) to understand its underlying causes, 2) to develop methods of early detection, 3) to improve treatment, and 4) to help patient's and their families better manage the disease.

A study completed several years ago examined the use of oxygen therapy for people who, because of COPD, cannot get enough oxygen into their blood by breathing air. This study has determined that continuous oxygen therapy is more beneficial in extending life than giving oxygen only for 12 hours at night.

Another clinical study compared inhalation therapy using a machine which administers medication to the lungs by intermittent positive pressure breathing (IPPB) with one that delivers the medicine by relying on the patient's own breathing. Although home use of IPPB machines is widespread, previous studies had not been able to show conclusively whether they were effective. In this study, 985 ambulatory patients with COPD were randomly assigned to a treatment group which received a bronchodilator aerosol solution by IPPB, or to a control group which received the medication via a compressor nebulizer. The only difference between the two groups was the positive pressure applied by the IPPB. There was no statistically significant difference between the two treatment groups in numbers of deaths, frequency and length of hospitalization, change in lung function tests, or in measurements of quality of life. This study suggests that the use of IPPB devices may be unnecessary.

An intervention trial called the Lung Health Study, which began in 1983, has enrolled approximately 6,000 smokers in a study to determine whether an intervention program incorporating smoking cessation and use of inhaled bronchodilators (to keep air passages open) in men and women at high risk of developing COPD can slow the decline in pulmonary function compared to a group receiving usual care. When this study is completed, it should help to determine the extent to which identification and treatment of asymptomatic subjects with early signs of obstructive lung disease would be useful as a preventive health measure. In addition, the study will test some of the current theories about behavior and smoking cessation. Early results indicate that cigarette smoking may be more harmful to women than to men. Furthermore, smoking cessation results in greater weight gain in women than in men, and to avoid weight gain women are less likely to quit smoking and more likely to revert to their smoking habit.

Because familial emphysema results from a deficiency of AAT in affected individuals, efforts to minimize the risk of emphysema have been directed at increasing the circulating AAT levels either by promoting or increasing the production of AAT within the individual, or augmenting it from the outside. One strategy for improving the production of AAT is by pharmacological means (e.g., by administration of drugs such as danazol or estrogen/progesterone combinations), but this has not been found to be effective. Genetic engineering to correct the defective gene or introduce the functional gene in the deficient individuals is being attempted by several NHLBI-supported investigators. The normal gene for AAT as well as the mutant genes causing AAT deficiency have been characterized and cloned, and animal models carrying the mutant gene have been developed. The resulting animals displayed many of the physical and histologic changes seen in human neonatal AAT deficiency. These studies should provide the groundwork for future development of gene replacement therapy for AAT deficiency.

In the meantime, attention is being focused on AAT augmentation therapy for familial emphysema. Studies have shown that intravenous infusion of AAT fractionated from blood is safe and biochemically effective, that is, the needed blood levels of AAT can be maintained by the continued administration of AAT at appropriate intervals.

Because of the practical and fiscal limitations to mounting a clinical trial for establishing the clinical efficacy of AAT augmentation therapy for emphysema, the NHLBI sponsored a national registry of patients with AAT deficiency to assess the natural history of severe AAT deficiency and to examine whether the disease course is altered by the augmentation therapy. This program is enrolling, at various medical centers both in the U.S. and Europe, at least 1,000 adult patients with AAT deficiency satisfying certain other eligibility criteria. The patients will be followed for 3 to 5 years (chest x rays, lung function, blood and urine analysis, etc.) at one of 37 participating clinical centers. The evaluation of the data and the release of the conclusions are expected by early 1995.

Methods to treat emphysema before it becomes disabling remain an important research objective of programs supported by NHLBI. Since it is believed that either excess protease (elastase), or too little useful antiprotease, can lead to development of the disease, scientists have also been attempting to use other approaches to develop animal models which will mimic the human condition of inherited alpha-1-protease inhibitor deficiency and using such models to test if natural or synthetic antiproteases can be used safely to prevent development of emphysema-like lesions in these animals. If found safe and effective in animals, these agents can be tried in humans.

For More Information

Additional information on COPD can be obtained from

National Heart, Lung, and Blood Institute
Division of Lung Diseases
Two Rockledge Center
6701 Rockledge Dr
MSC 7952
Ste 10018
Bethesda, MD 20892-7952
(301) 435-0230

Glossary

Aerosol: A solution of a drug that is made into a fine mist for inhalation.

Airway obstruction: A narrowing, clogging, or blocking of the passages that carry air to the lungs.

Alpha-1-antitrypsin: (See alpha-1-protease inhibitor.)

Alpha-1-protease inhibitor: A substance in blood transported to the lungs that inhibits the digestive activity of trypsin and other proteases which digest proteins. Deficiency of this substance is associated with emphysema.

Alveoli: Tiny sac-like air spaces in the lungs where transfer of carbon dioxide from blood into the lungs and oxygen from air into blood takes place.

Bronchi: Larger air passages of the lungs.

Bronchiole: Finer air passages of the lungs.

Broncho-constriction: Tightening of the muscles surrounding bronchi, the tubes that branch from the windpipe.

Bronchodilator: A drug that relaxes the smooth muscles and opens the constricted airway.

Capillaries: The smallest blood vessels in the body through which most of the oxygen, carbon dioxide, and nutrient exchanges take place.

Cor pulmonale: Heart disease due to lung problems.

Corticosteroids: A group of hormones produced by adrenal glands.

Continuous positive airway pressure (CPAP): A mechanical ventilation technique used to deliver continuous positive airway pressure.

Cyanosis: Bluish color of the skin associated with insufficient oxygen.

Dyspnea: Shortness of breath; difficult or labored breathing.

Elastin: An elastic substance in the lungs (and some other body organs) that support their structural framework.

Elastase inhibitors or antielastases: Substances in the blood transported to the lungs and other organs which prevent the digestive action of elastases.

Elastin degrading enzymes (elastases): Substances in the blood transported to the lungs and other organs which digest or breakdown elastin.

Gas exchange: A primary function of the lungs involving transfer of oxygen from inhaled air into blood and of carbon dioxide from blood into lungs.

Hypoventilation: A state in which there is an insufficient amount of air entering and leaving the lungs to bring oxygen into tissues and eliminate carbon dioxide.

Hypoxemia: Deficient oxygenation of the blood.

Hypoxia: A state in which there is oxygen deficiency.

Intermittent positive pressure breathing (IPPB) machine: A device that assists intermittent positive pressure inhalation of therapeutic aerosols without hand coordination required in the use of hand nebulizers or metered dose inhalers.

Laser: In the context of a therapeutic tool, it is a device that produces a high-intensity light that can generate extreme heat instantaneously when it hits a target.

Lavage: To wash a body organ.

Neonatal: Period up to the first 4 weeks after birth.

Pneumonia: Inflammation of the lungs.

Postural bronchial drainage: Draining of liquids from the lungs by placing the patient in postures (e.g., head below chest) which facilitate liquid flow.

Vaccination: Administration of weakened or killed bacteria or virus to stimulate immunity and protection against further exposure to that agent.

Ventilation: The process of exchange of air between the lungs and the atmosphere leading to exchange of gases in the blood.

■ **Document Source:**
U.S. Department of Health and Human Services, Public Health Service
Public Health Service
National Institutes of Health
National Heart, Lung, and Blood Institute
NIH Publication No. 95-2020
Originally Printed 1981; Previously Revised 1993; Reprinted November 1995

National Institute on Aging Age Page

PNEUMONIA PREVENTION: IT'S WORTH A SHOT

Pneumococcal (pronounced new-mo-KOK-al) disease is an infection caused by bacteria. These bacteria can attack different parts of the body. When they invade the lungs, they cause the most common kind of bacterial pneumonia. When the same bacteria attack blood cells, they cause an infection called bacteremia (bak-ter-E-me-ah). And in the brain, they cause meningitis. Pneumococcal pneumonia is a serious illness that kills thousands of older people in the United States each year.

Can pneumonia be prevented?

Yes. The pneumococcal vaccine is safe, it works, and one shot lasts most people a lifetime. People who get the vaccine are protected against almost all of the bacteria that cause pneumococcal pneumonia and other pneumococcal diseases as well. The shot, which is covered by Medicare, can be a lifesaver.

Some experts say it may be best to get the shot before age 65—anytime after age 50—since the younger you are, the better the results. They also say people should have this shot even if they have had pneumonia before. There are many different kinds of pneumonia, and having one kind does not protect against the others. The vaccine, however, does protect against 88 percent of the pneumococcal bacteria that cause pneumonia. It does not guarantee that you will never get pneumonia. It does not protect against viral pneumonia. Most people need to get the shot only once. However some older people may need a booster; check with your doctor to find out if this is necessary.

Are there side effects?

Some people have mild side effects from the shot, but these usually are minor and last only a very short time. In studies, about half of the people getting the vaccine had mild side effects—swelling and soreness at the spot where the shot was given, usually on the arm. A few people (less than 1 percent) had fever and muscle pain as well as more serious swelling and pain on the arm. The pneumonia shot cannot cause pneumonia because it is not made from the bacteria itself, but from an extract that is not infectious. The same is true of the flu shot; it cannot cause flu. In fact, people can get the pneumonia vaccine and a flu shot at the same time.

Who should get the vaccine?

According to the National Institute on Aging, one of the National Institutes of Health, everyone age 65 and older should get the pneumococcal vaccine. Some younger people should get it also.

Ask a doctor for the vaccine if you

- Are age 65 or older, or
- Have a chronic illness, such as heart or lung disease or diabetes, or
- Have a weak immune system (this can be caused by certain kidney diseases, some cancers, HIV infection, organ transplant medicines, and other diseases).

Key Facts

- Everyone age 65 and older should get the pneumococcal vaccine.
- Anyone with a chronic disease or a weak immune system should also get the vaccine.
- Most people need to get it only once.
- Most people have mild or no side effects.
- It is covered by Medicare.

About the Disease and the Vaccine

- There are two main kinds of pneumonia—viral pneumonia and bacterial pneumonia. Bacterial pneumonia is the most serious. One kind of bacteria causes pneumococcal pneumonia. In older people, this type of pneumonia is a common cause of hospitalization and death.
- About 20 to 30 percent of people over age 65 who have pneumococcal pneumonia develop bacteremia. At least 20 percent of those with bacteremia die from it, even though they get antibiotics.
- People age 65 and older are at high risk. They are two to three times more likely than people in general to get pneumococcal infections.
- A recent, large study by the National Institutes of Health shows that the vaccine prevents most cases of pneumococcal pneumonia.

The U.S. Public Health Service, the National Foundation for Infectious Diseases, and the American Lung Association now recommend that all people age 65 and older get this vaccine.

Resources

More information about adult immunizations is available from the following groups.

National Institute on Aging
PO Box 8057
Gaithersburg, MD 20898-8057
1-800-222-2225
1-800-222-4225 (TTY)

National Institute of Allergy and Infectious Diseases
9000 Rockville Pike
Rm 7A50
Bethesda, MD 20892
(301) 496-5717

Centers for Disease Control and Prevention
National Immunization Program
1600 Clifton Rd
Atlanta, GA 30333
(404) 639-1819

American Lung Association
1740 Broadway
New York, NY 10019-4374
1-800-LUNG-USA
(1-800-586-4872)

National Foundation for Infectious Diseases
Ste 750
4733 Bethesda Ave
Bethesda, MD 20814
(301) 656-0003

■ **Document Source:**
  U.S. Department of Health and Human Services, Public Health Service
  National Institutes of Health
  National Institute on Aging
  1994

SARCOIDOSIS

Usual Symptoms

Shortness of breath (dyspnea) and a cough that won't go away can be among the first symptoms of sarcoidosis. But sarcoidosis can also show up suddenly with the appearance of skin rashes. Red bumps (erythema nodosum) on the face, arms, or shins, and inflammation of the eyes are also common symptoms. It is not unusual, however, for sarcoidosis symptoms to be more general. Weight loss, fatigue, night sweats, fever, or just an overall feeling of ill health can also be clues to the disease.

Who gets sarcoidosis?

Sarcoidosis was once considered a rare disease. We now know that it is a common chronic illness that appears all over the world. Indeed, it is the most common of the fibrotic lung disorders, and occurs often enough in the United States for Congress to have declared a national Sarcoidosis Awareness Day in 1990.

Anyone can get sarcoidosis. It occurs in all races and in both sexes. Nevertheless, the risk is greater if you are a young black adult, especially a black woman, or of Scandinavian, German, Irish, or Puerto Rican origin. No one knows why.

Because sarcoidosis can escape diagnosis or be mistaken for several other diseases, we can only guess at how many people are affected. The best estimate today is that about 5 in 100,000 white people in the United States have sarcoidosis. Among black people, it occurs more frequently, in probably 40 out of 100,000 people.

Overall, there appear to be 20 cases per 100,000 in cities on the east coast and somewhat fewer in rural locations. Some scientists, however, believe that these figures greatly underestimate the percentage of the US population with sarcoidosis.

Sarcoidosis mainly affects people between 20 to 40 years of age. White women are just as likely as white men to get sarcoidosis, but the black female gets sarcoidosis two times as often as the black male.

Sarcoidosis also appears to be more common and more severe in certain geographic areas. it has long been recognized as a common disease in Scandinavian countries, where it is estimated to affect 64 out of 100,000 people. But it was not until the mid-1940s—when a large number of cases were identified during mass chest x-ray screening for the Armed Forces—that its high prevalence was recognized in North America.

What Sarcoidosis Is Not

Much about sarcoidosis remains unknown. Nevertheless, if you have the disease, you can be reassured about several things.

Sarcoidosis is usually not crippling. It often goes away by itself, with most cases healing in 24 to 36 months. Even when sarcoidosis lasts longer, most patients can go about their lives as usual.

Sarcoidosis is not a cancer. It is not contagious, and your friends and family will not catch it from you. Although it can occur in families, there is no evidence that sarcoidosis is passed from parents to children.

Some Things We Don't Know About Sarcoidosis

Sarcoidosis is currently thought to be associated with an abnormal immune response. Whether a foreign substance is the trigger; whether that trigger is a chemical, drug, virus, or some other substance; and how exactly the immune disturbance is caused are not known.

Researchers supported by the National Heart, Lung, and Blood Institute are trying to solve some of these mysteries. Among the research questions they are trying to answer are:

- Does sarcoidosis have many causes, or is it produced by a single agent?
- In which body organ does sarcoidosis actually start?
- How does sarcoidosis spread from one part of the body to another?
- Do heredity, environment, and lifestyle play any role in the appearance, severity, or length of the disease?
- Is the abnormal immune response seen in patients a cause or an effect of the disease?
- How can sarcoidosis be prevented?

Course of the Disease

In general, sarcoidosis appears briefly and heals naturally in 60 to 70 percent of the cases, often without the patient knowing or doing anything about it. From 20 to 30 percent of sarcoidosis patients are left with some permanent lung damage. In 10 to 15 percent of the patients, sarcoidosis can become chronic.

When either the granulomas or fibrosis seriously affect the function of a vital organ—sarcoidosis can be fatal. This occurs 5 to 10 percent of the time.

No one can predict how sarcoidosis will progress in an individual patient. But the symptoms the patient experiences, the doctor's findings, and the patient's race can give some clues.

For example, a sudden onset of general symptoms such as weight loss or feeling poorly are usually taken to mean that the course of sarcoidosis will be relatively short and mild. Dyspnea and possibly skin sarcoidosis often indicate that the sarcoidosis will be more chronic and severe.

White patients are more likely to develop the milder form of the disease. Black people tend to develop the more chronic and severe form.

Sarcoidosis rarely develops before the age of 10 or after the age of 60. However, the illness—with or without symptoms—has been reported in younger as well as in older people. When symptoms do appear in these age groups, the symptoms are those that are more general in nature, for example, tiredness, sluggishness, coughing, and a general feeling of ill health.

Diagnosis

Preliminary diagnosis is based on the patient's medical history, routine tests, a physical examination, and a chest x-ray.

The doctor confirms the diagnosis of sarcoidosis by eliminating other diseases with similar features. These include such granulomatous diseases as berylliosis (a disease resulting from exposure to beryllium metal), tuberculosis, farmer's lung disease (hypersensitivity pneumonitis), fungal infections, rheumatoid arthritis, rheumatic fever, and cancer of the lymph nodes (lymphoma).

Signs and Symptoms

In addition to the lungs and lymph nodes, the body organs more likely than others to be affected by sarcoidosis are the liver, skin, heart, nervous system, and kidneys, in that order of frequency. Patients can have symptoms related to the specific organ affected, they can have only general symptoms, or they can be without any symptoms whatsoever. Symptoms also can vary according to how long the illness has been under way, where the granulomas are forming, how much tissue has become affected, and whether the granulomatous process is still active.

Even when there are no symptoms, a doctor can sometimes pick up signs of sarcoidosis during a routine examination, usually a chest x-ray, or when checking out another complaint. The patient's age and race or ethnic group can raise an additional red flag that a sign or symptom of illness could be related to sarcoidosis. Enlargement of the salivary or tear glands and cysts in bone tissue are also among sarcoidosis signals.

Lungs. The lungs are usually the first site involved in sarcoidosis. Indeed, about 9 out of 10 sarcoidosis patients have some type of lung problem, with nearly one-third of these patients showing some respiratory symptoms—usually coughing, either dry or with phlegm, and dyspnea. Occasionally, patients have chest pain and a feeling of tightness in the chest.

It is thought that sarcoidosis of the lungs begins with alveolitis (inflammation of the alveoli), the tiny sac-like air spaces in the lungs where carbon dioxide and oxygen are exchanged. Alveolitis either clears up spontaneously or leads to granuloma formation. Eventually fibrosis can form, causing the lung to stiffen and making breathing even more difficult.

Eyes. Eye disease occurs in about 20 to 30 percent of patients with sarcoidosis, particularly in children who get the disease. Almost any part of the eye can be affected—the membranes of the eyelids, cornea, outer coat of the eyeball (sclera), retina, and lens. The eye involvement can start with no symptoms at all or with reddening or watery eyes. In a few cases, cataracts, glaucoma, and blindness can result.

Skin. The skin is affected in about 20 percent of sarcoidosis patients. Skin sarcoidosis is usually marked by small, raised patches on the face. Occasionally the patches are purplish in color and larger. Patches can also appear on limbs, face, and buttocks.

Other symptoms include erythema nodosum, mostly on the legs and often accompanied by arthritis in the ankles, elbows, wrists, and hands. Erythema nodosum usually goes away, but other skin problems can persist.

Nervous system. In an occasional case (1 to 5 percent), sarcoidosis can lead to neurological problems. For example, sarcoid granulomas can appear in the brain, spinal cord, and facial and optic nerves. Facial paralysis and other symptoms of nerve damage call for prompt treatment.

Laboratory Tests

No single test can be relied on for a correct diagnosis of sarcoidosis. X-rays and blood tests are usually the first procedures the doctor will order. Pulmonary function tests often provide clues to diagnosis. Other tests may also be used, some more often than others.

Many of the tests that the doctor calls on to help diagnose sarcoidosis can also help the doctor follow the progress of the disease and determine whether the sarcoidosis is getting better or worse.

Chest x-ray. A picture of the lungs, heart, as well as the surrounding tissues containing lymph nodes, where infection-fighting white blood cells form, can give the first indication of sarcoidosis. For example, a swelling of the lymph glands between the two lungs can show up on an x-ray. An x-ray can also show which areas of the lung are affected.

Pulmonary function tests. By performing a variety of tests called pulmonary function tests (PFT), the doctor can find out how well the lungs are doing their job of expanding the exchanging oxygen and carbon dioxide with the blood. The lungs of sarcoidosis patients cannot handle these tasks as well as they should; this is because granulomas and fibrosis of lung tissue decrease lung capacity and disturb the normal flow of gases between the lungs and the blood.

One PFT procedure calls for the patient to breathe into a machine, called a spirometer. It is a mechanical device that records changes in the lung size as air is inhaled and exhaled, as well as the time it takes the patient to do this.

Blood tests. Blood analyses can evaluate the number and types of blood cells in the body and how well the cells are functioning. They can also measure the levels of various blood proteins known to be involved in immunological activities, and they can show increases in serum calcium levels and abnormal liver function that often accompany sarcoidosis.

Blood tests can measure a blood substance called angiotensin-converting enzyme (ACE). Because the cells that make up granulomas secrete large amounts of ACE, the enzyme levels are often high in patients with sarcoidosis. ACE levels, however, are not always high in sarcoidosis patients, and increased ACE levels can also show up in other illnesses.

Bronchoalveolar lavage. This test uses an instrument called a bronchoscope—a long, narrow tube with a light at the end—to wash out, or lavage, cells and other materials from inside the lungs. This wash fluid is then examined for the amount of various cells and other substances that reflect inflammation and immune activity in the lungs. A high number of white blood cells in this fluid usually indicates an inflammation in the lungs.

Biopsy. Microscopic examination of specimens of lung tissue obtained with a bronchoscope, or of specimens of other tissues, can tell a doctor where granulomas have formed in the body.

Gallium scanning. In this procedure, the doctor injects the radioactive chemical element gallium-67 into the patient's vein. The gallium collects at places in the body affected by sarcoidosis and other inflammatory conditions. Two days after the injection, the body is scanned for radioactivity.

Increases in gallium uptake at any site in the body indicate that inflammatory activity has developed at the site and also give an idea of which tissue, and how much tissue, has been affected. However, since any type of inflammation causes gallium uptake, a positive gallium scan does not necessary mean that the patient has sarcoidosis.

Kveim test. This test involves injecting a standardized preparation of sarcoid tissue material into the skin. On the one hand, a unique lump formed at the point of injection is considered positive for sarcoidosis. On the other hand, the test result is not always positive even if the patient has sarcoidosis.

The Kveim test is not used often in the United States because no test material has been approved for sale by the U.S. Food and Drug Administration. However, a few hospitals and clinics may have some standardized test preparation prepared privately for their own use.

Slit-lamp examination. An instrument called a slit lamp, which permits examination of the inside of the eye, can be used to detect silent damage from sarcoidosis.

Management

Fortunately, many patients with sarcoidosis require no treatment. Symptoms, after all, are usually not disabling and do tend to disappear spontaneously.

When therapy is recommended, the main goal is to keep the lungs and other affected body organs working and to relieve symptoms. The disease is considered inactive once the symptoms fade. After many years of experience with treating the disease, corticosteroids remain the primary treatment for inflammation and granuloma formation. Prednisone is probably the corticosteroid most often prescribed today. There is no treatment at present to reverse the fibrosis that might be present in advanced sarcoidosis.

Occasionally, a blood test will show a high blood level of calcium accompanying sarcoidosis. The reasons for this are not clear. Some scientists believe that this condition is not common. When it does occur, the patient may be advised to avoid calcium-rich foods, vitamin D, or sunlight, or to take prednisone; this corticosteroid quickly reverses the condition.

Because sarcoidosis can disappear even without therapy, doctors sometimes disagree on when to start the treatment, what dose to prescribe, and how long to continue the medicine. The doctor's decision depends on the organ system involved and how far the inflammation has progressed. If the disease appears to be severe—especially in the lungs, eyes, heart, nervous system, spleen, or kidneys—the doctor may prescribe corticosteroids.

Corticosteroid treatment usually results in improvement. Symptoms often start up again, however, when it is stopped. Treatment, therefore, may be necessary for several years, sometimes for as long as the disease remains active or to prevent relapse.

Frequent checkups are important so that the doctor can monitor the illness and, if necessary, adjust the treatment. Corticosteroids, for example, can have side effects—mood swings, swelling, and weight gain because the treatment tends to make the body hold on to water; high blood pressure; high blood sugar; and craving for food. Long-term use can affect the stomach, skin, and bones. This situation can bring on stomach pain, an ulcer, or acne, or cause the loss of calcium from bones. However, if the corticosteroid is taken in carefully prescribed, low doses, the benefits from the treatment are usually far greater than the problems.

Besides corticosteroids, various other drugs have been tried, but their effectiveness has not been established in controlled studies. These drugs include chloroquine and D-penicillamine.

Several drugs such as chlorambucil, azathioprine, methotrexate, and cyclophosphamide, which might suppress alveolitis by killing the cells that produce granulomas, have also been used. None has been evaluated in controlled clinical trials, and the risk of using these drugs is high, especially in pregnant women.

Cyclosporine, a drug used widely in organ transplants to suppress immune reaction, has been evaluated in one controlled trial. it was found to be unsuccessful.

Research Status in Sarcoidosis: Goals of the National Heart, Lung, and Blood Institute

There are many unanswered questions about sarcoidosis. Identifying the agent that causes the illness, along with the inflammatory mechanisms that set the stage for the alveolitis, granuloma formation, and fibrosis that characterize the disease, is the major aim of the National Heart, Lung, and Blood Institute's program on sarcoidosis. Development of reliable methods of diagnosis, treatment, and eventually, the prevention of sarcoidosis is the ultimate goal.

Originally, scientists thought that sarcoidosis was caused by an acquired state of immunological inertness (anergy). This notion was revised a few years ago, when the technique of bronchoalveolar lavage provided access to a vast array of cells and cell-derived mediators operating in the lungs of sarcoidosis patients. Sarcoidosis is now believed to be associated with a complex mix of immunological disturbances involving simultaneous activation, as well as depression, of certain immunological functions.

Immunological studies on sarcoidosis patients show that many of the immune functions associated with thymus-derived white blood cells, called T-lymphocytes or T-cells, are depressed. The depression of this cellular component of systemic immune response is expressed in the inability of the patients to evoke a delayed hypersensitivity skin reaction (a positive skin test), when tested by the appropriate foreign substance, or antigen, underneath the skin.

In addition, the blood of sarcoidosis patients contains a reduced number of T-cells. These T-cells do not seem capable of responding normally when treated with substances known to stimulate the growth of laboratory-cultured T-cells. Neither do they produce their normal complement of immunological mediators, cytokines, through which the cells modify the behavior of other cells.

In contrast to the depression of the cellular immune response, humoral immune response of sarcoidosis patients is elevated. The humoral immune response is reflected by the production of circulating antibodies against a variety of exogenous antigens, including common viruses. This humoral component of systemic immune response is mediated by another class of lymphocytes known as B-lymphocytes, or B-cells, because they originate in the bone marrow.

In another indication of heightened humoral response, sarcoidosis patients seem prone to develop autoantibodies (antibodies against endogenous antigens) similar to rheumatoid factors.

With access to the cells and cell products in the lung tissue compartments through the bronchoalveolar technique, it also has become possible for researchers to complement the above investigations at the blood level with analysis of local inflammatory and immune events in the lungs.

In contrast to what is seen at the systemic level, the cellular immune response in the lungs seems to be heightened rather than depressed. The heightened cellular immune response in the diseased tissue is characterized by significant increases in activated T-lymphocytes with certain characteristic cell-surface antigens, as well as in activated alveolar macrophages.

This pronounced, localized cellular response is also accompanied by the appearance in the lung of an array of mediators that are thought to contribute to the disease process; these include interleukin-1, interleukin-2, B-cell growth factor, B-cell differentiation factor, fibroblast growth factor, and fibronectin.

Because a number of lung diseases follow respiratory tract infections, ascertaining whether a virus can be implicated in the events leading to sarcoidosis remains an important area of research. Some recent observations seem to provide suggestive leads on this question. In these studies, the genes of cytomegalovirus (CMV), a common disease-causing virus, were introduced into lymphocytes, and the expression of the viral genes was studied. It was found that the viral genes were expressed both during acute infection of the cells and when the virus was not replicating in the cells. However, this expression seemed to take place only when the T-cells were activated by some injurious event.

In addition, the product of a CMV gene was found capable of activating the gene in alveolar macrophage responsible for the production of interleukin-1. Since interleukin-1 levels are found to increase in alveolar macrophages from patients with sarcoidosis, this suggests that certain viral genes can enhance the production of inflammatory components associated with sarcoidosis. Whether these findings implicate viral infections in the disease process in sarcoidosis is unclear. Future research with viral models may provide clues to the molecular mechanisms that trigger alterations in lymphocyte and macrophage regulation leading to sarcoidosis.

In 1995, the National Heart, Lung, and Blood Institute started a multicenter case control study of the etiology of sarcoidosis. The investigation is planned to last six years and will collect information and specimen for use in investigation of environmental, occupational, lifestyle, and genetic risk factors for sarcoidosis. Examination of the natural history of sarcoidosis is planned in patients at early and late stages of the disease. Such information should improve our understanding of the cause(s) of sarcoidosis and provide insight into how to better prevent and treat the disease.

Living with Sarcoidosis

The cause of sarcoidosis still remains unknown, so there is at present no known way to prevent or cure this disease. However, doctors have had a great deal of experience in management of the illness.

If you have sarcoidosis, you can help yourself by following sensible health measures. You should not smoke. You should also avoid exposure to other substances such as dusts and chemicals that can harm your lungs.

Patients with sarcoidosis are best treated by a lung specialist or a doctor who has a special interest in sarcoidosis. Sarcoidosis specialists are usually located at major research centers.

If you have any symptoms of sarcoidosis, see your doctor regularly so that the illness can be watched and, if necessary, treated. if it heals naturally, sarcoidosis is unlikely to recur. Nevertheless, if you have had sarcoidosis, or are suspected of having the illness but have no symptoms now, be sure to have physical checkups every year, including an eye examination.

Although severe sarcoidosis can reduce the chances of becoming pregnant, particularly for older women, many young women with sarcoidosis have given birth to healthy babies while on treatment. Patients planning to have a baby should discuss the matter with their doctor. Medical checkups all through pregnancy and immediately thereafter are especially important for sarcoidosis patients. In some cases, bed rest is necessary during the last three months of pregnancy.

In addition to family and close friends, a number of local lung organizations, other nonprofit health organizations, and self-help groups are available to help patients cope with sarcoidosis. By keeping in touch with them, you can share personal feelings and experiences. Members also share specific information on the latest scientific advances, where to find sarcoidosis specialists, and how to improve one's self-image.

For More Information

Additional information on sarcoidosis is available from a number of sources.

For the names of US scientists working on sarcoidosis or physicians specializing in the disease, write to

National Heart, Lung, and Blood Institute Division of Lung Diseases
2 Rockledge Center
6701 Rockledge Drive
MSC 7952
Ste 10018
Bethesda, MD 20892-7952

If you are interested in participating in clinical studies of sarcoidosis ongoing at the NHLBI, **have your physician** write to

National Heart, Lung, and Blood Institute
Pulmonary Branch
9000 Rockville Pike
Building 10, Room 6D06
Bethesda, MD 20892

Information and publications for sarcoidosis patients and their families are available from

National Institute of Allergy and Infectious Diseases
9000 Rockville Pike
Building 31, Room 7A32
Bethesda, MD 20892

Sarcoidosis Family Aid and Research Foundation
460A Central Ave
East Orange, NJ 07018

Many local chapters of the American Lung Association host support groups for sarcoidosis patients. The address and telephone number of the chapter nearest to you should be in your local telephone directory. Or you can write or call the association's national headquarters

American Lung Association
1740 Broadway
New York, NY 10019-4374
(212) 315-8700

Listed below are addresses of organizations that provide additional information and patient support groups on sarcoidosis

Sarcoidosis Networking
13925 80th Street E
Puyallup, WA 98372
(206) 845-3108

National Sarcoidosis Resources Center
PO Box 1593
Piscataway, NJ 08855-1593
(907) 699-0733

Sarcoidosis Research Institute
3475 Central Ave
Memphis, TN 38111
(901) 327-5454

Glossary

ACE: Angiotensin-converting enzyme.

Alveoli: The tiny sac-like air spaces in the lung where carbon dioxide and oxygen are exchanged.

Alveolitis: Inflammation of the alveoli.

Anergy: Absence of immune response to particular substances.

Berylliosis: A lung disease resulting from exposure to beryllium metal.

Bronchoscope: A long, narrow tube with a light at the end that is used by the doctor for direct observation of the airways, as well as for suction of tissue and other materials.

Dyspnea: Shortness of breath.

Enzyme: Substance, made by living cells, that causes specific chemical changes.

Erythema nodosum: Red bumps that tend to appear on the face, arms, and shins.

Fibrotic tissue: Inflamed tissue that has become scarred.

Granulomas: Small lumps in tissues caused by inflammation.

Inflammation: A basic response of the body to injury, usually showing up in skin redness, warmth, swelling, and pain.

Lavage: To wash out a body organ.

Lymph nodes: Small, bean-shaped organs of the immune system distributed throughout the body tissue.

Lymphoma: Cancer of the lymph nodes.

PFT: Pulmonary function test.

Pneumonitis: A disease caused by inhaling a wide variety of substances such as dusts and molds. Also called "farmer's disease."

Sclera: Outer coat of the eyeball.

■ Document Source:
  U.S. Department of Health and Human Services, Public Health Service
  National Institutes of Health
  National Heart, Lung, and Blood Institute
  NIH Publication No. 95-3093
  Reprinted July 1995

SLEEP APNEA

What is sleep apnea?

Sleep apnea is a serious, potentially life-threatening condition that is far more common than generally understood. First described in 1965, sleep apnea is a breathing disorder characterized by brief interruptions of breathing during sleep. It owes its name to a Greek word, apnea, meaning "want of breath." There are two types of sleep apnea: central and obstructive. Central sleep apnea, which is less common, occurs when the brain fails to send the appropriate signals to the breathing muscles to initiate respirations. Obstructive sleep apnea is far more common and occurs when air cannot flow into or out of the person's nose or mouth although efforts to breathe continue.

In a given night, the number of involuntary breathing pauses or "apneic events" may be as high as 20 to 30 or more per hour. These breathing pauses are almost always accompanied by snoring between apnea episodes, although not everyone who snores has this condition. Sleep apnea can also be characterized by choking sensations. The frequent interruptions of deep, restorative sleep often lead to early morning headaches and excessive daytime sleepiness.

Early recognition and treatment of sleep apnea is important because it may be associated with irregular heartbeat, high blood pressure, heart attack, and stroke.

Who gets sleep apnea?

Sleep apnea occurs in all age groups and both sexes but is more common in men (it may be underdiagnosed in women) and possibly young African Americans. It has been estimated that as many as 18 million Americans have sleep apnea. Four percent of middle-aged men and 2 percent of middle-aged women have sleep apnea along with excessive daytime sleepiness. People most likely to have or develop sleep apnea include those who snore loudly and also are overweight, or have high blood pressure, or have some physical abnormality in the nose, throat, or other parts of the upper airway. Sleep apnea seems to run in some families, suggesting a possible genetic basis.

What causes sleep apnea?

Certain mechanical and structural problems in the airway cause the interruptions in breathing during sleep. In some people, apnea occurs when the throat muscles and tongue relax during sleep and partially block the opening of the airway. When the muscles of the soft palate at the base of the tongue and the uvula (the small fleshy tissue hanging from the center of the back of the throat) relax and sag, the airway becomes blocked, making breathing labored and noisy and even stopping it altogether. Sleep apnea also can occur in obese people when an excess amount of tissue in the airway causes it to be narrowed. With a narrowed airway, the person continues his or her efforts to breathe, but air cannot easily flow into or out of the nose or mouth. Unknown to the person, this results in heavy snoring, periods of no breathing, and frequent arousals (causing abrupt changes from deep sleep to light sleep). Ingestion of alcohol and sleeping pills increases the frequency and duration of breathing pause in people with sleep apnea.

How is normal breathing restored during sleep?

During the apneic event, the person is unable to breathe in oxygen and to exhale carbon dioxide, resulting in low levels of oxygen and increased levels of carbon dioxide in the blood. The reduction in oxygen and increase in carbon dioxide alert the brain to resume breathing and cause an arousal. With each arousal, a signal is sent from the brain to the upper airway muscles to open the airway; breathing is resumed, often with a loud snort or gasp. Frequent arousals, although necessary for breathing to restart, prevent the patient from getting enough restorative, deep sleep.

What are the effects of sleep apnea?

Because of the serious disturbances in their normal sleep patterns, people with sleep apnea often feel very sleepy during the day and their concentration and daytime performance suffer. The consequences of sleep apnea range from annoying to life-threatening. They include depression, irritability, sexual dysfunction, learning and memory difficulties, and falling asleep while at work, on the phone, or driving. It has been estimated that up to 50 percent of sleep apnea patients have high blood pressure. Although it is not known with certainty if there is a cause and effect relationship, it appears that sleep apnea contributes to high blood pressure. Risk for heart attack and stroke may also increase in those with sleep apnea. In addition, sleep apnea is sometimes implicated in sudden infant death syndrome.

When should sleep apnea be suspected?

For many sleep apnea patients, their spouses are the first ones to suspect that something is wrong, usually from their heavy snoring and apparent struggle to breathe. Coworkers or friends of the sleep apnea victim may notice that the individual falls asleep during the day at inappropriate times (such as while driving a car, working, or talking). The patient often does not know he or she has a problem and may not believe it when told. It is important that the person see a doctor for evaluation of the sleep problem.

How is sleep apnea diagnosed?

In addition to the primary care physician, pulmonologists, neurologists, or other physicians with specialty training in sleep disorders may be involved in making a definitive diagnosis and initiating treatment. Diagnosis of sleep apnea is not simple because there can be many different reasons for disturbed sleep. Several tests are available for evaluating a person for sleep apnea.

Polysomnography is a test that records a variety of body functions during sleep, such as the electrical activity of the brain, eye movement, muscle activity, heart rate, respiratory effort, air flow, and blood oxygen levels. These tests are used both to diagnose sleep apnea and to determine its severity.

The *Multiple Sleep Latency Test* (MSLT) measures the speed of falling asleep. In this test, patients are given several opportunities to fall asleep during the course of a day when they would normally be awake. For each opportunity, time to fall asleep is measured. People without sleep problems usually take an average of 10 to 20 minutes to fall asleep. Individuals who fall asleep in less than 5 minutes are likely to require some treatment for sleep disorders. The MSLT may be useful to measure the degree of excessive daytime sleepiness and to rule out other types of sleep disorders.

Diagnostic tests usually are performed in a sleep center, but new technology may allow some sleep studies to be conducted in the patient's home.

How is sleep apnea treated?

The specific therapy for sleep apnea is tailored to the individual patient based on medical history, physical examination, and the results of polysomnography. Medications are generally not effective in the treatment of sleep apnea. Oxygen administration may safely benefit certain patients but does not eliminate sleep apnea or prevent daytime sleepiness. Thus, the role of oxygen in the treatment of sleep apnea is controversial, and it is difficult to predict which patients will respond well. It is important that the effectiveness of the selected treatment be verified; this is usually accomplished by polysomnography.

Behavioral Therapy

Behavioral changes are an important part of the treatment program, and in mild cases behavioral therapy may be all that is needed. The individual should avoid the use of alcohol, tobacco, and sleeping pills, which make the airway more likely to collapse during sleep and prolonged the apneic periods. Overweight persons can benefit from losing weight. Even a 10 percent weight loss can reduce the number of apneic events for most patients. In some patients with mild sleep apnea, breathing pauses occur only when they sleep on their backs. In such cases, using pillows and other devices that help them sleep in a side position is often helpful.

Physical or Mechanical Therapy

Nasal *continuous positive airway pressure (CPAP)* is the most common effective treatment for sleep apnea. In this procedure, the patient wears a mask over the nose during sleep, and pressure from an air blower forces air through the nasal passages. The air pressure is adjusted so that it is just enough to prevent the throat from collapsing during sleep. The pressure is constant and continuous. Nasal CPAP prevents airway closure while in use, but apnea episodes return when CPAP is stopped or used improperly.

Variations of the CPAP device attempt to minimize side effects that sometimes occur, such as nasal irritation and drying, facial skin irritation, abdominal bloating, mask leaks, sore eyes, and headaches.

Some versions of CPAP vary the pressure to coincide with the person's breathing pattern, and others start with low pressure, slowly increasing it to allow the person to fall asleep before the full prescribed pressure is applied.

Dental appliances that reposition the lower jaw and the tongue have been helpful to some patients with mild sleep apnea or who snore but do not have apnea. Possible side effects include damage to teeth, soft tissues, and the jaw joint. A dentist or orthodontist is often the one to fit the patient with such a device.

Surgery

Some patients with sleep apnea may need surgery. Although several surgical procedures are used to increase the size of the airway, none of them is completely successful or without risks. More than one procedure may need to be tried before the patient realizes any benefits.

Some of the more common procedures include removal of adenoids and tonsils (especially in children), nasal polyps or other growths, or other tissue in the airway and correction of structural deformities. Younger patients seem to benefit from these surgical procedures more than older patients.

Uvulopalatopharyngoplasty (UPPP) is a procedure used to remove excess tissue at the back of the throat (tonsils, uvula, and part of the soft palate). The success of this technique may range from 30 to 50 percent. The long-term side effects and benefits are not known, and it is difficult to predict which patients will do well with this procedure.

Laser-assisted uvulopalatoplasty (LAUP) is done to eliminate snoring but has not been shown to be effective in treating sleep apnea. This procedure involves using a laser device to eliminate tissue in the back of the throat. Like UPPP, LAUP may decrease or eliminate snoring but not sleep apnea itself. Elimination of snoring, the primary symptom of sleep apnea, without influencing the condition may carry the risk of delaying the diagnosis and possible treatment of sleep apnea in patients who elect LAUP. To identify possible underlying sleep apnea, sleep studies are usually required before LAUP is performed.

Tracheostomy is used in persons with severe, life-threatening sleep apnea. In this procedure, a small hole is made in the windpipe and a tube is inserted into the opening. This tube stays closed during waking hours, and the person breathes and speaks normally. It is opened for sleep so that air flows directly into the lungs, bypassing any upper airway obstruction. Although this procedure is highly effective, it is an extreme measure that is poorly tolerated by patients and rarely used.

Other procedures. Patients in whom sleep apnea is due to deformities of the lower jaw may benefit from surgical reconstruction. Finally, surgical procedures to treat obesity are sometimes recommended for sleep apnea patients who are morbidly obese.

For More Information

Information about sleep disorders research can be obtained from the NCSDR. In addition, the NHLBI Information Center can provide you with sleep education materials as well as other publications relating to heart, lung, and blood diseases.

National Center on Sleep Disorders Research
Two Rockledge Centre, Ste 7024
6701 Rockledge Dr MSC 7920
Bethesda, MD 20892-7920
(301) 435-0199
(301) 480-3451 (fax)

NHLBI Information Center
PO Box 30105
Bethesda, MD 20824-0105
(301) 251-1222
(301) 251-1223 (fax)

■ **Document Source:**
U.S. Department of Health and Human Services, Public Health Service
National Institutes of Health
National Heart, Lung, and Blood Institute
NIH Publication No. 95-3798
September 1995

MENTAL AND EMOTIONAL HEALTH

■ ■ ■

ANXIETY DISORDERS

by Marilyn Dickey

Everybody knows what it's like to feel anxious—the butter-flies in your stomach before a first date, the tension you feel when your boss is angry, the way your heart pounds if you're in danger. Anxiety rouses you to action. It gears you up to face a threatening situation. It makes you study harder for that exam, and keeps you on your toes when you're making a speech. In general, it helps you cope.

But if you have an *anxiety disorder,* this normally helpful emotion can do just the opposite—it can keep you from coping and can disrupt your daily life. Anxiety disorders aren't just a case of "nerves." They are illnesses, often related to the biological makeup and life experiences of the individual, and they frequently run in families. There are several types of anxiety disorders, each with its own distinct features.

An anxiety disorder may make you feel anxious most of the time, without any apparent reason. Or the anxious feelings may be so uncomfortable that to avoid them you may stop some everyday activities. Or you may have occasional bouts of anxiety so intense they terrify and immobilize you.

Anxiety disorders are the most common of all the mental disorders. At the National Institute of Mental Health (NIMH), the federal agency that conducts and supports research related to mental disorders, mental health, and the brain, scientists are learning more and more about the nature of anxiety disorders, their causes, and how to alleviate them. NIMH also conducts educational outreach activities about anxiety disorders and other mental illnesses.

Many people misunderstand these disorders and think individuals should be able to overcome the symptoms by sheer willpower. Wishing the symptoms away does not work—but there are treatments that can help. That's why NIMH has produced this pamphlet—to help you understand these conditions, describe their treatments, and explain the role of research in conquering anxiety and other mental disorders.

This brochure gives brief explanations of generalized anxiety disorder, panic disorder (which is sometimes accompanied by agoraphobia), specific phobias, social phobias, obsessive-compulsive disorder, and post-traumatic stress dis-

order. More detailed information on some of these anxiety disorders is available through NIMH or other sources. (See the listings at the end of this pamphlet.)

Generalized Anxiety Disorder

I always thought I was just a worrier. I'd feel keyed up and unable to relax. At times it would come and go, and at times it would be constant. It could go on for days. I'd worry about what I was going to fix for a dinner party, or what would be a great present for somebody. I just couldn't let something go.

I'd have terrible sleeping problems. There were times I'd wake up wired in the morning or in the middle of the night. I had trouble concentrating, even reading the newspaper or a novel. Sometimes I'd feel a little lightheaded. My heart would race or pound. And that would make me worry more.

Generalized Anxiety Disorder (GAD) is much more than the normal anxiety people experience day to day. It's chronic and exaggerated worry and tension, even though nothing seems to provoke it. Having this disorder means always anticipating disaster, often worrying excessively about health, money, family, or work. Sometimes, though, the source of the worry is hard to pinpoint. Simply the thought of getting through the day provokes anxiety.

People with GAD can't seem to shake their concerns, even though they usually realize that their anxiety is more intense than the situation warrants. People with GAD also seem unable to relax. They often have trouble falling or staying asleep. Their worries are accompanied by physical symptoms, especially trembling, twitching, muscle tension, headaches, irritability, sweating, or hot flashes. They may feel lightheaded or out of breath. They may feel nauseated or have to go to the bathroom frequently. Or they might feel as though they have a lump in the throat.

Many individuals with GAD startle more easily than other people. They tend to feel tired, have trouble concentrating, and sometimes suffer depression, too.

Usually the impairment associated with GAD is mild and people with the disorder don't feel too restricted in social settings or on the job. Unlike many other anxiety disorders, people with GAD don't characteristically avoid certain situations as a result of their disorder. However, if severe, GAD can be very debilitating, making it difficult to carry out even the most ordinary daily activities.

GAD comes on gradually and most often hits people in childhood or adolescence, but can begin in adulthood, too. It's more common in women than in men and often occurs in relatives of affected persons. It's diagnosed when someone spends at least six months worried excessively about a number of everyday problems.

In general, the symptoms of GAD seem to diminish with age. Successful treatment may include a medication called buspirone. Research into the effectiveness of other medications, such as benzodiazepines and antidepressants, is ongoing. Also useful are cognitive-behavioral therapy, relaxation techniques, and biofeedback to control muscle tension.

Depression

Depression often accompanies anxiety disorders and, when it does, it needs to be treated as well. The feelings of sadness, apathy, or hopelessness, changes in appetite or sleep, and difficulty concentrating that often characterize depression can be effectively treated with antidepressant medications, or, depending on their severity, by psychotherapy. Some people respond best to a combination of medication and psychotherapy. Treatment can help the majority of people with depression.

Panic Disorder

It started 10 years ago. I was sitting in a seminar in a hotel and this thing came out of the clear blue. I felt like I was dying.

For me, a panic attack is almost a violent experience. I feel like I'm going insane. It makes me feel like I'm losing control in a very extreme way. My heart pounds really hard, things seem unreal, and there's this very strong feeling of impending doom.

In between attacks there is this dread and anxiety that it's going to happen again. It can be very debilitating, trying to escape those feelings of panic.

Panic Attack Symptoms

- Pounding heart
- Chest pains
- Lightheadedness or dizziness
- Nausea or stomach problems
- Flushes or chills
- Shortness of breath or a feeling of smothering or choking
- Tingling or numbness
- Shaking or trembling
- Feelings of unreality
- Terror
- A feeling of being out of control or going crazy
- Fear of dying
- Sweating

People with panic disorder have feelings of terror that strike suddenly and repeatedly with no warning. They can't predict when an attack will occur, and many develop intense anxiety between episodes, worrying when and where the next one will strike. In between times there is a persistent, lingering worry that another attack could come any minute.

When a panic attack strikes, most likely your heart pounds and you may feel sweaty, weak, faint, or dizzy. Your hands may tingle or feel numb, and you might feel flushed or chilled. You may have chest pain or smothering sensations, a sense of unreality, or fear of impending doom or loss of control. You may genuinely believe you're having a heart attack or stroke, losing your mind, or on the verge of death. Attacks can occur any time, even during nondream sleep. While most attacks average a couple of minutes, occasionally they can go on for up to 10 minutes. In rare cases, they may last an hour or more.

Panic disorder strikes between three and six million Americans, and is twice as common in women as in men. It can appear at any age—in children or in the elderly—but most often it begins in young adults. Not everyone who experiences panic attacks will develop panic disorder—for example, many people have on attack but never have another. For those who do have panic disorder, though, it's important to seek treatment. Untreated, the disorder can become very disabling.

Panic disorder is often accompanied by other conditions such as depression or alcoholism, and may spawn phobias, which can develop in places or situations where panic attacks have occurred. For example, in a panic attack strikes while you're riding an elevator, you may develop a fear of elevators and perhaps start avoiding them.

Some people's lives become greatly restricted—they avoid normal, everyday activities such as grocery shopping, driving, or in some cases even leaving the house. Or, they may be able to confront a feared situation only if accompanied by a spouse or other trusted person. Basically, they avoid any situation they fear would make them feel helpless if a panic attack occurs. When people's lives become so restricted by the disorder, as happens in about one-third of all people with panic disorder, the condition is called *agoraphobia*. A tendency toward panic disorder and agoraphobia runs in families. Nevertheless, early treatment of panic disorder can often stop the progression to agoraphobia.

Studies have shown that proper treatment—a type of psychotherapy called cognitive-behavioral therapy, medications, or possibly a combination of the two—helps 70 to 90 percent of people with panic disorder. Significant improvement is usually seen within six to eight weeks.

Cognitive-behavioral approaches teach patients how to view the panic situations differently and demonstrate ways to reduce anxiety, using breathing exercises or techniques to refocus attention, for example. Another technique used in cognitive-behavioral therapy, called exposure therapy, can often help alleviate the phobias that may result from panic disorder. In exposure therapy, people are very slowly exposed to the fearful situation until they become desensitized to it.

Some people find the greatest relief from panic disorder symptoms when they take certain prescription medications. Such medications, like cognitive-behavioral therapy, can help to prevent panic attacks or reduce their frequency and severity. Two types of medications that have been shown to be safe and effective in the treatment of panic disorder are antidepressants and benzodiazepines.

Phobias

Phobias occur in several forms. A *specific phobia* is a fear of a particular object or situation. *Social phobia* is a fear of being painfully embarrassed in a social setting. And *agoraphobia*, which often accompanies panic disorder, is a fear of being in any situation that might provoke a panic attack, or from which escape might be difficult if one occurred.

Specific Phobias

I'm scared to death of flying, and I never do it anymore. It's an awful feeling when that airplane door closes and I feel trapped. My heart pounds and I sweat bullets. If somebody starts talking to me, I get very stiff and preoccupied. When the airplane starts to ascend, it just reinforces that feeling that I can't get out. I picture myself losing control, freaking out, climbing the walls, but of course I never do. I'm not afraid of crashing or hitting turbulence. It's just that feeling of being trapped. Whenever I've thought about changing jobs, I've had to think, "Would I be under pressure to fly?" These days I only go places where I can drive or take a train. My friends always point out that I couldn't get off a train traveling at high speeds either, so why don't trains bother me? I just tell them it isn't a rational fear.

Many people experience specific phobias, intense, irrational fears of certain things or situations—dogs, closed-in places, heights, escalators, tunnels, highway driving, water, flying, and injuries involving blood are a few of the more common ones. Phobias aren't just extreme fear; they are irrational fear. You may be able to ski the world's tallest mountains with ease but panic going above the 10th floor of an office building. Adults with phobias realize their fears are irrational, but often facing, or even thinking about facing, the feared object or situation brings on a panic attack or severe anxiety.

Specific phobias strike more than one in 10 people. No one knows just what causes them, though they seem to run in families and are a little more prevalent in women. Phobias usually first appear in adolescence or adulthood. They start suddenly and tend to be more persistent than childhood phobias; only about 20 percent of adult phobias vanish on their own. When children have specific phobias—for example, a fear of animals—those fears usually disappear over time, though they may continue into adulthood. No one knows why they hang on in some people and disappear in others.

If the object of the fear is easy to avoid, people with phobias may not feel the need to seek treatment. Sometimes, though, they may make important career or personal decisions to avoid a phobic situation.

When phobias interfere with a person's life, treatment can help. Successful treatment usually involves a kind of cognitive-behavioral therapy called desensitization or exposure therapy, in which patients are gradually exposed to what frightens them until the fear begins to fade. Three-fourths of patients benefit significantly from this type of treatment. Relaxation and breathing exercises also help reduce anxiety symptoms.

There is currently no proven drug treatment for specific phobias, but sometimes certain medications may be prescribed to help reduce anxiety symptoms before someone faces a phobic situation.

Social Phobia

I couldn't go on dates or to parties. For a while, I couldn't even go to class. My sophomore year of college I had to come home for a semester.

My fear would happen in any social situation. I would be anxious before I even left the house, and it would escalate as I got closer to class, a party, or whatever. I would feel sick to my stomach—it almost felt like I had the flu. My heart would pound, my palms would get sweaty, and I would get this feeling of being removed from myself and from everybody else.

When I would walk into a room full of people, I'd turn red and it would feel like everybody's eyes were on me. I was too embarrassed to stand off in a corner by myself, but I couldn't think of anything to say to anybody. I felt so clumsy, I couldn't wait to get out.

Social phobia is an intense fear of becoming humiliated in social situations, specifically of embarrassing yourself in front of other people. It often runs in families and may be accompanied by depression or alcoholism. Social phobia often begins around early adolescence or even younger.

If you suffer form social phobia, you tend to think that other people are very competent in public and that you are not. Small mistakes you make may seem to you much more exaggerated than they really are. Blushing itself may seem painfully embarrassing, and you feel as though all eyes are focused on you. You may be afraid of being with people other than those closest to you. Or your fear may be more specific, such as feeling anxious about giving a speech, talking to a boss or other authority figure, or dating. The most common social phobia is a fear of public speaking. Sometimes social phobia involves a general fear or social situations such as parties. More rarely it may involve a fear of using a public restroom, eating out, talking on the phone, or writing in the presence of other people, such as when signing a check

Although this disorder is often thought of as shyness, the two are not the same. Shy people can be very uneasy around others, but they don't experience the extreme anxiety in anticipating a social situation, and they don't necessarily avoid circumstances that make them feel self-conscious. In contrast, people with social phobias aren't necessarily shy at all. They can be completely at ease with people most of the time, but particular situations, such as walking down an aisle in public or making a speech, can give them intense anxiety. Social phobia disrupts normal life, interfering with career or social relationships. For example, a worker can turn down a job promotion because he can't give public presentations. The dread of a social event can begin weeks in advance, and symptoms can be quite debilitating.

People with social phobia are aware that their feelings are irrational. Still, they experience a great deal of dread before facing the feared situation, and they may go out of their way to avoid it. Even if they manage to confront what they fear, they usually feel very anxious beforehand and are intensely uncomfortable throughout. Afterward, the unpleasant feelings may linger, as they worry about how they may have been judged or what others may have thought or observed about them..

Treatment for Anxiety Disorders

Many people with anxiety disorders can be helped with treatment. Therapy for anxiety disorders often involves medication or specific forms of psychotherapy.

Medications, although not cures, can be very effective at relieving anxiety symptoms. Today, thanks to research by scientists at NIMH and other research institutions, there are more medications available than ever before to treat anxiety disorders. So if one drug is not successful, there are usually others to try. In addition, new medications to treat anxiety symptoms are under development.

For most of the medications that are prescribed to treat anxiety disorders, the doctor usually starts the patient on a low dose and gradually increases it to the full dose. Every medication has side effects, but they usually become tolerated or diminish with time. If side effects become a problem, the doctor may advise the patient to stop taking the medication and to wait a week—or longer for certain drugs—before trying another one. When treatment is near an end, the doctor will taper the dosage gradually.

Research has also shown that behavioral therapy and cognitive-behavioral therapy can be effective for treating several of the anxiety disorders.

Behavioral therapy focuses on changing specific actions and uses several techniques to decrease or stop unwanted behavior. For example, one technique trains patients in *diaphragmatic breathing*, a special breathing exercise involving slow, deep breaths to reduce anxiety. This is necessary because people who are anxious often hyperventilate, taking rapid shallow breaths that can trigger rapid heartbeat, lightheadedness, and other symptoms. Another technique—*exposure therapy*—gradually exposes patients to what frightens them and helps them cope with their fears.

Like behavioral therapy, cognitive-behavioral therapy teaches patients to react differently to the situations and bodily sensations that trigger panic attacks and other anxiety symptoms. However, patients also learn to understand how their thinking patterns contribute to their symptoms and how to change their thoughts so that symptoms are less likely to occur. This awareness of thinking patterns is combined with exposure and other behavioral techniques to help people confront their feared situations. For example, someone who becomes lightheaded during a panic attack and fears he is going to die can be helped with the following approach used in cognitive-behavioral therapy. The therapist asks him to spin in a circle until he becomes dizzy. When he becomes alarmed and starts thinking, "I'm going to die," he learns to replace that thought with a more appropriate one, such as, "It's just a little dizziness—I can handle it."

About 80 percent of people who suffer from social phobia find relief from their symptoms when treated with cognitive-behavioral therapy or medications or a combination of the two. Therapy may involve learning to view social events differently; being exposed to a seemingly threatening social situation in such a way that it becomes easier to face; and learning anxiety-reducing technique, social skills, and relaxation techniques.

The medications that have proven effective include antidepressants called MAO inhibitors. People with a specific form of social phobia called performance phobia have been helped by drugs called beta-blockers. For example, musicians or others with this anxiety may be prescribed a beta-blocker for use on the day of a performance.

Obsessive-Compulsive Disorder

I couldn't do anything without rituals. They transcended every aspect of my life. Counting was big for me. When I set my alarm at night, I had to set it to a number that wouldn't add up to a "bad" number. If my sister was 33 and I was 24, I couldn't leave the TV on Channel 33 or 24. I would wash my hair three times as opposed to once because three was a good luck number and one wasn't. It took me longer to read because I'd count the lines in a paragraph. If I was writing a term paper, I couldn't have a certain number of words on a line if it added up to a bad number. I was always worried that if I didn't do something, my parents were going to die. Or I would worry about harming my parents, which was completely irrational. I couldn't wear anything that said Boston because my parents were from Boston. I couldn't write the word "death" because I was worried that something bad would happen.

Getting dressed in the morning was tough because I had a routine, and if I deviated from that routine, I'd have to get dressed again.

I knew the rituals didn't make sense, but I couldn't seem to overcome them until I had therapy.

Obsessive-compulsive disorder is characterized by anxious thoughts or rituals you feel you can't control. If you have OCD, as it's called, you may be plagued by persistent, unwelcome thoughts or images, or by the urgent need to engage in certain rituals.

You may be obsessed with germs or dirt, so you wash your hands over and over. You may be filled with doubt and feel the need to check things repeatedly. You might be preoccupied by thoughts of violence and fear that you will harm people close to you. You may spend long periods of time touching things or counting; you may be preoccupied by order or symmetry; you may have persistent thoughts of performing sexual acts that are repugnant to you; or you may be troubled by thoughts that are against your religious beliefs.

The disturbing thoughts or images are called obsessions, and the rituals that are performed to try to prevent or dispel them are called compulsions. There is no pleasure in carrying out the rituals you are drawn to, only temporary relief from the discomfort caused by the obsession.

A lot of healthy people can identify with having some of the symptoms of OCD, such as checking the stove several times before leaving the house. But the disorder is diagnosed only when such activities consume at least an hour a day, are very distressing, and interfere with daily life.

Most adults with this condition recognize that what they're doing is senseless, but they can't stop it. Some people, though, particularly children with OCD, may not realize that their behavior is out of the ordinary.

OCD strikes men and women in approximately equal numbers and afflicts roughly one in 50 people. It can appear in childhood, adolescence, or adulthood, but on the average it first shows up in the teens or early adulthood. A third of adults with OCD experienced their first symptoms as children. The course of the disease is variable—symptoms may come and go, they may ease over time, or they can grow progressively worse. Evidence suggests that OCD might run in families.

Depression or other anxiety disorders may accompany OCD. And some people with OCD have eating disorders. In addition, they may avoid situations in which they might have to confront their obsessions. Or they may try unsuccessfully to use alcohol or drugs to calm themselves. If OCD grows severe enough, it can keep someone from holding down a job or from carrying out normal responsibilities at home, but more often it doesn't develop to those extremes.

Research by NIMH-funded scientists and other investigators has led to the development of medications and behavioral treatments that can benefit people with OCD. A combination of the two treatments is often helpful for most patients. Some individuals respond best to one therapy, some to another. Two medications that have been found effective in treating OCD are clomipramine and fluoxetine. A number of others are showing promise, however, and may soon be available.

Behavioral therapy, specifically a type called *exposure and response prevention,* has also proven useful for treating OCD. It involves exposing the person to whatever triggers the problem and then helping him or her forego the usual ritual—for instance, having the patient touch something dirty and then not wash his hands. This therapy is often successful in patients who complete a behavioral therapy program, though results have been less favorable in some people who have both OCD and depression.

Post-Traumatic Stress Disorder

> I was raped when I was 25 years old. For a long time, I spoke about the rape on an intellectual level, as though it was something that happened to someone else. I was very aware that it had happened to me, but there just was no feeling. I kind of skidded along for a while.
>
> I started having flashbacks. They kind of came over me like a splash of water. I would be terrified. Suddenly I was reliving the rape. Every instant was startling. I felt like my entire head was moving a bit, shaking, but that wasn't so at all. I would get very flushed or a very dry mouth and my breathing changed. I was held in suspension. I wasn't aware of the cushion on the chair that I was sitting in or that my arm was touching a piece of furniture. I was in a bubble, just kind of floating. And it was scary. Having a flashback can wring you out. You're really shaken.
>
> The rape happened the week before Christmas, and I feel like a werewolf around the anniversary date. I can't believe the transformation into anxiety and fear.

Post-Traumatic Stress Disorder (PTSD) is a debilitating condition that follows a terrifying event. Often, people with PTSD have persistent frightening thoughts and memories of their ordeal and feel emotionally numb, especially with people they were once close to. PTSD, once referred to as shell shock or battle fatigue, was first brought to public attention by war veterans, but it can result from any number of traumatic incidents. These include kidnapping, serious accidents such as car or train wrecks, natural disasters such as floods or earthquakes, violent attacks such as a mugging, rape, or torture, or being held captive. The event that triggers it may be something that threatened the person's life or the life of someone close to him or her. Or it could be something witnessed, such as mass destruction after a plane crash.

Whatever the source of the problem, some people with PTSD repeatedly relive the trauma in the form of nightmares and disturbing recollections during the day. They may also experience sleep problems, depression, feeling detached or numb, or being easily startled. They may lose interest in things they used to enjoy and have trouble feeling affectionate. They may feel irritable, more aggressive than before, or even violent. Seeing things that remind them of the incident may be very distressing, which could lead them to avoid certain places or situations that bring back those memories. Anniversaries of the event are often very difficult.

PTSD can occur at any age, including childhood. The disorder can be accompanied by depression, substance abuse, or anxiety. Symptoms may be mild or severe—people may become easily irritated or have violent outbursts. In severe cases they may have trouble working or socializing. In general, the symptoms seem to be worse if the event that triggered them was initiated by a person—such as a rape, as opposed to a flood.

Ordinary events can serve as reminders of the trauma and trigger flashbacks or intrusive images. A flashback may make the person lose touch with reality and reenact the event for a period of seconds or hours or, very rarely, days. A person having a flashback, which can come in the form of images, sounds, smells, or feelings, usually believes that the traumatic event is happening all over again.

Not every traumatized person gets full-blown PTSD, or experiences PTSD at all. PTSD is diagnosed only if the symptoms last more than a month. In those who do have PTSD, symptoms usually begin within three months of the trauma, and the course of the illness varies. Some people recover within six months, others have symptoms that last much longer. In some cases, the condition may be chronic. Occasionally, the illness doesn't show up until years after the traumatic event.

Antidepressants and anxiety-reducing medications can ease the symptoms of depression and sleep problems, and psychotherapy, including cognitive-behavioral therapy, is an integral part of treatment. Being exposed to a reminder of the trauma as part of therapy—such as returning to the scene of a rape—sometimes helps. And, support from family and friends can help speed recovery.

How to Get Help for Anxiety Disorders

If you, or someone you know, has symptoms of anxiety, a visit to the family physician is usually the best place to start. A physician can help you determine if the symptoms are due to an anxiety disorder, some other medical condition, or both. Most often, the next step to getting treatment for an anxiety disorder is referral to a mental health professional.

Among the professionals who can help are psychiatrists, psychologists, social workers, and counselors. However, it's best to look for a professional who has *specialized training* in cognitive-behavioral or behavioral therapy and who is open to the use of medications, should they be needed.

Coexisting Conditions

Many people have a single anxiety disorder and nothing else, but it isn't unusual for an anxiety disorder to be accompanied by another illness, such as depression, an eating disorder, alcoholism, drug abuse, or another anxiety disorder. Often people who have panic disorder or social phobia, for example, also experience the intense sadness and hopelessness associated with depression or become dependent on alcohol. In such cases, these problems will need to be treated as well.

Psychologists, social workers, and counselors sometimes work closely with a psychiatrist or other physician, who will prescribe medications when they are required. For some people, group therapy or self-help groups are a helpful part of treatment. Many people do best with a combination of these therapies.

When you're looking for a health-care professional, it's important to inquire about what kinds of therapy he or she generally uses or whether medications are available. It's important that you feel comfortable with the therapy. If this is not the case, seek help elsewhere. However, if you've been taking medication, it's important not to quit certain drugs abruptly, but to taper them off under the supervision of your physician. Be sure to ask your physician about how to stop a medication.

Remember, though, that when you find a health-care professional you're satisfied with, the two of you are working as a team. Together you will be able to develop a plan to treat your anxiety disorder that may involve medications, behavioral therapy, or cognitive-behavioral therapy, as appropriate. Treatments for anxiety disorders, however, may not start working instantly. Your doctor or therapist may ask you to follow a specific treatment plan for several weeks to determine whether it's working.

For More Information

Anxiety Disorders Association of America
Dept. A
6000 Executive Blvd, Ste 513
Rockville, MD 20852
(301) 231-9350

Freedom from Fear
308 Seaview Ave
Staten Island, NY 10305
(718) 351-1717

National Anxiety Foundation
3135 Custer Drive
Lexington, KY 40157-4001
(606) 272-7166

Obsessive Compulsive (OC) Foundation, Inc.
PO Box 70
Milford, CT 06460
(203) 878-5669

American Psychiatric Association
1400 K Street, NW
Washington, DC 20005
(202) 682-6220

American Psychological Association
750 1st St, NE
Washington, DC 20002-4242
(202) 336-5500

Association for the Advancement of Behavior Therapy
305 7th Ave
New York, NY 10001
(212) 647-1890

National Alliance for the Mentally Ill
200 N Glebe Rd, Ste 1015
Arlington, VA 22203-3754
(800) 950-NAMI (-6264)

National Institute of Mental Health
Toll-free information services:
Depression: 1-800-421-4211
Panic and Other Anxiety Disorders: 1-800-647-2642

National Mental Health Association
1201 Prince St
Alexandria, VA 22314-2971
(703) 684-7722

National Mental Health Consumers' Self-Help Clearinghouse
1211 Chestnut St
Philadelphia, PA 19107
(800) 553-4539

Phobics Anonymous
PO Box 1180
Palm Springs, CA 92263
(619) 322-COPE (-2673)

Society for Traumatic Stress Studies
60 Revere Dr, Ste 500
Northbrook, IL 60062
(708) 480-9080

Related NIMH Brochures

The following brochures, giving more detailed information on various anxiety disorders and related topics, are available by contacting: NIMH, Room 7C-02, 5600 Fishers Lane, Rockville, MD 20857-8030.

- Understanding Panic Disorder (NIH Pub. No. 93-3482)
- Obsessive-Compulsive Disorder (NIH Pub. No. 94-3755)
- Medications (DHHS Pub. No. (ADM) 92-1509)
- Plain Talk About Depression (NIH Pub. No. 94-3561)

■ **Document Source:**
U.S. Department of Health and Human Services, Public Health Service
National Institutes of Health
National Institute of Mental Health
NIH Publication No. 95-3879
Printed 1994, Reprinted 1995

See also: Getting Treatment for Panic Disorder (page 328)

ATTENTION DEFICIT HYPERACTIVITY DISORDER

Imagine living in a fast-moving kaleidoscope, where sounds, images, and thoughts are constantly shifting. Feeling easily bored, yet helpless to keep your mind on tasks you need to complete. Distracted by unimportant sights and sounds, your mind drives you from one thought or activity to the next. Perhaps you are so wrapped up in a collage of thoughts and images that you don't notice when someone speaks to you.

For many people, this is what it's like to have Attention Deficit Hyperactivity Disorder, or ADHD. They may be unable to sit still, plan ahead, finish tasks, or be fully aware of what's going on around them. To their family, classmates, or coworkers, they seem to exist in a whirlwind of disorganized or frenzied activity. Unexpectedly—on some days and in some situations—they seem fine, often leading others to think the person with ADHD can actually control these behaviors. As a result, the disorder can mar the person's relationships with others in addition to disrupting their daily life, consuming energy, and diminishing self-esteem.

ADHA, once called hyperkinesis or minimal brain dysfunction, is one of the most common mental disorders among children. It affects 3 to 5 percent of all children, perhaps as many as two million American children. Two to three times more boys than girls are affected. On the average, at least one child in every classroom in the United States needs help for the disorder. ADHD often continues into adolescence and adulthood, and can cause a lifetime of frustrated dreams and emotional pain.

But there is help . . . and hope. In the last decade, scientists have learned much about the course of the disorder and are now able to identify and treat children, adolescents, and adults who have it. A variety of medications, behavior-changing therapies, and educational options are already available to help people with ADHD focus their attention, build self-esteem, and function in new ways.

Understanding the Problem

Mark

Mark, age 14, has more energy than most boys his age. But then, he's always been overly active. Starting at age three, he was a human tornado, dashing around and disrupting everything in his path. At home, he darted from one activity to the next, leaving a trail of toys behind him. At meals, he upset dishes and chattered nonstop. He was reckless and impulsive, running into the street with oncoming cars, no matter how many times his mother explained the danger or scolded him. On the playground, he seemed no wilder than the other kids. But his tendency to overreact—like socking playmates simply for bumping into him—had already gotten him into trouble several times. His parents didn't know what to do. Mark's doting grandparents reassured them, "Boys will be boys. Don't worry, he'll grow out of it." But he didn't.

Lisa

At age 17, Lisa still struggles to pay attention and act appropriately. But this has always been hard for her. She still gets embarrassed thinking about that night her parents took her to a restaurant to celebrate her 10th birthday. She had gotten so distracted by the waitress' bright red hair that her father called her name three times before she remembered to order. Then before she could stop herself, she blurted, "Your hair dye looks awful!"

In elementary and junior high school, Lisa was quiet and cooperative but often seemed to be daydreaming. She was smart, yet couldn't improve her grades no matter how hard she tried. Several times, she failed exams. Even though she knew most of the answers, she couldn't keep her mind on the test. Her parents responded to her low grades by taking away privileges and scolding, "You're just lazy. You could get better grades if you only tried." One day, after Lisa had failed yet another exam, the teacher found her sobbing, "What's wrong with me?"

Henry

Although he loves puttering around in his shop, for years Henry has had dozens of unfinished carpentry projects and ideas for new ones he knew he would never complete. His garage was piled so high with wood, he and his wife joked about holding a fire sale.

Every day Henry faced the real frustration of not being able to concentrate long enough to complete a task. He was fired from his job as stock clerk because he lost inventory and carelessly filled out forms. Over the years, afraid that he might be losing his mind, he had seen psychotherapists and tried several medications, but none ever helped him concentrate. He saw the same lack of focus in his young son and worried.

What are the symptoms of ADHD?

The three people you've just met, Mark, Lisa, and Henry, all have a form of ADHD—Attention Deficit Hyperactivity Disorder. ADHD is not like a broken arm, or strep throat. Unlike these two disorders, ADHD does not have clear physical signs that can be seen in an x-ray or a lab test. ADHD can only be identified by looking for certain characteristic behaviors, and as with Mark, Lisa, and Henry, these behaviors vary from person to person. Scientists have not yet identified a single cause behind all the different patterns of behavior—and they may never find just one. Rather, someday scientists may find that ADHD is actually an umbrella term for several slightly different disorders.

At present, ADHD is a diagnosis applied to children and adults who consistently display certain characteristic behaviors over a period of time. The most common behaviors fall into three categories: inattention, hyperactivity, and impulsivity.

Inattention. People who are inattentive have a hard time keeping their mind on any one thing and may get bored with a task after only a few minutes. They give effortless, automatic attention to activities and things they enjoy. But focusing deliberate, conscious attention to organizing and completing a task or learning something new is difficult.

For example, Lisa found it agonizing to do homework. Often, she forgot to plan ahead by writing down the assignment or bringing home the right books. And when trying to work, every few minutes she found her mind drifting to something else. As a result, she rarely finished and her work was full of errors.

Hyperactivity. People who are hyperactive always seem to be in motion. They can't sit still. Like Mark, they may dash around or talk incessantly. Sitting still through a lesson can be an impossible task. Hyperactive children squirm in their seat or roam around the room. Or they might wiggle their feet, touch everything, or noisily tap their pencil. Hyperactive teens and adults may feel intensely restless. They may be fidgety or, like Henry, they may try to do several things at once, bouncing around from one activity to the next.

Impulsivity. People who are overly impulsive seem unable to curb their immediate reactions or think before they act. As a result, like Lisa, they may blurt out inappropriate comments. Or like Mark, they may run into the street without looking. Their impulsivity may make it hard for them to wait for things they want or to take their turn in games. They may grab a toy from another child or hit when they're upset.

Not everyone who is overly hyperactive, inattentive, or impulsive has an attention disorder. Since most people sometimes blurt out things they didn't mean to say, bounce from one task to another, or become disorganized and forgetful, how can specialists tell if the problem is ADHD?

To assess whether a person has ADHD, specialists consider several critical questions: Are these behaviors excessive, long-term, and pervasive? That is, do they occur more often than in other people the same age? Are they a continuous problem, not just a response to a temporary situation? Do the behaviors occur in several settings or only in one specific place like the playground or the office? The person's pattern of behavior is compared against a set of criteria and characteristics of the disorder. These criteria appear in a diagnostic reference book called the DSM (short for the *Diagnostic and Statistical Manual for Mental Disorders*).

According to the diagnostic manual, there are three patterns of behavior that indicate ADHD. People with ADHD may show several signs of being consistently inattentive. They may have a pattern of being hyperactive and impulsive. Or they may show all three types of behavior.

According to the DSM, signs of **inattention** include

- becoming easily distracted by irrelevant sights and sounds
- failing to pay attention to details and making careless mistakes
- rarely following instruction carefully and completely
- losing or forgetting things like toys, or pencils, books, and tools needed for a task

Some signs of **hyperactivity** and **impulsivity** are

- feeling restless, often fidgeting with hands or feet, or squirming
- running, climbing, or leaving a seat, in situations where sitting or quiet behavior is expected
- blurting out answers before hearing the whole question
- having difficulty waiting in line or for a turn

Because everyone shows some of these behaviors at times, the DSM contains very specific guidelines for determining when they indicate ADHD. The behaviors must appear early in life, before age seven, and continue for at least six months. In children, they must be more frequent or severe than in others the same age. Above all, the behaviors must create a real handicap in at least two areas of a person's life, such as school, home, work, or social settings. So someone whose work or friendships are not impaired by these behaviors would not be diagnosed with ADHD. Nor would a child who seems overly active at school but functions well elsewhere.

Can any other conditions produce these symptoms?

The fact is, *many* things can produce these behaviors. Anything from chronic fear to mild seizures can make a child seem overactive, quarrelsome, impulsive, or inattentive. For example, a formerly cooperative child who becomes overactive and easily distracted after a parent's death is dealing with an emotional problem, not ADHD. A chronic middle ear infection can also make a child seem distracted and uncooperative. So can living with family members who are physically abusive or addicted to drugs or alcohol. Can you imagine a child trying to focus on a math lesson when his or her safety and well-being are in danger each day? Such children are showing the effects of other problems, not ADHD.

In other children, ADHD-like behaviors may be their response to a defeating classroom situation. perhaps the child has a learning disability and is not developmentally ready to learn to read and write at the time these are taught. Or maybe the work is too hard or too easy, leaving the child frustrated or bored.

Tyrone and Mimi are two examples of how classroom conditions can elicit behaviors that look like ADHD. For months, Tyrone shouted answers out in class, then became disruptive when the teacher ignored him. He certainly seemed hyperactive and impulsive. Finally, after observing Tyrone in other situations, his teacher realized he just wanted approval for knowing the right answer. She began to seek opportunities to call on him and praise him. Gradually, Tyrone became calmer and more cooperative.

Mimi, a fourth grader, made loud noises during reading group that constantly disrupted the class. One day the teacher realized that the book was too hard for Mimi. Mimi's disruptions stopped when she was placed in a reading group where the books were easier and she could successfully participate in the lesson.

Like Tyrone and Mimi, some children's attention and class participation improve when the class structure and lessons are adjusted a bit to meet their emotional needs, instructional level, or learning style. Although such children need a little help to get on track at school, they probably don't have ADHD.

It's also important to realize that during certain stages of development, the majority of children that age tend to be inattentive, hyperactive, or impulsive—but do not have ADHD. Preschoolers have lots of energy and run everywhere they go, but this doesn't mean they are hyperactive. And many teenagers go through a phase when they are messy, disorganized, and reject authority. This doesn't mean they will have a lifelong problem controlling their impulses.

ADHD is a serious diagnosis that may require long-term treatment with counseling and medication. So it's important that a doctor first look for and treat any other causes for these behaviors.

Can other disorders accompany ADHD?

One of the difficulties in diagnosing ADHD is that it is often accompanied by other problems. For example, many children with ADHD also have a specific learning disability (LD), which means they have trouble mastering language or certain academic skills, typically reading and math. ADHD is not in itself a specific learning disability. But because it can interfere with concentration and attention, ADHD can make it doubly hard for a child with LD to do well in school.

A very small proportion of people with ADHD have a rare disorder called Tourette's syndrome. People with Tourette's have tics and other movements like eye blinks or facial twitches that they cannot control. Others may grimace, shrug, sniff, or bark out words. Fortunately, these behaviors can be controlled with medication. Researchers at NIMH and elsewhere are involved in evaluating the safety and effectiveness of treatment for people who have both Tourette's syndrome and ADHD.

More serious, nearly half of all children with ADHD—mostly boys—tend to have another condition, called oppositional defiant disorder. Like Mark, who punched playmates for jostling him, these children may overreact or lash out when they feel bad about themselves. They may be stubborn, have outbursts of temper, or act belligerent or defiant. Sometimes this progresses to more serious conduct disorders. Children with this combination of problems are at risk of getting in trouble at school, and even with the police. They may take unsafe risks and break laws—they may steal, set fires, destroy property, and drive recklessly. It's important that children with these conditions receive help before the behaviors led to more serious problems.

At some point, many children with ADHD—mostly younger children and boys—experience other emotional disorders. About one-fourth feel anxious. They feel tremendous worry, tension, or uneasiness, even when there's nothing to fear. Because the feelings are scarier, stronger, and more frequent than normal fears, they can affect the child's thinking and behavior.. Others experience depression. Depression goes beyond ordinary sadness—people may feel so "down" that they feel hopeless and unable to deal with everyday tasks. Depression can disrupt sleep, appetite, and the ability to think.

Because emotional disorders and attention disorders so often go hand in hand, every child who has ADHD should be checked for accompanying anxiety and depression. Anxiety and depression can be treated, and helping children handle such strong, painful feelings will help them cope with and overcome the effects of ADHD.

Of course, not all children with ADHD have an additional disorder. Nor do all people with learning disabilities, Tourette's syndrome, oppositional defiant disorder, conduct disorder, anxiety, or depression have ADHD. But when they do occur together, the combination of problems can seriously complicate a person's life. For this reason, it's important to watch for other disorders in children who have ADHD.

What causes ADHD?

Understandably, one of the first questions parents ask when they learn their child has an attention disorder is *"Why? What went wrong?"*

Health professionals stress that since no one knows what causes ADHD, it doesn't help parents to look backward to search for possible reasons. There are too many possibilities to pin down the cause with certainty. It is far more important for the family to move forward in finding ways to get the right help.

Scientists, however, do need to study causes in an effort to identify better ways to treat, and perhaps some day, prevent ADHD. They are finding more and more evidence that ADHD does not stem from home environment, but from biological causes. When you think about it, there is no clear relationship between home life and ADHD. Not all children from unstable or dysfunctional homes have ADHD. And not all children with ADHD come from dysfunctional families. Knowing this can remove a huge burden of guilt from parents who might blame themselves for their child's behavior.

Over the last decades, scientists have come up with possible theories about what causes ADHD. Some of these theories have led to dead ends, some to exciting new avenues of investigation.

One disappointing theory was that all attention disorders and learning disabilities were caused by minor head injuries or undetectable damage to the brain, perhaps from early infection or complications at birth. Based on this theory, for many years both disorders were called "minimal brain damage" or "minimal brain dysfunction." Although certain types of head injury can explain some cases of attention disorder, the theory was rejected because it could explain only a very small number of cases. Not everyone with ADHD or LD has a history of head trauma or birth complications.

Another theory was that refined sugar and food additives make children hyperactive and inattentive. As a result, parents were encouraged to stop serving children foods containing artificial flavorings, preservatives, and sugars. However, this theory, too, came under question. In 1982, the National Institutes of Health (NIH), the federal agency responsible for biomedical research, held a major scientific conference to discuss the issue. After studying the data, the scientists concluded that the restricted diet only seemed to help about 5 percent of children with ADHD, mostly either young children or children with food allergies.

In recent years, as new tools and techniques for studying the brain have been developed, scientists have been able to test more theories about what causes ADHD.

Using one such technique, NIMH scientists demonstrated a link between a person's ability to pay continued attention and the level of activity in the brain. Adult subjects were asked to learn a list of words. As they did, scientists used a PET (positron emission tomography) scanner to observe the brain at work. The researchers measured the level of glucose used by the areas of the brain that inhibit impulses and control attention. Glucose is the brain's main source of energy, so measuring how much is used is a good indicator of the brain's activity level. The investigators found important differences between people who have ADHD and those who don't. In people with ADHD, the brain areas that control attention used less glucose, indicating that they were less active. It appears from this research that a lower level of activity in some parts of the brain may cause inattention.

The next step will be to research *why* there is less activity in these areas of the brain. Scientists at NIMH hope to compare the use of glucose and the activity level in mild and severe cases of ADHD. They will also try to discover why some medications used to treat ADHD work better than others, and if the more effective medications increase activity in certain parts of the brain.

Researchers are also searching for other differences between those who have and do not have ADHD. Research on how the brain normally develops in the fetus offers some clues about what may disrupt the process. Throughout pregnancy and continuing into the first year of life, the brain is constantly developing. It begins its growth from a few all-purpose cells and evolves into a complex organ made of billions of specialized, interconnected nerve cells. By studying brain development in animals and humans, scientists are gaining a better understanding of how the brain works when the nerve cells are connected correctly and incorrectly. Scientists at NIMH and other research institutions are tracking clues to determine what might prevent nerve cells from forming the proper connections. Some of the factors they are studying include drug use during pregnancy, toxins, and genetics.

Research shows that a mother's use of cigarettes, alcohol, or other drugs during pregnancy may have damaging effects on the unborn child. These substances may be dangerous to the fetus' developing brain. It appears that alcohol and the nicotine in cigarettes may distort developing nerve cells. For example, heavy alcohol use during pregnancy has been linked to fetal alcohol syndrome (FAS), a condition that can lead to low birth weight, intellectual impairment, and certain physical defects. Many children born with FAS show much the same hyperactivity, inattention, and impulsivity as children with ADHD.

Drugs such as cocaine—including the smokable form known as crack—seem to affect the normal development of brain receptors. These brain cell parts help to transmit incoming signals from our skin, eyes, and ears, and help control our responses to the environment. Current research suggests that drug abuse may harm these receptors. Some scientists believe that such damage may lead to ADHD.

Toxins in the environment may also disrupt brain development or brain processes, which may lead to ADHD. Lead is one such possible toxin. It is found in dust, soil, and flaking paint in areas where leaded gasoline and paint were once used. It is also present in some water pipes. Some animal studies suggest that children exposed to lead may develop symptoms associated with ADHD, but only a few cases have actually been found.

Other research shows that attention disorders tend to run in families, so there are likely to be genetic influences. Children who have ADHD usually have at least one close relative who also has ADHD. And at least one-third of all fathers who had ADHD in their youth bear children who have ADHD. Even more convincing: the majority of identical twins share the trait. At the National Institutes of Health, researchers are also on the trail of a gene that may be involved in transmitting ADHD in a small number of families with a genetic thyroid disorder.

Getting Help

Mark

In third grade, Mark's teacher threw up her hands and said, "Enough!" In one morning, Mark had jumped out of his seat to sharpen his pencil six times, each time accidentally charging into other children's desks and toppling books and papers. He was finally sent to the principal's office when he began kicking a desk he had overturned. In sheer frustration, his teacher called a meeting with his parents and the school psychologist.

But even after they developed a plan for managing Mark's behavior in class, Mark showed little improvement. Finally, after an extensive assessment, they found that Mark had an attention deficit that included hyperactivity. He was put on a medication called Ritalin to control the hyperactivity during school hours. Although Ritalin failed to help, another drug called Dexedrine did. With a psychologist's help, his parents learned to reward desirable behaviors, and to have Mark take "time out" when he became too disruptive. Soon Mark was able to sit still and focus on learning.

Lisa

Because Lisa wasn't disruptive in class, it took a long time for teachers to notice her problem. Lisa was first referred to the school evaluation team when her teacher realized that she was a bright girl with failing grades. The team ruled out a learning disability but determined that she had an attention deficit, ADHD without hyperactivity. The school psychologist recognized that Lisa was also dealing with depression.

Lisa's teachers and the school psychologist developed a treatment plan that included participation in a program to increase her attention span and develop her social skills. They also recommended that Lisa receive counseling to help her recognize her strengths and overcome her depression.

Henry

When Henry's son entered kindergarten, it was clear that he was going to have problems sitting quietly and concentrating. After several disruptive incidents, the school called and suggested that his son be evaluated for ADHD. As the boy was assessed, Henry realized that he had grown up with the same symptoms that specialists were now finding in his son. Fortunately, the psychologist knew that ADHD can persist in adults. She suggested that Henry be evaluated by a professional who worked with adults. For the first time, Henry was correctly diagnosed and given Ritalin to aid his concentration. What a relief! All the years that he had been unable to concentrate were due to a disorder that could be identified, and above all, treated.

How is ADHD identified and diagnosed?

Many parents see signs of an attention deficit in toddlers long before the child enters school. For example, as a three-year-old, Henry's son already displayed some signs of hyperactivity. He seemed to lose interest and dart off even during his favorite TV shows or while playing games. Once, during a game of "catch," he left the game before the ball even reached him!

Like Henry's son, a child may be unable to focus long enough to play a simple game. Or, like Mark, the child may be tearing around out of control. But because children mature at different rates, and are very different in personality, temperament, and energy level, it's useful to get an expert's opinion of whether the behaviors are appropriate for the child's age. Parents can ask their pediatrician, or a child psychologist or psychiatrist to assess whether their toddler has an attention disorder or is just immature, has hyperactivity or is just exuberant.

Seeing a child as a "a chip off the old block" or "just like his dad" can blind parents to the need for help. Parents may find it hard to see their child's behavior as a problem when it so closely resembles their own. In fact, like Henry, many parents first recognize their own disorder only when their children are diagnosed.

In many cases, the teacher is the first to recognize that a child is hyperactive or inattentive and may consult with the school psychologist. Because teachers work with many children, they come to know how "average" children behave in learning situations that require attention and self control. However, teachers sometimes fail to notice the needs of children like Lisa who are quiet and cooperative.

Types of Professionals Who Make the Diagnosis

School-age and preschool children are often evaluated by a school psychologist or a team made up of the school psychologist and other specialists. But if the school doesn't believe the student has a problem, or if the family wants another opinion, a family may need to see a specialist in private practice. In such cases, who can the family turn to? What kinds of specialists do they need?

Specialty	Can diagnose ADHD	Can prescribe medications, if needed	Provides counseling or training
Psychiatrists	yes	yes	yes
Psychologists	yes	no	yes
Pediatricians or family physicians	yes	yes	no
Neurologists	yes	yes	no

The family can start by talking with the child's pediatrician or their family doctor. Some pediatricians may do the assessment themselves, but more often they refer the family to an appropriate specialist they know and trust. In addition, state and local agencies that serve families and children, as well as some of the volunteer organizations listed in the back of this booklet, can help identify an appropriate specialist.

Knowing the differences in qualifications and services can help the family choose someone who can best meet their needs. Besides school psychologists, there are several types of specialists qualified to diagnose and treat ADHD. Child psychiatrists are doctors who specialize in diagnosing and treating childhood mental and behavioral disorders. A psychiatrist can provide therapy and prescribe any needed medications. Child psychologists are also qualified to diagnose and treat ADHD. They can provide therapy for the child and help the family develop ways to deal with the disorder. But psychologists are not medical doctors and must rely on the child's physician to do medical exams and prescribe medication. Neurologists, doctors who work with disorders of the brain and nervous system, can also diagnose ADHD and prescribe medicines. But unlike psychiatrists and psychologists, neurologists usually do not provide therapy for the emotional aspects of the disorder. Adults who think they may have ADHD can also seek a psychologist, psychiatrist, or neurologist. But at present, not all specialists are skilled in identifying or treating ADHD in adults.

Within each specialty, individual doctors and mental health professionals differ in their experience with ADHD. So in selecting a specialist, it's important to find someone with specific training and experience in diagnosing and treating the disorder.

Steps in Making a Diagnosis

Whatever the specialist's expertise, his or her first task is to gather information that will rule out other possible reasons for the child's behavior. In ruling out other causes, the specialist checks the child's school and medical records. The specialist tries to sense whether the home and classroom environments are stressful or chaotic, and how the child's parents and teachers deal with the child. They may have a doctor look for such problems as emotional disorders, undetectable (petit mal) seizures, and poor vision or hearing. Most schools automatically screen for vision and hearing, so this information is often already on record. A doctor may also look for allergies or nutrition problems like chronic "caffeine highs" that might make the child seem overly active.

Next the specialist gathers information on the child's ongoing behavior in order to compare these behaviors to the symptoms and diagnostic criteria listed in the DSM *(Diagnostic and Statistical Manual of Mental Disorders)*. This involves talking with the child and if possible, observing the child in class and in other settings.

The child's teachers, past and present, are asked to rate their observations of the child's behavior on standardized evaluation forms to compare the child's behaviors to those of other children the same age. Of course, rating scales are subjective—they only capture the teacher's personal perception of the child. Even so, because teachers get to know so many children, their judgment of how a child compares to others is usually accurate.

The specialist interviews the child's teachers, parents, and other people who know the child well, such as school staff and baby-sitters. Parents are asked to describe their child's behavior in a variety of situations. They may also fill out a rating scale to indicate how severe and frequent the behaviors seem to be.

In some cases, the child may be checked for social adjustment and mental health. Tests of intelligence and learning achievement may be given to see if the child has a learning disability and whether the disabilities are in all or only certain parts of the school curriculum.

In looking at the data, the specialist pays special attention to the child's behavior during noisy or unstructured situations, like parties, or during tasks that require sustained attention, like reading, working math problems, or playing a board game. Behavior during free play or while getting individual attention is given less importance in the evaluation. In such situations, most children with ADHD are able to control their behavior and perform well.

The specialist then pieces together a profile of the child's behavior. Which ADHD-like behavior listed in the DSM does the child show? How often? In what situations? How long has the child been doing them? How old was the child when the problem started? Are the behaviors seriously interfering with the child's friendships, school activities, or home life? Does the child have any other related problems? The answers to these questions help identify whether the child's hyperactivity, impulsivity, and inattention are significant and long-standing. If so, the child may be diagnosed with ADHD.

Adults are diagnosed for ADHD based on their performance at home and at work. When possible, their parents are asked to rate the person's behavior as a child. A spouse or roommate can help rate and evaluate current behaviors. But for the most part, adults are asked to describe their own experiences. One symptom is a sense of frustration. Since people with ADHD are often bright and creative, they often report feeling frustrated that they're not living up to their potential. Many also feel restless and are easily bored. Some say they need to seek novelty and excitement to help channel the whirlwind in their minds. Although it may be impossible to document when these behaviors first started, most adults with ADHD can give examples of being inattentive, impul-

sive, overly active, impatient, and disorganized most of their lives.

Until recent years, adults were not thought to have ADHD, so many adults with ongoing symptoms have never been diagnosed. People like Henry go for decades knowing that something is wrong, but not knowing what it is. Psychotherapy and medication for anxiety, depression, or manic-depression fail to help much, simply because the ADHD itself is not being addressed. Yet half the children with ADHD continue to have symptoms through adulthood. The recent awareness of adult ADHD means that many people can finally be correctly diagnosed and treated.

A correct diagnosis lets people move forward in their lives. Once the disorder is known, they can begin to receive whatever combination of educational, medical, and emotional help they need.

An effective treatment plan helps people with ADHD and their families at many levels. For adults with ADHD, the treatment plan may include medication, along with practical and emotional support. For children and adolescents, it may include providing an appropriate classroom setting, the right medication, and helping parents to manage their child's behavior.

What are the educational options?

Children with ADHD have a variety of needs. Some children are too hyperactive or inattentive to function in a regular classroom, even with medication and a behavior management plan. Such children may be placed in a special education class for all or part of the day. In some schools, the special education teacher teams with the classroom teacher to meet each child's unique needs. However, most children are able to stay in the regular classroom. Whenever possible, educators prefer not to segregate children, but to let them learn along with their peers.

Children with ADHD often need some special accommodations to help them learn. For example, the teacher may seat the child in an area with few distractions, provide an area where the child can move around and release excess energy, or establish a clearly posted system of rules and reward appropriate behavior. Sometimes just keeping a card or a picture on the desk can serve as a visual reminder to use the right school behavior, like raising a hand instead of shouting out, or staying in a seat instead of wandering around the room. Giving a child like Lisa extra time on tests can make the difference between passing and failing, and gives her a fairer chance to show what she's learned. Reviewing instructions or writing assignments on the board, and even listing the books and materials they will need for the task, may make it possible for disorganized, inattentive children to complete work.

Many of the strategies of special education are simply good teaching methods. Telling students in advance what they will learn, providing visual aids, and giving written as well as oral instructions are all ways to help students focus and remember the key parts of the lesson.

Students with ADHD often need to learn techniques for monitoring and controlling their own attention and behavior.

For example, Mark's teacher taught him several alternatives for when he loses track of what he's supposed to do. He can look for instructions on the blackboard, raise his hand, wait to see if he remembers, or quietly ask another child. The process of finding alternatives to interrupting the teacher has made him more self-sufficient and cooperative. And because he now interrupts less, he is beginning to get more praise than reprimands.

In Lisa's class, the teacher frequently stops to ask students to notice whether they are paying attention to the lesson or if they are thinking about something else. The students record their answer on a chart. As students become more consciously aware of their attention, they begin to see progress and feel good about staying better focused. The process helped make Lisa aware of when she was drifting off, so she could return her attention to the lesson faster. As a result, she became more productive and the quality of her work improved.

Because schools demand that children sit still, wait for a turn, pay attention, and stick with a task, it's no surprise that many children with ADHD have problems in class. Their minds are fully capable of learning, but their hyperactivity and inattention make learning difficult. As a result, many students with ADHD repeat a grade or drop out of school early. Fortunately, with the right combination of appropriate educational practices, medication, and counseling, these outcomes can be avoided.

Right to a Free Public Education

Although parents have the option of taking their child to a private practitioner for evaluation and educational services, most children with ADHD qualify for free services within the public schools. Steps are taken to ensure that each child with ADHD receives an education that meets his or her unique needs. For example, the special education teacher, working with parents, the school psychologist, school administrators, and the classroom teacher, must assess the child's strengths and weaknesses and design an Individualized Educational program (IEP). The IEP outlines the specific skills the child needs to develop as well as appropriate learning activities that build on the child's strengths. Parents play an important role in the process. They must be included in meetings and given an opportunity to review and approve their child's IEP.

Many children with ADHD or other disabilities are able to receive such special education services under the Individuals with Disabilities Education Act (IDEA). The Act guarantees appropriate services and a public education to children with disabilities from ages three to 21. Children who do not qualify for services under IDEA can receive help under an earlier law, the National Rehabilitation Act, Section 504, which defines disabilities more broadly. Qualifying for services under the National Rehabilitation Act is often called "504 eligibility."

Because ADHD is a disability that affects children's ability to learn and interact with others, it can certainly be a disabling condition. Under one law or another, most children can receive the services they need.

Some coping strategies for teens and adults with ADHD

When necessary, ask the teacher or boss to repeat instructions, rather than guess.

Break large assignments or job tasks into small, simple tasks. Set a deadline for each task and reward yourself as you complete each one.

Each day, make a list of what you need to do. Plan the best order for doing each task. Then make a schedule for doing them. Use a calendar or daily planner to keep yourself on track.

Work in a quiet area. Do one thing at a time. Give yourself short breaks.

Write things you need to remember in a notebook with dividers. Write different kinds of information—like assignments, appointments, and phone numbers—in different sections. Keep the book with you all of the time.

Post notes to yourself to help remind yourself of things you need to do. Tape notes on the bathroom mirror, on the refrigerator, in your school locker, or dashboard of your car—wherever you're likely to need the reminder.

Store similar things together. For example, keep all your Nintendo disks in one place and tape cassettes in another. Keep canceled checks in one place and bills in another.

Create a routine. Get yourself ready for school or work at the same time, in the same way, every day.

Exercise, eat a balanced diet, and get enough sleep.

Adapted from: Weinstein, C. "Cognitive Remediation Strategies." *Journal of Psychotherapy Practice and Research.* 3(1): 44–57, 1994.

What treatments are available?

For decades, medications have been used to treat the symptoms of ADHD. Three medications in the class of drugs known as stimulants seem to be the most effective in both children and adults. These are methylphenidate (Ritalin), dextroamphetamine (Dexedrine or Dextrostat), and pemoline (Cylert). For many people, these medicines dramatically reduce their hyperactivity and improve their ability to focus, work, and learn. The medications may also improve physical coordination, such as handwriting and ability in sports. Recent research by NIMH suggests that these medicines may also help children with an accompanying conduct disorder to control their impulsive, destructive behaviors.

Ritalin helped Henry focus on and complete tasks for the first time. Dexedrine helped Mark to sit quietly, focus his attention, and participate in class so he could learn. He also became less impulsive and aggressive. Along with these changes in his behavior, Mark began to make and keep friends.

Unfortunately, when people see such immediate improvement, they often think medication is all that's needed. But these medicines don't cure the disorder, they only temporarily control the symptoms. Although the drugs help people pay better attention and complete their work, they can't increase knowledge or improve academic skills. The drugs alone can't help people feel better about themselves or cope with problems. These require other kinds of treatment and support.

For lasting improvement, numerous clinicians recommend that medications should be used along with treatments that aid in these other areas. There are no quick cures. Many experts believe that the most significant, long-lasting gains appear when medication is combined with behavioral therapy, emotional counseling, and practical support. Some studies suggest that the combination of medicine and therapy may be more effective than drugs alone. NIMH is conducting a large study to check this.

Use of Stimulant Drugs

Stimulant drugs, such as Ritalin, Cylert, and Dexedrine, when used with medical supervision, are usually considered quite safe. Although they can be addictive to teenagers and adults if misused, these medications are not addictive in children. They seldom make children "high" or jittery. Nor do they sedate the child. Rather, the stimulants help children control their hyperactivity, inattention, and other behaviors.

Different doctors use the medications in slightly different ways. Cylert is available in one form, which naturally lasts five to 10 hours. Ritalin and Dexedrine come in short-term tablets that last about three hours, as well as longer-term preparations that last through the school day. The short-term dose is often more practical for children who need medication only during the school day or for special situations, like attending church or a prom, or studying for an important exam. The sustained-release dosage frees the child from the inconvenience or embarrassment of going to the office or school nurse every day for a pill. The doctor can help decide which preparation to use, and whether a child needs to take the medicine during school hours only or in the evenings and on weekends, too.

Nine out of 10 children improve on one of the three stimulant drugs. So if one doesn't help, the others should be tried. Usually a medication should be tried for a week to see if it helps. If necessary, however, the doctor will also try adjusting the dosage before switching to a different drug.

Other types of medication may be used if stimulants don't work or if the ADHD occurs with another disorder. Antidepressants and other medications may be used to help control accompanying depression or anxiety. In some cases, antihistamines may be tried. Clonidine, a drug normally used to treat hypertension, may be helpful in people with both ADHD and Tourette's syndrome. Although stimulants tend to be more effective, clonidine may be tried when stimulants don't work or can't be used. Clonidine can be administered either by pill or by skin patch and has different side effects than stimulants. The doctor works closely with each patient to find the most appropriate medication.

Sometimes, a child's ADHD symptoms seem to worsen, leading parents to wonder why. They can be assured that a drug that helps rarely stops working. However, they should work with the doctor to check that the child is getting the right dosage. Parents should also make sure that the child is actually getting the prescribed daily dosage at home or at school—it's easy to forget. They also need to know that new or exaggerated behaviors may also crop up when a child is under stress. The challenges that all children face, like changing schools or

entering puberty, may be even more stressful for a child with ADHD.

Some doctors recommend that children be taken off a medication now and then to see if the child still needs it. they recommend temporarily stopping the drug during school breaks and summer vacations, when focused attention and calm behavior are usually not as crucial. These "drug holidays" work well if the child can still participate at camp or other activities without medication.

Children on medications should have regular checkups. parents should also talk regularly with the child's teachers and doctor about how the child is doing. This is especially important when a medication is first started, restarted, or when the dosage is changed.

The Medication Debate

As useful as these drugs are, Ritalin and the other stimulants have sparked a great deal of controversy. Most doctors feel the potential side effects should be carefully weighed against the benefits before prescribing the drugs. While on these medications, some children may lose weight, have less appetite, and temporarily grow more slowly. Others may have problems falling asleep. Some doctors believe that stimulants may also make the symptoms of Tourette's syndrome worse, although recent research suggests this may not be true. Other doctors say if they carefully watch the child's height, weight, and overall development, the benefits of medication far outweigh the potential side effects. Side effects that do occur can often be handled by reducing the dosage.

Myths about Stimulant Medication

- Myth: Stimulants can lead to drug addiction later in life.
  Fact: Stimulants help many children focus and be more successful at school, home, and play. Avoiding negative experiences now may actually help prevent addictions and other emotional problems later.
- Myth: Responding well to a stimulant drug proves a person has ADHD.
  Fact: Stimulants allow many people to focus and pay better attention, whether or not they have ADHD. The improvement is just more noticeable in people with ADHD.
- Myth: Medication should be stopped when the child reaches adolescence.
  Fact: Not so! About 80 percent of those who needed medication as children still need it as teenagers. Fifty percent need medication as adults.

It's natural for parents to be concerned about whether taking a medicine is in their child's best interests. Parents need to be clear about the benefits and potential risks of using these drugs. The child's pediatrician or psychiatrist can provide advice and answer questions.

Another debate is whether Ritalin and other stimulant drugs are prescribed unnecessarily for too many children. Remember that many things, including anxiety, depression, allergies, seizures, or problems with the home or school environment can make children seem overactive, impulsive, or inattentive. Critics argue that many children who do not have a true attention disorder are medicated as a way to control their disruptive behaviors.

Medication and Self-esteem

When a child's schoolwork and behavior improve soon after starting medication, the child, parents, and teachers tend to applaud the drug for causing the sudden change. But these changes are actually the child's own strengths and natural abilities coming out from behind a cloud. Giving credit to the medication can make the child feel incompetent. The medication only makes these changes possible. The child must supply the effort and ability. To help children feel good about themselves, parents and teachers need to praise the child, not the drug.

It's also important to help children and teenagers feel comfortable about a medication they must take every day. They may feel that because they take medicine they are different from their classmates or that there's something seriously wrong with them. CHADD (which stands for Children and Adults with Attention Deficit Disorders), a leading organization for people with attention disorders, suggests several ways that parents and teachers can help children view the medication in a positive way:

- Compare the pills to eyeglasses, braces, and allergy medications used by other children in their class. Explain that their medicine is simply a tool to help them focus and pay attention.
- Point out that they're lucky their problem can be helped. Encourage them to identify ways the medicine makes it easier to do things that are important to them, like make friends, succeed at school, and play.

Treatments to help people with ADHD and their families learn to cope

Life can be hard for children with ADHD. They're the ones who are so often in trouble at school, can't finish a game, and lose friends. They may spend agonizing hours each night struggling to keep their mind on their homework, then forget to bring it to school.

It's not easy coping with these frustrations day after day. Some children release their frustration by acting contrary, starting fights, or destroying property. Some turn the frustration into body ailments, like the child who gets a stomachache each day before school. Others hold their needs and fears inside, so that no one sees how badly they feel.

It's also difficult having a sister, brother, or classmate who gets angry, grabs your toys, and loses your things. Children who live with or share a classroom with a child who has ADHD get frustrated, too. They may feel neglected as their parents or teachers try to cope with the hyperactive child. They may resent their brother or sister never finishing chores, or being pushed around by a classmate. They want to love their sibling and get along with their classmate, but sometimes it's so hard!

It's especially hard being the parent of a child who is full of uncontrolled activity, leaves messes, throws tantrums, and doesn't listen or follow instructions. Parents often feel powerless and at a loss. The usual methods of discipline, like reasoning and scolding, don't work with this child, because the child doesn't really *choose* to act in these ways. It's just that their self-control comes and goes. Out of sheer frustration, parents sometimes find themselves spanking, ridiculing, or screaming at the child, even though they know it's not appropriate. Their response leaves everyone more upset than before. Then they blame themselves for not being better parents. Once children are diagnosed and receiving treatment, some of the emotional upset within the family may fade.

Medication can help to control some of the behavior problems that may have led to family turmoil. But more often, there are other aspects of the problem that medication can't touch. Even though ADHD primarily affects a person's behavior, having the disorder has broad emotional repercussions. For some children, being scolded is the only attention they ever get. They have few experiences that build their sense of worth and competence. If they're hyperactive, they're often told they're bad and punished for being disruptive. If they are too disorganized and unfocused to complete tasks, others may call them lazy. If they impulsively grab toys, butt in, or shove classmates, they may lose friends. And if they have a related conduct disorder, they may get in trouble at school or with the law. Facing the daily frustrations that can come with having ADHD can make people fear that they are strange, abnormal, or stupid.

Often, the cycle of frustration, blame, and anger has gone on so long that it will take some time to undo. Both parents and their children may need special help to develop techniques for managing the patterns of behavior. In such cases, mental health professionals can counsel the child and the family, helping them to develop new skills, attitudes, and ways of relating to each other. In individual counseling, the therapist helps children or adults with ADHD learn to feel better about themselves. They learn to recognize that having a disability does not reflect who they are as a person. The therapist can also help people with ADHD identify and build on their strengths, cope with daily problems, and control their attention and aggression. In group counseling, people learn that they are not alone in their frustration and that others want to help. Sometimes only the individual with ADHD needs counseling support. But in many cases, because the problem affects the family as well as the person with ADHD, the entire family may need help. The therapist assists the family in finding better ways to handle the disruptive behaviors and promote change. If the child is young, most of the therapist's work is with the parents, teaching them techniques for coping with and improving their child's behavior.

Several intervention approaches are available and different therapists tend to prefer one approach or another. Knowing something about the various types of interventions makes it easier for families to choose a therapist that is right for their needs.

Psychotherapy works to help people with ADHD to like and accept themselves despite their disorder. In psychotherapy, patients talk with the therapist about upsetting thoughts and feelings, explore self-defeating patterns of behavior, and learn alternative ways to handle their emotions. As they talk, the therapist tries to help them understand how they can change. However, people dealing with ADHD usually want to gain control of their symptomatic behaviors more directly. If so, more direct kinds of intervention are needed.

Cognitive-behavioral therapy helps people work on immediate issues. Rather than helping people understand their feelings and actions, it supports them directly in changing their behavior. The support might be practical assistance, like helping Henry learn to think through tasks and organize his work. Or the support might be to encourage new behaviors by giving praise or rewards each time the person acts in the desired way. A cognitive-behavioral therapist might use such techniques to help a belligerent child like Mark learn to control his fighting, or an impulsive teenager like Lisa to think before she speaks.

Social skills training can also help children learn new behaviors. In social skills training, the therapist discusses and models appropriate behaviors like waiting for a turn, sharing toys, asking for help, or responding to teasing, then gives children a chance to practice. For example, a child might learn to "read" other people's facial expression and tone of voice, in order to respond more appropriately. Social skills training helped Lisa learn to join in group activities, make appropriate comments, and ask for help. A child like Mark might learn to see how his behavior affects others and develop new ways to respond when angry or pushed.

Support groups connect people who have common concerns. Many adults with ADHD and parents of children with ADHD find it useful to join a local or national support group. Many groups deal with issues of children's disorders, and even ADHD specifically. The national associations listed at the back of this booklet can explain how to contact a local chapter. Members of support groups share frustrations and successes, referrals to qualified specialists, and information about what works, as well as their hopes for themselves and their children. There is strength in numbers—and sharing experiences with others who have similar problems helps some know that they aren't alone.

Parenting skills training, offered by therapists or in special classes, gives parents tools and techniques for managing their child's behavior. One such technique is the use of "time out" when the child becomes too unruly or out of control. During time outs, the child is removed from the agitating situation and sits alone quietly for a short time to calm down. Parents may also be taught to give the child "quality time" each day, in which they share a pleasurable or relaxed activity. During this time together, the parent looks for opportunities to notice and point out what the child does well, and praise his or her strengths and abilities.

An effective way to modify a child's behavior is through a system of rewards and penalties. The parents (or teacher) identify a few desirable behaviors that they want to encourage in the child—such as asking for a toy instead of grabbing it, or completing a simple task. The child is told exactly what is expected in order to earn the reward. The child receives the reward when he performs the desired behavior and a mild penalty when he doesn't. A reward can be small, perhaps a token that can be exchanged for special privileges, but it should be something the child wants and is eager to earn. The penalty might be removal of a token or a brief "time out." The goal, over time, is to help children learn to control their own behavior and to choose the more desired behavior. The tech-

nique works well with all children, although children with ADHD may need more frequent rewards.

In addition, parents may learn to structure situations in ways that will allow their child to succeed. This may include allowing only one or two playmates at a time, so that their child doesn't get overstimulated. Or if their child has trouble completing tasks, they may learn to help the child divide a large task into small steps, then praise the child as each step is completed.

Parents may also learn to use stress management methods, such as meditation, relaxation techniques, and exercise to increase their own tolerance for frustration, so that they can respond more calmly to their child's behavior.

Controversial Treatments

Understandably, parents who are eager to help their children want to explore every possible option. Many newly touted treatments sound reasonable. Many even come with glowing reports. A few are pure quackery. Some are even developed by reputable doctors or specialists—but when tested scientifically, cannot be proven to help.

Here are a few types of treatment that have *not* been scientifically shown to be effective in treating the majority of children or adults with ADHD:

- biofeedback
- restricted diets
- allergy treatments
- medicines to correct problems in the inner ear
- megavitamins
- chiropractic adjustment and bone re-alignment
- treatment for yeast infection
- eye training
- special colored glasses

A few success stories can't substitute for scientific evidence. Until sound, scientific testing shows a treatment to be effective, families risk spending time, money, and hope on fads and false promises.

Sustaining Hope

Mark

Today, at age 14, Mark is doing much better in school. He channels his energy into sports and is a star player on the intramural football team. Although he still gets into fights now and then, a child psychologist is helping him learn to control his tantrums and frustration and he is able to make and keep friends. His grandparents point to him with pride and say, "We knew he'd turn out just fine!"

Lisa

Lisa is about to graduate from high school. She's better able to focus her attention and concentrate on her work, and now her grades are quite good. Overcoming her depression and learning to like herself have also given her more confidence to develop friendships and try new things.

Lately, she has been working with the school guidance counselor to identify the right kind of job to look for after graduation. She hopes to find a career that will bypass her attention problems and make the best use of her assets and skills. She is more alert and focused and is considering trying college in a year or two. Her counselor reminds her that she's certainly smart enough.

Henry

These days, Henry is successful and happy in his job as a shoe salesman. The work allows him to move around throughout the day, and the appearance of new customers provides the variety he needs to help him stay focused. He recently completed a course in time management, and now keeps lists, organizes his work, and schedules his day. Now that he has harnessed his energy, his ability to think about several things at once allows him to be creative and productive.

He is proud that he and his wife have developed important parenting skills for working with their son, so that he, too, is doing better at home and at school. Henry is also pleased with his new ability to follow through on projects. In fact, he just finished making his son a beautiful wooden toy chest for his birthday.

Can ADHD be outgrown or cured?

Even though most people don't outgrow ADHD, people do learn to adapt and live fulfilling lives. Mark, Lisa, and Henry are making good lives for themselves—not being cured, but by developing their personal strengths. With effective combinations of medicine, new skills, and emotional support, people with ADHD can develop ways to control their attention and minimize their disruptive behaviors. Like Henry, they may find that by structuring tasks and controlling their environment, they can achieve personal goals. Like Mark, they may learn to channel their excess energy into sports and other high energy activities. And like Lisa, they can identify career options that build on their strengths and abilities.

As they grow up, with appropriate help from parents and clinicians, children with ADHD become better able to suppress their hyperactivity and to channel it into more socially acceptable behaviors, like physical exercise or fidgeting. And although we know that half of all children with ADHD will still show signs of the problem into adulthood, we also know that the medications and therapy that help children also work for adults.

All people with ADHD have natural talents and abilities that they can draw on to create fine lives and careers for themselves. In fact, many people with ADHD even feel that their patterns of behavior give them unique, often unrecognized, advantages. People with ADHD tend to be outgoing and ready for action. Because of their drive for excitement and stimulation, many become successful in business, sports, construction, and public speaking. Because of their ability to think about many things at once, many have won acclaim as artists and inventors. Many choose work that gives them freedom to move around and release excess energy. But some find ways to be effective in quieter, more sedentary careers.

Sally, a computer programmer, found that she thinks best when she wears headphones to reduce distracting noises. Like Henry, some people strive to increase their organizational skills. Others who own their own business find it useful to hire support staff to provide day-to-day management.

What hope does research offer?

Although no immediate cure is in sight, a new understanding of ADHD may be just over the horizon. Using a variety of research tools and methods, scientists are beginning to uncover new information on the role of the brain in ADHD and effective treatments for the disorder. Such research will ultimately result in improving the personal fulfillment and productivity of people with ADHD.

For example, the use of new techniques like brain imaging to observe how the brain actually works is already providing new insights into the causes of ADHD. Other research is seeking to identify conditions of pregnancy and early childhood that may cause or contribute to these differences in the brain. As the body of knowledge grows, scientists may someday learn how to prevent these differences or at least how to treat them.

NIMH and the US Department of Education are cosponsoring a large national study—the first of its kind—to see which combinations of ADHD treatment work best for different types of children. During this five-year study, scientists at research clinics across the country will work together in gathering data to answer such questions as: Is combining stimulant medication with behavior modification more effective than either alone? Do boys and girls respond differently to treatment? How do family stresses, income, and environment affect the severity of ADHD and long-term outcomes? How does needing medicine affect children's sense of competence, self-control, and self-esteem? As a result of such research, doctors and mental health specialists may someday know who benefits most from different types of treatment and be able to intervene more effectively.

NIMH grantees are also trying to determine if there are different varieties of attention deficit. With further study researchers may find that ADHD actually covers a number of different disorders, each with its own cluster of symptoms and treatment requirements. For example, scientists are exploring whether there are any critical differences between children with ADHD who also have anxiety, depression, or conduct disorders and those who do not. Other researchers are studying slight physical differences that might distinguish one type of ADHD from another. If clusters of differences can be found, scientists can begin to distinguish the treatment each type needs.

Other NIMH-sponsored research is examining the long-term outcome of ADHD. How do children with ADHD turn out, compared to brothers and sisters without the disorder? As adults, how do they handle their own children? Still other studies seek to better understand ADHD in adults. Such studies give insights into what types of treatment or services make a difference in helping an ADHD child grow into a caring parent and a well-functioning adult.

Animal studies are also adding to our knowledge of ADHD in humans. Animal subjects make it possible to study some of the possible causes of ADHD in ways that can't be studied in people. In addition, animal research allows the safety and effectiveness of experimental new drugs to be tested long before they can be given to humans. One NIH-sponsored team of scientists is studying dogs to learn how new stimulant drugs that are similar to Ritalin act on the brain.

Piece by piece, through studies of humans and animals, scientists are beginning to understand the biological nature of attention disorders. New research is allowing us to better understand the inner workings of the brain as we continue to develop new medications and assess new forms of treatment.

As we learn more about what actually happens inside the brain, we approach a future where we can prevent certain brain and mental disorders, make valid diagnoses, and treat each effectively. This is the hope, mission, and vision of the National Institute of Mental Health.

What are sources of information and support?

Several publications, organizations, and support groups exist to help individuals, teachers, and families to understand and cope with attention disorders. The following resources provide a good starting point for gaining insight, practical solutions, and support. Other resources are outpatient clinics of children's hospitals, university medical centers, and community mental health centers. Additional printed information can be found at libraries and book stores.

Books for Children and Teens

Galvin, M. *Otto Learns about his Medication*. New York: Magination Press, 1988. (for young children)

Gehret, J. *Learning Disabilities and the Don't Give Up Kid*. Fairport, New York: Verbal Images Press, 1990. (for classmates and children with learning disabilities and attention difficulties, ages 7–12)

Gordon, M. *Jumpin' Johnny, Get Back to Work! A Child's Guide to ADHD/Hyperactivity*. De Witt, New York: GSI Publications, 1991. (for ages 7–12)

Meyer, D.; Vadasy, P.; and Fewell, R. *Living with a Brother or Sister with Special Needs: A book for Sibs*. Seattle: University of Washington Press, 1985.

Moss, D. *Shelly the Hyperactive Turtle*. Rockville, MD: Woodbine House, 1989. (for young children)

Nadeau, K., and Dixon, E. *Learning to Slow Down and Pay Attention*. Annandale, VA: Chesapeake Psychological Publications, 1993.

Parker, R. *Making the Grade: An Adolescent's Struggle with ADD*. Plantation, FL: Impact Publications, 1992.

Quinn, P., and Stern, J. *Putting on the Brakes: Young People's Guide to Understanding Attention Deficit Hyperactivity Disorder*. New York: Magination Press, 1991. (for ages 8–12)

Thompson, M. *My Brother Matthew*. Rockville, MD: Woodbine House, 1992.

Books for Adults with Attention Disorders

Adelman, P., and Wren, C. *Learning Disabilities, Graduate School, and Careers: the Student's Perspective*. Lake Forest, IL: Learning Opportunities program, Barat College, 1990.

Hallowell, E., and Ratey, J. *Driven to Distraction*. New York: Pantheon Books, 1994.

Hartmann, T. *Attention Deficit Disorder: A New Perception*. Lancaster, PA: Underwood-Miller, 1993.

Kelly, K., and Ramundo, P. *You Mean I'm Not Lazy, Stupid, or Crazy?!* Cincinnati, OH: Tyrell and Jeremy Press, 1993.

Weiss, G., and Hechtman, L. (eds). *Hyperactive Children Grown Up*. 2d ed. New York: Guilford Press, 1992.

Weiss, L. *Attention Deficit Disorder in Adults*. Dallas, TX: Taylor Pub. co., 1992.

Wender, P. *The Hyperactive Child, Adolescence, and Adult: Attention Deficit Disorder Through the Lifespan*. New York: Oxford University Press, 1987.

Books for Parents

Anderson, W.; Chitwood, S.; and Hayden D. *Negotiating the Special Education Maze: A Guide for Parents and Teachers*. 2d ed. Rockville, MD: Woodbine House, 1990.

Bain, L. *A parent's guide to Attention Deficit Disorders*. New York: Dell Publishing, 1991.

Barkley, R. *Defiant Children*. New York: Guilford Press, 1987.

Child Psychopharmacy Center, University of Wisconsin. *Stimulants and Hyperactive Children*. Madison: 1990. Order by calling (608) 263-6171.

Copeland, E., and Love, V. *Attention, Please!: A Comprehensive Guide for Successfully Parenting Children with Attention Disorders and Hyperactivity*. Atlanta, GA: SPI Press, 1991.

Fowler, M. *Maybe You Know My Kid: A Parent's Guide to Identifying, Understanding, and Helping Your Child with ADHD*. New York: Birch Lane Press, 1990.

Goldstein, S., and Goldstein, M. *Hyperactivity: Why Won't My Child Pay Attention?* New York: J. Wiley, 1992.

Greenberg, G.; Horn, S.; and Wasde F. *Attention Deficit Hyperactivity Disorder: Questions & Answers for Parents*. Champaign, IL: Research Press, 1991.

Ingersoll, B., and Goldstein, S. *Attention Deficit Disorder and Learning Disabilities: Realities, Myths, and Controversial Treatments*. New York: Doubleday, 1993.

Moss, R., and Dunlap, H. *Why Johnny Can't Concentrate: Coping with Attention Deficit Problems*. New York: Bantam Books, 1990.

Kennedy, P.; Terdal, L.; and Fusetti, L. *The Hyperactive Child Book*. New York: St. Martin's Press, 1993.

Silver, L. *Silver's Advice to Parents on Attention-Deficit Hyperactivity Disorder*. Washington, DC: American Psychiatric Press, 1993.

Vail, P. *Smart Kids with School problems*. New York: EP Dutton, 1987.

Wilson, N. *Optimizing Special Education: How Parents Can Make a Difference*. New York: Insight Books, 1992.

Windell, J. *Discipline: A Sourcebook of 50 Failsafe Techniques for Parents*. New York: Collier Books, 1991.

Other Resources

For individuals with a computer and modem, there are on-line bulletin boards where parents, adults with ADHD, and medical professionals share experiences, offer emotional support, and ask and respond to questions. Two such on-line services include CompuServe [(800) 848-8990] and America Online [(800) 837-6364]. You may also wish to check with other national and local on-line communications companies to see if they offer similar services.

Resources for Teachers and Specialists

Barkley, R. *Attention Deficit Hyperactivity Disorder* (four 40-minute videocassettes in VHS format). New York: Guilford Publications, 1990.

Copeland, E., and Love, V. *Attention Without Tension: A Teacher's Handbook on Attention Disorders*. Atlanta, GA: 3 C's of Childhood, 1992.

Haris, K., and Graham, S. *Helping Young Writers Master the Craft*. Cambridge, MA; Brookline Books, 1992.

Johnson, D. *I Can't Sit Still—Educating and Affirming Inattentive and Hyperactive Children: Suggestions for Parents, Teachers, and Other Care Providers of Children to Age 10*. Santa Cruz, CA: ETR Associates, 1992.

Parker, H. *The ADD Hyperactivity Handbook for Schools*. Plantation, FL: Impact Publications, 1992.

Related Materials Available from NIH

Attention Deficit Disorder Information packet and *Know Your Brain Fact Sheet*. Both are available from NIH Neurological Institute, PO Box 5801; Bethesda, MD 20824 (800) 352-9424

Learning Disabilities (NIH Pub. No. 93-3611) and *Plain Talk about Depression* (NIH Pub. No. 93-3561). These are available by contacting: NIMH, Room 7C-02, 5600 Fishers Lane, Rockville, MD 20857.

Support Groups and Organizations

Attention Deficit Information Network (Ad-IN)
475 Hillside Ave
Needham, MA 02194
(617) 455-9895

Provides up-to-date information on current research, regional meetings. Offers aid in finding solutions to practical problems faced by adults and children with an attention disorder.

ADD Warehouse
300 NW 70th Ave
Plantation, FL 33317
(800) 233-9273

Distributes books, tapes, videos, assessment on attention deficit hyperactivity disorders. A central location for ordering many of the books listed above. Call for catalog.

Center for Mental Health Services
Office of Consumer, Family, and Public Information
5600 Fishers Lane, Room 15-105
Rockville, MD 20857
(301) 443-2792

This national center, a component of the U.S. Public Health Service, provides a range of information on mental health, treatment, and support services.

Children and Adults with Attention Deficit Disorders (CH.A.D.D.)
499 NW 70th Ave, Ste 109
Plantation, FL 33317
(305) 587-3700

A major advocate and key information source for people dealing with attention disorders. Sponsors support groups and publishes two newsletters concerning attention disorders for parents and professionals.

Council for Exceptional Children
11920 Association Dr

Reston, VA 22091
(703) 620-3660

Provides publications for educators. Can also provide referral to ERIC (Educational Resource Information Center) Clearinghouse for Handicapped and Gifted children.

Federation of Families for Children's Mental Health
1021 Prince St
Alexandria, VA 22314
(703) 684-7710

Provides information, support, and referrals through federation chapters throughout the country. This national parent-run organization focuses on the needs of children with broad mental health problems.

HEALTH Resource Center
American Council on Education
1 Dupont Circle, Ste 800
Washington, DC 20036
(800) 544-3284

A national clearinghouse on post-high school education for people with disabilities.

Learning Disabilities Association of America
4156 Library Rd
Pittsburgh, PA 15234
(412) 341-8077

Provides information and referral to state chapters, parent resources, and local support groups. Publishes news briefs and a professional journal.

National Association of Private Schools for Exceptional Children
1522 K St, NW, Ste 1032
Washington, DC 20005
(202) 408-3338

Provides referrals to private special education programs.

National Center for Learning Disabilities
99 Park Ave, 6th Floor
New York, NY 10016
(212) 687-7211

Provides referrals and resources. Publishes "Their World" magazine describing true stories on ways children and adults cope with LD.

National Clearinghouse for Alcohol and Drug Information
PO Box 2345
Rockville, MD 20847
(800) 729-6686

Provides information on the risks of alcohol during pregnancy, and fetal alcohol syndrome.

National Information Center for Children and Youth with Disabilities (NICHCY)
PO Box 1492
Washington, DC 20013
(800) 695-0285

Publishes free, fact-filled newsletters. Arranges workshops. Advises parents on the laws entitling children with disabilities to special education and other services.

Sibling Information Network
A.J. Pappanikou Center
1776 Ellington Rd
South Windsor, CT 06074
(203) 648-1205

Publishes a newsletter for and about siblings of children with special needs.

Tourette Syndrome Association
42-40 Bell Blvd
Bayside, NY 11361
(718) 224-2999

State and local chapters provide national information, advocacy, research, and support.

Document Source:
U.S. Department of Health and Human Services, Public Health
Service
National Institutes of Health
National Institute of Mental Health
NIH Publication No. 94-3572
September 1994

BIPOLAR DISORDER

by Mary Lynn Hendrix

What is bipolar disorder?

Bipolar disorder—which is also known as manic-depressive illness and will be called by both names throughout this publication—is a mental illness involving episodes of serious mania and depression. The person's mood usually swings from overly "high" and irritable to sad and hopeless, and then back again, with periods of normal mood in between.

Bipolar disorder typically begins in adolescence or early adulthood and continues throughout life. It is often not recognized as an illness, and people who have it may suffer needlessly for years or even decades.

Effective treatments are available that greatly alleviate the suffering caused by bipolar disorder and can usually prevent its devastating complications. These include marital breakups, job loss, alcohol and drug abuse, and suicide.

Here are some facts about bipolar disorder.

Awareness

Manic-depressive illness has a devastating impact on many people.

- At least two million Americans suffer from manic-depressive illness. For those afflicted with the illness, it is extremely distressing and disruptive.
- Like other serious illnesses, bipolar disorder is also hard on spouses, family members, friends, and employers.
- Family members of people with bipolar disorder often have to cope with serious behavioral problems (such as wild spending sprees) and the lasting consequences of these behaviors.
- Bipolar disorder tends to run in families and is believed to be inherited in many cases. Despite vigorous research efforts, a specific genetic defect associated with the disease has not yet been detected.

D/ART: A National Educational Program

The National Institute of Mental Health (NIMH) has launched the Depression/Awareness, Recognition, and Treatment (D/ART) campaign to help people

- Recognize the symptoms of depressive disorders, including bipolar disorder
- Obtain an accurate diagnosis

- Obtain effective treatments

D/ART also

- Encourages and trains health care professionals to recognize the signs of manic-depressive illness and utilize the most up-to-date treatment approaches
- Organizes citizens' advocacy groups to extend the D/ART program
- Works with business and industry to improve recognition, treatment, and insurance coverage for depressive disorders

Recognition

Bipolar disorder involves cycles of mania and depression.

Signs and symptoms of mania include

- Extreme irritability and distractibility
- Excessive "high" and euphoric feelings
- A sustained period of behavior that is different from usual
- Increased energy, activity, restlessness, racing thoughts, and rapid talking
- Decreased need for sleep
- Unrealistic beliefs in one's abilities and powers
- Uncharacteristically poor judgment
- Increased sexual drive
- Abuse of drugs, particularly cocaine, alcohol, and sleeping medications
- Obnoxious, provocative, or intrusive behavior
- Denial that anything is wrong

Signs and symptoms of depression include

- Persistent sad, anxious, or empty mood
- Feelings of hopelessness or pessimism
- Feelings of guilt, worthlessness, or helplessness
- Loss of interest or pleasure in ordinary activities, including sex
- Decreased energy, a feeling of fatigue or of being "slowed down"
- Difficulty concentrating, remembering, making decisions
- Restlessness or irritability
- Sleep disturbances
- Loss of appetite and weight, or weight gain
- Chronic pain or other persistent bodily symptoms that are not caused by physical disease
- Thoughts of death or suicide; suicide attempts

It may be helpful to think of the various mood states in manic-depressive illness as a spectrum or continuous range. At one end is severe depression, which shades into moderate depression; then come mild and brief mood disturbances that many people call "the blues," then normal mood, then hypomania (a mild form of mania), and then mania.

Some people with untreated bipolar disorder have repeated depressions and only an occasional episode of hypomania (bipolar II). In the other extreme, mania may be the main problem and depression may occur only infrequently. In fact, symptoms of mania and depression may be mixed together in a single "mixed" bipolar state.

Descriptions provided by patients themselves offer valuable insights into the various mood states associated with bipolar disorder:

Depression: I doubt completely my ability to do anything well. It seems as though my mind has slowed down and burned out to the point of being virtually useless . . . [I am] haunt[ed] . . . with the total, the desperate hopelessness of it all. . . .Others say, "It's only temporary, it will pass, you will get over it," but of course they haven't any idea of how I feel, although they are certain they do. If I can't feel, move, think, or care, then what on earth is the point?

Hypomania: At first when I'm high, it's tremendous . . . ideas are fast . . . like shooting stars you follow 'til brighter ones appear . . . all shyness disappears, the right words and gestures are suddenly there . . . uninteresting people, things, become intensively interesting. Sensuality is pervasive, the desire to seduce and be seduced is irresistible. Your marrow is infused with unbelievable feelings of ease, power, well-being, omnipotence, euphoria. . .you can do anything. . .but, somewhere this changes.

Mania: The fast ideas become too fast and there are far too many. . .overwhelming confusion replaces clarity. . .you stop keeping up with it—memory goes. Infectious humor ceases to amuse. Your friends become frightened . . .everything is now against the grain . . . you are irritable, angry, frightened, uncontrollable, and trapped.

Recognition of the various mood states is essential so that the person who has manic-depressive illness can obtain effective treatment and avoid the harmful consequences of the disease, which include destruction of personal relationships, loss of employment, and suicide.

Manic-depressive illness is often not recognized by the patient, relatives, friends, or even physicians.

- An early sign of manic-depressive illness may be hypomania—a state in which the person shows a high level of energy, excessive moodiness or irritability, and impulsive or reckless behavior.
- Hypomania may feel good to the person who experiences it. Thus, even when family and friends learn to recognize the mood swings, the individual often will deny that anything is wrong.
- Also in its early stages, bipolar disorder may masquerade as a problem other than mental illness. For example, it may first appear as alcohol or drug abuse, or poor school or work performance.
- If left untreated, bipolar disorder tends to worsen, and the person experiences episodes of full-fledged mania and clinical depression.

Treatment

Most people with manic-depressive illness can be helped with treatment.

- Almost all people with bipolar disorder—even those with the most severe forms—can obtain substantial stabilization of their mood swings.
- One medications, lithium, is usually very effective in controlling mania and preventing the recurrence of both manic and depressive episodes.
- More recently, the anticonvulsants carbamazepine and valproate have also been found useful, especially in more refractory bipolar episodes.
- For depression, several types of antidepressants can be useful when combined with lithium, carbamazepine, or valproate.
- Electroconvulsive therapy (electroshock) is often helpful in the treatment of severe depression and/or mixed mania that does not respond to medications.
- As an adjunct to medications, psychotherapy is often helpful in providing support, education, and guidance to the patient and his or her family.

Getting Help

Anyone with bipolar disorder should be under the care of a psychiatrist skilled in the diagnosis and treatment of this disease.

Other mental health professionals, such as psychologists and psychiatric social workers, can assist in providing the patient and his or her family with additional approaches to treatment.

Help can be found at

- University- or medical school-affiliated programs
- Hospital departments of psychiatry
- Private psychiatric offices and clinics
- Health maintenance organizations
- Offices of family physicians, internists, and pediatricians

People with manic-depressive illness often need help to get help.

- Often people with this disorder do not recognize how impaired they are or blame their problems on some cause other than mental illness.
- People with bipolar disorder need strong encouragement from family and friends to seek treatment. Family physicians can play an important role for such referral.
- If this does not work, loved ones must take the patient for proper mental health evaluation and treatment.
- If the person is in the midst of a severe episode, he or she may have to be committed to a hospital for his or her own protection and for much needed treatment.
- Anyone who is considering suicide needs immediate attention, preferably from a mental health professional or a physician; school counselors and members of the clergy can also assist in detecting and/or making a referral for more definitive assessment or treatment.

With appropriate help and treatment, it is possible to overcome suicidal tendencies.

- It is important for patients to understand that bipolar disorder will not go away, and that continued compliance with treatment is needed to keep the disease under control.
- Ongoing encouragement and support are needed after the person obtains treatment, because it may take a while to discover what therapeutic regimen is best for that particular patient.
- Many people receiving treatment also benefit from joining mutual support groups such as those sponsored by the National Depressive and Manic Depressive Association (NDMDA), the National Alliance for the Mentally Ill (NAMI), and the National Mental Health Association.
- Families and friends of people with bipolar disorder can also benefit from mutual support groups such as those sponsored by NDMDA and NAMI.

For Further Information Contact

National Institutes of Mental Health
Public Inquiries, Room 7C-02
5600 Fishers Lane
Rockville, MD 20857

National Depressive and Manic Depressive Association
730 North Franklin St
Ste 501
Chicago, IL 60610
(312) 642-0049
(312) 642-7243 FAX
1-800-826-3632

National Alliance for the Mentally Ill
2101 Wilson Blvd., Ste 302
Arlington, VA 22201
(703) 524-7600
(703) 524-9094 FAX
1-800-950-NAMI (6264)

National Foundation for Depressive Illness
PO Box 2257
New York, NY 10116
(212) 268-4260
(212) 268-4434 FAX
1-800-248-4344

National Mental Health Association
1201 Prince St
Alexandria, VA 22314-2971
(703) 684-7722
(703) 684-5968 FAX
1-800-969-6942

■ **Document Source:**
U.S. Department of Health and Human Services, Public Health Service
National Institutes of Health
National Institute of Mental Health
NIH Publication No. 93-3679
September 1993

See also: Depression: What Every Woman Should Know (page 318)

DEPRESSION: WHAT EVERY WOMAN SHOULD KNOW

More Than the Blues

Life is full of emotional ups and downs and everyone experiences the "blues" from time to time. But when the "down" times are long-lasting or interfere with an individual's ability to function at home and at work, that person may be suffering from a common, serious illness—depression.

Clinical depression affects mood, mind, body, and behavior. Research has shown that in the United States more than 17 million people—one in 10 adults—experience depression each year, and nearly two-thirds do not get the help they need. Treatment can alleviate the symptoms in over 80 percent of cases. Yet, because it often goes unrecognized, depression continues to cause unnecessary suffering.

Women are disproportionately affected by depression, experiencing it at roughly twice the rate of men. Research continues to explore how the illness affects women and to identify new areas that hold promise of deepening our understanding. At the same time, it is important to increase women's awareness of what is already known about depression, so that they seek early and appropriate treatment. That is the purpose of this pamphlet.

To grasp the specifics of depression in women, it is essential to have a broad understanding of the illness itself. To this end, this pamphlet presents an overview of depression as a pervasive and impairing illness that affects women and men in similar fashion. It then focuses on special issues—biological, life cycle, and psychosocial—that are unique to women and may be associated with depression.

A Picture of Depression

Jane slowly walked into the house, as though her body ached in every muscle. Jeff had already tucked the kids in bed. When he asked why she was late, Jane told him she was trying to catch up at work. She was too tired to say more, and too scared to admit that she could hardly concentrate or remember what she was supposed to be doing. Jeff had cooked dinner—again—but Jane had no appetite. She felt guilty as she pushed away her plate, apologized, and went to bed.

Sitting in silence was familiar to Jeff. He was reluctant to speak because Jane often flew off the handle these days, so unlike the good humored woman she used to be. Jeff and her coworkers had noticed the change in Jane—the way she kept to herself, her forced smile, her pessimism and loss of interest in things. As she struggled through her days, neither Jane nor Jeff understood what was happening to her. She felt alone and empty, often plagued by negative thoughts and bad feelings about herself. One day she said she couldn't see the point in living anymore. That was when Jeff became alarmed and encouraged Jane to seek professional help. They found out that she had clinical depression.

What is depression?

Jane, our fictional patient, experienced many of the symptoms that characterize depressive illness. Her story depicts how depression alters not just mood but one's entire existence, and how it impacts not just the affected individual but family and coworkers. Most importantly, it illustrates the importance of awareness of the illness, so that early recognition and appropriate treatment can keep depressive symptoms and their impact to a minimum.

No two people become depressed in exactly the same way. Many have only some of the symptoms, varying in severity and duration. For some, symptoms occur in time-limited episodes; for others, symptoms can be present for long periods if no treatment is sought. The age at which depression first appears also varies. There is evidence that in individuals born after 1945, it occurs at a younger age than in previous generations. Common to all age groups, affecting rich and poor alike, depressive illness occurs most frequently in adults between the ages of 25 and 44.

The Symptoms of Depression and Mania

Depression

- Persistent sad, anxious, or "empty" mood
- Loss of interest or pleasure in activities, including sex
- Feelings of hopelessness, pessimism
- Feelings of guilt, worthlessness, helplessness
- Sleeping too much or too little, early-morning awakening
- Appetite and/or weight loss or overeating and weight gain
- Decreased energy, fatigue, feeling "slowed down"
- Thoughts of death or suicide, or suicide attempts
- Restlessness, irritability
- Difficulty concentrating, remembering, or making decisions
- Persistent physical symptoms that do not respond to treatment, such as headaches, digestive disorders, and chronic pain

Mania

- Abnormally elevated mood
- Irritability
- Severe insomnia
- Grandiose notions
- Increased talking
- Racing thoughts
- Increased activity, including sexual activity
- Markedly increased energy
- Poor judgement that leads to risk-taking behavior
- Inappropriate social behavior

A thorough diagnostic evaluation is needed if five or more of these symptoms persist for more than two weeks, or if they interfere with work or family life. An evaluation involves a complete physical checkup and information-gathering on family health history.

Having some depressive symptoms does not mean a person is clinically depressed. For example, it is not unusual for those who have lost a loved one to feel sad, helpless, and disinterested in regular activities. Only when these symptoms persists for an unusually long time is there reason to suspect that grief has become depressive illness. Similarly, living with the stress of potential layoffs, heavy workloads, or financial or family problems may cause irritability and "the blues". Up to a point, such feelings are simply a part of human experience. But when the symptoms increase in number, duration and intensity, so that an individual is unable to function as usual, a temporary mood has very likely become a clinical illness.

Types of Depressive Illness

Major Depression, Jane's illness emerges in episodes. Some people have one episode in a lifetime; others have recurrent episodes. While initial symptoms may not always seem significant, eventually the individual will experience emotional pain and misery, and impairment in productivity at work and home and in relationships with family and friends.

Sometimes the episodes appear seasonally—typically with depression occurring in fall and winter and diminishing in the spring. Women seem to be especially prone to this kind of depression, known as Seasonal Affective Disorder (SAD).

Manic-Depressive Illness, also called bipolar disorder, involves cycles similar to major depression alternating with inappropriate "highs." Unlike other depressions, women and men are equally vulnerable. During manic episodes, people become overly active, euphoric, irritable, talkative and may spend money irresponsibly and get involved in sexual misadventures.

Dysthymia involves symptoms similar to those of major depression. They are milder but longer lasting, with a minimum duration of two years. People with dysthymia are frequently lacking in zest and enthusiasm for life, living joyless and fatigued existences that seem almost natural outgrowths of their personalities. If, in addition, they have a major depressive episode, as often happens, they are sometimes referred to as having "double depression."

Causes of Depression

Genetic Factors

There is a risk for developing depression when there is a family history of the illness, indicating that a biological vulnerability may be inherited. The risk is somewhat higher for those with bipolar disorder. However, not everybody with a family history develops the illness. In addition, major depression can occur in people who have had no family members with the illness. This suggests that additional factors, possibly biochemistry, environmental stressors, and other psychosocial factors, are involved in the onset of depression.

Biochemical Factors

Evidence indicates that brain biochemistry is a significant factor in depressive disorders. It is known, for example, that individuals with major depressive illness typically have too little or too much of certain brain chemicals, called neurotransmitters. Additionally, sleep patterns, which are biochemically influenced, are typically different in people with mood disorders. Depression can be induced or alleviated with certain medications, and some hormones have mood-altering properties. What is not yet known is whether the "biochemical disturbances" of depression are of genetic origin, or are secondary to stress, trauma, physical illness, or some other environmental condition.

Environmental and Other Stressors

Significant loss, a difficult relationship, financial problems, or a major change in life pattern have all been cited as contributors to depressive illness. Sometimes the onset of depression is associated with acute or chronic physical illness. In addition, some form of substance abuse disorder occurs in about one third of people with any type of depressive disorder.

Other Psychosocial Factors

Persons with certain characteristics—pessimistic thinking, low self-esteem, a sense of having little control over life events, and proneness to excessive worrying—are more likely to develop depression. These attributes may heighten the effect of stressful events or interfere with taking action to cope with them or with getting well. Upbringing or sex role expectations may contribute to the development of these traits. It appears that negative thinking patterns typically develop in childhood or adolescence.

The Many Dimensions of Depression in Women

Women At Risk

Many factors that appear to contribute to depression are common to both women and men, while the specific causes of depression in women remain unclear. However, varied factors unique to women's lives are suspected to contribute to depression—developmental, reproductive, hormonal, genetic, and other biological factors; abuse and oppression; interpersonal factors; and certain psychological and personality characteristics.

Regardless of contributing factors, depression is a highly treatable illness and the types of treatment discussed later in this brochure are effective for a majority of women.

Developmental Roles

The Issues of Adolescence

The higher incidence of depression in females begins in adolescence, when there are dramatic changes in roles and expectations along with other physical, intellectual and hormonal changes. The added stresses of adolescence include forming an identity, confronting sexuality, separating from parents, and making decisions for the first time. These significant issues are generally different for boys and girls. Studies show that female high school students have significantly higher rates of depression, anxiety disorders, eating disor-

ders, and adjustment disorders than male students, who have higher rates of disruptive behavior disorders.

Adulthood: Relationships and Work Roles

Stress in general can contribute to depression in persons biologically vulnerable to the illness. Some have theorized that the higher incidence of depression in women is not due to greater vulnerability, but to the multidimensional stresses that many women face, such as major responsibilities at home and work, single parenthood, and caring for children and aging parents. How these factors uniquely affect women is not yet fully understood.

For both women and men, rates of major depression are highest among the separated and divorced, and lowest among the married, while remaining always higher for women than for men. The quality of a marriage, however, may contribute significantly to depression. Lack of an intimate, confiding relationship, as well as marital disputes, have been shown to be related to depression in women. In fact, rates of depression were shown to be highest among unhappily married women.

Reproductive Life Cycle

Significant events in women's reproductive life cycles include menstruation, pregnancy, the postpregnancy period, and menopause. These events bring fluctuations in mood that for some women include depression. Further, infertility and the decision not to have children can also bring about changes in mood. Researchers have confirmed that hormones have an effect on the brain chemistry that controls emotions and mood; a specific biological mechanism explaining hormonal involvement is not known, however.

Menstruation and Premenstrual Syndrome

Many women experience certain normal behavioral and physical changes associated with phases of their **menstrual cycles.** Some women, however, regularly experience a significant number of extreme changes, including depressed feelings, irritability, and other emotional and physical manifestations. Though not considered a disorder in the most recent diagnostic manual for psychiatry, these extreme changes are generally called **premenstrual syndrome** (PMS) or **premenstrual dysphoric disorder** (PMDD). The changes typically begin after ovulation and become gradually worse until menstruation starts. Scientists are exploring how the cyclical rise and fall of estrogen and other hormones may affect the brain chemistry that is associated with depressive illness.

Pregnancy

Pregnancy (if it is desired) seldom contributes to depression, and having an abortion does not appear to lead to a higher incidence of depression. Women with infertility problems may be subject to extreme anxiety or sadness, though it is unclear if this contributes to a higher rate of depressive illness.

Postpartum Depression

Following childbirth, women may experience sadness that ranges from transient "blues," to an episode of major depression to severe, incapacitating, psychotic depression. Studies suggest that women who experience depressive illness after childbirth very often have had prior depressive episodes, though they may not have been diagnosed and treated. For *most* women postpartum depressions are transient with no adverse consequences.

Maternal Depression

Because women typically carry the primary responsibility for child care, the impact of their depressive illness on their parenting ability is of particular concern. Evidence suggests that maternal depression may have a negative effect on a child's behavior, and psychological and social development. These findings give additional emphasis to the importance of women recognizing the need for and seeking treatment for depression.

Menopause

A definitive study has shown that, in general, menopause is not associated with an increased risk of depression. In fact, while once considered a unique disorder, research has shown that depressive illness at menopause is no different than at other ages. The women more vulnerable to change-of-life depression are those with a history of past depressive episodes.

Specific Cultural Considerations

As in depression in general, the prevalence rate of depression in African American and Hispanic women remains about twice that of men. There is some indication, however, that major depression and dysthymia may be diagnosed less frequently in African American and slightly more frequently in Hispanic than in Caucasion women. Prevalence information for other racial and ethnic groups is not definitive.

Possible differences in symptom presentation may effect the way depression is recognized and diagnosed among minorities. For example, African Americans are more likely to report somatic symptoms, such as appetite change. In addition, people from various cultural backgrounds may view depressive symptoms in different ways. Such factors should be considered when working with women from special populations.

Personality and Psychology

As mentioned earlier, persons with certain characteristics appear to be more likely to develop or have difficulty overcoming depression. Some experts have suggested that the traditional upbringing of girls might foster these traits and that may be a factor in the higher rate of depression.

Others have suggested that women are not more vulnerable to depression than men, but simply express or label their symptoms differently. Women may be more likely to admit feelings of depression, brood about their feelings, or seek professional assistance. Men, on the other hand, may be socially conditioned to deny such feelings or to bury them in alcohol, as reflected in the higher rates of alcoholism in men. There is currently insufficient scientific data to verify this theory.

Victimization

It is known that far more women than men are sexually abused as children. Studies show that women molested as children are more likely to have clinical depression at some time in their lives than those with no such history. In addition, there appears to be a higher incidence of depression among women who were raped as adults. Women who experience other, commonly occurring forms of abuse, such as physical abuse and sexual harassment on the job, also may experience higher rates of depression. It has been suggested that abuse may lead to depression by fostering low self-esteem, a sense of helplessness, self-blame, and social isolation. Research is needed to understand the connection between victimization and depression.

Poverty

Low economic status brings with it many stresses, including isolation, uncertainty, frequent negative events, and poor access to helpful resources. It is known that depressive feelings and demoralization are common among the poor, the deprived, and those lacking social supports, and yet it is not clear whether depressive illnesses are more prevalent among victims of such environmental stressors. In fact, one very large study has shown that these illnesses tend to equally effect the poor and the rich.

Depression in Later Adulthood

Close examination of the facts casts doubt on "the empty nest syndrome" as an explanation for depression in older women. The lack of increased rates of depression among women at this stage of life suggests that most women do *not* get depressed when children leave home.

As with younger age groups, more elderly women than men suffer from depressive illness. Similarly, for all age groups, being unmarried (which includes widowhood) is also a risk factor for depression. Despite this, depression should not be dismissed as a normal consequence of the physical, social, and economic problems of later life. In fact, studies show that the rate of clinical depression in older people is lower than that of the general population, and that most older people feel satisfied with their lives.

About 800,000 persons are widowed each year, most of them are older, female, and experience varying degrees of depressive symptomatology. Most do not need formal treatment, but many who are moderately or severely sad appear to benefit from self-help groups or various psychosocial treatments. Remarkably, a third of widows/widowers meet criteria for major depressive episodes in the first month after the death of a spouse, but only half of these remain clinically depressed one year later. These depressions respond to standard antidepressant medications, although the optimal timing of the intervention is a matter of clinical judgement.

Depression Is a Treatable Illness

Even severe depression can be highly responsive to treatment. Indeed, believing one's condition is "incurable" is often part of the hopelessness that accompanies serious depression. Such patients should be provided with the information about the effectiveness of treatments for depression. As with many illnesses, the earlier treatment begins, the more effective it is and the greater the likelihood of preventing serious recurrences. Of course, treatment will not eliminate life's inevitable stresses and ups and downs; but it can greatly enhance the ability to manage such challenges and lead to greater enjoyment of life.

As a first step, a thorough physical examination may be recommended to rule out any physical illnesses that may cause depressive symptoms.

Types of Treatment for Depression

The most commonly used treatments for depression are antidepressant medication, psychotherapy, or a combination of the two. Which of these is the right treatment for an individual case depends on the nature and severity of the depression and, to some extent, on individual preference. In mild or moderate depression, one or both of these treatments may be useful, while in severe or incapacitating depression, medication is generally recommended as a first step in treatment. In combined treatment, medication can relieve physical symptoms quickly, while psychotherapy allows the opportunity to learn more effective ways of handling problems.

Medications

The medications used to treat depression include tricyclic antidepressants, monoamine oxidase inhibitors (MAOIs), serotonin reuptake inhibitors (SRIs), and bupropion. Each acts on different chemical pathways of the brain related to moods. Antidepressant medications are not habit-forming. To be effective, medications must be taken for at least four to six months (in a first episode), carefully following the doctor's instructions. Medications must be monitored to ensure the most effective dosage and to minimize side effects.

The prescribing doctor will provide information about possible side-effects and dietary restrictions. In addition, other medications being used should be reviewed because some can interact negatively with antidepressant medication. There may be restrictions during pregnancy.

Psychotherapy

In mild to moderate cases, psychotherapy is also a treatment option. Some short-term (10-20 week) therapies have been very effective in several types of depression. "Talking" therapies help patients gain insight and resolve problems through verbal give-and-take with the therapist. "Behavioral" therapies help patients learn new behaviors that lead to more satisfaction in life and "unlearn" counter-productive behaviors.

Research has shown that two short-term psychotherapies, Interpersonal and Cognitive/Behavioral, are helpful for some forms of depression. Interpersonal therapy works to change interpersonal relationships that cause or exacerbate depression. Cognitive/Behavioral therapy helps change negative styles of thinking and behaving that may contribute to the depression.

Other Treatments

Despite the unfavorable publicity electroconvulsive therapy (ECT) has received, research has shown that there are circumstances in which its use is medically justified and can even save lives. This is particularly true for those at high risk for suicide or with psychotic agitation, severe weight loss or physical debilitation due to other physical illness. ECT may also be recommended for persons who cannot take or do not respond to medication.

People who experience Seasonal Affective Disorder (SAD) can also be helped by a new form of therapy using lights, called phototherapy.

Treating Recurrent Depression

Even when treatment is successful, depression may recur. Studies indicate that certain treatment strategies are very useful in this instance. Continuation of antidepressant medication at the same dosage that successfully treated the acute episode can often prevent recurrence. Monthly interpersonal psychotherapy can lengthen the time between episodes in patients not taking medication.

The Path to Healing

Reaping the benefits of treatment begins by recognizing the signs of depression. The list of symptoms can be used for this purpose.

The next step is to be evaluated by a qualified professional. Depression can be diagnosed and treated by psychiatrists, psychologists, clinical social workers, and other mental health professionals, as well as by primary care physicians.

Treatment is a partnership between the patient and the health care provider. An informed consumer knows her treatment options and discusses concerns with her provider as they arise.

If you don't feel some improvement after several weeks of treatment, or if symptoms worsen, discuss this with your treatment provider. Trying another treatment approach, or getting a second opinion from another health or mental health professional, may be in order.

Helping Resources

General

- Physicians
- Mental health specialists
- Health maintenance organizations
- Community mental health centers
- Hospital departments of psychiatry or outpatient psychiatric clinics
- University or medical school-affiliated programs

- State hospital outpatient clinics
- Family service/social agencies
- Private clinics and facilities
- Employee assistance programs
- Clergy

Professional Organizations

- American Psychiatric Association
- American Psychological Association
- National Association for Social Workers
- American Nurses Association
- American Mental Health Counselors Association
- American Orthopsychiatric Association

Advocacy Groups

- National Mental Health Association
- National Alliance for the Mentally Ill
- National Foundation for Depressive Illness
- National Depressive and Manic Depressive Association

Helping Yourself

Depressive illnesses make you feel exhausted, worthless, helpless and hopeless. Such feelings make some people want to give up. It is important to realize that these negative views are part of the depression and will fade as treatment begins to take effect.

Along with professional treatment, there are other things you can do to help yourself get better. Some people find participating in support groups very helpful. It may also help to spend some time with other people and to participate in activities that make you feel better, such as mild exercise. Just don't overdo it or expect too much from yourself right away. Feeling better takes time. Your treating professional can also suggest other self-help strategies.

Helping the Depressed Person

The most important thing anyone can do for the depressed person is to help him or her get appropriate diagnosis and treatment. This may involve encouraging the person to seek professional help or to stay in treatment once it is instituted.

The second most important thing is to offer emotional support. This involves understanding, patience, affection, and encouragement. Engage the depressed person in conversation or activities and be gently insistent if you meet with resistance. Remind that person that with time and help, he or she will feel better.

Remember. . .

Here, again, are the steps to healing:

- Check your symptoms against the list.
- Talk to a health or mental health professional.

- Consider yourself a partner in treatment and be an informed consumer.
- If you do not start to feel better after several weeks of treatment, discuss this with your provider. Different or additional treatment may be recommended.
- If you experience a recurrence, remember what you know about coping with depression, and don't shy away from seeking help again.

For further information on depression, call: 1-800-421-4211

References

Blehar, M.D. and Lozovsky, D.B. Guest Eds. (1993). Special edition: Toward a new psychobiology of depression in women. *Journal of Affective Disorders.* 29:75-211.

Frank, E., Karp, J.F., and Rush, A. J. (1993). Efficacy of treatments for major depression. *Psychopharmacology Bulletin,* 29:457-475.

Lewinsohn, P.M., Hyman, H., Roberts, R.E., Seeley, J.R., and Andrews, J.A. (1993) Adolescent psychopathology: I. prevalence and incidence of depression and other DSM-III-R disorders in high school students. *Journal of Abnormal Psychology,* 102:133-144.

NIH Consensus Development Panel on Depression in Late Life (1992). Diagnosis and treatment of depression in late life. *JAMA,* 268:1018-1024.

Regier, D.A., Narrow, W.E., Rae, D.S., Manderscheid, R.W., Locke, B.Z., and Goodwin, F.K. (1993). The de facto U.S. mental and addictive disorders service system: Epidemiologic Catchment Area prospective 1-year prevalence rates of disorders and services. *Archives of General Psychiatry,* 50:85-94.

Rosenthal, N.E. (1993). Diagnosis and treatment of Seasonal Affective Disorder. *JAMA,* 270:2717-2720.

Weissman, M. Epidemiology of depression: frequency, risk groups, and risk factors. *Perspectives on Depressive Disorders,* U.S. Department of Health and Human Services, National Institute of Mental Health, 1-21.

"Depression: What Every Women Should Know" was developed for the Depression Awareness, Recognition, and Treatment (D/ART) program. D/ART is a professional and public education program sponsored by NIMH in collaboration with private organizations and citizens. D/ART's goals include the alleviation of symptoms through effective treatment for the millions of Americans who suffer from depressive disorders each year. The program is based on more than 40 years of research on the diagnosis and treatment of depressive disorders.

For Further Information on Depression

Free Brochures:
1-800-421-4211
Program/Materials:
D/ART
National Institute of Mental Health
5600 Fishers Lane
Room 10-85
Rockville, MD 20857
(301) 443-4140

Acknowledgements: Production of this booklet was coordinated by Denise Juliano at the Depression Awareness, Recognition, and Treatment (D/ART) Program of the National Institute of Mental Health. Isabel Davidoff assisted with editing. The following people provided scientific information and review for this publication—Hagop Akiskal, MD; Mary Blehar, PhD; Deborah Dauphinais, MD, Freda Lewis-Hall, MD; Eve Moscicki, ScD; William Narrow, MD; Delores Parron, PhD; Darrel Regier, MD; and Myrna Weissman, PhD.

■ **Document Source:**
U.S. Department of Health and Human Services, Public Health Service
National Institutes of Health
National Institute of Mental Health
NIH Publication No 95-3871

EATING DISORDERS

Each year millions of people in the United States are affected by serious and sometimes life-threatening eating disorders. The vast majority—more than 90 percent—of those afflicted with eating disorders are adolescent and young adult women. One reason that women in this age group are particularly vulnerable to eating disorders is their tendency to go on strict diets to achieve an "ideal" figure. Researchers have found that such stringent dieting can play a key role in triggering eating disorders.

Approximately 1 percent of adolescent girls develop *anorexia nervosa,* a dangerous condition in which they can literally starve themselves to death. Another 2 to 3 percent of young women develop bulimia nervosa, a destructive pattern of excessive overeating followed by vomiting or other "purging" behaviors to control their weight. These eating disorders also occur in men and older women, but much less frequently.

The consequences of eating disorders can be severe. For example, one in ten cases of anorexia nervosa leads to death from starvation, cardiac arrest, other medical complications, or suicide. Fortunately, increasing awareness of the dangers of eating disorders—sparked by medical studies and extensive media coverage of the illness—has led many people to seek help. Nevertheless, some people with eating disorders refuse to admit that they have a problem and do not get treatment. Family members and friends can help recognize the problem and encourage the person to seek treatment.

This brochure provides valuable information to individuals suffering from eating disorders, as well as to family members and friends trying to help someone cope with the illness. The publication describes the symptoms of eating disorders, possible causes, treatment options, and how to take the first steps toward recovery.

Scientists funded by the National Institute of Mental Health (NIMH) are actively studying ways to treat and understand eating disorders. In NIMH-supported research, scientists have found that people with eating disorders who get early treatment have a better chance of full recovery than those who wait years before getting help.

Anorexia Nervosa

People who intentionally starve themselves suffer from an eating disorder called *anorexia nervosa.* The disorder, which usually begins in young people around the time of puberty, involves extreme weight loss—at least 15 percent below the individual's normal body weight. Many people with the disorder look emaciated but are convinced they are overweight. Sometimes they must be hospitalized to prevent starvation.

Deborah developed anorexia nervosa when she was 16. A rather shy, studious teenager, she tried hard to please everyone. She had an attractive appearance, but was slightly overweight. Like many teenage girls, she was interested in boys but concerned that she wasn't pretty enough to get their attention. When her father jokingly remarked that she would never get a date if she didn't take off some weight, she took him seriously and began to diet relentlessly—never believing she was thin enough even when she became extremely underweight.

Soon after the pounds started dropping off, Deborah's menstrual periods stopped. As anorexia tightened its grip, she became obsessed with dieting and food and developed strange eating rituals. Every day she weighed all the food she would eat on a kitchen scale, cutting solids into minuscule pieces and precisely measuring liquids. She would then put her daily ration in small containers, lining them up in neat rows. She also exercised compulsively, even after she weakened and became faint. She never took an elevator if she could walk up steps.

No one was able to convince Deborah that she was in danger. Finally, her doctor insisted that she be hospitalized and carefully monitored for treatment of her illness. While in the hospital, she secretly continued her exercise regimen in the bathroom, doing strenuous routines of sit-ups and knee-bends. It took several hospitalizations and a good deal of individual and family outpatient therapy for Deborah to face and solve her problems.

Deborah's case is not unusual. People with anorexia typically starve themselves, even though they suffer terribly from hunger pains. *One of the most frightening aspects of the disorder is that people with anorexia continue to think they are overweight even when they are bone-thin.* For reasons not yet understood, they become terrified of gaining any weight.

Food and weight become obsessions. For some, the compulsiveness shows up in strange eating rituals or the refusal to eat in front of others. It is not uncommon for people with anorexia to collect recipes and prepare gourmet feasts for family and friends, but not partake in the meals themselves. Like Deborah, they may adhere to strict exercise routines to keep off weight. Loss of monthly menstrual periods is typical in women with the disorder. Men with anorexia often become impotent.

Bulimia Nervosa

People with *bulimia nervosa* consume large amounts of food and then rid their bodies of the excess calories by vomiting, abusing laxatives or diuretics, taking enemas, or exercising obsessively. Some use a combination of all these forms of purging. Because many individuals with bulimia "binge and purge" in secret and maintain normal or above normal body weight, they can often successfully hide their problem from others for years.

> Lisa developed bulimia nervosa at 18. Like Deborah, her strange eating behavior began when she started to diet. She too dieted and exercised to lose weight, but unlike Deborah, she regularly ate huge amounts of food and maintained her normal weight by forcing herself to vomit. Lisa often felt like an emotional powder keg—angry, frightened, and depressed.
>
> Unable to understand her own behavior, she thought no one else would either. She felt isolated and lonely. Typically, when things were not going well, she would be overcome with an uncontrollable desire for sweets. She would eat pounds of candy and cake at a time, and often not stop until she was exhausted or in severe pain. Then, overwhelmed with guilt and disgust, she would make herself vomit.
>
> Her eating habits so embarrassed her that she kept them secret until, depressed by her mounting problems, she attempted suicide. Fortunately, she didn't succeed. While recuperating in the hospital, she was referred to an eating disorders clinic where she became involved in group therapy. There she received medications to treat the illness and the understanding and help she so desperately needed from others who had the same problem.

Family, friends, and physicians may have difficulty detecting bulimia in someone they know. Many individuals with the disorder remain at normal body weight or above because of their frequent binges and purges, which can range from once or twice a week to several times a day. Dieting heavily between episodes of binging and purging is also common. Eventually, half of those with anorexia will develop bulimia.

As with anorexia, bulimia typically begins during adolescence. The condition occurs most often in women but is also found in men. Many individuals with bulimia, ashamed of their strange habits, do not seek help until they reach their thirties or forties. By this time, their eating behavior is deeply ingrained and more difficult to change.

Binge Eating Disorder

An illness that resembles bulimia nervosa is *binge eating disorder*. Like bulimia, the disorder is characterized by episodes of uncontrolled eating or binging. However, binge eating disorder differs from bulimia because its sufferers do not purge their bodies of excess food.

Individuals with binge eating disorder feel that they lose control of themselves when eating. They eat large quantities of food and do not stop until they are uncomfortably full. Usually, they have more difficulty losing weight and keeping it off than do people with other serious weight problems. Most people with the disorder are obese and have a history of weight fluctuations. Binge eating disorder is found in about 2 percent on the general population—more often in women than men. Recent research shows that binge eating disorder occurs in about 30 percent of people participating in medically supervised weight control programs.

Medical Complications

Medical complications can frequently be a result of eating disorders. Individuals with eating disorders who use drugs to stimulate vomiting, bowel movements, or urination may be in considerable danger, as this practice increases the risk of heart failure.

In patients with anorexia, starvation can damage vital organs such as the heart and brain. To protect itself, the body shifts into "slow gear": monthly menstrual periods stop, breathing, pulse, and blood pressure rates drop, and thyroid function slows. Nails and hair become brittle; the skin dries, yellows, and becomes covered with soft hair called lanugo. Excessive thirst and frequent urination may occur. Dehydration contributes to constipation, and reduced body fat leads to lowered body temperature and the inability to withstand cold.

Mild anemia, swollen joints, reduced muscle mass, and light-headedness also commonly occur in anorexia. If the disorder becomes severe, patients may lose calcium from their bones, making them brittle and prone to breakage. They may also experience irregular heart rhythms and heart failure. In some patients, the brain shrinks, causing personality changes. Fortunately, this condition can be reversed when normal weight is reestablished.

In NIMH-supported research, scientists have found that many patients with anorexia also suffer from other psychiatric illnesses. While the majority have co-occurring clinical depression, others suffer from anxiety, personality or substance abuse disorders, and many are at risk for suicide. Obsessive-compulsive disorder (OCD), an illness characterized by repetitive thoughts and behaviors, can also accompany anorexia. Individuals with anorexia are typically compliant in personality but may have sudden outbursts of hostility and anger or become socially withdrawn.

Bulimia nervosa patients—even those of normal weight—can severely damage their bodies by frequent binge eating and purging. In rare instances, binge eating causes the stomach to rupture; purging may result in heart failure due to loss of vital minerals, such as potassium. Vomiting causes other less deadly, but serious, problems—the acid in vomit wears down the outer layer of the teeth and can cause scarring on the backs of hands when fingers are pushed down the throat to induce vomiting. Further, the esophagus becomes inflamed and glands near the cheeks become swollen. As in anorexia, bulimia may lead to irregular menstrual periods. Interest in sex may also diminish.

Some individuals with bulimia struggle with addictions, including abuse of drugs and alcohol, and compulsive stealing. Like individuals with anorexia, many people with bulimia suffer from clinical depression, anxiety, OCD, and other psychiatric illnesses. These problems, combined with their impulsive tendencies, place them at increased risk for suicidal behavior.

People with binge eating disorder are usually overweight, so they are prone to the serious medical problems associated with obesity, such as high cholesterol, high blood pressure, and diabetes. Obese individuals also have a higher risk for gallbladder disease, heart disease, and some types of cancer. Research at NIMH and elsewhere has shown that individuals with binge eating disorder have high rates of co-occurring psychiatric illnesses—especially depression.

Common Symptoms of Eating Disorders

Symptoms	Anorexia Nervosa*	Bulimia Nervosa*	Binge Eating Disorder
Excessive weight loss in relatively short period of time	X		
Continuation of dieting although bone thin	X		
Dissatisfaction with appearance; belief that body is fat, even though severely underweight	X		
Loss of monthly menstrual periods	X	X	
Unusual interest in food and development of strange eating habits	X	X	
Eating in secret	X	X	X
Obsession with exercise	X	X	
Serious depression	X	X	X
Binging—consumption of large amounts of food		X	X
Vomiting or use of drugs to stimulate vomiting, bowel movements, and urination		X	
Binging but no noticeable weight gain		X	
Disappearance into bathroom for long periods of time to induce vomiting		X	
Abuse of drugs or alcohol		X	X

*Some individuals suffer from anorexia and bulimia and have symptoms of both disorders.

Causes of Eating Disorders

In trying to understand the causes of eating disorders, scientists have studied the personalities, genetics, environments, and biochemistry of people with these illnesses. As is often the case, the more that is learned, the more complex the roots of eating disorders appear.

Personalities

Most people with eating disorders share certain personality traits: low self-esteem, feelings of helplessness, and a fear of becoming fat. In anorexia, bulimia, and binge eating disorder, eating behaviors seem to develop as a way of handling stress and anxieties.

People with anorexia tend to be "too good to be true." They rarely disobey, keep their feelings to themselves, and tend to be perfectionists, good students, and excellent athletes. Some researchers believe that people with anorexia restrict food—particularly carbohydrates—to gain a sense of control in some area of their lives. Having followed the wishes of others for the most part, they have not learned how to cope with the problems typical of adolescence, growing up, and becoming independent. Controlling their weight appears to offer two advantages, at least initially: they can take control of their bodies and gain approval from others. However, it eventually becomes clear to other that they are out-of-control and dangerously thin.

People who develop bulimia and binge eating disorder typically consume huge amounts of food—often junk food—to reduce stress and relieve anxiety. With binge eating, however, comes guilt and depression. Purging can bring relief, but it is only temporary. Individuals with bulimia are also impulsive and more likely to engage in risky behavior such as abuse of alcohol and drugs.

Genetic and Environmental Factors

Eating disorders appear to run in families—with female relatives most often affected. This finding suggests that genetic factors may predispose some people to eating disorders; however, other influences—both behavioral and environmental—may also play a role. One recent study found that mothers who are overly concerned about their daughters' weight and physical attractiveness may put the girls at increased risk of developing an eating disorder. In addition, girls with eating disorders often have father and brothers who are overly critical of their weight.

Although most victims of anorexia and bulimia are adolescent and young adult women, these illnesses can also strike men and older women. Anorexia and bulimia are found most often in Caucasians, but these illnesses also affect African Americans and other racial ethnic groups. People pursuing professions or activities that emphasize thinness—like modeling, dancing, gymnastics, wrestling, and long-distance running—are more susceptible to the problem. In contrast to other eating disorders, one-third to one-fourth of all patients with binge eating disorder are men. Preliminary studies also show that the condition occurs equally among African Americans and Caucasians.

Biochemistry

In an attempt to understand eating disorders, scientists have studied the biochemical on the neuroendocrine system—a combination of the central nervous and hormonal systems. Through complex but carefully balanced feedback mechanisms, the neuroendocrine system regulates sexual function, physical growth and development, appetite and digestion, sleep, heart and kidney function, emotions, thinking, and memory—in other words, multiple functions of the mind and body. Many of these regulatory mechanisms are seriously disturbed in people with eating disorders.

In the central nervous system—particularly the brain—key chemical messengers known as neurotransmitters control hormone production. Scientists have found that the neurotransmitters *serotonin* and *norepinephrine* function abnormally in people affected by depression. Recently, researchers funded by NIMH have learned that these neurotransmitters are also decreased in acutely ill anorexia and bulimia patients and long-term recovered anorexia patients. Because many people with eating disorders also appear to suffer from depression, some scientists believe that there may be a link between these two disorders. In fact, new research has suggested that some patients with anorexia may respond well to the antidepressant medication fluoxetine, which affects serotonin function in the body.

People with either anorexia or certain forms of depression also tend to have higher than normal levels of cortisol, a brain hormone released in response to stress. Scientists have been able to show that the excess levels of cortisol in both anorexia and depression are caused by a problem that occurs in or near a region of the brain called the hypothalamus.

In addition to connections between depression and eating disorders, scientists have found biochemical similarities between people with eating disorders and obsessive-compulsive disorder (OCD). Just as serotonin levels are known to be abnormal in people with depression and eating disorders, they are also abnormal in patients with OCD. Recently, NIMH researchers have found that many patients with bulimia have obsessive-compulsive behavior as severe as that seen in patients actually diagnosed with OCD. Conversely, patients with OCD frequently have abnormal eating behaviors.

The hormone *vasopressin* is another brain chemical found to be abnormal in people with eating disorders and OCD. NIMH researchers have shown that levels of this hormone are elevated in patients with OCD, anorexia, and bulimia. Normally released in response to physical and possibly emotional stress, vasopressin may contribute to the obsessive behavior seen in some patients with eating disorders.

NIMH-supported investigators are also exploring the role of other brain chemicals in eating behavior. Many are conducting studies in animals to shed some light on human disorders. For example, scientists have found that levels of neuropeptide Y and peptide YY, recently shown to be elevated in patients with anorexia and bulimia, stimulate eating behavior in laboratory animals. Other investigators have found that cholecystokinin (CCK), a hormone known to be low in some women with bulimia, causes laboratory animals to feel full and stop eating. This finding may possibly explain why women with bulimia do not feel satisfied after eating and continue to binge.

Treatment

Eating disorders are most successfully treated when diagnosed early. Unfortunately, even when family members confront the ill person about his or her behavior, or physicians make a diagnosis, individuals with eating disorders may deny that they have a problem. Thus, people with anorexia may not receive medical or psychological attention until they have already become dangerously thin and malnourished. People with bulimia are often normal weight and are able to hide their illness from others for years. Eating disorders in males may be overlooked because anorexia and bulimia are relatively rare in boys and men. Consequently, getting—and

keeping—people with these disorders into treatment can be extremely difficult.

In any case, it cannot be overemphasized how important treatment is—the sooner, the better. The longer abnormal eating behaviors persist, the more difficult it is to overcome the disorder and its effects on the body. In some cases, long-term treatment may be required. Families and friends offering support and encouragement can play an important role in the success of the treatment program.

If an eating disorder is suspected, particularly if it involves weight loss, the first step is a complete physical examination to rule out any other illnesses. Once an eating disorder is diagnosed, the clinician must determine whether the patient is in immediate medical danger and requires hospitalization. While most patients can be treated as outpatients, some need hospital care. Conditions warranting hospitalization include excessive and rapid weight loss, serious metabolic disturbances, clinical depression or risk of suicide, severe binge eating and purging, or psychosis.

The complex interaction of emotional and physiological problems in eating disorders calls for a comprehensive treatment plan, involving a variety of experts and approaches. Ideally, the treatment team includes an internist, a nutritionist, an individual psychotherapist, and a psychopharmacologist—someone who is knowledgeable about psychoactive medications useful in treating these disorders.

To help those with eating disorders deal with their illness and underlying emotional issues, some form of psychotherapy is usually needed. A psychiatrist, psychologist, or other mental health professional meets with the patient individually and provides ongoing emotional support, while the patient begins to understand and cope with the illness. Group therapy, in which people share their experiences with others who have similar problems, has been especially effective for individuals with bulimia.

Use of individual psychotherapy, family therapy, and cognitive-behavioral therapy—a form of psychotherapy that teaches patients how to change abnormal thoughts and behavior—is often the most productive. Cognitive-behavior therapists focus on changing eating behaviors usually by rewarding or modeling wanted behavior. These therapists also help patients work to change the distorted and rigid thinking patterns associated with eating disorders.

NIMH-supported scientists have examined the effectiveness of combining psychotherapy and medications. In a recent study of bulimia, researchers found that both intensive group therapy and antidepressant medications, combined or alone, benefited patients. In another study of bulimia, the combined use of cognitive-behavioral therapy and antidepressant medications was most beneficial. The combination treatment was particularly effective in preventing relapse once medications were discontinued. For patients with binge eating disorder, cognitive-behavioral therapy and antidepressant medications may also prove to be useful.

Antidepressant medications commonly used to treat bulimia include desipramine, imipramine, and fluoxetine. For anorexia, preliminary evidence shows that some antidepressant medications may be effective when combined with other forms of treatment. Fluoxetine has also been useful in treating some patients with binge eating disorder. These antidepressants may also treat any co-occurring depression.

The efforts of mental health professionals need to be combined with those of other health professionals to obtain the best treatment. Physicians treat any medical complications, and nutritionists advise on diet and eating regimens. The challenge of treating eating disorders is made more difficult by the metabolic changes associated with them. Just to maintain a stable weight, individuals with anorexia may actually have to consume more calories than someone of similar weight and age without an eating disorder.

This information is important for patients and the clinicians who treat them. Consuming calories is exactly what the person with anorexia wishes to avoid, yet must do to regain the weight necessary for recovery. In contrast, some normal weight people with bulimia may gain excess weight if they consume the number of calories required to maintain normal weight in others of similar size and age.

Helping the Person with an Eating Disorder

Treatment can save the life of someone with an eating disorder. Friends, relatives, teachers, and physicians all play an important role in helping the ill person start and stay with a treatment program. Encouragement, caring, and persistence, as well as information about eating disorders and their dangers, may be needed to convince the ill person to get help, stick with treatment, or try again.

Family members and friends can call local hospitals or university medical centers to find out about eating disorder clinics and clinicians experienced in treating the illnesses. For college students, treatment programs may be available in school counseling centers.

Family members and friends should read as much as possible about eating disorders, so they can help the person with the illness understand his or her problem. Many local mental health organizations and the self-help groups listed at the end of this brochure provide free literature on eating disorders. Some of these groups also provide treatment program referrals and information on local self-help groups. Once the person gets help, he or she will continue to need lots of understanding and encouragement to stay in treatment.

NIMH continues its search for new and better treatments for eating disorders. Congress has designated the 1990s as the Decade of the Brain, making the prevention, diagnosis, and treatment of all brain and mental disorders a national research priority. This research promises to yield even more hope for patients and their families by providing a greater understanding of the causes and complexities of eating disorders.

For Further Information

For additional information on eating disorders, check local hospitals or university medical centers for an eating disorders clinic, or contact:

National Association of Anorexia Nervosa and Associated Disorders (ANAD)
PO Box 7
Highland Park, IL 60035

(708) 831-3438

Anorexia Nervosa and Related Eating Disorders, Inc. (ANRED)
PO Box 5102
Eugene, OR 97405
(503) 344-1144

American Anorexia/Bulimia Association, Inc. (AABA)
425 E 61st St, 6th Fl
New York, NY 10021
(212) 891-8686

Center for the Study of Anorexia and Bulimia
1 W 91st St
New York, NY 10024
(212) 595-3449

National Eating Disorder Organization
445 E Grandille Rd
Worthington, OH 43085
(614) 436-1112

For information on Eating Disorders Awareness Week, contact:

Eating Disorder Awareness & Prevention Inc.
603 Stewart St, Ste 803
Seattle, WA 98101
(206) 382-3587

For information on other mental disorders, contact:

Information Resources and Inquiries Branch
National Institute of Mental Health
5600 Fishers Lane, Room 7C02
Rockville, MD 20857

This pamphlet was rewritten by Lee Hoffman, Office of Scientific Information (OSI), National Institute of Mental Health (NIMH). An earlier version was prepared by OSI staff member Marilyn Sargent. Scientific review was provided by NIMH staff, Susan J. Blumenthal, MD; Harold Goldstein, PhD; Harry E. Gwirtsman, MD; and Susan Z. Yanovski, MD.

■ Document Source:
**U.S. Department of Health and Human Services, Public Health Service
National Institutes of Health
National Institute of Mental Health
NIH Publication No. 943477
Printed 1993, Reprinted 1994**

GETTING TREATMENT FOR PANIC DISORDER

This brochure is for people who want to find out whether they or someone they know may have panic disorder and how it can be treated most effectively. It may be helpful to refer to this pamphlet when consulting with a health care professional.

Also in this brochure, three people with panic disorder comment on how treatment has helped them regain their lives.

Could you have panic disorder?

- Do you experience sudden episodes of intense and overwhelming fear that seem to come on for no apparent reason?
- During these episodes, do you also experience several of the following:
  - Racing, pounding, or skipping heartbeat
  - Chest pain, pressure, or discomfort
  - Difficulty catching your breath
  - Choking sensation or lump in your throat
  - Excessive sweating
  - Lightheadedness or dizziness
  - Nausea or stomach problems
  - Tingling or numbness in parts of your body
  - Chills or hot flashes
  - Shaking or trembling
  - Feelings of unreality, or being detached from your body
- During these episodes, do you have the urge to flee, or the feeling that you need to escape?
- During these episodes, do you think something terrible might happen—that you might die, have a heart attack, suffocate, lose control, or embarrass yourself?
- Do you worry a lot about these episodes or fear that they will happen again? And does this fear cause you to avoid places or situations that you think might have triggered the attack?

If you answered yes to most of these questions, chances are you are suffering from panic disorder. If so, you are not alone.

Panic disorder is very different from everyday anxiety. More than three million American adults have, or will have, panic disorder. Most frequently, it starts in young adulthood. Usually, it does not go away by itself. But with proper treatment, people with panic disorder can be helped.

Why Seeking Treatment Is Critical

Repeated episodes of fear—commonly called panic attacks—that are typical of panic disorder can be devastating. The panic attacks, or avoidance of them, can completely take control of your life.

- Without treatment, you may continue to have panic attacks for years. The disorder can seriously interfere with your relationships with family, friends, and co-workers.
- Without treatment, your life may become severely restricted. For example, you may start to avoid certain situations where you fear you will experience a panic attack—even normal, everyday activities, such as grocery shopping or driving. In extreme cases, people with untreated panic disorder grow afraid to leave the house, a condition known as agoraphobia.
- Without treatment, you may find it difficult to be productive at work. Your symptoms may keep you from getting to your job or staying there once you arrive. You may turn down promotions or job assignments that you believe will make you more likely to have panic attacks.

Some people with panic disorder even quit their jobs. Many can keep working, but otherwise rarely leave home.

- Without treatment, you may become severely depressed. You may try unsuccessfully to numb the symptoms of panic disorder or depression with alcohol or other drugs. You may even begin to have thoughts about suicide.

You do not have to live this way. You need to know that panic disorder is treatable. In fact, proper treatment reduces or completely prevents panic attacks in 70 to 90 percent of people. Many people feel substantial relief in just weeks or months.

Unfortunately, some people are reluctant to pursue treatment. Perhaps they think their condition is not serious. Perhaps they fell embarrassed. They may blame themselves or have trouble asking for help. Perhaps they dislike the idea of medication or therapy. Or, maybe they have sought help but are frustrated because their condition was not diagnosed or treated effectively.

Do not let these or any other reasons stop you from getting proper treatment. If you have panic disorder, you should get whatever help is necessary to overcome it, just as you would for any serious medical illness.

Do not be discouraged if some people say, "It's nothing to worry about," "It's just stress," "It's all in your head," or "Snap out of it." While they often mean well, the fact is that most people who do not have panic disorder do not understand that it is real and, therefore, tend to doubt its seriousness.

Most importantly, do not try to numb the effects of panic attacks with alcohol or other drugs. This will only make the problem worse.

Getting a Diagnosis

Since panic disorder can mimic a variety of medical conditions, such as heart problems and digestive complaints, the first thing you should do is have a full medical evaluation.

Although it is important for you and your doctor to concentrate on your physical symptoms, you should not overlook other aspects of your attacks. You may want to re-read the questions at the beginning of this pamphlet and tell your doctor anything you notice about how your attacks make you feel and when they usually occur.

Information on both the physical and emotional aspects of the attacks can be very useful to your doctor in making a diagnosis. For example, your doctor will want to know if your attacks, or fear of having attacks, keep you from carrying out any of your normal activities.

Many people with panic disorder also suffer from depression—feelings of intense sadness, even hopelessness. Depression is accompanied by an impaired ability to think, concentrate, and enjoy the normal pleasures of life. Be sure to make your doctor aware of these symptoms as well. If you have been drinking or using drugs to try to control your symptoms, let your doctor know about that too.

Once you have been properly diagnosed, your doctor—perhaps in consultation with a mental health specialist—can help you determine which treatment is best for you.

Effective Treatment for Panic Disorder

Treatment for panic disorder can consist of taking a medication to adjust the chemicals in your body—just as you might take medicine to correct a thyroid imbalance.

Or treatment might involve working with a psychotherapist to gain more control over your anxieties—just as some people work with specialists to learn techniques to control migraine headaches or lower their blood pressure.

Research shows that both kinds of treatment can be very effective. For many patients, the combination of medication and psychotherapy appears to be more effective than either treatment alone. Early treatment can help keep panic disorder from progressing.

Cognitive-Behavioral Therapy

Cognitive-behavioral therapy (CBT) teaches you to anticipate and prepare yourself for the situations and bodily sensations that may trigger panic attacks. CBT usually includes the following elements:

- A therapist helps you identify the thinking patterns that lead you to misinterpret sensations and assume "the worst" is happening. These patterns of thinking are deeply ingrained, and it will take practice to notice them and then to change them.
- A therapist can teach you breathing exercises that calm you and that can prevent the overbreathing, or hyperventilation, that often occurs during a panic attack.
- A therapist can help you gradually become less sensitive to the frightening bodily sensations and feelings of terror. This is done by helping you, step by step, to safely test yourself in the places and situations you've been avoiding.

CBT generally requires at least eight to 12 weeks. Some people may need a longer time in treatment to learn the skills and put them into practice. Most panic disorder patients are successful in controlling or preventing their panic attacks after completing treatment with CBT.

CBT required a motivated patient and a specially trained therapist. Make sure any therapist you work with has proper training and experience in this method of panic disorder treatment. Indeed, in some parts of the country, you may find limited access to professionals trained and experienced in CBT.

Medication

Several types of medication that alter the ways chemicals interact in the brain can reduce or prevent panic attacks and decrease anxiety. Two major categories of medication that have been shown to be safe and effective in the treatment of panic disorder are antidepressants and benzodiazepines.

Each medication works differently. Some work quickly and others more gradually. All of them have to be taken on a regular basis. Usually, treatment with medication lasts at least six months to a year. But within eight weeks, you and your doctor should be able to assess whether it's effectively blocking the panic attacks. More details on medications can be found in the brochure, "Understanding Panic Disorder." If you need a copy, call 1-800-64-PANIC.

Clinical experience suggests that for many patients with panic disorder, a combination of CBT and medication may be the best treatment. The National Institute of Mental Health (NIMH) is conducting a large study to confirm this and to help determine the kinds of patients most likely to need combined therapy.

How to Choose the Right Treatment for You

Various types of health professionals may have the training and experience needed to treat panic disorder. Sometimes panic disorder patients are treated by two health care professionals—one who prescribes and monitors medication and another who provides CBT.

Each professional will use the treatments with which he or she is most familiar and successful. It is vital to choose a professional who is trained and experienced in the treatment methods described earlier; it is equally important to choose someone with whom you feel comfortable.

Many people begin looking for treatment by visiting their family doctor or a local clinic or health maintenance organization. Other places to seek help include your local health department or community mental health clinic. If there is a university near you, you may wish to ask about participating in a panic disorder study. Many universities have ongoing treatment research programs in their psychology or psychiatry departments that may provide care at less expense.

To help you locate mental health professionals in your area, NIMH has available a Referral List, which gives the names and telephone numbers of organizations that can provide you with a referral. (You can receive a copy of this list by calling 1-800-64-PANIC.)

When seeking a health care professional to treat your panic disorder, you may want to ask the following questions:

- How many patients with panic disorder have you treated?
- Do you have any special training in panic disorder treatment?
- What is your basic approach to treatment—cognitive-behavioral therapy, medication, or both? If you provide only one type of treatment, how do I get the other if I need it?
- How long is a typical course of treatment?
- How frequent are treatment sessions? How long does each session last?
- What are your fees?
- Can you help me determine whether my health insurance will cover this?

How to Make Your Treatment Successful

From the beginning, it is important to be a full participant in your treatment. Be active and assertive. Ask questions. Maintain open communication with your treatment professional and let him or her know your concerns.

Every patient responds differently, but it is important to know that none of the treatments for panic disorder works instantly. So, you must stick with a particular treatment for at least eight weeks to see if it works. If you do not see significant improvement within that time, you and your treatment professional can adjust your treatment plan. It may take a bit of trial and error before you find what works best for you. Be patient and communicate with your treatment professional. Of course, if at any time you feel uncomfortable with the professional you have chosen or don't think your treatment is going well, you should feel free to consider seeking a second opinion or even changing providers.

If your treatment involves medication, talk with your doctor about how often and in what manner your dosage will be monitored. No matter what medication you are taking, your doctor is likely to start you on a low dose and gradually increase it to the full dose. You should know that every medication has side effects, but they usually become tolerated or diminish with time. If side effects become a problem, the doctor may advise you to stop taking the medication and to wait a week or so before trying another medication. When your treatment is near an end, your doctor will taper the dosage gradually.

Support Groups and Self-Help Tools

Patient-run support groups can be a rich source of information for people with panic disorder. These groups typically involve five to 10 people who meet weekly to talk about their experiences, encourage each other, and share tips on coping strategies and local treatment resources. Sometimes, family members are invited to attend.

The NIMH Referral List can help you find a support group in your area. If there are no groups near you, you may want to form your own. Some of the sources listed can aid you in doing this. NIMH also has a Resource List that provides some self-help information about panic disorder, including books, articles, and videotapes.

Another way to get help is to enlist the support of friends and family members. You may want to share this booklet and other materials with them so they can better understand panic disorder and its treatment.

Take the Next Step Today

Panic disorder is far too serious—and far too treatable—to delay getting help. Recognizing the situation is the first step to recovery.

Now take the next step. If you think you may have panic disorder, act now. See your health professional for a diagnosis and then follow the suggestions in this booklet for making your treatment successful. Educate yourself about your condition. The more you know about panic attacks and panic

disorder, the better you will understand your role in treatment. To obtain the materials referred to in this booklet, call 1-800-64-PANIC.

Remember, Panic Disorder Is Very Treatable. You Can Get Better.

■ Document Source:
   U.S. Department of Health and Human Services, Public Health Service
   National Institutes of Health
   National Institute of Mental Health
   NIH Publication No. 94-3641

See also: Anxiety Disorder (page 297)

MEDICATIONS

Introduction

Anyone can develop a mental illness—you, a family member, a friend, or the fellow down the block. Some disorders are mild, while others are serious and long-lasting. These conditions can be helped. One way—an important way—is with psychotherapeutic medications. Compared to other types of treatment, these medications are relative newcomers in the fight against mental illness. It was only 41 years ago that the first one, chlorpromazine, was introduced. But considering the short time they've been around, psychotherapeutic medications have made dramatic changes in the treatment of mental disorders. People who, years ago, might have spent many years in mental hospitals because of crippling mental illness may now only go in for brief treatment, or might receive all their treatment at an outpatient clinic.

Psychotherapeutic medications also may make other kinds of treatment more effective. Someone who is too depressed to talk, for instance, can't get much benefit from psychotherapy or counseling; but often, the right medication will improve symptoms so that the person can respond better.

Another benefit from these medications is an increased understanding of the causes of mental illness. Scientists have learned a great deal more about the workings of the brain as a result of their investigations into how psychotherapeutic medications relieve disorders such as psychosis, depression, anxiety, obsessive-compulsive disorder, and panic disorder.

Symptom Relief, Not Cure

Just as aspirin can reduce a fever without clearing up the infection that causes it, psychotherapeutic medications act by controlling symptoms. Like most drugs used in medicine, they correct or compensate for some malfunction in the body. Psychotherapeutic medications do not cure mental illness, but they do lessen its burden. In many cases, these medications can help a person get on with life despite some continuing mental pain and difficulty coping with problems. For example, drugs like chlorpromazine can turn off the "voices" heard by some people with schizophrenia and help them to perceive reality more accurately. And antidepressants can lift the dark, heavy moods of depression. The degree of response—ranging from little relief of symptoms to complete remission—depends on a variety of factors related to the individual and the particular disorder being treated.

How long someone must take a psychotherapeutic medication depends on the disorder. Many depressed and anxious people may need medication for a single period—perhaps for several months—and then never have to take it again. For some conditions, such as schizophrenia or manic-depressive illness, medication may have to be take indefinitely or, perhaps, intermittently.

Like any medication, psychotherapeutic medications do not produce the same effect in everyone. Some people may respond better to one medication than another. Some may need larger dosages than others do. Some experience annoying side effects, while others do not. Age, sex, body size, body chemistry, physical illnesses and their treatment, diet, and habits such as smoking, are some of the factors that can influence a medication's effect.

Questions for Your Doctor

To increase the likelihood that a medication will work well, patients and their families must actively participate with the doctor prescribing it. They must tell the doctor about the patient's past medical history, other medications being taken, anticipated life changes—such as planning to have a baby—and, after some experience with a medication, whether it is causing side effects. When a medication is prescribed, the patient or family member should ask the following questions recommended by the U.S. Food and Drug Administration (FDA) and professional organizations:

- What is the name of the medication, and what is it supposed to do?
- How and when do I take it, and when do I stop taking it?
- What foods, drinks, other medications, or activities should I avoid while taking the prescribed medication?
- What are the side effects, and what should I do if they occur?
- Is there any written information available about the medication?

In this booklet, medications are described by their generic (chemical) names and in italics by their trade names (brand names used by drug companies). They are divided into four large categories based on the symptoms for which they are primarily used—antipsychotic, antimanic, antidepressant, and antianxiety medications. In addition, stimulants used for attention-deficit/hyperactivity disorder are listed.

An index at the end of the booklet gives the trade name, and the generic name, of the most commonly prescribed medications and notes the section that contains information about each type.

---

* "He" is used here to refer to both men and women.

Treatment evaluation studies have established the efficacy of the medications described here; however, much remains to be learned about these medications. The National Institute of Mental Health, other federal agencies, and private research groups are sponsoring studies of these medications. Scientists are hoping to improve their understanding of how and why these medications work, how to control or eliminate unwanted side effects, and how to make the medications more effective.

Antipsychotic Medications

A person who is psychotic is out of touch with reality. He may "hear voices" or have strange and untrue ideas (for example, thinking that others can hear his thoughts, or are trying to harm him, or that he is the President of the United States or some other famous person). * He may get excited or angry for no apparent reason, or spend a lot of time off by himself, or in bed, sleeping during the day and staying awake at night. He may neglect his appearance, not bathing or changing clothes, and may become difficult to communicate with— saying things that make no sense, or barely talking at all.

These kinds of behaviors are symptoms of psychotic illness, the principal form of which is schizophrenia. All of the symptoms may not be present when someone is psychotic, but some of them always are. Antipsychotic medications, as their name suggests, act against these symptoms. These medications cannot "cure" the illness, but they can take away many of the symptoms or make them milder. In some cases, they can shorten the course of the illness as well.

There are a number of antipsychotic (neuroleptic) medications available. They all work; the main differences are in the potency—that is, the dosage (amount) prescribed to produce therapeutic effects—and the side effects. Some people might think that the higher the dose of medication, the more serious the illness, but this is not always true.

A doctor will consider several factors when prescribing an antipsychotic medication, besides how "ill" someone is. These include the patient's age, body weight, and type of medication. Past history is important, too. If a person took a particular medication before and it worked, the doctor is likely to prescribe the same one again. Some less potent drugs, like chlorpromazine *(Thorazine),* are prescribed in higher numbers of milligrams than others of high potency, like haloperidol *(Haldol).*

If a person has to take a large amount of a "high-dose" antipsychotic medication, such as chlorpromazine, to get the same effect as a small amount of a "low-dose" medication, such as haloperidol, why doesn't the doctor just prescribe "low-dose" medications? The main reason is the difference in their side effects (actions of the medication other than the one intended for the illness). These medications vary in their side effects, and some people have more trouble with certain side effects than others. A side effect may sometimes be desirable. For instance, the sedative effect of some antipsychotic medications is useful for patients who have trouble sleeping or who become agitated during the day.

Unlike some prescription drugs, which must be taken several times during the day, antipsychotic medications can usually be taken just once a day. Thus, patients can reduce daytime side effects by taking the medications once, before bed. Some antipsychotic medications are available in forms that can be injected once or twice a month, thus assuring that the medicine is being taken reliably.

Most side effects of antipsychotic medications are mild. Many common ones disappear after the first few weeks of treatment. These include drowsiness, rapid heartbeat, and dizziness when changing position.

Some people gain weight while taking antipsychotic medications and may have to change their diet to control their weight. Other side effects that may be caused by some antipsychotic medications include decrease in sexual ability or interest, problems with menstrual periods, sunburn, or skin rashes. If a side effect is especially troublesome, it should be discussed with the doctor who may prescribe a different medication, change the dosage level or schedule, or prescribe an additional medication to control the side effects.

Movement difficulties may occur with the use of antipsychotic medications, although most of them can be controlled with an anticholinergic medication. These movement problems include muscle spasms of the neck, eye, back, or other muscles; restlessness and pacing; a general slowing-down of movement and speech; and a shuffling walk. Some of these side effects may look like psychotic or neurologic (Parkinson's disease) symptoms, but aren't. If they are severe, or persist with continued treatment with an antipsychotic, it is important to notify the doctor, who might either change the medication or prescribe an additional one to control the side effects.

Just as people vary in their responses to antipsychotic medications, they also vary in their speed of improvement. Some symptoms diminish in days, while others take weeks or months. For many patients, substantial improvement is seen by the sixth week of treatment, although this is not true in every case. If someone does not seem to be improving, a different type of medication may be tried.

Even if a person is feeling better or completely well, he should not just stop taking the medication. Continuing to see the doctor while tapering off medication is important. Some people may need to take medication for an extended period of time, or even indefinitely. These people usually have chronic (long-term, continuous) schizophrenic disorders, or have a history of repeated schizophrenic episodes, and are likely to become ill again. Also, in some cases a person who has experienced one or two severe episodes may need medication indefinitely. In these cases, medication may be continued in as low a dosage as possible to maintain control of symptoms. This approach, called maintenance treatment, prevents relapse in many people and removes or reduces symptoms for others.

While maintenance treatment is helpful for many people, a drawback for some is the possibility of developing long-term side effects, particularly a condition called tardive dyskinesia. This condition is characterized by involuntary movements. These abnormal movements most often occur around the mouth, but are sometimes seen in other muscle areas such as the trunk, pelvis, or diaphragm. The disorder may range from mild to severe. For some people, it cannot be reversed, while others recover partially or completely. Tardive dyskinesia is seen most often after long-term treatment with antipsychotic medications. There is a higher incidence in women, with the risk rising with age. There is no way to determine whether someone will develop this condition, and if it develops, whether the patient will recover. At present, there is no effective treatment for tardive dyskinesia. The possible risks of long-term treatment with antipsychotic medications must be weighed against the benefits in each individual case by patient, family, and doctor.

Antipsychotic medications can produce unwanted effects when taken in combination with other medications. Therefore, the doctor should be told about all medicine being taken, including over-the-counter preparations, and the extent of the use of alcohol. Some antipsychotic medications interfere with the action of antihypertensive medications (taken for high blood pressure), anticonvulsants (taken for epilepsy), and medications used for Parkinson's disease. Some antipsychotic medications add to the effects of alcohol and other central nervous system depressants, such as antihistamines, antidepressants, barbiturates, some sleeping and pain medications, and narcotics.

Atypical Neuroleptics

In 1990, clozapine *(Clozaril)*, an "atypical neuroleptic," was introduced in the United States. In clinical trials, this medication was found to be more effective than traditional antipsychotic medications in individuals with treatment-resistant schizophrenia, and the risk of tardive dyskinesia is lower. However, because of the potential side effect of a serious blood disorder, agranulocytosis, patients who are on clozapine must have a blood test each week. The expense involved in this monitoring, together with the cost of the medication, has made maintenance on clozapine difficult for many persons with schizophrenia. However, five years after its introduction in the United States, approximately 58,000 persons are being treated with clozapine.

Early 1994 saw the introduction of another atypical neuroleptic, risperidone *(Risperdal)*. Risperidone, when taken in low dosage, has few clinically significant side effects. There have been no reported cases of agranulocytosis. Several other atypical neuroleptics are being investigated at present, and some will probably be approved within the next year or two.

Antimanic Medications

Bipolar disorder (manic-depressive illness) is characterized by cycling mood changes: severe highs (mania) and lows (depression). Cycles may be predominantly manic or depressive with normal mood between cycles. Mood swings may follow each other very closely, within hours or days, or may be separated by months to years. These "highs" and "lows" may vary in intensity and severity.

When someone is in a manic "high," he may be overactive, overtalkative, and have a great deal of energy. He will switch quickly from one topic to another, as if he cannot get his thoughts out fast enough; his attention span is often short, and he can be easily distracted. Sometimes, the "high" person is irritable or angry and has false or inflated ideas about his position or importance in the world. He may be very elated, full of grand schemes that might range from business deals to romantic sprees. Often, he shows poor judgment in these ventures. Mania, untreated, may worsen to a psychotic state.

Depression will show in a "low" mood, lack of energy, changes in eating and sleeping patterns, feelings of hopelessness, helplessness, sadness, worthlessness, and guilt, and sometimes thoughts of suicide.

Lithium

The medication used most often to combat a manic "high" is lithium. It is unusual to find mania without a subsequent or preceding period of depression. Lithium evens out mood swings in both directions, so that it is used not just for acute manic attacks or flare-ups of the illness, but also as an ongoing treatment of bipolar disorder.

Lithium will diminish severe manic symptoms in about five to 14 days, but it may be anywhere from days to several months until the condition is fully controlled. Antipsychotic medications are sometimes used in the first several days of treatment to control manic symptoms until the lithium begins to take effect. Likewise, antidepressants may be needed in addition to lithium during the depressive phase of bipolar disorder.

Someone may have one episode of bipolar disorder and never have another, or be free of illness for several years. However, for those who have more than one episode, continuing (maintenance) treatment on lithium is usually given serious consideration.

Some people respond well to maintenance treatment and have no further episodes, while others may have moderate mood swings that lessen as treatment continues. Some people may continue to have episodes that are diminished in frequency and severity. Unfortunately, some manic-depressive patients may not be helped at all. Response to treatment with lithium varies, and it cannot be determined beforehand who will or will not respond to treatment.

Regular blood tests are an important part of treatment with lithium. A lithium level must be checked periodically to measure the amount of the drug in the body. If too little is taken, lithium will not be effective. If too much is taken, a variety of side effects may occur. The range between an effective dose and a toxic one is small. A lithium level is routinely checked at the beginning of treatment to determine the best lithium dosage for the patient. Once a person is stable and on maintenance dosage, a lithium level should be checked every few months. How much lithium a person needs to take may vary over time, depending on how ill he is, his body chemistry, and his physical condition.

Anything that lowers the level of sodium (table salt is sodium chloride) in the body may cause a lithium buildup and lead to toxicity. Reduced salt intake, heavy sweating, fever, vomiting, or diarrhea may do this. An unusual amount of exercise or a switch to a low-salt diet are examples. It's important to be aware of conditions that lower sodium and to share this information with the doctor. The lithium dosage may have to be adjusted.

When a person first takes lithium, he may experience side effects, such as drowsiness, weakness, nausea, vomiting, fatigue, hand tremor, or increased thirst and urination. These usually disappear or subside quickly, although hand tremor may persist. Weight gain may also occur. Dieting will help, but crash diets should be avoided because they may affect the lithium level. Drinking low-calorie or no-calorie beverages will help keep weight down. Kidney changes, accompanied by increased thirst and urination, may develop during treatment. These conditions that may occur are generally manageable and are reduced by lowering the dosage. Because lithium may cause the thyroid gland to become underactive (hypothyroidism) or sometimes enlarged (goiter), thyroid function monitoring is a part of the therapy. To restore normal thyroid function, thyroid hormone is given along with lithium.

Because of possible complications, lithium may either not be recommended or may be given with caution when a person has existing thyroid, kidney, or heart disorders, epilepsy, or brain damage. Women of child-bearing age should be aware that lithium increases the risk of congenital malformations in babies born to women taking lithium. Special caution should be taken during the first three months of pregnancy.

Lithium, when combined with certain other medications, can have unwanted effects. Some diuretics—substances that remove water from the body—increase the level of lithium and can cause toxicity. Other diuretics, like coffee and tea, can lower the level of lithium. Signs of lithium toxicity may include nausea, vomiting, drowsiness, mental dullness, slurred speech, confusion, dizziness, muscle twitching, irregular heart beat, and blurred vision. A serious lithium overdose can be life-threatening. *Someone who is taking lithium should tell all the doctors—including dentists—he sees about all other medications he is taking.*

With regular monitoring, lithium is a safe and effective drug that enables many people, who otherwise would suffer from incapacitating mood swings, to lead normal lives.

Anticonvulsants

Not all patients with symptoms of mania benefit from lithium. Some have been found to respond to another type of medication, the anticonvulsant medications that are usually used to treat epilepsy. Carbamazepine *(Tegretol)* is the anticonvulsant that has been most widely used. Manic-depressive patients who cycle rapidly—that is, they change from mania to depression and back again over the course of hours or days, rather than months—seem to respond particularly well to carbamazepine.

Early side effects of carbamazepine, although generally mild, include drowsiness, dizziness, confusion, disturbed vision, perceptual distortions, memory impairment, and nausea. They are usually transient and often respond to temporary dosage reduction. Another common but generally mild adverse effect is the lowering of the white blood cell count which requires periodic blood tests to monitor against the rare possibility of more serious, even life-threatening, bone marrow depression. Also serious are the skin rashes that can occur in 15 to 20 percent of patients. These rashes are sometimes severe enough to require discontinuation of the medication.

In 1995, the anticonvulsant divalproex sodium *(Depakote)* was approved by the Food and Drug Administration for manic-depressive illness. Clinical trials have shown it to have an effectiveness in controlling manic symptoms equivalent to that of lithium; it is effective in both rapid-cycling and non-rapid-cycling bipolar.

Though divalproex can cause gastrointestinal side effects, the incidence is low. Other adverse effects occasionally reported are headache, double vision, dizziness, anxiety, or confusion. Because in some cases divalproex has caused liver disfunction, liver function tests should be performed prior to therapy and at frequent intervals thereafter, particularly during the first six months of therapy.

Antidepressant Medications

The kind of depression that will most likely benefit from treatment with medications is more than just "the blues." It's a condition that's prolonged, lasting two weeks or more, and interferes with a person's ability to carry on daily tasks and to enjoy activities that previously brought pleasure.

The depressed person will seem sad, or "down," or may show a lack of interest in his surroundings. He may have trouble eating and lose weight (although some people eat more and gain weight when depressed). He may sleep too much or too little, have difficulty going to sleep, sleep restlessly, or awaken very early in the morning. He may speak of feeling guilty, worthless, or hopeless. He may complain that his thinking is slowed down. He may lack energy, feeling "everything's too much," or he might be agitated and jumpy. A person who is depressed may cry. He may think and talk about killing himself and may even make a suicide attempt. Some people who are depressed have psychotic symptoms, such as delusions (false ideas) that are related to their depression. For instance, a psychotically depressed person might imagine that he is already dead, or "in hell," being punished.

Not everyone who is depressed has all these symptoms, but everyone who is depressed has at least some of them. A depression can range in intensity from mild to severe.

Antidepressants are used most widely for serious depressions, but they can also be helpful for some milder depressions. Antidepressants, although they are not "uppers" or stimulants, take away or reduce the symptoms of depression and help the depressed person feel the way he did before he became depressed.

Antidepressants are also used for disorders characterized principally by anxiety. They can block the symptoms of panic, including rapid heartbeat, terror, dizziness, chest pains, nausea, and breathing problems. They can also be used to treat some phobias.

The physician chooses the particular antidepressant to prescribe based on the individual patient's symptoms. When someone begins taking an antidepressant, improvement generally will not begin to show immediately. With most of these medications, it will take from one to three weeks before changes begin to occur. Some symptoms diminish early in treatment, others, later. For instance, a person's energy level or sleeping or eating patterns may improve before his depressed mood lifts. If there is little or no change in symptoms after five to six weeks, a different medication may be tried. Some people will respond better to one than another. Since there is no certain way of determining beforehand which medication will be effective, the doctor may have to prescribe first one, then another, until an effective one is found. Treatment is continued for a minimum of several months and may last up to a year or more.

While some people have one episode of depression and then never have another, or remain symptom-free for years, others have more frequent episodes or very long-lasting depressions that may go on for years. Some people find that their depressions become more frequent and severe as they get older. For these people, continuing (maintenance) treatment with antidepressants can be an effective way of reducing the frequency and severity of depressions. Those that are commonly used have no known long-term side effects and may be continued indefinitely. The prescribed dosage of the medication may be lowered if side effects become troublesome. Lithium can also be used for maintenance treatment of repeated depressions whether or not there is evidence of a manic or manic-like episode in the past.

Dosage of antidepressants varies, depending on the type of drug, the person's body chemistry, age, and, sometimes, body weight. Dosages are generally started low and raised gradually over time until the desired effect is reached without the appearance of troublesome side effects.

There are a number of antidepressant medications available. They differ in their side effects and, to some extent, in their level of effectiveness. Tricyclic antidepressants (named for their chemical structure) are more commonly used for treatment of major depressions than are monoamine oxidase inhibitors (MAOIs); but MAOIs are often helpful in so-called "atypical" depressions in which there are symptoms like oversleeping, anxiety, panic attacks, and phobias.

The last few years have seen the introduction of a number of new antidepressants. Several of them are called "selective serotonin reuptake inhibitors" (SSRIs). Those available at the present time in the United States are fluoxetine *(Prozac),* fluvoxamine *(Luvox),* paroxetine *(Paxil),* and sertraline *(Zoloft).* (The most recently marketed, *Luvox,* has been approved for obsessive-compulsive disorder only.) Though structurally different from each other, all the SSRIs' antidepressant effects are due to their action on one specific neurotransmitter, serotonin. Two other antidepressants that affect two neurotransmitters—serotonin and norepinephrine—have also been approved by the FDA. They are venlafaxine *(Effexor)* and nefazodone *(Serzone).* All of these newer antidepressants seem to have less bothersome side effects than the older tricyclic antidepressants.

The tricyclic antidepressant clomipramine *(Anafranil)* affects serotonin but is not as selective as the SSRIs. It was the first medication specifically approved for use in the treatment of obsessive-compulsive disorder (OCD). *Prozac* and *Luvox* have now been approved for use with OCD.

Another of the newer antidepressants, bupropion *(Wellbutrin),* is chemically unrelated to the other antidepressants.

It has more effect on norepinephrine and dopamine than on serotonin. *Wellbutrin* has not been associated with weight gain or sexual dysfunction. It is contraindicated for individuals with, or at risk for, a seizure disorder or who have been diagnosed with bulimia or anorexia nervosa.

Side Effects of Antidepressant Medications

1. Tricyclic Antidepressants

There are a number of possible side effects with tricyclic antidepressants that vary, depending on the medication. For example, amitriptyline *(Elavil)* may make people feel drowsy, while protriptyline *(Vivactil)* hardly does this at all and, in some people, may have an opposite effect, producing feelings of anxiety and restlessness. Because of this kind of variation in side effects, one antidepressant might be highly desirable for one person and not recommended for another. Tricyclics on occasion may complicate specific heart problems, and for this reason the physician should be aware of all such difficulties. Other side effects with tricyclics may include blurred vision, dry mouth, constipation, weight gain, dizziness when changing position, increased sweating, difficulty urinating, changes in sexual desire, decrease in sexual ability, muscle twitches, fatigue, and weakness. Not all these medications produce all side effects, and not everybody gets them. Some will disappear quickly, while others may remain for the length of treatment. Some side effects are similar to symptoms of depression (for instance, fatigue and constipation). For this reason, the patient or family should discuss all symptoms with the doctor, who may change the medication or dosage.

Tricyclics also may interact with thyroid hormone, antihypertensive medications, oral contraceptives, some blood coagulants, some sleeping medications, antipsychotic medications, diuretics, antihistamines, aspirin, bicarbonate of soda, vitamin C, alcohol, and tobacco.

An overdose of antidepressants is serious and potentially lethal. It requires immediate medical attention. Symptoms of an overdose of tricyclic antidepressant medication develop within an hour and may start with rapid heartbeat, dilated pupils, flushed face, and agitation, and may progress to confusion, loss of consciousness, seizures, irregular heartbeats, cardiorespiratory collapse, and death.

2. The Newer Antidepressants

The most common side effects of these antidepressants are gastrointestinal problems and headache. Others are insomnia, anxiety, and agitation. Because of potentially serious interaction between these medications and monoamine oxidase inhibitors, it is advisable to stop taking one medication from two to four or five weeks before starting the other, depending on the specific medications involved. In addition, some SSRIs have been found to affect metabolism of certain other medications in the liver, creating possible drug interactions.

3. Monoamine Oxidase Inhibitors (MAOIs)

MAOIs may cause some side effects similar to those of the other antidepressants. Dizziness when changing position and rapid heartbeat are common. MAOIs also react with certain foods and alcoholic beverages (such as aged cheeses, foods containing monosodium glutamate (MSG), Chianti and other red wines), and other medications (such as over-the-counter cold and allergy preparations, local anesthetics, amphetamines, insulin, some narcotics, and antiparkinsonian medications). These reactions often do not appear for several hours. Signs may include severe high blood pressure, headache, nausea, vomiting, rapid heartbeat, possible confusion, psychotic symptoms, seizures, stroke, and coma. For this reason, people taking MAOIs *must* stay away from restricted foods, drinks, and medications. They should be sure that they are furnished, by their doctor or pharmacist, a list of *all* foods, beverages, and other medications that should be avoided.

Precautions to Be Observed When Taking Antidepressants

When taking antidepressants, it is important to tell all doctors (and dentists) being seen—not just the one who is treating the depression—about all medications being used, including over-the-counter preparations and alcohol. Antidepressants should be taken only in the amount prescribed and should be kept in a secure place away from children. When used with proper care, following doctors' instructions, antidepressants are extremely useful medications that can reverse the misery of a depression and help a person feel like himself again.

Antianxiety Medications

Everyone experiences anxiety at one time or another—"butterflies in the stomach" before giving a speech or sweaty palms during a job interview are common symptoms. Other symptoms of anxiety include irritability, uneasiness, jumpiness, feelings of apprehension, rapid or irregular heartbeat, stomachache, nausea, faintness, and breathing problems.

Anxiety is often manageable and mild. But sometimes it can present serious problems. A high level or prolonged state of anxiety can be very incapacitating, making the activities of daily life difficult or impossible. Besides generalized anxiety, other anxiety disorders are panic, phobia, obsessive-compulsive disorder (OCD), and posttraumatic stress disorder.

Phobias, which are persistent, irrational fears and are characterized by avoidance of certain objects, places, and things, sometimes accompany anxiety. A panic attack is a severe form of anxiety that may occur suddenly and is marked with symptoms of nervousness, breathlessness, pounding heart, and sweating. Sometimes the fear that one may die is present.

Antianxiety medications help to calm and relax the anxious person and remove the troubling symptoms. There are a number of antianxiety medications currently available. The preferred medications for most anxiety disorders are the benzodiazepines. In addition to the benzodiazepines, a non-benzodiazepine, buspirone *(BuSpar),* is used for generalized anxiety disorders. Antidepressants are also effective for panic attacks and some phobias and are often prescribed for these conditions. They are also sometimes used for more generalized forms of anxiety, especially when it is accompanied by depression. The medications approved by the FDA for use in OCD are all antidepressants—clomipramine, fluoxetine, and fluvoxamine.

The most commonly used benzodiazepines are alprazolam *(Xanax)* and diazepam *(Valium)*, followed by chlordiazepoxide *(Librium, Librax, Libritabs)*. Benzodiazepines are relatively fast-acting medications; in contrast, buspirone must be taken daily for two or three weeks prior to exerting its antianxiety effect. Most benzodiazepines will begin to take effect within hours, some in even less time. Benzodiazepines differ in duration of action in different individuals; they may be taken two or three times a day, or sometimes only once a day. Dosage is generally started at a low level and gradually raised until symptoms are diminished or removed. The dosage will vary a great deal depending on the symptoms and the individual's body chemistry.

Benzodiazepines have few side effects. Drowsiness and loss of coordination are most common; fatigue and mental slowing or confusion can also occur. These effects make it dangerous to drive or operate some machinery when taking benzodiazepines—especially when the patient is just beginning treatment. Other side effects are rare.

Benzodiazepines combined with other medications can present a problem, notably when taken together with commonly used substances such as alcohol. It is wise to abstain from alcohol when taking benzodiazepines, as the interaction between benzodiazepines and alcohol can lead to serious and possibly life-threatening complications. Following the doctor's instructions is important. The doctor should be informed of all other medications the patient is taking, including over-the-counter preparations. Benzodiazepines increase central nervous system depression when combined with alcohol, anesthetics, antihistamines, sedatives, muscle relaxants, and some prescription pain medications. Particular benzodiazepines may influence the action of some anticonvulsant and cardiac medications. Benzodiazepines have also been associated with abnormalities in babies born to mothers who were taking these medications during pregnancy.

With benzodiazepines, there is a potential for the development of tolerance and dependence as well as the possibility of abuse and withdrawal reactions. For these reasons, the medications are generally prescribed for brief periods of time—days or weeks—and sometimes intermittently, for stressful situations or anxiety attacks. For the same reason, ongoing or continuous treatment with benzodiazepines is not recommended for most people. Some patients may, however, need long-term treatment.

Consult with the doctor before discontinuing a benzodiazepine. A withdrawal reaction may occur if the treatment is abruptly stopped. Symptoms may include anxiety, shakiness, headache, dizziness, sleeplessness, loss of appetite, and, in more severe cases, fever, seizures, and psychosis. A withdrawal reaction may be mistaken for a return of the anxiety, since many of the symptoms are similar. Thus, after benzodiazepines are taken for an extended period, the dosage is gradually tapered off before being completely stopped.

Although benzodiazepines, buspirone, tricyclic antidepressants, or SSRIs are the preferred medications for most anxiety disorders, occasionally, for specific reasons, one of the following medications may be prescribed: antipsychotic medications; antihistamines (such as *Atarax, Vistaril,* and others); barbiturates such as phenobarbital; and beta-blockers such as propranolol *(Inderal, Inderide.)* Propanediols such as meprobamate *(Equanil)* were commonly prescribed prior to the introduction of the benzodiazepines, but today rarely are used.

Children, the elderly, and pregnant and nursing women have special concerns and needs when taking psychotherapeutic medications. Some effects of medications on the growing body, the aging body, and the childbearing body are known, but much remains to be learned. Research in these areas in ongoing.

While, in general, what has been said in this booklet applies to these groups, below are a few special points to bear in mind.

Children, the Elderly, and Pregnant, Nursing, or Child-Bearing-Age Women: Special Considerations

Children

Studies consistently show that about 15 percent of the U.S. population below age 18, or over nine million children, suffer from a psychiatric disorder that compromises their ability to function. It is easy to overlook the seriousness of childhood mental disorders. In children, these disorders may present symptoms that are different or less clear-cut than the same disorders in adults. Younger children, especially, may not talk about what's bothering them, but this is sometimes a problem with older children as well. For this reason, having a doctor, other mental health professional, or psychiatric team examine the child is especially important.

There is an array of treatments that can help these children. These include medications and psychotherapy—behavioral therapy, treatment of impaired social skills, parental and family therapy, group therapy. The therapy used for an individual child is based on the child's diagnosis and individual needs.

When the decision is reached that a child should take medication, active monitoring by all caretakers (parents, teachers, others who have charge of the child) is essential. Children should be watched and questioned for side effects (many children, especially younger ones, do not volunteer information). They should also be monitored to see that they are actually taking the medication and taking the proper dosage.

One type of medication not covered elsewhere in this booklet is stimulants. Three stimulants, methylphenidate *(Ritalin)* dextroamphetamine *(Dexedrine,)* and pemoline *(Cylert)* are more commonly prescribed for children than adults. They are successfully used in the treatment of attention-deficit/hyperactivity disorder (ADHD). ADHD is a disorder usually diagnosed in early childhood in which the child exhibits such symptoms as short attention span, excessive activity, and impulsivity. A child with ADHD should take a stimulant medication only on the advice and under the careful supervision of a physician.

The use with children of the medications described in this booklet is more limited than with adults. In the list of medications, commonly used psychotropic medications that have specific indications and dose guidelines for children, as listed in the *Physicians' Desk Reference,* are indicated by a double asterisk (**).

The Elderly

Persons over the age of 65 make up 12 percent of the population of the United States, yet they receive 30 percent of prescriptions filled. The elderly generally have more medical problems and often are taking medications for more than one of these problems. In addition, they tend to be more sensitive to medications. Even healthy older people eliminate some medications from the body more slowly than younger persons and therefore require a lower or less frequent dosage to maintain an effective level of medication.

The elderly may sometimes accidentally take too much of a medication because they forget that they have taken a dose and take another dose. The use of a 7-day pill box is especially helpful to an elderly person.

The elderly and those close to them—friends, relatives, caretakers—need to pay special attention and watch for adverse (negative) physical and psychological responses to medication. Because they often take more medications—not only those prescribed but also over-the-counter preparations and home or folk remedies—the possibility of negative drug interactions is higher.

Pregnant, Nursing, or Child-Bearing-Age Women

In general, during pregnancy, all medications (including psychotherapeutic medications) should be avoided where possible, and other methods of treatment should be tried.

A woman who is taking a psychotherapeutic medication and plans to become pregnant should discuss her plans with her doctor; if she discovers that she is pregnant, she should contact her doctor immediately. During early pregnancy, there is a possible risk of birth defects with some of these medications, and for this reason:

1) Lithium is not recommended during the first three months of pregnancy.
2) Benzodiazepines are not recommended during the first three months of pregnancy.

The decision to use a psychotherapeutic medication should be made only after a careful discussion with the doctor concerning the risks and benefits to the woman and her baby.

Small amounts of medication pass into the breast milk; this is a consideration for mothers who are planning to breast-feed.

A woman who is taking birth-control pills should be sure that her doctor is aware of this. The estrogen in these pills may alter the breakdown of medications by the body, for example increasing side effects of some antianxiety medications and/or reducing their efficacy to relieve symptoms of anxiety.

For more detailed information, talk to your doctor or mental health professional, consult your local public library, or write to the pharmaceutical company that produces the medication or the U.S. Food and Drug Administration, 5600 Fishers Lane, Rockville, MD 20857.

Index of Medications

To find the section of the text that describes the medication you or a friend or family member is taking, find either the generic (chemical) name and look it up on the first list, or the trade name and look it up on the second list. If you do not find the name of the medication on the label, ask your doctor or pharmacist for it. (Note: some drugs, such as amitriptyline and chlordiazepoxide, are marketed under numerous trade names, not all of which can be mentioned in a brief publication such as this. If your medication's trade name does not appear in this list, look it up by its generic name or ask your doctor or pharmacist for more information.)

Alphabetical Listing of Medications by Generic Name

GENERIC NAME	TRADE NAME
Antipsychotic Medications	
chlorpromazine **	Thorazine
chlorprothixene	Taractan
clozapine	Clozaril
fluphenazine	Permitil
	Prolixin
haloperidol **	Haldol
loxapine	Daxolin
	Loxitane
mesoridazine	Serentil
molindone	Lidone
	Moban
perphenazine	Trilafon
pimozide (for Tourette's Syndrome) **	Orap
risperidone	Risperdal
thioridazine **	Mellaril
thiothixene	Navane
trifluoperazine	Stelazine
triflupromazine	Vesprin
Antimanic Medications	
carbamazepine	Tegretol
divalproex sodium	Depakote
lithium carbonate	Eskalith
	Lithane
	Lithobid
lithium citrate	Cibalith-S
Antidepressants	
amitriptyline	Elavil
amoxapine	Asendin
bupropion	Wellbutrin
desipramine	Norpramin
	Pertofrane
doxepin	Adapin
	Sinequan

clomipramine **	Anafranil
fluvoxamine (SSRI)	Luvox
fluoxetine (SSRI)	Prozac
imipramine **	Tofranil
isocarboxazid (MAOI)	Marplan
maprotiline	Ludiomil
nefazodone	Serzone
nortriptyline	Aventyl
	Pamelor
paroxetine (SSRI)	Paxil
phenelzine (MAOI)	Nardil
protriptyline	Vivactil
sertraline (SSRI)	Zoloft
tranylcypromine (MAOI)	Parnate
trazodone	Desyrel
trimipramine	Surmontil
venlafaxine	Effexor

Antianxiety Medications

(All of these antianxiety medications except buspirone are benzodiazepines)

alprazolam	Xanax
buspirone	BuSpar
chlordiazepoxide	Librax
	Libritabs
	Librium
clorazepate	Azene
	Tranxene
diazepam	Valium
halazepam	Paxipam
lorazepam	Ativan
oxazepam	Serax
prazepam	Centrax

Stimulants

(Given for Attention-Deficit/Hyperactivity Disorder)

d-amphetamine **	Dexedrine
methylphenidate **	Ritalin
pemoline **	Cylert

Alphabetical Listing of Medications by Trade Name

TRADE NAME	*GENERIC NAME*

Antipsychotic Medications

Clozaril	clozapine
Daxolin	loxapine
Haldol **	haloperidol
Lidone	molindone
Loxitane	loxapine
Mellaril **	thioridazine
Moban	molindone
Navane	thiothixene
Orap (for Tourette's Syndrome) **	pimozide
Permitil	fluphenazine
Prolixin	fluphenazine
Risperdal	risperidone
Serentil	mesoridazine
Stelazine	trifluoperazine
Taractan	chlorprothixene
Thorazine **	chlorpromazine
Trilafon	perphenazine
Vesprin	trifluopromazine

Antimanic Medications

Cibalith-S	lithium citrate
Depakote	divalproex sodium
Eskalith	lithium carbonate
Lithane	lithium carbonate
Lithobid	lithium carbonate
Tegretol	carbamazepine

Antidepressant Medications

Adapin	doxepin
Anafranil **	clomipramine
Asendin	amoxapine
Aventyl	nortriptyline
Desyrel	trazodone
Effexor	venlafaxine
Elavil	amitriptyline
Ludiomil	maprotiline
Luvox (SSRI)	fluvoxamine
Marplan (MAOI)	isocarboxazid
TRADE NAME	GENERIC NAME
Nardil (MAOI)	phenelzine
Norpramin	desipramine
Pamelor	nortriptyline
Parnate (MAOI)	tranylcypromine
Paxil (SSRI)	paroxetine
Pertofrane	desipramine
Prozac (SSRI)	fluoxetine
Serzone	nefazodone
Sinequan	doxepin
Surmontil	trimipramine
Tofranil **	imipramine
Vivactil	protriptyline
Wellbutrin	bupropion
Zoloft (SSRI)	sertraline

Antianxiety Medications

(All of these antianxiety medications except buspirone are benzodiazepines)

Ativan	lorazepam
Azene	clorazepate
BuSpar	buspirone
Centrax	prazepam
Paxipam	halazepam
Serax	oxazepam
Tranxene	clorazepate
Valium	diazepam
Xanax	alprazolam

Stimulants

(Given for Attention-Deficit/Hyperactivity Disorder)

Cylert **	pemoline
Dexedrine **	d-amphetamine
Ritalin **	methylphenidate

At one time, two combination medications not included in the above list were often prescribed, but are prescribed only occasionally today. They are: a combination of amitriptyline (antidepressant) and perphenazine (antipsychotic) marketed as *Triavil* or *Etrafon;* and a combination of amitriptyline (antidepressant) and chlordiazepoxide (antianxiety) marketed as *Limbitrol.*

References

AHFS Drug Information, 91. Gerald K. McEvoy, Editor. Bethesda, MD: American Society of Hospital Pharmacists, Inc., 1991.

Bohn J. and Jefferson J.W., *Lithium and Manic Depression: A Guide.* Madison, WI: Lithium Information Center, rev. ed. 1990.

Goodwin F.K. and Jamison K.R. *Manic-Depressive Illness.* NY: Oxford University Press, 1990.

Jensen P.S., Vitiello B., Leonard H., and Laughren T.P. Child and adolescent psychopharmacology: expanding the research base. *Psychopharmacology Bulletin,* Vol. 30, No. 1, 1994.

Johnston H.F. *Stimulants and Hyperactive Children: A Guide.* Madison, WI: Lithium Information Center, 1990.

Medenwald J.R., Greist J.H., and Jefferson J.W. *Carbamazepine and Manic Depression: A Guide.* Madison, WI: Lithium Information Center, rev. ed., 1990.

Physicians' Desk Reference, 48th edition. Montvale, NJ: Medical Economics Data Production Company, 1994.

New Developments in the Pharmacologic Treatment of Schizophrenia. Rockville, MD: National Institute of Mental Health, 1992.

This brochure was revised by Margaret Strock, staff member in the Information Resources and Inquiries Branch, Office of Scientific Information, National Institute of Mental Health (NIMH). Expert assistance was provided by John Hsiao, MD, Peter Jensen, MD, Matthew Rudorfer, MD, David Shore, MD, and Benedetto Vitiello, MD, NIMH staff members. Their help in assuring the accuracy of this pamphlet is gratefully acknowledged. An earlier version of the brochure was written under contract for NIMH by Brana Lobel.

■ **Document Source:**
U.S. Department of Health and Human Services, Public Health Service
National Institutes of Health
National Institute of Mental Health
NIH Publication No. 95-3929
Printed 1987, Revised 1992, 1995

OBSESSIVE-COMPULSIVE DISORDER

What is OCD?

Obsessive-compulsive disorder (OCD), one of the anxiety disorders, is a potentially disabling condition that can persist throughout a person's life. The individual who suffers from OCD becomes trapped in a pattern of repetitive thoughts and behaviors that are senseless and distressing but extremely difficult to overcome. OCD occurs in a spectrum from mild to severe, but if severe and left untreated, can destroy a person's capacity to function at work, at school, or even in the home.

The following three case histories are typical for those who suffer from obsessive-compulsive disorder—a disorder that can be effectively treated.

Isobel is intelligent, but she is failing her first period class in biology because she is either late to class or absent. She gets up at five o'clock, hoping to get to school on time. The next three hours are spent taking a long shower followed by changing clothes repeatedly until it "feels right." She finally packs and repacks her books until they are just right, opens the front door and prepares to walk down the front steps. She goes through a ritual of pausing on each step for a particular length of time. Even though she recognizes her thoughts and behaviors are senseless, she feels compelled to complete her rituals. Once she has completed these rituals, she makes a mad dash for school and arrives when first period is almost over.

Meredith's pregnancy was a time of joyous anticipation. If she had moments of trepidation about taking care of a new baby, these times passed quickly. She and her husband proudly brought a beautiful, perfect baby boy home from the hospital. Meredith bathed and fed the baby, comforted him when he was restless, and became a competent young mother. Then the obsessional thoughts began; she feared that she might harm her child. Over and over again she imagined herself stabbing the baby. She busied herself around the house, tried to think of other things, but the distressing thought persisted. She became terrified to use the kitchen knives or her sewing scissors. She knew she did not want to harm her child. Why did she have these distressing, alien thoughts?

During his last year at college, John became aware that he was spending more and more time preparing for classes, but he worked hard and graduated in the top ten percent of his class with a major in accounting. He accepted a position at a prestigious accounting firm in his hometown and began work with high hopes for the future. Within weeks, the firm was having second thoughts about John. Given work that should have taken two or three hours, he was going over and over the figures, checking and rechecking, spending a week or more on a task. He knew it was taking too long to get each job done, but he felt compelled to continue checking. When his probation period was over, the company let him go.

How common is OCD?

For many years, mental health professionals thought of OCD as a rare disease because only a small minority of their patients had the condition. The disorder often went unrecognized because many of those afflicted with OCD, in efforts to keep their repetitive thoughts and behaviors secret, failed to seek treatment. This led to underestimates of the number of people with the illness. However, a survey conducted in the early 1980s by the National Institute of Mental Health (NIMH)—the Federal agency that supports research nationwide on the brain, mental illnesses, and mental health—provided new knowledge about the prevalence of OCD. The

NIMH survey showed that OCD affects more than two percent of the population, meaning that OCD is more common than such severe mental illnesses as schizophrenia, bipolar disorder, or panic disorder. OCD strikes people of all ethnic groups. Males and females are equally affected. The social and economic costs of OCD were estimated to be $8.4 billion in 1990 (DuPont et al, 1994).

Although OCD symptoms typically begin during the teenage years or early adulthood, recent research shows that some children develop the illness at earlier ages, even during the preschool years. Studies indicate that at least one-third of cases of OCD in adults began in childhood. Suffering from OCD during early stages of a child's development can cause severe problems for the child. It is important that the child receive evaluation and treatment by a knowledgeable clinician to prevent the child from missing important opportunities because of this disorder.

Key Features of OCD

Obsessions

These are unwanted ideas or impulses that repeatedly well up in the mind of the person with OCD. Persistent fears that harm may come to self or a loved one, an unreasonable belief that one has a terrible illness, or an excessive need to do things correctly or perfectly, are common. Again and again, the individual experiences a disturbing thought, such as, "My hands may be contaminated—I must wash them"; "I may have left the gas on"; or "I am going to injure my child." These thoughts are intrusive, unpleasant, and produce a high degree of anxiety. Often the obsessions are of a violent or a sexual nature, or concern illness.

Compulsions

In response to their obsessions, most people with OCD resort to repetitive behaviors called compulsions. The most common of these are washing and checking. Other compulsive behaviors include counting (often while performing another compulsive action such as hand washing), repeating, hoarding, and endlessly rearranging objects in an effort to keep them in precise alignment with each other. These behaviors generally are intended to ward off harm to the person with OCD or others. Some people with OCD have regimented rituals while others have rituals that are complex and changing. Performing rituals may give the person with OCD some relief from anxiety, but it is only temporary.

Insight

People with OCD usually have considerable insight into their own problems. Most of the time, they know that their obsessive thoughts are senseless or exaggerated, and that their compulsive behaviors are not really necessary. However, this knowledge is not sufficient to enable them to stop obsessing or the carrying out of rituals.

Resistance

Most people with OCD struggle to banish their unwanted, obsessive thoughts and to prevent themselves from engaging in compulsive behaviors. Many are able to keep their obsessive-compulsive symptoms under control during the hours when they are at work or attending school. But over the months or years, resistance may weaken, and when this happens, OCD may become so severe that time-consuming rituals take over the sufferers' lives, making it impossible for them to continue activities outside the home.

Shame and Secrecy

OCD sufferers often attempt to hide their disorder rather than seek help. Often they are successful in concealing their obsessive-compulsive symptoms from friends and coworkers. An unfortunate consequence of this secrecy is that people with OCD usually do not receive professional help until years after the onset of their disease. By that time, they may have learned to work their lives—and family members' lives—around the rituals.

Long-Lasting Symptoms

OCD tends to last for years, even decades. The symptoms may become less severe from time to time, and there may be long intervals when the symptoms are mild, but for most individuals with OCD, the symptoms are chronic.

What causes OCD?

The old belief that OCD was the result of life experiences has given way before the growing evidence that biological factors are a primary contributor to the disorder. The fact that OCD patients respond well to specific medications that affect the neurotransmitter serotonin suggests the disorder has a neurobiological basis. For that reason, OCD is no longer attributed to attitudes a patient learned in childhood—for example, an inordinate emphasis on cleanliness, or a belief that certain thoughts are dangerous or unacceptable. Instead, the search for causes now focuses on the interaction of neurobiological factors and environmental influences.

OCD is sometimes accompanied by depression, eating disorders, substance abuse disorder, a personality disorder, attention deficit disorder, or another of the anxiety disorders. Co-existing disorders can make OCD more difficult both to diagnose and to treat.

In an effort to identify specific biological factors that may be important in the onset or persistence of OCD, NIMH-supported investigators have used a device called the positron emission tomography (PET) scanner to study the brains of patients with OCD. Several groups of investigators have obtained findings from PET scans suggesting that OCD patients have patterns of brain activity that differ from those of people without mental illness or with some other mental illness. Brain-imaging studies of OCD showing abnormal neurochemical activity in regions known to play a role in certain neurological disorders suggest that these areas may be crucial in the origins of OCD. There is also evidence that medications and cognitive/behavior therapy induce changes in the brain coincident with clinical improvement.

Symptoms of OCD are seen in association with some other neurological disorders. There is an increased rate of OCD in people with Tourette's syndrome, an illness characterized by involuntary movements and vocalizations. Investigators are currently studying the hypothesis that a genetic relationship exists between OCD and the tic disorders. Another illness that may be linked to OCD is trichotillomania (the repeated urge to pull out scalp hair, eyelashes, or eyebrows). Genetic studies of OCD and other related conditions may enable scientists to pinpoint the molecular basis of these disorders.

Do I have OCD?

A person with OCD has obsessive and compulsive behaviors that are extreme enough to interfere with everyday life. People with OCD should not be confused with a much larger group of individuals who are sometimes called "compulsive" because they hold themselves to a high standard of performance and are perfectionistic and very organized in their work and even in recreational activities. This type of "compulsiveness" often serves a valuable purpose, contributing to a person's self-esteem and success on the job. In that respect, it differs from the life-wrecking obsessions and rituals of the person with OCD.

Treatment of OCD: Progress Through Research

Clinical and animal research sponsored by NIMH and other scientific organizations has provided information leading to both pharmacologic and behavioral treatments that can benefit the person with OCD. A combination of the two therapies is often an effective method of treatment for most patients. Some individuals respond best to one therapy, some to another.

Pharmacotherapy

Clinical trials in recent years have shown that drugs that affect the neurotransmitter serotonin can significantly decrease the symptoms of OCD. Two serotonin reuptake inhibitors (SRIs), clomipramine (Anafranil) and fluoxetine (Prozac), have been approved by the Food and Drug Administration for the treatment of OCD. Other SRIs that have been studied in controlled clinical trials include sertraline (Zoloft) and fluvoxamine (Luvox). Paroxetine (Paxil) is also being used. All these SRIs have proved effective in treatment of OCD. If a patient does not respond well to one SRI, another SRI may give a better response. For patients who are only partially responsive to these medications, research is being conducted on the use of an SRI as the primary medication and one of a variety of medications as an additional drug (an augmenter). Medications are of great help in controlling the symptoms of OCD, but often, if the medication is discontinued, relapse will follow. Most patients can benefit from a combination of medication and behavioral therapy.

Behavior Therapy

Traditional psychotherapy, aimed at helping the patient develop insight into his or her problem, is generally not helpful for OCD. However, a specific behavior therapy approach called "exposure and response prevention" is effective for many people with OCD. In this approach, the patient is deliberately and voluntarily exposed to the feared object or idea, either directly or by imagination, and then is discouraged or prevented from carrying out the usual compulsive response. For example, a compulsive hand washer may be urged to touch an object believed to be contaminated, and then may be denied the opportunity to wash for several hours. When the treatment works well, the patient gradually experiences less anxiety from the obsessive thoughts and becomes able to do without the compulsive actions for extended periods of time.

Studies of behavior therapy for OCD have found it to produce long-lasting benefits. To achieve the best results, a combination of factors is necessary: The therapist should be well trained in the specific method developed; the patient must be highly motivated; and the patient's family must be cooperative. In addition to visits to the therapist, the patient must be faithful in fulfilling "homework assignments." For those patients who complete the course of treatment, the improvements can be significant.

With a combination of pharmacotherapy and behavioral therapy, the majority of OCD patients will be able to function well in both their work and social lives. The ongoing search for causes, together with research on treatment, promises to yield even more hope for people with OCD and their families.

How to Get Help for OCD

If you think that you have OCD, you should seek the help of a mental health professional. Family physicians, clinics, and health maintenance organizations usually can provide treatment or make referrals to mental health centers and specialists. Also, the department of psychiatry at a major medical center or the department of psychology at a university may have specialists who are knowledgeable about the treatment of OCD and are able to provide therapy or recommend another doctor in the area.

What the Family Can Do to Help

OCD affects not only the sufferer but the whole family. The family often has a difficult time accepting the fact that the person with OCD cannot stop the distressing behavior. Family members may show their anger and resentment, resulting in an increase in the OCD behavior. Or, to keep the peace, they may assist in the rituals or give constant reassurance.

Education about OCD is important for the family. Families can learn specific ways to encourage the person with OCD by supporting the medication regime and the behavior therapy. Self-help books are often a good source of information. Some families seek the help of a family therapist who is trained in the field. Also, in the past few years, many families have joined one of the educational support groups that have been organized throughout the country.

If You Have Special Needs

Individuals with OCD are protected under the Americans with Disabilities Act (ADA). Among organizations that offer information related to the ADA are the ADA Information Line at the U.S. Department of Justice, (202) 514-0301, and the Job Accommodation Network (JAN), part of the President's Committee on the Employment of People with Disabilities in the U.S. Department of Labor. JAN is located at West Virginia University, 809 Allen Hall, P.O. Box 6122, Morgantown, WV 26506, telephone (800) 526-7234 (voice or TDD), (800) 526-4698 (in West Virginia).

The Pharmaceutical Manufacturers Association publishes a directory of indigent programs for those who cannot afford medications. Physicians can request a copy of the guide by calling (800) PMA-INFO.

For Further Information

For further information on OCD, its treatment, and how to get help, you may wish to contact the following organizations:

Anxiety Disorders Association of America
6000 Executive Blvd, Ste 513
Rockville, MD 20852
(301) 231-9350

Makes referrals to professional members and to support groups. Has a catalog of available brochures, books, and audiovisuals.

Association for Advancement of Behavior Therapy
305 Seventh Ave
New York, NY 10001
(212) 647-1890

Membership listing of mental health professionals focusing in behavior therapy.

Dean Foundation
Obsessive Compulsive Information Center
8000 Excelsior Dr, Ste 302
Madison, WI 53717-1914
(608) 836-8070

Computer database of over 4,000 references updated daily. Computer searches done for nominal fee. No charge for quick reference questions. Maintains physician referral and support group lists.

Obsessive Compulsive Foundation
PO Box 70
Milford, CT 06460
(203) 878-5669

Offers free or at minimal cost brochures for individuals with the disorder and their families. In addition, videotapes and books are available. A bimonthly newsletter goes to members who pay an annual membership fee of $30. Has over 250 support groups nationwide.

Tourette Syndrome Association, Inc.
4240 Bell Blvd
New York, NY 11361-2874
(718) 224-2999

Publications, videotapes, and films available at minimal cost. Newsletter goes to members who pay an annual fee of $35.

Books Suggested for Further Reading

Baer, L. *Getting Control. Overcoming Your Obsessions and Compulsions.* Boston: Little, Brown & Co., 1991.

Foster, C.H. *Polly's Magic Games: A Child's View of Obsessive-Compulsive Disorder.* Ellsworth, ME: Dilligaf Publishing, 1994.

Greist, J.H. *Obsessive Compulsive Disorder: A Guide.* Madison, WI: Obsessive Compulsive Disorder Information Center. Rev. ed., 1992. (Thorough discussion of pharmacotherapy and behavior therapy)

Johnston, H.F. *Obsessive Compulsive Disorder in Children and Adolescents: A Guide.* Madison, WI: Child Psychopharmacology Information Center, 1993.

Livingston, B. *Learning to Live with Obsessive Compulsive Disorder.* Milford, CT: OCD Foundation, 1989. (Written for the families of those with OCD)

Rapoport, J.L. *The Boy Who Couldn't Stop Washing: The Experience and Treatment of Obsessive-Compulsive Disorder.* New York: E.P. Dutton, 1989.

Videotape

The Touching Tree. Jim Callner, writer/director, Awareness films. Distributed by the OCD Foundation, Inc., Milford, CT. (About a child with OCD)

References

DuPont, R.L.; Rice, D.P.; Shiraki, S.; and Rowland C. *Economic Costs of Obsessive Compulsive Disorder.* Unpublished, 1994.

Jenike, M.A. Obsessive-Compulsive Disorder: Efficacy of Specific Treatments as Assessed by Controlled Trials. *Psychopharmacology Bulletin* 29: 4: 487499, 1993.

Jenike, M.A. Managing the Patient with Treatment-Resistant Obsessive Compulsive Disorder: Current Strategies. *Journal of Clinical Psychiatry* 55: 3 (suppl): 1117, 1994.

Leonard, H.L.; Swedo, S.E.; Lenane, M.C.; Rettew, D.C.; Hamburger, S.D.; Bartko, J.J.; and Rapoport, J.L. A 2- to 7-Year Follow-up Study of 54 Obsessive-Compulsive Children and Adolescents. *Archives of General Psychiatry* 50: 429439, 1993.

March, J.S.; Mulle, K.; and Herbel, B. Behavioral Psychotherapy for Children and Adolescents with Obsessive-Compulsive Disorder: An Open Trial of a New Protocol-Driven Treatment Package. *Journal of the American Academy of Child and Adolescent Psychiatry* 33: 3: 333341, 1994.

Pato, M.T.; Zohar-Kadouch, R.; Zohar, J.; and Murphy, D.L. Return of Symptoms after Discontinuation of Clomipramine in Patients with Obsessive Compulsive Disorder. *American Journal of Psychiatry* 145: 15211525, 1988.

Swedo, S.E, and Leonard, H.L. Childhood Movement Disorders and Obsessive Compulsive Disorder. *Journal of Clinical Psychiatry* 55: 3 (suppl): 3237, 1994.

This brochure is a revision by Margaret Strock, staff member in the Information Resources and Inquiries Branch, Office of Scientific Information (OSI), National Institute of Mental Health (NIMH) of a publication originally written by Mary Lynn Hendrix, OSI. Expert assistance was provided by Henrietta Leonard, MD, and Jack Maser, PhD, NIMH staff members; Robert L. DuPont, MD, The Institute for Behavior and Health; Wayne Goodman, MD, University of Florida College of Medicine; and James Broatch, Obsessive Compulsive Foundation, Inc.

■ Document Source:
U.S. Department of Health and Human Services, Public Health Service
National Institutes of Health
National Institute of Mental Health
NIH Publication No. 943755
September 1994

PARANOIA

Paranoia—The Word

Paranoia is a term used by mental health specialists to describe suspiciousness (or mistrust) that is either highly exaggerated or not warranted at all. The word is often used in everyday conversation, often in anger, often incorrectly. Simple suspiciousness is not paranoia—not if it is based on past experience or expectations learned from the experience of others.

Paranoia can be mild and the affected person may function fairly well in society, or it can be so severe that the individual is incapacitated. Because many psychiatric disorders are accompanied by some paranoid features, diagnosis is sometimes difficult. Paranoias can be classified into three main categories—paranoid personality disorder, delusional (paranoid) disorder, and paranoid schizophrenia.

Paranoid Personality Disorder

Derek worked in a large office as a computer programmer. When another programmer received a promotion, Derek felt that the supervisor "had it in for him" and would never recognize his worth. He was sure that his co-workers were subtly downgrading him. Often he watched as others took coffee breaks together and imagined they spent this time talking about him. If he saw a group of people laughing, he knew they were laughing at him. He spent so much time brooding about the mistreatment he received that his work suffered and his supervisor told him he must improve or receive a poor performance rating. This action reinforced all Derek's suspicions, and he looked for and found a position in another large company. After a few weeks on his new job, he began to feel that others in the office didn't like him, excluded him from all conversations, made fun of him behind his back, and eroded his position. Derek has changed jobs six times in the last seven years. Derek has paranoid personality disorder.

Some people regularly become suspicious without cause—so much so that their paranoid thoughts disrupt their work and family life. Such people are said to have a *paranoid personality.* They are

Suspicious

An unmistakable sign of paranoia is continual mistrust. People with paranoid personality disorder are constantly on their guard because they see the world as a threatening place. They tend to confirm their expectations by latching on to any speck of evidence that supports their suspicions and ignore or mis-interpret any evidence to the contrary. They are ever watchful and may look around for signs of a threat.

Anyone in a new situation—beginning a job or starting a relationship, for example—is cautious and somewhat guarded until he or she learns that the fears are groundless. People suffering from paranoia cannot abandon their fears. They continue to expect trickery and to doubt the loyalty of others. In a personal relationship or marriage, this suspiciousness may take the form of pathological, unrealistic jealousy.

Hypersensitive

Because persons with paranoid personality disorder are hyperalert, they notice any slight and may take offense where none is intended. As a result, they tend to be defensive and antagonistic. When they are at fault, they cannot accept blame, not even mild criticism. Yet they are highly critical of others. Other people may say that these individuals make "mountains out of molehills."

Cold and Aloof

In addition to being argumentative and uncompromising, the people with paranoid personality disorder are often emotionally cut off from other people. They appear cold and, in fact, often avoid becoming intimate with others. They pride themselves on their rationality and objectivity. People with a paranoid outlook on life rarely come to the attention of clinicians—it is not in their nature to seek help. Many presumably function competently in society. They may seek out social niches in which a moralistic and punitive style is acceptable, or at least tolerated to a certain degree.

Delusional (Paranoid) Disorder

Psychiatrists make a distinction between the milder paranoid personality disorder described above and the more debilitating delusional (paranoid) disorder. The hallmark of this disorder is the presence of a persistent, nonbizarre delusion without symptoms of any other mental disorder.

Delusions are firmly held beliefs that are untrue, not shared by others in the culture, and not easily modifiable. Five delusional themes are frequently seen in delusional disorder. In some individuals, more than one of them is present.

Ruth is a clerk-typist who is efficient and helpful. Her employers and co-workers value her contribution to the office. But Ruth spends her evenings writing letters to state and federal officials. She feels that God has opened her mind and given her the cure for cancer. She wants some leading treatment center to use her cure on all its patients so that the world can see she is right. Many of her letters go unanswered, or she receives noncommittal replies that only make her feel that no one understands that she can save all cancer patients if only given the chance. When one of her letters is answered by an employee of the official to whom she wrote, she is sure that the official is being deliberately kept unaware of her knowledge and power. Sometimes she despairs that the world will never know how wonderful she is, but she doesn't give up. She just keeps writing. Ruth suffers from one of the delusional disorders, grandiose delusion.

The most common delusion in delusional disorder is that of *persecution*. While persons with paranoid personality might suspect their colleagues of joking at their expense, persons with delusional disorder may suspect others of participating in elaborate master plots to persecute them. They believe that they are being poisoned, drugged, spied upon, or are the targets of conspiracies to ruin their reputations or even to kill them. They sometimes engage in litigation in an attempt to redress imagined injustices.

Another theme seen frequently is that of *delusional jealousy*. Any sign—even a meaningless spot on clothing, or a short delay in arriving home—is summoned up as evidence that a spouse is being unfaithful.

Erotic delusions are based on the belief that one is romantically loved by another, usually someone of higher status or a well-known public figure. Individuals with erotic delusions often harass famous persons through numerous letters, telephone calls, visits, and stealthy surveillance.

Persons with *grandiose delusions* often feel that they have been endowed with special powers and that, if allowed to exercise these powers, they could cure diseases, banish poverty, ensure world peace, or perform other extraordinary feats.

Individuals with *somatic delusions* are convinced that there is something very wrong with their bodies—that they emit foul odors, have bugs crawling in or on their bodies, or are misshapen and ugly. Because of these delusions, they tend to avoid the society of other people and spend much time consulting physicians for their imagined condition.

Whether or not persons with delusional disorder are dangerous to others has not been systematically investigated, but clinical experience suggests that such persons are rarely homicidal. Delusional patients are commonly angry people, and thus they are perceived as threatening. In the rare instances when individuals with delusional disorder do become violent, their victims are usually people who unwittingly fit into their delusional scheme. The person in most danger from an individual with delusional disorder is a spouse or lover.

Paranoid Schizophrenia

Steven had not liked high school very much and was glad to graduate and get a job. But when he realized he needed more education to reach his goals, he applied for admission into a nearby college. He rented a house with several other young men and did well in his studies. Near the end of his second year, Steven stopped eating with the others and ate only food directly out of a can so he could be sure it wasn't poisoned. When he crossed the campus, he tried to avoid girls as he felt they shot poisoned webs at him that encompassed his body like a giant spider web. When he began to feel that his housemates had put poisoned gas in his room, he dropped out of school and returned home. He cleaned up his room at home and put a lock on the door so his parents could not enter it and contaminate it. He bought a small electric hot plate and prepared all his own food. If his mother urged him to eat a meal with the family, he accused her of wanting to poison him. His parents finally were able to convince him to see a psychiatrist who diagnosed "schizophrenia, subtype paranoia." With medication, individual and group therapy, Steven has improved enough to work in an office under the supervision of an understanding and supportive employer.

Paranoid thinking and behavior are hallmarks of the form of schizophrenia called "paranoid schizophrenia." Individuals with paranoid schizophrenia commonly have extremely bizarre delusions or hallucinations, almost always on a specific theme. Sometimes they hear voices that others cannot hear or believe that their thoughts are being controlled or broadcast aloud. Also, their performance at home and on the job deteriorates, often with a much diminished degree of emotional expressiveness.

In contrast, people with relatively milder paranoid disorders may have such symptoms as delusions of persecution or delusional jealousy, but not the prominent hallucinations or impossible, bizarre delusions of paranoid schizophrenia. Those with milder paranoid disorders are customarily able to work, and their emotional expression and behavior are appropriate to their delusional belief. Apart from their delusions, their thinking remains clear and orderly. On the other hand, those with paranoid schizophrenia are often intellectually disorganized and confused.

Causes of Paranoia

Genetic Contribution

Little research has been done on the role of heredity in causing paranoia. Scientists have found that the families of paranoid patients do not have higher than normal rates of either schizophrenia or depression. However, there is some evidence that paranoid symptoms in schizophrenia may be genetically influenced. Some studies have shown that when one twin of a pair of identical twins with schizophrenia has paranoid symptoms, the other twin usually does also. And, recent research has suggested that paranoid disorders are significantly more common in relatives of persons with schizophrenia than in the general population. Whether paranoid disorder—or a predisposition to it—is inherited is not yet known.

Biochemistry

The discovery that psychosis (a state in which the individual is out of touch with reality) is treatable with antipsychotic drugs has led scientists to look for the origins of severe mental disorders in abnormal brain chemistry. The search has become very complex, as more and more of the chemical substances that carry messages from one nerve cell to another—the neurotransmitters—have been discovered. So far, no clear-cut answers have been found. As with the genetic studies, biochemical studies have not examined paranoia except as a subtype of schizophrenia. There is, however, limited evidence that paranoid schizophrenia is biochemically distinct from nonparanoid forms of the disorder.

Abuse of drugs such as amphetamines, cocaine, marijuana, PCP, LSD, or other stimulants or "psychedelic" compounds may lead to symptoms of paranoid thinking or behavior. Patients with major mental disorders like paranoid schizophrenia may have their symptoms become worse under the influence of these drugs. Scientists are studying the biochemical actions of such drugs to determine how they produce their behavioral effects. This may help us to learn more about the neurochemistry of paranoid disorders, which is poorly understood at this time.

Stress

Some scientists believe paranoia may be a reaction to high levels of life stress. Lending support to this opinion is the evidence that paranoia is more prevalent among immigrants, prisoners of war, and others undergoing severe stress. Sometimes, when thrust into a new and highly stressful situation, people suffer an acute form—called "acute paranoia"—in which delusions develop over a short period of time and last only a few months.

Some studies indicate that paranoia has become more prevalent in the twentieth century. The connection between stress and paranoia does not, of course, rule out other contributing factors. A genetic defect, a brain abnormality, an information-processing disability—or all three—could predispose a person to paranoia; stress may merely act as a trigger.

Treatment of Paranoia

Paranoid people's mistrustfulness makes treatment of the condition difficult. Rarely will they talk casually in an interview. They are suspicious of the kind of open-ended questions many therapists rely on to learn about the patient's history (for example, "Tell me about your relationships with your co-workers."). They may try to avoid hospitalization and drugs, fearing a loss of control or other real or imagined dangers.

Drug Treatment

Treatment with appropriate antipsychotic drugs may help the paranoid patient overcome some symptoms. Although the patient's functioning may be improved, the paranoid symptoms often remain intact. Some studies indicate that symptoms improve following drug treatment, but the same results sometimes occur among patients who receive a placebo, a "sugar pill" without active ingredients. This finding suggests that in some cases the paranoia diminishes for psychological reasons rather than because of the drug's action. Paranoid patients receiving medication must be closely monitored. Their fearfulness and persecutory delusions often lead them to refuse or sabotage treatment—for example, by holding the drug in their cheek until they are alone and then spitting it out.

Psychotherapy

Reports on individual cases suggest that the regular opportunity to express suspicions and self-doubts afforded by psy-

chotherapy can help the paranoid patient function in the community. Although paranoid ideas do seem to persist, they may be less disruptive. Other types of psychotherapy that have reportedly led to improved social functioning without appreciably diminishing paranoid delusions are art therapy, family therapy, and group therapy.

Outlook for Paranoid Patients

In spite of the treatment difficulties, patients with a paranoid disorder may function quite well. Even though their paranoid views are apparently unshakable, various treatments appear effective in improving social functioning, so that they do not often require lengthy hospitalization. The symptoms are less bizarre than those associated with paranoid schizophrenia. Also, the paranoid disorders seem to cause less disorganization of the personality and disruptions in social and family life. Unlike schizophrenia, which can become progressively worse, paranoid disorder seems to reach a certain level of severity and stay there.

For Further Information

Kendler, K.S.; Spitzer, R.L.; and Williams, J.B.W. Psychotic disorders in DSM-III-R. *The American Journal of Psychiatry* 146:953-962, 1989.

Munro, A. Delusional (paranoid) disorders. *Canadian Journal of Psychiatry* Vol. 33(5):399-404, 1988.

Opjordsmoen, S. Long-term course and outcome in delusional disorder. *Acta Psychiatrica Scandinavica* Vol. 78(5):576-586, 1988. *Schizophrenia Bulletin* Vol 7, No. 4, 1981 (available in most medical libraries).

Sorensen, D.J.; Paul, G.L.; and Mariotto, M.J. Inconsistencies in paranoid functioning, premorbid adjustment, and chronicity: Question of diagnostic criteria. *Schizophrenia Bulletin* Vol. 14(2):323-336, 1988.

Williams, J.G. Cognitive intervention for a paranoid personality disorder. *Psychotherapy* Vol. 25(4):570-575, 1988.

This brochure was revised by Margaret Strock, staff member in the Office of Scientific Information, National Institute of Mental Health (NIMH). An earlier version was done under contract for NIMH by Wray Herbert. Expert assistance was provided by David Shore, MD, David Pickar, MD, and Darryl G. Kirch, MD, NIMH staff members. Their help in assuring the accuracy of this pamphlet is gratefully acknowledged.

■ **Document Source:**
U.S. Department of Health and Human Services, Public Health Service
National Institutes of Health
National Institute of Mental Health
NIH Publication No. 95-3927
Printed 1987; Revised 1989; Reprinted 1995

MUSCULOSKELETAL AND CONNECTIVE TISSUE DISORDERS

■ ■ ■

ABOUT LOW-BACK PAIN

Low-back pain is a common problem among people of just about any age. It is so common, in fact, that four out of five adult Americans will be bothered by it at one time or another.

This booklet has been prepared to tell you about low-back pain, what causes it, how to treat it, and when and why your doctor may recommend an operation as the best treatment for your back pain (usually after an adequate trial of nonoperative treatment).

It is important to remember that each individual is different, and the indications for nonoperative or operative treatment depend upon the individual patient's condition. This booklet is not intended to take the place of the professional advice of a qualified spinal surgeon* who is familiar with your symptoms. After reading this booklet, you will probably have further questions; you should discuss them openly and honestly with your surgeon.

About the Back

The back bears a heavy load; it supports the weight of the body, sustains the weight of objects that are lifted or carried, and absorbs the stresses that result when parts of the body move. The back is a complex combination of muscles, ligaments, tendons, and bones—all attached to the backbone. The backbone is a series of interconnected blocks of bone called vertebrae. They form a tubelike "vertebral canal" that contains and protects the spinal cord and its bundles of nerves. Each vertebra has a cylinder-shaped body, a vertebral arch, and several bony protuberances. The body of the vertebra rests on a cushion of tissue, known as an intervertebral disc, that can act as a shock absorber. The vertebral arch extends from the body of the vertebra up and over the spinal cord to safeguard the spinal nerves. The bony protuberances are the

places at which muscles, ligaments, tendons, and other bones join the backbone; they allow for normal flexibility of spinal movements.

Causes of Low-Back Pain

Low-back pain may be caused by abnormal development of the backbone, excessive stress on the back, injury, or any one of a number of physical disorders that affect the bones or the discs in the spine. The following are among the most common:

1. **Ruptured or Herniated Disc.** This is a frequent cause of low-back pain, and is sometimes called a "slipped" disc. Actually, an intervertebral disc cannot "slip" out of position. It can rupture, however, and when it does, some of the disc's fragments push backward (prolapse posteriorly) into the spinal canal and press on nearby nerves, causing pain, numbness, tingling, and sometimes weakness in the leg or foot.

    A disc may rupture after a relatively minor stress, such as bending over to pick up an object. Pain may occur immediately after the rupture occurs, or it may grow steadily worse over the next few minutes or hours. Pain from a ruptured disc may involve the center or one side of the back, and it spreads gradually to the leg. This leg pain, which may be accompanied by numbing or tingling sensations, may affect the thigh, the back or outside of the calf, or the edge or top of the foot. Called sciatica (si-at'- i-kah), leg pain or numbness is caused by the pressure that the ruptured disc's fragments exert on the components of the sciatic nerve, which runs from the spinal cord down the thigh to the calf and foot.

2. **Degeneration of the Vertebrae or Discs.** Low-back pain occurs when parts of the vertebrae or the intervertebral disc deteriorate. When vertebral joints be-

---

* Generally a neurosurgeon or orthopaedic surgeon

gin to wear down, the condition is called osteoarthritis. When the intervertebral discs start to degenerate, the spinal canal may become narrow and bone spurs can develop, a condition known as spondylosis (spon'd i-lo'sis). Osteoarthritis and spondylosis produce intermittent aching or stiffness in the low back. Such low-back pain may spread into the buttocks and the thighs and may be aggravated by exercise or poor posture. People with osteoarthritis or spondylosis often feel stiff when they try to bend forward or stretch backward, because with these diseases, the backbone loses its mobility.

3. **Spinal Stenosis.** Narrowing of the vertebral canal is known as spinal stenosis. It may be due to overgrowth of vertebral joints associated with backward bulging of the discs or to degenerative diseases such as osteoarthritis or spondylosis (accompanied by thickening of the normal spinal ligaments). Pain from spinal stenosis, which typically occurs during walking or other exercise, develops after a few minutes of activity, accompanied by numbness, tingling, or cramps in the legs, and eases after a few minutes of rest.

4. **Sprains.** Just as a sudden twist of the foot can cause a sprained ankle, an abrupt movement of the spine can sprain the muscles and ligaments of the back. A sprain is a partial tear of a ligament that has been overstretched. The pain from a sprain is located over the damaged ligament.

5. **Infection.** An infection in one part of the body, such as tuberculosis, can spread to the backbone and produce an inflammation of the bone or, occasionally, an abscess. Back pain from an infection develops slowly and eventually becomes severe. In addition to the back pain, a spinal infection raises the patient's temperature and brings on an overall feeling of weakness and bouts of chills. The pain is often associated with severe spasms and stiffness of the back.

6. **Tumors.** Spinal tumors are uncommon. They may arise in the vertebral column or within the spinal cord or nerve roots, or they may spread to the spine from cancer elsewhere in the body. Spinal tumors cause pain in the back and may produce weakness or numbness in the legs or lower part of the body. The back pain characteristically may be worse at night or at rest.

7. **Ankylosing Spondylitis.** Ankylosing spondylitis (ang'k i-lo'sing spon'd i-li'tis) is an inflammation of the backbone that causes stiffness. It occurs mainly in men between the ages of 15 and 25. In the most severe form of the disease, the backbone becomes completely rigid. Initially, the low back is stiff and painful, and the pain is aggravated by rest. A person with ankylosing spondylitis will often awake with an aching and stiff back and will gain relief only by exercising.

Before an Operation is Considered

Many of the conditions that bring about low-back pain (ankylosing spondylitis, sprains, osteoarthritis, and even a prolapsed disc) can be treated through rest, appropriate medication, and mild exercise. An operation is not considered, in fact, until these and sometimes other conservative measures have proved unsuccessful. If a trial period of conservative therapy produces unsatisfactory results and low-back pain continues to interfere with a person's day-to-day activities, an operation may be considered.

Even when an operation becomes a possibility, it will not be attempted until the spine has been carefully assessed. Before performing a surgical procedure, the surgeon must know the exact nature of the problem in the back. Consequently, he or she will study the back by means of X rays or other tests, such as myelography (mi'e-log'rah-fe), computerized axial tomography (CT), or magnetic resonance imaging (MRI).

In myelography, a radiopaque material is injected into the vertebral canal to outline any disorders that may be found in the vertebrae or discs. Usually, the patient is placed on a special table that makes it possible to change his or her position, thereby distributing the injected material up and down the vertebral canal. Because myelography may cause headaches, which can be aggravated by sitting up or standing, patients may be asked to remain in bed for a day after the test.

During CT, a patient is placed in a large, circular device that projects X rays through a cross-section of the body. The X rays outline the densities of various tissues, and by analyzing these densities, a physician can detect abnormalities.

Magnetic resonance imaging (MRI) is a relatively new technique for showing the bones and other tissues of the body. MRI scans do not involve the use of X rays, and they may or may not include the injection of a contrast agent in the vertebral canal to enhance the images seen by the physician. An advantage of this method is that soft tissues (such as ruptured discs) show up much better on an MRI scan than they do on an X ray or a CT scan. The test takes a longer time to perform than an X ray or CT, and the patient must lie quietly in a large magnetic tube for the time of the examination. However, this type of examination is proving to be a safe and highly effective way to diagnose spinal disorders. In addition, electrical studies of the muscles and nerves may be useful in diagnosing and managing spinal disorders.

About Operations on the Back

The type of operation a surgeon performs depends on the nature of a patient's back problem. However, most procedures involve a laminectomy (lam' i-nek'to-me), which may require the partial removal of the vertebral arch to gain access to the cause of the patient's low-back pain. If a disc has ruptured, a surgeon will perform a partial laminectomy to investigate the vertebral canal, identify the ruptured disc, and remove a good portion of the degenerated disc material, especially those fragments that press on the nerve roots. The surgeon may consider a second procedure—spinal fusion—if he or she feels that stabilization of the spine is necessary. A spinal fusion is performed by fusing the vertebrae together with bone grafts; sometimes, the grafts are combined with metal plates or other types of instruments.

Some types of herniated discs are suitable for treatment by microsurgery or by a technique known as percutaneous discectomy, in which the disc is repaired through the skin without making a surgical incision. For this technique, the surgeon uses an X ray as a guide for inserting a large bore needle into the center of the disc; the central portion of the disc is then removed by using fine instruments that are placed through the needle. Another procedure, chemonueclolysis, uses injections of enzymes into the discs. Although it has been used experimentally in this country for several years, chemoneuclolysis is *rarely recommended* at the present time. You should discuss with your surgeon the various treatment options to determine which is the most appropriate for your specific problems.

To treat spinal stenosis, the surgeon makes an incision that is long enough to allow inspection of all of the vertebrae that have contributed to narrowing of the vertebral canal. After performing a laminectomy, the surgeon performs a decompression operation by entering the vertebral canal and removing the material that is pressing on the spinal nerve roots. Occasionally, some form of spinal fusion or other type of stabilization may be indicated.

When a patient has a spinal tumor, the physician may opt to treat the patient with radiation or chemotherapy rather than a surgical operation. If an operation is needed, the surgeon performs a laminectomy, locates the tumor, and removes it from the spine, the spinal cord, and the nerve roots. Some tumors require that the operation be approached from the front of the spine, followed by spinal stabilization. Following the removal of a spinal tumor, the surgeon decides if further radiation therapy and/or chemotherapy should be given.

When a patient has a spinal infection with an abscess in the back part of the spinal canal, the surgeon removes the vertebral arch, locates the abscess, and drains away the pus. If the abscess is toward the front (anterior) in the disc space, the surgeon may make an anterior approach to the vertebral bodies. Appropriate antibodies will be given to cure the infection.

Recovering from the Operation

Recovering after back surgery varies with the type of operation that was performed. Following ordinary disc removal, most patients are able to get out of bed and move about in three or four days or sooner. Patients who have undergone a spinal fusion or an operation for stenosis take longer to become mobile, and these patients may remain in the hospital for longer periods of time after the operation. In addition, they may be required to wear a brace or cast for a few weeks to several months after surgery.

The length of stay for patients with spinal tumors depends on the type of tumor. Patients who have had an operation to drain an abscess of the spine stay in the hospital until the infection has been controlled.

A common problem after major back surgery is difficulty with urination. This problem usually subsides in three to four days. The insertion of a tube (catheter) into the bladder that will drain the urine may be necessary until the patient is able to void normally.

After discharge from the hospital, most back surgery patients will need some time to recuperate before returning to their usual activities. The types of activities the patient can safely resume should be outlined by the operating surgeon and should be followed carefully by the patient. The period of recuperation varies, but it may range from several weeks to several months, and a back brace or physical therapy program may be recommended

Surgery by Surgeons

A fully trained surgeon is a physician who, after medical school, has gone through years of training in an accredited residency program to learn the specialized skills of a surgeon. One good sign of a surgeon's competence is certification by a national surgical board approved by the American Board of Medical Specialties. All board-certified surgeons have satisfactorily completed an approved residency training program and have passed a rigorous specialty examination.

The letters F.A.C.S. (Fellow of the American College of Surgeons) after a surgeon's name are a further indication of a physician's qualifications. Surgeons who become Fellows of the College have passed a comprehensive evaluation of their surgical training and skills; they also have demonstrated their commitment to high standards of ethical conduct. This evaluation is conducted according to national standards that were established to ensure that patients receive the best possible surgical care.

Reviewed by Edward R. Laws, Jr., MD, FACS, Professor of Neurosurgery, University of Virginia Health Sciences Center, Charlottesville, VA, and David G. Murray, MD, FACS, Professor and Chairman, Department of Orthopaedic Surgery, State University of New York Health Science Center, Syracuse, NY.

■ **Document Source:**
American College of Surgeons
55 East Erie St
Chicago, IL 60611

See also: Understanding Acute Low Back Problems (page 361)

COPING WITH ARTHRITIS IN ITS MANY FORMS

by Carolyn J. Strange

It may begin as a slight morning stiffness. For the lucky person with arthritis, that's as far as it goes. But for millions of others, arthritis can become a disabling, even crippling, disease. Roman Emperor Diocletian exempted citizens with severe arthritis from paying taxes, no doubt realizing that the disease itself can be taxing enough.

One in seven Americans—nearly 40 million—have some form of arthritis. That number will climb as the baby boomers age. By 2020, about 60 million Americans will have arthritis, according to The National Arthritis Data Workgroup of the National Institute of Arthritis and Musculoskeletal and Skin Diseases. The disease is physical, but also exacts a mental, emotional, and economic toll.

"Chronic illness impacts a person's entire lifestyle—work, family and recreation," says Gail Wright, Ph.D., a rehabilitation psychologist at the University of Missouri, Columbia. To improve quality of life, doctors and health educators increasingly advise combining drug treatment with education, social support, and moderate forms of exercise.

Arthritis means joint inflammation. In a normal joint, where two bones meet, the ends are coated with cartilage, a smooth, slippery cushion that protects the bone and reduces friction during movement. A tough capsule lined with synovial membrane seals the joint and produces a lubricating fluid. Ligaments surround and support each joint, connecting the bones and preventing excessive movement. Muscles attach to bone by tendons on each side of a joint. Inflammation can affect any of these tissues.

Inflammation is a complex process that causes swelling, redness, warmth, and pain. It's the body's natural response to injury and plays an important role in healing and fighting infection. Joint injury can be caused by trauma or by the wear and tear of aging. But in many forms of arthritis, injury is caused by the uncontrolled inflammation of autoimmune disease, in which the immune system attacks the body's own tissues. In severe cases, all joint tissues, even bone, can be damaged.

The general term arthritis includes over 100 kinds of rheumatic diseases, most of which last for life. Rheumatic diseases are those affecting joints, muscle, and connective tissue, which makes up or supports various structures of the body, including tendons, cartilage, blood vessels, and internal organs. The Food and Drug Administration has approved a wide variety of drugs to treat the many forms of arthritis.

The most common type of arthritis is osteoarthritis, affecting more than 16 million Americans. This degenerative joint disease is common in people over 65, but may appear decades earlier. It begins when cartilage breaks down, sometimes eroding entirely to leave a bone-on-bone joint in extreme cases. Any joint can be affected, but the feet, knees, hips, and fingers are most common. It may appear in one or two joints and spread no further. Painful and knobby bone growths in the fingers are common, but usually not crippling. The disease is often mild, but can be quite severe.

Second most common is rheumatoid arthritis, which affects 2.5 million Americans. It can strike at any age, but usually appears between ages 20 and 50. The hands are most commonly affected, but it can affect most joints of the body. Inflammation begins in the synovial lining and can spread to the entire joint. Highly variable and difficult to control, the disease can severely deform joints. Some people become bedridden. Others continue to run marathons.

An autoimmune disease affecting the whole body, rheumatoid arthritis can also cause weakness, fatigue, loss of appetite, muscle pain, and weight loss. Blood tests may reveal anemia and the presence of an antibody called rheumatoid factor (RF). However, some people with RF never develop rheumatoid arthritis, and some people with the disease never have RF. In about one in six, the disease becomes severe and can shorten life. Researchers hope to find ways to predict which patients should be treated more aggressively.

Common Types of Arthritis

Of more than 100 different kinds of arthritis, these are the most common:

Osteoarthritis—Also called degenerative arthritis. Occurs when the cushioning cartilage in a joint breaks down. Commonly affects feet, knees, hips, and fingers. Affects 16 million Americans, mostly 45 and older. About half of those 65 and older have this form.

Rheumatoid Arthritis—Immune system attacks the lining, or synovial membrane, of the joints. Joint damage can become severe and deforming. Involves the whole body, and may also cause fatigue, weight loss and anemia, and affect the lungs, heart and eyes. Affects about 2.1 million Americans, three times more women than men.

Gout—Causes sudden, severe attacks, usually in the big toe, but any joint can be affected. A metabolic disorder in which uric acid builds up in the blood and crystals form in joints and other places. Drugs and attention to diet can control gout. Affects about 1 million Americans (70 to 80 percent men), with first attack starting between 40 and 50 years of age.

Ankylosing Spondylitis—A chronic inflammatory disease of the spine that can result in fused vertebrae and rigid spine. Often milder and harder to diagnose in women. Most people with the disease also have a genetic marker known as HLA-B27. Affects about 318,000 Americans, usually men between the ages of 16 and 35.

Juvenile Arthritis—The most common form is juvenile rheumatoid arthritis. Arthritis diagnosis, treatment, and disease characteristics are different in children and adults. Some children recover completely; others remain affected throughout their lives. Affects about 200,000 Americans.

Psoriatic Arthritis—Bone and other joint tissues become inflamed, and, like rheumatoid arthritis, it can affect the whole body. Affects about 5 percent of people with psoriasis, a chronic skin disease. Likely to affect fingers or spine. Symptoms are mild in most people but can be quite severe. Affects about 160,000 Americans.

Systemic Lupus Erythematosus—Involves skin, joints, muscles, and sometimes internal organs. Symptoms usually appear in women of childbearing age but can occur in anyone at any age. Also called lupus or SLE, it can be mild or life threatening. Affects at least 131,000 Americans, nine to ten times as many women as men.

Other forms—Arthritis can develop as a result of an infection. For example, bacteria that cause gonorrhea or Lyme disease can cause arthritis. Infectious arthritis can cause serious damage, but usually clears up completely with antibiotics. Scleroderma is a systemic disease that involves the skin, but may include problems with blood vessels, joints, and internal organs. Fibromyalgia syndrome is a soft-tissue rheumatism that doesn't lead to joint deformity, but affects an estimated 5 million Americans, mostly women.

Ups and Downs

With so many kinds of arthritis, which can appear and progress unpredictably, diagnosis and treatment can be trying for both physician and patient. Diagnosis depends on integrating a host of factors, including the possibility that a person may have two forms of the disease.

The normal ups and downs of chronic, painful disease further complicate matters. "Just about any painful condition will wax and wane on its own," says rheumatologist Dennis Boulware, M.D., University of Alabama, Birmingham.

A worsening or reappearance of the disease is called a flare. Remissions bring welcome relief, but can also obscure whether symptoms decreased on their own or due to treatment.

Proper treatment depends on correct diagnosis of the specific disease, and varies with severity and location, as well as from person to person. But treatment need not wait for a final diagnosis because initial treatment options, such as anti-inflammatory drugs and exercise, are similar for many forms of the disease. Treatment should begin early to reduce joint damage.

The drugs used for treating most types of arthritis are drawn from many categories, but can be thought of in a few broad groups, such as anti-inflammatory drugs and disease-modifying drugs. For treating gout, there are also drugs that reduce the amount of uric acid in the blood. More than one medication may be required for treating arthritis.

Anti-inflammatory agents generally work by slowing the body's production of prostaglandins, substances that play a role in inflammation. Many have an analgesic, or painkilling, effect at low doses. Usually, higher, sustained doses are required to see sufficient anti-inflammatory activity for treating arthritis. The most familiar anti-inflammatory agent is aspirin, often a good arthritis treatment. Like aspirin, nonsteroidal anti-inflammatory drugs (NSAIDs) fight pain and inflammation. More than a dozen NSAIDs are available, most by prescription only. At press time, FDA was considering whether labeling changes to prescription-strength NSAIDs are necessary, due to gastrointestinal side effects.

FDA has approved three NSAIDs for over-the-counter (OTC) marketing: ibuprofen (marketed as Advil, Nuprin, Motrin, and others), naproxen sodium (sold as Aleve), and ketoprofen (marketed as Actron and Orudis). Although these drugs are available OTC, a doctor should be consulted before taking any medication for arthritis symptoms.

"People shouldn't be mixing medications," says Linda Katz, M.D., of FDA's pilot drug evaluation staff, and anyone regularly taking NSAIDs should carefully read the labels of OTC products to make sure they don't contain similar drugs. For example, many cough and cold preparations contain analgesics such as aspirin, acetaminophen or ibuprofen.

The most potent anti-inflammatories are corticosteroids, synthetic versions of the hormone cortisone. Like prednisone and dexamethasone, the generic names often end in "-one." They're usually reserved for short periods of use during intense flares or when other drugs don't control unrelenting disease. Relief can be dramatic, but long-term use causes side effects, such as weight gain, high blood pressure, and thinning of bones and skin. Usually given orally, they can also be injected directly into a joint to reduce side effects.

Disease modifiers slow the disease process in autoimmune diseases such as rheumatoid arthritis or systemic lupus erythematosus. Patients taking these drugs are closely monitored. It may take weeks or months to learn if a drug works. During that wait, it's important to keep taking other medications such as NSAIDs. Gold salts have been used to treat rheumatoid arthritis for 60 years, although nobody knows why this treatment works. Penicillamine, methotrexate, and antimalarials such as hydroxychloroquine are also used. Doctors usually reserve other powerful drugs that suppress the immune system for extremely serious disease.

Most people with arthritis never need surgery, but when all else fails, it can dramatically improve independence and quality of life by reducing pain and improving mobility. The surgeon may remove damaged or chronically inflamed tissue, or replace the joint entirely. Artificial replacements are available for all of the most commonly affected joints.

Use It or Lose It

In the past, doctors often advised arthritis patients to rest and avoid exercise. Rest remains important, especially during flares. But doing nothing results in weak muscles, stiff joints, reduced mobility, and lost vitality. Now, rheumatologists routinely advise a balance of physical activity and rest. Exercise offers physical and psychological benefits that include improved overall fitness and well-being, increased mobility, and better sleep.

For example, twice a week for three years, Elsie Sequeira, 81, of Concord, Calif., has attended a water-based exercise class sponsored by the Arthritis Foundation. "It's helped me a lot," she says. Sequeira has rheumatoid arthritis in her shoulders and legs. She had also had a mild stroke and got to her first classes with the help of a walker and an attendant.

A few weeks passed before she saw any improvement, but within a few months she no longer needed either the walker or the attendant. "The warm water is very soothing and we can do things in the water that we couldn't do on land," Sequeira says. She enjoys the social contact, and feels better able to take care of herself. "I don't feel so hamstrung," she says.

Joints require motion to stay healthy. That's why doctors advise arthritis patients to do range-of-motion, or flexibility, exercises every day—even during flares. Painful or swollen joints should be moved gently, however.

Strengthening and endurance activities are also recommended, but should be limited or avoided during flares. Arthritis patients should consult their doctors before starting an exercise program, and begin gradually. Exercises must be individualized to work the right muscles while avoiding overstressing affected joints. Doctors or physical therapists can teach proper ways to move.

Muscle strength is especially important because strong muscles better support and protect joints. "Several studies show that if you improve muscle strength, you decrease pain," Boulware says. Joints will probably hurt during exercise, but shouldn't still hurt several hours later.

"There's a fine line between doing too much and too little," says rheumatologist William Ginsburg, M.D., of the Mayo Clinic, Jacksonville, Fla. "Sometimes people have to be reminded to slow down and listen to their disease."

Support groups and arthritis education can help people learn how to listen to their disease, and cope with it. "The psychological aspects are very important because that's what changes people's lives," Ginsburg says.

Participants learn practical things, such as how to: get up off the floor after a fall, protect joints with careful use and assistive devices, drive a car, get comfortable sleep, use heat and cold treatments, talk with their doctors, and cope with emotional aspects of pain and disability. They may also learn to acquire and maintain what health experts have long touted—a positive attitude.

Health education not only improves quality of life, but also lowers health-care costs, and the benefits are lasting, according to studies at Stanford University, Palo Alto, Calif. Four years after a short Arthritis Self-Management Program, participants still reported significantly less pain and made fewer physician visits, even though disability increased. The benefits came, not from the specifics taught, but from improved ability to cope with the consequences of arthritis—in other words, confidence. "It's the same thing that any good coach tries to instill," says Halsted R. Holman, M.D., Stanford University.

Normal Joint

In a normal joint (where two bones come together), the muscle, bursa and tendon support the bone and aid movement. The synovial membrane (an inner lining) releases a slippery fluid into the joint space. Cartilage covers the bones ends, absorbing shocks and keeping the bones from rubbing together when the joint moves.

Osteoarthritis

In osteoarthritis, cartilage breaks down and the bones rub together. The joint then loses shape and alignment. Bone ends thicken, forming spurs (bony growths). Bits of cartilage or bone float in the joint space.

Rheumatoid Arthritis

In rheumatoid arthritis, inflammation accompanies thickening of the synovial membrane or joint lining, causing the whole joint to look swollen due to swelling in the joint capsule. The inflamed joint lining enters and damages bone and cartilage, and inflammatory cells release an enzyme that gradually digests bone and cartilage. Space between joints diminishes, and the joint loses shape and alignment.

Avoiding Fraud

Learning to understand their disease can also help make people less likely to fall victim to fraud. Because they have a painful, incurable condition, people with arthritis are among the prime targets for fraud and spend nearly a billion dollars annually on unproved remedies, largely diets and supplements.

A claim describing the relationship between a nutrient or dietary ingredient and a disease, such as arthritis, cannot be made on the label or in labeling of a dietary supplement unless the claim is authorized by FDA. In order for FDA to consider authorizing the use of a health claim, there must be significant agreement among qualified experts that the health claim is scientifically valid. Frequently, however, dietary supplements are found on the market labeled in violation of these requirements.

"If the claim sounds too good to be true, it probably is. Talk to your doctor or other health professional," says Peggy Binzer, a consumer safety officer in FDA's Center for Food Safety and Applied Nutrition.

Consumers who have questions or who wish to report a company for falsely labeling its products should call FDA's Office of Consumer Affairs at (301) 443-3170 from 1 p.m. to 3:30 p.m. Eastern time. Consumers who have suffered from a serious adverse effect associated with the use of a dietary supplement should report the effect to their health-care professional or to MED WATCH at (1-800) FDA-1088.

Some remedies, such as vinegar and honey or copper bracelets, seem harmless. But they can become harmful if they cause people to abandon conventional therapy. Others, such as the solvent dimethyl sulfoxide (DMSO), can be outright dangerous.

It's tempting to conclude that arthritis pain gets better or worse because of what was added or eliminated from the diet the day or week before. However, gout is the only rheumatic disease known to be helped by avoiding certain foods. The unpredictable ups and downs of arthritis make it hard to establish a relationship between diet and disease. Scientists have only recently begun to study nutritional therapy for arthritis, and the American College of Rheumatology (ACR) urges continued research.

The ACR Position Statement on Diet and Arthritis advises, "Until more data are available, patients should continue to follow balanced and healthy diets, be skeptical of 'miraculous' claims and avoid elimination diets and fad nutritional practices."

Research under Way

New treatments are likely to stem from better understanding of the underlying causes and destructive processes of the disease. Overuse, injury and obesity are contributing factors in osteoarthritis, and researchers have implicated a faulty gene in the breakdown of cartilage. Heredity plays a role in other forms of arthritis, too, increasing susceptibility in some people. Potential genetic therapy approaches are still far off, however.

Increased knowledge of immunology and the inflammatory process offers more immediate promise. Researchers have developed a drug that blocks the effects of TNF-alpha, an inflammatory protein responsible for reactions resulting in joint damage. In short-term preliminary trials, the drug significantly reduced symptoms in rheumatoid arthritis patients.

Such results are encouraging, but the ultimate goal is to understand what starts the immune response in the first place.

"Until you know the real cause, you're not going to have the right drug," Ginsburg says.

That quest continues and offers hope. But short of a cure, enlightened coping may be the most promising avenue to a less taxing life for people with arthritis. Emperor Diocletian would be pleased.

■ Document Source:
U.S. Department of Health and Human Services; Public Health Service
Food and Drug Administration
FDA Consumer
March 1996

CORRECTING THE CURVED SPINE OF SCOLIOSIS

by Dixie Farley

When Laura Bradbard was 12, her mother noticed a lump on her back and was concerned it might be a tumor.

"It was my rib cage rotating," Bradbard says today, 38 and working as a secretary in Rockville, Md. "The lump was my shoulder blade and ribs protruding out the back. X-rays showed my spine was growing sideways, curving in the shape of an 'S.' The doctor said I should do something about it before it got worse."

Sideways curvature of the spine of 11 degrees or more is known as scoliosis. Bradbard's spine was off-center 36 degrees.

Bradbard has scoliosis—in her case, it's called "idiopathic," which means the cause is unknown. Some 80 percent of patients have this variety. Other cases are due to birth defects, spinal cord injuries, and nerve and muscle diseases such as muscular dystrophy.

Who gets scoliosis?

Showing up during the growth spurt at ages 10 to 15, scoliosis strikes 2 to 3 percent of adolescents. For unknown reasons, it affects more girls than boys—an inequality of about 3.6 to 1 overall, but 10 to 1 when curves are 30 degrees or more.

Very mild scoliosis curves, under 20 degrees, are nothing to worry about, doctors say. Even 20-degree curves sometimes improve on their own, with only 1 in 5 worsening, and only 3 in 1,000 worsening enough to need treatment.

When curvature gets worse, the spine twists on its center, slowly pulling the rib cage out of normal position. One side of the rib cage becomes higher at the back and sticks out. The ribs inside the curve scrunch together as those outside the curve spread apart. Although most scoliosis curves are "S" shaped like Bradbard's, some resemble a long "C."

"As a curve approaches 60 degrees," says Martin Yahiro, M.D., "the distorted rib cage restricts expansion of the lungs, causing breathing problems." Yahiro is an orthopedist (specialist in bone disorders) at the Food and Drug Administra-

tion's Center for Devices and Radiological Health, which regulates scoliosis treatment devices.

Why some scoliosis curves worsen and others don't is unknown. The larger the curve and the younger the patient when it's discovered, the greater the chance it will worsen, Yahiro says.

Curve Watch

Often, the first clue that scoliosis is developing is an uneven skirt hemline or a difference in pant-leg length. Other early warning signs, which might resemble poor posture to an untrained eye, include a hip or shoulder higher than the other, protruding shoulder blade, or tilted head.

After a thorough examination to rule out other problems, the orthopedist diagnoses scoliosis and orders one or more x-rays (see "X-Ray Safety") to determine the type and extent of the curve. (A person with scoliosis may also have other abnormal curvatures, which can be detected by x-ray and treated along with the scoliosis. If the normal rounding of the back is too great, the condition is called "hyperkyphosis." If the normal forward curving in the lower back is too great, the condition is called "hyperlordosis.")

The American Academy of Pediatrics recommends screening for scoliosis during routine doctor visits at ages 10, 12, 14, and 16. The American Academy of Orthopaedic Surgeons and the Scoliosis Research Society recommend screening girls at 10 and 12 and boys once at 13 or 14. Many states have scoliosis screening programs in schools.

Tailored Treatment

Decisions about scoliosis treatment depend on the person's age, gender, general health, and potential for growth, as well as severity and location of the curve.

For a very mild curve, the doctor may only advise monitoring checkups, with x-rays to detect worsening, every three or four months or maybe once a year.

Even moderate curves of 25 to 40 degrees may not warrant treatment, Yahiro says. "If an 18-year-old no longer growing has a 30-degree curve," he says, "I probably would do no more than monitor it. On the other hand, I'd immediately treat such a curve, and often a slighter one, in a 12-year-old just starting the growth spurt."

A severe curve of 40 to 50 degrees or more that's detected early, Yahiro says, would be expected to rapidly get much worse, so he would treat it even more aggressively.

Another important factor is the patient's attitude toward treatment. For instance, Yahiro says, a worsening 35-degree curve that could have been treated with bracing may, in fact, need surgery if the young person refuses to wear a brace.

Bracing for Prevention

A nonsurgical treatment for moderate curves (24 to 40 degrees) is a body brace. Not a cure, bracing is intended to check a curve until growth is completed. It can generally straighten a moderate curve. Unfortunately, as happened with

Bradbard, some curves return after the brace is no longer worn.

Bradbard wore a full torso brace, formed from a cast modeled from her body. It consisted of a molded leather girdle, straps, and a neck ring to hold support bars in position. Together, these parts held Bradbard in a position that kept her rigid from chin to hips. Bolts and buckles permitted adjustments as she grew.

"I wore it day and night for 23 hours from eighth grade through 10th," she says, "only taking it off for gym and showers. After a time, it was just part of me. I played neighborhood baseball and basketball and rode a bike wearing it."

But Bradbard's inability to bend meant she couldn't look down, and she had to adjust for this. "I couldn't see the stairs when I was walking," she says, "and I had to carry a desk frame from class to class to hold my books up where I could see them. I had several frames that had belonged to an older girl in school who didn't need her brace anymore."

Today, molded braces are available that generally don't show under clothing because they fit close and only come up to the underarms. Although underarm braces are effective for lower chest and lower back curves, a full torso brace works best for a high chest curve. Getting a young person to wear a full brace continuously isn't always successful, says Yahiro, "so it's not used as much as it could be."

An alternative treatment is stimulation of muscles alongside the spine during sleep with an electrical muscle stimulator, attached by electrodes placed on the skin. FDA approved stimulators for scoliosis in 1986.

But doctors may not want to use this alternative. One study, sponsored by the Scoliosis Research Society, reported success with bracing, but not stimulation. The study was summarized in the fall-winter 1993 newsletter of the National Scoliosis Foundation, Inc.

Surgery

Of the 30,000 to 70,000 spinal surgery procedures done each year, "about a third are probably for severe scoliosis," says Mark Melkerson, who reviews the medical devices used in these procedures for FDA's orthopedic devices branch. "Depending on the patient's age," he says, "doctors usually start considering surgery when a curve exceeds 40 to 50 degrees, to prevent breathing problems."

The surgeon attaches steel rods to vertebrae at the top and bottom of the curve with hooks, screws or wires, fusing the vertebrae with bone fragments taken from the hips, ribs, or the spine itself. The healed fusions harden in a straightened position, leaving the rest of the spine flexible.

Afterwards, most patients need a brace for about six weeks.

"It usually takes three months for everything to fuse," Yahiro says. "Still, we don't say a fusion has failed until after a year."

Bradbard had corrective surgery five years ago. She'd gone back to the doctor complaining of back pain, and x-rays showed her curve had progressed to 52 degrees.

X-Ray Safety

When teenagers have scoliosis x-rays taken, they (or their parents) can help keep their radiation exposure as low as possible by asking whether exposure-reducing techniques are being used. This is especially important for young women, because developing breast tissue has increased sensitivity to radiation, and repeated exposure in adolescence can increase the risk of breast cancer later on.

In addition to the general practice of narrowing the x-ray beam to the spinal area, the techniques are:

- Attaching a special filter to the x-ray tube that absorbs much of the x-ray beam, reducing exposure by two to five times.
- Using a fast screen-film combination to reduce exposure by two to six times.
- Using breast shields that reduce radiation exposure to breast tissue by three to 10 times. These include the x-ray tube shield that shades the breasts; a lead vest or stole-like garment with a lead insert, worn if x-rays are taken with the patient facing the x-ray machine; or facing away from the x-ray machine so that the x-rays enter the body from behind, and the body shields the breasts.
- Combinations of these methods.

Since someone past adolescence is no longer growing, why would a scoliosis curve worsen?

Yahiro says that doctors don't yet have a complete answer, but they do know that when the spine is already severely curved, the person's weight is distributed across the abnormal curve. Over time, this stress may make the curve worse.

Before Bradbard's surgery, her right hip and ribs practically sat on each other, she says, so that she essentially had no waist. Afterwards, she suddenly was 2 inches taller, thanks to straightening with 8 inches of rods and a fused spine.

"For the longest time," she says, "I kept hitting my head when I'd get in or out of the car."

When corrective surgery is done *before* growth is completed, Yahiro says, the patient both gains height from the straightening and loses height from the fusions, which stop growth. The gain and loss tend to cancel each other out, he says.

Bradbard's recovery required two weeks in the hospital. But with help, she was sitting for short periods by the second day, and standing for short periods by the third. Unlike patients undergoing scoliosis surgery 15 years ago, Bradbard didn't have to lie in a body cast for months. She didn't even have to wear a brace, though it took a full year before muscle strength returned.

The lower end of her curve couldn't be corrected, or she wouldn't be able to bend at all. As a result, one leg is a quarter of an inch shorter, which she compensates for by wearing a heel lift in her shoe.

The corrective method her surgeon used is called Cotrel-Dubousset, one of several newer systems for attaching rods to the spine with hooks and screws. Researchers report Cotrel-Dubousset has less than 2 percent loss of correction, compared with 10 to 25 percent loss from the older (Harrington Rod) system. The older system allowed the hooks to rotate, so a body cast was needed to prevent their movement until fusion.

"With many of the newer systems," Melkerson says, "the hooks are rigidly fixed to resist rotation."

Like any surgery, a scoliosis operation can have complications, such as infection or a bad reaction to anesthesia. Additional risks, though rare, are possibly dislodging a hook, fracturing a fused vertebra, or damaging the spinal cord.

Someone facing possible scoliosis surgery should ask the doctor to explain how it will help and how it poses risks, which vary with the patient and method of surgery.

For More Information

American Academy of Orthopaedic Surgeons
6300 N River Rd
Rosemont, IL 60018-4262
(1-800) 346-2267

National Scoliosis Foundation, Inc.
72 Mt Auburn St
Watertown, MA 02172
(617) 926-0390

Scoliosis Research Society
6300 N River Rd, Ste 727
Rosemont, IL 60018-4226
(708) 698-1627

The Scoliosis Association, Inc.
PO Box 811705
Boca Raton, FL 33481-1705
(1-800) 800-0669

■ **Document Source:**
U.S. Department of Health and Human Services, Public Health Service
Food and Drug Administration
FDA Consumer
July-August 1994

GETTING TO KNOW GOUT

by Ken Fliege

Say the word **gout** and some people will think of a bloated king surveying the remains of a sumptuous feast, wine glass in hand, swollen foot propped on a pillow—looking for all the world like the dismal product of a grossly overindulgent life.

There are a couple of flaws in that conventional image. We know, for example, that gout doesn't afflict only the privileged classes and that women, too, are susceptible, though a lot less than men.

But still there's a good deal right with that picture. It correctly reflects that:

• About 90 percent of people afflicted with gout are men over 40.
• Obesity in general, and in particular excessive weight gain in men between ages 20 and 40, has been shown to increase the risk of gout. In fact, about half of all gout sufferers are overweight.

• Alcohol abuse and so-called "binge" drinking are associated with gout, as is eating purine-rich foods such as brains, kidneys, liver, sardines, anchovies, and dried beans and peas.

In addition, careful scientific surveys have shown that occupational exposure to lead, the use of certain drugs to control high blood pressure, some surgical procedures, family history (possibly a genetic predisposition), and trauma are all linked to an increased risk of gout. Indeed, the prevalence of gout—the number of gout sufferers for each 100,000 people—is rising rapidly in the United States and other developed countries. Some authorities believe the increase is related to higher living standards.

Our fanciful image of a gouty Henry VIII (or other bloated monarch) can't show, however, the one common denominator that ties together this mixed bag of risk factors: failure of the metabolic process that controls the amount of uric acid in the blood. For most people, the process works just fine. But in some one million Americans, uric acid metabolism has gone seriously haywire. As a result, they suffer from gout.

And suffer they do. An Englishman, Thomas Sydenham, writing in the 17th century, left this unfortunately all-too-accurate description of a typical attack of gout:

> The victim goes to bed . . . in good health. About two o'clock in the morning, he is awakened by a severe pain in the great toe; more rarely in the heel, ankle, or instep. The pain is like that of a dislocation. [It] becomes more intense . . . . So exquisite and lively meanwhile is the feeling of the part affected, that it cannot bear the weight of the bed-clothes nor the jar of a person walking in the room. The night is passed in torture . . . .

A Crystal Culprit

In spite of the agony and havoc it can cause, uric acid is a normal constituent of the human body. Ordinarily about one-third of the uric acid in our system comes from food, especially foods like those noted earlier that are rich in purines. The rest we produce ourselves through ordinary metabolism.

The body converts purines to uric acid. The level of uric acid in the blood fluctuates in response to diet, fluid intake, overall health status, and other factors. Men normally have somewhat more uric acid than women do (although the difference begins to narrow after menopause), and in both sexes it tends to increase with advancing age.

Higher-than-normal amounts of uric acid in the blood, a condition called hyperuricemia, is quite common and only rarely warrants medical treatment. On the other hand, sustained hyperuricemia is the primary risk factor for gout. It's safe to say that, while not all people with hyperuricemia develop gout, virtually everyone with gout is hyperuricemic. It works this way:

At normal and even somewhat elevated levels, uric acid stays in solution in the blood. It moves through the circulation, gets filtered by the kidneys, and is excreted in the urine. When, however, blood uric acid levels rise above a certain concentration (which varies with temperature and blood acidity), it forms needle-like crystals that lodge in or around a joint.

In response to irritation caused by uric acid crystals, the skin covering the affected area rapidly becomes tight, inflamed, swollen, and red or purplish. These classical signs of inflammation, together with sudden and extreme pain (just as Thomas Sydenham described), strongly suggest an acute attack of gout. The diagnosis is confirmed by laboratory finding of uric acid crystals in fluid taken from the affected joint.

Why is the big toe the most common site for an initial gout attack? Perhaps because first, the extremities are a bit cooler than other parts of the body, and uric acid crystals form more readily at lower temperatures; and second, normal walking and standing subject the feet to considerable stress. Together, these factors might explain why the big toe, heel, instep, and Achilles tendon are among the places that gout attacks first. Other targets, especially in untreated patients who have recurrent attacks of gout, are the knee, elbow, wrist, fingers and, less often, the shoulder, pelvis, spine, and internal organs.

Gout is classified as a form of arthritis because it is initially and predominantly a disease of the joints. Other similar conditions exist; one called "pseudogout" is somewhat milder than true gout and is caused by calcium rather than uric acid crystals. Infection or trauma to the affected area can mimic gout and mislead both patients and health professionals. Accurate diagnosis is essential for appropriate treatment.

Without treatment, an initial acute attack of gout will run its painful course within several days or a few weeks, by which time all outward evidence of the disease disappears. The next acute attack—50 or more percent of gout sufferers will have a second attack—may not occur for months or years. Subsequent attacks, however, are likely to be more frequent, more severe, and more destructive to joints and other tissue unless the problem is treated. Over time, uric acid crystals accumulate in the body, causing gritty, chalky deposits called tophi that are sometimes visible under the skin, particularly around joints and in the edges of the ears. Tophi may also form inside bone near the joints, in the kidneys, and in other organs and tissues, causing permanent damage. Advances in treatment, fortunately, have made this kind of chronic gout extremely rare.

Treatment

As with most illnesses, effective treatment of gout depends on a correct diagnosis. Gout can be unequivocally diagnosed by telltale uric acid crystals in joint fluid. But appropriate treatment is often started after a "clinical" diagnosis based on painfully obvious signs and symptoms and other relevant factors, such as the patient's uric acid level, age, weight, gender, diet, and alcohol use. If this picture adds up to a strong suspicion of gout, treatment can be started with the immediate goal of arresting the acute attack.

Acute gout is treated with drugs that block the inflammatory reaction. One of the oldest agents known to be effective against acute gout is colchicine, which comes from a common European plant, the autumn crocus, and is marketed in this country primarily as a generic drug. An English clergyman,

Sidney Smith, said a century and a half ago that he had only to go into his garden and hold out his gouty toe to the plant to obtain a prompt cure. This may have been an exaggeration, but a rapid response to colchicine suggests that the patient does indeed have gout.

This old, powerful remedy is now used less often than it once was because it can be quite toxic, causing nausea, vomiting, diarrhea, and stomach cramps when taken by mouth and severe (even fatal) blood disorders when taken intravenously. Moreover, modern agents, specifically nonsteroidal anti-inflammatory drugs (NSAIDs) are highly effective against acute gout and less toxic than colchicine. To treat an acute case of gout, the first choice of many physicians is the NSAID Indocin (and other brands of indomethacin). Naprosyn (naproxen) is another NSAID commonly used in acute gout.

Steroid drugs, such as Deltasone (and other brands of prednisone) and Acthar (and other brands of adrenocorticotropic hormone), may be used if NSAIDs fail to control an acute attack. Steroids may be taken by mouth or by injection into the bloodstream or muscle.

Drug treatment usually relieves the symptoms of acute gout within 48 hours. Subsequent treatment, which may well be lifelong, is aimed at preventing further attacks by controlling uric acid in the blood—keeping it below concentrations at which crystals can form. Two main treatment approaches are used, in some cases simultaneously.

One approach is to slow the rate at which the body produces uric acid. Zyloprim (allopurinol) has been approved for the treatment of gout and is frequently prescribed for gout patients who have uric acid kidney stones or other kidney problems. Side effects include skin rash and upset stomach, both of which usually subside as the body becomes used to the drug. Zyloprim makes some patients drowsy, so they need to be cautious about driving or using machinery.

The other approach to controlling gout following an initial acute attack is to increase the amount of uric acid excreted in urine. Two so-called uricosuric drugs commonly used for this are Benemid (probenecid) and Anturane (sulfinpyrazone), both approved by FDA for gout treatment. In addition to lowering blood uric acid levels, these drugs help dissolve deposits of uric acid crystals around joints and in other tissue. Zyloprim is also used to dissolve tophaceous gout in uric acid over-producers. Uricosurics can cause nausea, stomach upset, headache, and a potentially serious skin rash.

Drugs to control uric acid levels may, paradoxically, prolong an acute attack. For this reason, Benemid, Anturane and Zyloprim are not used during the acute stage of gout. They may, in fact, induce gout flare-ups during the early part of long-term use. Accordingly, colchicine in a dose low enough to avoid toxic side effects is sometimes prescribed to prevent acute attacks during this phase of treatment.

Common-Sense Measures

Better understanding of what gout is, what causes it, and how to treat it has perhaps dispelled some of the traditional myths about what has been erroneously called "the disease of kings." Then, too, folk wisdom about gout, coupled with good science and medicine, points to measures that prudent people can take to prevent or at least lessen the severity of the condition.

Many authorities and the Arthritis Foundation, which supports research and public service programs relating to gout, advocate weight control as a logical aid to gout prevention. They point out, however, that people who are overweight should get professional guidance in planning a weight-reduction program, because fasting or severe dieting can actually increase uric acid levels.

Experts generally agree that people with gout can eat pretty much what they want, within limits. People who have kidney stones caused by uric acid may need to avoid purine-rich foods. But this problem can usually be handled effectively with drug treatment.

Curbing alcohol use and avoiding "binge" drinking can reduce the likelihood of acute attacks. So can drinking six or eight glasses of water a day, which dilutes uric acid and aids its removal by the kidneys. Some medicines—in particular the thiazide diuretics ("water pills") used to control high blood pressure—tend to increase uric acid levels. A gout patient taking one of these drugs may have to switch to another type of diuretic or blood pressure medicine.

Finally, although uncommon, it might be helpful to find out if an environmental or occupational exposure to lead is playing a role in a patient's problem with gout.

While a cure for gout—a treatment that gets rid of the condition once and for all—isn't on the horizon, reliable and effective ways of diagnosing gout and keeping it under control constitute one of the more impressive success stories of modern medical science.

There may be no sure-fire way to keep a person from having that first agonizing attack, but prompt treatment can minimize the risk of further attacks and virtually rule out the damaging and crippling effects of chronic gouty arthritis.

■ U.S. Department of Health and Human Services, Public Health Service
Food and Drug Administration
FDA Consumer
March 1995

LUPUS ERYTHEMATOSUS: WHAT IS LUPUS?

*Adapted from **Lupus Erythematosus**, edited by Daniel J. Wallace and Bevra Hannahs Hahn, 1993.*

What is lupus erythematosus?

LE usually appears in one of two forms: Discoid, or cutaneous lupus erythematosus (the skin form, called discoid LE) or systemic lupus erythematosus (the internal form, called systemic LE or SLE).

Discoid (or chronic cutaneous) LE has a particular type of skin rash with raised, red, scaly areas, often with healing in the centers or with scars. These eruptions are seen most commonly on the face and other light-exposed areas. Usually, patients with discoid LE have normal internal organs. A skin biopsy of the lesion may be helpful in confirming the diagnosis.

Subacute cutaneous lupus erythematosus is a non-scarring subset of lupus that is characterized by distinct immunologic abnormalities and some systemic features.

Systemic lupus erythematosus is classified as one of the autoimmune rheumatic diseases, in the same family as rheumatoid arthritis, and is usually considered a chronic, systemic, inflammatory disease of connective tissue. *Chronic* means that the condition lasts for a long period of time. *Inflammatory* describes the body's reaction to irritation with pain and swelling. LE involves changes in the immune system, so that elements of the system attack the body's own tissues. The organs effects are different in each person. Joints are usually inflamed. Inflammation can also involve the skin, kidney, blood cells, brain, heart, lung, and blood vessels. The inflammation can be controlled by medication.

SLE can be a mild condition but, because it can affect joints, skin, kidneys, blood, heart, lungs, and other internal organs, it can appear in different forms and with different intensities at different times in the same person. A large number of people with SLE have few symptoms and can live a nearly normal life. Therefore, while reading about the symptoms, you should not become unnecessarily worried, because all the symptoms probably do not occur in one person.

How serious lupus is varies greatly from a mild to a life-threatening condition. It depends on what parts of the body are affected. Even a mild case can become more serious if it is not properly treated. (The results are usually good with use of the more recently developed medicines.) The severity of your LE should be discussed with your physician.

LE is not infectious or contagious. It is not a type of cancer or malignancy. LE is not related to acquired immunodeficiency syndrome (AIDS).

What causes lupus erythematosus?

The cause of discoid LE is unknown. In most cases, the cause of SLE is also unknown, although it is believed that many factors may be involved, including genetic predisposition and environmental factors such as excessive sun exposure, certain medicines, and infections. In families of SLE patients, it is known that there is an increase in the number of relatives with SLE and rheumatoid arthritis compared with the normal population. Many of the relatives have abnormal proteins in their blood, such as antinuclear antibodies, although they may not have any symptoms of the disease.

Some of the genes that increase a person's risk for SLE are known. For example, in the United States, a gene called DR2 increases a person's risk of developing lupus nephritis, although the vast majority of individuals with the gene are healthy.

Many researchers suspect that a special type of immune reaction causes the disease. It is believed that patients develop antibodies against their own tissues, as if vaccinated against themselves. These antibodies are known as autoantibodies (auto means self), and the type of allergy is called *autoimmu-*

nity, or an allergy against oneself. Some of us possess lupus "genes." Certain viruses, drugs, chemicals in the environment, or extreme emotional stress might activate the gene. This gene encodes antibodies and/or other products that damage tissue, the net effect of which results in the white blood cells' (lymphocytes) surveillance system ultimately stimulating the formation of antibodies. Still, the basic question that remains unanswered is what events set off the mechanism that causes antibodies to be produced against one's own tissues. Answering this question may be an important step toward preventing and curing LE.

In perhaps 10% of patients with SLE, the disease may have been caused by medicine. The most common is procainamide (Pronestyl), which is often used to treat heart irregularities. It is essential that your physician be told of all medications you are taking, including birth control pills and estrogens for menopause.

Diagnosis of Lupus Erythematosus

The skin rash of discoid LE may be so typical that an experienced physician can make the diagnosis by the history and appearance of the rash. If there is any question, a skin biopsy usually helps. It is essential that each patient with discoid LE have a thorough physical examination, including laboratory tests, to check the possibility of systemic LE being present.

Diagnosing systemic LE is more difficult. Finding definite answers may take months of observation, many laboratory tests, and sometimes a trial of drugs. Because of many different symptoms, some patients are thought to have another disease, rheumatoid arthritis, with swelling of a few or many joints of the hands, feet, ankles, or wrists. If typical skin lesions are present, they are helpful in making the diagnosis. Other findings, such as fever, pleurisy (painful breathing), or kidney disease also point to the diagnosis of SLE.

In addition to a complete medical history and physical examination, routine tests are done to learn what internal organs are involved—for example, a blood count to see if there are too few red cells, white cells, or platelets (cells that are necessary for clotting). A routine analysis of the urine is always done and often a kidney function test, using all urine passed in a 24-hour period, is necessary. A chest x-ray and electrocardiogram may be recommended if clinical evidence of problems in the lung or heart is found.

To help confirm the diagnosis, special tests for SLE are performed that measure blood antibodies. These include examinations for antinuclear antibody (ANA), which is the most sensitive test for the disease. Serum complement (a protein that is decreased during active phases of autoimmune illness) is often measured. Anti-DNA antibody is a specific type of antinuclear antibody that is often present in the blood of SLE patients. Its presence is helpful in confirming the diagnosis of SLE. Moreover, when the disease is active, especially if the kidneys are affected in SLE, anti-DNA antibodies are usually present in high amounts in the blood. Thus, tests for anti-DNA antibody can be useful in monitoring disease activity in SLE. Again, none of these tests is specific for SLE. Different medical centers may use other diagnostic tests, depending on their individual experience. For example, the LE cell test is fairly specific for the disease but is technically difficult to perform. A small percentage of people without disease have positive ANA tests; consequently, obtaining such a result does not confirm the diagnosis of SLE. All tests must be evaluated by the physician in regard to the signs and symptoms of the patient.

Some patients with a negative ANA may still have SLE. Usually, these patients have anti-Ro/SSA antibody or a positive, nonlesional skin biopsy using immunofluorescence (lupus band test). Discoid LE patients often have a negative ANA and positive lesional lupus band test or typical light microscopic findings.

One problem in diagnosis is that there is no single set of symptoms or pattern of disease. Also, SLE can mimic symptoms of many other diseases and can strike many different parts of the body, sometimes confusing even the most experienced physicians. One out of six patients may have a false-positive blood test for syphilis as one of the first symptoms of LE. This is frequently found during a routine premarital examination, but does not mean that the patient has venereal disease or that there is any relationship between syphilis and SLE. This test is associated with the lupus anticoagulant and anticardiolipin antibody.

Symptoms and Course of Lupus Erythematosus

Symptoms of systemic LE are varied, and no two patients have exactly the same ones. Any part of the body can be involved, so symptoms may include one or more of these in any combination: joint and muscle pain, fever, skin rashes, chest pain, swelling of hands and feet, and hair loss. Joint involvement in SLE is usually less severe than that occurring in rheumatoid arthritis, and is usually nondeforming. You should remember that, in most patients, most of the symptoms disappear. This clearing of symptoms is called a remission. Medications are usually necessary to cause remissions, but sometimes they occur spontaneously—that is without treatment.

Physicians use the term "remission" or "controlled" rather than "cure" in speaking of the periods when patients are free of symptoms because both physician and patients can then be watchful for signs and symptoms, which may be a warning that a flare is beginning. Treatment can then be started, before unnecessary damage occurs.

Generalized aching, weakness, tiring easily, low-grade fever, and chills are commonly associated with active SLE. Although these symptoms are usually particularly noticeable during flare-ups of the disease, some patients give a life-long history of low energy, malaise (generalized discomfort), and inability to keep up an active work schedule. A low-grade rise in temperature (99.5 to 100.5 F), usually in the late afternoon, may be a sign of smoldering LE activity, and may appear several days before the patient feels really ill. In the patient with systemic LE, the loss of energy, development of weakness, low-grade fever, or tiring easily are each considered to be danger signs. They may indicate that new activity of the disease is developing. When any of these early warning signs develop, patients should consult their physician immediately, so that examination may be made and further treatment prescribed, if necessary.

Frequency of Lupus Erythematosus

No one has made an accurate estimate of the number of patients with discoid LE because many people have mild cases and probably don't know it. There may be as many as 1,000,000 people with systemic LE in the United States.

The number of new cases of systemic LE diagnosed by physicians is definitely increasing, for several reasons. After the LE cell test came into use, physicians were able to diagnose the illness correctly in patients who were believed to have other rheumatic diseases, or who were thought to have "neurotic" complaints. Tests for antinuclear and other antibodies, which are usually positive in systemic LE, have helped physicians discover even more patients with milder cases, but the test might be positive in patients without SLE. It has also been learned that certain medications, like procainamide (Pronestyl) and a number of other drugs, may cause systemic LE. Patients with this type of drug-caused lupus usually improve dramatically after stopping the offending medication. Therefore, some of the increase in the number of cases of LE is the result of better recognition by physicians, and some may be the result of increasing toxic changes in our environment, with greater exposure to drugs, chemicals, and possibly triggering agents.

Many patients have combined symptoms of SLE, scleroderma (thickening and hardening of the skin), and polymyositis (inflammation of muscles). These combinations may be called mixed connective tissue disease (MCTD), or cross-over or overlap syndrome, depending on certain laboratory features.

Seven of ten patients with discoid LE are women, half of them developing their first symptoms between the ages of 15 and 30 years. LE is rare in children under the age of five. It is found throughout the world, and affects all ethnic groups and religions.

SLE is more common than rheumatic fever, leukemia, cystic fibrosis, muscular dystrophy, multiple sclerosis, hemophilia, and several other well-known diseases.

For the address of the representative or Lupus Support Group near you, please contact the headquarters of

Lupus Foundation of America, Inc
1300 Piccard Dr, Ste 200
Rockville, MD 20850
(301) 670-9292
(800) 558-0121
(301) 670-9486 (FAX)

or

260 Maple Court, Ste 123
Ventura, CA 93003
(805) 339-0443
(800) 331-1802

■ **Document Source:**
Lupus Foundation of America, Inc
260 Maple Court, Suite 123
Ventura, California 93003
May 1996

OSTEOPOROSIS: A WOMAN'S GUIDE

Osteoporosis is a disease in which the skeleton becomes so weakened that the slightest injury can cause a broken bone. Many bones become more brittle and susceptible to fracture. Most typical are fractures of the hip and wrist and collapse or crush fractures of the spine, which can produce deformity and loss of height.

This painful, disfiguring and disabling disease is a major threat to 25 million Americans, 80 percent of whom are women. In the U.S. alone, 7-8 million people have osteoporosis, 17 million more have low bone mass, placing them at increased risk for the disease. Osteoporosis is the most common cause of hip fracture, a tragedy that can result in permanent disability, loss of independence, or death.

While it is normal to lose bone tissue gradually as you age, osteoporosis involves a degree of loss that endangers your health. This exaggerated loss of bone tissue produces no symptoms or warning signs until fractures occur. **Osteoporosis: A Woman's Guide,** will help you understand what you can do to reduce bone loss and prevent osteoporosis. If you already have osteoporosis, you should know that you can decrease your chances of breaking a bone.

Building Strong Bones

You may think of bone as hard and lifeless when, in fact, bone is complex, living tissue. Our bones provide structural support for muscles, protect vital organs, and store the calcium essential for bone density and strength.

Because bones are constantly changing, they can heal and may be affected by diet and exercise. Until the age of about 35, you build and store bone efficiently. Then, as part of the natural aging process, your bones begin to break down faster than new bone can be formed. Bone loss accelerates after menopause, when your ovaries stop producing estrogen—the hormone that protects against bone loss.

Think of your bones as a savings account. There is only as much bone mass in your account as you deposit. The critical years for building bone mass are prior to age 30. Some experts believe that young women can increase their bone mass by as much as 20 percent—a critical factor in protecting against osteoporosis.

Are you at risk?

There are many factors that determine who will develop osteoporosis. The first step in prevention is to determine whether you are at risk, since not everyone is. The risk factors are:

Age. The older you are, the greater your risk of osteoporosis. Your bones become less dense and weaker as you age.

Gender. Your chances of developing osteoporosis are greater if you are a woman. Women have less bone tissue and lose bone more rapidly than men because of the changes involved in menopause.

Race. Caucasian and Asian women are more likely to develop osteoporosis. However, African American and Hispanic women are at significant risk for developing the disease.

Bone Structure and Body Weight. Small-boned, thin women are at greater risk.

Menopause. Normal or early menopause (brought about naturally or because of surgery), increases your risk of developing osteoporosis. In addition, women who stop menstruating before menopause because of conditions such as anorexia or bulimia, or because of excessive physical exercise, may also lose bone tissue more rapidly than normal.

Lifestyle. By smoking, drinking too much alcohol, consuming an inadequate amount of calcium, or getting little or no weight-bearing exercise, you increase your chances of developing osteoporosis.

Medications and Disease. Osteoporosis is associated with certain medications (e.g., cortisone-like drugs), and is a recognized complication of a number of medical conditions, including endocrine disorders (having an overactive thyroid), rheumatoid arthritis, and immobilization.

Family History. Susceptibility to fracture may be, in part hereditary. Young women whose mothers have a history of vertebral fractures also seem to have reduced bone mass.

Preventing Osteoporosis

There is much you can do to protect yourself against osteoporosis and help yourself to better overall health at the same time

Estrogen

In national and international research conferences sponsored by the National Osteoporosis Foundation and the National Institutes of Health, experts recommended estrogen replacement therapy (ERT) for women at high risk for osteoporosis. ERT is especially recommended for women whose ovaries were removed before age 50. ERT should also be considered by women who have experienced natural menopause and have multiple osteoporosis risk factors, such as an early menopause, a blood relative with osteoporosis, or below normal bone mass for her age. ERT is not without risks. Because individual circumstances differ, you must discuss the pros and cons of estrogen replacement therapy with your doctor.

Diet

Making sure you get an adequate amount of calcium may help in protecting you against osteoporosis. The Foundation recommends that non-pregnant adults obtain 1,000 milligrams (mg) of elemental calcium each day to help maintain strong bones. For individuals at risk for osteoporosis, calcium intake should be increased to 1,500 mg a day.

Recent studies indicate that many adults get only half or less of their daily calcium requirement. An 8-ounce glass of whole or skim milk, 1 1/2 ounces of cheddar cheese, 2 cups of cottage cheese, and 1 cup of yogurt each contain an estimated 300 mg of calcium—nearly one-third of the recommended daily allowance before menopause. As you increase your calcium intake, try to eat foods that are low in fat. Keep track of your daily calcium intake for a week and discuss this record with your doctor. If your diet doesn't contain enough of this vital nutrient, supplement your intake with calcium tablets. Ask your doctor or pharmacist to recommend a supplement which is well absorbed by your body. If you're ill or if you've had kidney stones, talk to your doctor before taking any supplements.

Exercise

Weight-bearing exercise (e.g., walking, stairclimbing, and jogging) can help prevent osteoporosis. If you are older and have not been exercising regularly, check with your doctor before embarking on a more ambitious exercise program.

Vitamin D

You need normal levels of vitamin D to absorb calcium. Your body manufactures this vitamin as a result of exposure to sunlight, and it is also available in vitamin-enriched milk products. Too much vitamin D is harmful, so don't decide to take supplements without first consulting your doctor. However, you can safely take 400 units (the recommended daily allowance) in a multivitamin.

The Silent Thief

Osteoporosis has been called the "silent thief" because there are no early warning signs and few outward indications of the disease until a fracture occurs.

By using special methods, it is now possible to measure bone density in those areas subject to fracture. Medical experts agree that bone mass measurement tests are best used in conjunction with a complete clinical assessment and risk factor survey. A single measurement of bone mass around time of menopause may be helpful in deciding whether to initiate a treatment program. Your doctor can advise you whether and when you should be tested.

If You Have Osteoporosis

There are steps you can take to slow its progress.

Experts recommend 1,000 mg of calcium a day for women undergoing estrogen replacement therapy and 1,500 mg of calcium daily for women not receiving estrogen therapy.

Women with established osteoporosis who cannot take estrogen may be able to use calcitonin or alendronate. Nasal or injectable calcitonin is a hormone that has been shown to reduce bone loss. Alendronate, a bisphosphonate, has been shown to slow bone loss, increase bone density and reduce the risk of fractures. Both medications are approved by the Food and Drug Administration for the treatment of osteoporosis.

While exercise is good for someone with osteoporosis, it should not put any sudden or excessive strain on your bones. As extra insurance against fractures, your doctor can recommend specific exercises to strengthen and support your back.

Fall Prevention

If you have osteoporosis, it's important to minimize your chances of breaking a bone. This safety checklist can help you eliminate many common fracture hazards.

Floors. Remove all loose wires, cords, and throw rugs. Minimize clutter. Make sure rugs are anchored and smooth. Keep furniture in its accustomed place.

Bathrooms. Install grab bars and non-skid tape in the tub or shower.

Lighting. Make sure halls, stairways, and entrances are well lit. Install a night light in your bathroom. Turn lights on if you get up in the middle of the night.

Kitchen. Install non-skid rubber mats near sink and stove. Clean spills immediately.

Stairs. Make sure treads, rails, and rugs are secure.

Other Precautions. Wear sturdy, rubber-soled shoes. Keep your intake of alcoholic beverages to a minimum. Ask your doctor whether any of your medications might cause you to fall.

For more information on osteoporosis, contact the National Osteoporosis Foundation.
1150 17th St NW, Ste 500
Washington, DC 20036-4603
(202) 223-2226
(800) 223-9994

■ **Document Source:**
 National Osteoporosis Foundation
 1150 17th St NW, Ste 500
 Washington, DC 20036-4603

UNDERSTANDING ACUTE LOW BACK PROBLEMS

About the Back and Back Problems

The human spine (or backbone) is made up of small bones called vertebrae. The vertebrae are stacked on top of each other to form a column. Between each vertebra is a cushion known as a disc. The vertebrae are held together by ligaments, and muscles are attached to the vertebrae by bands of tissue called tendons.

Openings in each vertebra line up to form a long hollow canal. The spinal cord runs through this canal from the base of the brain. Nerves from the spinal cord branch out and leave the spine through the spaces between the vertebrae.

The lower part of the back holds most of the body's weight. Even a minor problem with the bones, muscles, ligaments, or tendons in this area can cause pain when a person stands, bends or moves around. Less often, a problem with a disc can pinch or irritate a nerve from the spinal cord, causing pain that runs down the leg, below the knee called sciatica.

Purpose

This booklet is about acute low back problems in adults. If you have a low back problem, you may have symptoms that include

- pain or discomfort in the lower part of the back
- pain or numbness that moves down the leg (sciatica)

Low back symptoms can keep you from doing your normal daily activities or doing things that you enjoy.

> A low back problem may come on suddenly or gradually. It is **acute** if it lasts a short while, usually a few days to several weeks. An episode that lasts longer than three months is not acute.

If you have been bothered by your lower back, you are not alone. Eight out of ten adults will have a low back problem at some time in their life. And most will have more than one episode of acute low back problems. In between episodes, most people return to their normal activities with little or no symptoms.

This booklet will tell you more about acute low back problems, what to do, and what to expect when you see a health care provider.

Causes of Low Back Problems

Even with today's technology, the exact reason or cause of low back problems can be found in very few people. Most times, the symptoms are blamed on poor muscle tone in the back, muscle tension or spasm, back sprains, ligament or muscle tears, joint problems. Sometimes nerves from the spinal cord can be irritated by "slipped" discs causing buttock or leg pain. This may also cause numbness, tingling, or weakness in the legs.

People who are in poor physical condition or do work that includes heavy labor or long periods of sitting or standing are at greater risk for low back problems. These people also get better more slowly. Emotional stress or long periods of inactivity may make back symptoms seem worse.

Low back problems are often painful. But the good news is that very few people turn out to have a major problem with the bones or joints of the back or a dangerous medical condition.

Things to Do About Low Back Problems

Seeing a Health Care Provider

Many people who develop mild low back discomfort may not need to see a health care provider right away. Often, within a few days, the symptoms go away without any treatment.

A visit to your health care provider is a good idea if

- your symptoms are severe

- the pain is keeping you from doing things that you do every day
- the problem does not go away within a few days

If you also have problems controlling your bowel or bladder, if you feel numb in the groin or rectal area, or if there is extreme leg weakness, call your health care provider right away.

Your health care provider will check to see if you have a medical illness causing your back problem (chances are you will not). Your health care provider can also help you get some relief from your symptoms.

Your health care provider will

- ask about your symptoms and what they keep you from doing
- ask about your medical history
- give you a physical exam

Talking About Your Symptoms

Your health care provider will want to know about your back problem. Here are some examples of the kinds of questions he or she may ask you.

- When did you back symptoms start?
- Which of your daily activities are you not able to do because of your back symptoms?
- Is there anything you do that makes the symptoms better or worse?
- Have you noticed any problem with your legs?
- Around the time your symptoms began, did you have a fever or symptoms of pain or burning when urinating?

Talking About Your Medical History

Be sure to tell your health care provider about your general health and about illnesses you have had in the past. Here are some questions your health care provider may ask you about your medical history.

- Have you had a problem with your back in the past? If so, when?
- What medical illnesses have you had (for example, cancer, arthritis, or diseases of the immune system)?
- Which medicines do you take regularly?
- Have you ever used intravenous (IV) drugs?
- Have you recently lost weight without trying?

You should also tell your health care provider about anything you may be doing for your symptoms: medicines you are taking, creams or ointments you are using, and other home remedies.

Having a Physical Exam

Your health care provider will examine your back. Even after a careful physical examination, it may not be possible for your health care provider to tell you the exact cause of your low back problem. But you most likely will find out that your symptoms are not being caused by a dangerous medical condition. Very few people (about 1 in 200) have low back symptoms caused by such conditions. You probably won't need special tests if you have had low back symptoms for only a few weeks.

Getting Relief

Your health care provider will help you get relief from your pain, discomfort, or other symptoms. A number of medicines and other treatments help with low back symptoms. The good news is that most people start feeling better soon.

Proven Treatments

Medicine often helps relieve low back symptoms. The type of medicine that your health care provider recommends depends on your symptoms and how uncomfortable you are.

- If your symptoms are mild to moderate, you may get the relief you need from an over-the-counter (non-prescription) medicine such as acetaminophen, aspirin, or ibuprofen. These medicines usually have fewer side effects than prescription medicines and are less expensive.
- If your symptoms are severe, your health care provider may recommend a prescription medicine.

For most people, medicine works well to control pain and discomfort. But any medicine can have side effects. For example, some people cannot take aspirin of ibuprofen because it can cause stomach irritation and even ulcers. Many medicines prescribed for low back pain can make people feel drowsy. These medicines should not be taken if you need to drive or use heavy equipment. Talk to your health care provider about the benefits and risks of any medicine recommended. If you develop side effects (such as nausea, vomiting, rash, dizziness), stop taking the medicine, and tell your health care provider right away.

Your health care provider may recommend one or more of the following to be used alone or along with medicine to help relieve your symptoms.

- **Heat or cold applied to the back.** Within the first 48 hours after your back symptoms start, you may want to apply a cold pack (or a bag of ice) to the painful area for 5 to 10 minutes at a time. If your symptoms last longer than 48 hours, you may find that a heating pad or hot shower or bath helps relieve your symptoms.
- **Spinal manipulation.** This treatment (using the hands to apply force to the back to "adjust" the spine) can be helpful for some people in the first month of low back symptoms. It should only be done by a professional with experience in manipulation. You should go back to your health care provider if your symptoms have not responded to spinal manipulation within four weeks.

Keep in mind that everyone is different. You will have to find what works best to relieve your own back symptoms.

Other Treatments

A number of other treatments are sometimes used for low back symptoms. While these treatments may give relief for a short time, none have been found to speed recovery or keep acute back problems from returning. They may also be expensive. Such treatments include

- traction
- TENS (transcutaneous electrical nerve stimulation)
- massage
- biofeedback
- acupuncture
- injections into the back
- back corsets
- ultrasound

Physical Activity

Your health care provider will want to know about the physical demands of your life (your job or daily activities). Until you feel better, your health care provider may need to recommend some changes in your activities. You will want to talk to your health care provider about your own personal situation. In general, when pain is severe, you should avoid

- heavy lifting
- lifting when twisting
- sitting for long periods of time

The most important goal is for you to return to your normal activities as soon as it is safe. Your health care provider and (if you work) your employer can help you decide how much you are able to do safely at work. Your schedule can be gradually increased as your back improves.

Bed Rest

If your symptoms are severe, your health care provider may recommend a short period of bed rest. However, bed rest should be limited to two or three days. Lying down for longer periods may weaken muscles and bones and actually slow your recovery. If you feel that you must lie down, be sure to get up every few hours and walk around—even if it hurts. Feeling a little discomfort as you return to normal activity is common and does not mean that you are hurting yourself.

About Work and Family

Back problems take time to get better. If your job or your normal daily activities make your back pain worse, it is important to communicate this to your family, supervisor, and coworkers. Put your energy into doing those things at work and at home that you are able to do comfortably. Be productive, but be clear about those tasks that you are not able to do.

Things You Can Do Now

While waiting for your back to improve, you may be able to make yourself more comfortable if you do the following:

- Wear comfortable, low-heeled shoes.
- Make sure your work surface is at a comfortable height for you.
- Use a chair with a good lower back support that may recline slightly.
- If you must sit for long periods of time, try resting your feet on the floor or on a low stool, whichever is more comfortable.
- If you must stand for long periods of time, try resting one foot on a low stool.
- If you must drive long distances, try using a pillow or rolled-up towel behind the small of your back. Also, be sure to stop often and walk around for a few minutes.
- If you have trouble sleeping, try sleeping on your back with a pillow under your knees, or sleep on your side with your knees bent and a pillow between your knees.

Exercises

A gradual return to normal activities, including exercise, is recommended. Exercise is important to your overall health and can help you to lose body fat (if needed). Even if you have mild to moderate low back symptoms, the following things can be done without putting much stress on your back:

- walking short distances
- using a stationary bicycle
- swimming

It is important to start any exercise program slowly and to gradually build up the speed and length of time that you do the exercise. At first, you may find that your symptoms get a little worse when you exercise or become more active. Usually, this is nothing to worry about. However, if your pain becomes severe, contact your health care provider. Once you are able to return to normal activities comfortably, your health care provider may recommend further aerobic and back exercises.

If You Are Not Getting Better

Most low back problems get better quickly, and usually within four weeks. If your symptoms are not getting better within this time period, you should contact your health care provider.

Special Tests

Your health care provider will examine your back again and may talk to you about getting some special tests. These may include x-rays, blood tests, or other special studies such as an MRI (magnetic resonance imaging) or CT (computerized tomography) scan of your back. These tests may help your health care provider understand why you are not getting better. Your health care provider may also want to refer you to a specialist.

Certain things, such as stress (extra pressure at home or work), personal or emotional problems, depression, or a problem with drug or alcohol use can slow recovery or make back symptoms seem worse. If you have any of these problems, tell your health care provider.

About Surgery

Even having a lot of back pain does not by itself mean you need surgery. Surgery has been found to be helpful in only 1 in 100 cases of low back problems. In some people, surgery can even cause more problems. This is especially true if your only symptom is back pain.

People with certain nerve problems or conditions such as fractures or dislocations have the best chance of being helped by surgery. In most cases, however, decisions about surgery do not have to be made right away. Most back surgery can wait for several weeks without making the condition worse.

If your health care provider recommends surgery, be sure to ask about the reason for the surgery and about the risks and benefits you might expect. You may also want to get a second opinion.

Prevention of Low Back Problems

The best way to prevent low back problems is to stay fit. If you must lift something, even after your back seems better, be sure to

- keep all lifted objects close to your body
- avoid lifting while twisting, bending forward, and reaching

You should continue to exercise even after your back symptoms have gone away. There are many exercises that can be done to condition muscles of your body and back. You should talk to your health care provider about the exercises that would be best for you.

When Low Back Symptoms Return

More than half of the people who recover from a first episode of acute low back symptoms will have another episode within a few years. Unless your back symptoms are very different from the first episode, or you have a new medical condition, you can expect to recover quickly and fully from each episode.

While Your Back Is Getting Better

It is important to remember that even though you are having a problem with your back now, most likely it will begin to feel better soon. It is important to keep in mind that you are the most important person in taking care of your back and in helping to get back to your regular activities.

It may also help you to remember that

- Most low back problems last for a short amount of time and the symptoms usually get better with little or no medical treatment.
- Low back problems can be painful. But pain rarely means that there is serious damage to your back.
- Exercise can help you to feel better faster and prevent more back problems. A regular exercise program adds to your general health care provider and may help you get back to the things you enjoy doing.

For Further Information

The information in this booklet was based on the *Clinical Practice Guideline, Acute Low Back Problems in Adults.* The *Guideline* was developed by a non-federal panel of experts sponsored by the Agency for Health Care Policy and Research. Other guidelines on common health problems are available, and more are being developed.

For more information about guidelines or to receive a free copy of *Understanding Acute Low Back Problems,* call toll-free, 800-358-9295, or write to

Agency for Health Care Provider Care Policy and Research
Publications Clearinghouse
PO Box 8547
Silver Spring, MD 20907

■ Document Source:
  U.S. Department of Health Care Provider and Human Services,
  Public Health Service
  Agency for Health Care Policy and Research
  Executive Office Center, Ste 501
  2101 East Jefferson St
  Rockville, MD 20852
  AHCPR Publication No. 95-0644
  December 1994

See also: About Low-Back Pain (page 347)

NEUROLOGIC DISORDERS

■ ■ ■

Information from PDQ for Patients

ADULT BRAIN TUMOR

Description

What is adult brain tumor?

Adult brain tumor is a disease in which cancer (malignant) cells begin to grow in the tissues of the brain. Your brain controls memory and learning, senses (hearing, sight, smell, taste, and touch), and emotion. It also controls other parts of the body, including muscles, organs, and blood vessels.

This PDQ statement covers tumors that start in the brain (primary brain tumors). Often cancer found in the brain has started somewhere else in the body and has spread (metastasized) to the brain. This is called brain metastasis (see the PDQ patient information statement on brain metastasis)

Like most cancer, adult brain tumor is best treated when it is found (diagnosed) early. You should see your doctor if you have headaches often, vomiting, or difficulty walking or speaking.

If you have symptoms, your doctor may order a computed tomographic scan, a special x-ray that uses a computer to make a picture of your brain. A magnetic resonance imaging scan, which uses magnetic waves to make a picture of your brain, may also be done. Often surgery is required to determine if you have a brain tumor and to see what type of tumor you have.

Your chance of recovery (prognosis) and choice of treatment depend on your general state of health and the type of brain tumor you have.

Stage Explanation

Types of Adult Brain Tumor

Once adult brain tumor is found, more tests will be done to find out the type of tumor you have. Your doctor will also need to know how different the tumor cells are from the cells that are near it, which is called the histologic grade of the tumor. To plan treatment, your doctor needs to know the type and grade of brain tumor you have. The following types are used to group adult brain tumors.

Astrocytomas

Astrocytomas are tumors that start in brain cells called astrocytes. There are different kinds of astrocytomas, which are defined by how the cancer cells look under a microscope.

Noninfiltrating astrocytoma

Noninfiltrating astrocytomas are tumors that grow slowly and usually do not grow into the tissues around them.

Well-differentiated mildly and moderately anaplastic astrocytoma

Well-differentiated mildly and moderately anaplastic astrocytomas are slow growing, but grow more quickly than noninfiltrating astrocytomas. They start to grow into other tissues around them.

Anaplastic astrocytoma

Anaplastic astrocytomas have cells that look very different from normal cells and that grow more rapidly.

Glioblastoma multiforme

Glioblastoma multiformes are tumors that grow very quickly and have cells that look very different from normal cells. Glioblastoma multiforme is also called grade IV astrocytoma.

Brain Stem Gliomas

Brain stem gliomas are tumors located in the bottom part of the brain that connects to the spinal cord (the brain stem).

Ependymal Tumors

Ependymal tumors are tumors that begin in the ependyma, the cells that line the passageways in the brain where special fluid that protects the brain and spinal cord (called cerebrospinal fluid) is made and stored. There are different kinds of ependymal tumors, which are defined by how the cells look under a microscope.

Well-differentiated ependymoma

Well-differentiated ependymomas have cells that look very much like normal cells and grow quite slowly.

Anaplastic ependymoma

Anaplastic ependymomas are ependymal tumors that do not look like normal cells and grow more quickly than well-differentiated ependymal tumors.

Ependymoblastoma

Ependymoblastomas are rare cancers that usually occur in children. They may grow very quickly.

Oligodendroglial Tumors

Oligodendroglial tumors begin in the brain cells called oligodendrocytes, which provide support and nourishment for the cells that transmit nerve impulses. There are different types of oligodendroglial tumors, which are defined by how the cells look under a microscope.

Well-differentiated oligodendroglioma

Well-differentiated oligodendrogliomas are slow-growing tumors that look very much like normal cells.

Anaplastic oligodendroglioma

Anaplastic oligodendrogliomas grow more quickly, and the cancer cells look very different from normal cells.

Other Brain Tumors

Mixed gliomas

Mixed gliomas are brain tumors that occur in more than one type of brain cell, including cells of astrocytes, ependymal cells, and/or oligodendrocytes.

Medulloblastoma

Medulloblastomas are brain tumors that begin in the lower part of the brain. They are almost always found in children or young adults. This type of cancer may spread from the brain to the spine.

Pineal parenchymal tumors

Pineal region tumors are tumors found in or around a tiny organ located near the center of the brain (the pineal gland). The tumors can be slow growing (pineocytomas) or fast growing (pineoblastomas). Astrocytomas may also start here.

Germ cell tumors

Germ cell tumors arise from the sex cells. There are different kinds of germ cells, including germinomas, embryonal carcinomas, choriocarcinomas, and teratomas.

Craniopharyngioma

Craniopharyngiomas are tumors that occur near the pituitary gland. The pituitary gland is a small organ about the size of a pea; this gland is located just above the back of the nose and controls many of the body's functions.

Meningioma

Meningiomas are tumors that occur in the membranes that cover and protect the brain and spinal cord (the meninges). Meningiomas usually grow slowly.

Malignant meningioma

Malignant meningioma is a rare tumor that grows more quickly than other meningiomas.

Recurrent

Recurrent disease means that the cancer has come back (recurred) after it has been treated. It may come back in the brain or in another part of the body.

Treatment Option Overview

How Adult Brain Tumors Are Treated

There are treatments for all patients with an adult brain tumor. Three kinds of treatment are used:
- surgery
- radiation therapy
- chemotherapy

Biological therapy (using your body's immune system to fight cancer) is being studied in clinical trials.

Surgery is the most common treatment for adult brain tumors. To take out the cancer from the brain, your doctor will cut a part of the bone from the skull to get to your brain. This operation is called a craniotomy. After your doctor removes the cancer, the bone will be put back or a piece of metal or fabric will be used to cover the opening in the skull.

Radiation therapy uses x-rays produced by a machine called a linear accelerator or a cobalt machine to kill cancer cells from the outside and shrink tumors (external-beam radiation therapy). Radiation therapy may also be used by putting materials that produce radiation (radioisotopes) through thin plastic tubes into the tumor to kill cancer cells from the inside (internal radiation therapy).

Chemotherapy uses drugs to kill cancer cells. Chemotherapy may be taken by pill, or it may be put into the body by a needle in the vein or muscle. Chemotherapy is called a systemic treatment because the drug enters the bloodstream, travels through the body, and can kill cancer cells throughout the body.

Biological therapy tries to get your own body to fight cancer. It uses materials made by your own body or made in a laboratory to boost, direct, or restore your body's natural defenses against disease. Biological therapy is sometimes called biological response modifier therapy or immunotherapy.

Treatment by Type

Treatment for adult brain tumor depends on the type and stage of your disease, your age, and your overall health.

You may receive treatment that is considered standard based on its effectiveness in a number of patients in past studies, or you may choose to go into a clinical trial. Not all patients are cured with standard therapy, and some standard treatments may have more side effects than are desired. For these reasons, clinical trials are designed to find better ways to treat cancer patients and are based on the most up-to-date information. Clinical trials are going on in most parts of the country for most types of adult brain tumor. If you want more information, call the Cancer Information Service at 1-800-4-CANCER (1-800-422-6237).

Adult Noninfiltrating Astrocytomas

Your treatment may be one of the following:
1. Surgery to remove the cancer.
2. Surgery followed by external-beam radiation therapy.

Adult Well-Differentiated Mildly and Moderately Anaplastic Astrocytoma

Your treatment may be one of the following:
1. Surgery followed by external-beam radiation therapy.
2. Surgery alone.
3. A clinical trial of surgery followed by radiation therapy and chemotherapy.

Adult Anaplastic Astrocytoma

Your treatment may be one of the following:
1. Surgery followed by external-beam radiation therapy.
2. Surgery followed by external-beam radiation therapy and chemotherapy.
3. A clinical trial of new forms of radiation therapy, such as internal radiation, radiation given during surgery, or radiation given with drugs to make the cancer cells more sensitive to radiation.
4. A clinical trial of chemotherapy or biological therapy following radiation therapy.

Adult Glioblastoma Multiforme

Your treatment may be one of the following:
1. Surgery followed by external-beam radiation therapy and chemotherapy.
2. Surgery followed by external-beam radiation therapy.
3. A clinical trial of new forms of radiation therapy, such as internal radiation, radiation given during surgery, or radiation given with drugs to make the cancer cells more sensitive to radiation.
4. A clinical trial of chemotherapy or biological therapy following radiation therapy.

Adult Brain Stem Glioma

Your treatment may be one of the following:
1. External-beam radiation therapy.
2. A clinical trial of chemotherapy or biological therapy.

Adult Well-Differentiated Ependymoma

Your treatment may be one of the following:
1. Surgery to remove the cancer.
2. Surgery to remove the cancer followed by external-beam radiation therapy.
3. A clinical trial of chemotherapy or biological therapy.

Adult Malignant Ependymoma

Your treatment may be one of the following:
1. Surgery to remove the cancer followed by external-beam radiation therapy.
2. A clinical trial of external-beam radiation therapy with chemotherapy.
3. A clinical trial of chemotherapy or biological therapy.

Adult Well-Differentiated Oligodendroglioma

Your treatment may be one of the following:
1. Surgery to remove the cancer followed by external-beam radiation therapy.
2. Surgery to remove the cancer.
3. A clinical trial of radiation therapy plus chemotherapy.

Adult Anaplastic Oligodendroglioma

Your treatment may be one of the following:
1. Surgery to remove the cancer followed by external-beam radiation therapy.
2. Surgery followed by external-beam radiation therapy and chemotherapy.
3. A clinical trial of new forms of radiation therapy, such as internal radiation, radiation given during surgery, or radiation given with drugs to make the cancer cells more sensitive to radiation.
4. A clinical trial of chemotherapy or biological therapy following radiation therapy.

Mixed Gliomas

Your treatment may be one of the following:
1. Surgery followed by external-beam radiation therapy.
2. Surgery followed by external-beam radiation therapy and chemotherapy.
3. A clinical trial of new forms of radiation therapy, such as internal radiation, radiation given during surgery, or radiation given with drugs to make the cancer cells more sensitive to radiation.
4. A clinical trial of chemotherapy or biological therapy following radiation therapy.

Adult Medulloblastoma

Your treatment may be one of the following:
1. Surgery to remove the cancer plus external-beam radiation therapy.
2. A clinical trial of surgery plus external-beam radiation therapy and chemotherapy.

See the PDQ patient information statement on childhood brain tumor for more information.

Adult Pineal Parenchymal Tumors

Your treatment may be one of the following:
1. Surgery plus external-beam radiation therapy.
2. Surgery plus external-beam radiation therapy plus chemotherapy.
3. A clinical trial of new forms of radiation therapy, such as internal radiation, radiation given during surgery, or radiation given with drugs to make the cancer cells more sensitive to radiation.
4. A clinical trial of chemotherapy or biological therapy following radiation therapy

Adult Central Nervous System Germ Cell Tumors

Treatment depends on whether the cancer can be removed in an operation, the kind of cells, the location of the tumor, and other factors.

Adult Craniopharyngioma

Your treatment may be one of the following:
1. Surgery to remove the cancer.
2. Surgery to remove the cancer followed by radiation therapy.

Adult Meningioma

Treatment usually consists of surgery to remove the tumor. If all of the tumor cannot be removed in an operation, you may also receive external-beam radiation therapy after surgery.

Adult Malignant Meningiomas

Your treatment may be one of the following:
1. Surgery followed by external-beam radiation therapy.
2. A clinical trial of new forms of radiation therapy, such as internal radiation, radiation given during surgery, or radiation given with drugs to make the cancer cells more sensitive to radiation.
3. A clinical trial of chemotherapy or biological therapy following radiation therapy.

Recurrent Adult Brain Tumor

Your treatment may be one of the following:
1. Surgery alone.
2. Surgery followed by chemotherapy.
3. External-beam radiation therapy alone, if not used during previous treatment, with or without chemotherapy.
4. Internal radiation therapy.
5. A clinical trial of chemotherapy.

To Learn More

To learn more about adult brain tumor, call the National Cancer Institute's Cancer Information Service at 1-800-4-CANCER (1-800-422-6237). By dialing this toll-free number, you can speak with someone who can answer your questions.

The Cancer Information Service can also send you free booklets. The following booklet about brain tumors may be helpful to you:

- What You Need To Know About Brain Tumors

The following general booklets on questions related to cancer may also be helpful:

- What You Need To Know About Cancer
- Taking Time: Support for People with Cancer and the People Who Care About Them
- What Are Clinical Trials All About?
- Chemotherapy and You: A Guide to Self-Help During Treatment
- Radiation Therapy and You: A Guide to Self-Help During Treatment
- Eating Hints for Cancer Patients
- Advanced Cancer: Living Each Day
- When Cancer Recurs: Meeting the Challenge Again

There are many other places where you can get material about cancer treatment and services to help you. You can check the social service office at your hospital for local and national agencies that may help with your finances, getting to and from treatment, care at home, and dealing with your problems. The American Cancer Society, for example, has many free services. Their local offices are listed in the white pages of the telephone book.

You can also write to the National Cancer Institute at this address:

National Cancer Institute
Office of Cancer Communications
31 Center Drive, MSC 2580
Bethesda, MD 20892-2580

■ **Document Source:**
U.S. Department of Health and Human Services, Public Health Service
National Institutes of Health
National Cancer Institute
May 1996

See also: Brain and Spinal Cord Tumors (page 371)

ALZHEIMER'S DISEASE: AN OVERVIEW

What is Alzheimer's disease?

Alzheimer's disease (pronounced Alz-himerz) is a progressive, degenerative disease that attacks the brain and results in impaired memory, thinking and behavior. It affects an estimated 4 million American adults.

When it was first diagnosed by German physician Alois Alzheimer in 1907, Alzheimer's disease was considered a rare disorder. Today, it is recognized as the most common cause of dementia.

Dementia is not a disease itself but a group of symptoms that characterize certain diseases and conditions. Dementia is commonly defined as a decline in intellectual functioning that is severe enough to interfere with the ability to perform routine activities.

The second most common form of dementia is multi-infarct dementia, which is caused by vascular disease and strokes. Other causes of dementia are Huntington's disease, Parkinson's disease, Pick's disease and Creutzfeldt-Jakob disease.

A number of other conditions can cause dementia or dementia-like symptoms: depression, drug reactions, thyroid disease, nutritional deficiencies, brain tumors, head injuries, alcoholism, infections (meningitis, syphilis, AIDS) and hydrocephalus.

In some cases, such symptoms or conditions may be reversible with appropriate treatment. Therefore, it is vitality important to seek a comprehensive diagnostic evaluation.

Alzheimer's disease is distinguished from other forms of dementia by characteristic changes in the brain that are visible only upon microscopic examination.

At autopsy, brains affected by Alzheimer's disease show the presence of fiber tangles within nerve cells (neurofibrillary tangles) and clusters of degenerating nerve endings (neuritic plaques) in areas that are important for memory and intellectual functions.

Another characteristic of Alzheimer's disease is the reduced production of certain brain chemicals, especially acetylcholine, but also including norepinephrine, serotonin and somatostatin. These chemicals are necessary for normal communication between nerve cells.

Who is affected by Alzheimer's disease?

Alzheimer's disease is more likely to occur as a person gets older. Approximately 10 percent of people age 65 and older are affected by Alzheimer's disease. This percentage rises to 47.2 percent for those age 85 or older. Alzheimer's can occur in middle age as well. The youngest documented case is that of a 28-year old individual.

Alzheimer's disease also affects the family of an Alzheimer patient. The emotional, social, and financial costs of caring for an Alzheimer patient are high. Family members often risk their own health in order to care for the Alzheimer patient at home.

What are the symptoms?

Alzheimer's disease has a gradual onset. Symptoms include difficulty with memory and loss of intellectual abilities severe enough to interfere with routine work or social activities. The Alzheimer patient may also experience confusion, language problems (such as trouble finding words), poor or decreased judgement, disorientation in place and time and changes in behavior or personality.

How quickly these changes occur in an Alzheimer patient will vary from person to person. Eventually, the disease leaves its victims totally unable to care for themselves. The course of the disease usually progresses an average of eight years from the time the symptoms first appear, although Alzheimer's disease has been known to last as long as 25 years.

How is Alzheimer's disease diagnosed?

At this time, there is no single diagnostic test for Alzheimer's disease. A complete physical, psychiatric and neurological evaluation by a physician (or team of physicians) experienced in diagnosing dementing disorders should be obtained when symptoms are noticed.

The examination should include a detailed medical history, mental status test, neuropsychological testing, blood work, urinalysis, chest x-ray, electroencephalography (EEG), computerized tomography (CT scan) and electrocardiogram (EKG). Such an evaluation is essential in determining whether the dementia is the result of a treatable illness.

When this kind of detailed examination is done, the accuracy of the diagnosis is about 90 percent. However, the only way to confirm a diagnosis of Alzheimer's disease is through autopsy at the time of death.

What causes Alzheimer's disease?

Scientists are still looking for the causes of Alzheimer's disease, and new clues are being uncovered rapidly through research.

For rare forms of the disease, which strikes people in their 30's and 40's and often runs in families, researchers believe there are at least three specific genes responsible. One is on Chromosome 21, another is on Chromosome 14, and the third is unknown.

However, for most Alzheimer patients the genetic involvement is less clear. Although there does seem to be genetic predisposition for the disease, and there is strong evidence that one predisposing gene is on Chromosome 19, other unknown factors also influence whether or not an individual develops Alzheimer's disease.

An increasing number of physicians believe that Alzheimer's disease is a complex disease, like heart disease and cancer, that can be caused by the interactions of several influences. Understanding any one of these influences would give researchers new targets for treatment.

Is Alzheimer's disease fatal?

From onset of symptoms, the life span of a person with Alzheimer's can range anywhere from three to 20 or more years. Unfortunately, it is always fatal.

Alzheimer's disease eventually leaves the patient less resistant to infections and other illnesses, which are often the ultimate cause of death.

Can Alzheimer's disease be treated or cured?

At this time there is no treatment available to stop or reverse the mental deterioration of Alzheimer's disease. However, new research findings give reason for hope. Several drugs are being studied in clinical trials to find out whether they can slow the progression of the disease or improve memory for a period of time.

One drug, Cognex r (a.k.a. tacrine or THA) was approved by the FDA in September 1993 for the treatment of mild to moderate Alzheimer's disease. In studies, some of the patients who tried the drug showed memory improvement, though only temporarily. The potential risks and benefits of this drug should be discussed with a doctor to decide whether a patient should try it.

Other medications are now available to assist in managing some of the most troubling symptoms of Alzheimer's disease. Under a doctor's supervision, medication can be used to control depression, behavioral disturbance and sleeplessness. Physical exercise and social activity are important, as are proper nutrition and health maintenance. A calm and well-structured environment will help the affected person maintain as much comfort and dignity as possible.

Can Alzheimer's disease be prevented?

Prevention is not possible at this time because the cause of the disease is unknown. Since no controllable risk factors for Alzheimer's disease are known, people are not yet able to reduce their chances of getting the disease. However, advances in science are bringing us closer to answers that can lead to treatments and effective strategies for prevention.

Meanwhile, focus on improved care and support for the patient and caregiver are helping to ease the burden of Alzheimer's disease. Although it is difficult for the person and their caregivers to cope with the symptoms of Alzheimer's disease, thoughtful care planning and modifications to the living environment can often relieve distress.

Is there help for people affected by Alzheimer's disease?

The Alzheimer's Association is the largest national voluntary organization dedicated to providing support and assistance to Alzheimer's patients and their families. The Alzheimer's Association is continuing research into the causes, treatment, prevention, and cure of Alzheimer's disease, as well as ways to improve the care and management of Alzheimer's patients.

The Alzheimer's Association has more than 3,000 support groups and 220 chapters nationwide. For more information on Alzheimer's disease and the Alzheimer's Association or to volunteer in the fight against Alzheimer's disease, call the Association's toll-free number (1-800-272-3900) for the location of the chapter nearest you.

Further Reading

The 36-Hour Day: A Family Guide to Caregiving for Persons with Alzheimer's Disease and Related Dementing Illnesses, and Memory Loss in Later Life by Nancy L. Mace, M.A. and Peter V. Rabins, MD Baltimore: Johns Hopkins University Press, 1991 (Revised Edition). *

The Loss of Self: A Family Resource for the Care of Alzheimer's Disease and Related Disorders by Donna Cohen, PhD and Carl Eisdorfer, PhD, MD N.Y.: W.W. Norton & Co., 1986.

Understanding Alzheimer's Disease by Miriam K. Aronson, Ed.D. (ed). N.Y.: Scribners, 1988. *

Guidelines for Dignity: Goals of Specialized Alzheimer/Dementia Care in Residential Settings. Alzheimer's Association, 1992. *

Family Guide for Alzheimer's Care in Residential Settings. Alzheimer's Association, 1992. *

* Available from the Alzheimer's Association national office and chapters.

Glossary

Dementia: This is not a disease in itself but a group of symptoms that characterize certain diseases and conditions. The major symptoms involve a decline in intellectual functioning that is severe enough to interfere with routine daily activities. Alzheimer's disease is the most common form of dementia.

Senility: This label often was used in the past to describe an individual 65 years or older with dementia. Senility used to be considered a normal part of aging. Today, physicians recognize that dementia is not a normal part of aging, but the result of an illness such as Alzheimer's disease.

Senile dementia/pre-senile dementia: Senile dementia is a label that was formerly applied to patients whose symptoms of dementia appeared after age 65. Pre-senile dementia is a description that used to be applied to dementia victims who were younger than age 65. These distinctions have largely been eliminated. Today, most cases of dementia in both groups of patients are diagnosed as Alzheimer's disease.

Chronic organic brain syndrome: This term is sometimes applied to patients with a collection of symptoms such as memory loss, disorientation, confusion, personality changes, and inability to carry out normal daily activities. The preferred term for these symptoms is dementia or dementing illness.

Hardening of the arteries: The correct medical term is arteriosclerosis. Dementia symptoms can be associated with arteriosclerosis, but only when multiple cerebral infarcts (strokes) have occurred. This condition is called multi-infarct dementia.

This brochure is made available by the Alzheimer's Association. For more information and an Association Materials Catalog, contact your local Alzheimer's Association chapter or call the Association's toll-free number.

Alzheimer's Disease: An Overview was reprinted with permission from the Alzheimer's Association. Contact the Alzheimer's Association at (800) 272-3900 for additional information or to locate the chapter in your area.

■ **Document Source:**
Alzheimer's Association
919 N Michigan Ave
Chicago, IL 60611-1676
312-335-8700
1-800-272-3900
TDD: 312-335-8882
ED 211Z
1994

BRAIN AND SPINAL CORD TUMORS

Introduction

The diagnosis of a brain or spinal cord tumor often comes as a shock, leaving confusion, uncertainty, fear, or even anger in its wake. After the diagnosis, a physician's explanation can fall on ears deafened by this blow. Although it cannot substitute for the advice and expertise of a physician, this brochure is designed to convey the latest research information on the diagnosis, course, and possible treatment of various brain and spinal cord tumors, so that patients and their families have the information they need to become active participants in their treatment.

What are brain and spinal cord tumors?

Brain and spinal cord tumors are abnormal growths of tissue found inside the skull or the bony spinal column. The word *tumor* is used to describe both abnormal growths that are new *(neoplasms)* and those present at birth *(congenital tumors)*. This brochure will focus primarily on neoplasms.

No matter where they are located in the body, tumors are usually classed as *benign* (or noncancerous) if the cells that make up the growth are similar to other normal cells, grow relatively slow, and are confined to one location. Tumors are called *malignant* (or cancerous) when the cells are very different from normal cells, grow relatively quickly, and can spread easily to other locations.

In most parts of the body, benign tumors are not particularly harmful. This is not necessarily true in the brain and spinal cord, which are the primary components of the central nervous system (CNS). Because the CNS is housed within rigid, bony quarters (that is, the skull and spinal column), any abnormal growth can place pressure on sensitive tissues and impair function. Also, any tumor located near vital brain structures or sensitive spinal cord nerves can seriously threaten health. A benign tumor growing next to an important blood vessel in the brain does not have to grow very large before it can block blood flow. Or, if a benign tumor is found deep inside the brain, surgery to remove it may be very risky because of the chances of damaging vital brain centers. On the other hand, a tumor located near the brain's surface can often be removed surgically.

An important difference between malignant tumors in the CNS and those elsewhere in the body lies with their potential to spread. While malignant cells elsewhere in the body can easily seed tumors inside the brain and spinal cord, malignant CNS tumors rarely spread out to other body parts. Laboratory and clinical investigators are exploring such unusual characteristics of CNS tumors because these unique properties may suggest new strategies to prevent or treat them.

What causes these tumors?

When newly formed tumors begin within the brain or spinal cord, they are called *primary tumors*. Primary CNS tumors rarely grow from neurons—nerve cells that perform the nervous system's important functions—because once neurons are mature they no longer divide and multiply. Instead, most tumors are caused by out-of-control growth among cells that surround and support neurons. Primary CNS tumors—such as gliomas and meningiomas—are named by the types of cells they contain, their location, or both. The appendix at the end of this brochure describes many types of primary CNS tumors, as well as other tumor-related conditions.

In a small number of individuals, primary tumors may result from specific genetic diseases—such as neurofibromatosis and tuberous sclerosis—or exposure to radiation or cancer-causing chemicals. Although smoking, alcohol consumption, and certain dietary habits are associated with some types of cancers, they have not been linked to primary brain and spinal cord tumors.

In fact, the cause of most primary brain and spinal cord tumors—and most cancers—remains a mystery. Scientists do not know exactly why and how cells in the nervous system or elsewhere in the body lose their normal identity as nerve, blood, skin, or other cell types and grow uncontrollably. Research scientists are looking for clues to this process with the goals of learning why and how cancer begins and developing new tools to stop it. Some of the possible causes under investigation include viruses and defective genes. Also, there is increasing interest in learning about the possible role played by environmental factors, such as chemicals and new technologies.

Metastatic tumors are caused by cancerous cells that shed from tumors in other parts of the body, travel through the bloodstream, burrow through the blood vessel walls, latch onto tissue, and spawn new tumors inside the brain or spinal cord.

For every four people who have cancer that has spread within the body, one develops metastatis within the CNS. The top two culprits that lead to these secondary CNS tumors are lung and breast cancer. Other, less frequent causes of CNS metastases include kidney (renal) cancer, lymphoma (a cancer affecting immune cells), prostate cancer, and melanoma, a form of skin cancer.

Brain and spinal cord tumors are not contagious or, at this time, preventable.

How many people have these tumors?

Research studies suggest that new brain tumors arise in more than 40,000 Americans each year. About half of these tumors are primary, and the remainder are metastatic.

Individuals of any age can develop a brain tumor. In fact, they are the second most common cause of cancer-related death in people up to the age of 35, with a slight peak in occurrence among children between the ages of 6 and 9. However, brain tumors are most common among middle-aged and older adults. People in their 60s face the highest risk—

each year one of every 5,000 people in this age group develops a brain tumor.

Spinal cord tumors are less common than brain tumors. About 10,000 Americans develop primary or metastatic spinal cord tumors each year. Although spinal cord tumors affect people of all ages, they are most common in young and middle-aged adults.

By studying the epidemiology of CNS tumors, scientists can learn if different tumors are more common at certain ages or in certain people. This information, in turn, may reveal environmental factors that are linked to tumors, connections between tumors and other disorders, or patterns of tumor occurrence, all of which offer clues about why tumors develop.

What are the symptoms?

Brain and spinal cord tumors cause many diverse symptoms, which can make detection tricky. Whatever specific symptoms a patient has, the symptoms generally develop slowly and worsen over time.

Brain Tumors

A 3.5-pound wrinkled mass of tissue, the brain orchestrates behavior, movement, feeling, and sensation. It controls automatic functions like breathing and heartbeat. Many of these important functions are controlled by specialized brain areas. For example, the brain's left and right hemispheres jointly control hearing and vision; the front part of each hemisphere controls voluntary movements, like writing, for the opposite side of the body; and the brain stem is responsible for basic life-sustaining functions, including blood pressure, heartbeat, and breathing.

As a result, brain tumors can cause a bewildering array of symptoms depending on their size, type, and location. Certain symptoms are quite specific because they result from damage to particular brain areas. Other, more general symptoms are triggered by increased pressure within the skull as the growing tumor encroaches on the brain's limited space or blocks the flow of *cerebrospinal fluid* (fluid that bathes the brain and spinal cord). Some of the more common symptoms of a brain tumor include

- **Headaches.** More than half of people with brain tumors experience headaches. Because the skull cannot expand, the growing mass places pressure on pain-sensitive areas. The headaches recur, often at irregular periods, and can last several minutes or hours. They may worsen when coughing, changing posture, or straining. As the tumor grows, headaches often last longer, become more frequent, and grow more severe.
- **Seizures.** The abnormal tissue found in a brain tumor can disrupt the normal flow of electricity through which brain cells communicate. The resulting bursts of electrical activity cause seizures with a variety of symptoms, such as convulsions, loss of consciousness, or loss of bladder control. Seizures that first start in adulthood (in a patient who has not been in an accident or had an illness that causes seizures) are a key warning

sign of brain tumors. Sometimes, seizures are the only sign of a slowly growing brain tumor.
- **Nausea and vomiting.** Increased pressure within the skull can cause nausea and vomiting. These symptoms sometimes accompany headaches.
- **Vision or hearing problems.** Increased intracranial pressure can also decrease blood flow in the eye and trigger swelling of the optic nerve, which in turn causes blurred vision, double vision, or partial visual loss. Tumors growing on or near sensory nerves often trigger visual or hearing disturbances, such as ringing or buzzing sounds, abnormal eye movements or crossed eyes, and partial or total loss of vision or hearing. Tumors that grow in the brain's occipital lobe, which interprets visual images, may also cause partial vision loss.
- **Behavioral and cognitive symptoms.** Because they strike at the core of the individual's identify, changes in behavior and personality can be the most frightening and devastating symptoms of a brain tumor. These symptoms usually occur when the tumor is located in the brain's cerebral hemispheres, which are responsible, in part, for personality, communication, thinking, behavior, and other vital functions. Examples include problems with speech, language, thinking, and memory, or psychotic episodes and changes in personality.
- **Motor problems.** When tumors affect brain areas responsible for command of body movement, they can cause motor symptoms, including weakness or paralysis, lack of coordination, or trouble with walking. Often, muscle weakness or paralysis affects only one side of the body.
- **Balance problems.** Brain tumors that disrupt the normal control of equilibrium can cause dizziness or difficulty with balance.

Spinal Cord Tumors

The spinal cord is, in part, like a living telephone cable. Lying protected inside the bony spine, it contains bundles of nerves that carry messages between the brain and the body's nerves, such as instructions from the brain to move an arm or information from the skin that signals pain.

A tumor that forms on or near the spinal cord can disrupt this communication. Often, these tumors exert pressure on the spinal cord or the nerves that exit from it; sometimes, they restrict the cord's supply of blood. Common symptoms that result from this include

- **Pain.** Normally, the spinal cord carries important warnings about pain from the body's nerves to the brain. By putting pressure on the spinal cord, a tumor can trigger these circuits and cause pain that feels as if it is coming from various parts of the body. This pain is often constant, sometimes severe, and can have a burning or aching quality.
- **Sensory changes.** Many people with spinal cord tumors suffer a loss of sensation. This usually takes the form of numbness and decreased skin sensitivity to temperature.

- **Motor problems.** Since the nerves control the muscles, tumors that affect nerve communication can trigger a number of muscle-related symptoms. Early symptoms include muscle weakness; *spasticity* in which the muscles stay stiffly contracted; and impaired bladder and/or bowel control. If untreated, symptoms may worsen to include muscle wasting and paralysis. In addition, some people develop an abnormal walking rhythm known as *ataxia*.

The parts of the body affected by these symptoms vary with tumor location along the spinal cord. In general, symptoms strike body areas at the same level or at a level below that of the tumor. For example, a tumor midway along the spinal cord (in the thoracic spine) can cause pain that spreads over the chest in a girdle-shaped pattern and gets worse when the individual coughs, sneezes, or lies down. A tumor that grows in the top fourth of the spinal column (or cervical spine) can cause pain that seems to come from the neck or arms. And a tumor that grows in the lower spine (or lumbar spine) can trigger back or leg pain.

In some cases, one or more tumors extend over several sections of the spinal cord. This results in symptoms that are spread over various parts of the body. Sometimes sensory symptoms occur in a patchy, confusing pattern in which some parts of the body are unaffected even though they lie between affected areas.

Doctors divide spinal cord tumors into three major groups based on where they are found. Extradural tumors grow between the bony spinal canal and the tough membrane called *dura mater* that protects the spinal cord. Tumors inside the dura (intradural tumors) are further divided into those outside the spinal cord (extramedullary tumors) and those inside the spinal cord (intramedullary tumors).

How are CNS tumors diagnosed?

Research has made major strides in the ability to detect and diagnose CNS tumors. When a doctor suspects a brain or spinal cord tumor because of a patient's medical history and symptoms, he or she can turn to a number of specialized tests and techniques to confirm the diagnosis. However, the first test is often a traditional neurological exam. A neurological exam checks

- **Eye movement, eye reflexes, and pupil reaction.** For example, the doctor can shine a pen light into the eye to see if the pupil contracts normally or ask the patient to follow a moving object, such as a finger.
- **Reflexes.** Tests like tapping below the knee with a rubber hammer can identify changes in reflexes.
- **Hearing.** Using a tuning fork, the physician can check for changes in hearing.
- **Sensation.** The doctor can use something sharp like a pin to test the sense of touch.
- **Movement.** Problems with movement are often tested by asking the patient to move his or her tongue, head, or facial muscles—as in smiling—and to perform tasks with the arms and legs.

- **Balance and coordination.** Typical tests include maintaining balance with the eyes closed, walking heel-to-toe in a straight line, or touching the nose with the eyes closed.

The next step in diagnosing brain tumors often involves X-rays or special imaging techniques and laboratory tests that can detect the presence of a tumor and provide clues about its location and type.

Imaging and X-rays

Special imaging techniques developed through recent research, especially *computed tomography* (CT) and *magnetic resonance imaging* (MRI), have dramatically improved the diagnosis of CNS tumors in recent years. In many cases, these scans can detect the presence of a tumor even if it is less than half an inch across.

CT uses a sophisticated X-ray machine and a computer to create a detailed picture of the body's tissues and structures. Often, doctors will inject a special dye into the patient before performing a CT scan. The dye, also called contrast material, makes it easier to see abnormal tissue. A CT scan often gives doctors a good idea of where the tumor is located in the brain or spinal cord and can sometimes help them determine the tumor's type. It can also help doctors detect swelling, bleeding, and other associated conditions. In addition, CT scans can help doctors check the results of treatment and watch for tumor recurrence.

MRI is a relatively new imaging technique that is rapidly gaining widespread use in diagnosing CNS tumors. This technique uses a magnetic field and radio waves, rather than X-rays, and can often distinguish more accurately between healthy and diseased tissue. MRI gives better pictures of tumors located near bone than CT, does not use radiation as CT does, and provides pictures from various angles that can enable doctors to construct a three-dimensional image of the tumor.

A third imaging technique, *positron emission tomography,* (PET) provides a picture of brain activity rather than structure by measuring levels of injected glucose (sugar) that has been labeled with a radioactive tracer. Glucose is used by the brain for energy. Detectors placed around the head can spot the labeled glucose, and a computer uses the pattern of glucose distribution to form an image of the brain. Since malignant tissue uses more glucose than normal, it shows up on the scan as brighter or lighter than surrounding tissue. Currently, PET is not widely used in tumor diagnosis, in part because the technique requires very elaborate, expensive equipment, including a cyclotron to create the radioactive glucose.

Although it is not widely used for diagnosis now that CT and MRI scans are possible, *angiography* continues to help doctors distinguish certain types of brain tumors and make decisions about surgery. In angiography, doctors inject dye into a major blood vessel, usually one of the large arteries in the neck. This dye deflects X-rays and makes it possible for doctors to see the network of blood vessels by taking a series of X-ray pictures as the dye flows through the brain. Since some tumors have a characteristic pattern of blood vessels and blood flow, the pictures can provide clues about the tumor's type. Information from angiography can also tell physicians if a tumor is located close to important, normal blood vessels that must be avoided during surgery.

Widesprad use of CT and MRI has also largely displaced use of traditional X-rays for diagnosis of brain and spinal cord tumors, since X-rays do not provide very useful images of brain tissue. They are occasionally helpful when tumors cause changes in the skull or spinal cord or when they contain tiny deposits of bone-like material made of calcium.

Physicians may also use a specialized X-ray technique, called a *myelogram,* when diagnosing spinal cord tumors. In myelography, a special dye that absorbs X-rays is injected into the spinal cord. This dye outlines the spinal cord but will not pass through a tumor. The resulting X-ray picture shows a dark area or narrowing that reveals the tumor's location.

Laboratory Tests

Laboratory tests commonly used include the *electroencephalogram* (or EEG) and *lumbar puncture,* also known as the spinal tap. The EEG uses special patches placed on the scalp or fine needles placed in the brain to record electrical currents inside the brain. This recording can help the doctor see telltale patterns in the brain's electrical activity that suggests a brain tumor. Repeated EEG recordings can be particularly helpful in deciding if an abnormality in brain activity is getting worse.

In lumbar puncture, doctors obtain a small sample of cerebrospinal fluid. This fluid can be examined for abnormal cells or unusual levels of various compounds that suggest a brain or spinal cord tumor.

In the future, diagnosis of brain tumors should grow more accurate as additional techniques—including new ways to image the CNS and advanced laboratory tests—are developed through basic laboratory studies and clinical research.

What is a biopsy and how is it used?

A *biopsy* is a surgical procedure in which a small sample of tissue is taken from the suspected tumor, often during surgery aimed at removing as much tumor as possible.

A biopsy gives doctors the clues they need to specifically diagnose the type of tumor. By examining the sample under a microscope, the pathologist—a physician who specializes in understanding how disease affects the body's tissues—can tell what kinds of cells are in a tumor. Pathologists also look carefully for certain changes that signal cancer. These signs include abnormal growths or changes in the cell membranes and telltale problems in the cell nuclei, which normally control cell characteristics and growth. For example, cancerous cells may grow small finger-like projections on their normally smooth surface or have extra nuclei.

Using this information, the pathologist provides a diagnosis of the tumor type. The tumor may also be classified as benign or malignant and given a numbered score that reflects how malignant it is. This score can help doctors determine how to treat a tumor and predict the likely outcome, or *prognosis,* for the patient.

Although biopsy has long been a mainstay of brain tumor diagnosis, it is still an important research area. Scientists continue to look for better ways to identify and classify types of abnormal cells in order to improve the best possible information for treatment decisions.

How are brain and spinal cord tumors treated?

The three most commonly used treatments—surgery, radiation, and chemotherapy—are largely the result of recent research. For some patients, doctors may suggest a new treatment still being tested. In any case, the doctor will recommend a treatment or a combination of treatments based on the tumor's location and type, any previous treatment the patient may have received, and the patient's medical history and general health.

Surgery

Surgery to remove as much tumor as possible is usually the first step in treating an *accessible tumor*—that is, a tumor that can be removed without unacceptable risk of neurological damage. Fortunately, research has led to advances in neurosurgery that make it possible for doctors to reach many tumors that were previously considered inaccessible. These new techniques and tools equip neurosurgeons to operate in the tight, vulnerable confines of the CNS. Some recently developed approaches in use in the operating room include:

- **Microsurgery.** In this widely used technique, the surgeon looks through a high-powered microscope to get a magnified view of the operating area. This makes it easier to see—and remove—tumor tissue while sparing surrounding healthy tissue.
- **Stereotactic procedures.** In these procedures, a computer uses information from CT or MRI to create a three-dimensional map of the operation site. The computer uses the map to help the surgeon guide special, computer-assisted tools. This makes it possible for surgeons to approach certain difficult-to-reach tumors with greater precision. Many procedures can be performed using this approach, including biopsy, certain types of surgery, and planting radiation pellets in a tumor.
- **Lasers.** Lasers release a beam of concentrated light energy that can destroy tissue. Lasers are occasionally helpful for tasks traditionally performed with a scalpel. For example, surgeons can use a laser to remove an entire tumor. Or, once most of a tumor is removed through surgery, they can destroy remaining tumor tissue with the laser's intense beam of energy.
- **Ultrasonic aspirators.** Ultrasonic aspirators use sound waves to vibrate tumors and break them up. Like a vacuum, the aspirator then sucks up the tumor fragments.
- **Evoked potentials.** Doctors use this test during surgery to determine the role of specific nerves and thus avoid damage. In this technique, small electrodes are used to

stimulate a nerve so its electrical response, or evoked potential, can be measured.

- **Shunts.** Shunts are flexible tubes used to reroute and drain fluid. Doctors sometimes insert a shunt into the brain when a tumor blocks the flow of cerebrospinal fluid and causes *hydrocephalus*. Shunting of the fluid can relieve headaches, nausea, and other symptoms caused by too much pressure inside the skull.

Surgery may be the beginning and end of treatment if the biopsy shows a benign tumor. If the tumor is malignant, however, doctors often recommend additional treatment following surgery, including radiation, chemotherapy, or experimental treatments. Sometimes, if a tumor is very large, radiation is used before surgery to reduce the tumor's size.

An *inaccessible* or *inoperable tumor* is one that cannot be removed surgically because of the risk of severe nervous system damage. These tumors are frequently located deep within the brain or near vital structures such as the brain stem—the part of the brain that controls many crucial functions including breathing and heart rate. Malignant, multiple tumors may also be inoperable. Doctors treat most malignant, inaccessible, or inoperable CNS tumors with radiation and/or chemotherapy.

Among patients who have metastatic CNS tumors, doctors usually focus on treating the original cancer first. However, when a metastatic tumor causes serious disability or pain, doctors may recommend surgery or other treatments to reduce symptoms even if the original cancer has not been controlled.

Radiation Therapy

In radiation therapy, the tumor is bombarded with beams of energy that kill tumor cells. Traditional radiation therapy delivers radiation from outside the patient's body, usually begins a week or two after surgery, and continues for about six weeks. The dosage is fairly uniform throughout the treated areas, making it especially useful for tumors that are large or have infiltrated into surrounding tissue.

However, when traditional radiation therapy is given to the brain, it may also cause damage to healthy tissue. Depending on the type of tumor, doctors may be able to choose a modified form of radiation therapy to help prevent this and to improve the effectiveness of treatment. Modifying therapy can be as simple as changing the dosage schedule and amount of radiation that a patient receives. For example, an approach called hyperfractionation uses smaller, more frequent doses. Neurological investigators are also testing several other, more complex techniques to improve radiation therapy.

Chemotherapy

Chemotherapy uses tumor-killing drugs that are given orally or injected into the bloodstream. Because not all tumors are vulnerable to the same anticancer drugs, doctors often use a combination of drugs for chemotherapy.

Chemotherapeutic drugs generally kill cells that are growing or dividing. This property makes them more deadly to malignant tissue, which contains a high proportion of growing and dividing cells, than to most normal cells. It also causes some of the side effects that can accompany chemotherapy—such as skin reactions, hair loss, or digestive problems—because a high proportion of these normal cell types are also growing and dividing at any given time. The drugs most commonly used for CNS tumors are known by the initials BCNU (sometimes called carmustine) and CCNU (or lomustine). Research scientists are also testing many promising drugs to learn if they can improve treatment for brain and spinal cord tumors and reduce side effects.

Other Drugs

Tumors, surgery, and radiation therapy can all result in swelling inside the CNS. Doctors may prescribe steroids for short or long periods to reduce this swelling. Examples of such drugs include dexamethasone, methylprednisolone, and prednisone.

Whether new treatment approaches involve surgery, radiation therapy, chemotherapy, or completely new avenues to treating CNS tumors, carefully planned clinical trials of new and experimental therapies are vital for identifying promising treatments and learning the best applications of current therapies. Experimental treatments, in turn, would not be possible without research by basic and clinical scientists who identify new approaches.

Where should patients go for treatment?

Brain and spinal cord tumors are often difficult to diagnose, and surgery to remove them demands great skill. Experience, therefore, is probably the most important factor in choosing among physicians. Brain and spinal cord tumors are also relatively rare. Many physicians see only a few patients with CNS tumors each year. Others, however, have made treating brain and spinal cord tumors their specialty. Patients should consider how many patients a physician treats each year. Because many patients are understandably perplexed or frightened by a CNS tumor diagnosis, it is also important that they choose a physician who will answer questions and describe treatment options clearly and fully.

Patients should also learn what techniques and tools are available at the physician's hospital. Teaching hospitals affiliated with a medical college or university are more likely to be involved in research, and, thus, have the equipment and specialists necessary to offer experimental treatments. Finally, if a patient is dissatisfied with a physician or a physician's recommendations, he or she may wish to seek another opinion.

The voluntary organizations listed on the pocket card at the back of this publication may be able to help in locating physicians who specialize in treating brain tumors, as well as provide information about CNS tumors.

What research is being done?

Scientists are attacking CNS tumors through biomedical research to improve medical understanding and treatment. CNS tumor research ranges from bench-side studies on the origins and characteristics of tumors to bedside studies that test new tumor-killing drugs and other innovative treatments. Much of this work is supported by the National Institute of Neurological Disorders and Strokes (NINDS) and by the National Cancer Institute (NCI), as well as other agencies within the federal government, non-profit groups, and private institutions.

Some key areas of brain tumor research include:

- **Brachytherapy.** In brachytherapy, which is also known as interstitial radiation, doctors implant small, radioactive pellets directly into the tumor. The pellets may be left in permanently or for a few days, weeks, or months. This technique can deliver a large dose of radiation to the tumor while minimizing radiation of normal tissue. Through research, scientists thus far have found that brachytherapy is most useful for small tumors that are difficult to remove surgically. Research scientists continue to examine whether this technique can help patients with other tumor types as well.

- **Drugs and techniques for chemotherapy.** Dozens of new chemotherapeutic drugs are in various stages of development. Scientists are testing these drugs in animals and patients to determine what side effects they cause, what doses are appropriate, and whether they can improve survival and recovery. Patients interested in up-to-date information on current trials are encouraged to contact the resources listed on the pocket card at the end of the brochure.

  Scientists are also working to overcome an obstacle to effective chemotherapy for brain and spinal cord tumors—the *blood-brain barrier*. The blood-brain barrier—an elaborate meshwork of fine blood vessels and cells that filters blood reaching the CNS—normally helps protect the sensitive tissues of the CNS from potentially dangerous compounds in the bloodstream and changes in its environment. But the blood-brain barrier also stymies many efforts to deliver anticancer drugs that may help patients with CNS tumors. Investigators are testing drugs, such as the chemical leukotriene, that may help open the barrier. If these drugs prove useful and safe in animal models and humans, then physicians would be equipped to test promising anticancer drugs that normally cannot cross the blood-brain barrier.

  Another experimental path aimed at improving drug delivery into the CNS is called interstitial chemotherapy. In this technique, doctors place disc-shaped wafers soaked with chemotherapeutic drugs directly into tumor tissue. This technique may help physicians increase the dose of life-prolonging drugs while limiting side effects—since less of the drug spreads elsewhere in the body. Most trials of this technique currently involve patients with recurrent gliomas.

- **Drugs to improve radiation therapy.** Many scientists are testing the usefulness of drugs known as radiosensitizers that make tumor tissue more vulnerable to radiation. Early results with the two most commonly studied radiosensitizers, metronidazole and misonidazole, have been mixed; some trials suggest these drugs may improve survival in certain patients, while other trials have shown little benefit. In addition, other scientist are looking at whether another family of drugs known as barbiturates may improve radiation therapy by protecting normal brain tissue. Early studies have shown these sedating drugs can slow down the metabolism of healthy brain tissue, possibly shielding it from radiation damage.

- **Gamma knife.** The gamma knife, used for a procedure known technically as stereotractic gamma knife radiosurgery, combines precise stereotactic guidance and a sharply focused beam of radiation energy to deliver a single, precise dose of radiation. Despite its name, the gamma knife does not require a surgical incision. Investigators using this tool have found it can help them reach and treat some small tumors that are not accessible through surgery.

- **Gene therapy.** Gene therapy, an innovative approach to treating CNS cancer, is in the early stages of research in laboratories around the country. Genes are the blueprints the body's cells use to make proteins and other vital substances. In gene therapy, scientists insert a new gene into specific cells. In the case of gene therapy for brain tumors, this inserted gene could make the tumor cells sensitive to certain drugs, program the cancerous cells to self-destruct, or instruct them to manufacture substances that would slow their growth. Scientists are using tumor cells and animal models to learn how various genes, once introduced, hinder cancer growth and to identify the best methods for inserting new genes into tumor cells. Human trials are just beginning.

- **Hyperthermia.** Tumors are more sensitive to heat than normal tissue, partly because they have less blood flow to cool them. Research scientists testing hyperthermia take advantage of this sensitivity by placing special heat-producing antennae into the tumor region after surgery. Most often, these antennae send out microwaves that raise the temperature in nearby tissues. Hyperthermia is a new treatment for tumors in the brain, and scientists are still testing its effectiveness. They are also looking at heat sources that may be more effective than microwaves, including electromagnetic energy and radiofrequencies.

- **Immunotherapy.** The body's immune system normally seeks out and destroys foreign tissue such as cancerous cells by detecting antigens, telltale proteins found on foreign cells that alert the body to the foreign cells' presence. Stimulated by the antigens, the body manufacturers a variety of immune cells and special proteins called antibodies. These antibodies then latch onto the antigens, working as tiny flags that alert immune cells to attack and destroy the foreign cells. In immunotherapy—an exciting and very new field of CNS tumor research—scientists are looking for ways to duplicate or enhance the body's immune response to fight against brain and spinal cord cancer.

  Some scientists are testing the effectiveness of giving the body's immune system a general boost. Much like the way coffee can stimulate the nervous system, certain naturally occurring body chemicals trigger immune cells to grow and divide. In numerous studies, researchers have supplied patients with extra amounts of immune stimulants, such as interleuekin-2, in the hope that they will improve the body's ability to fight CNS cancer. However, this technique has produced mixed results. A second type of general immunotherapy involves removing immune cells from a patient, growing and activating these cells, and then returning them to the patient where they can work against the cancer. This approach has also yielded mixed results.

Another, still more recent approach in immunotherapy research specifically targets tumor cells using monoclonal antibodies. Like duplicate keys for the same lock, monoclonal antibodies are multiple copies of a single antibody; they fit one—and only one—antigen. Scientists are now producing monoclonal antibodies against tumor cell antigens and testing their usefulness. For example, scientists at the NINDS and elsewhere are linking these antibodies to toxins that can kill tumor cells. The armed monoclonal antibodies then function like guided missiles; they seek out the tumor cells with a matching antigen, bind to these tumor cells, and deliver their toxin. Early experiments with this therapy suggest it has more promise for treating widespread cancer cells than solid tumors. Studies are underway to corroborate these early results and to learn if this therapy has promise for other types of CNS tumors. Monoclonal antibodies may also prove helpful in improving brain tumor diagnosis, because they can be attached to special tracers to make tumor cells more visible.

- **Intraoperative ultrasound.** This technique, which uses sound waves, provides the surgeon with an image of brain tissues during the operation. Ultrasound is less expensive and complex than other imaging techniques. Some scientists conducting research on intraoperative ultrasound have found the technique makes it easier for the surgeon to locate the outer edges of tumor tissue, which can be hard to find. Thus, this technique may help improve tumor surgery by increasing the amount of tumor that can be safely removed.
- **Oncogenes.** The body contains a number of genes that are important in normal cell growth and development. Changes in some of these genes—which might be triggered by such events as exposure to chemicals or radiation—can transform them into dangerous, cancer-causing oncogenes. A number of oncogenes have already been found, and scientists continue to look for more. They are also working to identify specific events that can create oncogenes and to learn if there may be ways to prevent oncogenes from forming or to impair oncogene function in cancerous cells.
- **PET.** Based on recent research, some scientists believe that PET scans offer important clues for diagnosis of brain tumors. For example, physicians sometimes have trouble detecting recurrent tumors with CT or MRI scans. Recent studies have shown that PET may make it easier to detect recurrent brain tumors. Scientists are also examining whether PET can help physicians tell the difference between benign and malignant tumors before performing a biopsy or surgery.

- **Physiological mapping.** Mapping brain functions has promise for improving the safety and effectiveness of brain tumor surgery, particularly among children with tumors in critical brain regions. In physiological mapping, the physician locates brain areas responsible for key functions, such as language or sensation. The surgeon then has a map to help avoid these critical areas, thus reducing the change of serious complications.
- **Photodynamic therapy.** Photodynamic therapy uses drugs that collect in tumor cells and can be turned on or activated by special light. The drugs may be given by injection or placed directly into the tumor during an initial surgery. In order to activate the tumor-killing drug, the physician must expose the tumor tissue to light during surgery. Thus far, this technique has been found useful only for small amounts of tumor tissue, although researchers continue the search for new light-sensitive drugs and better light sources that can penetrate tumors.
- **Tumor growth factors.** Cancerous tumors are often rich in an array of substances, called growth factors, that enable them to grow and spread rapidly. In recent years, scientists have identified a number of these factors, including one that triggers growth of nerve tissue and another that stimulates blood vessels to grow. Many investigators continue the search for more such factors. Meanwhile, other researchers have begun testing antibodies that can block these factors. Early results in animals have shown that blocking growth factors with antibodies may help slow tumor growth, suggesting this research arena could lead to new therapies for brain tumors.

Although many new approaches to treatment thus appear promising, it is important to remember that all potential therapies must stand the test of well-designed, carefully controlled clinical trials and long-term follow-up of treated patients before any conclusion can be drawn about their safety or effectiveness.

Past research has led to improved tumor treatments and techniques, providing longer survival and richer lives for many CNS tumor patients. Current research promises to generate further improvements. In the years ahead, physicians and patients can look forward to new forms of therapy developed through an understanding of the unique traits of CNS tumors.

What can I do to help?

The NINDS and the National Institute of Mental Health jointly support two national brain specimen banks. These banks supply research scientists around the world with nervous system tissue from patients with neurological and psychiatric disorders. They need tissue from patients with CNS tumors so that scientists can study and understand these tumors. Those who may be interested in donating should write to

Dr. Wallace W. Tourtellotte, Director
Human Neurospecimen Bank
VA Wadsworth Medical Center
Wilshire and Sawtelle Blvds
Los Angeles, CA 90073
(310) 824-4307

Dr. Edward D. Bird, Director
Brain Tissue Bank, Mailman Research Center
McLean Hospital
115 Mill St
Belmont, MA 02178
1-800-BRAIN-BANK (1-800-272-4622)
(617) 855-2400

Where can I find more information?

The NINDS is the Federal Government's leading supporter of biomedical research on nervous system disorders, including brain and spinal cord tumors. The NINDS conducts research on brain tumors in its own laboratories at the National Institutes of Health (NIH) in Bethesda, MD, and supports research at institutions worldwide. The Institute also sponsors an active public information program. Other NINDS publications that may be of interest to those concerned about brain and spinal cord tumors include "Epilepsy: Hope Through Research" and the fact sheets "Neurofibromatosis" and "Tuberous Sclerosis."

The Institute's address and phone number, as well as information on other organizations that offer various services to those affected by brain and spinal cord tumors, are provided on the information resources card enclosed in the back pocket of this brochure.

Glossary

accessible tumor: a tumor that can be reached and removed using surgical tools without unreasonable risk of severe damage.

anaplastic: cancerous, malignant *(see below)*.

angiography: an imaging technique that provides an X-ray picture of blood vessels.

benign: non-malignant or non-cancerous. Often used to describe tumor cells that are similar to other normal cells, grow relatively slowly, and are confined to one location. Benign CNS tumors can nevertheless be dangerous.

biopsy: diagnostic test in which a sample of a patient's tissue is examined for disease.

blood-brain barrier: an elaborate meshwork of fine blood vessels and cells that filters blood reaching the central nervous system.

central nervous system (CNS): the brain and spinal cord.

cerebrospinal fluid: clear liquid that bathes the brain and spinal cord.

computed tomography (CT): an imaging technique that uses X-rays and computer analysis to create a picture of body tissues and structures.

congenital tumor: an abnormal growth present at birth.

dura mater: a tough, fibrous membrane covering the brain and spinal cord. The dura mater is located inside the spinal bones and skull.

electroencephalogram: a written recording of the brain's electrical activity.

hydrocephalus: abnormal accumulation of cerebrospinal fluid within the skull.

inaccessible or inoperable tumor: a tumor that cannot be reached surgically without unreasonable risk of severe damage to nearby tissue.

lumbar puncture: a diagnostic procedure in which a sample of cerebrospinal fluid is removed from the spinal cord using a needle.

magnetic resonance imaging (MRI): an imaging technique which uses radio waves, magnetic fields, and computer analysis to create a picture of body tissues and structures.

malignant: harmful, cancerous. Often used to describe tumor cells that are very different from normal cells, grow relatively quickly, and can easily spread to other locations.

meninges: membranes that cover the brain and spinal cord.

metastatic tumors: tumors caused by cancerous cells that have spread from other parts of the body.

myelogram: a diagnostic test that uses injected dye and X-rays to create a picture of the spinal cord.

neoplasms: new, abnormal growths in the body.

positron emission tomography (PET): an imaging technique that provides a visual measure of metabolism, or activity, within body tissues.

primary tumors: as opposed to metastatic tumors, these are abnormal growths that originated in the location where they have been diagnosed.

prognosis: the likely outcome of a situation, especially for an individual with a disease.

reflexes: automatic movements that the body makes in response to a given stimulus.

spasticity: abnormal, involuntary stiffness or contraction of the body's muscles.

Primary CNS Tumors and Tumor-Related Conditions

Chordomas

Chordomas, which are more common in people in theirs 20s and 30s, develop from remnants of the flexible spine-like structure that forms and dissolves early in fetal development and is later replaced by the spinal cord. Although these tumors are often slow-growing, they can metastasize or recur after treatment. They are usually treated with a combination of surgery and radiation.

Craniopharyngiomas

Craniopharyngiomas are brain tumors that usually affect infants and children. Like chordomas, they develop from cells left over from early fetal development. Craniopharyngiomas are often located near the brain's pituitary gland, a gland that releases chemicals important for the body's growth and metabolism. Treatment for these tumors usually includes surgery and, in some patients, radiation therapy.

Gliomas

About half of all primary brain tumors and about one-fifth of all primary spinal cord tumors are gliomas, meaning that they grow from glial cells. Within the brain, gliomas usually occur in the cerebral hemispheres but may also strike other areas, especially the optic nerve, the brain stem, and, particularly among children, the cerebellum. Gliomas are classified into several groups because there are different kinds of glial cells.

astrocytomas

These are the most common types of glioma. They develop from star-shaped glial cells called astrocytes. Doctors will often assign one of three grades to an astrocytomas following biopsy. The types of graded astrocytomas include:

- **well-differentiated**

  Also known as low-grade astrocytomas or grade I astrocytomas, these tumors contain cells that are relatively normal and are less malignant than the other two grades. They grow relatively slowly and may sometimes be completely removed through surgery. However, even well-differentiated astrocytomas are life-threatening if they are inaccessible.

- **anaplastic**

  Anaplastic astrocytomas, also called mid-grade astrocytomas or grade II astrocytomas, grow more rapidly than well-differentiated astrocytomas and contain cells with some malignant traits. Surgery followed by radiation and, sometimes, chemotherapy is used to treat anaplastic astrocytomas.

- **glioblastoma multiforme**

  These tumors, sometimes called high-grade or grade III astrocytomas, grow rapidly, invade nearby tissue, and contain cells that are very malignant. Glioblastoma multiforme are among the most common and devastating primary brain tumors that strike adults. Doctors usually treat glioblastomas with surgery followed by radiation therapy, and, sometimes, chemotherapy.

ependymomas

Ependymomas usually affect children and develop from cells that line both the hollow cavities of the brain and the canal containing the spinal cord. About 85 percent of ependymomas are benign. Treatment usually includes surgery followed by radiation therapy. Chemotherapy is sometimes used, especially for recurrent tumors.

oligodendrogliomas

These tumors, which develop from glial cells called eligodendroglia, represent about 5 percent of all gliomas. They occur most often in young adults, within the brain's cerebral hemispheres. Doctors often treat these tumors with surgery followed by radiation therapy.

ganglioneuromas

The rarest form of glioma, these tumors contain both glial cells and mature neurons. They grow relatively slowly and may occur in the brain or spinal cord. These tumors are usually treated with surgery.

mixed gliomas

Mixed gliomas contain more than one type of glial cell, usually astrocytes and other glial cell types. Treatment focuses on the most malignant cell type found within the tumor.

brain stem gliomas

Named by their location at the base of the brain rather than the cells they contain, brain stem gliomas are most common in children and young adults. Surgery is not usually used to treat brain stem gliomas because of their vulnerable location. Radiation therapy sometimes helps to reduce symptoms and improve survival by slowing tumor growth.

optic nerve gliomas

These tumors are found on or near the nerves that travel between the eye and brain vision centers and are particularly common in individuals who have neurofibromatosis. Treatment usually includes surgery or radiation.

Meningiomas

Meningiomas are tumors that develop from the thin membranes, or *meninges,* that cover the brain and spinal cord. Meningiomas account for about 15 percent of all brain tumors and about 25 percent of all primary spinal cord tumors. They affect people of all ages, but are most common among those in their 40s. Meningiomas usually grow slowly, generally do not invade surrounding normal tissue, and rarely spread to other parts of the CNS or body. Surgery is the preferred treatment for accessible meningiomas and is more successful for these tumors than for most tumor types.

Pineal Tumors

Tumors in the pineal gland, a small structure deep within the brain, account for about 1 percent of brain tumors. When possible, physicians will begin a treatment with surgery or perform a biopsy to confirm the tumor type. They may also recommend radiation or chemotherapy, or both, for malignant pineal tumors. The three most common types of pineal region tumors are gliomas, germ cell tumors, and pineal cell tumors.

Pituitary Tumors

The pituitary gland, a small oval-shaped structure located at the base of the brain, releases several chemical messengers known as hormones, which help control the body's other glands and influence the body's growth, metabolism, and maturation. Tumors that affect the pituitary gland, also called pituitary adenomas, account for about 10 percent of brain tumors. Doctors classify pituitary tumors into two groups—secreting and nonsecreting. Secreting tumors release unusually high levels of pituitary hormones, triggering a constellation of symptoms, which can include impotence, abnormal body growth, Cushing's syndrome, or hyperthyroidism depending on which hormone is involved. Surgery or the drug bromocriptine is used to treat most pituitary tumors.

Primitive Neuroectodermal Tumors

Primitive neuroectodermal tumors (PNETs) usually affect children and young adults. Their name reflects the belief, held by many scientists, that these tumors spring from primitive cells left over from early development of the nervous system. PNETs are usually very malignant, growing rapidly and spreading easily within the brain and spinal cord. In rare cases, they cause cancer outside the CNS. Medulloblastomas, the most common PNET, represent more than 25 percent of all childhood brain tumors. Other, more rare PNETs include neuroblastomas, pineoblastomas, medulloepitheliomas, ependymoblastomas, and polar songioblastomas. Because their malignant cells often spread in a scattered, patchy pattern, PNETs are difficult to remove totally through surgery. Doctors usually remove as much tumor as possible with surgery, then prescribe high doses of radiation, and, in some cases, chemotherapy.

Schwannomas

These tumors arise from the cells that form a protective sheath around the body's nerve fibers. They are usually benign and are surgically removed when possible. One of the more common forms of schwannoma affects the eighth cranial nerve, which contains nerve cells important for balance and hearing. Also known as vestibular schwannomas or acoustic neuromas, these tumors may grow on one or both sides of the brain.

Vascular Tumors

These rare, noncancerous tumors arise from the blood vessels of the brain and spinal cord. The most common vascular tumor is the hemangioblastoma, which is linked in a small number of people to a genetic disorder called Von Hippel-Lindau disease. Hemangioblastomas do not usually spread, and doctors typically treat them with surgery.

Other Tumor-Related Conditions

CNS lymphoma

CNS lymphoma occurs when cells from the body's immune system grow out of control. A type of cancer, CNS lymphoma affects a small number of otherwise healthy people and a larger fraction of those who have an impaired immune system, whether from organ transplants, infection with the AIDS virus, or other causes.

CNS lymphoma can be primary or secondary. In both cases, doctors usually treat the disorder with radiation. Chemotherapy may also be used and, if lymphoma affects the meninges, doctors often deliver chemotherapy directly into the cerebrospinal fluid. Although most lymphomas respond well to radiation therapy, they often recur.

meningeal carcinomatosis

This condition strikes when individual cells from cancer outside the CNS enter into the cerebrospinal fluid and grow like seeds. These cells travel with the fluid and can form colonies or small tumors in many places, including the roots of nerves, the surface of the brain, the brain stem, and the spinal cord. Treatment usually involves radiation, which can sometimes slow growth of the cells.

neurofibromatosis

Neurofibromatosis is a genetic disorder that can cause tumors in various parts of the nervous system. Neurofibromatosis type 2 causes multiple CNS tumors (including neurofibromas, bilateral vestibular schwannomas, and an increased risk of optic nerve gliomas.) Treatment usually consists of surgery to remove tumors that are causing symptoms. The more common form of this disorder, neurofibromatosis type 1, usually causes benign tumors outside the CNS.

pseudotumor cerebri

This condition can easily be confused with a brain tumor because its symptoms closely mimic those of brain tumors, possibly because abnormal buildup of cerebrospinal fluid places pressure on the brain. Pseudotumor cerebri is diagnosed by ruling out all other possible causes for symptoms and confirming that the cerebrospinal fluid pressure is increased. Doctors may treat this condition by lumbar puncture to release cerebrospinal fluid, special drugs to correct fluid levels, shunts to drain fluid, or, in severe cases, surgery to relieve pressure on the brain.

tuberous sclerosis

This genetic disorder causes numerous neurological and physical symptoms, including tumors of the kidneys, eyes, and CNS. About half of those with tuberous sclerosis develop benign astrocytomas.

Information Resources

NIH Neurological Institute
PO Box 5801
Bethesda, MD 20824
(301) 496-5751 or 1-800-352-9424

The National Institute of Neurological Disorders and Stroke, a component of the National Institutes of Health, is the leading federal supporter of research on disorders of the brain and nervous system. The Institute also sponsors an active public information program and can answer questions about diagnosis, treatment, and research related to brain and spinal cord tumors.

Office of Cancer Communications
National Cancer Institute
Building 31, Room 10A-24
Bethesda, MD 20892
1-800-4-CANCER (1-800-422-6237)

The NCI, also a part of the NIH and the primary federal supporter of cancer-related biomedical research, offers a variety of publications and a toll-free cancer information service.

Private organizations that offer information include the following:

American Brain Tumor Association
2720 River Rd, Ste 146
Des Plaines, IL 60018
(708) 827-9910 or 1-800-886-2282

This association provides referrals and information and publishes a newsletter and brochures on various tumor types and treatments.

American Cancer Society
1599 Clifton Rd, NE
Atlanta, GA 30329
1-800-ACS-2345 (1-800-227-2345)

The ACS supports research, conducts educational programs, and offers patient and family services.

Brain Tumor Information Service
(312) 684-1400

This 24-hour service provides information on diagnosis and treatment for patients and families.

The Brain Tumor Society
60 Leo Birmingham Parkway
Boston, MA 02135-1116
(617) 783-0340

The society distributes information, publishes a newsletter, and provides referrals to resources, as well as sponsoring research, a patient-family telephone network, and professional education programs.

The Children's Brain Tumor Foundation
35 Alpine Lane
Chappaqua, NY 10514
(914) 238-1656

The foundation funds research and professional training, sponsors support groups, publishes a newsletter, and provides services for children with brain tumors and their families.

National Brain Tumor Foundation
323 Geary St, Ste 510
San Francisco, CA 94102
(415) 296-0404
1-800-93-4-CURE (1-800-934-2873)

The foundation sponsors support groups and offers a variety of publications, including a newsletter, a booklet for newly diagnosed tumor patients, and a guide to employment, support groups, insurance, and other resources. The foundation also offers audiocassettes of their annual brain tumor conference.

■ **Document Source:**
U.S. Department of Health and Human Services, Public Health Service
National Institutes of Health
National Institute of Neurological Disorders and Stroke
Bethesda, MD 20892
NIH Publication No. 93-504
March 1993, Revised June 1993

See also: Adult Brain Tumor (page 365)

CEREBRAL PALSY

Introduction

In the 1860s, an English surgeon named William Little wrote the first medical descriptions of a puzzling disorder that struck children in the first years of life, causing stiff, spastic muscles in their legs and, to a lesser degree, their arms. These children had difficulty grasping objects, crawling, and walking, They did not get better as they grew up nor did they become worse. Their condition, which was called Little's disease for many years, is now known as *spastic diplegia.* It is just one of several disorders that affect control of movement and are grouped together under the term cerebral palsy.

Because it seemed that many of these children were born following complicated deliveries, Little suggested their condition resulted from a lack of oxygen during birth. This oxygen shortage damaged sensitive brain tissues controlling movement, he proposed. But in 1897, the famous physician Sigmund Freud disagreed. Noting that children with cerebral palsy often had other problems such as mental retardation, visual disturbances, and seizures, Freud suggested that the disorder might sometimes have roots earlier in life, during the brain's development in the womb. "Difficult birth, in certain cases," he wrote, "is merely a symptom of deeper effects that influence the development of the fetus."

Despite Freud's observation, the belief that birth complications cause most cases of cerebral palsy was widespread among physicians, families, and even medical researchers until very recently. In the 1980s, however, scientists analyzed extensive data from a government study of more than 35,000 births and were surprised to discover that such complications account for only a fraction of cases—probably less than 10 percent. In most cases of cerebral palsy, no cause could be found. These findings from the National Institute of Neurological Disorders and Stroke (NINDS) perinatal study have profoundly altered medical theories about cerebral palsy and have spurred today's researchers to explore alternative causes.

At the same time, biomedical research has also led to significant changes in understanding, diagnosing, and treating persons with cerebral palsy. Identification of infants with cerebral palsy very early in life gives youngsters the best opportunity for developing to their full capacity. Biomedical research has led to improved diagnostic techniques—such as advanced brain imaging and modern gait analysis—that are making this easier. Certain conditions known to cause cerebral palsy, such as *rubella* (German measles) and *jaundice,* can now be prevented or treated. Physical, psychological, and behavioral therapy that assist with such skills as movement and speech and foster social and emotional development can help children who have cerebral palsy to achieve and succeed. Medications, surgery, and braces can often improve nerve and muscle coordination, help treat associated medical problems, and either prevent or correct deformities.

Much of the research to improve medical understanding of cerebral palsy has been supported by the NINDS, one of the Federal Government's National Institutes of Health. The NINDS is America's leading supporter of biomedical research into cerebral palsy and other neurological disorders. Through this publication, the NINDS hopes to help the more than 4,500 American babies and infants diagnosed each year, their families, and others concerned about cerebral palsy benefit from these research results.

What is cerebral palsy?

Cerebral palsy is an umbrella-like term used to describe a group of chronic disorders impairing control of movement that appear in the first few years of life and generally do not worsen over time. The term *cerebral* refers to the brain's two halves, or hemispheres, and *palsy* describes any disorder that impairs control of body movement. Thus, these disorders are not caused by problems in the muscles or nerves. Instead, faulty development or damage to motor areas in the brain disrupts the brain's ability to adequately control movement and posture.

Symptoms of cerebral palsy lie along a spectrum of varying severity. An individual with cerebral palsy may have difficulty with finer motor tasks, such as writing or cutting with scissors; experience trouble with maintaining balance and walking; or be affected by involuntary movements, such as uncontrollable writing motion of the hands or drooling. The symptoms differ from one person to the next, and may even change over time in the individual. Some people with cerebral palsy are also affected by other medical disorders, including seizures or mental impairment. Contrary to common belief, however, cerebral palsy does not always cause profound handicaps. While a child with severe cerebral palsy might be unable to walk and need extensive, lifelong care, a child with mild cerebral palsy might only be slightly awkward and require no special assistance. Cerebral palsy is not contagious nor is it usually inherited from one generation to the next. At this time, it cannot be cured, although scientific research continues to seek improved treatments and methods of prevention.

How many people have this disorder?

The United Cerebral Palsy Associations estimate that more than 500,000 Americans have cerebral palsy. Despite advances in preventing and treating certain causes of cerebral palsy, the number of children and adults it affects has remained essentially unchanged or perhaps risen slightly over the past 30 years. This is partly because more critically premature and frail infants are surviving through improved intensive care. Unfortunately, many of these infants have developmental problems of the nervous system or suffer neurological damage. Research is under way to improve care for these infants, as in ongoing studies of technology to alleviate troubled breathing and trials of drugs to prevent bleeding in the brain before or soon after birth.

What are the different forms?

Spastic diplegia, the disorder first described by Dr. Little in the 1860s, is only one of several disorders called cerebral palsy. Today doctors classify cerebral palsy into four broad categories—spastic, athetoid, ataxic, and mixed forms—according to the type of movement disturbance.

Spastic Cerebral Palsy

In this form of cerebral palsy, which affects 70 to 80 percent of patients, the muscles are stiffly and permanently contracted. Doctors will often describe which type of spastic cerebral palsy a patient has based on which limbs are affected. The names given to these types combine a Latin description of affected limbs with the term *plegia* or *paresis*.

When both legs are affected by spasticity, they may turn in and cross at the knees. This abnormal leg posture, called scissoring, can interfere with walking.

Individuals with spastic hemiparesis may also experience *hemiparetic tremors*, in which uncontrollable shaking affects the limbs on one side of the body. If these tremors are severe, they can seriously impair movement.

Athetoid, or Dyskinetic, Cerebral Palsy

This form of cerebral palsy is characterized by uncontrolled, slow, writhing movements. These abnormal movements usually affect the hands, feet, arms, or legs and, in some cases, the muscles of the face and tongue, causing grimacing or drooling. The movements often increase during periods of emotional stress and disappear during sleep. Patients may also have problems coordinating the muscle movements needed for speech, a condition known as *dysarthria*. Athetoid cerebral palsy affects about 10 to 20 percent of patients.

Ataxic Cerebral Palsy

This rare form affects balance and coordination. Affected persons may walk unsteadily with a wide-based gait, placing their feet unusually far apart, and experience difficulty when attempting quick or precise movements, such as writing or buttoning a shirt. They may also have intention tremor. In this form of tremor, beginning a voluntary movement, such as reaching for a book, causes a trembling that affects the body part being used. The tremor worsens as the individual gets nearer to the desired object. The ataxic form affects an estimated 5 to 10 percent of cerebral palsy patients.

Mixed Forms

It is common for patients to have symptoms of more than one form of cerebral palsy mentioned above. The most common combination includes spasticity and athetoid movements but other combinations are possible.

What other medical disorders are associated with cerebral palsy?

Many individuals who have cerebral palsy have no associated medical disorders. However, disorders that involve the brain and impair its motor function can also cause seizures and impair an individual's intellectual development, attentiveness to the outside world, activity and behavior, and vision and hearing. medical disorders associated with cerebral palsy include

- **Mental impairment.** About one-third of children who have cerebral palsy are mildly intellectually impaired, one-third are moderately or severely impaired, and the remaining third are intellectually normal. Mental impairment is more commonly seen in children with spastic quadriplegia.
- **Seizures or epilepsy.** As many as half of all children with cerebral palsy have seizures. During a seizure, the normal, orderly pattern of electrical activity in the brain is disrupted by uncontrolled bursts of electricity. When seizures recur without a direct trigger, such as fever, the condition is called epilepsy. In the person who has cerebral palsy and epilepsy, this disruption may be spread throughout the brain and cause varied symptoms all over the body—as in tonic-clonic seizures—or may be confined to just one part of the brain and cause more specific symptoms—as in partial seizures.

  Tonic-clonic seizures are classified as simple or complex. In simple partial seizures, the individual has localized symptoms, such as muscle twitches, numbness, or tingling. In complex partial seizures, the individual may hallucinate, stagger, perform automatic and purposeless movements, or experience impaired consciousness or confusion.
- **Growth problems.** A syndrome called *failure to thrive* is common in children with moderate-to-severe cerebral palsy, especially those with spastic quadriparesis. Failure to thrive is a general term physicians use to describe children who seem to lag behind in growth and

development despite having enough food. In babies, this lag usually takes the form of too little weight gain; in young children, it can appear as abnormal shortness; in teenagers, it may appear as a combination of shortness and lack of sexual development. Failure to thrive probably has several causes, including, in particular, poor nutrition and damage to the brain centers controlling growth and development.

In addition, the muscles and limbs affected by cerebral palsy tend to be smaller than normal. This is especially noticeable in some patients with spastic hemiplegia, because limbs on the affected side of the body may not grow as quickly or as large as those on the more normal side. this condition usually affects the hand and foot most severely. Since the involved foot in hemiplegia is often smaller than the unaffected foot even among patients who walk, this size difference is probably not due to lack of use. Scientists believe the problem is more likely to result from disruption of the complex process responsible for normal body growth.

- **Impaired vision or hearing.** *A large number of children with cerebral palsy have strabismus,* a condition in which the eyes are not aligned because of differences in the left and right eye muscles. In an adult, this condition causes double vision. In children, however, the brain often adapts to the condition by ignoring signals from one of the misaligned eyes. Untreated, this can lead to very poor vision in one eye and can interfere with certain visual skills, such as judging distance. In some cases, physicians may recommend surgery to correct strabismus.

  Children with hemiparesis may have *hemianopia,* which is defective vision or blindness that impairs the normal field of vision. For example, when hemianopia affects the right field of vision, a child looking straight ahead might have perfect vision except on the far right. In homonymous hemianopia, the impairment affects the same part of the visual field of both eyes.

  Impaired hearing is also more frequent among those with cerebral palsy than in the general population.

- **Abnormal sensation and perception.** Some children with cerebral palsy have impaired ability to feel simple sensations like touch and pain. They may also have *stereognosia,* or difficulty perceiving and identifying objects using the sense of touch. A child with stereognosia, for example, would have trouble identifying a hard ball, sponge, or other object placed in his hand, without looking at the object.

What causes cerebral palsy?

Cerebral palsy is not one disease with a single cause, like chicken pox or measles. It is a group of disorders that are related but have different causes. When physicians try to uncover the cause of cerebral palsy in an individual child, they look at the form of cerebral palsy, the mother's and child's medical history, and onset of the disorder.

About 10 to 20 percent of children who have cerebral palsy acquire the disorder after birth. Acquired cerebral palsy results from brain damage in the first few months or years of life and often follows brain infections, such as bacterial meningitis or viral encephalitis, or results from head injury—most often from a motor vehicle accident, a fall, or child abuse.

Congenital cerebral palsy, on the other hand, is present at birth, although it may not be detected for several months. In most cases, the cause of congenital cerebral palsy is unknown. Thanks to research, however, scientists have pinpointed some specific events during pregnancy or around the time of birth that can damage motor centers in the developing brain. Some of these causes of congenital cerebral palsy include

- **Infections during pregnancy.** German measles, or rubella, is caused by a virus that can infect pregnant women and, therefore, the fetus in the uterus, to cause damage to the developing nervous system. Other infections that can cause brain injury in the developing fetus include cytomegalovirus and toxoplasmosis.

- **Jaundice in the infant.** *Bile pigments,* compounds that are normally found in small amounts in the bloodstream, are produced when blood cells are destroyed. When many blood cells are destroyed in a short time, as in the condition called Rh incompatibility (see below), the yellow-colored pigments can build up and cause jaundice. Severe, untreated jaundice can damage brain cells.

- **Perinatal asphyxia.** During labor and delivery, a shortage of oxygen in the blood, reduced brain blood flow, or both, can impair the supply of oxygen to the newborn's brain, causing the condition known as perinatal asphyxia. When asphyxia is severe enough to put the newborn at risk for long-term brain damage, it immediately causes problems with brain function (as in moderate-to-severe hyposic-ischemic encephalopathy). Asphyxia this severe is very uncommon, is always linked to dysfunction of other body organs, and is often accompanied by seizures.

- **Rh incompatibility.** In this blood condition, the mother's body produces immune cells called antibodies that destroy the fetus's blood cells, leading to a form of jaundice in the newborn.

  In the past, physicians and scientists attributed most cases of cerebral palsy to asphyxia or other complications during birth if they could not identify another cause. However, extensive research by NINDS scientists and others has shown that very few babies who experience asphyxia during birth develop encephalopathy after birth. Research also shows that most babies who experience asphyxia do not grow up to have cerebral palsy or other neurological disorders. In fact, current evidence suggests that cerebral palsy is associated with asphyxia and other birth complications in no more than 10 percent of cases.

- **Stroke/intracranial hemorrhage.** Bleeding in the brain (intracranial hemorrhage) has several causes—including broken blood vessels in the brain, clogged blood vessels, or abnormal blood cells—and is one form of stroke. Newborn respiratory distress, a breathing disorder that is particularly common in premature infants, is one cause. Although strokes are better known for their effects on older adults, they can also occur in the fetus during pregnancy or the newborn around the time of birth, damaging brain tissue and causing neurological problems. Ongoing research is testing potential treatments that may one day help prevent stroke in fetuses and newborns.

What are the risk factors?

Research scientists have examined thousands of expectant mothers, followed them through childbirth, and monitored their children's early neurological development. As a result, they have uncovered certain characteristics, called risk factors, that increase the possibility that a child will later be diagnosed with cerebral palsy:

- **Breech presentation.** Babies with cerebral palsy are more likely to present feet first, instead of head first, at the beginning of labor.
- **Complicated labor and delivery.** Vascular or respiratory problems of the baby during labor and delivery may sometimes be the first sign that a baby has suffered brain damage or that a baby's brain has not developed normally during the pregnancy. Such complications can cause permanent brain damage.
- **Inborn malformations outside the nervous system.** Babies with physical birth defects—including faulty formation of the spinal bones, hernia (a protrusion of organs through an abnormal opening inside the body) in the groin area, or an abnormally small jaw bone—are at an increased risk for cerebral palsy.
- **Low Apgar score.** The *Apgar score* (named for anesthesiologist Virginia Apgar) is a numbered rating that reflects a newborn's condition. To determine an Apgar score, doctors periodically check the baby's heart rate, breathing, muscle tone, reflexes, and skin color in the first minutes after birth. They then assign points; the higher the score, the more normal the baby's condition. A low score at 10-20 minutes after delivery is often considered an important sign of potential problems.
- **Low birth weight and premature birth.** The risk of cerebral palsy is higher among babies who weigh less than 2500 grams (5 lbs., 7 oz.) at birth and among babies who are born less than 37 weeks into pregnancy. This risk increases as birth weight falls.
- **Multiple births.** Twins, triplets, and other multiple births are linked to an increased risk of cerebral palsy.
- **Nervous system malformations.** Some babies born with cerebral palsy have visible signs of nervous system malformation, such as an abnormally small head (microphaly). This suggests that problems occurred in the development of the nervous system while the baby was in the womb.
- **Maternal bleeding or severe proteinuria late in pregnancy.** Vaginal bleeding during the sixth to ninth months of pregnancy and severe proteinuria (the pres-

ence of excess proteins in the urine) are linked to a higher risk of having a baby with cerebral palsy.
- **Maternal hyperthyroidism, mental retardation, or seizures.** Mothers with any of these conditions are slightly more likely to have a child with cerebral palsy.
- **Seizures in the newborn.** An infant who has seizures faces a higher risk of being diagnosed, later in childhood, with cerebral palsy.

Knowing these warning signs helps doctors keep a close eye on children who face a higher risk for long-term problems in the nervous system. However, parents should not become too alarmed if their child has one or more of these factors. Most such children do not have and do not develop cerebral palsy.

Can cerebral palsy be prevented?

Several of the causes of cerebral palsy that have been identified through research are preventable or treatable:

- **Head injury** can be prevented by regular use of child safety seats when driving in a car and helmets during bicycle rides, and elimination of child abuse. In addition, common sense measures around the household—like close supervision during bathing and keeping poisons out of reach—can reduce the risk of accidental injury.
- **Jaundice** of newborn infants can be treated with phototherapy. In phototherapy, babies are exposed to special blue lights that break down bile pigments, preventing them from building up and threatening the brain. In the few cases in which this treatment is not enough, physicians can correct the condition with a special form of blood transfusion.
- **Rh incompatibility** is easily identified by a simple blood test routinely performed on expectant mothers and, if indicated, expectant fathers. This incompatibility in blood types does not usually cause problems during a woman's first pregnancy, since the mother's body generally does not produce the unwanted antibodies until after delivery. In most cases, a special serum given after each childbirth can prevent the unwanted production of antibodies. In unusual cases, such as when a pregnant woman develops the antibodies during her first pregnancy or antibody production is not prevented, doctors can help minimize problems by closely watching the developing baby and, when needed, performing a transfusion to the baby while in the womb or an exchange transfusion (in which a large volume of the baby's blood is removed and replaced) after birth.
- **Rubella,** or German measles, can be prevented if women are vaccinated against this disease *before* becoming pregnant.

In addition, it is always good to work toward a healthy pregnancy through regular prenatal care and good nutrition and by eliminating smoking, alcohol consumption, and drug abuse. Despite the best efforts of parents and physicians, however, children will still be born with cerebral palsy. Since in most cases the cause of cerebral palsy is unknown, little can currently be done to prevent it. As investigators learn more about the causes of cerebral palsy through basic and clinical research, doctors and parents will be better equipped to help prevent this disorder.

What are the early signs?

Early signs of cerebral palsy usually appear before three years of age, and parents are often the first to suspect that their infant is not developing motor skills normally. Infants with cerebral palsy are frequently slow to reach developmental milestones, such as learning to role over, sit, crawl, smile, or walk. This is sometimes called developmental delay.

Some affected children have abnormal muscle tone. Decreased muscle tone is called *hypotonia;* the baby may seem flaccid and relaxed, even floppy. Increased muscle tone is called *hypertonia,* and the baby may seem stiff or rigid. In some cases, the baby has an early period of hypotonia that progresses to hypertonia after the first two to three months of life. Affected children may also have unusual posture or favor one side of their body.

Parents who are concerned about their baby's development for any reason should contact their physician, who can help distinguish normal variation in development from a developmental disorder.

How is cerebral palsy diagnosed?

Doctors diagnose cerebral palsy by testing an infant's motor skills and looking carefully at the infant's medical history. In addition to checking for those symptoms described above—slow development, abnormal muscle tone, and unusual posture—a physician also tests the infant's reflexes and looks for early development of hand preference.

Reflexes are movements that the body makes automatically in response to a specific cue. For example, if a newborn baby is held on its back and tilted so the legs are above its head, the baby will automatically extend its arms in a gesture, called the Moro reflex, that looks like an embrace. Babies normally lose this reflex after they reach six months, but those with cerebral palsy may retain it for abnormally long periods. This is just one of several reflexes that a physician can check.

Doctors can also look for hand preference—a tendency to use either the right or left hand more often. When the doctor holds an object in front and to the side of the infant, an infant with hand preference will use the favored hand to reach for the object, even when it is held closer to the opposite hand. During the first 12 months of life, babies do not usually show hand preference. But infants with spastic hemiplegia, in particular, may develop a preference much earlier, since the hand on the unaffected side of their body is stronger and more useful.

The next step in diagnosing cerebral palsy is to rule out other disorders that can cause movement problems. Most important, doctors must determine that the child's condition is not getting worse. Although its symptoms may change over time, cerebral palsy by definition is not progressive. If a child is continuously losing motor skills, the problem is probably due to other causes—including genetic diseases, muscle dis-

eases, disorders of metabolism, or tumors in the nervous system. The child's medical history, special diagnostic tests, and, in some cases, repeated check-ups can help confirm that other disorders are not the cause.

The doctor may also order specialized tests to learn more about the possible cause of cerebral palsy. One such test is *computed tomography,* or CT, a sophisticated imaging technique that uses X rays and a computer to create an anatomical picture of the brain's tissues and structures. A CT scan may reveal brain areas that are underdeveloped, abnormal cysts (sacs that are often filled with liquid) in the brain, or other physical problems. With the information from CT scans, doctors may be better equipped to judge the long-term outlook for an affected child.

Magnetic resonance imaging, or MRI, is a relatively new brain imaging technique that is rapidly gaining widespread use for identifying brain disorders. This technique uses a magnetic field and radio waves, rather than X rays. MRI gives better pictures of structures or abnormal areas located near bone than CT.

A third test that can expose problems in brain tissues is *ultrasonography.* This technique bounces sound waves off the brain and uses the pattern of echoes to form a picture, or sonogram, of its structures. Ultrasonography can be used in infants before the bones of the skull harden and close. Although it is less precise than CT and MRI scanning, this technique can detect cysts and structures in the brain, is less expensive, and does not require long periods of immobility.

Finally, physicians may want to look for other conditions that are linked to cerebral palsy, including seizure disorders, mental impairment, and vision or hearing problems.

When the doctor suspects a seizure disorder, an *electroencephalogram,* or EEG, may be ordered. An EEG uses special patches called electrodes placed on the scalp to record the natural electrical currents inside the brain. This recording can help the doctor see telltale patterns in the brain's electrical activity that suggest a seizure disorder.

Intelligence tests are often used to determine if a child with cerebral palsy is mentally impaired. Sometimes, however, a child's intelligence may be underestimated because problems with movement, sensation, or speech due to cerebral palsy make it difficult for him or her to perform well on these tests.

If problems with vision are suspected, the doctor may refer the patient to an ophthalmologist for examination; if hearing impairment seems likely, an etiologist may be called in.

Identifying these accompanying conditions is important and is becoming more accurate as ongoing research yields advances that make diagnosis easier. Many of these conditions can then be addressed through specific treatments, improving the long-term outlook for those with cerebral palsy.

How is cerebral palsy managed?

Cerebral palsy can not be cured, but treatment can often improve a child's capabilities. In fact, progress due to medical research now means that many patients can enjoy near-normal lives if their neurological problems are properly managed. There is no standard therapy that works for all patients. Instead, the physician must work with a team of health care professionals first to identify a child's unique needs and impairments and then to create an individual treatment plan that addresses them.

Some approaches that can be included in this plan are drugs to control seizures and muscle spasms, special braces to compensate for muscle imbalance, surgery, mechanical aids to help overcome impairments, counseling for emotional and psychological needs, and physical, occupational, speech, and behavioral therapy. In general, the earlier treatment begins, the better chance a child has of overcoming developmental disabilities or learning new ways to accomplish difficult tasks.

The members of the treatment team for a child with cerebral palsy should be knowledgeable professionals with a wide range of specialties. A typical treatment team might include

- a *physician,* such as a pediatrician, a pediatric neurologist, or a pediatric physiatrist, trained to help developmentally disabled children. This physician, often the leader of the treatment team, works to synthesize the professional advice of all team members into a comprehensive treatment plan, implements treatments, and follows the patient's progress over a number of years.
- *an orthopedist,* a surgeon who specializes in treating the bones, muscles, tendons, and other parts of the body's skeletal system. An orthopedist might be called on to predict, diagnose, or treat muscle problems associated with cerebral palsy.
- a *physical therapist,* who designs and implements special exercise programs to improve movement and strength.
- *an occupational therapist,* who can help patients learn skills for day-to-day living, school, and work.
- *a speech and language pathologist,* who specializes in diagnosing and treating communication problems.
- *a social worker,* who can help patients and their families locate community assistance and education programs.
- *a psychologist,* who helps patients and their families cope with the special stresses and demands of cerebral palsy. In some cases, psychologists may also oversee therapy to modify unhelpful or destructive behaviors or habits.
- *an educator,* who may play an especially important role when mental impairment or learning disabilities present a challenge to education.

Individuals who have cerebral palsy and their family or caregivers are also key members of the treatment team, and they should be intimately involved in all steps of planning, making decisions, and applying treatments. Studies have shown that family support and personal determination are two of the most important predictors of which individuals who have cerebral palsy will achieve long-term goals.

Too often, however, physicians and parents may focus primarily on an individual symptom—especially the inability to walk. While mastering specific skills is an important focus of treatment on a day-to-day basis, the ultimate goal is to help individuals grow to adulthood and have maximum independence in society. In the words of one physician, "After all, the real point of walking is to get from point A to point B. Even if a child needs a wheelchair, what's important is that they're able to achieve this goal."

What specific treatments are available?

Physical, Behavioral, and Other Therapies

Therapy—whether for movement, speech, or practical tasks—is a cornerstone of cerebral palsy treatment. The skills a 2-year-old needs to explore the world are very different from those that a child needs in the classroom or a young adult needs to become independent. Cerebral palsy therapy should be tailored to reflect these changing demands.

Physical therapy usually begins in the first few years of life, soon after the diagnosis is made. Physical therapy programs use specific sets of exercises to work toward two important goals: preventing the weakening or deterioration of muscles that can follow lack of use (called disuse atrophy) and avoiding *contracture,* in which muscles become fixed in a rigid, abnormal position.

Contracture is one of the most common and serious complications of cerebral palsy. A contracture is a chronic shortening of a muscle due to abnormal tone and weakness associated with cerebral palsy. A muscle contracture limits movement of a bony joint, such as the elbow, and can disrupt balance and cause loss of previous motor abilities. Physical therapy alone, or in combination with special braces (sometimes called *orthotic devices*), works to prevent this complication by stretching spastic muscles. For example, if a child has spastic hamstrings (tendons located behind the knee), the therapist and parents should encourage the child to sit with the legs extended to stretch them.

A third goal of some physical therapy programs is to improve the child's motor development. A widespread program of physical therapy that works toward this goal is the Bobath technique, named for a husband and wife team who pioneered this approach in England. This program is based on the idea that the primitive reflexes retained by many children with cerebral palsy present major roadblocks to learning voluntary control. A therapist using the Bobath technique tries to counteract these reflexes by positioning the child in an opposing movement. So, for example, if a child with cerebral palsy normally keeps his arm flexed, the therapist would repeatedly extend it.

A second such approach to physical therapy is "patterning," which is based on the principle that motor skills should be taught in more or less the same sequence that they develop normally. In this controversial approach, the therapist guides the child with movement problems along the path of normal motor development. For example, the child is first taught elementary movements like pulling himself to a standing position and crawling before he is taught to walk—regardless of his age. Some experts and organizations, including the American Academy of Pediatrics, have expressed strong reservations about the patterning approach, because studies have not documented its value.

Physical therapy is usually just one element of an infant development program that also includes efforts to provide a varied and stimulating environment. Like all children, the child with cerebral palsy needs new experiences and interactions with the world around him in order to learn. Simulation programs can bring this valuable experience to the child who is physically unable to explore.

As the child with cerebral palsy approaches school age, the emphasis of therapy shifts away from early motor development. Efforts now focus on preparing the child for the classroom, helping the child master activities of daily living, and maximizing the child's ability to communicate.

Physical therapy can now help the child with cerebral palsy prepare for the classroom by improving his or her ability to sit, move independently or in a wheelchair, or perform precise tasks, such as writing. In **occupational therapy,** the therapist works with the child to develop such skills as feeding, dressing, or using the bathroom. This can help reduce demands on caregivers and boost self-reliance and self-esteem. For the many children who have difficulty communicating, **speech therapy** works to identify specific difficulties and overcome them through a program of exercises. For example, if a child has difficulty saying words that begin with "b," the therapist may suggest daily practice with a list of "b" words, increasing their difficulty as each list is mastered. Speech therapy can also work to help the child learn to use special communication devices, such as a computer with voice synthesizers.

Behavioral therapy provides yet another avenue to increase a child's abilities. This therapy, which uses psychological theory and techniques, can complement physical, speech, or occupational therapy. For example, behavioral therapy might include hiding a toy inside a box to reward a child for learning to reach into the box with his weaker hand. Likewise, a child learning to say his "b" words might be given a balloon for mastering the word. In other cases, therapists may try to discourage unhelpful or destructive behaviors, such as hair-pulling or biting, by selectively presenting a child with rewards and praise during other, more positive activities.

As a child with cerebral palsy grows older, the need for and types of therapy and other support services will continue to change. Continuing physical therapy addresses movement problems and is supplemented by vocational training, recreation and leisure programs, and special education when necessary. Counseling for emotional and psychological challenges may be needed at any age, but is often most critical during adolescence. Depending on their physical and intellectual abilities, adults may need attendant care, living accommodations, transportation, or employment opportunities.

Regardless of the patient's age and which forms of therapy are used, treatment does not end when the patient leaves the office or treatment center. In fact, most of the work is often done at home. The therapist functions as a coach, providing parents and patients with the strategy and drills that can help improve performance at home, at school, and in the world. As research continues, doctors and parents can expect new forms of therapy and better information about which forms of therapy are most effective for individuals with cerebral palsy.

Drug Therapy

Physicians usually prescribe drugs for those who have seizures associated with cerebral palsy, and these medications are very effective in preventing seizures in many patients. In general, the drugs given to individual patients are chosen based on the type of seizures, since no one drug controls all types. However, different people with the same type of seizure may do better on different drugs, and some individuals may need a combination of two or more drugs to achieve good seizure control.

Drugs are also sometimes used to control spasticity, particularly following surgery. The three medications that are used most often are diazepam, which acts as a general relaxant of the brain and body; baclofen, which blocks signals sent from the spinal cord to contract the muscles; and dantrolene, which interferes with the process of muscle contraction. Given by mouth, these drugs can reduce spasticity for short periods, but their value for long-term control of spasticity has not been clearly demonstrated. They may also trigger significant side effects, such as drowsiness, and their long-term effects on the developing nervous system are largely unknown. One possible solution to avoid such side effects may lie in current research to explore new routes for delivering these drugs.

Patients with athetoid cerebral palsy may sometimes be given drugs that help reduce abnormal movements. Most often, the prescribed drug belongs to a group of chemicals called anticholinergics that work by reducing the activity of acetylcholine. Acetylcholine is a chemical messenger that helps some brain cells communicate and that triggers muscle contraction. Antichonlinergic drugs include trihexyphenidyl, benztropine, and procyclidine hydrochloride.

Occasionally, physicians may use alcohol "washes"—or injections of alcohol into a muscle—to reduce spasticity for a short period. This technique is most often used when physicians want to correct a developing contracture. Injecting alcohol into a muscle that is too short weakens the muscle for several weeks and gives physicians time to work on lengthening the muscle through bracing, therapy, or casts. In some cases, if the contracture is detected early enough, this technique may avert the need for surgery. In addition, a number of experimental drug therapies are under investigation.

Surgery

Surgery is often recommended when contractures are severe enough to cause movement problems. In the operating room, surgeons can lengthen muscles and tendons that are proportionately too short. First, however, they must determine the exact muscles at fault, since lengthening the wrong muscle could make the problem worse,

Finding problem muscles that need correction can be a difficult task. To walk two strides with a normal gait, it takes more than 30 major muscles working at exactly the right time and exactly the right force. A problem in any one muscle can cause abnormal gait. Furthermore, the natural adjustments the body makes to compensate for muscle problems can be misleading. A new tool that enables doctors to spot gait abnormalities, pinpoint problem muscles, and separate real problems from compensation is called *gait analysis.* Gait analysis combines cameras that record the patient while walking, computers that analyze each portion of the patient's gait, force plates that detect when feet touch the ground, and a special recording technique that detects muscle activity (known as *electromyography*). Using these data, doctors are better equipped to intervene and correct significant problems. They can also use gait analysis to check surgical results.

Because lengthening a muscle makes it weaker, surgery for contractures is usually followed by months of recovery. For this reason, doctors try to fix all of the affected muscles at once when it is possible or, if more than one surgical procedure is unavoidable, they may try to schedule operations close together.

A second surgical technique, known as *selective dorsal root rhizotomy,* aims to reduce spasticity in the legs by reducing the amount of stimulation that reaches leg muscles via nerves. In the procedure, doctors try to locate and selectively sever some of the overactivated nerve fibers that control leg muscle tone. Although there is scientific controversy over how selective this technique actually is, recent research results suggest it can reduce spasticity in some patients, particularly those who have spastic diplegia. Ongoing research is evaluating this surgery's effectiveness.

Experimental surgical techniques include chronic cerebella stimulation and stereotaxic thalamotomy. In chronic cerebellar stimulation, electrodes are implanted on the surface of the cerebellum—the part of the brain responsible for coordinating movement—and are used to stimulate certain cerebellar nerves. While it was hoped that this technique would decrease spasticity and improve motor function, results of this invasive procedure have been mixed. Some studies have reported improvements in spasticity and function, others have not.

Stereotaxic thalamotomy involves precise cutting of parts of the thalamus, which serves as the brain's relay station for messages from the muscles and sensory organs. This has been shown effective only for reducing hemiparetic tremors (*see* Glossary).

Mechanical Aids

Whether they are as humble as velcro shoes or as advanced as computerized communication devices, special machines and gadgets in the home, school, and workplace can help the child or adult with cerebral palsy overcome limitations.

The computer is probably the most dramatic example of a new device that can make a difference in the lives of those with cerebral palsy. For example, a child who is unable to speak or write but can make head movements may be able to learn to control a computer using a special light pointer that attaches to a headband. Equipped with a computer and voice synthesizer, this child could communicate with others. In other cases, technology has led to new versions of old devices, such as the traditional wheelchair and its modern offspring that runs on electricity.

What other major problems are associated with cerebral palsy?

A common complication is **incontinence,** caused by faulty control over the muscles that keep the bladder closed. Incontinence can take the form of bed-wetting (also known as enuresis), uncontrolled urination during physical activities (or stress incontinence), or slow leaking of urine from the bladder. Possible medical treatments for incontinence include special exercises, biofeedback, prescription drugs, surgery, or surgically implanted devices to replace or aid muscles. Specially designed undergarments are also available.

Poor control of the muscles of the throat, mouth, and tongue sometimes leads to **drooling.** Drooling can cause severe skin irritation and, because it is socially unacceptable, can lead to further isolation of affected children from their peers. Although numerous treatments for **drooling** have been tested over the years, there is no one treatment that always helps. Drugs called anticholinergics can reduce the flow of saliva but may cause significant side effects, such as mouth dryness and poor digestion. Surgery, while sometimes effective, carries the risk of complications, including worsening of swallowing problems. Some patients benefit from a technique called biofeedback that can tell them when they are drooling or having difficulty controlling muscles that close the mouth. This kind of therapy is most likely to work if the patient has a mental age of more than two or three years, is motivated to control drooling, and understands that drooling is not socially acceptable.

Difficulty with eating and swallowing—also triggered by motor problems in the mouth—can cause **poor nutrition.** Poor nutrition, in turn, may make the individual more vulnerable to infections and cause or aggravate "failure to thrive"—a lag in growth and development that is common among those with cerebral palsy. When eating is difficult, a therapist trained to address swallowing problems can help by instituting special diets and teaching new feeding techniques. In severe cases of swallowing problems and malnutrition, physicians may recommend tube feeding, in which a tube delivers food and nutrients down the throat and into the stomach, or *gatrostomy*, in which a surgical opening allows a tube to be placed directly into the stomach.

What research is being done?

Investigators from many arenas of medicine and health are using their expertise to help improve treatment and prevention of cerebral palsy. Much of their work is supported through the National Institute of Neurological Disorders and Stroke (NINDS), the National Institute of Child Health and Human Development, other agencies within the Federal government, nonprofit groups such as the United Cerebral Palsy Research and Educational Foundation, and private institutions.

The ultimate hope for overcoming cerebral palsy lies with prevention. In order to prevent cerebral palsy, however, scientists must first understand the complex process of normal brain development and what can make this process go awry.

Between early pregnancy and the first months of life, one cell divides to form first a handful of cells, and then hundreds, millions, and, eventually, billions of cells. Some of these cells specialize to become brain cells. These brain cells specialize into different types and migrate to their appropriate site in the brain. They send out branches to form crucial connections with other brain cells. Ultimately, the most complex entity known to us is created: a human brain with its billions of interconnected neurons.

Mounting evidence is pointing investigators toward this intricate process in the womb for clues about cerebral palsy. For example, a group of researchers has recently observed that more than one-third of children who have cerebral palsy also have missing enamel on certain teeth. This tooth defect can be traced to problems in the early months of fetal development, suggesting that a disruption at this period in development might be linked both to this tooth defect and to cerebral palsy.

As a result of this and other research, many scientists now believe that a significant number of children develop cerebral palsy because of mishaps early in brain development. They are examining how brain cells specialize, how they know where to migrate, how they form the right connections—and they are looking for preventable factors that can disrupt this process before or after birth.

Scientists are also scrutinizing other events—such as bleeding in the brain, seizures, and breathing and circulation problems—that threaten the brain of the newborn baby. Through this research, they hope to learn how these hazards can damage the newborn's brain and to develop new methods for prevention.

Some newborn infants, for example, have life-threatening problems with breathing and blood circulation. A recently introduced treatment to help these infants is extracorporeal membrane oxygenation (ECMO), in which blood is routed from the patient to a special machine that takes over the lungs' task of removing carbon dioxide and adding oxygen. Although this technique can dramatically help many such infants, some scientists have observed that a substantial fraction of treated children later experience long-term neurological problems, including developmental delay and cerebral palsy. Investigators are studying infants through pregnancy, delivery, birth, and infancy, and are tracking those who undergo this treatment. By observing them at all stages of development, scientists can learn whether their problems developed before birth, result from the same breathing problems that made them candidates for the treatment, or spring from errors in the treatment itself. Once this is determined, they may be able to correct any existing problems or develop new treatment methods to prevent brain damage.

Other scientists are exploring how brain insults like hypoxic-ischemic encephalopathy (brain damage from a shortage of oxygen or blood flow), bleeding in the brain, and seizures can cause the abnormal release of brain chemicals and trigger brain damage. For example, research has shown that bleeding in the brain unleashes dangerously high amounts of a brain chemical called glutamate. While glutamate is normally used in the brain for communication, too much glutamate overstimulates the brain's cells and causes a cycle of destruction. Scientists are now looking closely at glutamate to detect how its release harms brain tissue and spreads the damage from stroke. By learning how such brain chemicals that normally help us function can hurt the brain, scientists may be equipped to develop new drugs that block their harmful effects.

In related research, some investigators are already conducting studies to learn if certain drugs can help prevent neonatal stroke. Several of these drugs seem promising because they appear to reduce the excess production of potentially dangerous chemicals in the brain and may help control brain blood flow and volume. Earlier research has linked sudden changes in blood flow and volume to stroke in the newborn.

Low birth-weight itself is also the subject of extensive research. In spite of improvements in health care for some pregnant women, the incidence of low birth-weight babies born each year in the United States remains at about 7 percent. Some scientists currently investigating this serious health problem are working to understand how infections, hormonal problems, and genetic factors may increase a woman's chances of giving birth prematurely. They are also conducting more applied research that could yield: 1) new drugs that can safely delay labor, 2) new devices to further improve medical care for premature infants, and 3) new insight into how smoking and alcohol consumption can disrupt fetal development.

While this research offers hope for preventing cerebral palsy in the future, ongoing research to improve treatment brightens the outlook for those who must face the challenges of cerebral palsy today. An important thrust of such research is the evaluation of treatments already in use so that physicians and parents have the information they need to choose the best therapy. A good example of this effort is an ongoing NINDS-supported study that promises to yield new information about which patients are most likely to benefit from selective dorsal root rhizotomy, a recently introduced surgery that is becoming increasingly in demand for reduction of spasticity.

Similarly, although physical therapy programs are a popular and widespread approach to managing cerebral palsy, little scientific evidence exists to help physicians, other health professionals, and parents determine how well physical therapy works or to choose the best approach among many. Current research on cerebral palsy aims to provide this information through careful studies that compare the abilities of children who have had physical and other therapy with those who have not.

As part of this effort, scientists are working to create new measures to judge the effectiveness of treatment, as in ongoing research to precisely identify the specific brain areas responsible for movement. Using such techniques as magnetic pulses, researchers can locate brain areas that control specific actions, such as raising an arm or lifting a leg, and construct detailed maps. By comparing charts made before and after therapy among children who have cerebral palsy, researchers may gain new insights into how therapy affects the brain's organization and new data about its effectiveness.

Investigators are also working to develop new drugs—and new ways of using existing drugs—to help relieve cerebral palsy's symptoms. In one such set of studies, early research results suggest that doctors may improve the effectiveness of the anti-spasticity drug called baclofen by giving the drug through spinal injections, rather than by mouth. In addition, scientists are also exploring the use of tiny implanted pumps that deliver a constant supply of anti-spasticity drugs into the fluid around the spinal cord, in the hope of improving these drugs' effectiveness and reducing side effects, such as drowsiness.

Other experimental drug development efforts are exploring the use of minute amounts of the familiar toxin called botulinum. Ingested in large amounts, this toxin is responsible for botulism poisoning, in which the body's muscles become paralyzed. Injected in tiny amounts into specific muscles, however, this toxin has shown early promise in reducing local spasticity.

A large research effort is also directed at producing more effective, nontoxic drugs to control seizures. Through its Antiepileptic Drug Development Program, the NINDS screens new compounds developed by industrial and university laboratories around the world for toxicity and anticonvulsant activity and coordinates clinical studies of efficacy and safety. To date, this program has screened more than 13,000 compounds and, as a result, five new antiepileptic drugs—carbamazepine, clonazepam, valproate, clorazepate, and felbamate—have been approved for marketing. A new project within the program is exploring how the structure of a given antiseizure medication relates to its effectiveness. If successful, this project may enable scientists to design better antiseizure medications more quickly and cheaply.

As researchers continue to explore new treatments for cerebral palsy and to expand our knowledge of brain development, we can expect significant medical advances to prevent cerebral palsy and many other disorders that strike in early life.

Where can I find more information?

The NINDS is the Federal Governments' leading support of biomedical research on brain and nervous system disorders, including cerebral palsy. The NINDS conducts research in its own laboratories at the National Institutes of Health in Bethesda, MD, and supports research at institutions worldwide. The Institute also sponsors an active public information program. Other NINDS publications that may be of interest to those concerned about cerebral palsy include "Epilepsy: Hope Through Research" and "The Dystonias." The Institute's address and phone number, as well as information on other organizations that offer various services to those affected by cerebral palsy, are provided on the information resources card enclosed in the back pocket of this brochure.

Glossary

Apgar score: a numbered score doctors use to assess a baby's physical state at the time of birth.

asphyxia: interference with oxygen delivery to the brain and other vital organs.

bile pigments: yellow-colored substances produced by the human body as a byproduct of digestion and red blood cell destruction.

cerebral: relating to the two hemispheres of the human brain.

computer tomography (CT): an imaging technique that uses X rays and a computer to create a picture of the brain's tissues and structures.

congenital: present at birth.

contracture: chronic shortening of a muscle that limits movement of a bony joint, such as the knee.

dysarthria: problems with speaking caused by difficulty moving or coordinating the muscles needed for speech.

electroencephalogram (EEG): a technique for recording the pattern of electrical currents inside the brain.

electromyography: a special recording technique that detects muscle activity.

failure to thrive: a condition characterized by lag in physical growth and development.

gait analysis: a technique that uses camera recording, force plates, electromyography, and computer analysis to objectively measure an individual's pattern of walking.

gastrostomy: a surgical procedure to create an artificial opening in the stomach.

hemianopia: defective visionary blindness that impairs half of the normal field of vision.

hemiparetic tremors: uncontrollable shaking affecting the limbs on the spastic side of the body in those who have spastic hemiplegia.

hypertonia: increased tone.

hypotonia: decreased tone.

hypoxic-ischemic encephalopathy: brain damage caused by poor blood flow or insufficient oxygen supply to the brain.

jaundice: a blood disorder caused by the abnormal buildup of bile pigments in the bloodstream.

magnetic resonance imaging (MRI): an imaging technique which uses radio waves, magnetic fields, and computer analysis to create a picture of body tissues and structures.

orthotic devices: special devices, such as splints or braces, used to treat problems of the muscles, ligaments, or bones.

palsy: paralysis, or problems in the control of voluntary movement.

paresis or plegia: weakness or paralysis. In cerebral palsy, these terms are typically combined with another phrase that describes the distribution of paralysis and weakness, e.g., paraparesis.

reflexes: movements that the body makes automatically in response to a specific cue.

Rh incompatibility: a blood condition in which antibodies in a pregnant woman's blood can attach fetal blood cells, impairing the fetus's supply of oxygen.

rubella: also known as German measles, rubella is a viral infection that can damage the nervous system in the developing fetus.

selective dorsal root rhizotomy: a surgical procedure in which selected nerve fibers are severed to reduce spasticity in the legs.

spastic diplegia: a form of cerebral palsy in which both arms and both legs are affected, the legs being more severely affected.

spastic hemiplegia (or hemiparesis): a form of cerebral palsy in which spasticity affects the arm and leg on one side of the body.

spastic paraplegia (or paraparesis): a form of cerebral palsy in which spasticity affects both legs but the arms are relatively or completely spared.

spastic quadriplegia (or quadriparesis): a form of cerebral palsy in which all four limbs are affected equally.

stereognosia: difficulty perceiving and identifying objects using the sense of touch.

strabismus: misalignment of the eyes.

ultrasonography: a technique that bounces sound waves off of tissues and structures and uses the pattern of echoes to form an image, called a sonogram.

Information Resources

NIH Neurological Institute
PO Box 5801
Bethesda, MD 20824
(301) 496-5751
(800) 352-9424

The National Institute of Neurological Disorders and Stroke, a component of the National Institutes of Health, is the leading federal supporter of research on brain and nervous system disorders. The Institute also sponsors an active public information program and can answer questions about diagnosis, treatment, and research related to cerebral palsy.

In addition, a number of private organizations offer a variety of services and information that can help those affected by cerebral palsy. They include:

March of Dimes Birth Defects Foundation
1275 Mamaroneck Ave
White Plains, NY 10605
(914) 428-7100

This foundation funds research, medical services, public education, and genetic counseling. Resources include fact sheets, brochures, educational kits, and audiovisual materials.

National Easter Seal Society
230 W Monroe, 18th Fl
Chicago, IL 60606
(312) 726-6200
(312) 726-4258 (TDD)

This organization includes state and local affiliates and operates facilities and programs across the country. They offer a range of rehabilitation services, research and public education programs, and assertive technology services. Their programs also include therapy, counseling, training, social clubs, camping, transportation, and referrals. In addition, the society sponsors a grants program for research on disabling conditions and rehabilitation, provides low-cost booklets and pamphlets to the public, and publishes a bimonthly journal.

United Cerebral Palsy Associations and
The United Cerebral Palsy Research and Educational Foundation
1522 K St, NW, Ste 1112
Washington, DC 20005
(202) 842-1266
(800) USA-5UCP (outside Washington, DC)

This coalition of associations provides family support, legislative advocacy, public information and education, and training, specifically for issues of importance to those who have cerebral palsy. It also publishes newsletters and various brochures and pamphlets. the UCP Research and Educational Foundation supports research to prevent cerebral palsy and develop therapies to improve the quality of life for those affected by this disorder.

More information about seizures and epilepsy is available from

Epilepsy Foundation of America
4351 Garden City Dr
Landover, MD 20785
(301) 459-3700
(800) EFA-1000

This foundation sponsors programs for patient and public education, legal and government affairs, and employment training and placement. The foundation also supports research, maintains the National Epilepsy Library (800-EFA-4050), publishes a variety of patient/family and professional education materials, and sponsors affiliates.

■ **Document Source:**
U.S. Department of Health and Human Services, Public Health Service
National Institutes of Health
National Institute of Neurological Disorders and Stroke
Bethesda, MD 20892
NIH Publication No. 93-159
September 1993

FEBRILE SEIZURES

What are febrile seizures?

Febrile seizures are convulsions brought on by a fever in infants or small children. During a febrile seizure, a child often loses consciousness and shakes, moving limbs on both sides of the body. Less commonly, the child becomes rigid or has twitches in only a portion of the body, such as an arm or a leg, or on the right or the left side only. Most febrile seizures last a minute or two, although some can be as brief as a few seconds while others last for more than 15 minutes.

The majority of children with febrile seizures have rectal temperatures greater than 102° F. Most febrile seizures occur during the first day of a child's fever.

Children prone to febrile seizures are not considered to have epilepsy, since epilepsy is characterized by recurrent seizures that are *not* triggered by fever.

How common are febrile seizures?

Approximately one in every 25 children will have at least one febrile seizure, and more than one-third of these children will have additional febrile seizures before they outgrow the tendency to have them. Febrile seizures usually occur in children between the ages of six months and five years and are particularly common in toddlers. Children rarely develop their first febrile seizure before the age of six months or after three years of age. The older a child is when the first febrile seizure occurs, the less likely that child is to have more.

What makes a child prone to recurrent febrile seizures?

A few factors appear to boost a child's risk of having recurrent febrile seizures, including young age (less than 15 months) during the first seizure, frequent fevers, and having immediate family members with a history of febrile seizures. If the seizure occurs soon after a fever has begun or when the temperature is relatively low, the risk of recurrence is higher. A long initial febrile seizure does not substantially boost the risk of recurrent febrile seizures, either brief or long.

Are febrile seizures harmful?

Although they can be frightening to parents, the vast majority of febrile seizures are harmless. During a seizure, there is a small chance that the child may be injured by falling or may choke from food or saliva in the mouth. Using proper first aid for seizures can help avoid these hazards (see section entitled "What should be done for a child having a febrile seizure?").

There is no evidence that febrile seizures cause brain damage. Large studies have found that children with febrile seizures have normal school achievement and perform as well on intellectual tests as their siblings who don't have seizures. Even in the rare instances of very prolonged seizures (more than one hour), most children recover completely.

Between 95 and 98 percent of children who have experienced febrile seizures do not go on to develop epilepsy. However, although the absolute risk remains very small, certain children who have febrile seizures face an increased risk of developing epilepsy. These children include those who have febrile seizures that are lengthy, that affect only part of the body, or that recur within 24 hours, and children with cerebral palsy, delayed development, or other neurological abnormalities. Among children who don't have any of these risk factors, only one in 100 develops epilepsy after a febrile seizure.

What should be done for a child having a febrile seizure?

Parents should stay calm and carefully observe the child. To prevent accidental injury, the child should be placed on a protected surface such as the floor or ground. The child should not be held or restrained during a convulsion. To prevent choking, the child should be placed on his or her side or stomach. When possible, the parent should gently remove all objects in the child's mouth. The parent should never place anything in the child's mouth during a convulsion. Objects placed in the mouth can be broken and obstruct the child's airway. If the seizure lasts longer than 10 minutes, the child should be taken immediately to the nearest medical facility for further treatment. Once the seizure has ended, the child should be taken to his or her doctor to check for the source of the fever. This is especially urgent if the child shows symptoms of stiff neck, extreme lethargy, or abundant vomiting.

How are febrile seizures diagnosed and treated?

Before diagnosing febrile seizures in infants and children, doctors sometimes perform tests to be sure that seizures are not caused by something other than simply the fever itself. For example, if a doctor suspects the child has meningitis (an infection of the membranes surrounding the brain), a spinal tap may be needed to check for signs of the infection in the cerebrospinal fluid (fluid that bathes the brain and spinal cord). If there has been severe diarrhea or vomiting, dehydration could be responsible for seizures. Also, doctors often perform other tests such as examining the blood and urine to pinpoint the cause of the child's fever.

A child who has a febrile seizure usually doesn't need to be hospitalized. If the seizure is prolonged or is accompanied by a serious infection, or if the source of the infection cannot be determined, a doctor may recommend that the child be hospitalized for observation.

How are febrile seizures prevented?

If a child has a fever most parents will use fever-lowering drugs such as acetaminophen or ibuprofen to make the child more comfortable, although there are no studies that prove that this will reduce the risk of a seizure. One preventive measure would be to try to reduce the number of febrile illnesses, although this is often not a practical possibility.

Prolonged daily use of oral anticonvulsants, such as phenobarbital or valproate, to prevent febrile seizures is usually not recommended because of their potential for side effects and questionable effectiveness for preventing such seizures.

Children especially prone to febrile seizures may be treated with the drug diazepam, orally or rectally, whenever they have a fever. The majority of children with febrile seizures do not need to be treated with medication, but in some cases a doctor may decide that medicine given only while the child has a fever may be the best alternative. This medication may lower the risk of having another febrile seizure. It is usually well tolerated, although it occasionally can cause drowsiness, a lack of coordination, or hyperactivity. Children vary widely in their susceptibility to such side effects.

What research is being done on febrile seizures?

The National Institute of Neurological Disorders and Stroke (NINDS), a part of the National Institutes of Health (NIH), sponsors research on febrile seizures in medical centers throughout the country. NINDS-supported scientists are exploring what environmental and genetic risk factors make children susceptible to febrile seizures. Some studies suggest that women who smoke or drink alcohol during their pregnancies are more likely to have children with febrile seizures, but more research needs to be done before this link can be clearly established. Scientists are also working to pinpoint factors that can help predict which children are likely to have recurrent or long-lasting febrile seizures.

Investigators continue to monitor the long-term impact that febrile seizures might have on intelligence, behavior, school achievement, and the development of epilepsy. For example, scientists conducting studies in animals are assessing the effects of seizures and anticonvulsant drugs on brain development.

Investigators also continue to explore which drugs can effectively treat or prevent febrile seizures and to check for side effects of these medicines.

Where can I get more information?

Additional information for patients, families, and physicians is available from:

Epilepsy Foundation of America
4351 Garden City Drive
Landover, MD 20785
(301) 459-3700
(800) EFA-1000 (332-1000)

For more information on research on febrile seizures, you may with to contact:

Office of Scientific and Health Reports
NIH Neurological Institute
PO Box 5801
Bethesda, MD 20824
(301) 496-5751
(800) 352-9424

■ Document Source:
U.S. Department of Health and Human Services, Public Health Service
National Institutes of Health
National Institute of Neurological Disorders and Stroke
Bethesda, MD 20892-2540
NIH Publication No. 95-3930
September 1995

GUIDE TO THE DIAGNOSIS AND TREATMENT OF TOURETTE SYNDROME

Ruth Dowling Bruun, MD; Donald J. Cohen, MD; James F. Leckman, MD

Tourette Syndrome and Other Tic Disorders

Introduction

This publication is the third edition of *A Physician's Guide to the Diagnosis and Treatment of Tourette Syndrome*. It has been revised substantially to include up-to-date clinical information for physicians treating patients with this complex, frequently misunderstood neurobehavioral (neurobiological) disorder.

Definitions of Tic Disorders

Tics are involuntary, rapid, repetitive and stereotyped movements of individual muscle groups. They are more easily recognized than precisely defined. Tic disorders are generally categorized according to age of onset, duration of symptoms, severity of symptoms and the presence of vocal and/or motor tics.

Transient tic disorders often begin during the early school years and can occur in up to 18% of all children. Common tics include eye blinking, nose puckering, grimacing and squinting. Transient vocalizations are less common and include various throat sounds, humming or other noises. Childhood tics may be bizarre—palm licking, poking and/or pinching the genitals are examples. Transient tics last only a few weeks or months and are usually not associated with specific behavioral or school problems. They are especially noticeable during times of heightened excitement or fatigue. As with all tic syndromes, boys are three to four times more often affected than girls. While transient tics by definition do not persist for more than a year, it is not uncommon for a child to have recurrent episodes of transient tics over the course of several years.

Chronic tic disorders are differentiated from transient tic disorders not only by their duration over many years, but by their relatively unchanging character. While transient tics come and go (sniffing may be replaced by forehead furrowing and the furrowing may become finger snapping), chronic tics—such as facial contortions or blinking—may persist unchanged for years.

Chronic multiple tics suggest that an individual has several chronic motor tics (or, in rare cases, several chronic vocal tics). Often it is not an easy task to draw distinctions between transient tics, chronic tics and chronic multiple tics.

Tourette Syndrome (TS), first described by Gilles de la Tourette, can be the most debilitating tic disorder and is characterized by multiform, frequently changing motor and phonic tics. The current diagnostic criteria, as defined by the *Diagnostic and Statistical Manual of Mental Disorders IV* are as follows:

A. Both multiple motor and one or more vocal tics have been present at some time during the illness, although not necessarily concurrently.
B. The tics occur many times a day (usually in bouts) nearly every day or intermittently throughout a period of more than one year, and during this period there was never a tic-free period of more than three consecutive months.
C. The disturbance causes marked distress or significant impairment in social, occupational, or other important areas of functioning.
D. The onset is before age 18.
E. The disturbance is not due to the direct physiological effects of a substance (e.g. stimulants) or a general medical condition (e.g. Huntington's disease or postviral encephalitis).

While the criteria appear basically valid, they are not absolute. First, there have been rare cases of TS which have emerged later than age 18. Second, the concept of "involuntary" may be hard to define operationally, since many patients experience their tics as having a volitional component—either a capitulation to an internal sensory urge for motor discharge, or a more generalized psychological tension and anxiety, or both. Finally, the diagnostic criteria do not adequately portray the full range of behavioral difficulties that are commonly observed in patients with TS, such as attentional problems, compulsions and obsessions.

Differential Diagnosis

Today the full-blown case of TS is unlikely to be confused with any other disorder. In the past, however, TS was frequently misdiagnosed or undiagnosed.

The differentiation of TS from other tic syndromes may be no more than semantic, especially since recent genetic evidence links TS with multiple and transient tics of childhood and can only be defined in retrospect.

At times it may be difficult to distinguish children with extreme attention deficit hyperactivity disorder (ADHD) from those with TS. On close examination, many ADHD children have a few phonic or motor tics, grimace, or produce noises similar to those with TS. Since at least half of patients with TS also have had attention deficits and hyperactivity as children, a physician may well be confused. However, the treating doctor should be aware of the potential complications of treating a possible case of TS with stimulant medication.

On rare occasions, the differentiation between TS and a seizure disorder may be difficult. The symptoms of TS sometimes occur in a rather sharply separated paroxysmal manner and may resemble automatisms. Patients with TS, however, retain a clear consciousness during such paroxysms. If the diagnosis is in doubt, an EEG may be useful.

We have seen TS in association with a number of developmental and other neurological disorders. It is possible that central nervous system injury from trauma or disease may cause a child to be vulnerable to the expression of the disorder, particularly if there is a genetic predisposition. Autistic and retarded children may display the entire gamut of TS symptoms. Whether an autistic or retarded individual requires the additional diagnosis of TS may remain an open question until testing (biological or otherwise) is available for a definitive diagnosis of TS.

In older patients, conditions such as Wilson's disease, tardive dyskinesia, Meige's syndrome, chronic amphetamine abuse and the sterotypic movements of schizophrenia must be considered in the differential diagnosis. The distinction can usually be made by taking a good history or by blood tests.

Since more physicians are now aware of TS, there is a growing danger of over-diagnosis or over-treatment. It is up to the clinician to consider the effect that the symptoms have on the patient's ability to function (as well as the severity of associated symptoms) before deciding to treat with medication or other approaches.

Symptomatology

The varied symptoms of TS can be divided into motor, vocal and behavioral manifestations (Table 1). Simple motor tics are fast, darting, meaningless muscular events. They can be embarrassing or even painful (such as jaw snapping). They are easily distinguished from simple muscular twitches or rapid fasciculations, e.g., of the eyelid or lip. Complex motor tics may be slower or more purposeful in appearance and more easily described by terms used for deliberate actions (Table 2).

Complex motor tics can be virtually any type of movement that the body can produce including gyrating, hopping, clapping, tensing arm or neck muscles, touching people or things and obscene gesturing.

At some point in the continuum of complex motor tics, the term "compulsion" seems appropriate for capturing the organized, ritualistic character of the actions. The need to do and then redo or undo the same action a certain number of times (e.g., to stretch out an arm 10 times before writing, to "even up," or to stand up and push a chair into "just the right position") is compulsive in quality and accompanied by considerable internal discomfort. Complex motor tics may greatly impair school work, e.g., when a child must stab at a workbook with a pencil or must go over the same letter so many times that the paper is worn thin. Self-destructive behaviors, such as head banging, eye poking and lip biting also may occur. The distinction between complex tics and compulsions may be a difficult one for the physician to make and some "complex tics" may be alleviated by medications used for obsessive-compulsive disorder.

Table 1. Range Of Symptoms Of TS

Motor

- **Simple motor tics:** fast, darting and meaningless.
- **Complex motor tics:** may be slower or may consist of stereotyped series of movements and may appear purposeful (includes copropraxia and echopraxia).

Vocal

- **Simple vocal tics:** meaningless sounds and noises.
- **Complex vocal tics:** linguistically meaningful utterances such as words and phrases (including coprolalia, echolalia and palilalia), interruptions in the flow of speech, sudden alterations in pitch or volume.

Behavioral and Developmental

Often associated with attention deficit hyperactivity disorder, obsessions and compulsions, emotional lability, irritability, impulsivity, aggressivity and self-injurious behaviors; various learning disabilities, social difficulties including peer rejection.

Vocal tics extend over a similar spectrum of complexity and disruption as do motor tics (Table 3). With simple vocal tics, patients emit linguistically meaningless sounds or noises, such as hissing, coughing or barking. Complex vocal tics involve linguistically meaningful words, phrases or sentences, e.g., "wow," "Oh boy, now you've said it," "Yup, that's it," "but, but...." Vocal symptoms may interfere with the smooth flow of speech and resemble a stammer, stutter or other speech irregularity. Often, but not always, vocal symptoms occur at points of linguistic transition, such as at the beginning of a sentence where there may be speech blocking at the initiation of speech or at phrase transitions. Patients suddenly may alter speech volume, slur a phrase, emphasize a word or assume an accent.

The most socially distressing complex vocal symptom is coprolalia, the explosive utterance of foul or "dirty" words or more elaborate sexual, aggressive or insulting statements (e.g., racial slurs). Coprolalia is not simply obscene speech spoken in anger or to offend. Rather it is often sudden speech (typically just the first syllable of an inappropriate word) that interrupts an otherwise appropriate flow of words. While coprolalia occurs in only a minority of patients with TS (from 5-30%, depending on the clinical series), it remains the most well known TS symptom. A diagnosis of TS does not require that coprolalia be present and the majority of patients do not ever exhibit this symptom.

Some patients with TS may have a tendency to imitate what they have just seen (echopraxia), heard (echolalia), or said (palilalia). For example, the patient may feel an impulse to imitate another's body movements, to speak with an odd inflection or to accent a syllable in just the same manner as another person. Such modeling or repetition may lead to the onset of new specific symptoms that will wax and wane in the same way as other TS symptoms. Some patients also describe "triggers" that almost invariably prompt a tic, e.g., another person coughing in a certain way.

Table 2. Examples Of Motor Symptoms

Simple Motor Tics

Eye blinking, grimacing, nose twitching, lip pouting, shoulder shrugging, arm jerking, head jerking, abdominal tensing, kicking, finger movements, jaw snapping, tooth clicking, frowning, tensing parts of the body and the rapid jerking of any part of the body.

Complex Motor Tics

Hopping, clapping, touching objects (or others or self), throwing, twirling, gyrating, bending, "dystonic" postures, biting the mouth, the lip or the arm, head banging, picking scabs, writhing movements, rolling eyes upwards or side-to-side, making funny expressions, kissing, pinching, pulling back on a pencil while writing and tearing paper or books.

Copropraxia

"Giving the finger," grabbing genitals and other obscene gestures.

Echopraxia

Imitating gestures or movements of other people.

The symptoms of TS can be characterized as mild, moderate or severe by their frequency, their complexity and the degree to which they cause impairment or disruption of the patient's ongoing activities and daily life. For example, extremely frequent tics that occur 20-30 times a minute, such as blinking, nodding or arm flexion, may be less disruptive than an infrequent tic that occurs several times an hour, such as loud barking, coprolalic utterances or touching tics. The premonitory sensory urges tend to be present by 9 to 10 years of age. They are most commonly reported in the shoulder girdle, hands, throat and abdomen.

There may be tremendous variability over short and long periods of time in symptomatology, frequency and severity. Tics typically occur in "bouts" with many tics over a short interval of time. Patients may be able to inhibit or not feel a great need to emit their symptoms while at school or work. When they arrive home, however, the tics may erupt with violence and remain at a distressing level throughout the remainder of the day.

It is not unusual for patients to "lose" their tics as they enter the doctor's office. Parents may plead with a child to "show the doctor what you do at home," only to be told that the youngster, "just doesn't feel like doing them" or "can't do them" on command. Adults will say, "I only wish you could see me outside of your office," and family members will heartily agree.

Often a patient with minimal symptoms may display more severe tics when the examination is over. Thus, for example, the doctor may often see a nearly symptom-free patient who then leaves the office and begins to hop, flail or bark as soon as he or she reaches the street.

In addition to the moment-to-moment or short-term changes in symptom intensity, many patients have oscillations in severity over the course of weeks and months. The waxing and waning of severity may be triggered by changes in the patient's life; for example, around holidays, children may develop exacerbations that take weeks to subside. Other patients report that their symptoms show seasonal fluctuation. However, there are no rigorous data on whether life events, stresses or seasons do, in fact, influence the onset or offset of a period of exacerbation. Once a patient enters a phase of waxing symptomatology, a process seems to be triggered that will run its course for weeks or months.

In its most severe forms, patients may have uncountable motor and vocal tics during all their waking hours with paroxysms of full body movements, shouting or self-mutilation. At times the tics seem organized in orchestrated patterns that are characteristic of that individual. Despite this, many patients with severe tics manage to achieve adequate social adjustment in adult life, although usually with considerable emotional pain. More than the severity of motor and vocal tics, the factors that appear to be of importance with regard to social adaptation include the seriousness of attentional problems, obsessive-compulsive symptoms, the degree of family acceptance and support, intelligence and ego strength.

In adolescence and early adulthood, patients with TS frequently come to feel that their social isolation, vocational or academic failure and embarrassing symptoms are more than they can bear. At times, a small number may consider and attempt suicide. Conversely, some patients with the most bizarre and disruptive symptomatology may achieve excellent social, academic and vocational adjustment. Fortunately, in many cases, tics diminish during the course of adolescence. However, in other cases (less that 10 percent), the tic symptoms can become even more severe in adulthood.

Associated Behaviors and Cognitive Difficulties

Many, though not all patients with TS experience a variety of behavioral and psychological difficulties in addition to tics. These behavioral features have placed TS on the border between neurology and psychiatry and require an understanding of both disciplines to comprehend the complex problems faced by many patients.

Table 3. Examples Of Vocal Symptoms

Simple Vocal Tics

Coughing, spitting, screeching, barking, grunting, gurgling, clacking, whistling, hissing, sucking sounds, and syllable sounds such as "uh, uh," "eee," and "bu."

Complex Vocal Tics

"Oh boy," "you know," "shut up," "you're fat," "all right," and "what's that."

Rituals

Repeating a phrase until it sounds "just right" and saying something over three times.

Speech Atypicalities

Unusual rhythms, tone, accents, loudness and very rapid speech.

Coprolalia

Obscene, aggressive or otherwise socially unacceptable words or phrases.

Palilalia

Repeating one's own words or parts of words.

Echolalia

Repeating sounds, words, or parts of words of others.

The most frequently reported behavioral problems are attentional deficits, obsessions, compulsions, impulsivity, irritability, aggressivity, immaturity, self-injurious behaviors and depression. Some of the behaviors (e.g., obsessive-compulsive behavior and certain forms of ADHD) may be an integral part of TS, while others may be common in patients with TS because of certain biological vulnerabilities. Still others may represent responses to the social stresses associated with a multiple tic disorder or a combination of biological and psychological reactions.

Obsessions and Compulsions

Although TS may present itself purely as a disorder of multiple motor and vocal tics, many TS patients also have obsessive-compulsive (OC) symptoms that may be as disruptive to their lives as the tics—sometimes even more so. There is recent evidence that obsessive-compulsive symptomatology may be another expression of the TS gene and, therefore, an integral part of the disorder. Whether this is true or not, it has been well documented that a high percentage of patients with TS have OC symptoms, that these symptoms tend to appear somewhat later than the tics, and that they may be seriously impairing.

The nature of OC symptoms in patients with TS is quite variable. Conventionally, obsessions are defined as thoughts, images or impulses that intrude on consciousness, are involuntary and distressful and while perceived as silly or excessive, cannot be abolished. Compulsions consist of the actual behaviors, often carried out in response to the obsessions or

in an effort to ward them off. Typical OC behaviors include rituals of counting, repetitively checking things over and washing or cleaning excessively. While many patients with TS do have such behaviors, there are other typical TS symptoms that seem to straddle the border between tics and OC symptoms. Examples are the need to "even things up," to touch things a certain number of times, to perform tasks over and over until they "feel right," and self-injurious behaviors. Although patients with TS can have the full range of OC symptoms, some symptoms such as contamination worries occur less frequently than among OCD patients without tics or TS.

Attention Deficit Hyperactivity Disorder (ADHD)

Up to 50 percent of all children with TS who come to the attention of a physician also have attention deficit hyperactivity disorder (ADHD), which is manifested by problems with attention span, concentration, distractibility, impulsivity and motoric hyperactivity. Attentional problems often precede the onset of TS symptoms and may worsen as the tics develop. The increasing difficulty with attention may reflect an underlying biological dysfunction involving inhibition, and may be exacerbated by the strain of attending to the outer world while working hard to remain quiet and still. Attentional problems and hyperactivity can profoundly affect school achievement. At least 30-40 percent of children with TS have serious school performance handicaps that require special intervention and children with both TS and ADHD are especially vulnerable to serious, long term educational impairment.

Attention deficits may persist into adulthood and together with compulsions and obsessions, can seriously impair job performance.

Emotional Lability, Impulsivity and Aggressivity

Some patients with TS (percentages vary greatly in different studies) have significant problems with labile emotions, impulsivity and aggression directed at others. Fits of temper that include screaming, punching holes in walls, threatening others, hitting, biting and kicking are common in such patients. Often they will be the patients who also have ADHD, making impulse control a considerable problem. At times, the temper outbursts can be seen as reactions to the internal and external pressures of having TS. A specific etiology for such behavioral problems is, at present, not well understood. Nevertheless, they create much consternation in teachers and great anguish for the patients and their families. The treating physician or counselor is often asked whether these behaviors are as involuntary as the tics, or whether they can be controlled. *Rather than trying to make such a distinction, it is perhaps more helpful to think of such patients as having a "thin barrier" between aggressive thoughts and the expression of those thoughts through actions.* These patients may think of themselves as being out of control, a concept that is as frightening to them as it is to others.

Management of these behaviors is often difficult and may involve adjustment of medications, individual therapy, family therapy or behavioral retraining. The intensity of these behaviors sometimes increases as the tics wax and decreases as the tics wane. Along with the tics and ADHD symptoms, these additional disruptive symptoms can cause major social difficulties.

Self-Injurious Behaviors

These may consist of complex tics (e.g., hitting or biting oneself) or may be compulsions (e.g., moving a sore joint over and over in order to achieve a certain painful sensation).

Learning Difficulties

There are many reasons why children with TS have difficulties in school and may require special educational assistance. Tics may interfere with writing, listening (as trying to control tics may require all of the student's concentration), or may be disruptive in the classroom. Associated symptoms such as ADD, ADHD or obsessions and compulsions may impair attention. Medications may also impair attention and concentration. Finally, there are a number of specific learning disabilities which have been found to be frequently associated with TS. These include impairments in visual-perceptual and visual-motor skills, wide discrepancies between verbal and performance IQs and other specific learning disabilities.

Etiology

The most intensive research in relation to etiology has focused on genetic factors and neurochemical alterations in the brain.

Multiple neurochemical systems have been implicated by pharmacologic and metabolic evidence. The most convincing evidence for dopaminergic involvement has come from the dramatic response to haloperidol and other neuroleptics such as pimozide, fluphenazine and penfluridol, as well as exacerbations produced by stimulant medications.

Serotonergic mechanisms have been suggested on the basis of the beneficial effects of serotonin reuptake inhibitors (SRIs) in the treatment of OCD. Since systems relying on neurotransmitters send projections to the substantia nigra and the striatum, they could play an important role in the pathophysiology of TS. Medications affecting that system seem somewhat effective for obsessions but have inconsistent effects on tics.

The role of the cholinergic system is clouded by contradictory reports. Enhancing cholinergic function by use of physostigmine has been associated both with the improvement and the worsening of TS. Investigators have reported that nicotine gum can be helpful to symptomatic patients by potentiating neuroleptics such as haloperidol.

Investigation of the GABAergic system suggests that it may be implicated. The proximity and connections between the GABA and dopamine systems support the possibility of an interrelationship. Response to clonazepam (a GABAergic agent) has been positive in some cases.

Noradrenergic mechanisms have been most persuasively implicated by observations that clonidine, a drug that inhibits noradrenergic functioning by the stimulation of an autoreceptor, may improve motor and phonic symptoms. Noradrenergic involvement has also been suggested by the exacerbation of the syndrome by stress and anxiety.

Magnetic resonance imaging (MRI) has provided evidence of alteration in the volume of parts of the brain involved in the regulation of movement and associated behavioral systems (basal ganglia). The use of functional neuroimaging techniques such as positron emission tomography may help clarify many physiologic relationships and identify important anatomical areas in the near future.

Stimulant Medications

A much debated risk factor in tics and TS is the use of stimulant medication. Over 25 percent of all patients with TS in some cohorts have had a course of stimulant medication early in the emergence of their behavioral or tic symptoms because they were diagnosed as having ADHD. Over the last several years, a series of cases has been reported in which the use of stimulants (methylphenidate, dextroamphetamine and pemoline) has been correlated with the onset of motor and phonic tics. There is also chemical evidence to support the observation that stimulants will increase the severity of tics in 25-50 percent of patients with TS.

While there has been concern that stimulant medications might actually cause TS, the prevailing information at present indicates that while tics may be provoked or worsened by these medications, there is little or no indication that this will be permanent. Thus, while it is prudent to first try other medications for attentional problems (e.g., tricyclics or clonidine) when treating patients or members of families with a TS history, stimulants need not be withheld if they are deemed necessary. When attentional difficulties are more severe than tics, it may be appropriate to treat with stimulants even at the cost of a moderate increase in tics.

Children and parents should be educated concerning the risks versus benefits in each case prior to being treated with stimulants. Behavioral management and environmental manipulation should be used either as alternatives or in conjunction with medication.

Epidemiology and Genetics

While once thought to be rare, TS is now seen as a relatively common childhood onset disorder affecting up to one person in every 2,500 in its complete form and three times that number in its partial expressions which include chronic motor tics and some forms of obsessive-compulsive disorder.

Based on available information, it is now clear that TS is a familial and genetic disorder. The vulnerability to TS is transmitted from one generation to another. When we speak of "vulnerability," we imply that the child receives the genetic or constitutional basis for developing a tic disorder; the precise type of disorder or severity may be different from one generation to another; that vulnerability is transmitted by either mothers or fathers and can be passed on to either sons or daughters. When one parent is a carrier or has TS, it appears that there is about a 50-50 chance that a child will receive the genetic vulnerability from that parent. That pattern of inheritance is described as **autosomal dominant**. In addition to such a gene of major effect, other genes of minor effect may also play an important role in shaping an individual's genetic vulnerability.

However, not everyone who inherits the genetic vulnerability will express any of the symptoms of TS. There is a 70 percent chance that female gene carriers will express any of the symptoms of TS. For a male gene carrier, there is a 90 percent or higher chance of showing some clinical expression of the gene. The degree of expression is described as **penetrance.** In males, the penetrance is higher than in females: thus, males are more likely to have some form of expression of the genetic vulnerability. There is a full 30 percent chance of female gene carriers showing no symptoms at all. For males, the figure is probably below 10 percent.

There is a range of forms in which the vulnerability may be expressed that includes full-blown TS, chronic multiple tics, and, as most recently recognized, obsessive-compulsive disorder. Some individuals have TS (or chronic tics) and obsessive-compulsive disorder together; others may have the conditions singly. There are also differences between the sexes in the TS gene's form of expression. Males are more likely to have TS or tics; females are more likely to have obsessive-compulsive disorder; however, both males and females may have any combination or severity. The severity of the disorder is also highly variable. **Most individuals who inherit the TS genetic vulnerability have very mild conditions for which they do not seek medical attention.**

Researchers are actively engaged in searching for the chromosomal location of the TS gene of affected individuals. At present, there is no genetic or biochemical test to determine if a person with TS or an unaffected individual carries the gene. There is no prenatal test for the vulnerability to TS. When scientists succeed in locating the gene, such tests may become available.

Non-genetic Contributions

The individual variations in character, course and degree of severity by which TS is manifested cannot be explained by genetic hypotheses alone. Furthermore, it appears that about 10-15 percent of patients with TS do not acquire the disorder genetically. Thus, non-genetic factors are also responsible, both as causes and as modifiers of TS. Non-genetic factors that have been implicated include such stressful processes or events during the prenatal, perinatal, or early life periods as fetal compromise and exposure to drugs (stimulants, steroids) or other toxins. Findings from two studies in which decreased birth weights were observed in affected co-twins of discordant monozygotic pairs lend further support for the influence of early environmental factors active during brain development.

Clinical Assessment of Tourette Syndrome

Assessment of a case of TS involves far more than simple diagnosis. Since symptoms may fluctuate in severity and character from hour to hour, a thorough understanding of the patient may take a considerable amount of time. As the patient becomes more comfortable with the doctor, there will be less likelihood of symptom suppression or inhibition. Only when confidence in the physician exists is the patient likely to acknowledge the most frightening or bizarre symptoms.

The nature, severity, frequency and degree of disruption produced by the motor and vocal tics, need careful assessment from the time of their emergence to the present. Inquiries should be made about factors that may have worsened or ameliorated symptom severity. A critical question concerns the degree to which the tics have interfered with the patient's social, familial and school/work experiences. In all these respects, interviews with family members may be revealing and informative.

During the evaluation of a patient with TS, the clinician must assess all areas of functioning to fully understand both difficulties and strengths. It is important to explore the presence of attentional and learning disabilities, a history of school and/or work performance, and relationships with family and peers. Before being given a diagnosis, the patient and/or family members may have thought they were "going crazy." The patient may have become extremely distressed by his or her experiences and by the often negative responses evoked by the symptoms. Parents may have scolded, cajoled, ridiculed, threatened and perhaps beaten the child to stop the "weird" and embarrassing behavior. The emotional sequelae may affect the patient far beyond the period of childhood.

During the evaluation of a child therefore, family issues (including parental guilt) need to be addressed. Relevant factors elicited through careful diagnostic evaluation can be approached through clarification, education and therapeutic discussion with the youngster and the family. Careful assessment of cognitive functioning and school achievement is indicated for children who have problems in school. Children with TS who exhibit school performance difficulties often do not have clearly delineated learning disorders and the average IQ of patients with TS is normal. Rather, their problems tend to be in the areas of attentional deployment, perseverance and their ability to organize themselves and their work. Many have difficulties with penmanship (graphomotor skills) and compulsions that interfere with writing. Determining specific problem areas will help in the recommendation of alternatives (e.g., extended periods of time for tests, computer use or the emphasis on oral rather than written reports.)

The neurological examination should include documentation of neuro-maturational difficulties and other neurological findings. About half of patients with TS have non-localizing, so called "soft," neurological findings suggesting disturbances in the body scheme and integration of motor control. While such findings have no specific therapeutic implications, they are worth noting as "baseline" data because the use of medications such as haloperidol may cloud the neurological picture.

The EEG is often abnormal in TS, but findings are nonspecific. Clinical use of magnetic resonance imaging or computed tomography of the brain produce normal results in people with TS. Thus, unless there is some doubt about the diagnosis or some complicating neurological factors, these tests are not necessary parts of the clinical evaluation.

Brain imaging studies (MRIs, etc.) are frequently read as within normal limits although researchers have found consistent subtle differences in the volume and symmetry of certain sub-cortical brain structures.

Additional tests which may be considered in the biological workup include serum electrolytes, calcium, phosphorous, copper, ceruloplasmin and liver function tests—all related to movement disorders of various types. In practice, however, they are rarely needed for a TS diagnosis.

A behavioral pedigree of the extended family, including tics, compulsions, attentional problems and the like is useful.

Previous medications must be reviewed in detail during assessment. If a child has received stimulant medications, it is important to determine what the indications for the medications were, whether there were any pre-existing tics or compulsions and the temporal relation between the stimulants and the new symptoms. Catecholaminergic agonists are contained in other drugs such as in the decongestant combinations used in treating allergies and in medications used for asthma. If a patient with TS is on a stimulant or a drug containing an ephedrine-like agent, discontinuation should be considered if possible.

If the physician examines a previously diagnosed patient, a complete medication history is essential to determine what medications were used, what the initial positive and negative responses to the drugs were and why the medications were discontinued. A patient or a parent may report that haloperidol was not useful or that there were unacceptable side effects. A careful history may reveal that the patient improved on haloperidol but then developed akathisia which was not recognized, or that the side effects were dose-related and probably controllable.

Concepts to consider might include the following: was the medication used at the correct dosage, with good enough monitoring, for a long enough time? Were any behavioral changes noted during the use of the medication that might represent unrecognized side effects? Patients and families may be excellent at identifying and reporting side effects, but they also may not appreciate that symptoms such as depression or school phobia may be related to neuroleptic treatment rather than to psychological issues.

If a patient is currently on an appropriate medication but still has serious difficulties, the clinician must decide whether to: increase the medication and look for improvement; decrease or discontinue the medication and observe the patient's response; or switch to an alternative medication. These are difficult clinical judgments.

Rapid discontinuation from drugs such as haloperidol, pimozide and fluphenazine may lead to severe withdrawal effects including dyskinesia and choreiform movements. In general, abrupt discontinuation of medication may lead to two to three months of increased symptoms. Thus, if these medications are withdrawn, it cannot be expected that the patient's "real" status will be visible for quite a while. Withdrawal emergent dyskinesias may further complicate the picture and threaten the possibility of permanent tardive dyskinesia. Although permanent dyskinesias or dystonias are relatively rare in patients with TS, the physician who is treating tics with neuroleptic medications must always keep these conditions in mind.

Side effects such as cognitive blunting, memory problems, feelings of dullness, poor motivation, school and social phobias, excessive appetite and sedation may lift rather quickly (from days to several weeks), but emergent tic symptoms can remain or become worse. Thus, the decision to discontinue neuroleptics, particularly haloperidol, may be harder than their initiation. Withdrawal must be planned so that the patient's life is disrupted as little as possible. Often, patients and their families will have great difficulty in tolerating the discontinuation and will need a good deal of support from the physician.

If a patient is not benefiting from clonidine, it should be tapered gradually. Even so, a short exacerbation period may occur. When clonidine is withdrawn abruptly, rebound hypertension may follow and exacerbation of tics lasting as long as six to eight weeks has been reported. Gradual withdrawal of other medications sometimes used in the treatment of TS (clonazepam, fluoxetine, clomipramine, etc.) is also important.

Treatment of Tourette Syndrome

The decision about whether to treat and, if so, what form the treatment should take, will depend on the degree to which the TS symptoms are interfering with the child's normal development or the adult patient's ability to function productively. When treating a child, the primary emphasis must be on helping the youngster to navigate the normal developmental tasks—to feel competent in school, develop friendships, experience trust in his or her parents and enjoy life's adventures. Many children with multiple tics and TS do well in moving onward with their lives. For them, treatment to ameliorate the tics generally is not indicated. Natural parental upset about the tics requires lengthy, calm discussion and education about available treatments. When treatment is decided upon by the child, family and physician, developmental issues must constantly be reassessed.

There are several approaches to treatment.

Monitoring

Unless there is a state of emergency, the clinician can usually follow a patient for some time before a specific treatment plan is organized. Ideally, the goals of first stage treatment are to establish a baseline of symptoms; define associated difficulties in school, family and peer relationships; obtain necessary medical tests; through check lists and interviews, monitor the range and fluctuations in symptoms and the specific contexts of greatest difficulties, and; establish a relationship. Unfortunately, it is often a crisis which brings a patient in for diagnosis and/or treatment so that a delay in prescribing medication is not practical or even desirable. In most cases, symptoms are at their worst in the years preceding puberty.

Education and Reassurance

It may become apparent that the child's tics are of minimal functional significance. Even if a youngster satisfies the criteria for TS, no treatment may be necessary because of good peer relations, school achievement and self image. If parents have read about TS, they may be worried about the child's future. In the majority of cases, the severity of TS becomes apparent within two or three years of its first appearance. For milder cases, we tend to tell families that while their child has been diagnosed as having TS, the severity is less than TS cases they may have heard about in the media, and that "in the old days," their child probably would have been called simply "a nervous child." We also explain that, in many instances, TS symptoms are spontaneously ameliorated in the late teens. However, even if they are assured about the nature of their child's disorder, families deserve to know about the emerging information related to genetic and other issues, to the degree that they desire such knowledge. Although scientifically rigorous long term outcome studies have yet to be performed, most experts agree that tics generally improve by early adulthood. Speaking directly with teachers and others involved in the child's care can also be very beneficial in reducing anxiety and "explaining" the tics.

Treatment of adult patients with TS requires much of the same kind of reassurance and education. A well informed patient is much better able to make a wise decision about the need for drugs and to be cooperative in adjusting the dosage if medication is decided upon.

Pharmacologic Treatment of Tourette Syndrome

Although some behavior therapies show promise, pharmacologic intervention is the only proven effective treatment for simple and complex motor and vocal tics. Up to 70% of patients report a history of beneficial treatment with some medication.

The basic principles governing treatment of TS with medication are:

- Start patients on the smallest dose of medication that is possible and reasonable.
- Increase the dosage gradually, paying close attention to the development of side effects as well as the diminution of symptoms. A slow increase will usually result in fewer and milder side effects.
- Assure an adequate duration of any drug trial on sufficient dosage. An adequate length of drug trial may be difficult for the clinician who is faced with his patient's urgent need for effective symptom control. However, it is important since premature discontinuation of a medication trial will only result in failure and a series of such "failures" will make the patient feel that he or she is incurable.
- Maintain the lowest effective dosage.
- Do not "chase" tic symptoms (i.e. continue to raise the dose of medication as tics reappear)—you will never win and the patient will most likely be over medicated.
- Make changes in regimens as sequences of single steps.
- When discontinuing medication, be careful not to confuse withdrawal reactions with the need for more potent medication.

Haloperidol

Since the 1960s, haloperidol (Haldol r) has been the mainstay of treatment for TS. Haloperidol is usually most effective at quite low doses. Patients generally are started at 0.25 to 0.50 mg/day and slowly increased every four to five days up to an average of three to four mg/day. Impressive benefits are seen at those low doses and patients may have almost complete

remissions with few side effects. Some may benefit from as little as 1 mg/day or less. Those who do not respond to low doses of haloperidol may sustain a reduction of symptoms at higher doses (10-15 mg), but results are rarely as satisfying and side effects interfere to limit the drug's usefulness.

Up to 80 percent of patients with TS initially benefit from haloperidol, sometimes dramatically. However, our long term follow-up suggests that only a smaller number, perhaps 20-30 percent, continue haloperidol for an extended period of time. Patients often discontinue the drug because of the emergence of side effects. These side effects may include excessive fatigue, weight gain, dysphoria, parkinsonian symptoms, intellectual dulling, memory problems, personality changes, feeling like a "zombie," akathisia, school and social phobias, loss of libido, sexual dysfunction, and, especially after chronic use of high doses, tardive dyskinesia (TD). There is a diversity of opinion about the use of anti-parkinsonian agents with haloperidol. Some clinicians prefer to initiate treatment with both haloperidol and low doses of anti-parkinsonian medication (e.g., 0.5 mg/day of benztropine). Others will not use anti-parkinsonian medication until side effects warrant them. Most parkinsonian and acute dystonic reactions can be controlled with one to two mg/day of benztropine or an equivalent medication. Akathisia may be harder to manage and may require the use of other medications (e.g., clonidine, propranolol or diazepam).

School phobias may appear during the first weeks of treatment even with low doses of haloperidol while the tic symptoms are improving. In adults, social phobias and dysphorias may cause acute anxiety about going to work or performing at work and can be extremely disabling. When such phobias are not recognized as drug side effects, they can continue for months; they remit within weeks of haloperidol discontinuation. Intellectual dulling leads to marked worsening of school and work performance. Children who are "A" students and have friends may become "C" students, dysphoric and isolated.

The long term use of medication often complicates the understanding of the emergence of social and personality difficulties. Side effects of neuroleptics may have considerable impact on a child's sense of self control, autonomy, self esteem, and cognitive and social competence. In addition to the way that psychoactive medication may alter how a child's body feels to him or her and how he or she experiences the working of his or her mind, the use of any medication may single out a child in school, alter the daily schedule and focus too much parental and other adult concern on small changes in symptoms and side effects.

Education of the patient and/or family about the possibility of developing TD is essential, as are periodic assessments for dyskinetic movements that the patient or family may mistake for TS symptoms. Because of the frequency and potential gravity of side effects associated with haloperidol, many clinicians experienced in the treatment of TS prefer to try other medications first and reserve haloperidol for more severe and refractory cases.

It should be emphasized that withdrawal from haloperidol and other neuroleptics may produce confusing symptoms.

Pimozide

Pimozide (Orap) was approved in the United States for treatment of TS in 1984 and is now in fairly common use. Pimozide is a diphenylbutylpiperidine, chemically distinctive from haloperidol or phenothiazines, with potent dopamine blocking properties. Its side effects are similar to haloperidol, but may be less severe and appear in fewer patients. In general, it is better tolerated than haloperidol and probably is of equal efficacy. Concern about cardiotoxicity was raised by initial reports in early studies of EKG abnormalities (U waves, inverted T waves, and Q-T prolongation). Further investigations with larger numbers of patients have not justified those early concerns. Nevertheless, routine EKG studies before and periodically during treatment are still advised.

Treatment with pimozide is usually initiated at 1 mg/day and dosage is gradually increased, on clinical indications, to a maximum of 6-10 mg/day for children and 20 mg/day for adults. (The *Physicians' Desk Reference* indicates that doses greater than 0.2 mg/kg or 10 mg/day are not recommended.) Because of its long half-life (55 hours), a single daily dosage may be feasible. Major side effects are similar to haloperidol and, as with haloperidol, tardive dyskinesia is a possibility.

Other Neuroleptics

Phenothiazines, particularly fluphenazine, may be effective alternatives to haloperidol and pimozide. Fluphenazine's side effects are potentially the same as those associated with haloperidol, but, as with pimozide, some patients tolerate them better. The recommended dose range is similar to haloperidol and the same principles (lowest possible starting dose and gradual increases) are applicable. Other neuroleptics that have been reported to be effective in a few patients include thiothixene, chlorpromazine and trifluoperazine.

A neuroleptic currently being evaluated for TS is risperidone. This appears to have some effectiveness in controlling tics, possibly with fewer side effects than the neuroleptics mentioned above. More studies need to be done, however, before any definitive statements can be made about this medication. Most children and adults will achieve maximum benefit with doses under six mg per day.

Clonidine

Clonidine (Catapres) is an imidazoline compound with alpha-adrenergic agonist activity. In low doses it "down-regulates" alpha-adrenergic neurons in the locus ceruleus, decreasing the release of central norepinephrine. Since 1979, it has been considered to be of benefit for the treatment of TS although the response rate is lower than that of either haloperidol or pimozide. In general, it is of advantage because of the low incidence of side effects associated with its use. Perhaps of greatest importance is that it does not have the potential of causing tardive dyskinesia. Clonidine has been approved by the FDA only for use in hypertension, but clinicians can prescribe it for TS without special government approval as long as they understand its indications and share the basis for their decision with the family and child.

In addition to reducing the simple motor and phonic symptoms in TS, clonidine seems especially useful in improving attentional problems and ameliorating complex motor and phonic symptoms.

In general, clonidine is started at low doses of 0.05 mg/day and slowly titrated over several weeks to 0.15-0.30 mg/day. Since clonidine has a six hour half-life, it is important that patients take small doses three to four times each day. (An alternative to multiple doses is the transdermal patch that needs to be changed only once a week.) Doses of 0.4 mg daily are not infrequent, but doses above 0.5 to 0.6 mg/day are more likely to produce side effects. When the medication is working effectively, patients may feel the need for their next dose by sensing increased anxiety, frequency of symptoms or irritability. Unlike haloperidol, which may lead to clear improvement within a few days, clonidine tends to have a slower onset of action. When larger doses are prescribed earlier, improvement may occur sooner but there may be more sedation. With slower titration to therapeutic levels, clonidine may take three weeks or longer to show a beneficial effect.

The patient may experience a reduction in tension, a feeling of being calm, or a sense of having a "longer fuse" before tics are reduced. A gradual decrease in complex motor tics and compulsions also may precede clear improvement in simple tics. In the most successful cases, attentional, behavioral and complex phenomena seem more responsive than the simpler tics. Evaluation of the medication's effectiveness may not be possible prior to three or four months of treatment. When there is a positive response, improvement may progress over many months and up to a year or more later. Patients gain confidence in themselves, adjust better to school, feel less irritable and have fewer tic symptoms. These therapeutic benefits reinforce each other.

The major side effect of clonidine is sedation, which appears early in the course of treatment, especially if the dose is increased quickly, but tends to abate after several weeks. A few patients have dry mouth, with children experiencing this symptom less often than adults. There are occasional reports of patients feeling that things are "too bright," perhaps because of the impairment of pupillary contraction. At high doses, there may be hypotension and dizziness, particularly if clonidine is prescribed at high doses quite early or if it is increased to over 0.4 or 0.5 mg/day. At lower doses, blood pressure is not clinically affected, although a fall of several mm mercury in diastolic and systolic pressure can be detected. Slight prolongation of the PR interval on the electrocardiogram has been noted, but this has not been considered to be of significance. Increased irritability, nightmares and insomnia have also been reported.

When clonidine is withdrawn, it should be tapered gradually.

Treatment of Obsessions and Compulsions in TS

It is now recognized that obsessive-compulsive symptoms occur in about half of patients with Tourette Syndrome. Current evidence suggests a genetic relationship between obsessive-compulsive disorder (OCD) and TS. Symptoms of OCD may be even more disabling than motor and vocal tics for some patients, resulting in impaired school or job performance, abnormal psychosocial development or disrupted family life. Furthermore, obsessive thought patterns and/or compulsive activities may contribute to impaired attention—another behavioral problem of TS.

Clomipramine

Among pharmacological interventions for OCD, antidepressant medications have shown the greatest clinical efficacy. A widely studied antidepressant drug for the treatment of primary OCD in psychiatric populations is clomipramine (Anafranil), a potent serotonin reuptake inhibitor. Controlled clinical trials have confirmed superior efficacy of clomipramine over other tricyclic antidepressants in adult patients with primary OCD. Experience indicates that the drug can be effective for OCD associated with TS as well.

Clomipramine is administered in capsules of either 25 mg, 50 mg or 75 mg. The drug is initiated at 25 mg daily and can be titrated to a maximum daily dosage of 250 mg in adults (three mg/kg in children) as needed. Each patient is brought to his or her optimal dosage level as determined by clinical response and side effects encountered. Clomipramine should be administered with meals to reduce gastrointestinal side effects or at bedtime to minimize daytime sedation. The maintenance dose for all patients should be the lowest effective dose, usually 50-150 mg per day. The clinical response to clomipramine may be delayed by several weeks. Side effects observed during clomipramine therapy are those typical of tricyclic antidepressant drugs, such as sedation, dry mouth, dizziness, tremor, constipation and sexual dysfunction. As with other tricyclic antidepressant drugs, clomipramine may lower seizure threshold.

Fluoxetine

Fluoxetine (Prozac) is a selective serotonin reuptake inhibitor (SSRI) marketed widely as an antidepressant. It has also been proven to be effective for the treatment of OCD. This medication is initiated at 10-20 mg each morning and may be adjusted as required to 60-80 mg per day, divided into two or three doses. Clinical response to fluoxetine may also be delayed by several weeks.

Fluoxetine produces fewer and less toxic side effects than clomipramine. In addition to those side effects typical of antidepressant medications, dyspepsia, nausea, skin rash and hypomanic behavior may occur. The drug appears to suppress appetite for some patients. Fluoxetine has been used safely in children with TS. However, many children experience agitation or over-arousal at levels needed for clinical improvement.

Other SSRI Medications

Sertraline (Zoloft) and **paroxetine (Paxil)** are other SSRI medications with effects and side effects that are similar to fluoxetine. They are also used in the treatment of OCD. **Fluvoxamine (Luvox)** another medication in the OCD armamentarium has shown promise as an effective drug, perhaps with fewer side effects than fluoxetine.

In addition to medications, behavioral treatments, such as "exposure and response prevention" can be quite helpful for some patients with TS and concomitant OCD.

Combinations of Medications

Some clinicians prefer to use combinations of medications when a single agent is only partially effective. There is some clinical evidence to indicate that haloperidol (or another of the neuroleptics mentioned previously) plus clonidine may have synergistic effects. There is also some evidence that clonidine may reduce akathisia caused by neuroleptics. The combination of haloperidol and clonidine has been used in two clinical situations: (1) for patients whose symptoms are not fully controlled on haloperidol, or who are having serious side effects when medication is increased, yet who cannot have their haloperidol fully discontinued because of the severity of symptoms or the emergence of an exacerbation with tapering; and (2) for patients who are on clonidine but are still having motor and phonic symptoms. It appears that patients can be managed with smaller doses of haloperidol if clonidine is added to the regimen, and, on the other hand, that haloperidol may improve the tic control for some patients on clonidine. In general, quite small doses of both medications have been used when the drugs are combined and no serious side effects have been reported beyond what is seen when each drug is used individually.

Other combinations such as a neuroleptic plus fluoxetine or a tricyclic antidepressant may be helpful for patients with tics and OC symptoms in which both are severe. Clonazepam has been used in combination with either clonidine or neuroleptics, but there is little evidence of the improved efficacy of these combinations. While there may be justification for using various combinations of medications in individual patients, the best recommendation would be to thoroughly explore the use of single pharmacologic agents before resorting to polypharmacy.

Clonazepam has been found to be effective in some cases for mild tic symptoms. It may also be used in conjunction with another of the previously discussed medications. However, it has the disadvantage of being a habit-forming drug.

Choice of Medication

The clinician's choice of a first drug is a difficult decision. Haloperidol and pimozide have long "track records," and their therapeutic benefits and side effects are well defined. Another major contender as a first drug is clonidine, which is less well defined and less likely to be dramatically effective. Clinicians who lean toward clonidine as a first drug do so because of its limited side effects and positive effect on attention; however, where a rapid response is needed, haloperidol or pimozide are more effective.

When treating a child with both ADHD and TS, it is advisable to carefully consider the alternatives to stimulant medications. Alternative medications for ADHD include various antidepressants, clonidine and neuroleptics.

When used alone, antidepressant medications are not useful in the treatment of tics. However, a patient with TS may develop serious depression and then the use of antidepressant medication should be considered when this occurs. In such situations, antidepressants have been added to ongoing TS treatment (haloperidol, pimozide and clonidine) with good results. Complicating the assessment of depression in TS is the fact that pimozide, haloperidol and clonidine may elicit lowered spirits or dysphoria. Therefore, a trial of no medication might be considered before the addition of an antidepressant, especially if the depression emerges soon after the use of another medication and with no apparent psychosocial precipitant.

Various minor tranquilizers have been used in the treatment of TS with questionable benefit on tic symptomatology. Individual patients seem to have benefitted from medications such as benzodiazepines (e.g., diazepam and alprazolam) when used to help alleviate anxiety or to improve sleep. As such, their use for patients with TS should follow the usual guidelines.

Psychodynamic Psychotherapy

Although psychotherapy will not eliminate tics, it may be beneficial to some patients with TS who require treatment of the psychological sequelae of this difficult illness. The inability to control one's own body and even one's own thoughts, which is taken for granted by most people, often is a great source of anxiety, guilt, fear, helplessness, anger and depression. Some patients react by withdrawal, others by aggressivity, and still others by perfectionism and excessive efforts to be in control. Since virtually all patients with TS are subjected to some form of negative social reaction, self-esteem problems are common. In addition, the person with TS experiences all the difficulties related to growing up with a chronic illness. For these reasons, rather than for the primary symptoms of TS, psychodynamic psychotherapeutic treatment may well be indicated.

Family Treatment

As with any chronic illness, TS causes a great strain on the family as well as on the individual patient. Parents often have a harder time accepting their children's symptoms than the children themselves. Part of the trouble may lie in the guilt associated with the genetic nature of the disorder. Another major problem for parents is understanding which behaviors are beyond the control of the child with TS and which can and should be controlled. Also, preoccupation with the "sick" child may lead to a situation where scant attention is paid to the impact on siblings without TS. Often, spouses of patients with TS do not appreciate the complex problems of TS and its effect on a loving relationship until some time after the marriage.

Family therapy for TS should focus on the role that the patient with TS plays in the family. Is he or she overprotected, treated punitively, misunderstood or a source of embarrassment? Does the illness dominate the family's interrelationships or is it taken more "in stride?" If the family can learn to accept the member with TS along with the symptoms — not despite them—it can provide the sense of security necessary for a healthy approach to the "outside world."

Usually, the first task of family therapy is to educate family members about various aspects of the disorder. It is often found that the family and even the patient do not thoroughly understand the range of symptomatology or how they might be expected to handle it. Following an understanding of the symptoms, an effort should be made to understand how the symptoms impact on each member of the family. Ultimate goals for the family member with TS include: the promotion of self-esteem, competency and support in the challenges of work, school and peer group relationships. The goal for family members is to develop the flexibility to give special help when needed but not to overprotect.

Genetic Counseling

With the recognition that TS is familial and genetic, families naturally have become interested in the possibility of genetic counseling. Such counseling must be provided by knowledgeable clinicians who can impart accurate information about the mode of transmission and work with families in dealing with the complex feelings which are aroused. Until the precise gene (or genes) responsible for TS is determined, physicians can only give possibilities and probabilities to guide patients and their families.

Academic and Occupational Interventions

Children with attentional and learning problems require educational intervention similar to the approaches used in the treatment of other forms of ADHD and learning disabilities. Depending on the severity of the school and associated behavioral problems, patients with TS may require special tutoring, a learning laboratory, a self-contained classroom, a special or residential school. It may be difficult to convince a school district of the need for special school provisions for a bright student with TS who does not have specific learning disabilities, but whose attentional problems limit optimal functioning.

Since TS is an uncommon disorder, schools need to be informed about the nature of TS and the ways it affects attention and learning. Sometimes, the physician must actively serve as a child's advocate.

Children with TS sometimes are kept as homebound students because their symptoms are thought to be too disruptive for the classroom. Vocal tics are usually the most difficult for teachers to handle. However, the homebound child is deprived of his or her legal rights for the least restrictive educational environment and adequate education.

When children stay at home instead of attending school, their TS symptoms are likely to be exacerbated as they exert less control, are exposed to a tedious lack of diversion and sometimes interact with parents in a negative and ambivalent manner. A chain reaction may be set up in which bad symptoms lead to worse symptoms and increased isolation.

Some further specific recommendations for teachers may be found in the "Additional Resources" section.

Many adults with TS require special modifications in their work situation. Often, an explanation to the employer about special needs will receive a positive response. Flexibility, compassion and productivity in the workplace can be increased to everyone's benefit with appropriate interventions for a very symptomatic patient or for a patient who is having difficulty adjusting to a new medication.

References

American Psychiatric Association (1987). *Diagnostic and Statistical Manual of Mental Disorders (DSM-III-R)*. Washington, D.C.: American Psychiatric Association.

Cohen, D.J., Bruun, R.D., Leckman, J.F., eds. (1988). *Tourette's Syndrome and Tic Disorders: Clinical Understanding and Treatment*. New York: John Wiley & Sons.

Cohen, D.J., Leckman, J.F., Towbin, K.E. (1989). "Tic Disorders." In: *Treatments of Psychiatric Disorders: A Task Force Report of the American Psychiatric Association*. T.B. Karasu (ed). Washington, D.C.: American Psychiatric Association Press, pp. 683-711.

Cohen, D.J., Towbin, K.E., Leckman, J.F. (1989). *Tourette's Syndrome: A Model Developmental Neuropsychiatric Disorder*. Paris: Presse Universitaire de France.

Friedhoff, A.J., Chase, T.N., eds. (1982). "Gilles de la Tourette Syndrome." *Advances in Neurology, Vol. 35*. New York: Raven Press.

Kurlan, R., Caine, E. (1988). *Current Pharmacology of Tourette Syndrome*. Bayside, New York: Tourette Syndrome Association.

Mini-Conference on Tourette Syndrome and Associated Behaviors (1989). Bayside, New York: Tourette Syndrome Association.

Shapiro, A., Shapiro, E., Bruun, R.D., Sweet, R.D. (1978). *Gilles de la Tourette's Syndrome*. New York: Raven Press.

Shapiro, A., Shapiro, E., Young, J.G., Feinberg, T.E. (1988). Second Edition. *Gilles de la Tourette Syndrome*. New York: Raven Press.

Stefl, M.E. (1984). "Mental Health Needs Associated with Tourette Syndrome." *American Journal of Public Health, Vol. 74* pp. 1310-1313.

Bruun, R., Bruun, B., (eds.) (1994). *A Mind of Its Own: Tourette Syndrome: A Story and A Guide*. New York: Oxford University Press.

Cohen, D.J., Leckman, J.F. (1994). "Developmental Psychopathology and Neurobiology of Tourette's Syndrome." *Journal of The American Academy of Child and Adolescent Psychiatry*. 33(1):2-15.

Chase, T.N., Friedhoff, A.J., Cohen, D.J. (1992). *Tourette's Syndrome and Tic Disorders: Clinical Understanding and Treatment*. New York: John Wiley & Sons, Inc.

Cicchetti, D., Cohen, D.J. (eds.) (1995). *Manual of Developmental Psychopathology. Volume I: Theory and Method. Volume II: Risk, Disorder and Adaptation*. New York: John Wiley & Sons, Inc.

Erenberg, G. (1992). "Tourette's Syndrome and Other Tic Disorders." In: *Child and Adolescent Neurology for Psychiatrists*. Kaufman, D.J., Solomon, G.E., Pfeffer, C.R. (eds.). Baltimore: Williams and Wilkins, pp. 67-78.

Kurlan, R. (ed.) (1993). *Handbook of Tourette's Syndrome and Related Tic and Behavioral Disorders*. New York: Marcel Dekker.

Kurlan, R. (1989). "Tourette's Syndrome: Current Concepts." *Neurology*. 39:1625-1630.

Leckman, J.F., Pauls, D.L., Cohen, D.J. (1995). "Tic Disorders." In: *Psychopharmacology: The Fourth Generation of Progress*. F.E. Bloom, D. Kupfer (eds.). In press.

Leckman, J.F., Riddle, M.A., Hardin, M.T., Ort, S.I., Swartz, K.L., Stevenson, J., Cohen, D.J. (1989). "The Yale Global Tic Severity Scale (YGTSS): Initial Testing of a Clinician-Rated Scale of Tic Severity." *Journal of the American Academy of Child and Adolescent Psychiatry*. 28:566-573.

Singer, H.S. (1994). "Neurobiological Issues in Tourette Syndrome." *Brain and Development*. 16:353-364.

Singer, H.S., Walkup, J.T. (1991). "Tourette Syndrome and Other Tic Disorders: Diagnosis, Patho-physiology and Treatment." *Medicine*. 70:15-32.

Additional Resources

VHS Films

Tourette Syndrome: Guide to Diagnosis—A video for interested medical professionals who have not seen substantial numbers of patients with TS. This film presents seven individuals who exhibit the full range of movements, vocalizations and behavioral patterns associated with the disorder. Descriptions and demonstrations of other movement disorders are also presented for the purpose of differential diagnosis. (Developed by Drs. R. Bruun, J. Jankovic and G. Erenberg.) 30 min.

- 2:03 Motor tics
- 3:09 Vocal tics
- 3:44 Other tic symptoms
- 6:20 Diagnostic criteria
- 7:10 Natural progression
- 9:05 Symptom suppression/situations and severity
- 10:33 Difficulties of diagnosis
- 10:54 Behavioral aspects
- 21:16 Differential diagnosis
- 26:45 Other sources of information

Talking About TS—A psychiatrist with TS leads an in-depth discussion with a brother and sister, both of whom have TS. 45 min.

I'm a Person Too—Prize winning documentary featuring five people from diverse backgrounds talking about living with TS; depicts the broad range of symptoms. Viewers can obtain a better understanding of the disorder and its manifestations. Narrated by Cliff Robertson. 22 min.

An Inservice Film for Educators: A Regular Kid, That's Me—A new aid for teachers to help understand the complexities of teaching children with TS. Includes explanation of the disorder and suggests interventions that work. (Depicts 19 children interacting in a classroom setting.) 45 min.

Literature

Current Pharmacology of TS—R. Kurlan, MD. Covers medications used currently to treat TS. Includes specific information about clinical evaluation, dosages, side effects, testing. 12 pgs.

Consumer's Guide to TS Medications—G. Erenberg, MD. This brochure has been written for the lay reader. Covers common medications used for the control of TS motor and vocal tics as well as those traditionally prescribed for associated behaviors. Starting and maximum dosages as well as possible side effects are covered. 12 pgs.

The Genetics of Tourette Syndrome—Covers mode of inheritance, penetrance degrees in males and females, other related conditions, non-genetic factors. Pamphlet.

Discipline and the TS Child: A Guide for Parents and Teachers—R. Fisher-Collins, M.Ed. Helps children redirect impulses and compulsions through teaching cause and effect relationships. Included are techniques about disciplining children without the use of aggression or intimidation. 15 pgs.

An Educator's Guide to Tourette Syndrome—S. Bronheim, PhD. Covers symptoms, techniques for classroom management, attentional, writing and language problems. 16 pgs.
To obtain an up-to-date Catalog of Publications and Films, including order form, write to:

Tourette Syndrome Association, Inc.
42-40 Bell Blvd
Bayside, NY 11361-2874
(718) 224-2999
Fax: (718) 279-9596

The Tourette Syndrome Association is a national voluntary health organization dedicated to identifying the cause, finding the cure and controlling the effects of TS.

■ **Document Source:**
   Tourette Syndrome Association, Inc
   42-40 Bell Boulevard
   Bayside, NY 11361-2874
   3rd Revision IOM/1995

GUILLAIN-BARRÉ SYNDROME

What is Guillain-Barré syndrome?

Guillain-Barré *(ghee-yan bah-ray)* syndrome is a disorder in which the body's immune system attacks part of the nervous system. The first symptoms of this disorder include varying degrees of weakness or tingling sensations in the legs. In many instances the weakness and abnormal sensations spread to the arms and upper body. These symptoms can increase in intensity until the muscles cannot be used at all and the patient is almost totally paralyzed. In these cases the disorder is life threatening—potentially interfering with blood pressure, heart rate, and breathing—and is considered a medical emergency. The patient is often put on a respirator to assist with breathing and is watched closely for problems such as an abnormal heart beat, infections, blood clots, and high or low blood pressure. Most patients, however, recover from even the most severe cases of Guillain-Barré syndrome, although some continue to have minor problems.

Guillain-Barré syndrome can affect anybody. It can strike at any age and both sexes are equally prone to the disorder. The syndrome is rare, however, afflicting only about one person in 100,000. Usually Guillain-Barré occurs a few days or weeks after the patient has had symptoms of a respiratory or gastrointestinal viral infection. Occasionally pregnancy, surgery, or vaccinations will trigger the syndrome. The disorder can develop over the course of hours or days, or it may take up to 3 to 4 weeks. Most people reach the stage of greatest weakness within the first 2 weeks after symptoms appear, and by the third week of the illness 90 percent of all patients are at their weakest.

What causes Guillain-Barré syndrome?

No one yet knows why Guillain-Barré strikes some people and not others. Nor does anyone know exactly what sets the disease in motion. What scientists do know is that the body's immune system begins to attack the body itself, causing what is known as an *autoimmune disease.* Usually the cells of the immune system attack only foreign material and invading organisms. In Guillain-Barré syndrome, however, the immune system starts to destroy the myelin sheath that surrounds the axons of many nerve cells, or even the axons themselves (axons are long, thin extensions of the nerve cells; they carry nerve signals). The myelin sheath surrounding the axon speeds up the transmission of nerve signals and allows the transmission of signals over long distances.

In diseases in which the nerve cells' myelin sheaths are injured or degraded, the nerves cannot transmit signals efficiently. That is why the muscles begin to lose their ability to respond to the brain's commands, commands that must be carried through the nerve network. The brain also receives fewer sensory signals from the rest of the body, resulting in an inability to feel textures, heat, pain, and other sensations. Alternately, the brain may receive inappropriate signals that result in tingling, "crawling-skin," or painful sensations. Because the signals to and from the arms and legs must travel the longest distances they are most vulnerable to interruption. Therefore, muscle weakness and tingling sensations usually first appear in the hands and feet.

When Guillain-Barré is preceded by a viral infection, it is possible that the virus has changed the nature of cells in the nervous system so that the immune system treats them as foreign cells. It is also possible that the virus has changed the nature of cells in the nervous system so that the immune system treats them as foreign cells. It is also possible that the virus makes the immune system itself less discriminating about what cells it attacks. Scientists are investigating these possibilities and others to find why the immune system goes awry in Guillain-Barré syndrome and other autoimmune diseases, The cause and course of Guillain-Barré syndrome is an active area of neurological investigation, incorporating the cooperative efforts of neurological scientists, immunologists, and virologists.

How is Guillain-Barré syndrome diagnosed?

Guillain-Barré is called a syndrome rather than a disease because it is not clear that a specific disease-causing agent is involved. A syndrome is a medical condition characterized by a collection of symptoms (what the patient feels) and signs (what a doctor can observe or measure). Because the signs and symptoms of the syndrome can be quite varied, doctors may find it difficult to diagnose Guillain-Barré in its earliest stages.

Several disorders have symptoms similar to those found in Guillain-Barré, so doctors examine and question patients carefully before making a diagnosis. Collectively, the signs and symptoms form a certain pattern that helps doctors differentiate Guillain-Barré from other disorders. For example, physicians will note whether the symptoms appear on both sides of the body (most common in Guillain-Barré) and the quickness with which the symptoms appear (in other disorders muscle weakness may progress over months rather than days or weeks). In Guillain-Barré, reflexes such as knee jerks are usually lost. Because the signals traveling along the nerve are slower, a nerve conduction velocity (NCV) test can give a doctor clues to aid the diagnosis. In Guillain-Barré patients, the cerebrospinal fluid that bathes the spinal cord and brain contains more protein than usual. Therefore a physician may decide to perform a spinal tap. a procedure in which the doctor inserts a needle into the patient's spinal column. Laboratory scientists, working with clinical neurologists, are conducting research that may help provide physicians with more precise and reliable diagnostic tests for this disorder.

How is Guillain-Barré treated?

There is no known cure for Guillain-Barré syndrome. However, there are therapies that lessen the severity of the illness in most patients, and there are a number of ways to read the complications of the disease.

Currently, plasmapheresis and high-dose immunoglobulin therapy are used in the more serious cases of Guillain-Barré syndrome. Plasmapheresis is a method by which whole-blood is removed from the body and processed so that the red and white blood cells are separated from the plasma, or liquid portion of the blood. The blood cells are then returned to the patient without the plasma, which the body quickly replaces. Scientists still don't know exactly why plasmapheresis works, but the technique seems to reduce the severity and duration of the Guillain-Barré episode. This may be because the plasma portion of the blood contains elements that the immune system needs to function. When these elements are removed along with the plasma, the immune system is not able to attack the nervous system as effectively.

In high-dose immunoglobulin therapy, doctors give intravenous injections of the proteins that the immune system uses to attack invading organisms. Investigators have found that these immunoglobulins, when given to Guillain-Barré patients, can lessen the immune attack on the nervous system. Investigators don't know why this is, but some suggest that the immunoglobulins may overwhelm the immune system and keep it from attacking the nerve cells and their myelin sheaths.

The use of steroid hormones has also been tried as a way to reduce the severity of Guillain-Barré, but controlled clinical trails have not demonstrated that this treatment is effective.

Much of the treatment for this syndrome consists of keeping the patient's body functioning during recovery of the nervous system. This can sometimes require placing the patients on a respirator, a heart monitor, or other machines that assist body function. The need for this sophisticated machinery is one reason why Guillain-Barré syndrome patients are usually treated in hospitals, often in an intensive care ward. In the hospital, doctors can also look for and treat the many problems that can afflict any paralyzed patient— complications such as pneumonia or bed sores.

Often, even before recovery begins, caregivers may be instructed to manually move the patient's limbs to help keep the muscles flexible and strong. Later, as the patient begins to recover limb control, physical therapy begins,

Carefully planned clinical trials of new and experimental therapies are the key to improving the treatment of patients with Guillain-Barré syndrome. Such clinical trials begin with the research of basic and clinical scientists who, working with clinicians, identify new approaches to treating patients with the disease.

What is the long-term outlook for those with Guillain-Barré syndrome?

Guillian-Barré syndrome can be a devastating disorder because of its sudden and unexpected onset. In addition, recovery is not necessarily quick. As noted previously, patients usually reach the point of greatest weakness or paralysis days or weeks after the first symptoms occur. Symptoms then stabilize at this level for a period of days, weeks, or, sometimes, months. The recovery period may be as little as a few weeks or as long as a few years. About 30 percent of those with Guillain-Barré still feel a residual weakness after 3 years. About 3 to 5 percent may suffer a relapse of muscle weakness and tingling sensations many years after the initial attack.

Guillain-Barré syndrome patients face not only physical difficulties, but emotionally painful periods as well. It is often extremely difficult for patients to adjust to sudden paralysis and dependence on others for help with routine daily activities. Patients sometimes need psychological counseling to help them adapt.

What research is being done?

Scientists are concentrating on finding new treatments and refining existing ones. Scientists are also looking at the workings of the immune system to find which cells are responsible for beginning and carrying out the attack on the nervous system. The fact that so many cases of Guillain-Barré begin after a viral infection suggests that certain characteristics of these viruses may activate the immune system inappropriately. Investigators are searching for those characteristics. As noted previously, neurological scientists, immunologists, virologists, and pharmacologists are all working collaboratively to learn how to prevent this disorder and to make better therapies available when it strikes.

Where can I go for more information?

The National Institute of Neurological Disorders and Stroke conducts and supports a wide range of research on neurological disorders, including Guillain-Barré syndrome. For more information on this or other neurological disorders, or on the Institute and its research programs, contact:

Office of Scientific and Health Reports
Neurological Institute
PO Box 5801
Bethesda, MD 20824
(301) 496-5751
(800) 352-9424

The organization listed below provides printed information and assistance to Guillain-Barré patients and other interested parties.

Guillain-Barré Syndrome Foundation International
PO Box 262
Wynnewood, PA 19096
(215) 667-0131

■ Document Source:
**U.S. Department of Health and Human Services, Public Health
Service
National Institute of Health
National Institute of Neurological Disorders and Stroke
Behesda, MD 20892
NIH Publication No. 92-2902
September 1992**

INSOMNIA

What is insomnia?

Insomnia is the perception or complaint of inadequate or
poor-quality sleep because of one or more of the following:

- difficulty falling asleep
- waking up frequently during the night with difficulty
  returning to sleep
- waking up too early in the morning
- unrefreshing sleep

Insomnia is not defined by the number of hours of
sleep a person gets or how long it takes to fall asleep.
Individuals vary normally in their need for, and their satisfaction with, sleep. Insomnia may cause problems during the
day, such as tiredness, a lack of energy, difficulty concentrating, and irritability.

Insomnia can be classified as transient (short term), intermittent (on and off), and chronic (constant). Insomnia
lasting from a single night to a few weeks is referred to as
transient. If episodes of transient insomnia occur from time
to time, the insomnia is said to be intermittent. Insomnia is
considered to be chronic if it occurs on most nights and lasts
a month or more.

What causes it?

Certain conditions seem to make individuals more likely to
experience insomnia. Examples of these conditions include:

- advanced age (insomnia occurs more frequently in
  those over age 60)
- female gender
- a history of depression

If other conditions (such as stress, anxiety, a medical problem, or the use of certain medications) occur along with the
above conditions, insomnia is more likely.

There are many causes of insomnia. Transient and intermittent insomnia generally occur in people who are temporarily experiencing one or more of the following:

- stress
- environmental noise
- extreme temperatures

- change in the surrounding environment
- sleep/wake schedule problems such as those due to jet lag
- medication side effects

Chronic insomnia is more complex and often results
from a combination of factors, including underlying physical or mental disorders. One of the most common causes
of chronic insomnia is depression. Other underlying causes
include arthritis, kidney disease, heart failure, asthma,
sleep apnea, narcolepsy, restless legs syndrome, Parkinson's disease, and hyperthyroidism. However, chronic insomnia may also be due to behavioral factors, including the
misuse of caffeine, alcohol, or other substances; disrupted
sleep/wake cycles as may occur with shift work or other
nighttime activity schedules; and chronic stress.

In addition, the following behaviors have been shown to
perpetuate insomnia in some people:

- expecting to have difficulty sleeping and worrying
  about it
- ingesting excessive amounts of caffeine
- drinking alcohol before bedtime
- smoking cigarettes before bedtime
- excessive napping in the afternoon or evening
- irregular or continually disrupted sleep/wake schedules

These behaviors may prolong existing insomnia, and
they can also be responsible for causing the sleeping problem
in the first place. Stopping these behaviors may eliminate the
insomnia altogether.

Who gets insomnia?

Insomnia is found in males and females of all age groups,
although it seems to be more common in females (especially
after menopause) and in the elderly. The ability to sleep,
rather than the need for sleep, appears to decrease with
advancing age.

How is it diagnosed?

Patients with insomnia are evaluated with the help of a medical history and a sleep history. The sleep history may be
obtained from a sleep diary filled out by the patient or by an
interview with the patient's bed partner concerning the quantity and quality of the patient's sleep. Specialized sleep studies may be recommended, but only if there is suspicion that
the patient may have a primary sleep disorder such as sleep
apnea or narcolepsy.

How is it treated?

Transient and intermittent insomnia may not require treatment since episodes last only a few days at a time. For
example, if insomnia is due to a temporary change in the
sleep/wake schedule, as with jet lag, the person's biological
clock will often get back to normal on its own. However, for
some people who experience daytime sleepiness and impaired performance as a result of transient insomnia, the use

of short-acting sleeping pills may improve sleep and next-day alertness. As with all drugs, there are potential side effects. The use of over-the-counter sleep medicines is not usually recommended for the treatment of insomnia.

Other Sleep Publications Available from the National Heart, Lung, and Blood Institute Information Center

Facts About Sleep Apnea. A four-page brochure that discusses sleep apnea and how it is treated. (NIH Publication No. 95-3798)
Test Your Sleep I. Q. This quiz tests your knowledge about sleep and sleep-related disorders. (NIH Publication No. 95-3797)

Treatment for chronic insomnia consists of:

- First, diagnosing and treating underlying medical or psychological problems.
- Identifying behaviors that may worsen insomnia and stopping (or reducing) them.
- Possibly using sleeping pills, although the long-term use of sleeping pills for chronic insomnia is controversial. A patient taking any sleeping pill should be under the supervision of a physician to closely evaluate effectiveness and minimize side effects. In general, these drugs are prescribed at the lowest dose and for the shortest duration needed to relieve the sleep-related symptoms. For some of these medicines, the dose must be gradually lowered as the medicine is discontinued because, if stopped abruptly, it can cause insomnia to occur again for a night or two.
- Trying behavioral techniques to improve sleep, such as relaxation therapy, sleep restriction therapy, and reconditioning.

Relaxation Therapy

There are specific and effective techniques that can reduce or eliminate anxiety and body tension. As a result, the person's mind is able to stop "racing," the muscles can relax, and restful sleep can occur. It usually takes much practice to learn these techniques and to achieve effective relaxation.

Sleep Restriction

Some people suffering from insomnia spend too much time in bed unsuccessfully trying to sleep. They may benefit from a sleep restriction program that at first allows only a few hours of sleep during the night. Gradually the time is increased until a more normal night's sleep is achieved.

Reconditioning

Another treatment that may help some people with insomnia is to recondition them to associate the bed and bedtime with sleep. For most people, this means not using their beds for any activities other than sleep and sex. As part of the reconditioning process, the person is usually advised to go to bed only when sleepy. If unable to fall asleep, the person is told to get up, stay up until sleepy, and then return to bed.

Throughout this process, the person should avoid naps and wake up and go to bed at the same time each day. Eventually the person's body will be conditioned to associate the bed and bedtime with sleep.

Where to Get More Information

Talk to your doctor if you are having trouble getting good, refreshing sleep each night. Together you can identify possible reasons for your sleeping difficulty and then try appropriate measures to correct the problem. For additional information on sleep and sleep disorders, contact the following offices of the National Heart, Lung, and Blood Institute of the National Institutes of Health.

The National Center on Sleep Disorders Research (NCSDR), located within the National Heart, Lung, and Blood Institute, supports research, scientist training, dissemination of health information, and other activities on sleep disorders and related concerns. The NCSDR also coordinates sleep research activities with other federal agencies and with public and non-profit organizations.

National Center on Sleep Disorders Research
Two Rockledge Centre Ste 7024
6701 Rockledge Dr, MSC 7920
Bethesda, MD 20892-7920
(301) 435-0199
(301) 480-3451 (FAX)

National Heart, Lung, and Blood Institute Information Center acquires, analyzes, promotes, maintains, and disseminates programmatic and educational information related to sleep disorders and sleep-disordered breathing. Write for a list of available publications or to order additional copies of this fact sheet.

NHLBI Information Center
PO Box 30105
Bethesda, MD 20824-0105
(301) 251-1222
(301) 251-1223 (FAX)

■ **Document Source:**
U.S. Department of Health and Human Services, Public Health Service
National Institutes of Health
National Heart, Lung, and Blood Institute
NIH Publication No. 95-3801
October 1995

See also: The Nature of Sleep (page 413)

LIVING WITH MS

by Debra Frankel, M.S., O.T.R. Special Projects Manager, National Multiple Sclerosis Society Massachusetts Chapter, with Hettie Jones

Stop

If you've just found out you've got MS you're probably overwhelmed. Before you read any further, remember you're not alone. In the United States, more than a third of a million people are living with MS. Much has already been discovered about this disease, and research continues to offer new treatments and better management, which means a better quality of life for people with MS.

Begin Here

Here are the 28 most commonly asked questions about MS. They can start you on your own investigation. Learning as much as you can is the best way to address your concerns and prepare to work with the health professionals involved in your care.

The Key Idea

Living with MS is a challenge, but it's a challenge that can be met. Keeping yourself well, both emotionally and physically, is the key. How and what you do for yourself—how you take control—will play a big part.

1. What is multiple sclerosis?

MS is a disease of the central nervous system, which has two major parts, the brain and the spinal cord. Surrounding and protecting the nerve fibers of the central nervous system is a fatty tissue called myelin, which helps nerve fibers conduct electrical impulses. In MS, myelin is lost in *multiple* areas, leaving scars called *sclerosis*. These damaged areas are also known as *plaques* or *lesions*.

Myelin not only protects nerve fibers, it also makes their job possible. When myelin is destroyed or damaged, the ability of the nerves to conduct electrical impulses to and from the brain is disrupted, and this produces the various symptoms of MS.

MS is not contagious. No one in your family will catch it from you.

2. What causes this disease?

While the exact cause of MS is unknown, many researchers believe that the damage to myelin results from an abnormal response by the body's immune system. Normally, the immune system defends the body against foreign "invaders" such as viruses or bacteria. In *autoimmune* diseases, the body inadvertently attacks its own tissue. In the case of MS, the substance that is attacked is myelin.

Scientists do not yet know what triggers the immune system to attack myelin. Most agree that several factors are involved.

3. What are the symptoms of MS?

Because these depend on which areas of the central nervous system have been attacked, not all people are affected the same way. Symptoms are not only different for different people, but different in the same person from time to time. They also vary in severity and duration.

A person with MS will usually experience more than one symptom, but not all people have all of them.

Symptoms include weakness, tingling, numbness or impaired sensation, poor coordination, fatigue, problems with balance, visual disturbances, involuntary rapid eye movement (also called *nystagmus*), tremors, spasticity or muscle stiffness, slurred speech, bowel or bladder problems, unstable walking (*ataxia*), problems with sexual function, sensitivity to heat, and problems with short-term memory, judgment, or reasoning (*cognitive problems*). In extreme cases, MS can cause partial or complete paralysis.

Remember, the majority of people with MS do not have all these symptoms.

4. How is MS diagnosed?

Because no single test can diagnose MS, several tests and procedures are needed. They are likely to include:

- A medical history, in which the physician will look for evidence of past signs and symptoms.
- A thorough neurological exam.
- Studies—called "evoked potentials"—that measure the response of the central nervous system to specific stimulation.
- MRI (magnetic resonance imaging), a relatively new form of imaging that produces precise and highly detailed pictures of the brain and spinal cord.

Other tests, less commonly used but helpful where diagnosis is unusually difficult, are:

- CAT scan (computerized axial tomography), which uses X-rays to produce images of the central nervous system.
- Lumbar puncture or spinal tap, which looks at the composition of the fluid that surrounds the spinal cord (cerebrospinal fluid or CSF).

5. Are second opinions—to confirm diagnosis—a good idea?

If you've seen only one doctor, it's certainly reasonable to get a second opinion. Your original doctor should not be insulted or hurt because you want to confirm your diagnosis. You might ask your family doctor, or call the National MS Society, for a referral to a specialist in your area.

6. What will happen next?

No one really knows, but you and your doctor can and should talk over your particular situation.

The words you will hear most often are "unpredictable" and "variable." MS not only varies widely from person to person, it varies in the same person from time to time. Living with this unpredictability is part of living with MS.

Many people go through periods of *exacerbation*. These are attacks, often called *relapses*, during which new symptoms appear or existing symptoms become more severe. Exacerbations are usually followed by *remissions* which may bring you back to your pre-relapse level or may leave you with some remaining disability. This form of MS is usually called *relapsing-remitting MS.*

Not all MS is the same. Some people have few severe attacks but instead experience a worsening of symptoms and disability over time without abrupt changes. This steady pattern can follow an earlier period of relapsing-remitting MS, in which case it is called *secondary progressive MS,* or this pattern may exist from the outset in which case it is called *primary progressive MS.* MS may stabilize at any time, regardless of pattern.

Your first several years of experience with MS are likely to be the best guide you and your physician have to your long-term outlook. If your physician has a history of caring for other people with MS, he/she may have additional insights about your situation.

7. Is MS inherited?

MS is not directly inherited, although studies do reveal *familial predisposition.* This means that siblings or other close relatives are somewhat more likely to develop the disease. However, 80 percent of people with MS do *not* have a close relative with MS.

8. Who gets MS?

Women develop MS at a rate almost double that of men. Diagnosis is usually made sometime between ages 20 and 40. It's estimated that in the United States some 350,000 people are living with MS. Some complicated cases of MS are difficult to diagnose, and because it isn't contagious, reporting of cases is not required. So the actual number of people with MS can only be estimated.

Worldwide, MS occurs more frequently in temperate than tropical climates, and is more common among Caucasians, especially those of northern European ancestry. African Americans, Hispanic Americans, Asian Americans, and Native Americans all get MS, but at lower rates than people of European ancestry.

9. Are there any therapies that will stop or cure MS?

There is no known cure. But there are treatments that lessen the frequency or severity of attacks.

Because treatment for MS is changing so rapidly, it's a good idea to be in contact with your doctor for up-to-date advice. The National MS Society is also a source of information on new developments. Call 1-800-FIGHT-MS or your local chapter.

10. Are there any therapies to relieve symptoms?

Yes. Talk to your doctor about your problems. For example, stiffness in the muscles (*spasticity*) may be reduced by prescription drugs such as baclofen (Lioresal®), dantrolene (Dantrium®), or diazepam (Valium®). Fatigue may be reduced with amantadine (Symmetrel®) or pemoline

(Cylert®). Spasticity and fatigue may also be treated with physical and occupational therapies.

Bladder problems sometimes improve with oxybutynin (Ditropan®) or propantheline (Pro-Banthine®). Techniques such as self-catheterization can be easily learned. Prompt treatment of urinary tract infections and adequate intake of fluids may help prevent other bladder complications. Bowel problems may be managed with diet to increase bulk, suppositories, or medications. Burning, painful, or unusual sensations (called *paresthesias*) may be managed with medications such as carbamazepine (Tegretol®) or amitriptyline (Elavil®). Cognitive problems may be handled through rehabilitation and training.

11. What can rehabilitation offer?

Physical therapy (PT) can help strengthen weakened or uncoordinated muscles. PT might include range-of-motion exercises, stretching, training in walking and best ways to use canes, walkers, or other assistive devices, transfer training (which means learning how to move from wheelchairs to cars, for example), and strengthening exercises to increase overall function and stamina.

Occupational therapy (OT) is geared to improving independence in daily living. OT teaches techniques for dressing, grooming, eating, and driving, and may also provide exercises for coordination and strength. An occupational therapist can recommend equipment and ways to adapt the home or workplace for safety and independence.

Speech therapy improves communication skills for those who may have difficulty speaking or swallowing due to weakness or poor coordination of the muscles. Techniques used by speech therapists (also called speech pathologists) might include exercise, voice training, or the use of special devices. Ask your doctor what will work best for you, or call your chapter of the National MS Society for information and referrals.

12. Does exercise help?

Exercise alone cannot alter MS, but it can improve overall health and it may prevent complications from disuse or inactivity. Because exercise helps to regulate appetite and sleep patterns, and contributes to feelings of well-being, there are psychological as well as physical advantages to be gained from a regular exercise program.

You and your doctor or therapist can work out a combination of activities that will benefit you the most.

13. What about work? What do employers need to know?

MS varies from person to person, and so will its impact on your work situation.

Keep in mind that it's not a good idea to make major decisions about employment while you're in the midst of a crisis—either right after diagnosis, or during a flare-up of symptoms. First, give yourself time to recover from immediate problems. Then gather information that will help you understand your options.

It's up to you whether or not to disclose your diagnosis to co-workers and your employer. Legally, you're *not* required to reveal this information.

If you have been offered a job that requires a medical examination, you should be honest about your diagnosis and/or symptoms. However, a job offer may not be withdrawn on the basis of your diagnosis alone.

If you need any accommodations such as flex time, a modified telephone, or other equipment, you should discuss this with your employer. The Americans with Disabilities Act (ADA) requires your employer to provide reasonable accommodations for you.

The ADA contains many other provisions to protect you. For information, call your local chapter of the National MS Society.

14. Does MS affect sexuality?

Everything connected to MS—from its physical symptoms to its emotional impact—can affect sexual expression. But this doesn't mean that sexual problems can't be managed successfully. People with MS can and do have fulfilling sex lives.

Several important suggestions:

- Work at sharing feelings with your partner.
- Communicate honestly.
- Be flexible about sexual expression.
- Seek medical treatment for physical symptoms.
- For non-physical problems, consider consulting a psychotherapist or counselor who specializes in sex therapy.

15. Is depression common for someone with MS?

It's common to feel fear, confusion, loss of control, and grief at a diagnosis or worsening of MS. At one time or another, 30 to 40 percent of people with MS experience what doctors define as mild or moderate depression. Depression can also be a direct result of the damage this disease causes. Depression is treatable, with medications and with counseling.

If emotions trouble you, remember that asking for help is not weakness but strength. Many chapters of the National MS Society have peer counseling programs. Or ask your doctor to refer you to a professional.

16. Can family counseling help?

The whole family lives with MS. It may change family routines for work, play—almost everything—and everyone is affected. Counseling may help the whole family to adjust.

Many National MS Society chapters offer family-oriented programs. Contact your local chapter for information or for referral to a counselor:

17. What's the best way to tell children about MS?

Young children need basic, simple explanations. Discussing rather than hiding issues benefits children of any age—usually they're more resilient and able to accept painful realities than their parents assume. All children, of course, need reassurance that they will be safe and cared for regardless of what MS may bring.

18. Does pregnancy have an impact on MS?

Studies show that pregnancy doesn't appear to alter the long-term course of MS. However, many women experience a remission during pregnancy, and then, after delivery, a temporary increase in symptoms.

19. Does stress make MS worse?

There's no evidence that stress either causes MS or makes it worse. But people with MS can benefit from stress management techniques:

- Keep as active as possible—mentally and physically.
- Manage time to conserve energy.
- Simplify life—set priorities.
- Learn relaxation/meditation exercises.
- Get help with hard-to-solve problems.
- Make time for fun and maintain your sense of humor.
- Set realistic goals and expectations.
- Accept what cannot be changed.

20. Does smoking or drinking affect MS?

There's no evidence that smoking makes MS worse. But smoking can cause shortness of breath, susceptibility to lung infections, and heartbeat irregularities—symptoms that could add to disability. And because of weakness and incoordination, a smoker with these symptoms may be a fire waiting to happen!

Drinking causes incoordination, poor balance, and slurred speech. It also impairs judgment and alters behavior. All this adds to existing neurological symptoms, although, again, there's no evidence that alcohol makes MS worse.

21. How does heat affect MS?

Heat doesn't make MS worse permanently. But many, though not all, people with MS find that hot and humid weather, a hot bath or shower, or a fever temporarily makes their symptoms worse. It's a good idea to avoid the heat of day and to bathe in warm rather than hot water: Many people with MS find that cooling, with ice packs, iced drinks, and cool baths, helps to reduce symptoms.

An air conditioner may be an essential piece of equipment and may even be tax deductible if your doctor recommends it.

22. Is dental or surgical anesthesia dangerous?

The risks of *general* anesthesia for a person with MS are about the same as for everyone else, with one exception: those who have severe, advanced MS may have respiratory problems that require caution.

There is no reason to avoid such common *local* anesthetics as novocaine unless you know you're allergic to them.

Spinal anesthetics, such as the epidural anesthetic used during childbirth, are more problematic. Although most people with MS tolerate epidural anesthesia well, some neurologists feel that there are potential complications in the method and don't recommend it.

23. What about vaccination against the flu?

Flu vaccination is controversial. Flu shots may cause an increase in MS symptoms for some people. However, there is currently no evidence to support the idea that flu shots cause an increased number of exacerbations. On the other hand, there is good evidence of a relationship between viral infections such as flu and exacerbations. People who are frail or who have had an exacerbation that followed a case of the flu may want to consider flu shots. As a rule, people on immune-suppressing medications should avoid any vaccinations. You should discuss the individual pros and cons with your doctor.

24. Are there any diet recommendations for someone with MS?

There is no scientific evidence that MS has a dietary cause, so there's no reason for a special diet. Many "MS diets" exist—but none has proved effective over the long term.

Well-balanced meals are the key to general good health, so it's essential to pay attention to what you eat.

25. Will "alternative" therapies help?

Acupuncture, yoga, visualization and relaxation techniques, or dietary supplements (including vitamins) have not had a proven effect on MS. However, some people find alternative therapies help them feel better about themselves.

As a person with MS, you may choose any technique that helps you. But before deciding to pursue an alternative therapy, it's wise to investigate its potential risks, benefits, and especially its costs. Discuss it with your doctor.

26. Are there recommendations about seeing the doctor?

Your doctor is your ally in managing MS. You should feel comfortable discussing *all* practical questions, especially what changes to report and anything you should be watching. Always report a worsening of symptoms or the start of new ones.

However, it's possible that a problem may not be connected to MS at all. Beware of attributing all medical problems to MS!

27. What does coping with MS mean?

Everyone copes differently. Here are some general tips:

- Take care of yourself. Eat well, exercise, and get enough rest. Listen to your body.
- Take control of your emotional well-being. Find people with whom you can talk and share feelings, and who will offer support.
- Your MS is unique to you. Some people find it helpful to keep a diary, tracking what happens and when.
- Live one day at a time. MS poses uncertainties about the future. Direct your energy to today and try not to worry about tomorrow's potential problems.
- Examine your priorities. Try to make sense of MS within your own world view, according to your personal values and insights. You might seek support from clergy, spiritual organizations, or counselors.
- Use the National MS Society for information, referral, and support. Call the chapter nearest you and find out about their programs.

28. How can the National Multiple Sclerosis Society help?

Through its chapters, the National MS Society offers counseling, education, social and recreational activities, information and referral, equipment assistance, and more.

The Society, founded in 1946, serves people with MS, their families, health professionals, and the interested public. It also provides funding for MS research, public and professional education, advocacy, and the design of community and client programs.

The National Multiple Sclerosis Society is proud to be a source of information about multiple sclerosis. Our comments are based on professional advice, published experience, and expert opinion, but do not represent therapeutic recommendations or prescription. For specific information and advice, consult your personal physician.

The Society publishes many other pamphlets and articles about various aspects of MS. To ask for these or for other information, contact the chapter nearest you or call the National MS Society at 1-800-FIGHT-MS [1-800-344-4867].

Some of our popular pamphlets include

- Research Directions in Multiple Sclerosis
- Food for Thought: MS and Nutrition
- Things I Wish Someone Had Told Me: Practical Thoughts for People Newly Diagnosed with Multiple Sclerosis
- The Rehab Outlook
- The ADA and People with MS

■ Document Source:
National Multiple Sclerosis Society
733 Third Ave
New York, NY 10017-3288
(212) 986-3240
Fax (212) 986-7981

THE NATURE OF SLEEP

Sleep. It's a basic necessity of life, as fundamental to our health and well-being as air, food and water. When we sleep well, we wake up feeling refreshed, alert, ready to face the day. When we don't, every aspect of our lives can suffer.

A National Sleep Debt

Sleep problems have become a modern epidemic that is taking a catastrophic toll on our bodies and our minds. According to a Gallup Poll conducted for the National Sleep Foundation, one out of every three people suffers from sleeplessness at some point in their lives, many of them chronically. It's estimated that 30-40 million Americans suffer from serious sleep disorders that undermine their sleep quality and their health. For the victims of disordered sleep, the night is a source of anguish, not rest.

For millions more, the body's need to sleep is treated as a waste of time. In our 24-hour society, we steal nighttime hours for daytime activities, cheating ourselves of precious sleep. In the past century, we have reduced our average time asleep by 20 percent and, in the past 25 years, added a month to our average annual work/commute time. Our national sleep debt is on the rise. Our society has changed, but our bodies have not, and we are paying the price.

The Cost of Sleeplessness Is High

What happens when we're deprived of the restful sleep we need? We're less alert and attentive, more inclined to irritability and other mood problems that can make our relationships with family, friends and co-workers difficult. Our concentration and judgment suffer, our ability to perform even simple tasks declines, our productivity is sabotaged. Sleeplessness, whether it's the result of a sleep disorder or an overextended lifestyle, invites diminished quality of life and deteriorating health.

When we lose sleep or our sleep is poor, we also put ourselves and those around us at high risk for accidents. Major industrial catastrophes such as the Three Mile Island incident have been attributed to human error that occurred during times when the body is at its sleepiest. If we ignore our sleep needs and get behind the wheel of a car, lives may be at stake. It only takes a few seconds—just long enough for a tired body to steal a needed "microsleep"—to run off the road or into an oncoming car.

What is a good night's sleep?

The amount of sleep you need to be at your best is as individual as the amount of food you need. It isn't simply how many hours of sleep time you're logging in that matters, but how good you feel and how well you're able to perform each day.

Unfortunately, too many of us think we're getting adequate sleep, but really aren't. Do you routinely roll over and snatch a few extra Zzzz before rolling out of bed? Do you look forward to "catching up" on your sleep over the weekends? Do long meetings, overheated rooms or heavy meals "put you right to sleep"? If you're getting the right amount and quality of sleep, your answer should be "no."

On your next vacation, go to bed when you feel tired and get up whenever you're ready, with no alarm clock. Sleep until you're slept out. You may spend the first few days getting rid of the sleep debt you've been accumulating, then your body should tell you how much sleep you need on a regular basis. If vacation plans don't allow this experiment, try getting up at the same time every day (even on weekends), but varying your bedtime until you've discovered the amount of sleep that seems to be the most restorative for you. Listen to your body and adjust your schedule accordingly.

What happens during sleep?

Sleep is a dynamic process with a complex "architecture" all its own. You begin your nightly journey by descending into Stage 1, a light sleep. Your muscles relax, your brain waves are irregular and rapid. In Stage 2, brain waves become larger, with bursts of electrical activity. Then you move into deep sleep, Stages 3 and 4, in which the brain produces large, slow waves (sometimes called "delta" or slow-wave sleep). You're more difficult to awaken in slow-wave sleep.

After an hour or so, you shift into a highly active stage characterized by rapid eye movements, hence the name REM sleep. Suddenly your brain waves are almost the same as if you were awake. You're in the dreaming stage, which occurs several times across the course of the night.

About 75 percent of your night is spent in non-REM sleep and about 25 percent dreaming. REM periods tend to become longer and more plentiful as the night wears on. Fortunately for your partners and neighbors, you're essentially paralyzed during REM so that you're not acting out your dreams no matter how real they may seem. Occasionally, you may awaken before this paralysis has entirely ended — don't be alarmed, it will pass in a matter of moments.

Sleeping Through the Ages

Sleep patterns change as we age. Newborns and children spend more time in deep sleep than adults. As we grow older, sleep tends to become more fragmented and we spend more time in the lighter stages. We'll probably need to turn in earlier and get up earlier.

It's myth that we need less sleep in our senior years. But it's a fact that most of us sleep less at a stretch than we did when we were younger. Changes in sleep patterns can be dramatic, and sleep problems are more common among the elderly.

Watching Nature's Clock

Sleep needs and patterns are regulated by an internal biological "clock" that's located in the brain. Most people's clock runs on a cycle of about 24 hours, but some of us are morning people, or "larks," and some of us "owls," who find ourselves more alert late in the day.

Almost everyone's clock is set for sleep at night, especially in the early morning hours between midnight and dawn. If you really listen to your body, you'll also discover that it gets sleepy in the middle of the day, between about 1 pm and 4 pm, as well. Some call this the "Siesta Zone," but if your daytime schedule won't permit a siesta, try to reserve this period of less alertness for less critical activities. This may not be the best time to start on a long drive, and it's especially important to stay off the roads between the hours of 2:00 am and 6:00 am when your internal clock makes sleep almost irresistible. Crashes are most likely to happen in these hours.

When our lives force us to work against our biological clocks, sleep problems are inevitable.

Jet Lag

You may become acutely aware of your biological clock when you travel from one time zone to another. Jet lag is what happens when your clock is out of sync with the new environment. You try to sleep when your body is not sleepy and struggle to stay awake while the sun is shining. You can't prevent jet lag, but you may be able to minimize the effects by easing yourself into the new time zone for a few days before you depart, resting as much as possible in transit, and planning a relaxed schedule for your first day or two after arrival.

Shiftwork

For the 20 percent of American employees who work non-traditional schedules, getting enough sleep is a common problem. Shiftworkers need to sleep when their clocks are set for wakefulness, so they tend to sleep badly and not enough. They're more prone to falling asleep on the job than the 9-to-5 worker and at high risk for crashes while driving home in the morning. Maintaining a rigorously regular schedule (for both sleeping and waking activities), even on the weekends, can help the body to adapt.

To Nap or Not?

The mid-afternoon slump most of us experience, even when we've slept well, suggests that the human body may be meant to nap. A regular afternoon siesta isn't likely to become a part of N American culture, but an occasional restorative nap may be a very good idea, particularly if you need to tap into an alertness reserve and a longer period of sleep isn't an option.

There's increasing evidence that a 15-20 minute nap can improve alertness, sharpen memory and generally reduce the symptoms of fatigue. If you're coping with the impact of lost sleep from last night or you know you're going to lose sleep tonight, a nap can help you through. In fact, it could be the difference between life and death if you're planning on a long drive with less than your regular quotient of sleep.

A few cautions. First, a nap is not a substitute for a full night's sleep; it is only a short-term solution. Second, if getting to sleep or staying asleep at night is a problem, naps are probably not for you.

Insomnia: When It Seems Sleep Will Never Come

It isn't unusual to have trouble sleeping — a third of Americans do. Insomnia has many causes and is often viewed as a symptom of some underlying problem, much like a stomach-ache. Doctors have identified three basic categories:

Transient insomnia lasts only a few nights and is usually brought on by stress, excitement, or a change in sleep timing or environment.

Short-term insomnia is poor sleep spanning two or three weeks and can be caused by ongoing stress, as well as medical or psychiatric problems. Alleviating the source will usually return sleep to normal. Recurring episodes are common.

Chronic insomnia lasts more than two weeks and can be related to underlying medical, behavioral or psychiatric problems, such as depression.

Insomnia's impact on waking hours can be significant and includes a decreased sense of well-being, and impaired concentration and memory. Sleep specialists recommend practicing good sleep hygiene to minimize episodes.

Keeping a sleep log for a few weeks may be helpful in identifying behaviors that are contributing to your sleep problem. Record when you wake up, go to sleep, drink caffeinated beverages, exercise, eat and any other suspected sleep-stealers. Simple changes in daily routine may be surprisingly effective in improving sleep quality.

How good is your sleep hygiene?

Following a few simple guidelines, and changing a few bad habits, can do wonders for troubled sleep. Your doctor can help identify the best sleep hygiene routine for you, but here are some basics:

- Avoid caffeinated beverages for at least six hours before bedtime.
- Avoid alcohol and nicotine for at least two hours before bedtime.
- Exercise regularly, but not too close to bedtime.
- Get up at the same time every day regardless of when you went to sleep.

Can sleeping pills help?

Sleeping pills have a role in the treatment of transient and short-term insomnia, where a medication can be useful in breaking the sleeplessness cycle. Once the source of the stress or disruption is dealt with or improved sleep hygiene shows positive effects, medications are discontinued, usually within two weeks. Sleeping pills have a limited role in chronic insomnia and are not intended for long-term use.

Prescription sleeping pills come in both shorter and longer-acting forms. The shorter-acting drugs help to induce and solidify sleep, but wear off faster. The longer-acting drugs help maintain sleep through the night, but may cause sleepiness the next day.

Non-prescription, or over-the-counter (OTC) sleep aids use antihistamines to induce drowsiness. Be sure to allow enough time for the drug to work through your system so there's no risk of sleepiness during the day.

If you decide to use sleeping medications, even an OTC product, be sure to talk to your doctor about the type and dosage that's best for you, as well as any cautions or side effects you should be aware of.

Sleep Apnea: Snoring That Takes Your Breath Away

For more than 10 million Americans, loud, habitual snoring is no joke. It can be a symptom of a potentially life-threatening disorder. Sleep apnea is literally a "lack of breath."

Doctors have identified three basic types of apnea:

Obstructive apnea is the most common and severe. The muscles at the back of the throat relax to the point of obstructing the upper airway. Breathing can actually stop for 10 seconds or more causing mini-awakenings (usually not remembered) several hundred times a night as the sleeper gasps for air. Loud snoring is common.

Central apnea is when the airways stay open but the diaphragm and chest muscles stop working and the sleeper must awaken several times a night to resume breathing, sometimes with a gasp. Sufferers of this relatively uncommon disorder may complain of insomnia or restless sleep. Snoring may not be a symptom.

Mixed apnea is a combination of the two, usually a brief period of central apnea followed by a longer period of obstructive apnea. The combination is common.

Sleep apnea is more common in middle-aged men and overweight people. Sufferers often experience excessive daytime sleepiness, and impaired memory and concentration. Complications arising from sleep apnea can include high blood pressure, increased risk of heart attacks and stroke, and even heart failure in severe cases.

Not all snoring indicates a serious problem, but if you suspect that you or your partner may have sleep apnea, you should seek prompt medical attention. Obstructive apnea is often treated with a device known as a CPAP (Continuous Positive Airway Pressure), in which a small compressor is used to maintain airflow during the night. Dental appliances worn at night to reposition the tongue and/or jaw may be useful in mild to moderate cases. Surgical corrections of physical abnormalities are other options, but the results of these are variable and need to be discussed with a specialist.

Narcolepsy: Irresistible Daytime Sleep Attacks

For sufferers of narcolepsy, the need for sleep is frequent and irresistible. "Sleep attacks" can happen anytime, during a conversation or even while driving, and last a few seconds or more than 30 minutes.

Narcolepsy affects the part of the brain that regulates sleep and wakefulness, resulting in the sudden onset of REM (dreaming) sleep. Symptoms typically begin between puberty and age 25. They may develop slowly over months or years, and excessive daytime sleepiness is generally the earliest sign.

Cataplexy, or sudden loss of muscle control, is a common characteristic of narcolepsy. Cataplexy can be brought on by strong emotions, like anger, laughter or surprise, and it may make narcoleptics so weak at the knees that they literally fall to the ground. Also, some narcoleptics experience sleep paralysis, an inability to move or speak, during the transition into sleep or wakefulness.

Many people with narcolepsy experience vivid, dreamlike images called hypnagogic hallucinations as they are drifting off to sleep or immediately upon awakening. The images can be mundane or nightmarish and often cause great anxiety.

Narcolepsy afflicts about one in every 2,000 people — as many as other, better-known diseases, including multiple sclerosis. Currently, no cure exists, but its symptoms can be controlled through lifestyle management and medications.

Restless Legs Syndrome: The Need to Move Keeps Sleep Away

For those with restless legs syndrome (RLS), the sensation of discomfort is so acute, it can only be relieved by moving or stimulating the legs. These tingling, crawling or prickling sensations are most pronounced during inactivity, particularly while trying to fall asleep.

RLS sufferers find staying asleep is a problem as well. Rubbing the legs, getting up and walking around, or taking a hot shower usually offer only temporary relief. The sensations return with the return to bed. The discomfort and sleeplessness that accompany RLS can lead to serious psychological distress and depression.

Most people with RLS also have periodic limb movement disorder (PLMD), characterized by a periodic jerking of the legs during sleep. The movements cause multiple sleep interruptions that are often so brief that the sleeper isn't aware of them, although the sleep partner may be. Unlike RLS, PLMD is not uncomfortable for the sufferer, but it can cause excessive daytime sleepiness.

RLS and PLMD rarely appear in people under age 30 and are more common in people over 65. There aren't any cures for these related disorders, but a number of prescription medications are being used to treat them.

Parasomnias: Things That Go Bump in the Night

Parasomnias are disorders that intrude on our sleep, and often the sleep of those around us, in very active, sometimes dramatic ways.

Sleepwalking causes people, usually children, to take nocturnal trips they don't remember, but navigate surprisingly well. It seems to be a temporary sleep mechanism malfunction that occurs during the deeper stages of sleep, and it tends to run in families. Since most will leave their nighttime wandering behind at puberty, there's usually no need for medical intervention, but it is important to protect habitual sleepwalkers from harm by keeping doors and windows closed.

Sleep talking can range from a word or two of gibberish to an entire speech, but except for the distress it causes others, it's harmless. The sleeper has no memory of it, and the condition is usually temporary, brought on by stress or illness. It can also be associated with sleep apnea or sleep terrors.

Sleep terrors are marked by a sudden awakening with physical behavior associated with intense fear. Screaming and fighting to escape are not uncommon, and harm to the sleeper or others can occur. Episodes last about 15 minutes, after which the person returns to sleep, unable to recall anything in the morning. Like sleepwalking, sleep terrors are more common in children and typically do not continue into adulthood. Until then, parental reassurance that "everything's OK" is the only treatment.

REM movement disorder is when the paralysis that normally occurs during rapid eye movement (REM) sleep is incomplete or absent, allowing the sleeper to "act out" dreams. Most common in older men, it may result in violent behavior and injuries. Unlike those who experience sleep terrors, the victims recall vivid dreams. Medication is usually very effective in treating this disorder.

Getting Help

Most sleep disorders can be successfully treated or controlled once properly diagnosed. If you sleep poorly for a month or more, or if you find sleepiness during the day interferes with normal tasks, see your doctor or ask for a referral to a sleep disorders specialist. *A listing of accredited sleep disorders centers in your region of the United States is also available on request from the National Sleep Foundation, publishers of this booklet.*

Sleep disorders centers are staffed by physicians and other medical professionals specializing in sleep-wake problems. During your first visit, a sleep history is assembled by asking questions about sleep and daytime habits. Family members may also be asked to provide important clues that you yourself may not be able to supply, such as information about snoring or gasping for air while asleep. Your regular doctor should also provide any relevant medical history in advance of the first visit.

After the initial consultation, you may be asked to spend a night or two at the center so your sleep can be monitored. Before you go to sleep, dime-sized sensors will be placed on your head and body to record brain waves, muscle activity, limb movements, heartbeat, breathing and other body functions. This test, called a "polysomnogram," isn't painful and doesn't hamper movement during sleep. You may also be given the Multiple Sleep Latency Test to see how quickly you fall asleep, a good measure of daytime sleepiness.

Once the study is complete, the sleep specialist will do a through evaluation and recommend treatment, either directly to you or to the referring physician.

Where to Learn More

The National Sleep Foundation offers individual booklets on specific sleep problems and issues, including: insomnia, sleep apnea, narcolepsy, restless legs syndrome, parasomnias, sleep as we grow older, children's sleep, and the dangers of drowsy driving. Write to the Foundation to request a copy or for more information on available booklets.

Further Reading

No More Sleepless Nights, by Peter J. Hauri, PhD, and Shirley Linde, PhD, John Wiley & Sons, Inc., New York 1990.

Sleep Disorders: America's Hidden Nightmare, by Roger Fritz, PhD, National Sleep Alert, Inc., Naperville, IL 1993.

Encyclopedia of Sleep and Dreaming, by Mary A. Carskadon, PhD, Macmillan, New York 1993.

The Sleep Book: Understanding and Preventing Sleep Problems in People Over 50 by Ernest Hartmann, MD, American Association of Retired Persons, Washington, D.C. 1987.

Solve Your Child's Sleep Problems, by Richard Ferber, MD, Simon & Schuster, New York 1985.

The National Sleep Foundation

The National Sleep Foundation is a nonprofit organization dedicated to improving the quality of life for the millions of Americans who suffer from sleep disorders and to the prevention of catastrophic accidents related to sleep deprivation or sleep disorders. Funded by charitable contributions, the Foundation supports sleep research, education, training, and public information programs.

■ **Document Source:**
National Sleep Foundation
1367 Connecticut Ave, NW, Ste 200
Washington, DC 20036
Copyright 1995

See also: Insomnia (page 407); Sleep and the Traveler (page 439)

THE PARKINSON HANDBOOK: A GUIDE FOR PARKINSON PATIENTS AND THEIR FAMILIES

Message of Hope

Each individual who comes to consult the National Parkinson Foundation and its clinic is given individual treatment. In addition to physical and neurological examinations, a psychologist looks at the way the individual is adapting. An evaluation is made of the patient's lifestyle and methods for coping with problems. Counselling is available to help patients work out better ways of adapting to the illness.

What the Patient Should Know

This booklet is intended only to give general background about Parkinson's disease. Your doctor can give you more details and answer your specific questions.

What is Parkinson's disease?

Parkinson's disease is a serious illness named after Dr. James Parkinson, a London physician, who was the first to describe it in 1817. Parkinson's disease (or PD) is a slowly progressive disease that affects a small area of cells in the middle part of the brain. These cells gradually degenerate and die. Their loss produces a reduction in a vital chemical called "dopamine", causing symptoms that include tremor, stiffness of muscles (rigidity), slowness of movement (bradykinesia), and loss of balance (postural dysfunction).

Patients with PD may have stooped posture, a slow shuffling gait, a tendency to keep their arms fixed at their sides when walking, and difficulty with fine movements of the hands. The condition may affect one or both sides of the body.

What are some other signs of Parkinson's disease?

Although tremor, muscle rigidity, and slowness of movement are the most common symptoms, others that occur less frequently include:

1. Episodes of "freezing" in which there is sudden difficulty in walking, particularly in turning or moving through a doorway.
2. Dementia, characterized particularly by decreased memory for recent events.
3. Depression.
4. Feelings of hot or cold, excessive sweating, oily skin.
5. Cramps or a burning sensation, particularly in the thighs or legs.
6. Low backache, accompanied by poor posture.
7. Small crowded handwriting.
8. Lessened facial expression and smiling (masked face).
9. Decreased blinking and the appearance of staring; and
10. Loss of voice power.

Is this a rare disease?

A patient, J.B., writes in: "For what reason and why, of 200,000,000 people in this country, was I picked out to be afflicted with this illness?"

The fact is that up to a million and a half Americans have Parkinson's disease.

PD affects about one out of every 100 people over the age of 60 and has become one of the most common ailments in the United States. There are several reasons for this:

1. People are living longer. The life span in the United States has increased from an average of 50 years in 1900 to 75 years in 1989. Since Parkinson's disease is generally an illness of the middle and later years,

more and more elderly people are likely to have symptoms of Parkinson's, unless some means of prevention is found.
2. There is, as yet, no cure for the illness.
3. Parkinson's disease is not a fatal illness; therefore, there is a continuing increase in the number of Parkinson's patients.

Can an accident, injury or shock produce Parkinson's disease?

Not likely. This is often the basis of medical-legal suits. A man develops Parkinson's disease two years after being stricken on the head by a falling object. There is no scientific basis for attributing the illness to the head injury.

Some patients trace Parkinson's disease to previous automobile accidents, surgical operations, or to emotional shocks.

However, millions of people suffer accidents, operations and emotional shocks, yet never develop Parkinson's disease.

What is the likely cause of Parkinson's disease?

The cause of Parkinson's disease remains a mystery.

Some people suggest that a virus may be involved. They give as an example the worldwide epidemic of influenza that took place from 1917 to 1927 and caused sleeping sickness (encephalitis) in hundreds of thousands of people. This illness affected the brain and left many of its victims with a form of secondary Parkinsonism. However, there is no evidence linking primary cases of Parkinson's disease with viral infections of any known type.

Another type of secondary Parkinsonism—fortunately, it's reversible—can be caused by the use of drugs which interfere with dopamine in the brain. These drugs include some tranquilizers (haloperidol, thioridazine or chlorpromazine) and high blood pressure drugs which contain reserpine.

Studies of this drug-induced Parkinsonism have led to better understanding of the role of dopamine in normal motor activities such as walking, writing and dressing.

There are many patients with "hardening of the arteries" who have suffered one or more strokes, and who also have symptoms of Parkinsonism. Even so, hardening of the arteries is not generally accepted as a cause of primary Parkinson's disease.

All that is known to date is that Parkinson's disease is a degenerative disorder of unknown cause.

Further research by the National Parkinson Foundation and other interested agencies into the cause, prevention, and cure of the illness will ultimately provide new approaches to treating Parkinson's disease.

Is Parkinson's disease contagious or inherited?

Parkinson's disease is definitely not a contagious disease. Cases do exist in which a husband and wife or other family member develops PD, but they do not catch it from each other. Although investigators have believed that there are occasional families in which Parkinson's disease appears to be inherited, there is little evidence to support this view.

A recent National Institutes of Health study examined the incidence of PD in identical twins. If PD is inherited, then in cases where one twin develops PD, the other twin eventually would develop it also.

But this did not occur in the NIH study. The researchers concluded there is no evidence of a hereditary role in the development of Parkinson's disease.

Often patients and their families report that a relative also has Parkinson's disease. Frequently, once this is checked out, it's found that the affected relative does not have Parkinson's disease, but some other neurological ailment.

As of the present, there is no evidence that Parkinson's disease is inherited.

Is there a cure for Parkinson's disease?

As yet, there are no means—medical or surgical—to cure Parkinson's disease, nor is there any way to prevent the disease.

Some patients drift from clinic to clinic and doctor to doctor looking for a "miracle" drug that will "cure" the illness.

PD patients would do well to have faith in their doctors and to avoid those who promise "cures" through years of useless injections or by other means.

What doctors do have today is a much better understanding of the illness and ways to treat it, than was available only a decade or two ago.

Good treatment can help recover many of the lost functions of the body, can protect patients against the disabilities and secondary symptoms that develop from neglect, and can maintain most patients in an independent useful condition for many, many years.

There are several medications which are very useful in treating Parkinson's disease. These drugs are often used alone or in combination and can affect quite remarkable changes in the patient's conditions.

It is important for the patient to be treated by a doctor who is well acquainted with Parkinson's disease and with these various medications so that the proper combination of therapy can be arrived at.

How does the disease start and progress?

In many patients, Parkinson's disease begins with an occasional tremor in a finger, which in time becomes more frequent. With time, the tremor may spread to involve the entire arm and may be accompanied by stiffness or rigidity in the arm. Skilled finger movements, as in buttoning clothes and writing, become more difficult. In time, the leg on the same side no longer moves freely, and the foot tends to drag and scuff.

As more years pass, the tremor and, especially the rigidity, may spread to the other side of the body and lead to a slowing down of movement in the body and limbs. The face may become somewhat frozen in appearance and the speech poorly enunciated.

In other people, the disease may begin with a heaviness and stiffness in both legs, which the patient often ascribes to tiredness and "old age," as time passes, walking presents a

challenge, and there is increasing difficulty in rising out of a soft chair and getting in and out of bed.

The stiffness of the legs, the slowness of body movement, and the shuffling gait are the outstanding features of PD in many elderly patients. Variations may occur, and some patients may begin with pronounced tremor of both arms, with rigidity not appearing until years later and in mild form.

Thus, the primary symptoms of Parkinson's disease are tremor, rigidity, slowness of movement (akinesia), and postural difficulties.

While tremor may prove annoying and embarrassing to the patient, it rarely leads to serious consequences in the years ahead.

Rigidity on the other hand can lead to serious complications in later years. Shortening of the muscles (contractures) can develop.

Slowness of movement and, in more severe cases, lack of movement are the most troublesome and disabling symptoms of Parkinson's disease. They prevent the patient from carrying out activities of daily living (eating, toilet activities) at a normal pace.

A major feature of Parkinson's disease is postural and gait trouble. Difficulty in turning around and in walking through doorways, a tendency to fall at the slightest provocation, and inability to stop after taking a step backwards, or a tendency to move forward in ever-quickening steps, are some of the problems that arise.

What methods of treatment are available for Parkinson's disease?

There is much the doctor can offer a patient with Parkinson's disease in treatment and support. The patient-doctor relationship should reflect genuine interest on the part of the doctor, since without this, the patient can lose confidence, discontinue his medication, and fail to keep active.

Patients must be informed that their basic symptoms can be controlled with success by means of

1. Drugs.
2. Rehabilitative measures like physical therapy.
3. Persistence by the patient in carrying out home exercise, a more productive and comfortable life may be expected.

The doctor should emphasize that the patient should keep busy in all phases of daily life and work for as long as possible.

Medication

Presently L-Dopa (specifically in the form of Sinemet®) is, for most people, the most effective medication in the treatment of Parkinson's disease. L-Dopa enters the brain and is converted to dopamine, the chemical in the brain that is lost in Parkinson's disease.

In addition to L-Dopa, Sinemet® also contains another ingredient called "carbidopa" which improves the action of L-Dopa in the brain. The use of carbidopa also decreases certain side effects, particularly nausea, that are common when L-Dopa alone is used.

Other medication may also be useful, when used alone or in combination with Sinemet®. These drugs help improve the biochemical balance of the brain and include amantadine (Symmetrel®), anticholinergics (Artane®, Congentin®), and antihistamines (Benadryl®).

Drugs that act very similarly to dopamine itself (dopamine agonists) such as bromocriptine (Parlodel) and pergolide (Permax) are useful in a number of situations. As the illness worsens, and the effectiveness of Sinemet diminishes, dopamine agonists are very useful in prolonging the duration of beneficial effects. Also, dopamine agonists may be useful when excessive involuntary movements (known as dyskinesias) are elicited by Sinemet. When a dopamine agonist such as pergolide is added, the dosage of Sinemet may be reduced and often the dyskinesias improve. Recently a reformulation of Sinemet, known as controlled release Sinemet (Sinemet CR) was made available to prolong the duration of benefit without producing dyskinesias.

Other experimental medications under development include Lisuride, Ropinirole, Pramipexole and Tolcapone. These medications are designed to improve the function of the dopamine system of the brain.

Parkinson medications may have side effects. Common side effects of Sinemet® include: confusion, visual hallucinations, and inadvertent jerking or squirming movements (such as a leg suddenly dancing out of control or facial grimacing; doctors call this "dyskinetic or choretic movement").

Clozapine (Clozaril) is a medication that is useful for hallucinations induced by anti-Parkinson drugs. It is the only medication of this sort that will not worsen the symptoms of PD and in fact may even help the tremor. Unfortunately, it may produce a serious aplastic anemia and so cannot be prescribed by a doctor without weekly blood tests for as long as the medication is being taken.

Cisapride (Propulsid) was developed to promote gastric emptying and is an excellent medication for promoting movement of the bowels. By virtue of enhancing gastric emptying, the absorption of Sinemet® and other anti-PD medicines is improved resulting in less motor fluctuation.

After using Sinemet® for several years, some patients develop an "on-off' effect in which symptoms of Parkinson's may suddenly switch "on" or "off" unexpectedly.

Some doctors believe that the "on-off" effect depends on how long the patient has taken Sinemet®. These doctors try not to use Sinemet® at the onset of Parkinson's disease if the patient's symptoms are mild. They reserve the medication until the symptoms become pronounced and the patient really needs it.

Another concern some doctors have about starting treatment with Sinemet® early in the course of the disease is the possibility that the drug may become less effective with time. Some evidence of this is the fact that some patients appear to get a better effect from Sinemet® after being taken off the drug for a while on a "drug holiday".

Other doctors do not feel that Sinemet® loses effectiveness with time, or that the side effects are necessarily related to the patient's length of time on the medication. These doctors believe that the main reason why a patient does not do as well after a few years on medications is that the disease continues to get worse.

This difference in medical opinion about when to start drug therapy for Parkinson's is still unresolved.

Almost all doctors agree that there is no point in using PD medication if it does not make the patient actually function better.

In Parkinson's disease, medication only treats the symptoms; it cannot cure the disease, nor can it stop the progression of the condition.

A new medication has recently become available to alleviate clinical fluctuation in response to Sinemet®. This medication Eldepryl® (deprenyl), also shows promise as an agent which may slow the progression of Parkinson's disease in its early stages.

The hope is that research will develop a cure for Parkinson's and that curative medication will replace the drugs that today are used only to make the patient live more comfortably with his or her symptoms.

There is a recent renewed interest in surgical procedures to relieve symptoms in PD patients who no longer respond to medication. Transplantation or grafting of fetal cells is currently under intensive investigation but these procedures are highly experimental and are not available at this time for routine therapy.

Physical Therapy

Treatment of the symptoms of Parkinson's disease requires a program designed to meet the individual needs of the patient.

Postural abnormalities, deformities of the extremities, and gait disturbances must be controlled by every possible effort on the part of the patient and physical therapist. Treatment should consist of the following:

1. Therapeutic exercise, divided into active and passive exercise. Active exercise should consist of movements by the patient to maintain joint range, improve coordination, and increase speed of movement. Passive exercise should consist of stretching and manipulation of the patient's limbs by the physical therapist to prevent or relieve shortening of the muscles caused by muscle rigidity.
2. Gait training to encourage proper foot placement, arm swing, and better balance control.
3. Practice in the functions of daily life if the patient is having trouble with everyday actions such as getting in and out of chairs or bed, getting in or out of cars, crossing streets, or going up and down stairs. The patient needs special instruction to overcome his or her problems in moving.
4. Use of heat treatments, electrical stimulation, hydrotherapy, or cold packs, depending on special needs of the patient.

Occupational Therapy

The use of crafts can help patients maintain coordination and as much manual dexterity as possible. Through crafts, patients may also be drawn into more active group participation, enabling them to broaden their interests and contact with others. Each patient should be encouraged to engage in all pursuits that are suited to his or her physical and emotional resources.

Speech Therapy

Patients who suffer problems in speaking can often benefit from speech therapy. The most common speech problems for PD patients are a nasal monotone and loss of speech volume. Exercises and techniques designed to overcome these and other speech problems can be ordered by the physician according to the patient's needs.

Exercise and Activities for PD Patients

Some patients, even when retired and disabled by Parkinson's disease, find more things to occupy themselves than they can possibly handle. Others find time hanging heavily on their hands, with no place to go and nothing to do. They feel forgotten, frustrated and unhappy, and become depressed.

It is to these patients that this message is particularly addressed, although others may also find it helpful.

It is essential for every PD patient to look at the illness practically and realistically. It is not a disease that is caused by any action of its victims.

There are a million or more victims of Parkinson's disease in the U.S. No one is immune to Parkinson's; it can come to anyone between 20 and 80 years of age.

Almost everyone is subject to one or another ailment during their life, some acute and of short duration, others lasting throughout life, and still others ending life very quickly. Some illnesses are mild and others severe. There are many worse ailments than Parkinson's disease.

At least with Parkinson's disease, the problems are clear—tremor, rigidity, slowness or lack of movement, and postural difficulties.

Tremor, while annoying, is not serious and does not cause muscle weakness or physical damage.

It can impair job performance for people whose work requires physical dexterity. But for most people, the greatest problem caused by tremor is embarrassment.

The symptoms of Parkinson's disease which may cause serious trouble are muscle rigidity and slowness of movement.

As muscle rigidity becomes more severe, many patients develop the habit of not using certain joints. In time, these joints may become physically difficult to move, or even frozen in place.

Another problem is that muscles which are unused over time gradually tend to shrink, further limiting motion. If the finger muscles are affected, for instance, they may shorten to the point where it becomes difficult or impossible to make the fine movements needed to button a shirt, tie shoes, or write.

What can help? Proper medication, physical therapy, and above all, activity and exercise by the patient can help keep the joints from freezing and muscles from shortening, as they do under conditions of disuse and inactivity.

Every form of work or activity is good for the muscles and helps to keep them mobile and alive. Even playing cards or checkers, visiting a friend, polishing furniture, or shopping for food is exercise.

More effective forms of exercise may be obtained at a rehabilitation center, a gymnasium, "Y", or through the use of special equipment at home such as stationary bicycles, rowing machines, overhead pulleys, beach balls for finger and arm exercise, or broom handles to draw across the back several times a day to straighten the spine and loosen the shoulders.

Functional Activities

Varied techniques of treatment are used at the Parkinson Rehabilitation and Research Institute after each patient is evaluated by the multidisciplinary team. Our goal is rehabilitation of the total patient, and in this case, the development of social contacts and group participation is an important therapeutic objective.

Patients are given a program of activities best suited to their needs and interests. Movement, strength, and endurance are enhanced by regular exercises. Patients relearn lost or diminished skills important to their total function. They are encouraged in every way to resume former activities in order to live as full and satisfying a life as possible.

Exercise

There are several categories of exercise that are helpful for PD patients, depending on the stage of their illness, their age, their physical strength, and their past interest and experiences.

Basic exercise. This consists of the daily activities of the patient—work, house chores, personal hygiene (dressing, bathing, grooming), eating, shopping, and attending family and community activities.

Special exercise. These are usually prescribed by the doctor, either to prevent complications as a result of muscle rigidity, to protect affected parts of the body from getting worse, or to recover functions that may already have been lost.

Preventive exercises. Exercises to prevent potential problems with walking can be particularly valuable. It is important, for example, that the PD patient make it a practice to walk with eyes looking straight ahead, instead of fixing them downward to watch the feet. If the eyes are continually cast down, the head will tend to be carried lower and lower.

Also, the PD patient should make it a practice to walk and turn with feet deliberately held wide apart, in order to insure the steadiest possible gait and prevent falling.

Corrective exercises. These must be used regularly without fail, if the patient is to overcome limitations in movement at particular joints as the result of severely tightened and shortened muscles. For example, if getting out of a chair is a struggle, the practice of quickly rising out of the chair many times a day will often ease the difficulty.

Recreational exercises. These may include a wide range of activities that help to keep muscles and joints free and mobile. Some of these activities involve group participation, such as ball games, bowling, golf, dancing, or singing in a choir.

Other activities can be done alone, such as swimming or hitting balls at a golf range. Some people take leisurely walks for recreation; others visit clubs or museums. Still others take trips to the country or seashore.

Special Exercises

Bar exercises. Move up, down, forward, then turn your trunk, sideways from the waist. Hold bar up, bend trunk to the right, then to the left. Hold bar behind back, raise, lower. Hold bar across shoulder. Bend trunk sideways from waist to right, then left.

Swing exercises. Swing both arms. As one arm swings forward, swing the other one backward. Walk with another person behind you, both of you holding the same bars in both hands and keeping in step. As your right arm moves forward, swing your left leg forward.

Air exercises. Stand up; sit down. Lift legs, one at a time. Make bicycling motions with your legs while seated. Walk quickly around chair three times. Hold onto back of chair. Raise right leg at side, return to normal position. Repeat with left leg. Hold chairback with one hand. Circle one leg clockwise, then counterclockwise. Turn around, hold chairback with other hand and circle other leg.

Club exercises. Stand with feet apart. Hold wooden club in hand and turn wrist forward and backward. Put club across shoulders. Bend sideways from waist to the right and then the left. Keeping elbows straight, circle club above shoulders.

Shoulder exercises. Shrug shoulders up to your ears. As you let your shoulders drop down, shift them forward and then draw them back.

Trunk exercises. Stand with feet apart. Breathe out as you bend forward, and then straighten again. Stand with feet apart, hands at waist, and bend sideways from the waist. Standing with feet apart, circle from the waist clockwise, then counterclockwise.

Arm exercises. Cross forearms in front of your chest. Lift them up over your head as far as you can and then bring back to your chest. Stand with feet apart. Swing arms forward, upward and then downward.

Leg exercises. Leaning against a wall or a sturdy piece of furniture, move legs forward and upward, alternating left and right legs. Holding onto furniture for support, do the same, moving legs back and up.

Parkinson's exercises: Relaxation. To precede EACH exercise session. Lie on your back with one or two pillows under your knees.

Breathing. Inhale through your nose. Blow out slowly and gently through pursed lips. Repeat 10 times.

Head wobble. Gently roll your head from side to side a few times until you feel relaxed. The head should be allowed to drop to each side using no muscular effort to hold it in any one position.

Shoulder shrug. Bring shoulders up toward ears; then drop shoulders completely. Repeat 10 times.

Hobbies

For those fully ambulatory. Many hobbies that involve the whole body in activity can be learned and developed. Consider gardening, carpentry, boating, fishing, travelling, birdwatching, shopping for collectibles, piano playing, sculpting.

For patients partially disabled but capable of activities outside of the house. Hobbies for this group of patients could include photography, participation in adult education courses, woodworking, painting.

Other activities could serve a similar purpose, such as volunteer hospital work involving greeting and directing visitors, assisting in feeding patients, or playing games with children.

For patients more or less confined to the home. If the fingers are sufficiently mobile, ceramics, painting and other arts and crafts deserve consideration, as well as sewing, collecting stamps, and playing cards, chess or checkers.

Whatever hobby is chosen as a sparetime activity, it should never be compared with work formerly done for income, but really as therapy.

Planning a Daily Program of Activity

Some patients are always at loose ends to find something to do, only because they have not planned a regular program of activities.

It's best to plan for a month ahead if possible, so that each day, as you go over your list of activities, you can fill in more and more things to be done.

Some patients prefer to type out their programs of activity, and if this is possible, it's a splendid exercise for the fingers and arms. Activities that could be listed for a day include

Arising, washing, bathing
Shaving
Brushing teeth
Dressing
Breakfast and medication
House chores, painting, repairs
Barber, tailor, shopping
Special exercises
Going for a newspaper
Gardening
Hobby work
Lunch and medication
Short nap, if needed
Walk of 5 to 10 blocks
Visit to church
Volunteer at a hospital
Gymnasium or "Y"
Senior citizen club
Writing a letter to a friend
Special exercises
Some work on hobby
Dinner and medication
Listening to records or radio
Watching television
Reading to family
Special exercise
Checkers or cards with family or friend
Special exercises
Neighborhood movie

Finger exercises with coins
Washing and brushing teeth
Medication
Preparing for bed

Patient Exercises

For Tight Muscles and Poor Posture

Standing

1. Stand facing a wall, about eight inches in front of it. Raise your arms and reach as high as possible toward the ceiling, then lean toward the wall and stretch.
2. With your back to the wall, alternate raising your legs as high as possible by bending your hip and knee, as if marching in place.
3. Holding on to something secure, bend knees and squat down as far as possible; then straighten up.

Sitting

1. Sitting in a straight back chair, place your arms behind the chair and bring your shoulders back as far as possible, raise your head up, and look at the ceiling.
2. Sitting in the same chair, place one leg at a time on another chair directly in front of you and press each knee straight. Try both legs together.
3. Sitting on the chair, raise your leg up from the hip by bending the knees alternately as if stamping your feet.

Lying on a Firm Bed or Floor

1. Lie on the floor or bed, flat on your back; try to press your body to the floor as flat as possible. Move your head from right to left as far as possible. Make sure your head, shoulders, back and back of knees touch the floor or bed.
2. Lie on the floor or bed on your abdomen. Do the following, one by one.
   - Put your hands behind your back, look up, and try to raise your chest.
   - With knees straight, kick your legs from each hip alternately, as if swimming.
   - Turn your head from right to left.

For Balance Difficulty

1. Standing, your hands on your hips and feet spread apart, or holding on to a support if your balance is poor:
   - Practice marching in place.
   - Practice raising each leg straight to the rear with the knee straight, but do not touch foot to floor.
2. Standing with your hands at your side and your feet spread apart:
   - Lean forward and back.
   - Lean to both sides.
   - Lean in a circular motion and reverse the motion.

For Walking

1. When walking, take as large a step as possible, raising your toes as you step forward and hitting the ground on your heel. Keep your legs apart and your posture straight. Let your legs do the walking, swing your arms, look straight ahead.
2. To practice proper swinging of the arms, walk holding folded magazines in both hands and keep your elbows straight. Your right arm should swing with your left leg; your left arm should swing with your right leg.
3. Practice walking sidewards, backwards and in circles.

For Turning

1. When practicing turning, use small steps, raising your feet from the floor. Keep feet spread apart and head high, rock from side to side.
2. If you feel glued to the floor, try the following: Relax back on your heels and raise your toes. Raise your head and shoulders and try again. Tap the hip of the leg you want to move. Rock from side to side or bend your knees and straighten up. Raise your arms in a sudden short motion.

For Getting in or out of a Chair

1. Approach the chair as closely as possible. Then back up to the chair and as you reach it, sit down.
2. To sit down, bend forward as far as possible and sit down slowly. Make sure you are close to the chair.
3. To get up—put both feet under the chair, bend forward and push up vigorously. Using your arms, try to count 1-2-3-GO! Then get up. If you have a favorite armchair, raise the back legs with four-inch blocks. this will help you get up more easily. Don't let people drag you up by your arms, but do permit assistance with a slight push up on your back.

For Getting out of Bed

1. Throw your arms back and forward vigorously, extending your legs toward the side of the bed as if to rock yourself to a sitting position.
2. A knotted rope tied to the foot of the bed can help you pull yourself up.
3. Place blocks under the legs of the head of the bed. This will elevate the bed, making it easier to get up.

For Using Your Arms and Hands

1. Practice buttoning and unbuttoning your clothes; practice cutting food and writing.
2. Bounce a large ball with your hand open if your fingers won't straighten; throw a beach or basketball back and forth against a wall or to another person.
3. Always try to dress yourself completely. Use a shoehorn, elastic shoelaces, or extra long laces to get a better grip. Dress sitting or standing in the most

comfortable position. Make sure you are in a safe position.

4. To keep your elbows straight and your shoulders loose, install a pulley in a doorway. Place a chair directly under the pulley or slightly in front of it. Stretch your arms and shoulders in all directions by working the pulley. If you are seated, you can get a more vigorous pull.

Safety in Using the Bathtub and Bathroom

1. If it is difficult for you to sit down in the bathtub, try the following:
   - Place a stool or kitchen chair in the tub; saw off the legs to tub edge height. You can sit on the chair and soap yourself. Use the shower to rinse or get a rubber shower extension.
   - Bathtub grab bars are available for purchase. Make sure the ones you get attach securely.
   - Raised toilet seats are commercially available.
   - Toilet arm rests for getting on and off the toilet are available.

For Speech Difficulties

1. Practice singing and reading aloud with forceful lip and tongue motion.
2. Practice making faces in front of a mirror, recite the alphabet, and count numbers with exaggerated facial motions.
3. When chewing food, chew hard and move the food around; avoid just swallowing.

Summary

Additional equipment for home exercise is available, including stationary bicycles, wall pulleys, rowing machines, dumbbells, etc. Exercise programs for specific problems should be undertaken only on the recommendation of your doctor.

Don't hesitate to engage in all possible activities: work, walking, shopping, house chores, gardening, visiting, senior club and church organizations, theatre, travel, and exercise.

Suggestions to Remember

1. Bring your toes up with every step you take.
2. Spread your legs 12 to 15 inches apart when walking or turning, to provide a wide base and better stance, and prevent falling. It may not look beautiful, but neither is falling.
3. For greater safety in turning, use small steps, with feet widely separated. Never cross one leg over the other or pivot when turning. Practice walking a few yards and turn; walk in the opposite direction and turn again.
4. Practice walking into tight corners of a room, to overcome any fear of closed places.
5. To ensure good body balance, practice rapid movements of the body, backward, forward and to the right and left, five minutes, several times a day. Don't look for a wall when you think you are falling. It may not be there. Your body will protect you, if you practice balance daily.
6. If your legs feel frozen or "glued" to the floor, a lift of the toes eliminates muscle spasm and the fear of falling. You are free to walk again. In addition, shift your weight from side to side in order to start moving again.
7. Swing your arms freely when walking. It helps to maintain balance, lessen fatigue, and loosen your arms and shoulders.
8. If getting out of a chair is difficult, try rising as quickly as possible to overcome the pull of gravity. Sitting down should be done slowly, with your body bent sharply forward until you touch the seat. Practice this at least a dozen times a day.
9. If you need assistance while walking, your helper should walk by your side, never pull from the front.
10. Any task that is difficult, such as buttoning a shirt or getting out of bed, should be practiced daily.
11. Rubber or crepe-soled shoes are not recommended since they grip the floor and may cause forward falling.

Speech Impairment in Parkinson's Disease

Almost half of all PD patients may expect to experience some difficulty with their speech. The degree to which speech is impaired varies; some patients are affected only minimally, and others may have severe impairment.

The medical term used to describe the symptoms of speech impairment in Parkinson's syndrome is "hypokinetic dysarthria." This occurs when Parkinson's disease affects the muscles that are necessary for speech production. These muscles are in the mouth, cheeks, jaw, lips, soft palate, voice-box, throat, windpipe, and chest.

Symptoms that may occur when these muscles are affected by PD include:

1. Rigidity of the facial muscles.
2. Reduced breath support for speech, causing low volume and a weak-sounding voice.
3. Lack of vocal variety—monotonous speech.
4. Frequent repetitions of syllables or words (palilalia).
5. Rapid rate of speech and/or a tendency to gradually talk faster and faster.

In addition, the PD patient may experience swallowing difficulties resulting from rigidity of the tongue, palate, and throat muscles. This makes it more difficult to manage food as it is being chewed and to control the normal pooling of saliva in the mouth. In these instances, drooling may occur.

The first step in treating speech problems if you have them, after you are under the medical management of your doctor, is to get a complete speech and language evaluation by a certified speech/language pathologist. This is necessary to accurately assess your difficulties and to get appropriate recommendations for improving your speech.

Following are exercises that may help you reduce rigidity and regain control of the muscles involved with speech. These exercises should be done daily in front of a mirror so that you can be sure you are doing them correctly.

Deep Breathing

1. Take five deep breaths, stretching out your abdominal/stomach muscles as you inhale, and tightening these muscles as you exhale. Remember to exhale as long as possible before you start the next breath.
2. It may help to add sound as you exhale. Repeat step 1, but say vowel sounds ("ah..." "oh...") aloud as you exhale.
3. Practice automatic speech, watching to be sure you have good breath support for your speech. Count to five, recite the days of the week, months of the year, etc., making sure to pause and take additional breaths as necessary. You may then go on to practice short phrases and sentences.

Mouth Exercises

1. Open and close your mouth five times, making certain to stretch your muscles as much as possible.
2. Smile five times, making certain to stretch your lips back as far as possible.
3. Practice these movements with nonsense syllables ("ma, ma, me, me") and alternate these syllables ("ma, me, mi, mo").
4. Stick your tongue out five times, making certain it protrudes straight from your mouth. Pushing against the back of a spoon with your tongue may also be helpful.
5. Move your tongue from side to side and around your mouth five times.
6. Pucker, (pushing your lips out as if you were kissing a baby) five times.

Now, use all those muscles together and make faces in the mirror. Show a) happiness, b) anger, c) surprise, d) sorrow. **Exaggerate your articulation.** If you have a too rapid rate of speech, try slowing down your speech by exaggerating every sound in every syllable of every word. Practice this by reading aloud from newspapers, books, magazines.

The use of a tape recorder may help make you aware of any changes in your speech. As you read aloud, try to vary the pitch and inflection of your voice.

Treatment of speech impairment resulting from Parkinson's can be effective. The key to managing your speech difficulty is the ability to replace what you have done automatically all your life with conscious control. What was second nature in the past must now be done with full awareness and resolution.

For Additional Information

The use of an augmented communication system may be recommended for some patients.

Sometimes amplifiers are helpful for patients who have reduced volume only. However, if a patient has other difficul-

ties besides reduced volume, an amplifying device would make things worse, since it would also amplify the other distortions.

You may obtain a list of certified centers and/or speech/language pathologists in your area by writing to the American Speech/Language and Hearing Association in Rockville, MD.

Parkinson's Disease and Psychology

Emotional factors are an important part of Parkinson's syndrome. The traumatic effect of the disease can create great confusion and anxiety.

We hope this chapter will be helpful both to PD patients and to members of their families, since adjustment is necessary in the home as part of the treatment program for Parkinson's disease.

The Importance of Attitude

A diagnosis of Parkinson's disease is a serious event in a person's life. How the individual interprets it is very important. On this will depend how he or she feels and what he or she does. Naturally, the patient's feelings and actions will also affect family members and friends.

Parkinson's disease is primarily physical, but the mind may also be affected. PD requires that the patient learn to cope with it mentally as well as physically. Most PD sufferers have continued capacity to enjoy life for a long period of time.

Attitudes of Early Stages

Because in the early stages, the symptoms of Parkinson's disease are usually so slight they may go unnoticed. There may be a tremor of the thumb which comes and goes, or a feeling of inner tremor, or the handwriting may become very small.

But even those who recognize early symptoms and seek help promptly may find their concern dismissed by doctors who cannot diagnose the presence of Parkinson's disease at this early stage.

Many people report that the diagnosis of early PD was overlooked during consultation with excellent, well-known diagnostic centers. The doctors there were not at fault. The signs of the illness were just too slight for an accurate diagnosis.

Naturally, diagnoses are missed most often when the symptoms do not appear externally. Inner tremors are not readily observable. People with these conditions frequently are misdiagnosed as neurotic. They often are given tranquilizers or referred for psychotherapy.

On the other hand, there are people who notice shakiness in themselves and believe they have Parkinson's, only to find out from a doctor that they do not.

These people may have something else which in some way resembles it. Some drugs, for instance, produce side effects which look like symptoms of Parkinson's disease.

People who ignore their symptoms may postpone the recognition that they have Parkinson's disease. When the diagnosis does come, they are amazed at how they could have overlooked their condition until it was forced on their attention.

In one case, for example, the illness in an easily observed stage was diagnosed at a distance by a doctor, who, while playing golf, observed the rapid gait and shuffling walk of a player. "You've got Parkinson's," he said. The man was shocked. "How could you know?" He had not noticed the gross changes in his posture and his movements.

Several patients have reported statements by observers that their arms did not swing, but hung stiffly at their sides when they walked. This is very typical of Parkinsonism.

Adaptation Necessary

Whether diagnosis is made early in the case of those who attend to minor physical problems immediately, or very late in the case of those who ignore even serious symptoms, it becomes necessary for everyone with the illness to adapt to it.

Those who accept the condition and seek helpful information are better able to plan their existence with it intelligently.

Those who try to hide it from people around them and even from themselves face a long series of mentally painful episodes.

In such instances, the battle to deny what is actually taking place may produce years of tension and anxiety.

The way an individual reacts to a diagnosis of Parkinson's disease depends in large measure upon what his or her thinking and outlook on life was before the illness.

It's important to recognize, however, that Parkinson's disease is a unique experience. It cannot be reacted to as if it were a minor problem. It does not disappear and is likely to get worse with time.

While some cases progress extremely slowly, others become severe very rapidly. No case can be predicted in advance. Whatever happens, the patient with Parkinson's disease needs to accept it as part of his or her life.

Major Types of Adaptation

Focusing on the disaster element of Parkinson's disease may be hard to avoid doing at times. But this causes added emotional pain and may intensify the symptoms themselves.

As much as possible, it will help the patient to concentrate on the positives in life, to adopt the attitude, "I will do the best I can."

Many PD patients find that their lives are still enjoyable even though the illness prevents them from acting in ways they previously did.

It is very important for close relatives to understand this, because their attitudes and reactions often influence the one who has the disease.

A positive and accepting attitude in the patient's spouse or other family members and friends can do much to maintain a spirit of well-being and relieve many of the fears and anxieties that may overtake the PD patient.

Attitudes about Information

PD patients generally have one of three attitudes toward obtaining information about the illness.

First is an attitude of not wanting to know about the illness at all, trying not to have anything to do with it by covering it up. There is an effort to deny it exists.

Second is an attitude of just letting things be, not trying to cover up, but not trying to do anything positive either, just taking things as they come.

A third attitude is to search out all possible information, to consult, to plan ahead.

An example of the first attitude may be a person who, on the job, finds that his writing is getting smaller, or that he cannot fill in forms as he used to.

One man, a superintendent of a steel mill, retired a year or two earlier than may have been necessary because he was ashamed that he couldn't fill out forms.

Another man also reacted to the knowledge that he had Parkinson's disease tragically. An airplane mechanic, he felt that his livelihood was in jeopardy and tried to escape by denying and hiding his condition. He wouldn't even allow his wife and children to mention the word "Parkinson's" in his presence. Soon he went into a very serious depression for which he had to be hospitalized.

It was only after a psychologist said to him, "You have to face the fact that you have Parkinson's disease," that he began to straighten up. From then on, he and his wife and family started to talk about it.

They began to plan for their circumstance. Among the things they did was pay off their house mortgage faster so as to reduce possible later expenditures. They took out job compensation insurance. They put themselves in a position to provide better for their needs.

This case illustrates how important attitude is when dealing with a serious illness such as PD. Denying the facts prevents you from coping to your best advantage.

The attitude of "do nothing and take things as they come" can hurt the PD patient over the long term, too. It can lead to situations in which important information is learned too late, or important actions are delayed too long.

PD patients need to be encouraged to gather the information they need to plan and adapt in the best possible way.

Grouping Together

Asking questions of others and talking things over can be very helpful.

The National Parkinson Foundation creates an atmosphere of togetherness in group discussions of patients and relatives. In addition, many of the Parkinsonian families at the National Parkinson Foundation were brought together at a time when the Foundation provided residential quarters called, "The M.L. Seidman-Parkinson Tower." This provided an opportunity for the patients and their families to enjoy being together.

They devised means of helping and advising each other. Their daily discussions proved tremendously fruitful. Even when "The M.L. Seidman-Parkinson Tower" was no longer available as a residence, some of this group maintained their free and open communication with each other.

Reviewing and discussing their situations resulted in shared understanding of the problems of coping with the illness. Their joint efforts led to accurate knowledge of the latest developments and to means for obtaining all the most recent relevant information. Thus, by adapting to the illness as a condition of life, they reinforced each other. The patients in this group fared much better than most others.

Physical Adaptations

Above all, anyone afflicted with Parkinson's disease must learn to cope with physical changes in his or her body.

Symptoms develop, some muscles may become rigid, tremors may appear, posture may change, walking may be affected, speech may become difficult, the ability to handle objects may be impaired. These physical changes require adjustments both immediately and over the long term.

Value of Trying

It is natural for the patient with Parkinson's disease to try to control his or her symptoms, for instance, tremor. Sometimes, such efforts are successful, and the exercise is good both physically and mentally.

It is important for the patient to realize, however, that a permanent victory over the symptom will not be possible.

But the value of trying to keep active, to the best of the patient's ability, is that it helps to keep the muscles as fluid as possible, and when successful, helps to keep the spirits up, too.

An example of a physical incident and the value of reporting it

It is important for a patient to explain to those around him what he's doing if he's making a special effort to control a symptom.

For example, one man illustrated how he could quiet a violently shaking right hand while eating, by deeply inhaling his breath.

This method enabled him to bring a forkful of food successfully to his mouth. He did this many times during the course of a meal. When his wife saw him take such deep breaths however, she thought he was sighing and that he was in distress.

In the effort to help him, she started to advise him to take it easy so he wouldn't feel bad and wouldn't have to react by sighing. Her reaction annoyed him, and her lack of understanding made him even more distressed.

Once the wife learned that his deep breaths were not expressions of anguish but were his efforts to help himself to stop shaking long enough to bring his food to his mouth, she was more at ease and so was he.

Physical Symptoms

Some symptoms of Parkinson's disease become very clear cut.

These signs include pill rolling tremors, in which the hand makes movements as if it were rolling pills, and cogwheeling, which you can feel if you take the relaxed arm of a PD patient and pump it up and down and feel with the fingers on the inside of the elbow.

In a normal person, you feel the arm move up and down smoothly. In the PD patient you feel the arm move as if there's a cogwheel that stops it at times.

However, there are more subtle symptoms which usually the patient does not recognize, and doctors may forget to tell about.

One of these is lack of some important reflexes. For example, when a normal person rises from a chair or begins to walk or run, he has reflexes which straighten out his posture so he doesn't tip over.

Such reflexes often do not come into play quickly enough or at all in some patients with Parkinson's disease. When they get up out of a chair suddenly, they tend to lean forward and cannot correct their posture. Therefore, they tend to pitch forward and fall.

Sometimes patients with Parkinson's disease are unable to correct their posture when they begin to lean backwards. The normal person's reflex to straighten out immediately comes into play. But the PD patient may lean backwards more and more to the point of falling. This is because the normal reflexes are not operating properly.

Try to Avoid Sudden Movements

In order to overcome the sluggishness or absence of normal reflexes, it's important for the PD patient to avoid sudden movements as much as possible. This is easier said than done, however, because often, PD patients can change from one position to another, like getting out of a chair, only by a sudden start. However, with practice, sometimes it is possible to bring stronger muscles into play and move without too sudden a change.

Simplifying Coordination

Another problem is that when some PD patients try to do two things at once, they find that their coordinating reflexes are not operating. It may be necessary for them to stop when they are walking in order to talk to someone or to see something.

They may find that if they walk and look at something at the same time, their walking will be impaired.

A normal person can walk up to a door, open it and walk through the doorway in one coordinated movement without having any difficulty. Some patients with Parkinson's disease may have trouble doing this. As they approach a door, they begin to do the movements that are necessary to open it. In the effort to make this coordination, they may "freeze".

Such difficulties may become manageable by special approaches.

For example, when they approach a door, these patients should keep walking, without any effort to open the door, until they are very close. Then they should stop walking, open the door, and then walk through. Thus, the action is broken into separate components each of which the patient can handle by itself.

Freezing also takes place frequently when obstacles are in the path. If someone stands in the path where a PD patient is to walk, he may freeze and be unable to get going again. He may also be unable to go around the obstacle smoothly as a normal person would do.

The most frequent occurrence of freezing is when the PD patient begins to move, either to start walking, or to get in or out of a chair. In such instances, just a bit of intervention on the part of someone else may be very effective.

If a PD patient cannot get out of a chair, for instance, someone may just touch him to release the tension of freezing so that movement is more easily achieved.

Slowness

It may sometimes be very difficult for patients with PD to cope with their physical symptoms because of both a lack of energy and a lack of control.

Often there is a continuing battle to exercise greater control. Some patients find it easier to accept their limitation; others continue to have strong and unhappy feelings about their condition.

It's very natural for PD patients to be upset about such things as taking 15 or 20 minutes to do what they used to do quickly and easily.

Some PD patients have trouble following conversations. They cannot take in as many messages at one time, or marshall their responses fast enough to continue with the conversation's flow. Slowness in perceiving and responding is one of the major symptoms of Parkinson's disease.

It is especially difficult on those whose characteristic responses before the illness were fast. Unless they understand that the illness itself produces a slowing up of all activity, they become angry with themselves.

These patients need reassurance and help in maintaining a positive self-image.

Fear of Falling

Many patients with Parkinson's disease look down at the floor as they walk to prevent themselves from tripping and falling. This actually can lead to more falling. In such cases, it often helps to train these patients to walk with their heads up and eyes looking straight ahead.

A simple experiment may be reassuring. Have the patient stand facing you about two or three feet away looking straight into your eyes. Lift one of your feet and jiggle it and ask him to tell you, without looking down, what your foot is doing. He will tell you that your foot is moving.

This will show that he has enough peripheral vision to see what is on the ground, or if anything is in the path without looking down. He can then more confidently walk with his eyes up. But it is difficult for many PD patients to feel comfortable walking with their eyes up. Frequent gentle reminders from those close to them may help.

Touching and Holding On

Many PD patients are afraid to bump into things. They have taught themselves not to lean on objects, or touch furniture, door jambs, railings, or other things they could lean on. But for many it can be helpful to use objects as supports and guides.

Here's an experiment for a patient who has difficulty in walking. Ask him to follow you as you walk backwards around a chair, keeping his eyes on yours as you go along. He may touch the chair, move it, shove it aside. This is a way of helping the patient become more confident in leaning on, touching, or holding chairs, tables, or other stabilizing objects. It reduces the tension the patient may feel in trying to avoid contact with objects and helps him get through narrow spaces.

Personality Adaptations

It's not difficult to understand that people with serious physical problems react by changes in personality.

For example, people who are used to having a feeling of control over events and other people may try, even after their symptoms become a problem, to maintain this control.

At first they may deny that there is anything wrong. Or they may make excuses for events which did not turn out as expected. Or, they may become resentful, particularly if others refer to their symptoms.

Some patients may become highly emotional and unstable. Others may become more aggressive. Still others may become resigned.

In some cases, professional guidance and counselling can help in achieving the most positive attitude possible.

Apathy

It is not unusual for some PD patients, before they work out better techniques of adapting to their illness, to seek to avoid company.

One churchgoer, who for 30 years had never missed a Sunday, suddenly refused to go because he didn't want "all those people staring at him." He disliked calling attention to himself. He felt that his shaking drew people's eyes to him and that they pitied him.

He was correct in that the shaking of PD does command attention. But such attention is not always accompanied by pity. Nor need pity be rejected, if that is the reaction of others. There is no need to be ashamed. Perhaps the patient may even help others see that pity is inappropriate to their condition.

Some patients withdraw from all activities—they no longer want to go out to restaurants, visit friends, or participate in social events.

These patients need help in finding new ways of adapting and new activities.

Pride

Some PD patients may show loss of will, a lack of desire to finish things once started. They no longer care for doing things with the quality they used to find necessary.

Their approach to problems may change in that they may seek out what is just adequate, rather than what is excellent. Their drive to accomplish seems to become dulled.

They may have concluded that what they do is not necessarily a reflection of their worth as people.

Or they may feel pride of performance is no longer important to them. This illustrates the significant changes in personality that often occur in Parkinson's disease.

Good Days and Bad Days

All of us have times when we feel that there is something wrong but we can't put our finger on it. Very often people who have Parkinson's disease have this kind of inner feeling. They get used to some of their physical symptoms, rigidity or difficulty in walking. But sometimes they just feel ill at ease, not quite themselves.

Very often patients will report that they have "good days" or "bad days," or "good times" or "bad times." Some patients function better in the morning, some in the afternoon. In one case, a person functioned well all morning and retreated to bed after three in the afternoon.

But all fluctuate in how well they feel. Sometimes someone who is suffering from even an advanced stage of Parkinsonism may say, "Well, today I feel very good," and even though he is tremendously handicapped, he feels fine. It is also possible to see the same person on another day saying, "Oh, I feel terrible." Those who are close to these patients need to understand and accept these fluctuations.

Activity is Essential

A general rule for all PD patients is to keep as active as possible so that the muscles can be as fluid as possible.

Mental activity is important, too, even though it may be an effort for the patient to engage in conversation, to respond.

Many people do not like to put forth this effort. Those who never liked to put forth effort in the first place attempt a more complete withdrawal.

Individuals who have been active and aggressive all their lives often carry on in heroic ways. One man continued to play handball for several years after the onset of Parkinson's disease. It was difficult for him to play, yet somehow or other he maintained his handball-playing ability.

Another patient continued walking long distances and swimming. Another maintained an active interest in her business affairs.

Sometimes a very great change in personality overtakes a PD patient who formerly was lively and vibrant. Difficulties in speech may play a large part in this change. As one patient said, "I don't enter into discussions as much as I used to because it is difficult for me to explain that I can't raise my voice enough to be heard. And it's too much of an effort for me to talk."

PD speech problems are especially hard for people who formerly were great talkers and enjoyed every opportunity to verbalize in the past. Repeated failures in conversation discourage these patients. For many, practice and speech therapy can lead to some improvement.

Changing Values

One of the great personal difficulties that PD patients have reported is being unable to carry on activities which mean a lot to them.

One man who had good mechanical ability and prided himself on being able to fix anything found that as he lost the use of his fingers, one of his greatest pleasures was taken away. He could no longer fix automobile engines and things that he had tinkered with. Such losses are frequently accompanied by depression.

One woman who spent several hours a day playing the piano and had a great deal of gratification from it, found she could no longer excel as she previously had. She, too, experienced depression.

Another woman who used to attend club meetings and was very active, being the president of various organizations, found that she could not conduct all the meetings in the way that she used to. She found herself becoming depressed upon her inability to do these things.

It is important for such people to reorganize their thinking and their values. Most fortunate is the person who can switch and say, "Well, up to this point I was able to contribute this way. Now I can't make the same contribution or achievement. But I can still contribute or achieve in other ways."

Aging is a fact of life, and no one can maintain peak strength or maximum abilities forever. Parkinson's disease generally occurs in the later years, usually after age 50. For PD patients, the illness becomes part of the aging process.

Feeling Threatened

Many psychological problems beset patients on first learning they have Parkinson's disease.

They are bewildered because they do not know what it is and what is going to happen. It's very natural to fear and imagine the worst.

Words like "incurable" and "progressive" sound very frightening. "Will I be able to continue to work?" "Will it affect my relationship with other people?" "Must I give up participation in events and activities that I enjoy?" "To what extent will it disrupt all things in my life?"

These are natural concerns and must be faced. They are normal questions for an individual who, due to the onset of such a severe illness, faces serious disruptions in life.

At the Foundation, there are some patients with severe affliction. For other patients who fear that they will develop the same condition, it is necessary to give reassurance candidly and openly. They need to know that they may not reach that stage, that their illness may not progress that far.

Other Problems

Many people who suffer from Parkinson's disease also have additional conditions, types of illnesses or incapacities which may have no specific relation to the Parkinson illness, but which also affect their ability to cope.

There may be some sort of psychological problem, for instance, which may have existed before PD occurred and which continues even while the Parkinson condition develops further. But taken together with Parkinson's disease, such problems usually become more complex.

Sometimes it is advisable to send a PD patient or someone in his family for psychotherapy, not for the Parkinson condition itself, but for handling other non-related conditions which may affect the situation. Likewise the physician is frequently called upon to handle various other conditions which a PD sufferer may have.

Working with the Doctor

In every illness, it is necessary to get good medical advice. This is usually easy to do, as most doctors know how to communicate with their patients so they can get the most benefit from their advice.

However, some PD patients may not work along with their doctors as well as they should.

Shy people may have special difficulty. They may be afraid to communicate clearly with their doctors and ask necessary questions.

The patient or the one caring for him needs to get all the information necessary to carry through with proper treatment.

Outlook

It is natural to ask, since PD is as yet an incurable, progressive disease, what is the outlook for anyone having it.

Although the future cannot be predicted, it should be remembered that not so long ago levodopa was not available.

The coming of L-Dopa brought tremendous improvements. To quote Mrs. Jeanne Levey, "It is the best thing that has happened for Parkinson's disease in 160 years."

The Foundation maintains contact with many of the people engaged in drug research for Parkinson's disease. It is very heartening to talk to some of these people in connection with their research. They convey great enthusiasm.

Research as to why people get Parkinson's disease is also going on. It is hoped that in the near future someone will come up with such a discovery.

False Information

People with the illness and their relatives naturally tend to develop an absorbing interest in any news item or report concerning Parkinson's disease. Occasionally they are misinformed.

Some years ago, in the Miami area, a local newspaper gave much publicity to a doctor who read a paper at a convention. The newspaper said that he had a cure for Parkinson's disease. Many patients immediately tried to contact this doctor and many relatives of patients insisted that they should consult him.

The fact is that this doctor did not say he had a cure for PD.

Sometimes a patient who hears about a medication prescribed for another patient will insist on having the same medication. Such self-prescribing is not in the best interest of the patient. Since individuals vary greatly in their reactions to medications, only a doctor can know what is most suitable for any one case.

When a patient finds some approach or medication which works well, it is best to report this to the doctor. Regard your physician as an ally with the special information needed to judge what is the most desirable treatment.

Misconceptions

Just as false rumors, beliefs, and fantasies play a part in confusing and misleading people on any subject, so it is with Parkinson's disease. One such erroneous statement is that certain races of people, such as blacks, are immune. The fact is that cases of Parkinson's disease in blacks have been seen at the Foundation, but in a percentage far smaller than their numbers in the general population.

Proportionately larger percentages of Spanish-speaking and Jewish people are seen at the Foundation. Perhaps these population figures are influenced by the greater incidence of such people in the local community and by the fact that many South Americans come here for evaluation and therapy.

Pain

Pain is not usual in Parkinson's disease. When a patient complains of pain, it may be from some condition directly associated with the illness, but more likely it results from some other source. Arthritis or some other condition may exist along with the PD. Although the muscles do get rigid in Parkinson's disease, there are surprisingly few instances of pain.

Mental Changes

With the patient in our experience, it appears that a large percentage show mental changes or some deterioration.

These patients are not as fully capable mentally as they were. Fortunately, this condition does not usually affect most ordinary activities.

Usually the deficiency is not even noticed. Performance may still be sharp, but gaps may occur. In some cases, confusion may occur.

Mental changes may also be the result of some medicines taken by patients. Some patients, for example, begin to hallucinate with certain drugs. If mental changes of this type occur suddenly, the patient's doctor must be notified promptly.

Memory

Often PD patients report interruptions of memory. They walk into a room to get something and forget what they came for, or they cannot recall a name they know very well, or they forget where they put something they had in their hands just a moment before. These lapses of immediate memory occur in younger people, but the frequency as people get older is much greater.

Unfortunately, there are some patients with PD who develop severe memory dysfunction.

Sex

Sexual desires and functions are highly individual. Coming later in life, PD may coincide with a decline in sexual interest and/or activity in some patients. Others, however, retain interest in sex and remain sexually active.

Since L-Dopa became widely publicized, there has been speculation about its effects on sexual desire and potency. Some newspapers carried glowing reports of restored sexual prowess. When such a side effect did show up, it proved to be short lived. The reports were of very few cases and in most instances created the wrong impression. L-Dopa is not an aphrodisiac.

The largest number of patients taking L-Dopa for any length of time have no such reaction, although many experience restoration of sex and other physical and mental powers.

The exhilaration or well-being felt by patients on L-Dopa may help renew their interest in sex, too.

Such interest may be difficult to satisfy in some instances. Renewed masturbation has been reported. Also, there may be an intensification of emotions related to sex, such as jealousy or love.

Hypnosis, Acupuncture

One strange phenomenon that people with Parkinson's disease encounter is the fact that tremors stop during sleep.

Some people claim that hypnosis can also stop tremors. Such experiments have been tried without any permanent results. It is possible to have someone with Parkinson's disease hypnotized to stop the shaking. Just as in sleep, the tremors will stop. But when the person is active again, the symptoms recur. Hypnosis is not an answer for Parkinson's disease.

Some persons have tried acupuncture. The results are not impressive.

Surgery

One approach used to alleviate some of the symptoms of Parkinson's disease, particularly tremor, is cryosurgery. This involves brain surgery in which certain tissue is destroyed by exposure to extreme cold.

In some instances tremor has been alleviated for a number of years by such surgery. In other cases, the tremor has returned in time. In still others, new tremors have appeared in different parts of the body.

Experience with patients who have had surgery indicates that this is not the answer for most patients. It is certainly not any cure. In any event, since the advent of L-Dopa, surgery is rarely performed for PD, and only after medications fail to relieve tremor or rigidity.

Driving

Should a person with Parkinson's disease drive a car? For many patients, the answer is obvious one way or the other. However, there are people who continue to drive long after they should have stopped and have suffered injuries as a result. Where there is a question, the doctor should be the judge.

Split-second judgments about when to lift the foot from the accelerator and put it on the brakes have to be made when driving. Muscle rigidity and impaired coordination can endanger the driver, passengers, and others on the road.

The doctor will take into consideration the conditions under which the driving is to be done and the condition of the patient.

Relationships

Relatives can play an important part in encouraging patients to seek help. Very often it is a relative who insists that a patient come to the National Parkinson Foundation for study and advice or go to a doctor or follow the doctor's therapy program.

Relatives can help set up exercise apparatus in the apartments or homes of patients, install railings in bathrooms and wall bars for patients to pull themselves up out of bed.

When a relative shows an interest in the patient's treatment, a team effort is established which helps the patient to function far better than he or she could have done alone.

Relationships with relatives may change for patients with PD. Individuals who were formerly very independent may become tremendously dependent and demanding.

Some PD patients may show impatience or anger. Hostilities suppressed in the past may surface. Other patients insist on trying everything for themselves, even things they cannot do.

Family members and friends will need to judge when to step in and help and when not to. The usual rule is to strongly encourage the patient to try as much as possible.

Motivation is very important for PD patients, and a supportive, positive attitude on the part of their family and friends can be a big factor in sustaining their motivation to remain active and reach out to others.

Family

Family structure is often very seriously affected by Parkinson's disease. Some spouses show great dedication. Husbands have devoted the major portions of their lives to their wives who are striken. Wives have given the understanding, sympathy, and help to husbands who need care.

On the other hand, there are some spouses who become annoyed, are unable to endure the suffering, or, for other reasons, are unable to respond, gradually they stay away from home more often, and perhaps even seek divorce.

The reaction of the spouse, when patients are married, is a key factor in patient care. Where a spouse or close relative attends to a patient, he or she needs to discuss the illness openly with the doctor.

Every once in a while, a spouse does too much and does not follow the doctor's orders to let the patient do as much as possible. By having groups of spouses meet and discuss their joint problems, such persons can be helped to accept a change in approach.

In one instance, a patient reports he is enjoying a new relationship with his wife. Before his illness, he was a very active person who was always in control and attentive to her. Now he is learning how rewarding it is to experience her devotion and dedication. She has taken control, become attentive to him, and as a result, he is experiencing a new closeness in their relationship.

One of the hardest problems faced by relatives of PD patients is knowing how much to go on with their regular activities and how much to sacrifice for the sake of the patient. One man, who formerly was very active, stopped going out at night to be with his wife, who was incapacitated by Parkinson's disease. After advice, however, he found that when he started to go out a few nights a week, and came back and told his wife the things that happened, both were happier.

These examples show that there are positive aspects of existence that can be experienced, even with Parkinson's disease.

Summary

This booklet has attempted to summarize the most frequently encountered experiences of Parkinson's disease.

Not all the facts about the disease are presented, nor are the problems discussed fully. We hope this will lead to further discussion and to better approaches for therapy.

Information provided in reference to medical diagnosis, treatment, and research reflects the views of the authors and should not be taken as an endorsement by the National Parkinson Foundation.

In cases of medical questions, individual patients should always check with their doctors.

National Parkinson Foundation, Inc
National Headquarters
Bob Hope Parkinson Research Center
Parkinson Diagnostic Rehabilitation Treatment Center and Care Institute
1501 NW 9th Ave, Bob Hope Rd
Miami, FL 33136-1494
Telephone: (305) 547-6666
Toll Free Nat'l: 1-800-327-4545, Toll Free in Florida: 1-800-433-7022

Washington Office
National Parkinson Foundation
1250 24th St, NW, Ste 300
Washington, DC 20037
Telephone: (202) 466-0550, Fax: (202) 466-0585

California Office
15840 Ventura Blvd, Ste 215
Encino, CA 91436
Telephone: (818) 981-2233
Toll Free in California: 1-800-400-8448

■ **Document Source:**
   National Parkinson Foundation, Inc
   NPF-1002 9th Printing
   January 1996

A PRACTICAL GUIDE TO MYASTHENIA GRAVIS

by John C. Keesey, MD and Rena Sonshine

The following summary has been prepared to provide information written in lay language about myasthenia gravis (**MG**). This is not "the official version," but just a personal view of a complicated and sometimes controversial subject. Each person's experience with it is in some way unique, and this guide can approach the topic only in a general way.

What is MG?

The distinctive feature of MG is fluctuating weakness of muscles, made worse by use of those muscles and improved at least partially by rest of the same muscles. The muscles affected are called voluntary or striated muscles. Involuntary heart muscle and smooth muscles of the gut, blood vessels, and uterus are not involved in MG.

Muscles which we use all the time, such as the six muscles which move each eyeball and those which hold the eyelids open, are often but not always involved. The muscles of facial expression, smiling, chewing, talking, or swallowing can be selectively affected in some people with MG. We take these muscles for granted until they don't work!

Other muscles which may be affected include those of the neck and limbs. Although MG is said to be painless, pain in the back of the neck and head may be present if neck muscles which hold up the head are weak and in spasm. Symmetrical limb weakness occurs in many other nerve and muscle diseases, but in MG, limb weakness is often not symmetrical, one side being weaker than the other. Shoulder weakness is demonstrated by trouble holding up an arm to comb or shampoo one's hair, or to shave or put on makeup. The grip may become weak opening jars (and child-proof medicine bottles), hips may be weak getting out of deep chairs or the bathtub, and legs may tire climbing stairs or when walking distances.

The "gravis" or seriousness of myasthenia is particularly noticeable when muscles we use in breathing are affected. If breathing or coughing becomes insufficient, the patient is said to be in **"crisis,"** and mechanical breathing assistance in a hospital may be necessary. It is seldom useful to try to determine whether the respiratory insufficiency is a "myasthenic crisis" (weakness from MG exacerbation) or a "cholinergic crisis" (weakness from too much anticholinesterase medication), because most crises have multiple causes and the treatment for any crisis is respiratory assistance. Patients with trouble swallowing and talking are the ones most likely to have trouble breathing also, and usually before a crisis happens there are progressive warning signs that swallowing, talking, and breathing are becoming compromised.

Different muscle groups are affected in different patients with MG. Some have only **ocular myasthenia** involving the eye muscles and eyelids; others have mainly swallowing difficulties or slurred speech; others have **generalized MG** affecting many muscle groups. Even though specific muscle fatigue is the hallmark of MG, patients with MG do not often complain of non-specific or general fatigue. Skin sensation is normal.

MG remains confined to the eye muscles in about 15% of patients who initially present with only ocular myasthenia. Within the first year after onset about half of the ocular MG patients will go on to experience involvement of other muscles, and another 30% do so during the next 2 years.

The maximum extent of involvement in an individual patient usually manifests itself within the first 5 to 7 years, and thereafter it tends not to be progressive, even though muscle involvement and severity of weakness may still fluctuate from hour-to-hour and day-to-day. The typical untreated patient may feel strong on awakening from a night's rest or a nap, but experiences increasing muscle fatigue as the day progresses. Although MG can be fatal if a respiratory crisis is not immediately treated, normal life expectancy is the rule with proper treatment.

MG occurs throughout the world and in all ethnic groups. Its onset can occur at any age from birth to the ninth decade, although women usually notice it first in the child-bearing ages and men in middle-age. Rarely, infants born to non-myasthenic mothers have myasthenic symptoms on the basis of a genetic defect in neuromuscular transmission. These infants are said to have **congenital myasthenia.**

However, the vast majority of MG cases are **autoimmune,** in which the body's immune system mistakenly attacks and destroys special proteins located on the muscle surface where the nerve attaches to the muscle. These proteins respond to the chemical acetylcholine which is released by the stimulated nerve, and this response starts the process which causes the muscle to contract. These special proteins are called **acetylcholine receptors.**

No one knows what sets off the autoimmune reaction, but if some acetylcholine receptors are missing because of it, the response of the muscle to nerve impulses is poor and weakness may occur.

Twelve percent of babies born to mothers with autoimmune MG develop a feeble cry, poor sucking, respiratory distress and "floppiness" which can be reversed by anticholinesterase medication or blood exchange. These signs of **neonatal myasthenia** spontaneously disappear over the first few months of life, and no well-documented case exists of autoimmune MG occurring in a child of a mother with autoimmune MG.

Autoimmune diseases such as MG, thyroid disease, lupus, rheumatoid arthritis and juvenile diabetes seem to run in families, and these families statistically (but not invariably) share certain tissue markers. New and promising experimental treatments for autoimmune diseases are based upon the presence of such markers.

How is the diagnosis of MG confirmed?

Weakness and fatigue are such common complaints from a variety of causes that it is not surprising that the diagnosis of myasthenia gravis is often missed in people in whom the weakness is mild or restricted to only a few muscles. Once the possibility occurs to a doctor, however, there are several approaches to confirming the diagnosis.

One way is to test for specific muscle fatigue by repetitive movements of the eyes, arms or legs. This can be done without equipment, or it can be done electrically by recording a weakening muscle response when a nerve to that muscle is electrically stimulated repetitively. Not every person with the disease will show a characteristic response to this **repetitive nerve stimulation.** A much more sensitive electrical test called **single fiber electromyography** is more likely to show evidence of neuromuscular malfunction (not specific for MG), but it requires special equipment and skills which are not widely available.

A very specific test for MG is a blood test to look for **serum antibodies** to acetylcholine receptor. Eighty percent of all patients with MG have abnormally elevated serum levels of these antibodies, but positive test results are less likely in patients with mild or purely ocular forms. The chance of receiving a falsely positive test result from a reputable laboratory is small, although borderline tests should be repeated.

A third approach to MG diagnosis is pharmacological, using drugs which may worsen or improve the weakness. At one time the native South American poison curare was used in very small doses to test for worsening of MG, but this can be dangerous and has fallen out of fashion. Nowadays the short-acting drug **edrophonium chloride** (brand-name **"Tensilon"**) is used intravenously to try to make the diagnosis of MG by reversing some obvious and measurable weakness, such as a drooping eyelid or a low breathing capacity.

Sometimes all these tests are negative or equivocal in someone whose story and examination still seem to point to a diagnosis of myasthenia gravis. The positive clinical findings should probably take precedence over negative confirmatory tests, each of which has its weaknesses. Some people, therefore, have to be followed by their doctors with a diagnosis of "possible MG" or "probable MG" until the situation clarifies itself. Under such circumstances both the patient and the doctor have to keep an open mind.

How is MG treated?

A lot of common-sense things can be very effective in coping with MG. Plenty of rest and a well-balanced diet actually help reverse the weakness. Preference should be given to foods high in **potassium,** such as oranges, tomatoes, apricots and their juices, bananas, broccoli and white meat of fowl. If possible, one should try to avoid exposure to infections and all forms of stress, but of course that's easier said than done.

It is very important that patients try to pace their activities so that they don't fatigue themselves unnecessarily. This may mean resting the eyes by closing them for a few minutes each hour or lying down briefly several times during the day. Each patient is different and by experience can adopt a daily schedule which optimizes the good times and minimizes the weak times. Support groups of MG patients offer many practical ideas for coping with this condition.

Avoid Exacerbations

Many things can exacerbate myasthenic weakness temporarily, including infections (such as a cold, pneumonia, or even a tooth abscess), fever, excessive heat or cold, over-exertion, and emotional stress. Some women notice increasing severity of their MG during a particular time of the menstrual cycle, during pregnancy, or after delivery. Either too little or too much thyroid activity can worsen MG, as can too little potassium in the body, such as is brought on by diuretics or frequent vomiting. The stress of surgery or radiation therapy can make MG temporarily worse.

The effect of **pregnancy** on MG follows the "one-third rule": One-third of pregnant myasthenics get better and one-third get worse at some time during their pregnancy, while one-third do not change. The course of MG during previous pregnancies does not predict the course of subsequent pregnancies. MG frequently manifests itself for the first time during a pregnancy. Standard drugs used to treat MG such as anticholinesterase medications or prednisone (see below) are not associated with significant risk for congenital defects, and plasmapheresis (see below) has been carried out safely during pregnancy. Obstetrical problems with myasthenics are uncommon because the uterus, a smooth muscle, is unaffected in myasthenia. Only during the second stage of labor when voluntary "striated" abdominal muscles are used does myasthenic weakness become noticeable. Even many non-myasthenic woman notice increased weakness after delivery, and this may be exaggerated in MG.

People with MG should make sure that their doctors and dentist are aware that many **drugs** can adversely affect some people with MG. The most common offenders are the very medications used to treat MG (too much anticholinesterase, steroids, or thyroid medication; see below), but anesthetic agents, muscle relaxants, magnesium salts, anticonvulsants and other membrane stabilizers for irregular heart rate, as well as aminoglycoside antibiotics, are other drugs generally accepted to unmask or exacerbate MG. The table includes drugs which have been reported in medical journals to cause weakness in humans.

Common sense dictates that sometimes an irregular heart beat, for instance, or a severe infection sensitive only to one of the antibiotics on the list will take precedence over the MG, and one of these drugs will have to be used, cautiously. A medical alert bracelet can alert medical personnel to use drug precautions in case of an accident or crisis.

Short-Term Treatments

In addition to the above common-sense approaches towards improving health and avoiding trouble, there are some well-known medications and newer treatments which can be tried to counteract the bothersome symptoms of MG.

Anticholinesterases, which boost the body's neuromuscular transmitter acetylcholine by blocking the enzyme which usually breaks it down, include **neostigmine** (brand-name **"Prostigmin"**) and **pyridostigmine** (brand-name **"Mestinon".**) Another drug in this category **ambenonium chloride** (brand-name **"Mytelase"**), is used much less frequently. These medicines don't do anything to cure MG, but they can provide a temporary crutch to help patients function better. Some muscles may improve for a few hours while others may be unresponsive or even get weaker on these medications.

Because muscle involvement and severity vary so much among patients with MG, there is no fixed dose or time schedule for anticholinesterases. For infants and children the dose is based on body weight, starting at one milligram per kilogram for "Mestinon" and 0.3 milligrams per kilogram for "Prostigmin." Generally it is a good idea to try to keep the adult dose somewhere between 1/2 and 2 of the 60 milligram tablets of "Mestinon" or a similar amount of the 15 milligram tablets of "Prostigmin," and to take the medication no closer than every three hours, always keeping on the low side to avoid tolerance (the drug may become less effective with time) or overdosing. These medications produce their maximal effects (good and bad) about one to two hours after ingestion, and these effects wear off after about three hours or sometimes longer. Therefore, patients who have trouble chewing or swallowing are advised to take their medication at a time which will produce optimal strength during meals.

These medicines can cause stomach cramps and gut hyperactivity, so they should be taken with bland food such as crackers or milk to minimize these problems. Increased perspiration, salivation, muscle twitching and muscle cramps are other unpleasant side effects sometimes experienced with this type of medication. The presence of these symptoms may be an indication of taking too much medication, in which case Mestinon should be taken at longer intervals or in lesser amounts.

"Mestinon" also comes as an 180 milligram **"Mestinon Timespan"** in which 60 milligrams is released immediately and the remaining 120 milligrams are released over several hours. Timespan is used for patients who require medication throughout the night, but the uneven release by Mestinon Timespan provides less predictable results than with ordinary Mestinon. There is also a liquid **"Mestinon" syrup** for children and adults who have trouble swallowing pills.

Historically, the drug **ephedrine sulfate** was discovered to improve myasthenic weakness a decade before the use of anticholinesterases, and it may still come in handy as an auxiliary medication, added to anticholinesterases, for those MG patients who need a little extra strength and are not bothered by its possible side effects of nervousness, palpitations or insomnia. It is taken as 25 milligram capsules two or three times a day.

Plasmapheresis (the drawing off of plasma) is an expensive short-term treatment in which several liters of blood are removed from the patient's vein, spun in a centrifuge, and the red blood cells are returned intravenously in artificial plasma (albumin and saline solution). Plasmapheresis is used repetitively (every other day) for two weeks when short-term benefit is critical to the patient, such as in impending respiratory crisis or prior to surgery or irradiation. Some patients get stronger several days following this procedure, but the benefit lasts only weeks.

Another expensive short-term treatment, **intravenous human immune globulin** or **IVIG,** may be thought of as the opposite of plasmapheresis. Instead of drawing off the offending antibodies, IVIG swamps the body with pooled gamma globulin antibodies from many donors. HIV and hepatitis viruses are removed completely during the preparation of IVIG. IVIG is thought to have a nonspecific suppressive effect upon the immune system. Like plasmapheresis, the beneficial effects if they occur last only weeks in MG patients. Therefore, its appropriate use at the present time is to avoid or curtail a stay in the even more expensive intensive care unit of a hospital. Allergic reactions sometimes occur, so the first treatment should be given in a hospital or doctor's office. Plenty of fluids should accompany the treatments to minimize the severe headache which can occur.

TABLE: Drugs and Myasthenia Gravis

A. Drugs generally accepted to unmask or exacerbate MG:
Excessive anticholinesterases
Adrenocorticosteroids & ACTH
Thyroid preparations
Neuromuscular blocking agents (including botox)
Anesthetic agents (including alcohol)
Magnesium salts, Epson salts
Antiarrhythmics:

- lidocaine (Xylocaine) intravenously but not locally
- quinidine (Quinaglute, Quinidex, Quinora, Cardioquin)
- procainamide (Procamide, Procan SR, Pronestyl)
- phenytoin (Dilantin)

Antibiotics

- Aminoglycosides
    - gentamicin (Garamycin)
    - tobramycin (Nebcin)
    - amikacin (Amikin)
    - kanamycin (Kantrex)
    - neomycin (Mycifradin, Neobiotic)
    - streptomycin
    - paromomycin (Humatin)
- Polypeptides
    - polymyxin B (Aerosporin)
    - colistin (Coly-Mycin, Mycin)
    - colistimethate (parenteral Coly-Mycin)
- Tetracyclines
    - chlortetracycline (Aureomycin)
    - oxytetracycline (Terramycin)
    - tetracycline (Achromycin, Tetracyn)
    - demeclocycline (Declomycin)
    - methacycline (Rondomycin)
    - doxycycline (Vibramycin, Doryx)
    - minocycline (Minocin, Vectrin)
- Miscellaneous
    - clindamycin (Cleocin)
    - ciprofloxacin (Cipro)
    - ampicillin (very high doses)
    - intravenous erythromycin (E-Mycin, Erythrocin)

B. Drugs or toxins which can induce MG by precipitating an autoimmune reaction:

- D-penicillamine (Cuprimine)
- trimethadione (Tridione)
- wasp stings
- coral snake bite

C. Other drugs implicated in isolated instances of MG exacerbations (Not every patient with MG is expected to react adversely to these medications):

- cimetidine (Tagamet)
- citrate
- chloroquine (Aralen, Avloclor, Rosochin)
- cocaine
- diazepam (Valium)
- lithium (Lithotabs, Eskalith, Lithane)
- meglumide diatrizoate (Reno-M-dip)
- propanolol (Inderal)
- quinine
- timolol maleate drops (Timoptic)
- trihexyphenidyl (Artane)

Long-Term Treatments

Usually the short-term treatments above do not *completely* relieve the symptoms of MG even temporarily, and eventually the patient with more than just mild disease must discuss with her/his doctor the controversial aspects of what to do next to attempt to obtain a long-term remission. This is especially true for patients with serious trouble swallowing or breathing, for whom long-term treatments may protect against rapid deterioration of these functions.

One approach is to do nothing more, and hope to be one of up to 20 percent of MG patients who go into a natural, spontaneous remission which lasts longer than one year. No one knows why MG fluctuates or why natural remissions occur.

Without spontaneous remission, the patient seeking more lasting improvement of generalized MG is faced with two choices: (A) Major thoracic surgery (thymectomy), or (B) Potentially dangerous drugs. Each approach has advantages and disadvantages.

(A) Thymectomy: About 15 percent of patients with MG are found by chest x-ray, computed tomography (CT), or magnetic resonance imaging (MRI) of the chest to have a tumor of the thymus gland called a **thymoma.** Although most thymomas are benign, they are usually removed surgically because of a perceived potential for malignancy. This has led to thymectomy as well for MG patients without thymoma. If most of the thymus gland is removed at surgery, myasthenic symptoms usually lessen and in some individuals go away completely.

The thymus gland is an organ involved in the development of the immune system. It migrates from the neck into the chest during formation of the fetus, and in adults it lies beneath the breast-bone (sternum). Like tonsils and adenoids, the thymus is large in infants and gets smaller, to be replaced by fat, as we get older. The thymus gland is not enlarged in patients with myasthenia, but often under the microscope it contains more cells than normal (the pathology term is "hyperplasia"), especially if myasthenia has been present several years.

Some neurologists do not think thymectomy adds to other treatments for MG, but most neurologists recommend it for some patients. In the past, thymectomy was not performed on patients who were over 25 years old (or, more recently, over 45 years old), nor was it offered to MG patients who have had their disease for more than five years. Yet some older patients and some long-standing MG patients have benefited from thymectomy, so now the recommendation for this procedure has to be considered on an individual basis.

Another question regarding thymectomy is, "Which surgical technique is best"? Most surgeons split the breastbone in a transsternal thymectomy, but a few surgical groups have championed a less traumatic approach through the neck, called a transcervical thymectomy. A patient who wants to shop around the country can find practically any surgical gradation between these two techniques, or even (at Columbia University in New York City) both a transsternal and a transcervical thymectomy on the same MG patient.

The results of this double approach are good, but so far not really better than a careful removal of all discernible thymic tissue through a transsternal approach. About 30% of

MG patients without a thymoma who undergo thymectomy eventually go into complete drug-free remission and another 50% experience marked improvement. This improvement usually does not occur immediately after surgery, but may take up to several months or years to reach its peak effect. We are unable to predict beforehand who will benefit from thymectomy, and even after benefit occurs there is still a small possibility of subsequent relapse. However, thymectomy itself rarely worsens the long-term course of MG.

Even invasive thymomas are not always detected with imaging tests and have been discovered serendipitously during thymectomy surgery. Such experiences would argue in favor of eventual thymectomy over immunosuppressive drug therapy in otherwise healthy young or middle-aged MG patients, once the patient is up to the surgery. The possibility of an eventually complete symptom-free remission after thymectomy without the need to take any drugs, compared to a remission dependent upon the continued treatment with immunosuppressive drugs, is another significant advantage of thymectomy.

(B) Immunosuppressive Drug Therapy: These drug alternatives consist of a group of general suppressants of the body's immune system, although no one really knows how they work in MG. In decreasing order of their frequency of use in MG, they are prednisone, azathioprine ("Imuran"), cyclophosphamide ("Cytoxan") and cyclosporine ("Sandimmune"). Except for prednisone, none of these drugs is endorsed by its manufacturer specifically for treatment of MG.

Prednisone is a synthetic drug taken by mouth which resembles natural hormones produced by the cortex of human adrenal glands. The body depends upon these hormones, called corticosteroids or "steroids," during stress. When prednisone is taken in doses higher that 20 milligrams daily for longer than a week, the body's natural production of adrenal hormones begins to decrease. This is called "adrenal suppression," and is an undesirable but inevitable effect of taking high doses of a synthetic steroid. Once this occurs, prednisone cannot be stopped all at once but must be slowly tapered down over several months to give the adrenal glands a chance to "wake up" and begin producing natural adrenal hormones again.

Prednisone has a great many potential undesirable effects, usually related to dose and duration of drug use. It can cause mood changes, weight gain, decreased resistance to infection, increased susceptibility to diabetes, high blood pressure, osteoporosis, glaucoma, lens cataracts and stomach ulcers, as well as a host of uncommon "side" effects. Unique to MG is the possibility of increasing weakness during the first two weeks of prednisone therapy. This necessitates close medical supervision of MG patients when prednisone is instituted, either on an out-patient or in-hospital basis.

Some physicians try to avoid this initial weakening by starting with a low dose of prednisone and gradually working up to a recommended amount of 50 to 60 milligrams every day for several months. Onset of improvement in muscle strength usually occurs within 2 weeks but may take as long as 2 months. In order to lessen the chance of undesirable effects, a gradual transition to alternate-day therapy is made after about two months of daily therapy, so that eventually twice the usual dose is given every other day for several more months. As soon as is feasible (3 to 12 months), the drug is very slowly tapered over many months to a long-term maintenance dosage (ideally, 5 to 10 milligrams every other day) sufficient enough to keep myasthenic symptoms in abeyance. The choice of prednisone therapy is thus a long-term commitment lasting several years.

Thirty percent of MG patients on high-dose prednisone therapy experience a drug-dependent symptom-free remission, and another 50 percent obtain marked improvement on prednisone. One out of four MG patients also experiences serious complications from this drug. Patients on prednisone should watch their weight, keep as active as possible, eat a balanced diet (high in protein, calcium and potassium but low in salt, free sugar and fat), stay out of crowds in enclosed areas in order to avoid people with infections, and see their physicians regularly.

Azathioprine (brand-name **Imuran**) was used to treat MG in Europe for years, but U S. experience is relatively recent, since it was introduced as an accompaniment to plasmapheresis. It is being used mainly for patients who cannot tolerate or do not respond to prednisone, or as an aid to decreasing the dosage of prednisone which a patient requires. The undesirable effects of azathioprine are less varied than those of prednisone but they can be very serious. Young women who may want to have children should avoid this drug, because it has a known potential for producing fetal deformities. Complete blood counts must be obtained periodically at the beginning of azathioprine therapy to detect rapid drops in the number of white and red cells in the blood, and periodic liver function tests must also be obtained to detect potential toxicity to the liver. Sometimes a systemic reaction occurs in the first few weeks of azathioprine therapy, consisting of fever, nausea, vomiting, loss of appetite, and abdominal pain. The drug must then be discontinued.

While most of the undesirable effects of azathioprine make themselves known early on, the beneficial effects seem to take months to occur and often emerge so slowly and subtly that they are apparent only in retrospect. Remissions which occur on azathioprine, like prednisone, are drug-dependent, and symptoms of MG recur when the drug is discontinued. There is still much to learn about azathioprine, including answers to such worrisome questions as whether it may increase the risk for cancer many years later.

Cyclophosphamide (brand-name **Cytoxan**) is considered only for the most severe cases of MG when other therapies have failed. Hair loss is an almost universal occurrence on the drug, and the risk of bladder hemorrhage and bladder cancer are of great concern. However, experience from the Philippines reported complete drug-free remission for a year and a half in three out of four MG patients who were treated with cyclophosphamide.

Experimental regimens in which cyclophosphamide is given intravenously or orally once a week—instead of daily—may reduce the occurrence of adverse effects. This drug usually requires the assistance of a rheumatologist or oncologist who is more familiar with it than are most neurologists.

Cyclosporine (brand-name **Sandimmune**) has recently been tested in clinical trials at one-third the dose which is used for immunosuppression during organ transplantation. It was tested for its potential ability to allow MG patients on prednisone to take less prednisone (a "steroid-sparing" effect). The results of this study are not yet available, although a preliminary study without prednisone suggested that such a dose of cyclosporine could produce significant improvement in some MG patients if they could tolerate the side effects of this medication, the most prominent of which are elevated blood pressure, headaches, and increased body hair.

Although cyclosporine is currently the gold standard for evaluating several new immunosuppressive agents, current pharmacologic approaches to nonspecific immune suppression of MG leave much to be desired. It is hoped that future treatment strategies will employ more specific regulation of immunity focused on selected molecules or cells, approaches which are at present experimental.

There is still much to learn about myasthenia gravis, its diagnosis and its treatment. There is no one recipe for all situations, so the choice of treatment for an individual patient requires judgment and experience. Patients and their doctors are often required to make decisions even when the evidence is inconclusive. Patients need all the support which doctors, family and friends can offer.

Myasthenia Gravis Foundation of America, Inc.

The Myasthenia Gravis Foundation of America is a National voluntary health agency whose mission is patient services, medical education, public awareness and research. The Foundation has chapters throughout the U.S. Other Foundation publications include:

- Practical Guide to MG, by John Keesey, MD
- Nurses Manual, Physician's Manual
- Mestinon, Imuran, Plasmapheresis, Nutrition, Thymectomy
- Emergency Management of MG
- Survival Guide by Jeanne Rhynsburger, RN

Myasthenia Gravis Foundation Of America, Inc.
222 S Riverside Plaza, Ste 1540
Chicago, IL 60606
(800) 541-5454
(312) 258-0522
(312) 258-0461 fax
Email: MGFA@aol.com

This publication has been approved by the Myasthenia Gravis Foundation Medical Advisory Board. John Keesey is Professor of Neurology at UCLA School of Medicine, a member of the National Medical Advisory Board and Chairman of the Medical Advisory Board of the California Chapter of the Myasthenia Gravis Foundation, Inc. He is the Director of the Myasthenia Gravis Clinic at Memorial Medical Center of Long Beach, California. Rena Sonshine is a technical editor and has MG.

Acknowledgments: Special thanks are due to the Director of Pharmacy, Horace B. Williams, Jr, PhD, and the Assistant Director of Pharmacy, Donald J. DeFazio, PharmD, at Methodist Hospital of Sern California, Arcadia, California, for their assistance with the Table of Drugs which affect myasthenia.

■ Document Source:
  Myasthenia Gravis Foundation of America, Inc.
  Copyright 1994, John C. Keesey, MD
  Myasthenia Gravis Foundation, 1996

PROGRESSIVE SUPRANUCLEAR PALSY

What is Progressive Supranuclear Palsy?

Progressive Supranuclear Palsy(PSP) is a rare brain disorder that causes serious and permanent problems with control of gait and balance. The most obvious sign of the disease is an inability to aim the eyes properly, which occurs because of lesions in the area of the brain that coordinates eye movements. Some patients describe this effect as a blurring. PSP patients often show alterations of mood and behavior, including depression and apathy as well as progressive mild dementia.

The disorder's long name indicates that the disease begins slowly and continues to get worse (*progressive*), causes damage in the brain above certain pea-sized structures called nuclei (*supranuclear*), and produces paralysis (*palsy*). However, PSP patients do not experience a true paralysis.

PSP was first described as a distinct disorder in 1964, when three scientists published a paper that distinguished the condition from Parkinson's disease. It is sometimes referred to as Steele-Richardson-Olszewski syndrome, reflecting the combined names of the scientists who defined the disorder. Although PSP gets progressively worse, no one dies from PSP itself.

Who gets PSP?

Approximately 20,000 Americans have PSP, making it much less common than Parkinson's disease, which affects more than 500,000 Americans. Patients are usually middle-aged or elderly, and men are affected more often than women. PSP is often difficult to diagnose because its symptoms can be very much like those of other, more common movement disorders, and because some of the most characteristics symptoms may develop late or not at all.

What are the symptoms?

The most frequent first symptom of PSP is a loss of balance while walking. Patients may have unexplained falls or a stiffness and awkwardness in gait. Sometimes the falls are described by the person experiencing them as attacks of dizziness. This often prompts suspicion of an inner ear problem.

Other common early symptoms are changes in personality such as a loss of interest in ordinary pleasurable activities or increased irritability, cantankerousness, and forgetfulness. Patients may suddenly laugh or cry for no apparent reason, they may be apathetic, or they may have occasional angry outbursts, also for no apparent reason. It must be emphasized that the pattern of signs and symptoms can be quite different from person to person.

As the disease progresses, most patients will begin to develop a blurring of vision and problems controlling eye movement. In fact, eye problems usually offer the first definitive clue that PSP is the proper diagnosis. PSP patients have trouble voluntarily shifting their gaze downward, and also can have trouble controlling their eyelids. This can lead to involuntary closing of the eyes, prolonged or infrequent blinking, or difficulty in opening the eyes.

Another common visual problem is an inability to maintain eye contact during a conversation. This can give the mistaken impression that the patient is hostile or uninterested.

Speech usually becomes slurred and swallowing solid foods or liquids can be difficult. In rare cases, some patients will notice shaking of the hands.

What causes PSP?

We know that the symptoms of PSP are caused by a gradual deterioration of brain cells in a few tiny but important places at the base of the brain, in the region called the brainstem. One of these areas, the substantia migra, is also affected in Parkinson's disease, and damage to this region of the brain accounts for the motor symptoms that PSP and Parkinson's have in common.

Scientists do not know what causes these brain cells to degenerate. There is no evidence that PSP is contagious, and genetic factors have not been implicated. No ethnic or racial groups have been affected more often than any others, and PSP is no more likely to occur in some geographic areas than in others.

There are, however, several theories about PSP's cause. One possibility is that an unconventional virus-like agent infects the body and takes years or decades to start producing visible effects. Creutzfeldt-Jakob disease is one disease known to be caused by such an agent. Another possibility is that random genetic mutations, of the kind that occur in all of us all the time, happen to occur in particular cells or certain genes, in just the right combination to injure these cells. A third possibility is that there is exposure to some unknown chemical in the food, air, or water which slowly damages certain vulnerable areas of the brain. This theory stems from a clue found on the Pacific island of Guam, where a common neurological disease occurring only there and on a few neighboring islands shares some of the characteristics of PSP, Alzheimer's disease, Parkinson's disease, and amyotrophic lateral sclerosis (Lou Gehrig's disease). Its cause is thought to be a dietary factor or toxic substance found only in that area.

Another possible cause of PSP is cellular damage caused by free radicals, unstable molecules produced continuously by all cells during normal metabolism. Although the body has built-in mechanisms for clearing free radicals from the system, scientists suspect that, under certain circumstances, free radicals can react with and damage other molecules. A great deal of research is directed at understanding the role of free radical damage in human diseases.

How is PSP diagnosed?

Initial complaints in PSP are typically vague and an early diagnosis is always difficult. The primary complaints fall into these categories: 1) symptoms of dysequilibrium, such as unsteady walking or abrupt and unexplained falls without loss of consciousness; 2) visual complaints, including blurred vision, difficulties in looking up or down, double vision, light sensitivity, burning eyes, or other eye trouble; 3) slurred speech; and 4) various mental complaints such as slowness of thought, impaired memory, personality changes, and changes in mood.

PSP is often misdiagnosed because some of its symptoms are very much like those of Parkinson's disease, Alzheimer's disease, and more rare neurodegenerative disorders, such as Creutzfeldt-Jakob disease. In fact, PSP is most often misdiagnosed as Parkinson's disease early in the course of the illness. Memory problems and personality changes may also lead a physician to mistake PSP for depression, or even attribute symptoms to some form of dementia. The key to establishing the diagnosis of PSP is the identification of early gait instability and difficulty moving the eyes, the hallmark of the disease, as well as ruling out other similar disorders, some of which are treatable.

How is PSP different from Parkinson's disease?

Both PSP and Parkinson's disease cause stiffness, movement difficulties, and clumsiness. However, patients with PSP usually stand straight or occasionally even tilt their heads backward (and tend to fall backward), while those with Parkinson's disease usually bend forward. Problems with speech and swallowing are much more common and severe in PSP than in Parkinson's disease, and tend to show up earlier in the course of the disease. Both diseases share other features: onset in late middle age, bradykinesia (slow movement), and rigidity of muscles. Tremor, almost universal in Parkinson's patients, is rare in PSP. Although Parkinson's patients markedly benefit from the drug levodopa, patients with PSP respond poorly and only transiently to this drug.

What is the prognosis?

PSP gets progressively worse but is not itself directly life-threatening. It does, however, predispose patients to serious complications such as pneumonia secondary to difficulty in swallowing (dysphagia). The most common complications are choking and pneumonia, head injury, and fractures caused by falls. The most common cause of death is pneumonia. With good attention to medical and nutritional needs, however, most PSP patients live well into their 70s and beyond.

Is there any treatment?

There is currently no effective treatment for PSP, although scientists are searching for better ways to manage the disease. In some patients the slowness, stiffness, and balance problems of PSP may respond to antiparkinsonian agents such as levodopa, but the effect is usually temporary. The speech, vision, and swallowing difficulties usually do not respond to any drug treatment.

Another group of drugs that has been of some modest success in PSP are antidepressant medications. The most commonly used of these drugs are fluoxetine (Prozac), amitriptyline (Elavil), and imipramine (Tofranil). The anti-PSP benefit of these drugs seems not to be related to their ability to relieve depression.

Non-drug treatment for PSP can take many forms. Patients frequently use weighted walking aids because of their tendency to fall backward. Bifocals or special glasses called prisms are sometimes prescribed for PSP patients to remedy the difficulty of looking down. Formal physical therapy is of no proven benefit in PSP, but certain exercises can be done to keep the joints limber.

A surgical procedure that may be necessary when there are swallowing disturbances is a gastrostomy. A gastrostomy (or a jejunostomy) is a minimally invasive procedure which is performed when the patient has difficulty swallowing or when severe choking is a definite risk. This surgery involves the placement of a tube through the skin of the abdomen into the stomach (intestine) for feeding purposes. Surgical procedures such as fetal brain cell implantation and pallidotomy, which are being tested as treatments for Parkinson's disease, are not effective in PSP.

What research is being done?

Studies to improve the diagnosis of PSP have recently been conducted at the National Institute of Neurological Disorders and Stroke (NINDS). Experiments to find the cause or causes of PSP are currently under way. Therapeutic trials with free radical scavengers (agents that can get rid of potentially harmful free radicals) are being planned for the future.

In addition, there is a great deal of ongoing research on Parkinson's and Alzheimer's diseases at the National Institutes of Health and at university medical centers throughout the country. Better understanding of those common related disorders will go a long way toward solving the problems of PSP, just as studying PSP may help shed light on Parkinson's and Alzheimer's diseases.

How can I help research?

The NINDS supports two national human brain specimen banks. These banks supply investigators around the world with tissue from patients with neurological diseases. Both banks need brain tissue from PSP patients to enable scientists to study this disorder more intensely. Prospective donors or their families should contact:

Dr. Wallace W. Tourtellotte, Director
Human Neurospecimen Bank
VA Wadsworth Medical Center
Wilshire and Sawtelle Blvds
Los Angeles, CA 90073
(310) 824-4307

Dr. Edward D. Bird, Director
Brain Tissue Bank, Mailman Research Center
McLean Hospital
115 Mill St
Belman, MA 02178
800-BRAIN-BANK (800-27246-2265)
(617) 855-2400

Two organizations not funded by the NINDS also provide research scientists with nervous system tissue from patients with neurological disorders. Interested donors should write or call:

National Disease Research Interchange (NDRI)
1880 JFK Blvd, 6th Fl
Philadelphia, PA 19103
(215) 557-7361
(800) 222-NDRI (800-222-6374)

University of Miami Brain Endowment Bank
Department of Neurology (D4-5)
1501 NW 9th Ave
Miami, FL 33101
(305) 547-6219
(800) UM-BRAIN (800-862-7246)

Is there help available?

The following voluntary agency promotes research, provides information, and helps affected families:

Society for Progressive Supranuclear Palsy, Inc.
Johns Hopkins Hospital Outpatient Center
Ste 5065
601 N. Caroline St
Baltimore, MD 21287
(410) 955-2954
(800) 457-4777

For more information on research programs of the National Institute of Neurological Disorders and Stroke contact:

NIH Neurological Institute
Office of Scientific and Health Reports
PO Box 5801
Bethesda, MD 20824
(301) 496-5751
(800) 352-9424

■ Document Source:
   U.S. Department of Health and Human Services, Public Health Service
   National Institutes of Health
   National Institute of Neurological Disorders and Stroke
   Bethesda, MD 20892-2540
   NIH Publication No. 95-3997
   October 1995

SLEEP AND THE TRAVELER: HOW TO GET THE MOST OUT OF SLEEP WHEN TRAVELING

Putting Together the Sleep Puzzle

Amazingly, we spend about 24 years (one-third) of our lives sleeping, yet relatively little is known about this critical daily routine. In fact, in relation to other biological research, it is only recently that scientists have begun to unlock some of the many mysteries of sleep.

As part of a cooperative effort between Hilton Hotels Corporation and the National Sleep Foundation (NSF), a group of some of the nation's top sleep experts gathered in Chicago recently for a first-ever discussion on sleep, its effect on travelers and potential information-based solutions for the general public. Much remains to be studied and learned. And with the development of unique partnerships such as these, new insights will be obtained to help people sleep more comfortably when traveling.

This brochure incorporates the group's findings and shares its advice on what travelers can do now to help get a better night's sleep.

Jet Lag: The Traveling Sleep Disorder

Every day, millions of travelers struggle against one of the most common sleep disorders—jet lag. For years, jet lag was considered merely a state of mind. Now, studies have shown that the condition actually results from an imbalance in our body's natural "biological clock" caused by traveling to different time zones.

Basically, our bodies work on a 24-hour cycle called "circadian rhythms." These rhythms are measured by the distinct rise and fall of body temperature, plasma levels of certain hormones and other biological conditions. All of these are influenced by our exposure to sunlight and help determine when we sleep and when we wake.

When traveling to a new time zone, our circadian rhythms are slow to adjust and remain on their original biological schedule for several days. This results in our bodies telling us it is time to sleep, when it's actually the middle of the afternoon, or it makes us want to stay awake when it is late at night. This experience is known as jet lag.

Taking the Air out of Jet Lag

Some simple behavioral adjustments before, during and after arrival at your destination can help minimize some of the side effects of jet lag.

- Select a flight that allows early evening arrival and stay up until 10 p.m. local time. (If you must sleep during the day, take a short nap in the early afternoon, but no longer than two hours. Set an alarm to be sure not to oversleep.)

- Anticipate the time change for trips by getting up and going to bed earlier several days prior to an eastward trip and later for a westward trip.
- Upon boarding the plane, change your watch to the destination time zone.
- Avoid alcohol or caffeine at least three to four hours before bedtime. Both act as "stimulants" and prevent sleep.
- Upon arrival at a destination, avoid heavy meals (a snack — not chocolate — is okay).
- Avoid any heavy exercise close to bedtime. (Light exercise earlier in the day is fine.)
- Bring earplugs and blindfolds to help dampen noise and block out unwanted light while sleeping.
- Try to get outside in the sunlight whenever possible. Daylight is a powerful stimulant for regulating the biological clock. (Staying indoors worsens jet lag.)

Contrary to popular belief, the type of foods we eat have no effect on minimizing jet lag.

Worrying About Sleep

According to experts, stress or the potential for stress is another problem that can lead to sleeplessness. Two common travel-related stress conditions are the "First Night Effect" and the "On-Call Effect." The first condition occurs when trying to sleep in a new or unfamiliar environment. The second is caused by the nagging worry that something just *might* wake you up, such as the possibility of a phone ringing, hallway noise or another disruption.

> Try these tips on your next trip to help avoid travel-related stress and subsequent sleeplessness:
> - Bring elements or objects from home (like a picture of the family, favorite pillow, blanket or even a coffee mug) to ease the feeling of being in a new environment.
> - Check with the hotel to see if voice mail services are available to guests. Then, whenever possible, have your calls handled by the service.
> - Check your room for potential sleep disturbances that may be avoided, e.g., light shining through the drapes, unwanted in-room noise, etc.
> - Request two wake-up calls in case you miss the first one.

Quiet Please! The Sleep Environment

The most common environmental elements affecting sleep are noise, sleep surface, temperature or climate, and altitude. Your age and gender also play a part in determining the level of sleep disturbance caused by these factors. One study found that women are more easily awakened than men by sonic booms and aircraft noise, while other research indicates that men may be more noise sensitive. Children are generally insensitive to extreme noise levels. However, this high threshold declines with age.

Noise

We have all experienced that dripping faucet, the barking dog or that blaring stereo next door that has kept us awake. Indeed, experts say the intensity, abruptness, regularity, intrusiveness, familiarity and regularity of noises all affect sleep.

Noises at levels as low as 40 decibels or as high as 70 decibels generally keep us awake. Interestingly, however, the absence of a familiar noise can also disrupt sleep. City dwellers may have trouble falling asleep without the familiar sounds of traffic. Or a traveler may find it difficult to sleep without the familiar tick, tick, tick of the alarm clock at home.

Some noises — although annoying at first — can gradually be ignored, allowing sleep to follow. Studies show people can get used to noises such as city traffic in about one week. However, important noises, like a parent's baby crying, a smoke alarm or even one's own name being called, are not easily assimilated and generally snap us awake.

Experts are also studying the ability of certain sounds to *induce* sleep. "White noise," such as caused by a fan, air conditioner, or radio static, can often block out unwanted noise and encourage sleep.

Sleep Surface

Little research is available—and not surprisingly—on how much sleeping surfaces affect our slumber. For the most part, we know people sleep better when horizontal and not cramped by space. As with noise, however, women and more mature people appear more sensitive to variations in sleep surfaces.

Temperature/Climate

The point at which sleep is disturbed due to temperature or climate conditions varies from person to person. Generally, temperatures above 75 degrees Fahrenheit and below 54 degrees will awaken people.

Altitudes

The higher the altitude, the greater the sleep disruption. Generally, sleep disturbance becomes greater at altitudes of 13,200 feet or more. The disturbance is thought to be caused by diminished oxygen levels and accompanying changes in respiration. Most people adjust to new altitudes in approximately two to three weeks.

Snooze Cues

Behavioral

Modifying your behavior and taking sleeping pills are both commonly accepted measures used to minimize certain sleep disorders.

As mentioned, certain behaviors can help your body better adjust to new time zones and surroundings. Although there are no guarantees to a fast and sound sleep, simple adjustments in your behavior when traveling may help you get the quality of rest needed to start the day refreshed.

Over-the-Counter Sleeping Pills

According to a recent Gallup survey, more than one-fourth (29 percent) of people with sleeping problems take over-the-counter (OTC) sleeping pills. In addition, many people use prescription drugs. While pills do not resolve the biological imbalance caused by jet lag, they may help manage short-term insomnia brought on by travel.

Be sure to discuss the use of sleeping pills with your doctor before you try them. Sleep medication can cause side effects.

Melatonin

One OTC product receiving a lot of attention lately is melatonin. Melatonin is a naturally secreted hormone in humans that affects the body's circadian rhythms. There is some evidence that when administered during the day, melatonin increases the tendency to sleep, but at night, the amount of sleep is unaffected. Currently, melatonin is largely available only in health food stores and is not regulated. Therefore, melatonin is, at present, an experimental approach to sleep problems and travelers should consult their physicians before using it.

The Business of Sleep

Because hotels are directly connected to the idea of sleep and traveling, some of the nation's preeminent hospitality companies, such as Hilton Hotels, are now working to learn more about the mysteries of sleep and discover new ways to maximize the sleep potential of guests. It is estimated that more than 125 million Americans crisscross the country every year on business or leisure trips, so it is no wonder that discovering the secret to better sleep has tremendous implications for the hospitality industry.

Many airlines are also examining travel-related sleep disorders and the impact they have on their customers, as well as on their own pilots and flight attendants who face time-zone travel on a regular basis.

One of the most interesting areas of sleep study involves the effect of sleeplessness on the body's mental and physical performance. As more is learned about the impact of sleep in this area, businesses that require their employees to travel a great deal will ultimately begin seeking ways to obtain peak performance from executives when they are on the road.

What's the future of sleep?

Although experts agree that a variety of analytical and anecdotal data exists about sleep, significant gaps still remain. Few definitive studies exist in the area of travel and sleep, making it impossible to know how prevalent travel-related sleep disorders are—or who is most susceptible to them. In addition, more research is needed in the sleep-related areas of environmental and stress effects.

Through the support of corporations like Hilton Hotels Corporation, which has extensive data and experience regarding travelers and their sleep needs, the NSF plans to expand its research and unravel more mysteries locked in the realm of sleep.

Don't Go to Bed Yet...

Since we spend a good portion of our lives sleeping, this quiz should be easy. Answer **true** or **false** to the following statements:

1. Jet lag can be controlled by carefully managing your dietary intake several hours before a flight.
2. "White noise," such as that caused by a fan or radio static, can block out noise and actually promote sleep in some cases.
3. According to sleep experts, sleeping pills are not an accepted method of sleep control and should be avoided.
4. Small amounts of alcohol prior to bedtime can be an effective way to induce sleep.
5. Due to the most recent research and studies regarding sleep, many of the mysteries surrounding that field have been solved.

Answers:

1. **False.** There is no conclusive evidence that diet can in any way minimize jet lag.
2. **True.** Studies indicate that "white noise" may help induce sleep.
3. **False.** Experts say, if taken as directed, sleeping pills can be an effective sleep manager. However, they have no effect on re-aligning the body's biological imbalance caused by traveling to a different time zone.
4. **False.** Although alcohol may initially cause sleepiness, later in the evening it acts as a "stimulant" and can keep you awake.
5. **False.** Scientists agree that more studies are needed to confirm or disaffirm what relatively little is known about sleep.

■ **Document Source:**
National Sleep Foundation
1367 Connecticut Ave, NW, Ste 200
Washington, DC 20036

See also: Insomnia (page 407)

NUTRITION AND WEIGHT CONTROL

■ ■ ■

CHOOSING A SAFE AND SUCCESSFUL WEIGHT-LOSS PROGRAM

Almost any of the commercial weight-loss programs can work, but only if they motivate you sufficiently to decrease the amount of calories you eat or increase the amount of calories you burn each day (or both). What elements of a weight-loss program should an intelligent consumer look for in judging its potential for safe and successful weight loss? A responsible and safe weight-loss program should be able to document for you the five following features:

- The diet should be safe. It should include all of the Recommended Daily Allowances (RDAs) for vitamins, minerals, and protein. The weight-loss diet should be low in *calories* (energy) only, not in essential foodstuffs.
- The weight-loss program should be directed towards a *slow, steady* weight loss unless your doctor feels your health condition would benefit from more rapid weight loss. Expect to lose only about a pound a week after the first week or two. With many calorie-restricted diets there is an initial rapid weight loss during the first one to two weeks, but this loss is largely fluid. The initial rapid loss of fluid also is regained rapidly when you return to a normal-calorie diet. Thus, a reasonable goal of weight loss must be expected.
- If you plan to lose more than 15 to 20 pounds, have any health problems, or take medication on a regular basis, you should be evaluated by your doctor before beginning your weight-loss program. A doctor can assess your general health and medical conditions that might be affected by dieting and weight loss. Also, a physician should be able to advise you on the need for weight loss, the appropriateness of the weight-loss program, and a sensible goal of weight loss for you. If you plan to use a very-low-calorie diet (a special liquid formula diet that replaces all food intake for one to four months), you definitely should be examined and monitored by a doctor.

- Your program should include plans for weight maintenance after the weight loss phase is over. It is of little benefit to lose a large amount of weight only to regain it. Weight maintenance is the most difficult part of controlling weight and is not consistently implemented in weight-loss programs. The program you select should include help in permanently changing your dietary habits and level of physical activity, to alter a lifestyle that may have contributed to weight gain in the past. Your program should provide behavior modification help, including education in healthy eating habits and long-term plans to deal with weight problems. One of the most important factors in maintaining weight loss appears to be increasing daily physical activity, often by sensible increases in daily activity, as well as incorporating an individually tailored exercise program.
- A commercial weight-loss program should provide a detailed statement of fees and costs of additional items such as dietary supplements.

Obesity is a chronic condition. Too often it is viewed as a temporary problem that can be treated for a few months with a strenuous diet. However, as most overweight people know, weight control must be considered a life-long effort. To be safe and effective, any weight-loss program must address the long-term approach or else the program is largely a waste of money and effort.

> Obesity affects about one in four adult Americans, and during any one year, over half of Americans go on a weight-loss diet or are trying to maintain their weight. For many people who try to lose weight, it is difficult to lose more than a few pounds and few succeed in remaining at the reduced weight. The difficulty in losing weight and keeping it off leads many people to turn to a professional or commercial weight-loss program for help. These programs are quite popular and are widely advertised in newspapers and on television. What is the evidence that any of these programs is worthwhile, that they will help you lose weight and keep it off and that they will do it safely?

This statement was developed with the advice of the National Task Force on Prevention and Treatment of Obesity, a subcommittee of the National Digestive Diseases Advisory Board.

■ **Document Source:**
   U.S. Department of Health and Human Services, Public Health Service
   National Institutes of Health
   National Institute of Diabetes and Digestive and Kidney Diseases
   NIH Publication No. 94-3700
   December 1993

See also: Gastric Surgery for Severe Obesity (page 443); Understanding Adult Obesity (page 459)

GASTRIC SURGERY FOR SEVERE OBESITY

Severe obesity is a chronic condition that is very difficult to treat. Surgery to promote weight loss by restricting food intake or interrupting digestive processes is an option for severely obese people. A body mass index (BMI) above 40—which means about 100 pounds of overweight for men and about 80 pounds for women—indicates that a person is severely obese and therefore a candidate for surgery. Surgery also may be an option for people with a BMI between 35 and 40 who suffer from life-threatening cardiopulmonary problems (for example, severe sleep apnea or obesity-related heart disease) or diabetes. However, as in other treatments for obesity, successful results depend mainly on motivation and behavior.

The Normal Digestive Process

Normally, as food moves along the digestive tract, appropriate digestive juices and enzymes arrive at the right place at the right time to digest and absorb calories and nutrients. After we chew and swallow our food, it moves down the esophagus to the stomach, where a strong acid continues the digestive process. The stomach can hold about three pints of food at one time. When the stomach contents move to the duodenum, the first segment of the small intestine, bile and pancreatic juice speed up digestion. Most of the iron and calcium in the foods we eat is absorbed in the duodenum. The jejunum and ileum, the remaining two segments of the nearly 20 feet of small intestine, complete the absorption of almost all calories and nutrients. The food particles that cannot be digested in the small intestine are stored in the large intestine until eliminated.

How does surgery promote weight loss?

The concept of gastric surgery to control obesity grew out of results of operations for cancer or severe ulcers that removed large portions of the stomach or small intestine.

Because patients undergoing these procedures tended to lose weight after surgery, some physicians began to use such operations to treat severe obesity. The first operation that was widely used for severe obesity was the intestinal bypass. This operation, first used 40 years ago, produces weight loss by causing malabsorption. The idea was that patients could eat large amounts of food, which would be poorly digested or passed along too fast for the body to absorb many calories. The problem with this surgery was that it caused a loss of essential nutrients and its side effects were unpredictable and sometimes fatal. The original form of the intestinal bypass operation is no longer used.

Surgeons now use techniques that produce weight loss primarily by limiting how much the stomach can hold. These restrictive procedures are often combined with modified gastric bypass procedures that somewhat limit calorie and nutrient absorption and may lead to altered food choices.

Two ways that surgical procedures promote weight loss are:

1. By decreasing food intake (restriction). Gastric banding, gastric bypass, and vertical-banded gastroplasty are surgeries that limit the amount of food the stomach can hold by closing off or removing parts of the stomach. These operations also delay emptying of the stomach (gastric pouch).
2. By causing food to be poorly digested and absorbed (malabsorption). In the gastric bypass procedures, a surgeon makes a direct connection from the stomach to a lower segment of the small intestine, bypassing the duodenum, and some of the jejunum.

Although results of operations using these procedures are more predictable and manageable, side effects persist for some patients.

What are the surgical options?

Restriction Operations

Restriction operations are the surgeries most often used for producing weight loss. Food intake is restricted by creating a small pouch at the top of the stomach where the food enters from the esophagus. The pouch initially holds about 1 ounce of food and expands to 2-3 ounces with time. The pouch's lower outlet usually has a diameter of about 1/4 inch. The small outlet delays the emptying of food from the pouch and causes a feeling of fullness.

After an operation, the person usually can eat only a half to a whole cup of food without discomfort or nausea. Also, food has to be well chewed. For most people, the ability to eat a large amount of food at one time is lost, but some patients do return to eating modest amounts of food without feeling hungry.

Restriction operations for obesity include gastric banding and vertical banded gastroplasty. Both operations serve only to restrict food intake. They do not interfere with the normal digestive process.

- Gastric banding. In this procedure, a band made of special material is placed around the stomach near its upper end, creating a small pouch and a narrow passage into the larger remainder of the stomach. In the future, it may be possible to perform gastric banding with smaller incisions through a laparoscope, a flexible fiberoptic tube and light source through which some surgical instruments may be passed. Laparoscopic gastric banding has not yet been approved by the Food and Drug Administration.

- Vertical banded gastroplasty (VBG). This procedure is the most frequently used restrictive operation for weight control. Both a band and staples are used to create a small stomach pouch.

Restrictive operations lead to weight loss in almost all patients. However, weight regain does occur in some patients. About 30 percent of persons undergoing vertical banded gastroplasty achieve normal weight, and about 80 percent achieve some degree of weight loss. However, some patients are unable to adjust their eating habits and fail to lose the desired weight. In all weight-loss operations, successful results depend on your motivation and behaviors.

A common risk of restrictive operations is vomiting caused by the small stomach being overly stretched by food particles that have not been chewed well. Other risks of VBG include erosion of the band, breakdown of the staple line, and, in a small number of cases, leakage of stomach juices into the abdomen. The latter requires an emergency operation. In a very small number of cases (less than 1 percent) infection or death from complications can occur.

Gastric Bypass Operations

These operations combine creation of small stomach pouches to restrict food intake and construction of bypasses of the duodenum and other segments of the small intestine to cause malabsorption.

- Roux-en-Y gastric bypass (RGB). This operation is the most common gastric bypass procedure. First, a small stomach pouch is created by stapling or by vertical banding. This causes restriction in food intake. Next, a Y-shaped section of the small intestine is attached to the pouch to allow food to bypass the duodenum (the first segment of the small intestine) as well as the first portion of the jejunum (the second segment of the small intestine). This causes reduced calorie and nutrient absorption.
- Extensive gastric bypass (biliopancreatic diversion). In this more complicated gastric bypass operation, portions of the stomach are removed. The small pouch that remains is connected directly to the final segment of the small intestine, thus completely bypassing both the duodenum and jejunum. Although this procedure successfully promotes weight loss, it is not widely used because of the high risk for nutritional deficiencies.

Gastric bypass operations that cause malabsorption and restrict food intake produce more weight loss than restriction operations that only decrease food intake. Patients who have bypass operations generally lose two-thirds of their excess weight within two years.

The risks for pouch stretching, band erosion, breakdown of staple lines, and leakage of stomach contents into the abdomen are about the same for gastric bypass as for vertical banded gastroplasty. However, because gastric bypass operations cause food to skip the duodenum, where most iron and calcium are absorbed, risks for nutritional deficiencies are higher in these procedures. Anemia may result from malabsorption of vitamin B12 and iron in menstruating women, and decreased absorption of calcium may bring on osteoporosis and metabolic bone disease. Patients are required to take nutritional supplements that usually prevent these deficiencies.

Gastric bypass operations also may cause "dumping syndrome," whereby stomach contents move too rapidly through the small intestine. Symptoms include nausea, weakness, sweating, faintness, and, occasionally, diarrhea after eating, as well as the inability to eat sweets without becoming so weak and sweaty that the patient must lie down until the symptoms pass.

The more extensive the bypass operation, the greater is the risk for complications and nutritional deficiencies. Patients with extensive bypasses of the normal digestive process require not only close monitoring, but also life-long use of special foods and medications.

Explore Benefits and Risks

Surgery to produce weight loss is a serious undertaking. Each individual should clearly understand what the proposed operation involves. Patients and physicians should carefully consider the following benefits and risks:

Benefits

- Immediately following surgery, most patients lose weight rapidly and continue to do so until 18 to 24 months after the procedure. Although most patients then start to regain some of their lost weight, few regain it all.
- Surgery improves most obesity-related conditions. For example, in one study, blood sugar levels of most obese patients with diabetes returned to normal after surgery. Nearly all patients whose blood sugar levels did not return to normal were older or had had diabetes for a long time.

Risks

- Ten to 20 percent of patients who have weight-loss operations require followup operations to correct complications. Abdominal hernias are the most common complications requiring followup surgery. Less common complications include breakdown of the staple line and stretched stomach outlets.
- More than one-third of obese patients who have gastric surgery develop gallstones. Gallstones are clumps of cholesterol and other matter that form in the gallbladder. During rapid or substantial weight loss a person's risk of developing gallstones is increased. Gallstones can be prevented with supplemental bile salts taken for the first six months after surgery.

- Nearly 30 percent of patients who have weight-loss surgery develop nutritional deficiencies such as anemia, osteoporosis, and metabolic bone disease. These deficiencies can be avoided if vitamin and mineral intakes are maintained.
- Women of childbearing age should avoid pregnancy until their weight becomes stable because rapid weight loss and nutritional deficiencies can harm a developing fetus.

Is the surgery for you?

For patients who remain severely obese after nonsurgical approaches to weight loss have failed, or for patients who have an obesity-related disease, surgery may be the best next step. But for other patients, greater efforts toward weight control, such as changes in eating habits, behavior modification, and increasing physical activity, may be more appropriate. Answers to the following questions may help in your decision to undergo surgery for weight loss.

Are you

- unlikely to lose weight successfully with (further) non-surgical measures?
- well informed about the surgical procedure and the effects of treatment?
- determined to lose weight and improve your health?
- aware of how your life may change after the operation (adjustment to the side effects of the surgery, including need to chew well and inability to eat large meals)?
- aware of the potential for serious complications, the associated dietary restrictions, and the occasional failures?
- committed to lifelong medical followup?

Do you

- have a BMI of 40 or more?
- have an obesity-related physical problem (such as body size that interferes with employment, walking, or family function)?
- have high-risk obesity-related health problems (such as severe sleep apnea or obesity-related heart disease)?

Remember: There are no guarantees for any method, including surgery, to produce and maintain weight loss. Success is possible only with your fullest cooperation and commitment to behavioral change and medical followup—and this cooperation and commitment should be carried out for the rest of your life.

Additional Reading

Gastrointestinal Surgery for Severe Obesity. Consensus Statement, NIH Consensus Development Conference, March 25-27, 1991; Public Health Service, National Institutes of Health, Office of Medical Applications of Research, Building 1, Room 260, Bethesda, MD 20892. This publication, written for health professionals, summarizes the findings of a conference discussing treatments for severe obesity. Available from WIN.

Understanding Adult Obesity. NIH Publication No. 94-3680. This fact sheet describes what obesity is, its causes, how it is measured, and associated health risks. Available from WIN.

Weight-Control Information Network

1 WIN Way
Bethesda, MD 20892-3665
(301) 570-2177
FAX: (301) 570-2186
Internet: WIN@matthewsgroup.com
Toll-free Number: (800) WIN-8098

The Weight-Control Information Network (WIN) is a service of the National Institute of Diabetes and Digestive and Kidney Diseases, part of the National Institutes of Health. Authorized by Congress (Public Law 103-43). WIN assembles and disseminates to health professionals and the general public information on weight control, obesity, and nutritional disorders. WIN responds to requests for information; develops, reviews, and distributes publications; and develops communication strategies to encourage individuals to achieve and maintain a health weight.

Publications produced by WIN are reviewed for scientific accuracy, content, and readability. Materials produced by other sources are also reviewed for scientific accuracy and are distributed, along with WIN publications, to answer requests.

■ **Document Source:**
U.S. Department of Health and Human Services, Public Health Service
National Institutes of Health
National Institute of Diabetes and Digestive and Kidney Diseases
NIH Publication No. 96-4006
April 1996

See also: Choosing a Safe and Successful Weight Loss Program (page 442); Understanding Adult Obesity (page 459)

NUTRITION AND YOUR HEALTH: DIETARY GUIDELINES FOR AMERICANS

What should Americans eat to stay healthy?

These guidelines are designed to help answer this question. They provide advice for healthy Americans age two years and over about food choices that promote health and prevent disease. To meet the Dietary Guidelines for Americans, choose a diet with most of the calories from grain products, vegetables, fruits, lowfat milk products, lean meats, fish, poultry, and dry beans. Choose fewer calories from fats and sweets.

Eating is one of life's greatest pleasures.

Food choices depend on history, culture, and environment, as well as on energy and nutrient needs. People also eat foods for enjoyment. Family, friends, and beliefs play a major role in the ways people select foods and plan meals. This booklet describes some of the many different and pleasurable ways to combine foods to make healthful diets.

Diet is important to health at all stages of life.

Many genetic, environmental, behavioral, and cultural factors can affect health. Understanding family history of disease or risk factors—body weight and fat distribution, blood pressure, and blood cholesterol, for example—can help people make more informed decisions about actions that can improve health prospects. Food choices are among the most pleasurable and effective of these actions.

Healthful diets help children grow, develop, and do well in school. They enable people of all ages to work productively and feel their best. Food choices also can help to reduce the risk for chronic diseases, such as heart disease, certain cancers, diabetes, stroke, and osteoporosis, that are leading causes of death and disability among Americans. Good diets can reduce major risk factors for chronic diseases—factors such as obesity, high blood pressure, and high blood cholesterol.

Foods contain energy, nutrients, and other components that affect health. People require energy and certain other essential nutrients. These nutrients are essential because the body cannot make them and must obtain them from food. Essential nutrients include vitamins, minerals, certain amino acids, and certain fatty acids. Foods also contain other components such as fiber that are important for health. Although each of these food components has a specific function in the body, all of them together are required for overall health. People need calcium to build and maintain strong bones, for example, but many other nutrients also are involved.

The carbohydrates, fats, and proteins in food supply energy, which is measured in calories. Carbohydrates and proteins provide about four calories per gram. Fat contributes more than twice as much—about nine calories per gram. Alcohol, although not a nutrient, also supplies energy—about seven calories per gram. Foods that are high in fat are also high in calories. However, many lowfat or nonfat foods can also be high in calories.

Physical activity fosters a healthful diet.

Calorie needs vary by age and level of activity. Many older adults need less food, in part due to decreased activity, relative to younger, more active individuals. People who are trying to lose weight and eating little food may need to select more nutrient-dense foods in order to meet their nutrient needs in a satisfying diet. Nearly all Americans need to be more active, because a sedentary lifestyle is unhealthful. Increasing the calories spent in daily activities helps to maintain health and allows people to eat a nutritious and enjoyable diet.

What is a healthful diet?

Healthful diets contain the amounts of essential nutrients and calories needed to prevent nutritional deficiencies and excesses. Healthful diets also provide the right balance of carbohydrate, fat, and protein to reduce risks for chronic diseases, and are a part of a full and productive lifestyle. Such diets are obtained from a variety of foods that are available, affordable, and enjoyable.

The Recommended Dietary Allowances refer to nutrients.

Recommended Dietary Allowances (RDAs) represent the amounts of nutrients that are adequate to meet the needs of most healthy people. Although people with average nutrient requirements likely eat adequately at levels below the RDAs, diets that meet RDAs are almost certain to ensure intake of enough essential nutrients by most healthy people. The Dietary Guidelines describe food choices that will help you meet these recommendations. Like the RDAs, the Dietary Guidelines apply to diets consumed over several days and not to single meals or foods.

The Dietary Guidelines describe food choices that promote good health.

The Dietary Guidelines are designed to help Americans choose diets that will meet nutrient requirements, promote health, support active lives, and reduce chronic disease risks. Research has shown that certain diets raise risks for chronic diseases. Such diets are high in fat, saturated fat, cholesterol, and salt and they contain more calories than the body uses. They are also low in grain products, vegetables, fruit, and fiber. This bulletin helps you choose foods, meals, and diets that can reduce chronic disease risks.

Food labels and the Food Guide Pyramid are tools to help you make food choices.

The Food Guide Pyramid and the Nutrition Facts Label serve as educational tools to put the Dietary Guidelines into practice. The Pyramid translates the RDAs and the Dietary Guide-

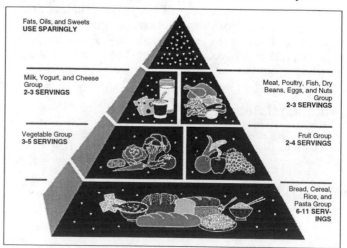

lines into the kinds and amounts of food to eat each day. The Nutrition Facts Label is designed to help you select foods for a diet that will meet the Dietary Guidelines. Most processed foods now include nutrition information. However, nutrition labels are not required for foods like coffee and tea (which contain no significant amounts of nutrients), certain ready-to-eat foods like unpackaged deli and bakery items, and restaurant food. Labels are also voluntary for many raw foods—your grocer may supply this information for the fish, meat, poultry, and raw fruits and vegetables that are consumed most frequently. Use the Nutrition Facts Label to choose a healthful diet.

Eat a variety of foods.

To obtain the nutrients and other substances needed for good health, vary the foods you eat.

Foods contain combinations of nutrients and other healthful substances. No single food can supply all nutrients in the amounts you need. For example, oranges provide vitamin C but no vitamin B12; cheese provides vitamin B12 but no vitamin C. To make sure you get all of the nutrients and other substances needed for health, choose the recommended number of daily servings from each of the five major food groups displayed in the Food Guide Pyramid.

Use foods from the base of the Food Guide Pyramid as the foundation of your meals.

Americans do choose a wide variety of foods. However, people often choose higher or lower amounts from some food groups than suggested in the Food Guide Pyramid. The Pyramid shows that foods from the grain products group, along with vegetables and fruits, are the basis of healthful diets. Enjoy meals that have rice, pasta, potatoes, or bread at the center of the plate, accompanied by other vegetables and fruit, and lean and low-fat foods from the other groups. Limit fats and sugars added in food preparation and at the table. Compare the recommended number of servings in Box 1 with what you usually eat.

BOX 1: Choose foods from each of five food groups.

The Food Guide Pyramid illustrates the importance of balance among food groups in a daily eating pattern. Most of the daily servings of food should be selected from the food groups that are the largest in the picture and closest to the base of the Pyramid.

- Choose most of your foods from the grain products group (6-11 servings), the vegetable group (3-5 servings), and the fruit group (2-4 servings).
- Eat moderate amounts of foods from the milk group (2-3 servings) and the meat and beans group (2-3 servings).
- Choose sparingly foods that provide few nutrients and are high in fat and sugars.

Note: A range of servings is given for each food group. The smaller number is for people who consume about 1,600 calories a day, such as many sedentary women. The larger number is for those who consume about 2,800 calories a day, such as active men.

What counts as a "serving"?

See Box 2 for suggested serving sizes in the Food Guide Pyramid food groups. Notice that some of the serving sizes are smaller than what you might usually eat. For example, many people eat a cup or more of pasta in a meal, which equals two or more servings. So, it is easy to eat the number of servings recommended.

BOX 2: What counts as a serving?*

Grain Products Group (bread, cereal, rice, and pasta)
- 1 slice of bread
- 1 ounce of ready-to-eat cereal
- 1/2 cup of cooked cereal, rice, or pasta

Vegetable Group
- 1 cup of raw leafy vegetables
- 1/2 cup of other vegetables — cooked or chopped raw
- 3/4 cup of vegetable juice

Fruit Group
- 1 medium apple, banana, orange
- 1/2 cup of chopped, cooked, or canned fruit
- 3/4 cup of fruit juice

Milk Group (milk, yogurt, and cheese)
- 1 cup of milk or yogurt
- 1-1/2 ounces of natural cheese
- 2 ounces of processed cheese

Meat and Beans Group (meat, poultry, fish, dry beans, eggs, and nuts)
- 2-3 ounces of cooked lean meat, poultry, or fish
- 1/2 cup of cooked dry beans or 1 egg counts as 1 ounce of lean meat.
- Two tablespoons of peanut butter or 1/3 cup of nuts count as 1 ounce of meat.

*Some foods fit into more than one group. Dry beans, peas, and lentils can be counted as servings in either the meat and beans group or vegetable group. These "cross over" foods can be counted as servings from either one or the other group, but not both. Serving sizes indicated here are those used in the Food Guide Pyramid and based on both suggested and usually consumed portions necessary to achieve adequate nutrient intake. They differ from serving sizes on the Nutrition Facts Label, which reflect portions usually consumed.

Choose different foods within each food group.

You can achieve a healthful, nutritious eating pattern with many combinations of foods from the five major food groups. Choosing a variety of foods within and across food groups improves dietary patterns because foods within the same group have different combinations of nutrients and other beneficial substances. For example, some vegetables and fruits are good sources of vitamin C or vitamin A, while others are high in folate; still others are good sources of calcium or iron. Choosing a variety of foods within each group also helps to make your meals more interesting from day to day.

What about vegetarian diets?

Some Americans eat vegetarian diets for reasons of culture, belief, or health. Most vegetarians eat milk products and eggs, and as a group, these lacto-ovo-vegetarians enjoy excellent health. Vegetarian diets are consistent with the Dietary Guidelines for Americans and can meet Recommended Dietary Allowances for nutrients. You can get enough protein from a vegetarian diet as long as the variety and amounts of foods consumed are adequate. Meat, fish, and poultry are major contributors of iron, zinc, and B vitamins in most American diets, and vegetarians should pay special attention to these nutrients.

Vegans eat only food of plant origin. Because animal products are the only food sources of vitamin B12, vegans must supplement their diets with a source of this vitamin. In addition, vegan diets, particularly those of children, require care to ensure adequacy of vitamin D and calcium, which most Americans obtain from milk products.

Foods vary in their amounts of calories and nutrients.

Some foods such as grain products, vegetables, and fruits have many nutrients and other healthful substances but are relatively low in calories. Fat and alcohol are high in calories. Foods high in both sugars and fat contain many calories but often are low in vitamins, minerals, or fiber.

People who do not need many calories or who must restrict their food intake need to choose nutrient-rich foods from the five major food groups with special care. They should obtain most of their calories from foods that contain a high proportion of essential nutrients and fiber. Growing children, teenage girls, and women have higher needs for some nutrients.

Many women and adolescent girls need to eat more calcium-rich foods to get the calcium needed for healthy bones throughout life. By selecting lowfat or fat-free milk products and other lowfat calcium sources, they can obtain adequate calcium and keep fat intake from being too high (Box 3). Young children, teenage girls, and women of child-bearing age should also eat enough iron-rich foods, such as lean meats and whole-grain or enriched white bread, to keep the body's iron stores at adequate levels (Box 4).

Box 3: Some Good Sources of Calcium*

- Most foods in the milk group**
  - milk and dishes made with milk, such as puddings and soups made with milk
  - cheeses such as Mozzarella, Cheddar, Swiss, and Parmesan
  - yogurt
- Canned fish with soft bones such as sardines, anchovies, and salmon**
- Dark-green leafy vegetables, such as kale, mustard greens, and turnip greens, and bak-choi
- Tofu, if processed with calcium sulfate. Read the labels.
- Tortillas made from lime-processed corn. Read the labels.

*Does not include complete list of examples. You can obtain additional information from "Good Sources of Nutrients," USDA, January 1990. Also read food labels for brand-specific information.

**Some foods in this group are high in fat, cholesterol, or both. Choose lower fat, lower cholesterol foods most often. Read the labels.

Box 4: Some Good Sources of Iron*

- Meats—beef, pork, lamb, and liver and other organ meats**
- Poultry—chicken, duck, and turkey, especially dark meat; liver**
- Fish—shellfish, like clams, mussels, and oysters; sardines; anchovies; and other fish**
- Leafy greens of the cabbage family, such as broccoli, kale, turnip greens, collards
- Legumes, such as lima beans and green peas; dry beans and peas, such as pinto beans, black-eyed peas, and canned baked beans
- Yeast-leavened whole-wheat bread and rolls
- Iron-enriched white bread, pasta, rice, and cereals. Read the labels.

*Does not include complete list of examples. You can obtain additional information from "Good Sources of Nutrients," USDA, January 1990. Also read food labels for brand-specific information.

**Some foods in this group are high in fat, cholesterol, or both. Choose lean, lower fat, lower cholesterol foods most often. Read the labels.

Enriched and fortified foods have essential nutrients added to them.

National policy requires that specified amounts of nutrients be added to enrich some foods. For example, enriched flour and bread contain added thiamin, riboflavin, niacin, and iron; skim milk, lowfat milk, and margarine are usually enriched with vitamin A; and milk is usually enriched with vitamin D. Fortified foods may have one or several nutrients added in extra amounts. The number and quantity of nutrients added vary among products. Fortified foods may be useful for meeting special dietary needs. Read the ingredient list to know which nutrients are added to foods. How these foods fit into your total diet will depend on the amounts you eat and the other foods you consume.

Where do vitamin, mineral, and fiber supplements fit in?

Supplements of vitamins, minerals, or fiber also may help to meet special nutritional needs. However, supplements do not supply all of the nutrients and other substances present in foods that are important to health. Supplements of some nutrients taken regularly in large amounts are harmful. Daily vitamin and mineral supplements at or below the Recommended Dietary Allowances are considered safe, but are usually not needed by people who eat the variety of foods depicted in the Food Guide Pyramid.

Sometimes supplements are needed to meet specific nutrient requirements. For example, older people and others with little exposure to sunlight may need a vitamin D supplement. Women of childbearing age may reduce the risk of certain birth defects by consuming folate-rich foods or folic acid supplements. Iron supplements are recommended for pregnant women. However, because foods contain many nutrients and other substances that promote health, the use of supplements cannot substitute for proper food choices.

Advice for Today

Enjoy eating a variety of foods. Get the many nutrients your body needs by choosing among the varied foods you enjoy from these groups: grain products, vegetables, fruits, milk and milk products, protein-rich plant foods (beans, nuts), and protein-rich animal foods (lean meat, poultry, fish, and eggs). Remember to choose lean and lowfat foods and beverages most often. Many foods you eat contain servings from more than one food group. For example, soups and stews may contain meat, beans, noodles, and vegetables.

Balance the food you eat with physical activity: Maintain or improve your weight.

Many Americans gain weight in adulthood, increasing their risk for high blood pressure, heart disease, stroke, diabetes, certain types of cancer, arthritis, breathing problems, and other illness. Therefore, most adults should not gain weight. If you are overweight and have one of these problems, you should try to lose weight, or at the very least, not gain weight. If you are uncertain about your risk of developing a problem associated with overweight, you should consult a health professional.

How to Maintain Your Weight

In order to stay at the same body weight, people must balance the amount of calories in the foods and drinks they consume with the amount of calories the body uses. Physical activity is an important way to use food energy. Most Americans spend much of their working day in activities that require little energy. In addition, many Americans of all ages now spend a lot of leisure time each day being inactive, for example, watching television or working at a computer. To burn calories, devote less time to sedentary activities like sitting. Spend more time in activities like walking to the store or around the block. Use stairs rather than elevators. Less sedentary activity and more vigorous activity may help you reduce body fat and disease risk. Try to do 30 minutes or more of moderate physical activity on most—preferably all—days of the week.

The kinds and amounts of food people eat affect their ability to maintain weight. High-fat foods contain more calories per serving than other foods and may increase the likelihood of weight gain. However, even when people eat less high-fat food, they still can gain weight from eating too much of foods high in starch, sugars, or protein. Eat a variety of foods, emphasizing pasta, rice, bread, and other whole-grain foods as well as fruits and vegetables. These foods are filling, but lower in calories than foods rich in fats or oils.

The pattern of eating may also be important. Snacks provide a large percentage of daily calories for many Americans. Unless nutritious snacks are part of the daily meal plan, snacking may lead to weight gain. A pattern of frequent binge-eating, with or without alternating periods of food restriction, may also contribute to weight problems.

Box 5: To increase calorie expenditure by physical activity

Remember to accumulate 30 minutes or more of moderate physical activity on most—preferably all—days of the week. Examples of moderate physical activities for healthy US adults:

- walking briskly (3-4 miles per hour)
- conditioning or general calisthenics
- home care, general cleaning
- racket sports such as table tennis
- mowing lawn, power mower
- golf—pulling cart or carrying clubs
- home repair, painting
- fishing, standing/casting
- jogging
- swimming (moderate effort)
- cycling, moderate speed (10 miles per hour or less)
- gardening
- canoeing leisurely (2.0-3.9 miles per hour)
- dancing

Source: Adapted from Pate, et al., Journal of the American Medical Association, 1995, Vol. 273, p. 404.

Maintaining weight is equally important for older people who begin to lose weight as they age. Some of the weight that is lost is muscle. Maintaining muscle through regular activity helps to keep older people feeling well and helps to reduce the risk of falls and fractures.

How to Evaluate Your Body Weight

Healthy weight ranges for adult men and women of all ages are shown in the following figure. See where your weight falls on the chart for people of your height. The health risks due to excess weight appear to be the same for older as for younger adults. Weight ranges are shown in the chart because people of the same height may have equal amounts of body fat but different amounts of muscle and bone. However, the ranges do not mean that it is healthy to gain weight, even within the same weight range. The higher weights in the healthy weight range apply to people with more muscle and bone.

Weights above the healthy weight range are less healthy for most people. The further you are above the healthy weight range for your height, the higher your weight-related risk. Weights slightly below the range may be healthy for some people but are sometimes the result of health problems, especially when weight loss is unintentional.

Location of Body Fat

Research suggests that the location of body fat also is an important factor in health risks for adults. Excess fat in the abdomen (stomach area) is a greater health risk than excess fat in the hips and thighs. Extra fat in the abdomen is linked to high blood pressure, diabetes, early heart disease, and certain types of cancer. Smoking and too much alcohol increase abdominal fat and the risk for diseases related to obesity. Vigorous exercise helps to reduce abdominal fat and decrease the risk for these diseases. The easiest way to check your body fat distribution is to measure around your waistline with a tape measure and compare this with the measure around your hips or buttocks to see if your abdomen is larger. If you are in doubt, you may wish to seek advice from a health professional.

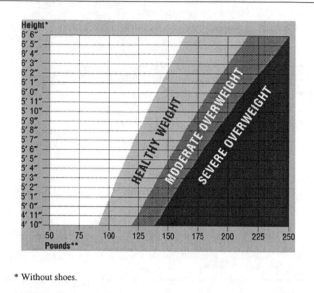

Height*

Pounds**

* Without shoes.

** Without clothes. The higher weights apply to people with more muscle and bone, such as many men.

Source: Report of the Dietary Guidelines Advisory Committee on the Dietary Guidelines for Americans, 1995, pages 23-24.

Problems with Excessive Thinness

Being too thin can occur with anorexia nervosa, other eating disorders, or loss of appetite, and is linked to menstrual irregularity and osteoporosis in women, and greater risk of early death in both women and men. Many people—especially women—are concerned about body weight, even when their weight is normal. Excessive concern about weight may cause or lead to such unhealthy behaviors as excessive exercise, self-induced vomiting, and the abuse of laxatives or other medications. These practices may only worsen the concern about weight. If you lose weight suddenly or for unknown reasons, see a physician. Unexplained weight loss may be an early clue to a health problem.

If You Need to Lose Weight

You do not need to lose weight if your weight is already within the healthy range in the figure, if you have gained less than 10 pounds since you reached your adult height, and if you are otherwise healthy. If you are overweight and have excess abdominal fat, a weight-related medical problem, or a family history of such problems, you need to lose weight. Healthy diets and exercise can help people maintain a healthy weight, and may also help them lose weight. It is important to recognize that overweight is a chronic condition which can only be controlled with long-term changes. To reduce caloric intake, eat less fat and control portion sizes (Box 6). If you are not physically active, spend less time in sedentary activities such as watching television, and be more active throughout the day. As people lose weight, the body becomes more efficient at using energy and the rate of weight loss may

decrease. Increased physical activity will help you to continue losing weight and to avoid gaining it back.

Box 6: To decrease calorie intake

- Eat a variety of foods that are low in calories and high in nutrients — check the Nutrition Facts Label.
- Eat less fat and fewer high-fat foods.
- Eat smaller portions and limit second helpings of foods high in fat and calories.
- Eat more vegetables and fruits without fats and sugars added in preparation or at the table.
- Eat pasta, rice, breads, and cereals without fats and sugars added in preparation or at the table.
- Eat less sugars and fewer sweets (like candy, cookies, cakes, soda).
- Drink less or no alcohol.

Many people are not sure how much weight they should lose. Weight loss of only 5-10 percent of body weight may improve many of the problems associated with overweight, such as high blood pressure and diabetes. Even a smaller weight loss can make a difference. If you are trying to lose weight, do so slowly and steadily. A generally safe rate is 1/2-1 pound a week until you reach your goal. Avoid crash weight-loss diets that severely restrict calories or the variety of foods. Extreme approaches to weight loss, such as self-induced vomiting or the use of laxatives, amphetamines, or diuretics, are not appropriate and can be dangerous to your health.

Weight Regulation in Children

Children need enough food for proper growth. To promote growth and development and prevent overweight, teach children to eat grain products; vegetables and fruits; lowfat milk products or other calcium-rich foods; beans, lean meat, poultry, fish or other protein-rich foods; and to participate in vigorous activity. Limiting television time and encouraging children to play actively in a safe environment are helpful steps. Although limiting fat intake may help to prevent excess weight gain in children, fat should not be restricted for children younger than two years of age. Helping overweight children to achieve a healthy weight along with normal growth requires more caution. Modest reductions in dietary fat, such as the use of lowfat milk rather than whole milk, are not hazardous. However, major efforts to change a child's diet should be accompanied by monitoring of growth by a health professional at regular intervals.

Advice for Today

Try to maintain your body weight by balancing what you eat with physical activity. If you are sedentary, try to become more active. If you are already very active, try to continue the same level of activity as you age. More physical activity is better than less, and any is better than none. If your weight is not in the healthy range, try to reduce health risks through better eating and exercise habits. Take steps to keep your weight within the healthy range (neither too high nor too low). Have children's heights and weights checked regularly by a health professional.

Choose a diet with plenty of grain products, vegetables, and fruits.

Grain products, vegetables, and fruits are key parts of a varied diet. They are emphasized in this guideline because they provide vitamins, minerals, complex carbohydrates (starch and dietary fiber), and other substances that are important for good health. They are also generally low in fat, depending on how they are prepared and what is added to them at the table. Most Americans of all ages eat fewer than the recommended number of servings of grain products, vegetables, and fruits, even though consumption of these foods is associated with a substantially lower risk for many chronic diseases, including certain types of cancer.

Most of the calories in your diet should come from grain products, vegetables, and fruits.

These include grain products high in complex carbohydrates—breads, cereals, pasta, rice—found at the base of the Food Guide Pyramid, as well as vegetables such as potatoes and corn. Dry beans (like pinto, navy, kidney, and black beans) are included in the meat and beans group of the Pyramid, but they can count as servings of vegetables instead of meat alternatives.

Plant foods provide fiber.

Fiber is found only in plant foods like whole-grain breads and cereals, beans and peas, and other vegetables and fruits. Because there are different types of fiber in foods, choose a variety of foods daily. Eating a variety of fiber-containing plant foods is important for proper bowel function, can reduce symptoms of chronic constipation, diverticular disease, and hemorrhoids, and may lower the risk for heart disease and some cancers. However, some of the health benefits associated with a high-fiber diet may come from other components present in these foods, not just from fiber itself. For this reason, fiber is best obtained from foods rather than supplements.

Plant foods provide a variety of vitamins and minerals essential for health.

Most fruits and vegetables are naturally low in fat and provide many essential nutrients and other food components important for health. These foods are excellent sources of vitamin C, vitamin B6, carotenoids, including those which form vitamin A (Box 7), and folate (Box 8). The antioxidant nutrients found in plant foods (e.g., vitamin C, carotenoids, vitamin E, and certain minerals) are presently of great interest to scientists and the public because of their potentially beneficial role in reducing the risk for cancer and certain other chronic diseases. Scientists are also trying to determine if other substances in plant foods protect against cancer.

Folate, also called folic acid, is a B vitamin that, among its many functions, reduces the risk of a serious type of birth defect (Box 8). Minerals such as potassium, found in a wide variety of vegetables and fruits, and calcium, found in certain vegetables, may help reduce the risk for high blood pressure (see Boxes 3 and 14).

Box 7: Some Good Sources of Carotenoids*

- Dark-green leafy vegetables (such as spinach, collards, kale, mustard greens, turnip greens), broccoli, carrots, pumpkin and calabasa, red pepper, sweet potatoes, and tomatoes
- Fruits like mango, papaya, cantaloupe

*Does not include complete list of examples. You can obtain additional information from "Good Sources of Nutrients," USDA, January 1990. Also read food labels for brand-specific information.

Box 8: Some Good Sources of Folate*

- Dry beans (like red beans, navy beans, and soybeans), lentils, chickpeas, cow peas, and peanuts
- Many vegetables, especially leafy greens (spinach, cabbage, brussel sprouts, romaine, loose leaf lettuce), peas, okra, sweet corn, beets, and broccoli
- Fruits such as blackberries, boysenberries, kiwifruit, oranges, plantains, strawberries, orange juice, and pineapple juice

*Does not include complete list of examples. You can obtain additional information from "Good Sources of Nutrients," USDA, January 1990. The Nutrition Facts Label may also provide brand-specific information on this nutrient.

The availability of fresh fruits and vegetables varies by season and region of the country, but frozen and canned fruits and vegetables ensure a plentiful supply of these healthful foods throughout the year. Read the Nutrition Facts Label to help choose foods that are rich in carbohydrates, fiber, and nutrients, and low in fat and sodium.

Advice for Today

Eat more grain products (breads, cereals, pasta, and rice), vegetables, and fruits. Eat dry beans, lentils, and peas more often. Increase your fiber intake by eating more of a variety of whole grains, whole-grain products, dry beans, fiber-rich vegetables and fruits such as carrots, corn, peas, pears, and berries (Box 9).

Choose a diet low in fat, saturated fat, and cholesterol.

Some dietary fat is needed for good health. Fats supply energy and essential fatty acids and promote absorption of the fat-soluble vitamins A, D, E, and K. Most people are aware that high levels of saturated fat and cholesterol in the diet are linked to increased blood cholesterol levels and a greater risk for heart disease. More Americans are now eating less fat, saturated fat, and cholesterol-rich foods than in the recent past, and fewer people are dying from the most common form of heart disease. Still, many people continue to eat high-fat diets, the number of overweight people has increased, and the risk of heart disease and certain cancers (also linked to fat intake) remains high. This guideline emphasizes the continued importance of choosing a diet with less total fat, saturated fat, and cholesterol.

Box 9: For a diet with plenty of grain products, vegetables, and fruits, eat daily

- 6-11 servings* of grain products (breads, cereals, pasta, and rice)
  - Eat products made from a variety of whole grains, such as wheat, rice, oats, corn, and barley.
  - Eat several servings of whole-grain breads and cereals daily.
  - Prepare and serve grain products with little or no fats and sugars.
- 3-5 servings* of various vegetables and vegetable juices
  - Choose dark-green leafy and deep-yellow vegetables often.
  - Eat dry beans, peas, and lentils often.
  - Eat starchy vegetables, such as potatoes and corn.
  - Prepare and serve vegetables with little or no fats.
- 2-4 servings* of various fruits and fruit juices
  - Choose citrus fruits or juices, melons, or berries regularly.
  - Eat fruits as desserts or snacks.
  - Drink fruit juices.
  - Prepare and serve fruits with little or no added sugars.

* See Box 2 for what counts as a serving.

Foods high in fat should be used sparingly.

Some foods and food groups in the Food Guide Pyramid are higher in fat than others. Fats and oils, and some types of desserts and snack foods that contain fat provide calories but few nutrients. Many foods in the milk group and in the meat and beans group (which includes eggs and nuts, as well as meat, poultry, and fish) are also high in fat, as are some processed foods in the grain group. Choosing lower fat options among these foods allows you to eat the recommended servings from these groups and increase the amount and variety of grain products, fruits, and vegetables in your diet without going over your calorie needs.

Choose a diet low in fat.

Fat, whether from plant or animal sources, contains more than twice the number of calories of an equal amount of carbohydrate or protein. Choose a diet that provides no more than 30 percent of total calories from fat. The upper limit on the grams of fat in your diet will depend on the calories you need (Box 10). Cutting back on fat can help you consume fewer calories. For example, at 2,000 calories per day, the suggested upper limit of calories from fat is about 600 calories. Sixty-five grams of fat contribute about 600 calories (65 grams of fat x 9 calories per gram = about 600 calories). On the Nutrition Facts Label, 65 grams of fat is the Daily Value for a 2,000-calorie intake.

Box 10: Maximum Total Fat Intake at Different Calorie Levels

Calories	1,600	2,200	2,800
Total fat (grams)	53	73	93

Choose a diet low in saturated fat.

Fats contain both saturated and unsaturated (monounsaturated and polyunsaturated) fatty acids. Saturated fat raises blood cholesterol more than other forms of fat. Reducing saturated fat to less than 10 percent of calories will help you lower your blood cholesterol level. The fats from meat, milk, and milk products are the main sources of saturated fats in most diets. Many bakery products are also sources of saturated fats. Vegetable oils supply smaller amounts of saturated fat. On the Nutrition Facts Label, 20 grams of saturated fat (9 percent of caloric intake) is the Daily Value for a 2,000-calorie diet.

Monounsaturated and Polyunsaturated Fat

Olive and canola oils are particularly high in monounsaturated fats; most other vegetable oils, nuts, and high-fat fish are good sources of polyunsaturated fats. Both kinds of unsaturated fats reduce blood cholesterol when they replace saturated fats in the diet. The fats in most fish are low in saturated fatty acids and contain a certain type of polyunsaturated fatty acid (omega-3) that is under study because of a possible association with a decreased risk for heart disease in certain people. Remember that the total fat in the diet should be consumed at a moderate level—that is, no more than 30 percent of calories. Mono- and polyunsaturated fat sources should replace saturated fats within this limit.

Partially hydrogenated vegetable oils, such as those used in many margarines and shortenings, contain a particular form of unsaturated fat known as trans-fatty acids that may raise blood cholesterol levels, although not as much as saturated fat.

Choose a diet low in cholesterol.

The body makes the cholesterol it requires. In addition, cholesterol is obtained from food. Dietary cholesterol comes from animal sources such as egg yolks, meat (especially organ meats such as liver), poultry, fish, and higher fat milk products. Many of these foods are also high in saturated fats. Choosing foods with less cholesterol and saturated fat will help lower your blood cholesterol levels (Box 11). The Nutrition Facts Label lists the Daily Value for cholesterol as 300 mg. You can keep your cholesterol intake at this level or lower by eating more grain products, vegetables and fruits, and by limiting intake of high cholesterol foods.

Advice for Children

Advice in the previous sections does not apply to infants and toddlers below the age of two years. After that age, children should gradually adopt a diet that, by about five years of age, contains no more than 30 percent of calories from fat. As they begin to consume fewer calories from fat, children should replace these calories by eating more grain products, fruits, vegetables, and lowfat milk products or other calcium-rich foods, and beans, lean meat, poultry, fish, or other protein-rich foods.

Box 11: For a diet low in fat, saturated fat, and cholesterol

Fats and Oils
- Use fats and oils sparingly in cooking and at the table.
- Use small amounts of salad dressings and spreads such as butter, margarine, and mayonnaise. Consider using lowfat or fat-free dressings for salads.
- Choose vegetable oils and soft margarines most often because they are lower in saturated fat than solid shortenings and animal fats, even though their caloric content is the same.
- Check the Nutrition Facts Label to see how much fat and saturated fat are in a serving; choose foods lower in fat and saturated fat.

Grain Products, Vegetables, and Fruits
- Choose lowfat sauces with pasta, rice, and potatoes.
- Use as little fat as possible to cook vegetables and grain products.
- Season with herbs, spices, lemon juice, and fat-free or lowfat salad dressings.

Meat, Poultry, Fish, Eggs, Beans, and Nuts
- Choose two to three servings of lean fish, poultry, meats, or other protein-rich foods, such as beans, daily. Use meats labeled "lean" or "extra lean." Trim fat from meat; take skin off poultry. (Three ounces of cooked lean beef or chicken without skin—a piece the size of a deck of cards—provides about 6 grams of fat; a piece of chicken with skin or untrimmed meat of that size may have as much as twice this amount of fat.) Most beans and bean products are almost fat-free and are a good source of protein and fiber.
- Limit intake of high-fat processed meats such as sausages, salami, and other cold cuts; choose lower fat varieties by reading the Nutrition Facts Label.
- Limit the intake of organ meats (three ounces of cooked chicken liver have about 540 mg of cholesterol); use egg yolks in moderation (one egg yolk has about 215 mg of cholesterol). Egg whites contain no cholesterol and can be used freely.

Milk and Milk Products
- Choose skim or lowfat milk, fat-free or lowfat yogurt, and lowfat cheese.
- Have two to three lowfat servings daily. Add extra calcium to your diet without added fat by choosing fat-free yogurt and lowfat milk more often. [One cup of skim milk has almost no fat, 1 cup of 1 percent milk has 2.5 grams of fat, 1 cup of 2 percent milk has 5 grams (one teaspoon) of fat, and 1 cup of whole milk has 8 grams of fat.] If you do not consume foods from this group, eat other calcium-rich foods (Box 3).

Advice for Today

To reduce your intake of fat, saturated fat, and cholesterol, follow these recommendations, as illustrated in the Food Guide Pyramid, which apply to diets consumed over several days and not to single meals or foods.

- Use fats and oils sparingly.

- Use the Nutrition Facts Label to help you choose foods lower in fat, saturated fat, and cholesterol.
- Eat plenty of grain products, vegetables, and fruits.
- Choose lowfat milk products, lean meats, fish, poultry, beans, and peas to get essential nutrients without substantially increasing calorie and saturated fat intakes.

Choose a diet moderate in sugars.

Sugars come in many forms.

Sugars are carbohydrates. Dietary carbohydrates also include the complex carbohydrates starch and fiber. During digestion, all carbohydrates except fiber break down into sugars. Sugars and starches occur naturally in many foods that also supply other nutrients. Examples of these foods include milk, fruits, some vegetables, breads, cereals, and grains. Americans eat sugars in many forms, and most people like their taste. Some sugars are used as natural preservatives, thickeners, and baking aids in foods; they are often added to foods during processing and preparation or when they are eaten. The body cannot tell the difference between naturally occurring and added sugars because they are identical chemically.

Sugars, Health, and Weight Maintenance

Scientific evidence indicates that diets high in sugars do not cause hyperactivity or diabetes. The most common type of diabetes occurs in overweight adults. Avoiding sugars alone will not correct overweight. To lose weight, reduce the total amount of calories from the food you eat and increase your level of physical activity.

If you wish to maintain your weight when you eat less fat, replace the lost calories from fat with equal calories from fruits, vegetables, and grain products, found in the lower half of the Food Guide Pyramid. Some foods that contain a lot of sugars supply calories but few or no nutrients (Box 12). These foods are located at the top of the Pyramid. For very active people with high calorie needs, sugars can be an additional source of energy. However, because maintaining a nutritious diet and a healthy weight is very important, sugars should be used in moderation by most healthy people and sparingly by people with low calorie needs. This guideline cautions about eating sugars in large amounts and about frequent snacks of foods and beverages containing sugars that supply unnecessary calories and few nutrients.

Sugar Substitutes

Sugar substitutes such as sorbitol, saccharin, and aspartame are ingredients in many foods. Most sugar substitutes do not provide significant calories and therefore may be useful in the diets of people concerned about calorie intake. Foods containing sugar substitutes, however, may not always be lower in calories than similar products that contain sugars. Unless you reduce the total calories you eat, the use of sugar substitutes will not cause you to lose weight.

Box 12: On a food label, sugars include

- brown sugar
- corn sweetener
- corn syrup
- fructose
- fruit juice concentrate
- glucose (dextrose)
- high-fructose corn syrup
- honey
- invert sugar
- lactose
- maltose
- molasses
- raw sugar
- [table] sugar (sucrose)
- syrup

A food is likely to be high in sugars if one of the above terms appears first or second in the ingredients list, or if several of them are listed.

Sugars and Dental Caries

Both sugars and starches can promote tooth decay. The more often you eat foods that contain sugars and starches, and the longer these foods are in your mouth before you brush your teeth, the greater the risk for tooth decay. Thus, frequent eating of foods high in sugars and starches as between-meal snacks may be more harmful to your teeth than eating them at meals and then brushing. Regular daily dental hygiene, including brushing with a fluoride toothpaste and flossing, and an adequate intake of fluoride, preferably from fluoridated water, will help you prevent tooth decay (Box 13).

Box 13: For healthier teeth and gums

- Eat fewer foods containing sugars and starches between meals.
- Brush and floss teeth regularly.
- Use a fluoride toothpaste.
- Ask your dentist or doctor about the need for supplemental fluoride, especially for children.

Advice for Today

Use sugars in moderation—sparingly if your calorie needs are low. Avoid excessive snacking, brush with a fluoride toothpaste, and floss your teeth regularly. Read the Nutrition Facts Label on foods you buy. The food label lists the content of total carbohydrate and sugars, as well as calories.

Choose a diet moderate in salt and sodium.

Sodium and salt are found mainly in processed and prepared foods Sodium and sodium chloride—known commonly as salt—occur naturally in foods, usually in small amounts. Salt and other sodium-containing ingredients are often used in food processing. Some people add salt and salty sauces, such as soy sauce, to their food at the table, but most dietary sodium or salt comes from foods to which salt has already been added during processing or preparation. Although many people add salt to enhance the taste of foods, their preference may weaken with eating less salt.

Sodium is associated with high blood pressure.

In the body, sodium plays an essential role in regulation of fluids and blood pressure. Many studies in diverse populations have shown that a high sodium intake is associated with higher blood pressure. Most evidence suggests that many people at risk for high blood pressure reduce their chances of developing this condition by consuming less salt or sodium. Some questions remain, partly because other factors may interact with sodium to affect blood pressure.

Other factors affect blood pressure.

Following other guidelines in the Dietary Guidelines for Americans may also help prevent high blood pressure. An important example is the guideline on weight and physical activity. The role of body weight in blood pressure control is well documented. Blood pressure increases with weight and decreases when weight is reduced. The guideline to consume a diet with plenty of fruits and vegetables is relevant because fruits and vegetables are naturally lower in sodium and fat and may help with weight reduction and control. Consuming more fruits and vegetables also increases potassium intakes which may help to reduce blood pressure (Box 14). Increased physical activity helps lower blood pressure and control weight. Alcohol consumption has also been associated with high blood pressure. Another reason to reduce salt intake is the fact that high salt intakes may increase the amount of calcium excreted in the urine and, therefore, increase the body's need for calcium.

Box 14: Some Good Sources of Potassium*

- Vegetables and fruits in general, especially
  - potatoes and sweet potatoes
  - spinach, swiss chard, broccoli, winter squashes, and parsnips
  - dates, bananas, cantaloupes, mangoes, plantains, dried apricots, raisins, prunes, orange juice, and grapefruit juice
  - dry beans, peas, lentils
- Milk and yogurt are good sources of potassium and have less sodium than cheese; cheese has much less potassium and usually has added salt.

*Does not include complete list of examples. You can obtain additional information from "Good Sources of Nutrients," USDA, January 1990. The Nutrition Facts Label may also provide brand-specific information on this nutrient.

Most Americans consume more salt than is needed.

Sodium has an important role in the body. However, most Americans consume more sodium than is needed. The Nutrition Facts Label lists a Daily Value of 2,400 mg per day for sodium [2,400 mg sodium per day is contained in 6 grams of sodium chloride (salt)]. In household measures, one level teaspoon of salt provides about 2,300 milligrams of sodium. Most people consume more than this amount.

There is no way at present to tell who might develop high blood pressure from eating too much sodium. However, consuming less salt or sodium is not harmful and can be recommended for the healthy normal adult (Box 15).

Box 15: To consume less salt and sodium

- Read the Nutrition Facts Label to determine the amount of sodium in the foods you purchase. The sodium content of processed foods—such as cereals, breads, soups, and salad dressings—often varies widely.
- Choose foods lower in sodium and ask your grocer or supermarket to offer more low-sodium foods. Request less salt in your meals when eating out or traveling.
- If you salt foods in cooking or at the table, add small amounts. Learn to use spices and herbs, rather than salt, to enhance the flavor of food.
- When planning meals, consider that fresh and most plain frozen vegetables are low in sodium.
- When selecting canned foods, select those prepared with reduced or no sodium.
- Remember that fresh fish, poultry, and meat are lower in sodium than most canned and processed ones.
- Choose foods lower in sodium content. Many frozen dinners, packaged mixes, canned soups, and salad dressings contain a considerable amount of sodium. Remember that condiments such as soy and many other sauces, pickles, and olives are high in sodium. Ketchup and mustard, when eaten in large amounts, can also contribute significant amounts of sodium to the diet. Choose lower sodium varieties.
- Choose fresh fruits and vegetables as a lower sodium alternative to salted snack foods.

Advice for Today

Fresh fruits and vegetables have very little sodium. The food groups in the Food Guide Pyramid include some foods that are high in sodium and other foods that have very little sodium, or can be prepared in ways that add flavor without adding salt. Read the Nutrition Facts Label to compare and help identify foods lower in sodium within each group. Use herbs and spices to flavor food. Try to choose forms of foods that you frequently consume that are lower in sodium and salt.

If you drink alcoholic beverages, do so in moderation.

Alcoholic beverages supply calories but few or no nutrients. The alcohol in these beverages has effects that are harmful when consumed in excess. These effects of alcohol may alter judgment and can lead to dependency and a great many other serious health problems. Alcoholic beverages have been used to enhance the enjoyment of meals by many societies throughout human history. If adults choose to drink alcoholic beverages, they should consume them only in moderation (Box 16).

Current evidence suggests that moderate drinking is associated with a lower risk for coronary heart disease in some individuals. However, higher levels of alcohol intake raise the risk for high blood pressure, stroke, heart disease, certain cancers, accidents, violence, suicides, birth defects, and over-

all mortality (deaths). Too much alcohol may cause cirrhosis of the liver, inflammation of the pancreas, and damage to the brain and heart. Heavy drinkers also are at risk of malnutrition because alcohol contains calories that may substitute for those in more nutritious foods.

Box 16: What is moderation?

Moderation is defined as no more than one drink per day for women and no more than two drinks per day for men.
Count as a drink—
- 12 ounces of regular beer (150 calories)
- 5 ounces of wine (100 calories)
- 1.5 ounces of 80-proof distilled spirits (100 calories)

Who should not drink?

Some people should not drink alcoholic beverages at all. These include

- Children and adolescents.
- Individuals of any age who cannot restrict their drinking to moderate levels. This is a special concern for recovering alcoholics and people whose family members have alcohol problems.
- Women who are trying to conceive or who are pregnant. Major birth defects, including fetal alcohol syndrome, have been attributed to heavy drinking by the mother while pregnant. While there is no conclusive evidence that an occasional drink is harmful to the fetus or to the pregnant woman, a safe level of alcohol intake during pregnancy has not been established.
- Individuals who plan to drive or take part in activities that require attention or skill. Most people retain some alcohol in the blood up to 2-3 hours after a single drink.
- Individuals using prescription and over-the-counter medications. Alcohol may alter the effectiveness or toxicity of medicines. Also, some medications may increase blood alcohol levels or increase the adverse effect of alcohol on the brain.

Advice for Today

If you drink alcoholic beverages, do so in moderation, with meals, and when consumption does not put you or others at risk.

Acknowledgments

The US Department of Health and Human Services and the US Department of Agriculture acknowledge the recommendations of the Dietary Guidelines Advisory Committee—the basis for this edition. The Committee consisted of Doris Howes Calloway, PhD (chair), Richard J. Havel, MD (vice-chair), Dennis M. Bier, MD, William H. Dietz, MD, PhD, Cutberto Garza, MD, PhD, Shiriki K. Kumanyika, PhD, RD, Marion Nestle, PhD, MPH, Irwin H. Rosenberg, MD, Sachiko T. St. Jeor, PhD, RD, Barbara O. Schneeman, PhD, and John W. Suttie, PhD The Departments also acknowledge the staff work of the executive secretaries to the committee: Karil Bialostosky, MS, and Linda

Meyers, PhD, from HHS; Eileen Kennedy, DSc, RD, and Debra Reed, MS, from USDA.

For Additional Information on Nutrition

Center for Nutrition Policy and Promotion
USDA
1120 20th St, NW, Ste 200 North Lobby
Washington, DC 20036

Food and Nutrition Information Center
USDA/National Agricultural Library
Room 304, 10301 Baltimore Blvd
Beltsville, MD 20705-2351
E-mail: fnic@nalusda.gov

Cancer Information Service
Office of Cancer Communications
National Cancer Institute
Building 31, Room 10A16, 9000 Rockville Pike
Bethesda, MD 20892.
E-mail: icic@aspensys.com

National Heart, Lung, and Blood Institute Information Center
PO Box 30105
Bethesda, MD 20824-0105.
Gopher: gopher://gopher.nhlbi.nih.gov/
E-mail: nhlbic@dgs.dgysys.com

Weight-Control Information Network (WIN) of the National Institute of Diabetes and Digestive and Kidney Diseases
1 WIN Way
Bethesda, MD 20892.
E-mail: winniddk@aol.com

National Institute on Alcohol Abuse and Alcoholism
600 Executive Blvd, Ste 409
Bethesda, MD 20892-7003.

National Institute on Aging Information Center
National Institutes of Health
Building 31, Room 5C27
Bethesda, MD 20892.

Office of Food Labeling
Food and Drug Administration (HFS-150)
200 C St, SW
Washington, DC 20204.

Contact your county extension home economist (cooperative extension system) or a nutrition professional in your local public health department, hospital, American Red Cross, dietetic association, diabetes association, heart association, or cancer society.

Persons with disabilities who require alternative means for communication of program information (Braille, large print, audiotape, etc.) should contact the USDA Office of Communications at 202-720-2791.

■ **Document Source:**
U.S. Department of Health and Human Services, Public Health Service and the
Department of Agriculture
Home and Garden Bulletin No. 232
Fourth Edition, December 1995

PHYSICAL ACTIVITY AND WEIGHT CONTROL

Regular physical activity is an important part of effective weight loss and weight maintenance. It also can help prevent several diseases and improve your overall health. It does not matter what type of physical activity you perform—sports, planned exercise, household chores, yard work, or work-related tasks—all are beneficial. Studies show that even the most inactive people can gain significant health benefits if they accumulate 30 minutes or more of physical activity per day. Based on these findings, the U.S. Public Health Service has identified increased physical activity as a priority in Healthy People 2000, our national objectives to improve the health of Americans by the year 2000.

Research consistently shows that regular physical activity, combined with healthy eating habits, is the most efficient and healthful way to control your weight. Whether you are trying to lose weight or maintain it, you should understand the important role of physical activity and include it in your lifestyle.

How can physical activity help control my weight?

Physical activity helps to control your weight by using excess calories that otherwise would be stored as fat. Your body weight is regulated by the number of calories you eat and use each day. Everything you eat contains calories, and everything you do uses calories, including sleeping, breathing, and digesting food. Any physical activity in addition to what you normally do will use extra calories.

Balancing the calories you use through physical activity with the calories you eat will help you achieve your desired weight. When you eat more calories than you need to perform your day's activities, your body stores the extra calories and you gain weight (a). When you eat fewer calories than you use, your body uses the stored calories and you lose weight (b). When you eat the same amount of calories as your body uses, your weight stays the same (c).

Any type of physical activity you choose to do—strenuous activities such as running or aerobic dancing or moderate-intensity activities such as walking or household work—will increase the number of calories your body uses. The key to successful weight control and improved overall health is making physical activity a part of your daily routine.

What are the health benefits of physical activity?

In addition to helping to control your weight, research shows that regular physical activity can reduce your risk for several diseases and conditions and improve your overall quality of life. Regular physical activity can help protect you from the following health problems.

- Heart Disease and Stroke. Daily physical activity can help prevent heart disease and stroke by strengthening your heart muscle, lowering your blood pressure, raising your high-density lipoprotein (HDL) levels (good cholesterol) and lowering low-density lipoprotein (LDL) levels (bad cholesterol), improving blood flow, and increasing your heart's working capacity.
- High Blood Pressure. Regular physical activity can reduce blood pressure in those with high blood pressure levels. Physical activity also reduces body fatness, which is associated with high blood pressure.
- Noninsulin-Dependent Diabetes. By reducing body fatness, physical activity can help to prevent and control this type of diabetes.
- Obesity. Physical activity helps to reduce body fat by building or preserving muscle mass and improving the body's ability to use calories. When physical activity is combined with proper nutrition, it can help control weight and prevent obesity, a major risk factor for many diseases.
- Back Pain. By increasing muscle strength and endurance and improving flexibility and posture, regular exercise helps to prevent back pain.
- Osteoporosis. Regular weight-bearing exercise promotes bone formation and may prevent many forms of bone loss associated with aging.

Studies on the psychological effects of exercise have found that regular physical activity can improve your mood and the way you feel about yourself. Researchers also have found that exercise is likely to reduce depression and anxiety and help you to better manage stress.

Keep these health benefits in mind when deciding whether or not to exercise. And remember, any amount of physical activity you do is better than none at all.

How much should I exercise?

For the greatest overall health benefits, experts recommend that you do 20 to 30 minutes of aerobic activity three or more times a week and some type of muscle strengthening activity and stretching at least twice a week. However, if you are unable to do this level of activity, you can gain substantial health benefits by accumulating 30 minutes or more of moderate-intensity physical activity a day, at least five times a week.

If you have been inactive for a while, you may want to start with less strenuous activities such as walking or swimming at a comfortable pace. Beginning at a slow pace will allow you to become physically fit without straining your body. Once you are in better shape, you can gradually do more strenuous activity.

Moderate-Intensity Activity

Moderate-intensity activities include some of the things you may already be doing during a day or week, such as gardening and housework. These activities can be done in short spurts—10 minutes here, 8 minutes there. Alone, each action does not have a great effect on your health, but regularly accumulating

30 minutes of activity over the course of the day can result in substantial health benefits.

To become more active throughout your day, take advantage of any chance to get up and move around. Here are some examples:

- Take a short walk around the block
- Rake leaves
- Play actively with the kids
- Walk up the stairs instead of taking the elevator
- Mow the lawn
- Take an activity break — get up and stretch or walk around
- Park your car a little farther away from your destination and walk the extra distance

The point is not to make physical activity an unwelcome chore, but to make the most of the opportunities you have to be active.

Aerobic Activity

Aerobic activity is an important addition to moderate-intensity exercise. Aerobic exercise is any extended activity that makes you breathe hard while using the large muscle groups at a regular, even pace. Aerobic activities help make your heart stronger and more efficient. They also use more calories than other activities. Some examples of aerobic activities include:

- Brisk walking
- Jogging
- Bicycling
- Swimming
- Aerobic dancing
- Racket sports
- Rowing
- Ice or roller skating
- Cross-country or downhill skiing
- Using aerobic equipment (i.e., treadmill, stationary bike)

To get the most health benefits from aerobic activity, you should exercise at a level strenuous enough to raise your heart rate to your target zone. Your target heart rate zone is 50 to 75 percent of your maximum heart rate (the fastest your heart can beat). To find your target zone, look for the category closest to your age in the chart below and read across the line. For example, if you are 35 years old, your target heart rate zone is 93-138 beats per minute.

Age	Target Heart Rate Zone 50-75%	Average Maximum Heart Rate 100%
20-30 years	98-146 beats per min	195
31-40 years	93-138 beats per min.	185
41-50 years	88-131 beats per min	175
51-60 years	83-123 beats per min.	165
61+ years	78-116 beats per min.	155

To see if you are exercising within your target heart rate zone, count the number of pulse beats at your wrist or neck for 15 seconds, then multiply by four to get the beats per minute. Your heart should be beating within your target heart rate zone. If your heart is beating faster than your target heart rate, you are exercising too hard and should slow down. If your heart is beating slower than your target heart rate, you should exercise a little harder.

When you begin your exercise program, aim for the lower part of your target zone (50 percent). As you get into better shape, slowly build up to the higher part of your target zone (75 percent). If exercising within your target zone seems too hard, exercise at a pace that is comfortable for you.

You will find that, with time, you will feel more comfortable exercising and can slowly increase to your target zone.

Stretching and Muscle Strengthening Exercises

Stretching and strengthening exercises such as weight training should also be a part of your physical activity program. In addition to using calories, these exercises strengthen your muscles and bones and help prevent injury.

Tips to a Safe and Successful Physical Activity Program

Make sure you are in good health. Answer the following questions* before you begin exercising.

1. Has a doctor ever said you have heart problems?
2. Do you frequently suffer from chest pains?
3. Do you often feel faint or have dizzy spells?
4. Has a doctor ever said you have high blood pressure?
5. Has a doctor ever told you that you have a bone or joint problem, such as arthritis, that has been or could be aggravated by exercise?
6. Are you over the age of 65 and not accustomed to exercise?
7. Are you taking prescription medications, such as those for high blood pressure?
8. Is there a good medical reason, not mentioned here, why you should not exercise?

*Source: British Columbia Department of Health

If you answered "yes" to any of these questions, you should see your doctor before you begin an exercise program.

- Follow a gradual approach to exercise to get the most benefits with the fewest risks. If you have not been exercising, start at a slow pace and as you become more fit, gradually increase the amount of time and the pace of your activity.
- Choose activities that you enjoy and that fit your personality. For example, if you like team sports or group activities, choose things such as soccer or aerobics. If you prefer individual activities, choose things such as swimming or walking. Also, plan your activities for a time of day that suits your personality. If you are a morning person, exercise before you begin the rest of your day's activities. If you have more energy in the evening, plan activities that can be done at the end of the day. You will be more likely to stick to a physical activity program if it is convenient and enjoyable.

- Exercise regularly. To gain the most health benefits it is important to exercise as regularly as possible. Make sure you choose activities that will fit into your schedule.
- Exercise at a comfortable pace. For example, while jogging or walking briskly you should be able to hold a conversation. If you do not feel normal again within 10 minutes following exercise, you are exercising too hard. Also, if you have difficulty breathing or feel faint or weak during or after exercise, you are exercising too hard.
- Maximize your safety and comfort. Wear shoes that fit and clothes that move with you, and always exercise in a safe location. Many people walk in indoor shopping malls for exercise. Malls are climate controlled and offer protection from bad weather.
- Vary your activities. Choose a variety of activities so you don't get bored with any one thing.
- Encourage your family or friends to support you and join you in your activity. If you have children, it is best to build healthy habits when they are young. When parents are active, children are more likely to be active and stay active for the rest of their lives.
- Challenge yourself. Set short-term as well as long-term goals and celebrate every success, no matter how small.

Whether your goal is to control your weight or just to feel healthier, becoming physically active is a step in the right direction. Take advantage of the health benefits that regular exercise can offer and make physical activity a part of your lifestyle.

Additional Resources

The following organizations have materials on physical activity and weight control available to the public.

President's Council on Physical Fitness and Sports
701 Pennsylvania Ave, NW
Ste 250
Washington, DC 20004
Phone: (202) 272-3421

National Heart, Lung, and Blood Institute Information Center
PO Box 30105
Bethesda, MD 20824-0105
Phone: (301) 251-1222

American College of Sports Medicine P.O. Box 1440
Indianapolis, IN 46206-1440
Phone: (317) 637-9200

Weight-control Information Network
1 WIN WAY
Bethesda, MD 20892-3665
Internet: WIN@matthewsgroup.com
Toll-free Number: (800) WIN-8098

The Weight-Control Information Network (WIN) is a service of the National Institute of Diabetes and Digestive and Kidney Diseases, part of the National Institutes of Health. Authorized by Congress (Public Law 103-43). WIN assembles and disseminates to health professionals and the general public information on weight control, obesity, and nutritional disorders. WIN responds to requests for information; develops, reviews, and distributes publications; and develops communication strategies to encourage individuals to achieve and maintain a healthy weight.

Publications produced by WIN are reviewed for scientific accuracy, content, and readability. Materials produced by other sources are also reviewed for scientific accuracy and are distributed, along with WIN publications, to answer requests.

■ Document Source:
U.S. Department of Health and Human Services, Public Health Service
National Institutes of Health
National Institute of Diabetes and Digestive and Kidney Diseases
NIH Publication No. 96-4031
April 1996

UNDERSTANDING ADULT OBESITY

Many Americans are at increased health risk because they are obese. The US Surgeon General, in a 1988 report on nutrition and health, estimated that one-fourth of adult Americans are overweight. Obesity is a known risk factor for chronic diseases including heart disease, diabetes, high blood pressure, stroke, and some forms of cancer.

This fact sheet provides basic information about obesity: what it is, what causes it, how to measure it. Companion fact sheets provide more in-depth information about some aspects addressed briefly here, such as health risks of obesity and treatment options for the condition.

How is obesity measured?

Everyone needs a certain amount of body fat for stored energy, heat insulation, shock absorption, and other functions. As a rule, women have more fat than men. Doctors generally agree that men with more than 25 percent body fat and women with more than 30 percent body fat are obese. Precisely measuring a person's body fat, however, is not easy. The most accurate method is to weigh a person underwater—a procedure limited to laboratories with sophisticated equipment.

There are two simpler methods for estimating body fat, but they can yield inaccurate results if done by an inexperienced person or if done on someone with severe obesity. One is to measure skinfold thickness in several parts of the body. The second involves sending a harmless amount of electric current through a person's body (bioelectric impedance analysis). Both methods are commonly used in health clubs and in commercial weight-loss programs, but results should be viewed skeptically.

Because measuring a person's body fat is tricky, doctors often rely on other means to diagnose obesity. Two widely used measurements are weight-for-height tables and body mass index. While both measurements have their limitations, they are reliable indicators that someone may have a weight problem. They are easy to calculate and require no special equipment.

Weight-for-Height Tables

Most people are familiar with weight-for-height tables. Doctors have used these tables for decades to determine whether a person is overweight. The tables usually have a range of acceptable weights for a person of a given height.

One problem with using weight-for-height tables is that doctors disagree over which is the best table to use. Many versions are available, all with different weight ranges. Some tables take a person's frame size, age, and sex into account; others do not. A limitation of all weight-for-height tables is that they do not distinguish excess fat from muscle. A very muscular person may appear obese, according to the tables, when he or she is not. Still, weight-for-height tables can be used as general guidelines.

The table printed here is from the 1990 edition of *Dietary Guidelines for Americans,* a pamphlet printed jointly by the U.S. Departments of Agriculture and Health and Human Services. This table has a wide range for what the pamphlet calls "healthy" or "suggested" weights.

In this table, the higher weights generally apply to men, who tend to have more muscle and bone. The lower weights more often apply to women, who have less muscle and bone. The table also shows higher weights for people age 35 and older, which some experts question.

Height[1]	Weight in pounds[2,3]	
	19 to 34 years	35 years and over
5'0"	97–128	108–138
5'1"	101–132	111–143
5'2"	104–137	115–148
5'3"	107–141	119–152
5'4"	111–146	122–157
5'5"	114–150	126–162
5'6"	118–155	130–167
5'7"	121–160	134–172
5'8"	125–164	138–178
5'9"	129–169	142–183
5'10"	132–174	146–188
5'11"	136–179	151–194
6'0"	140–184	155–199
6'1"	144–184	159–199
6'2"	148–195	164–210
6'3"	152–200	168–216
6'4"	156–205	173–222
6'5"	160–211	177–228
6'6"	164–216	182–234

[1]Without shoes.
[2]Without clothes.
[3]The higher weights in the ranges generally apply to men, who tend to have more muscle and bone; the lower weights more often apply to women, who have less muscle and bone.

Body Mass Index (BMI)

Body mass index, or BMI, is a new term to most people. However, it is the measurement of choice for many physicians and researchers studying obesity. BMI uses a mathematical formula that takes into account both a person's height and weight. BMI equals a person's weight in kilograms divided by height in meters squared. (BMI = kg/m2).

In general, a person age 35 or older is obese if he or she has a BMI of 27 or more. For people age 34 or younger, a BMI of 25 or more indicates obesity. A BMI of more than 30 usually is considered a sign of moderate to severe obesity.

The BMI measurement poses some of the same problems as the weight-for-height tables. Doctors don't agree on the cutoff points for "healthy" versus "unhealthy" BMI ranges. BMI also does not provide information on a person's percentage of body fat. However, like the weight-for-height table, BMI is a useful general guideline.

Body Fat Distribution: 'Pears' vs. 'Apples'

Doctors are concerned with not only how much fat a person has but where the fat is on the body.

Women typically collect fat in their hips and buttocks, giving their figures a "pear" shape. Men, on the other hand, usually build up fat around their bellies, giving them more of an "apple" shape. This is not a hard and fast rule, though. Some men are pear-shaped and some women become apple-shaped, especially after menopause.

People whose fat is concentrated mostly in the abdomen are more likely to develop many of the health problems associated with obesity.

Doctors have developed a simple way to measure whether someone is an apple or a pear. The measurement is called waist-to-hip ratio.

Waist-to-Hip Ratio

To find out someone's waist-to-hip ratio, measure the waist at its narrowest point, then measure the hips at the widest point. Divide the waist measurement by the hip measurement. A woman with a 35-inch waist and 46-inch hips would do the following calculation: 35 divided by 46 = 0.76

Women with waist-to-hip ratios of more than 0.8 or men with waist-to-hip ratios of more than 1.0 are "apples." They are at increased health risk because of their fat distribution.

What causes obesity?

In scientific terms, obesity occurs when a person's calorie intake exceeds the amount of energy he or she burns. What causes this imbalance between consuming and burning calories is unclear. Evidence suggests that obesity often has more than one cause. Genetic, environmental, psychological, and other factors all may play a part.

Genetic Factors

Obesity tends to run in families, suggesting that it may have a genetic cause. However, family members share not only genes but also diet and lifestyle habits that may contribute to obesity. Separating these lifestyle factors from genetic ones is often difficult. Still, growing evidence points to heredity as a strong determining factor of obesity. In one study of adults who were adopted as children, researchers found that the subjects' adult weights were closer to their biological parents' weights than their adoptive parents'. The environment provided by the adoptive family apparently had less influence on the development of obesity than the person's genetic makeup.

Nevertheless, people who feel that their genes have doomed them to a lifetime of obesity should take heart. As discussed in the next section, many people genetically predisposed to obesity do not become obese or manage to lose weight and keep it off.

Environmental Factors

Although genes are an important factor in many cases of obesity, a person's environment also plays a significant part. Environment includes lifestyle behaviors such as what a person eats and how active he or she is.

Americans tend to have high-fat diets, often putting taste and convenience ahead of nutritional content when choosing meals. Most Americans also don't get enough exercise.

People can't change their genetic makeup, of course, but they can change what they eat and how active they are. Some people have been able to lose weight and keep it off by:

- Learning how to choose more nutritious meals that are lower in fat.
- Learning to recognize environmental cues (such as enticing smells) that may make them want to eat when they are not hungry.
- Becoming more physically active.

Psychological Factors

Psychological factors also may influence eating habits. Many people eat in response to negative emotions such as boredom, sadness, or anger.

While most overweight people have no more psychological disturbance than normalweight people, about 30 percent of the people who seek treatment for serious weight problems have difficulties with binge eating. During a binge eating episode, people eat large amounts of food while feeling they can't control how much they are eating. Those with the most severe binge eating problems are considered to have binge eating disorder. These people may have more difficulty losing weight and keeping the weight off than people without binge eating problems. Some will need special help, such as counseling or medication, to control their binge eating before they can successfully manage their weight.

Other Causes of Obesity

Some rare illnesses can cause obesity. These include hypothyroidism, Cushing's syndrome, depression, and certain neurologic problems that can lead to overeating. Certain drugs, such as steroids and some antidepressants, may cause excessive weight gain. A doctor can determine if a patient has any of these conditions, which are believed to be responsible for only about 1 percent of all cases of obesity.

What are the consequences of obesity?

Health Risks

Obesity is not just a cosmetic problem. It's a health hazard. Someone who is 40 percent overweight is twice as likely to die prematurely as an average-weight person. (This effect is seen after 10 to 30 years of being obese.)

Obesity has been linked to several serious medical conditions, including diabetes, heart disease, high blood pressure, and stroke. It is also associated with higher rates of certain types of cancer. Obese men are more likely than nonobese men to die from cancer of the colon, rectum, and prostate. Obese women are more likely than nonobese women to die from cancer of the gallbladder, breast, uterus, cervix, and ovaries.

Other diseases and health problems linked to obesity include

- Gallbladder disease and gallstones.
- Osteoarthritis, a disease in which the joints deteriorate, possibly as a result of excess weight on the joints.
- Gout, another disease affecting the joints.
- Pulmonary (breathing) problems, including sleep apnea, in which a person can stop breathing for a short time during sleep.

Doctors generally agree that the more obese a person is, the more likely he or she is to have health problems.

Psychological and Social Effects

One of the most painful aspects of obesity may be the emotional suffering it causes. American society places great emphasis on physical appearance, often equating attractiveness with slimness, especially in women. The messages, intended or not, make overweight people feel unattractive. Many people assume that obese people are gluttonous, lazy, or both. However, more and more evidence contradicts this assumption.

Obese people often face prejudice or discrimination at work, at school, while looking for a job, and in social situations. Feelings of rejection, shame, or depression are common.

Who should lose weight?

Doctors generally agree that people who are 20 percent or more overweight, especially the severely obese person, can gain significant health benefits from weight loss.

Many obesity experts believe that people who are less than 20 percent above their healthy weight should try to lose weight if they have any of the following risk factors.

Risk Factors

- Family history of certain chronic diseases. People with close relatives who have had heart disease or diabetes are more likely to develop these problems if they are obese.

- Pre-existing medical conditions. High blood pressure, high cholesterol levels, or high blood sugar levels are all warning signs of some obesity-associated diseases.
- "Apple" shape. People whose weight is concentrated around their abdomens may be at greater risk of heart disease, diabetes, or cancer than people of the same weight who are pear-shaped.

Fortunately, even a modest weight loss of 10 to 20 pounds can bring significant health improvements, such as lowering one's blood pressure and cholesterol levels.

How is obesity treated?

Treatment options for obesity are explored in depth in other fact sheets. The method of treatment will depend on how obese a person is. Factors such as an individual's overall health and motivation to lose weight are also important considerations. Treatment may include a combination of diet, exercise, and behavior modification. In some cases of severe obesity, gastrointestinal surgery may be recommended.

Research on Obesity

The National Institute of Diabetes and Digestive and Kidney Diseases (NIDDK) is the part of the National Institutes of Health chiefly responsible for obesity research. NIDDK supports the study of obesity in its own labs and clinics and at universities, hospitals, and research centers across the United States. NIDDK-funded research has helped scientists learn more about the role of genes and metabolism in obesity. Other NIDDK-supported studies have examined the relationship between obesity and various medical conditions. Ongoing NIDDK research efforts include better ways to define and treat the various types of obesity and understanding how the body stores and uses fat.

NIDDK also oversees the National Task Force on Prevention and Treatment of Obesity. The task force comprises leading obesity and nutrition experts who gather and assess the latest information on obesity treatment and prevention. The task force also helps guide basic and clinical research on obesity. Scientific papers and general-interest brochures and pamphlets approved by the task force are available from the NIDDK's Obesity Resource Information Center.

In addition to NIDDK, other sections of the NIH sponsor obesity research. They include

- The National Heart, Lung, and Blood Institute (NHLBI)
- The National Center for Research Resources (NCRR)
- The National Institute of Child Health and Human Development (NICHD)
- The National Institute on Mental Health (NIMH)
- The National Cancer Institute (NCI)
- The National Institute on Aging (NIA)
- The National Institute of Nursing Research (NINR)
- The National Institute of Arthritis and Musculoskeletal and Skin Diseases (NIAMS)

- The National Institute of Neurological Diseases and Stroke (NINDS)
- The National Institute of Environmental and Health Sciences (NIEHS).

Additional Reading on Obesity

"Are You Eating Right?" *Consumer Reports,* October 1992. This article summarizes advice from 68 nutrition experts, including a discussion on weight control and health risks of obesity. Available in public libraries.

Bray, G.A. "Pathophysiology of Obesity." *American Journal of Clinical Nutrition.* 1992; Supplement to Vol. 55 (2): 488S-494S. This article comes from the proceedings of an NIH Consensus Development Conference on Gastrointestinal Surgery for Severe Obesity. Written for health professionals in technical language. Available in medical libraries.

"Dietary Guidelines for Americans." Fourth Edition, 1995. Home and Garden Bulletin No. 232. This pamphlet, issued by the U.S. Agriculture and Health and Human Services Departments, contains information about maintaining a healthy weight, as well as dietary and nutrition recommendations. Available through the Government Printing Office.

"Exercise and Weight Control." The President's Council on Physical Fitness and Sports, Department of Health and Human Services. This brochure discusses the difference between being "overweight" and "overfat" and the role diet and exercise can play in a weight loss program. Copies can be obtained from the President's Council on Physical Fitness and Sports, Dept. No. 176, 701 Pennsylvania Ave NW, Washington, DC 20004.

"The Facts About Weight Loss Products and Programs." This brochure, produced by the Federal Trade Commission in conjunction with the Food and Drug Administration and the National Association of Attorneys General, has tips on evaluating diet claims and weight loss programs. Copies can be obtained from the FTC, Public Affairs Branch, Room 130, Sixth St. and Pennsylvania Ave NW, Washington, DC 20580.

"Getting Slim." *U.S. News & World Report,* May 14, 1990. This article, written for the general public, discusses definitions of obesity, the role of genes, body mass index, and apple/pear weight distribution patterns. Available in public libraries.

Long, P. "The Great Weight Debate." *Health.* February/March, 1992, pp. 42-47. This article, written for the general public, discusses the controversy over which weight-for-height table is best to use. It also provides some simple guidelines for determining whether someone needs to lose weight. Available in public libraries.

"Methods for Voluntary Weight Loss and Control." National Institutes of Health Technology Assessment Conference Statement, March 30-April 1, 1992. This publication, written for health professionals, summarizes findings of a conference discussing success rates of various methods of weight loss, short-term and long-term effects of losing weight, and related topics. Copies are available from the Office of Medical Applications Research, National Institutes of Health, Federal Building, Room 618, Bethesda, MD 20892.

Yanovski, S.Z. "A Practical Approach to Treatment of the Obese Patient." *Archives of Family Medicine.* 1993; Vol. 2, No. 3, pp 309-316. Written for health professionals, this article provides guidance on evaluating overweight patients and developing plans for treatment.

■ **Document Source:**
U.S. Department of Health and Human Services, Public Health Service
National Institutes of Health
National Institute of Diabetes and Digestive and Kidney Diseases
NIH Publication No. 94-3680
November 1993

See also: Choosing a Safe and Successful Weight-Loss Program (page 442); Gastric Surgery for Severe Obesity (page 443); Physical Activity and Weight Control (page 456)

SKIN DISEASES AND DISORDERS

■ ■ ■

A GUIDE TO UNDERSTANDING PSORIASIS

Introduction

The National Psoriasis Foundation (NPF) of the United States is dedicated to educating people about psoriasis. The NPF published "A Guide To Understanding Psoriasis" to give you a basic awareness of psoriasis and its treatments. But each person's psoriasis is unique, and it is difficult to address every issue in this booklet. Most likely, you will discover topics that you wish to explore further and new questions will arise. That's why the NPF offers numerous educational booklets to answer your questions. Most of these booklets are highlighted throughout the "Guide" so that you are aware of this supplemental information. The NPF welcomes your inquiries and stands ready to assist you.

What is psoriasis?

Psoriasis is a chronic skin disorder and no one knows what causes it. We do know, however, that you cannot "catch" psoriasis; psoriasis is not contagious. There are many treatments for psoriasis but, to date, there isn't a cure. Psoriasis affects one to two percent of the population in the United States.

The most common form of psoriasis is called plaque psoriasis. It is characterized by raised, inflamed (red) lesions covered with a silvery white buildup of dead skin cells, called scale. The technical name for plaque psoriasis is psoriasis vulgaris (vulgaris means common). Though this booklet's focus is on plaque psoriasis, there are other forms of psoriasis. They are pustular, guttate, inverse, and erythrodermic psoriasis. The NPF publishes a booklet "Specific Forms of Psoriasis" that describes these forms of psoriasis.

What does psoriasis look like?

The initial lesions of plaque psoriasis might appear as red, dot-like spots and may be very small. These initial eruptions gradually enlarge and produce a silvery white surface scale. Surface scales come off easily and are shed constantly, but those below the surface of the skin are quite adherent. When forcibly removed, they may leave tiny bleeding points known as the Auspitz's sign.

The plaques may cover large areas of skin and merge into each other. Often, the lesions appear in the same place on the right and left sides of the body. Lesions vary in size and in shape from individual to individual.

How is psoriasis diagnosed?

Typically, psoriasis is diagnosed simply through observation—the inflamed lesion topped with silvery white scale. There are no blood tests for psoriasis; the diagnosis is made by a physician's examination of the skin lesions and occasionally by looking at a skin biopsy under a microscope. Sometimes, small pits in the fingernails can aid in diagnosing psoriasis.

African-Americans may not have the typical red, scaly patches. Their psoriasis may be the same color as the rest of their skin. The treatment is the same, however, for all races.

Who gets psoriasis?

Anyone can develop psoriasis, though heredity seems to play a role. There is a family association in one out of three cases.

Psoriasis appears in men and women in equal number. It can appear at any age, but appears most often between the ages of 15 and 35. In approximately 10-15 percent of individuals with psoriasis, the disease first appears before the age of ten. The disease is also reported in infants.

There are no personality types that have been identified as being more likely to develop psoriasis.

What causes psoriasis?

The cause of psoriasis is unknown. It is thought that some type of biochemical stimulus triggers the abnormal cell growth that characterizes psoriasis.

A normal skin cell matures in 28-30 days. In psoriasis, cells move to the top of the skin in three or four days. The excessive skin cells that are produced "heap up" and form the elevated, red, scaly lesions that characterize psoriasis. The white scale that covers the red lesion is composed of dead cells that are continually being cast off. The redness of the plaques is caused by the increased blood supply necessary to feed this area of dividing skin cells.

Skin injury, emotional stress, and some forms of infection are thought to help trigger its development. For example, psoriasis will sometimes appear at the site of a surgical incision, or may follow a drug reaction, or streptococcal throat infection. When injury to the skin leads to the appearance of psoriasis, it is known as the Koebner phenomenon.

The NPF's booklet "Psoriasis Research" provides detailed information on what is known about the biochemical nature of psoriasis and environmental factors that affect its course.

How serious is psoriasis?

The severity of psoriasis is measured in terms of its physical and its emotional impact. In physical terms, psoriasis is evaluated by the extent of body surface affected and its location on the body. If 10 percent of the body surface is involved, the case is usually considered mild. Ten to 30 percent is considered moderate; and more than 30 percent, severe. The palm of the hand equals one percent.

However, psoriasis can involve a small area of the body and have a serious impact on the person's ability to function. Psoriasis confined to the palms of the hands and soles of the feet, for example, can be severe enough to be physically disabling.

For most people, psoriasis remains limited to one or a few patches on the skin. The most common areas for psoriasis to appear are the scalp, elbow, knees, and trunk, though it can appear anywhere on the body.

When the disease affects major body surfaces, various physical problems can occur such as intense itching, skin pain, dry and cracking skin, and swelling. Body movement and flexibility can be affected.

In a few cases, severe types of psoriasis, such as pustular or erythrodermic psoriasis, can elevate body temperature to the point of placing strain on internal organs such as the heart and kidneys. In these instances, hospitalization is required to avoid complications which may threaten the person's life.

The emotional impact of psoriasis is as important to understand as the physical impact. Psoriasis can be unsightly and cause, or contribute to, low self-confidence and self-esteem. It may induce feelings of embarrassment, anger, depression, and guilt. Learning about psoriasis is the first step in coping effectively with this skin disorder. The NPF booklet that thoroughly discusses the emotional impact of psoriasis is "Psoriasis: How It Makes You Feel."

What is the normal course of psoriasis?

Normally, psoriasis goes through cycles of improvement and flares. Psoriasis can go into spontaneous remissions for reasons that are not understood. One study showed that two out of five patients indicated they had experienced remissions from the disease, lasting from 1 to 64 years.

One other consideration is psoriatic arthritis. About 10 percent of people with psoriasis develop this form of arthritis, which is similar to rheumatoid arthritis but generally milder. It causes inflammation and stiffness and frequently involves the fingers and toes. Psoriatic arthritis is treated by a derma-tologist, but sometimes the patient will be referred to a physician who specializes in treating arthritic disorders.

The NPF's booklet "Psoriatic Arthritis" specifically describes the symptoms and treatment for this condition.

Treatments for Psoriasis

There is not a cure for psoriasis at this time, but there are treatments that can, in most cases, temporarily clear the plaques or significantly improve the skin's appearance. The goal of psoriasis treatment is to clear psoriasis lesions from the skin. Once the treatment works, it is generally discontinued and resumed if the psoriasis returns.

The treatment used will depend upon several things: the type of psoriasis, location on the body, severity, the patient's age, and medical history.

Topical medications are used for mild to moderate psoriasis. These include emollients (moisturizers), steroids (cortisone-type medications), anthralin, various coal tar preparations, and vitamin D 3. These may be used alone, in combination, or with ultraviolet light (UVB). Regular sunbathing can clear psoriasis for some people because of the exposure to natural ultraviolet light.

Treatments for moderate to severe psoriasis include the topical medications already mentioned for mild to moderate psoriasis, ultraviolet light type B (UVB); PUVA (an oral or topical medication [psoralen] plus ultraviolet light type A); an oral or injected medication called methotrexate (MTX); and oral retinoid medications (Tegison and Accutane). These treatments may be used alone or in combination with each other. Systemic treatments for severe psoriasis are more toxic than topical treatments and their benefits must be weighed against their risks.

A rule of thumb in psoriasis therapy is to use the most effective therapy for an individual that poses the least amount of side effects. Generally, physicians will start with the least potent therapy and work up until one is found that will clear the psoriasis for the patient.

There is no single treatment that works for everyone who has psoriasis. Reactions to psoriasis treatments will vary from individual to individual. Often experimentation is required before an effective approach is discovered for the patient.

A treatment regimen may need periodic adjustment. A once-effective treatment can cease working which will necessitate switching to another therapy.

It is important to remember not to give up on treatment because of slow results. A commitment to lengthy treatment may be necessary to achieve clearance.

Emollients

The use of a lubricant on a regular schedule will help to restore moisture and flexibility to psoriatic skin. It can also help to reduce scaling, itching, and inflammation. There are a wide variety of emollients on the market. Generally, people select those that do not contain heavy perfumes, but are very mild.

Topical Steroids

Topical steroids are the most commonly prescribed therapy for treating localized areas of psoriasis. They come in various strengths, from very mild to very potent. The higher the strength the more effective the medication may be, but the possibility of side effects increases as well.

Steroids used to treat psoriasis are prescription medications. There are very low-strength hydrocortisone preparations that can be purchased over-the-counter (OTC) but they are not generally helpful in treating psoriasis.

Steroids are not usually effective in producing remission of severe psoriasis and can result in a "rebound" (the psoriasis comes back as bad or worse than before the treatment) of the disorder if used in large amounts.

Systemic (Internal) Steroids

Systemically administered steroids (internal administration of steroid medication by pill or muscular injection) are generally avoided in the treatment of psoriasis because of potentially serious side effects. Systemic steroids can also cause psoriasis to worsen, and, at times, precipitate life-threatening pustular forms of psoriasis.

Injected Intralesional Steroids

Injections of steroid medication directly into an isolated lesion (plaque) of psoriasis (called intralesional steroid injections) can be effective in clearing psoriasis lesions and seldom produce side effects. Also, a physician may give small doses of an oral steroid (such as prednisone) for a brief time to control a sudden flare.

Steroid medications are thoroughly discussed in the NPF's booklet of the same name.

Occlusion

Covering psoriasis lesions with a tape dressing, plastic wrap, or a special suit is called occlusion. Occlusion is sometimes used in conjunction with topical steroid medications. Sometimes lesions are covered with just a special tape dressing. Occasionally, if there is extensive psoriasis on the body and limbs, a special suit may be worn to enhance the effects of psoriasis medications or moisturizers.

Coal Tar

Crude coal tar or coal tar solutions are commonly used in the treatment of psoriasis. They may be prescription or over-the-counter medications.

Tar for the body can be applied directly to the affected area or it may be added to bath water to soak the whole body. It can also be used in combination with a topical steroid medication.

The tar preparation may be used in combination with ultraviolet light, type B (UVB). When coal tar is used in conjunction with UVB, the tar is left on the involved skin for a period of time, ranging from a couple of hours to overnight, prior to exposing the skin to the UVB light. The tar is removed from the skin prior to exposing the skin to the UVB light.

The NPF's booklet "Tar" details the use of coal tar for treating psoriasis on the body and scalp. Its use is also discussed in the booklet "Scalp Psoriasis."

Anthralin

Anthralin is a topical prescription compound that can be effective in clearing psoriasis. It is used in different concentrations. The higher-strength compounds cause staining of the skin and irritation, effects which make it difficult to use in the home. But lower-strength anthralin compounds have been developed which have made this therapy more tolerable. These new anthralin preparations can be used on both the body and scalp.

Anthralin is applied topically to the affected area and can be left on for a short period of time or overnight depending on the doctor's orders. Anthralin preparations are also used in combination with UVB. The NPF publishes a booklet on the use of anthralin that specifically details its use.

Vitamin D 3

Vitamin D 3, or calcipotriene, is the newest topical medication available for mild-moderate psoriasis. It was approved for use in the United States in 1994. It is a prescription medication that has few side effects if used as directed. It is odorless and nonstaining. Generally, it is applied to the lesions twice a day. This medication should not be used on the face or genitals because it can be irritating. It is not recommended for children or for use during pregnancy.

Vitamin D 3 is not the same as that found in commercial vitamin supplements taken orally. These commercial vitamin supplements should not be used to treat psoriasis, as ingesting large doses of over-the-counter vitamin D can lead to serious side effects.

Currently, the only available brand name of this medication is Dovonex. For more information, refer to the NPF booklet "Topical Vitamin D 3."

Other Topical Preparations

Salicylic acid is used to help remove scales and is often combined with steroids, anthralin, and tar to enhance their effectiveness. Salicylic acid is a prescription compound in higher strengths.

Oatmeal baths can be helpful in making the skin more comfortable and reducing the itching that might accompany psoriasis.

Ultraviolet Light, Type B (UVB)

UVB is a common choice for treating psoriasis. If the psoriasis is fairly extensive, physicians will generally initiate UVB treatments because it is considered to be effective and pose limited side effects. UVB has been used to treat psoriasis for many years.

UVB occurs naturally in sunlight, and it is that spectrum of the sunlight which causes sunburns. Artificial UVB is used to treat many skin disorders, including psoriasis.

UVB therapy can produce a temporary clearance in most psoriasis patients. The length of remission varies among individuals. Recent studies indicate that the remission is prolonged by maintenance UVB treatments.

The UVB can be administered to a particular area of the body or the entire body surface. The UVB can be given in a physician's office or home light units can be purchased.

UVB can be used alone, with emollients like petrolatum, or with over-the-counter or prescription tar preparations. Combined UVB and tar therapy is known as the Goeckerman regimen or modified Goeckerman regimen.

The NPF publishes booklets specifically on the use of "UVB" and "Home UVB." The Goeckerman regimen is fully described in the NPF's booklet on "Tar."

PUVA (Psoralen and Ultraviolet Light, Type A)

PUVA involves the combined use of a photosensitizing medication called psoralen and a long-wave ultraviolet light, UVA. The patient takes an oral dose of the psoralen medication (available only by prescription), which makes the skin sensitive to UVA light, and a short time later, exposes their skin to UVA light. There are also ways to use the psoralen medication topically, though the topical use isn't as common as the oral use.

PUVA is effective in 85-90 percent of patients and the length of remission varies from a few weeks to a year or more. In an NPF survey of PUVA patients, 68 percent said PUVA was the first therapy to clear their psoriasis. Once a person is clear, periodic treatment may be given to maintain a clearance, or treatments may resume only when the psoriasis returns.

The NPF's booklet on PUVA provides a detailed report about the ways in which PUVA is administered.

Methotrexate (MTX)

Methotrexate is a prescription, systemic drug used in small doses to clear severe and/or disabling psoriasis. Methotrexate is taken orally or given by injection.

Methotrexate is generally recommended only if other psoriasis therapies have not been effective or if other therapies are not tolerated by the patient for some reason. It is a potent drug that can cause serious side effects.

The NPF provides more detailed information about methotrexate in a booklet entitled "Methotrexate (MTX)."

Retinoid Therapy (Tegison and Accutane)

Tegison (generic name etretinate) is a prescription medication for treating severe, recalcitrant (stubbornly resistant) psoriasis. It is indicated when patients with severe psoriasis are unresponsive to standard therapies or, for some reason, cannot use other therapies. It is generally used in combination with other psoriasis treatments such as PUVA.

Because Tegison can cause birth defects, women of childbearing potential must use effective contraception throughout treatment and for an indefinite period of time after stopping Tegison. In fact, it is highly recommended that women DO NOT take this drug until their childbearing is absolutely completed.

Another form of this medication called acetretin (Soriatane) is awaiting approval by the FDA. Acetretin may pose fewer risks to women of childbearing age.

Accutane is another oral prescription medication sometimes used to control psoriasis. It, too, has the potential to cause birth defects, though childbearing is acceptable once the drug is discontinued and the woman has complied with a specific waiting period.

These childbearing side effects do not apply to males and conception. The NPF booklet "Retinoid Therapy: Tegison & Accutane" outlines the side effects of retinoids for both men and women. The NPF booklet "Conception, Pregnancy & Psoriasis" sheds further light on treatments to avoid when childbearing is an issue.

Other Treatments

New treatment developments are always featured in the NPF's national newsletter the *Bulletin*. If a treatment is prescribed for you that is not mentioned in this booklet, you may always contact the NPF about that specific treatment. The NPF has information on other less commonly used therapies, nontraditional treatments, and experimental medications as well.

Commonly-Asked Questions

Can psoriasis itch?

Yes, psoriasis often causes the skin to itch, sometimes intensely. It has been estimated that about 50 percent of those with psoriasis experience itching.

Various oral antihistamines and baths are often recommended to reduce the itching. The only guaranteed way to eliminate itching is to eliminate its cause—the psoriasis itself.

Can diet affect psoriasis?

To date, no specific dietary or herbal regimen has been identified through scientific investigation that will clear or improve psoriasis. More specific information can be obtained by requesting NPF's booklet "Your Diet & Psoriasis."

Does pregnancy and nursing have an effect on psoriasis?

Psoriasis sometimes goes into remission during pregnancy; other women experience a flare during pregnancy.

Women should talk to their doctor about the safety of anti-psoriasis therapies while nursing. There has been concern reported in medical journals that steroids can be excreted in milk and can adversely affect your baby. Therefore, the use of topical steroids when nursing must be carefully supervised.

The NPF's booklet "Conception, Pregnancy & Psoriasis" provides complete information about this aspect of psoriasis.

Does weather affect psoriasis?

The lesions can be affected by the seasons. Most people who have psoriasis get worse during the winter months and improve in the summer. It is presumed this is a result of the availability of natural sunlight.

What can cause psoriasis to worsen?

Psoriasis will often appear following physical and/or emotional trauma. Drug reactions and infections can lead to an appearance or worsening of psoriasis. Drugs that have been identified as having the potential to worsen psoriasis in some cases are: antimalarial drugs; Inderal and other beta blocker medications to control high blood pressure; lithium; Quinidine (a heart medication), and prolonged use of topical and systemic steroids. More information on these drugs is provided in the NPF's booklet "Practical Information About Psoriasis."

If someone plans to spend long hours in the sun, it is recommended that a sunscreen be used on the unaffected areas of skin. Also, avoid burning as that can cause psoriasis to worsen.

Does emotional stress cause psoriasis?

There is no evidence that stress is a direct cause of psoriasis, but studies have shown that psoriasis can be aggravated by emotional stress in some individuals.

Can suntan parlors be used to treat psoriasis?

Consult a dermatologist before using the lights in a suntan parlor. There are various medications that make people sensitive to ultraviolet light and which can produce burns. Some diseases, such as lupus erythematosus, are worsened by ultraviolet light and people with those diseases should not be exposed to UVB light. UVA light used alone is not very effective against psoriasis. Ask the parlor operators what light spectrums you will be receiving. You want the most UVB available. Some states have laws banning UVB from suntan parlors.

Is someone who has psoriasis protected from job discrimination?

Depending on the type of employment and the particular state in which someone lives, there are generally state and federal laws that protect an employee from being terminated for reasons not related to job performance or job qualifications.

Can psoriasis be disabling?

Psoriasis can result in job disability. The Social Security Administration (SSA) will grant job disability because of psoriasis under certain circumstances. These circumstances, as defined by the SSA, are when the skin is:

"with extensive lesions, including involvement of the hands and feet, which impose a severe limitation of function and which are not responding to prescribed treatment."

The NPF provides informal guidelines on things to consider in applying for disability.

Can someone with psoriasis serve in the military?

Psoriasis normally disqualifies an individual from military service.

Can alcohol consumption worsen psoriasis?

There does not seem to be any pattern. Studies have not discovered a link between alcohol consumption and flares of psoriasis. Individuals have observed a worsening of psoriasis with alcohol consumption; others note it does not seem to make a difference.

Can psoriasis be associated with any other disease?

To date, no other disease, with the exception of psoriatic arthritis, has been associated with psoriasis. Psoriasis, however, can appear simultaneously with any other disease.

Should scales be removed before applying topical medications?

Yes. It is important to remove the scales from psoriasis since they block the penetration of medications and ultraviolet light. The scales should be removed carefully either by hydration (use of water) or by medication that softens the skin. Hydration can be done simply by soaking in a tub of water. Softening medications include creams containing one or more of the following common ingredients: propylene glycol, glycerin, salicylic acid, lactic acid and urea.

Tips to Help Your Skin

- Keep your skin lubricated. Oils, creams, and petroleum jelly preparations are good moisturizers or emollients. During the winter months, low temperatures and humidity draw moisture from the skin, and can result in discomfort and itching.
- Use a humidifier in the home. When the air is dry from home heating, a humidifier may be helpful.
- Take advantage of the sunshine when possible. Sunlight will clear psoriasis for some people if obtained in sufficient doses on a regular basis. The use of oils and lubricants may enhance the effects of the natural ultraviolet light. For more information about treating psoriasis with sunlight, request the NPF's educational booklet "Sunshine & Psoriasis."
- Bathing in hot water may help reduce scaling. Some people report a flattening of their plaques or reduced scaling from soaking in hot water.
- Minimize contact with soap and chemicals. Use mild soaps or soap-free cleansers. Consult your physician or pharmacist for guidance.
- Minimize stress. Though NPF is not aware of any study on the benefits of exercise, some people observe that their psoriasis improves when they exercise regularly. The relaxing effects of exercise may lead to the skin's improvement. Consult a professional to develop an appropriate exercise program for you.

- Protect against skin injuries. This includes skin irritations like soap under a ring, tight waistbands or shaving with a dull razor. Harsh chemicals and cosmetics, such as depilatories (preparations used to remove hair from the body), can increase redness and scaling.
- Protect yourself from infections. Children, especially, should try to avoid exposure to throat infections which may make psoriasis worse.
- Check in with the NPF or your physician occasionally if you are not actively treating your psoriasis. Many people with psoriasis drop out of treatment and just learn to live with it. By staying informed, you know about new treatment options, are more likely to find something you've never tried, and/or discover a treatment that didn't work once, will work now. It is worthwhile to keep an open mind.
- Call or write the NPF. The NPF is a valuable resource for people who have psoriasis and their families. If you need information, a physician recommendation, or just want to compare notes with someone else who has psoriasis, don't hesitate to write or call. NPF is here for you.

How to Stay Informed

A Guide To Understanding Psoriasis, provides basic information about psoriasis, but continuing education is a vital part of living with a chronic skin disease. The NPF keeps members informed about treatment choices and psoriasis research. Members benefit from others' experiences, make fact-based decisions, and have a genuine understanding of their skin disorder.

Join the NPF by making a yearly donation of any amount. The NPF's mission is to meet the needs of people with psoriasis and to support psoriasis research to find a cure. We need your help to continue our efforts.

National Psoriasis Foundation® *A Guide To Understanding Psoriasis* is published as an educational service and is not intended to replace the counsel of a physician. NPF advises that you consult a physician before initiating any treatment. The NPF does not endorse any medications, products, or treatments for psoriasis.

The NPF is a 501(c)(3) nonprofit, lay organization working to improve the quality of life of people with psoriasis. Tax-deductible donations support the NPF's public education and research programs. The NPF's annual report is available by writing or calling NPF.

■ **Document Source:**
National Psoriasis Foundation
6600 SW 92nd Ave, Ste 300
Portland, OR 97223-7195
(503) 244-7404
Fax (503) 245-0626
Copyright, National Psoriasis Foundation, Inc.
1995

TREATING ACNE

by John Henkel

Acne.

The very word is enough to halt most teenagers in their tracks. Yet rare is the adolescent who can escape the skin disorder completely.

"It is almost universal," says Alan R. Shalita, MD, chairman of the dermatology department at State University of New York. Shalita and other experts estimate that 85 percent of the U.S. population between the ages of 12 and 25 suffers from some form of acne vulgaris, the medical term for the condition.

Though acne often is a simple case of pimples, it sometimes can erupt as unsightly pus-filled sores with the potential to disfigure. Acne may fracture self-esteem in the teen years, but this dermatological rite of passage generally is history by early adulthood.

But not always. Cases of the ailment occur occasionally in pre-teens and in older adults. Sometimes women experience acne flare-ups at certain stages of the menstrual cycle or after discontinuing oral contraceptives. Experts say stress and heredity also can play a part.

The American Academy of Dermatology says it's a good idea for acne sufferers to check with a dermatologist to ensure the skin condition really is acne. Rashes from other sources such as makeup and oral medicine can create acne-like symptoms.

Severe acne requires a doctor's attention to prevent permanent scarring. But milder cases often yield to treatment with over-the-counter (OTC) products. Dozens of products are available in varying strengths as creams, lotions, gels, and cleansers. In its review of OTC drugs, the Food and Drug Administration approved sulfur, resorcinol, and salicyclic acid for OTC treatment of acne. The agency determined that more safety studies are needed for another ingredient, benzoyl peroxide. All these ingredients were on the market before 1972, when FDA began a review of OTC drug products.

Some Unanswered Questions

Benzoyl peroxide products have been sold for more than 25 years. FDA and the dermatological community have long considered the drug to be an effective nonprescription acne medicine.

But FDA officials are concerned about what happens when skin treated with benzoyl peroxide is exposed to the sun. Study data are inconclusive at this time.

Scientists call chemicals and radiation that can start tumor growth "initiators." The sun's ultraviolet light is a known initiator. Substances that increase tumor development when an initiator is present are called "promotors." Benzoyl peroxide is considered a promotor.

Researchers have observed that benzoyl peroxide has a tumor-promoting effect in mice exposed to a chemical initiator. They don't know yet what effect the sun may have specifically on skin treated with benzoyl peroxide. Until research can establish or disprove a link, FDA plans to require extra warning and direction statements on benzoyl peroxide product labels. The agency published a *Federal Register* notice on Feb. 17 to solicit comments on its proposed labeling changes. Deadline for comments is May 18.

Though studies in mice showed that benzoyl peroxide did not cause the growth of tumors initiated by the sun, these studies did not resolve the issue, say FDA officials. The research used an inadequate number of mice and did not show conclusively whether benzoyl peroxide actually increased tumors. Another study in progress with more than 100 mice should allow scientists to make more valid conclusions.

Researchers also are conducting tests to determine what effect benzoyl peroxide has on mice and rats for the lifetime of the animal. When these tests are completed, FDA will evaluate results and decide how the information will affect the use of benzoyl peroxide products.

Other existing studies further cloud the association between the drug and cancer. For example, a recent Canadian survey-type study queried benzoyl peroxide users to find out if they had developed skin cancer. Results showed that users of these products did not have a higher risk of developing tumors or cancer. Though the study generally was well-designed and furnished useful information, FDA officials say, it did not group subjects for skin cancer risk by duration of use and time since last use of the drug. The survey also did not consider the reasons for benzoyl peroxide therapy and users' ages. FDA found the study to be limited in how well it can determine the effects of benzoyl peroxide over long periods for persons who have greater exposure in locations where the sun is more intense than in Canada.

Benzoyl peroxide continues to be available over the counter and by prescription in a number of strengths while researchers perform the additional studies. FDA considers benzoyl peroxide safe for treating acne while tests proceed.

The proposed warning is in two parts:

- In boldface type as the first sentence under the "Warnings" heading is the statement: "When using this product, avoid unnecessary sun exposure and use a sunscreen."
- In the "Directions" section of the labeling is the statement: "If going outside, use a sunscreen [the preceding sentence is in boldface type]. Allow (product name) to dry, then follow directions in the sunscreen labeling. If irritation or sensitivity develops, discontinue use of both products and consult a doctor."

Under FDA's proposal, manufacturers would put the new labeling on boxes or inserts for OTC products. Prescription acne treatments containing benzoyl peroxide would have the labeling in patient package inserts.

Benzoyl peroxide is found in more than a dozen OTC medications. Among them: Acne 10, Benoxyl 10, Clear By Design, Clearasil B.P., Fostex 10% BPO, Loxoide, Nutrogena Acne Mask, Noxzema Clear Up Acne Medicated Maximum Strength, Oxy-10, Oxy-5, Pan Oxyl 10 bar, Vanoxide .5%, and Zerac BP10.

FDA's concerns involve only benzoyl peroxide-based products. They do not apply to other OTC acne formulations, including

- *Sulfur*—Xerac-4% gel, Acne-Aid 10% lotion, Fostex Medicated Cover-Up Cream, Sulray 10% bar, and Cuticura ointment.
- *Sulfur/salicylic acid*—Aveenobar, Klaron lotion, Pernox Regular cleanser, and Sastid soap.
- *Sulfur/resorcinol*—Acnomel cream, Rezamid lotion, pHisoAc cream, and Clearasil Adult Care.
- *Salicyclic acid*—Dry & Clear cleanser 0.5%, Listerex Herbal Lotion, Saligel 5%, AquaGlyde cleanser, and Stri-Dex Maximum Strength Pads.

Acne's Origins

Acne starts when glands in hair canals (follicles) just below the skin's surface make an oily substance called sebum. Normally, sebum empties through follicle openings onto the skin surface, where it is washed away. In people of both sexes who get acne, the adrenal glands secrete male-type hormones that trigger excess production of sebum. Experts believe sebum stimulates the lining of the follicle wall, causing cells to shed, stick together, and plug up the follicle opening. If this plug remains below the surface, it is usually light in color and called a whitehead, or closed comedo. An enlarged plug that emerges from the follicle typically has a dark tip and is called a blackhead (an open comedo). The mixture of cells and oil creates a breeding ground for bacteria, which produce chemicals that can break down the follicle wall and create pimples or more serious inflammation.

OTC drugs work in similar ways. Benzoyl peroxide, resorcinol, salicylic acid, and sulfur are all "peeling agents," technically known as keratolytics. They cause a superficial irritation and drying that helps the body loosen plugs in the follicle and slough off dead cells. These drugs also keep bacteria from forming in the follicle. This, in turn, reduces fatty acids that contribute to plugs. A number of OTC acne drug products combine sulfur with resorcinol.

In severe acne cases, doctors prescribe other drugs either separately or in tandem with OTC preparations.

The American Academy of Dermatology cautions against scratching or squeezing acne sores, which can lead to more inflammation and scarring. The academy offers a free brochure about acne and its treatment. For a copy, send a stamped, business-size envelope to:

American Academy of Dermatology
PO Box 681069
Schaumburg, IL 60168-1069

■ **Document Source:**
U.S. Department of Health and Human Services Public Health Service
Food and Drug Administration
FDA Consumer
May 1995

STROKE
■■■

RECOVERING AFTER A STROKE

What is a stroke?

A stroke is a type of brain injury. Symptoms depend on the part of the brain that is affected. People who survive a stroke often have weakness on one side of the body or trouble with moving, talking, or thinking.

Most strokes are ischemic (is-KEE-mic) strokes. These are caused by reduced blood flow to the brain when blood vessels are blocked by a clot or become too narrow for blood to get through. Brain cells in the area die from lack of oxygen. In another type of stroke, called hemorrhagic (hem-or-AJ-ic) stroke, the blood vessel isn't blocked; it bursts, and blood leaks into the brain, causing damage.

Strokes are more common in older people. Almost three-fourths of all strokes occur in people 65 years of age or over. However, a person of any age can have a stroke.

A person may also have a transient ischemic attack (TIA). This has the same symptoms as a stroke, but only lasts for a few hours or a day and does not cause permanent brain damage. A TIA is not a stroke but it is an important warning signal. The person needs treatment to help prevent an actual stroke in the future.

> A stroke may be frightening to both the patient and family. It helps to remember that stroke survivors usually have at least some spontaneous recovery or natural healing and often recover further with rehabilitation.

Purpose of this Booklet

This booklet is about stroke rehabilitation. Its goal is to help the person who has had a stroke achieve the best possible recovery. Its purpose is to help people who have had strokes and their families get the most out of rehabilitation.

Note that this booklet sometimes uses the terms "stroke survivor" and "person" instead of "patient" to refer to someone who has had a stroke. This is because people who have had a stroke are patients for only a short time, first in the acute care hospital and then perhaps in a rehabilitation program. For the rest of their lives, they are people who happen to have had a stroke. The booklet also uses the word "family" to include those people who are closest to the stroke survivor, whether or not they are relatives.

Rehabilitation works best when stroke survivors and their families work together as a team. For this reason, both stroke survivors and family members are encouraged to read all parts of the booklet.

Recovering from Stroke

The process of recovering from a stroke usually includes treatment, spontaneous recovery, rehabilitation, and the return to community living. Because stroke survivors often have complex rehabilitation needs, progress and recovery are different for each person.

Treatment for stroke begins in a hospital with "acute care." This first step includes helping the patient survive, preventing another stroke, and taking care of any other medical problems.

Spontaneous recovery happens naturally to most people. Soon after the stroke, some abilities that have been lost usually start to come back. This process is quickest during the first few weeks, but it sometimes continues for a long time.

Rehabilitation is another part of treatment. It helps the person keep abilities and gain back lost abilities to become more independent. It usually begins while the patient is still in acute care. For many patients, it continues afterward, either as a formal rehabilitation program or as individual rehabilitation services. Many decisions about rehabilitation are made by the patient, family, and hospital staff before discharge from acute care.

The last stage in stroke recovery begins with the person's return to community living after acute care or rehabilitation. This stage can last for a lifetime as the stroke survivor and family learn to live with the effects of the stroke. This may include doing common tasks in new ways or making up for damage to or limits of one part of the body by greater activity of another. For example, a stroke survivor can wear shoes with velcro closures instead of laces or may learn to write with the opposite hand.

How Stroke Affects People

Effects on the Body, Mind, and Feelings

Each stroke is different depending on the part of the brain injured, how bad the injury is, and the person's general health. Some of the effects of stroke are:

- Weakness (hemiparesis—hem-ee-par-EE-sis) or paralysis (hemiplegia—hem-ee-PLEE-ja) on one side of the body. This may affect the whole side or just the arm or the leg. The weakness or paralysis is on the side of the body opposite the side of the brain injured by the stroke. For example, if the stroke injured the left side of the brain, the weakness or paralysis will be on the right side of the body.
- Problems with balance or coordination. These can make it hard for the person to sit, stand, or walk, even if muscles are strong enough.
- Problems using language (aphasia and dysarthria). A person with aphasia (a-FAY-zha) may have trouble understanding speech or writing. Or, the person may understand but may not be able to think of the words to speak or write. A person with dysarthria (dis-AR-three-a) knows the right words but has trouble saying them clearly.
- Being unaware of or ignoring things on one side of the body (bodily neglect or inattention). Often, the person will not turn to look toward the weaker side or even eat food from the half of the plate on that side.
- Pain, numbness, or odd sensations. These can make it hard for the person to relax and feel comfortable. Problems with memory, thinking, attention, or learning (cognitive problems). A person may have trouble with many mental activities or just a few. For example, the person may have trouble following directions, may get confused if something in a room is moved, or may not be able to keep track of the date or time.
- Being unaware of the effects of the stroke. The person may show poor judgment by trying to do things that are unsafe as a result of the stroke.
- Trouble swallowing (dysphagia—dis-FAY-ja). This can make it hard for the person to get enough food. Also, care must sometimes be taken to prevent the person from breathing in food (aspiration—as-per-AY-shun) while trying to swallow it.
- Problems with bowel or bladder control. These problems can be helped with the use of portable urinals, bedpans, and other toileting devices.
- Getting tired very quickly. Becoming tired very quickly may limit the person's participation and performance in a rehabilitation program.
- Sudden bursts of emotion, such as laughing, crying, or anger. These emotions may indicate that the person needs help, understanding, and support in adjusting to the effects of the stroke.
- Depression. This is common in people who have had strokes. It can begin soon after the stroke or many weeks later, and family members often notice it first.

Depression After Stroke

It is normal for a stroke survivor to feel sad over the problems caused by stroke. However, some people experience a major depressive disorder, which should be diagnosed and treated as soon as possible. A person with a major depressive disorder has a number of symptoms nearly every day, all day, for at least two weeks. These always include at least one of the following:

- Feeling sad, blue, or down-in-the-dumps.
- Loss of interest in things that the person used to enjoy.

A person may also have other physical or psychological symptoms, including:

- Feeling slowed down or restless and unable to sit still.
- Feeling worthless or guilty.
- Increase or decrease in appetite or weight.
- Problems concentrating, thinking, remembering, or making decisions.
- Trouble sleeping or sleeping too much.
- Loss of energy or feeling tired all of the time.
- Headaches.
- Other aches and pains.
- Digestive problems.
- Sexual problems.
- Feeling pessimistic or hopeless.
- Being anxious or worried.
- Thoughts of death or suicide.

If a stroke survivor has symptoms of depression, especially thoughts of death or suicide, professional help is needed right away. Once the depression is properly treated, these thoughts will go away. Depression can be treated with medication, psychotherapy, or both. If it is not treated, it can cause needless suffering and also makes it harder to recover from the stroke.

Disabilities After Stroke

A "disability" is difficulty doing something that is a normal part of daily life. People who have had a stroke may have trouble with many activities that were easy before, such as walking, talking, and taking care of "activities of daily living" (ADLs). These include basic tasks such as bathing, dressing, eating, and using the toilet, as well as more complex tasks called "instrumental activities of daily living" (IADLs), such as housekeeping, using the telephone, driving, and writing checks.

Some disabilities are obvious right after the stroke. Others may not be noticed until the person is back home and is trying to do something for the first time since the stroke.

What Happens During Acute Care

The main purposes of acute care are to:

- Make sure the patient's condition is caused by a stroke and not by some other medical problem.
- Determine the type and location of the stroke and how serious it is.

- Prevent or treat complications such as bowel or bladder problems or pressure ulcers (bed sores).
- Prevent another stroke.
- Encourage the patient to move and perform self-care tasks, such as eating and getting out of bed, as early as medically possible. This is the first step in rehabilitation.

Stroke survivors and family members may find the hospital experience confusing. Hospital staff are there to help, and it is important to ask questions and talk about concerns.

Before acute care ends, the patient and family, with the hospital staff, decide what the next step will be. For many patients, the next step will be to continue rehabilitation.

Preventing Another Stroke

People who have had a stroke have an increased risk of another stroke, especially during the first year after the original stroke. The risk of another stroke goes up with older age, high blood pressure (hypertension), high cholesterol, diabetes, obesity, having had a transient ischemic attack (TIA), heart disease, cigarette smoking, heavy alcohol use, and drug abuse. While some risk factors for stroke (such as age) cannot be changed, the risk factors for the others can be reduced through use of medicines or changes in lifestyle.

Patients and families should ask for guidance from their doctor or nurse about preventing another stroke. They need to work together to make healthy changes in the patient's lifestyle. Patients and families should also learn the warning signs of a TIA (such as weakness on one side of the body and slurred speech) and see a doctor immediately if these happen.

Deciding About Rehabilitation

Some people do not need rehabilitation after a stroke because the stroke was mild or they have fully recovered. Others may be too disabled to participate. However, many patients can be helped by rehabilitation. Hospital staff will help the patient and family decide about rehabilitation and choose the right services or program.

Types of Rehabilitation Programs

There are several kinds of rehabilitation programs:

- Hospital programs. These programs can be provided by special rehabilitation hospitals or by rehabilitation units in acute care hospitals. Complete rehabilitation services are available. The patient stays in the hospital during rehabilitation. An organized team of specially trained professionals provides the therapy. Hospital programs are usually more intense than other programs and require more effort from the patient.
- Nursing facility (nursing home) programs. As in hospital programs, the person stays at the facility during rehabilitation. Nursing facility programs are very different from each other, so it is important to get specific information about each one. Some provide a complete range of rehabilitation services; others provide only limited services.
- Outpatient programs. Outpatient programs allow a patient who lives at home to get a full range of services by visiting a hospital outpatient department, outpatient rehabilitation facility, or day hospital program.
- Home-based programs. The patient can live at home and receive rehabilitation services from visiting professionals. An important advantage of home programs is that patients learn skills in the same place where they will use them.

Individual Rehabilitation Services

Many stroke survivors do not need a complete range of rehabilitation services. Instead, they may need an individual type of service, such as regular physical therapy or speech therapy. These services are available from outpatient and home care programs.

Paying for Rehabilitation

Medicare and many health insurance policies will help pay for rehabilitation. Medicare is the federal health insurance program for Americans 65 years of age or over and for certain Americans with disabilities. It has two parts: hospital insurance (known as Part A) and supplementary medical insurance (known as Part B). Part A helps pay for home health care, hospice care, inpatient hospital care, and inpatient care in a skilled nursing facility. Part B helps pay for doctors' services, outpatient hospital services, durable medical equipment, and a number of other medical services and supplies not covered by Part A. Social Security Administration offices across the country take applications for Medicare and provide general information about the program.

In some cases, Medicare will help pay for outpatient services from a Medicare-participating comprehensive outpatient rehabilitation facility. Covered services include physicians' services; physical, speech, occupational, and respiratory therapies; counseling; and other related services. A stroke survivor must be referred by a physician who certifies that skilled rehabilitation services are needed.

Medicaid is a federal program that is operated by the states, and each state decides who is eligible and the scope of health services offered. Medicaid provides health care coverage for some low-income people who cannot afford it. This includes people who are eligible because they are older, blind, or disabled, or certain people in families with dependent children.

These programs have certain restrictions and limitations, and coverage may stop as soon as the patient stops making progress. Therefore, it is important for patients and families to find out exactly what their insurance will cover. The hospital's social service department can answer questions about insurance coverage and can help with financial planning.

Choosing a Rehabilitation Program

The doctor and other hospital staff will provide information and advice about rehabilitation programs, but the patient and family make the final choice. Hospital staff know the patient's disabilities and medical condition. They should also be familiar with the rehabilitation programs in the community and should be able to answer questions about them. The patient and family may have a preference about whether the patient lives at home or at a rehabilitation facility. They may have reasons for preferring one program over another. Their concerns are important and should be discussed with hospital staff.

Things to Consider When Choosing a Rehabilitation Program

- Does the program provide the services the patient needs?
- Does it match the patient's abilities or is it too demanding or not demanding enough?
- What kind of standing does it have in the community for the quality of the program?
- Is it certified and does its staff have good credentials?
- Is it located where family members can easily visit?
- Does it actively involve the patient and family members in rehabilitation decisions?
- Does it encourage family members to participate in some rehabilitation sessions and practice with the patient?
- How well are its costs covered by insurance or Medicare?
- If it is an outpatient or home program, is there someone living at home who can provide care?
- If it is an outpatient program, is transportation available?

A person may start rehabilitation in one program and later transfer to another. For example, some patients who get tired quickly may start out in a less intense rehabilitation program. After they build up their strength, they are able to transfer to a more intense program.

When Rehabilitation Is Not Recommended

Some families and patients may be disappointed if the doctor does not recommend rehabilitation. However, a person may be unconscious or too disabled to benefit. For example, a person who is unable to learn may be better helped by maintenance care at home or in a nursing facility. A person who is, at first, too weak for rehabilitation may benefit from a gradual recovery period at home or in a nursing facility. This person can consider rehabilitation at a later time. It is important to remember that

- Hospital staff are responsible for helping plan the best way to care for the patient after discharge from acute care. They can also provide or arrange for needed social services and family education.
- This is not the only chance to participate in rehabilitation. People who are too disabled at first may recover enough to enter rehabilitation later.

What Happens During Rehabilitation

In hospital or nursing facility rehabilitation programs, the patient may spend several hours a day in activities such as physical therapy, occupational therapy, speech therapy, recreational therapy, group activities, and patient and family education. It is important to maintain skills that help recovery. Part of the time is spent relearning skills (such as walking and speaking) that the person had before the stroke. Part of it is spent learning new ways to do things that can no longer be done the old way (for example, using one hand for tasks that usually need both hands).

Setting Rehabilitation Goals

The goals of rehabilitation depend on the effects of the stroke, what the patient was able to do before the stroke, and the patient's wishes. Working together, goals are set by the patient, family, and rehabilitation program staff. Sometimes, a person may need to repeat steps in striving to reach goals.

If goals are too high, the patient will not be able to reach them. If they are too low, the patient may not get all the services that would help. If they do not match the patient's interests, the patient may not want to work at them. Therefore, it is important for goals to be realistic. To help achieve realistic goals, the patient and family should tell program staff about things that the patient wants to be able to do.

Rehabilitation Goals

- Being able to walk, at least with a walker or cane, is a realistic goal for most stroke survivors.
- Being able to take care of oneself with some special equipment is a realistic goal for most.
- Being able to drive a car is a realistic goal for some.
- Having a job can be a realistic goal for some people who were working before the stroke. For some, the old job may not be possible but another job or a volunteer activity may be.

Reaching treatment goals does not mean the end of recovery. It just means that the stroke survivor and family are ready to continue recovery on their own.

Rehabilitation Specialists

Because every stroke is different, treatment will be different for each person. Rehabilitation is provided by several types of specially trained professionals. A person may work with any or all of these:

- Physician. All patients in stroke rehabilitation have a physician in charge of their care. Several kinds of doctors with rehabilitation experience may have this role. These include family physicians and internists (primary care doctors), geriatricians (specialists in working with older patients), neurologists (specialists in the brain and nervous system), and physiatrists (specialists in physical medicine and rehabilitation).
- Rehabilitation nurse. Rehabilitation nurses specialize in nursing care for people with disabilities. They pro-

vide direct care, educate patients and families, and help the doctor to coordinate care.

- Physical therapist. Physical therapists evaluate and treat problems with moving, balance, and coordination. They provide training and exercises to improve walking, getting in and out of a bed or chair, and moving around without losing balance. They teach family members how to help with exercises for the patient and how to help the patient move or walk, if needed.
- Occupational therapist. Occupational therapists provide exercises and practice to help patients do things they could do before the stroke such as eating, bathing, dressing, writing, or cooking. The old way of doing an activity sometimes is no longer possible, so the therapist teaches a new technique.
- Speech-language pathologist. Speech-language pathologists help patients get back language skills and learn other ways to communicate. Teaching families how to improve communication is very important. Speech-language pathologists also work with patients who have swallowing problems (dysphagia).
- Social worker. Social workers help patients and families make decisions about rehabilitation and plan the return to the home or a new living place. They help the family answer questions about insurance and other financial issues and can arrange for a variety of support services. They may also provide or arrange for patient and family counseling to help cope with any emotional problems.
- Psychologist. Psychologists are concerned with the mental and emotional health of patients. They use interviews and tests to identify and understand problems. They may also treat thinking or memory problems or may provide advice to other professionals about patients with these problems.
- Therapeutic recreation specialist. These therapists help patients return to activities that they enjoyed before the stroke such as playing cards, gardening, bowling, or community activities. Recreational therapy helps the rehabilitation process and encourages the patient to practice skills.
- Other professionals. Other professionals may also help with the patient's treatment. An orthotist may make special braces to support weak ankles and feet. A urologist may help with bladder problems. Other physician specialists may help with medical or emotional problems. Dietitians make sure that the patient has a healthy diet during rehabilitation. They also educate the family about proper diet after the patient leaves the program. Vocational counselors may help patients go back to work or school.

> Rehabilitation professionals, the patient, and the family are vitally important partners in rehabilitation. They must all work together for rehabilitation to succeed.

Rehabilitation Team

In many programs, a special rehabilitation team with a team leader is organized for each patient. The patient, family, and rehabilitation professionals are all members. The team has regular meetings to discuss the progress of treatment. Using a team approach often helps everyone work together to meet goals.

Getting the Most Out of Rehabilitation

What the Patient Can Do

If you are a stroke survivor in rehabilitation, keep in mind that you are the most important person in your treatment. You should have a major say in decisions about your care. This is hard for many stroke patients. You may sometimes feel tempted to sit back and let the program staff take charge. If you need extra time to think or have trouble talking, you may find that others are going ahead and making decisions without waiting. Try not to let this happen.

- Make sure others understand that you want to help make decisions about your care.
- Bring your questions and concerns to program staff.
- State your wishes and opinions on matters that affect you.
- Speak up if you feel that anyone is "talking down" to you; or, if people start talking about you as if you are not there.
- Remember that you have the right to see your medical records.

To be a partner in your care, you need to be well informed about your treatment and how well you are doing. It may help to record important information about your treatment and progress and write down any questions you have.

If you have speech problems, making your wishes known is hard. The speech-language pathologist can help you to communicate with other staff members, and family members may also help to communicate your ideas and needs.

Most patients find that rehabilitation is hard work. They need to maintain abilities at the same time they are working to regain abilities. It is normal to feel tired and discouraged at times because things that used to be easy before the stroke are now difficult. The important thing is to notice the progress you make and take pride in each achievement.

How the Family Can Help

If you are a family member of a stroke survivor, here are some things you can do:

- Support the patient's efforts to participate in rehabilitation decisions.
- Visit and talk with the patient. You can relax together while playing cards, watching television, listening to the radio, or playing a board game.
- If the patient has trouble communicating (aphasia), ask the speech-language pathologist how you can help.
- Participate in education offered for stroke survivors and their families. Learn as much as you can and how you can help.

- Ask to attend some of the rehabilitation sessions. This is a good way to learn how rehabilitation works and how to help.
- Encourage and help the patient to practice skills learned in rehabilitation.
- Make sure that the program staff suggests activities that fit the patient's needs and interests.
- Find out what the patient can do alone, what the patient can do with help, and what the patient can't do. Then avoid doing things for the patient that the patient is able to do. Each time the patient does them, his or her ability and confidence will grow.
- Take care of yourself by eating well, getting enough rest, and taking time to do things that you enjoy.

To gain more control over the rehabilitation process, keep important information where you can find it. One suggestion is to keep a notebook with the patient. Some things to include are

- Rehabilitation Goals
- Name, phone number, and job of each person on the program staff who works with the patient
- Schedule of rehabilitation activities
- Treatment instructions
- The patient's goals or planned activities for the week (include check marks showing which plans have been carried out and which goals have been reached)
- Other things accomplished during each day (include small steps in reaching goals)
- Questions and concerns to talk about with the program staff

Discharge Planning

Discharge planning begins early during rehabilitation. It involves the patient, family, and rehabilitation staff. The purpose of discharge planning is to help maintain the benefits of rehabilitation after the patient has been discharged from the program. Patients are usually discharged from rehabilitation soon after their goals have been reached.

Some of the things discharge planning can include are to

- Make sure that the stroke survivor has a safe place to live after discharge.
- Decide what care, assistance, or special equipment will be needed.
- Arrange for more rehabilitation services or for other services in the home (such as visits by a home health aide).
- Choose the health care provider who will monitor the person's health and medical needs.
- Determine the caregivers who will work as a partner with the patient to provide daily care and assistance at home, and teach them the skills they will need.
- Help the stroke survivor explore employment opportunities, volunteer activities, and driving a car (if able and interested).

- Discuss any sexual concerns the stroke survivor or husband/wife may have. Many people who have had strokes enjoy active sex lives.

Preparing a Living Place

Many stroke survivors can return to their own homes after rehabilitation. Others need to live in a place with professional staff such as a nursing home or assisted living facility. An assisted living facility can provide residential living with a full range of services and staff. The choice usually depends on the person's needs for care and whether caregivers are available in the home. The stroke survivor needs a living place that supports continuing recovery.

It is important to choose a living place that is safe. If the person needs a new place to live, a social worker can help find the best place.

During discharge planning, program staff will ask about the home and may also visit it. They may suggest changes to make it safer. These might include changing rooms around so that a stroke survivor can stay on one floor, moving scatter rugs or small pieces of furniture that could cause falls, and putting grab bars and seats in tubs and showers.

It is a good idea for the stroke survivor to go home for a trial visit before discharge. This will help identify problems that need to be discussed or corrected before the patient returns.

Deciding About Special Equipment

Even after rehabilitation, some stroke survivors have trouble walking, balancing, or performing certain activities of daily living. Special equipment can sometimes help. Here are some examples:

- Cane. Many people who have had strokes use a cane when walking. For people with balancing problems, special canes with three or four "feet" are available.
- Walker. A walker provides more support than a cane. Several designs are available for people who can only use one hand and for different problems with walking or balance.
- Ankle-foot orthotic devices (braces). Braces help a person to walk by keeping the ankle and foot in the correct position and providing support for the knee.
- Wheelchair. Some people will need a wheelchair. Wheelchairs come in many different designs. They can be customized to fit the user's needs and abilities. Find out which features are most important for the stroke survivor.
- Aids for bathing, dressing, and eating. Some of these are safety devices such as grab bars and nonskid tub and floor mats. Others make it easier to do things with one hand. Examples are velcro fasteners on clothes and placemats that won't slide on the table.
- Communication aids. These range from small computers to homemade communication boards. The stroke survivor, family, and rehabilitation program staff should decide together what special equipment is needed. Program staff can help in making the best

choices. Medicare or health insurance will often help pay for the equipment.

Preparing Caregivers

Caregivers who help stroke survivors at home are usually family members such as a husband or wife or an adult son or daughter. They may also be friends or even professional home health aides. Usually, one person is the main caregiver, while others help from time to time. An important part of discharge planning is to make sure that caregivers understand the safety, physical, and emotional needs of the stroke survivor, and that they will be available to provide needed care.

Since every stroke is different, people have different needs for help from caregivers. Here are some of the things caregivers may do:

- Keep notes on discharge plans and instructions and ask about anything that is not clear.
- Help to make sure that the stroke survivor takes all prescribed medicines and follows suggestions from program staff about diet, exercise, rest, and other health practices.
- Encourage and help the person to practice skills learned in rehabilitation.
- Help the person solve problems and discover new ways to do things.
- Help the person with activities performed before the stroke. These could include using tools, buttoning a shirt, household tasks, and leisure or social activities.
- Help with personal care, if the person cannot manage alone.
- Help with communication, if the person has speech problems. Include the stroke survivor in conversations even when the person cannot actively participate.
- Arrange for needed community services.
- Stand up for the rights of the stroke survivor.

If you expect to be a caregiver, think carefully about this role ahead of time. Are you prepared to work with the patient on stroke recovery? Talk it over with other people who will share the caregiving job with you. What are the stroke survivor's needs? Who can best help meet each of them? Who will be the main caregiver? Does caregiving need to be scheduled around the caregivers' jobs or other activities? There is time during discharge planning to talk with program staff about caregiving and to develop a workable plan.

Going Home

Adjusting to the Change

Going home to the old home or a new one is a big adjustment. For the stroke survivor, it may be hard to transfer the skills learned during rehabilitation to a new location. Also, more problems caused by the stroke may appear as the person tries to go back to old activities. During this time, the stroke survivor and family learn how the stroke will affect daily life and can make the necessary adjustments.

These adjustments are a physical and emotional challenge for the main caregiver as well as the stroke survivor. The caregiver has many new responsibilities and may not have time for some favorite activities. The caregiver needs support, understanding, and some time to rest. Caregiving that falls too heavily on one person can be very stressful. Even when family members and friends are nearby and willing to help, conflicts over caregiving can cause stress.

> A stroke is always stressful for the family, but it is especially hard if one family member is the only caregiver. Much time may be required to meet the needs of the stroke survivor. Therefore, the caregiver needs as much support as possible from others. Working together eases the stress on everyone.

Tips for Reducing Stress

The following tips for reducing stress are for both caregivers and stroke survivors.

- Take stroke recovery and caregiving one day at a time and be hopeful.
- Remember that adjusting to the effects of stroke takes time. Appreciate each small gain as you discover better ways of doing things.
- Caregiving is learned. Expect that knowledge and skills will grow with experience.
- Experiment. Until you find what works for you, try new ways of doing activities of daily living, communicating with each other, scheduling the day, and organizing your social life.
- Plan for "breaks" so that you are not together all the time. This is a good way for family and friends to help on occasion. You can also plan activities that get both of you out of the house.
- Ask family members and friends to help in specific ways and commit to certain times to help. This gives others a chance to help in useful ways.
- Read about the experiences of other people in similar situations. Your public library has life stories by people who have had a stroke as well as books for caregivers.
- Join or start a support group for stroke survivors or caregivers. You can work on problems together and develop new friendships.
- Be kind to each other. If you sometimes feel irritated, this is natural and you don't need to blame yourself. But don't "take it out" on the other person. It often helps to talk about these feelings with a friend, rehabilitation professional, or support group.
- Plan and enjoy new experiences and don't look back. Avoid comparing life as it is now with how it was before the stroke.

Followup Appointments

After a stroke survivor returns to the community, regular followup appointments are usually scheduled with the doctor and sometimes with rehabilitation professionals. The purpose of followup is to check on the stroke survivor's medical condition and ability to use the skills learned in rehabilitation. It is also important to check on how well the stroke survivor and family are adjusting. The stroke survivor and caregiver can be prepared for these visits with a list of questions or concerns.

Where to Get Help

Many kinds of help are available for people who have had strokes and their families and caregivers. Some of the most important are:

- Information about stroke. A good place to start is with the books and pamphlets available from national organizations that provide information on this subject. Many of their materials are available free of charge. A list of these organizations is at the end of this document.
- Local stroke clubs or other support groups. These are groups where stroke survivors and family members can share their experiences, help each other solve problems, and expand their social lives.
- Home health services. These are available from the Visiting Nurses Association (VNA), public health departments, hospital home care departments, and private home health agencies. Services may include nursing care, rehabilitation therapies, personal care (for example, help with bathing or dressing), respite care (staying with the stroke survivor so that the caregiver can take a vacation or short break), homemaker services, and other kinds of help.
- Meals on Wheels. Hot meals are delivered to the homes of people who cannot easily shop and cook.
- Adult day care. People who cannot be completely independent sometimes spend the day at an adult day care center. There they get meals, participate in social activities, and may also get some health care and rehabilitation services.
- Friendly Visitor (or other companion services). A paid or volunteer companion makes regular visits or phone calls to a person with disabilities.
- Transportation services. Most public transportation systems have buses that a person in a wheelchair can board. Some organizations and communities provide vans to take wheelchair users and others on errands such as shopping or doctor's visits.

Many communities have service organizations that can help. Some free services may be available or fees may be on a "sliding scale" based on income. It takes some work to find out what services and payment arrangements are available. A good way to start is to ask the social workers in the hospital or rehabilitation program where the stroke survivor was treated. Also, talk to the local United Way or places of worship. Another good place to look is the Yellow Pages of the telephone book, under "Health Services," "Home Health Care," "Senior Citizen Services," or "Social Service Organizations." Just asking friends may turn up useful information. The more you ask, the more you will learn.

Additional Resources

ACTION
1100 Vermont Ave, NW
Washington, DC 20525
(202) 606-4855 (call for telephone number of regional office)

Sponsors older American volunteer programs.

Administration on Aging
330 Independence Ave, SW
Washington, DC 20201
Toll-free (800) 677-1116 (call for list of community services for older Americans in your area)

AHA Stroke Connection (formerly the Courage Stroke Network)
American Heart Association
7272 Greenville Ave
Dallas, TX 75231
Toll-free (800) 553-6321 (or check telephone book for local AHA office)

Provides prevention, diagnosis, treatment, and rehabilitation information to stroke survivors and their families.

American Dietetic Association/National Center for Nutrition and Dietetics
216 W Jackson Blvd
Chicago, IL 60606
Toll-free (800) 366-1655 (Consumer Nutrition Hotline)

Consumers may speak to a registered dietitian for answers to nutrition questions, or obtain a referral to a local registered dietitian.

American Self-Help Clearinghouse
St. Clares-Riverside Medical Center
Denville, NJ 07834
(201) 625-7101 (call for name and telephone number of state or local clearinghouse)

Provides information and assistance on local self-help groups.

National Aphasia Association
PO Box 1887 Murray Hill Station
New York, NY 10156
Toll-free (800) 922-4622

Provides information on the partial or total loss of the ability to speak or comprehend speech, resulting from stroke or other causes.

National Easter Seal Society
230 W Monroe St, Ste 1800
Chicago, IL 60606
(312) 726-6200 (or check telephone book for local Easter Seal Society)

Provides information and services to help people with disabilities.

National Stroke Association
8480 E Orchard Rd, Ste 1000
Englewood, CO 80111
(303) 771-1700
Toll-free (800) STROKES (787-6537)

Serves as an information referral clearinghouse on stroke. Offers guidance on forming stroke support groups and clubs.

Rosalynn Carter Institute
Georgia Southwestern College
600 Simmons St
Americus, GA 31709

Provides information on caregiving. Reading lists, video products, and other caregiver resources are available by writing to the address listed above.

Stroke Clubs International
805 12th St
Galveston, TX 77550
(409) 762-1022 (call for the name of a stroke club located in your area)

Maintains list of over 800 stroke clubs throughout the United States.

The Well Spouse Foundation
PO Box 801
New York, NY 10023
(212) 724-7209
Toll-free (800) 838-0879

Provides support for the husbands, wives, and partners of people who are chronically ill or disabled.

Medicare Information

Consumer Information Center
Department 59
Pueblo, CO 81009

By writing to this address, you can receive a free copy of The Medicare Handbook (updated and published annually). This handbook provides information about Medicare benefits, health insurance to supplement Medicare, and limits to Medicare coverage. It is also available in Spanish.

For Further Information

Information in this booklet is based on *Post-Stroke Rehabilitation. Clinical Practice Guideline,* Number 16. It was developed by a non-federal panel sponsored by the Agency for Health Care Policy and Research (AHCPR), an agency of the Public Health Service. Other guidelines on common health problems are available, and more are being developed.

Four other patient guides are available from AHCPR that may be of interest to stroke survivors and their caregivers:

- *Preventing Pressure Ulcers: Patient Guide* gives detailed information about how to prevent pressure sores (AHCPR Publication No. 92-0048).
- *Treating Pressure Sores: Patient Guide* gives detailed information about treating pressure sores (AHCPR Publication No. 95-0654).
- *Urinary Incontinence in Adults: Patient Guide* describes why people lose urine when they don't want to and how that can be treated (AHCPR Publication No. 92-0040).
- *Depression Is a Treatable Illness: Patient Guide* discusses major depressive disorder, which most often can be successfully treated with the help of a health professional (AHCPR Publication No. 93-0053).

For more information about these and other guidelines, or to get more copies of this booklet, call toll-free: 800-358-9295 or write to

Agency for Health Care Policy and Research Publications Clearinghouse
PO Box 8547
Silver Spring, MD 20907

■ **Document Source:**
U.S. Department of Health and Human Services, Public Health Service
Agency for Health Care Policy and Research
Executive Office Center, Ste 501
2101 E Jefferson St
Rockville, MD 20852
AHCPR Publication No. 95-0664
May 1995

See also: Stroke Treatment and Recovery (page 480)

STROKE PREVENTION: ATRIAL FIBRILLATION & STROKE

AF Increases Your Risk

What is atrial fibrillation?

Atrial fibrillation—abbreviated as "AF"—is the name of a particular type of irregular heartbeat affecting more than one million Americans. In AF, the left *atrium* (left upper chamber) of the heart beats rapidly and unpredictably. Normally, all four chambers of your heart beat in the same rhythm somewhere between 60 and 100 times every minute. In someone who has AF, the left atrium may beat as many as 400 times a minute. If left untreated, AF can increase your stroke risk from four to six times. Long-term untreated AF can also weaken the heart, leading to potential heart failure.

What does AF have to do with stroke?

Your heart's chambers work together to pump blood throughout your body. A healthy heart's normal rhythm is highly effective at emptying the heart's chambers of incoming blood and moving it on. In AF, the irregular contractions of the left atrium make it hard for all the blood in that chamber to be emptied. As the blood remains in the left atrium, it tends to form clots. These clots can break loose and travel through the bloodstream to the brain. Once in the brain, a clot can plug an artery and cause a stroke. Deprived of blood, brain cells in the area of the stroke will die. Stroke can cause permanent disability, coma, or death.

Who has AF?

AF is relatively rare in healthy people, but it can occur. AF is found most often in people over age 65 and in people who have heart disease or thyroid disorders.

How can I tell if I have AF?

The only way to know for sure is to have your doctor perform a painless test called an *electrocardiogram* (ECG). During an ECG, sensitive electrodes are placed on your chest. These electrodes pick up the electrical impulses generated by your body that cause your heart to beat. The impulses are then transmitted to a device that records them on a piece of paper called an *ECG strip*. By examining the specific pattern of electrical impulses recorded on the ECG strip, your doctor can tell for certain whether you have AF. An ECG is the only reliable way to know if you have AF. That's because AF often has no strong outward symptoms. Some people with AF will experience heart palpitations—often described as a "pounding," "racing," or "fluttering" heartbeat. In other people, the only symptom of AF may be dizziness, faintness or lightheadedness. Others may experience chest pain ranging from mild discomfort to severe pain. And for yet another group, AF has no symptoms at all.

What can I do if I have AF?

Doctors have several options for managing your AF. Whenever possible, the first treatment efforts will be directed at *cardioversion*—restoring your heart's normal rhythm. This can be done either through the use of electrical stimulation or through pharmacologic (drug-based) therapy. For many people, one or the other of these measures will work to permanently convert the heart to normal rhythm. For others, however, these measures are not successful.

When cardioversion efforts fail or are not appropriate, AF treatment concentrates on protecting you from stroke-causing blood clots. Either warfarin (brand name Coumadin) or aspirin is generally prescribed. The choice of drug will depend on the presence and type of other cardiovascular risk factors you may have.

If your doctor has prescribed medication for you for AF, it's important for you to **take your medicine exactly as directed.** Failure to take your AF medication properly can significantly increase your stroke risk.

Contact the National Stroke Association for more information on

- NSA and Stroke Data
- Prevention
- Acute Care
- Rehabilitation
- Survivor & Caregiver Resources
- Research

■ **Document Source:**
National Stroke Association
8480 East Orchard Rd, Ste 1000
Englewood, CO 80111-5015
(303) 771-1700
FAX (303) 771-1886, TDD (303) 771-1887
1-800-STROKES (1-800-787-6537)
1995

See also: About Carotid Endarterectomy (page 227); Stroke Prevention: Reducing Risk & Recognizing Symptoms (page 479)

STROKE PREVENTION: REDUCING RISK & RECOGNIZING SYMPTOMS

Stroke is a Brain Attack!

Stroke is a "brain attack," cutting off vital supplies of blood and oxygen to the brain cells that control everything we do—from speaking, to walking, to breathing. A stroke happens when an artery becomes blocked or ruptured. Most strokes occur when arteries are blocked by blood clots (formed in the heart or elsewhere in the body) or by the gradual build-up of plaque and other fatty deposits. Arteries can rupture when weak spots on the blood vessel wall break. In rare cases, a brain artery may rupture because of a malformation present since birth.

Every year, stroke strikes nearly 500,000 Americans—killing 150,000 and forever changing the lives of the 350,000 who survive. Everyone has some stroke risk—*even you.* The good news is this—most strokes can be prevented by reducing risk and recognizing the symptoms.

> Important: The information in this brochure is not a substitute for medical guidance. Always consult your physician with questions about your health.

Reducing Risk

Stroke risk factors are the things about you that make you more likely to have a stroke. Several stroke risk factors (such as age, gender, race, diabetes, and family history of stroke) are beyond your control. Stroke risk factors you *can* control are generally divided into two categories: medical and lifestyle-related. Through a combination of medical attention and lifestyle changes, you can significantly reduce your risk of stroke.

Medical stroke risk factors include

- Previous stroke (increases stroke risk 10 times)
  If your first stroke was caused by blood clots or blocked arteries, medication and/or surgery may reduce your risk of having another stroke.
- Previous episode of stroke symptoms—known as a *transient ischemic attack* or "TIA" (increases stroke risk 10 times)
  If the underlying cause of the TIA is related to blood clots or blocked arteries, medication and/or surgery may reduce your risk of having a full stroke.
- High blood pressure—consistently higher than 140/90 (increases stroke risk four to six times)
  For most people, high blood pressure can be controlled through diet, exercise, weight loss, medication, or a combination of these.
- Heart disease—especially a specific type of irregular heartbeat known as atrial fibrillation or "AF," which can cause blood clots to form and travel to the brain (increases stroke risk four to six times)
  AF can be treated with medication. Other heart disease may be helped by surgery, medication, diet, exercise, or a combination of these.
- Carotid artery disease, in which the carotid arteries—the main blood supply between the heart and the brain—become blocked by the build-up of plaque and other fatty deposits (increases stroke risk three times)
  Depending on the degree of blockage, surgery to clear blocked arteries may be indicated. Medication and diet may also help reduce risk.

Lifestyle-related stroke risk factors include

- Smoking—injures blood vessel walls, speeds up hardening of the arteries, raises blood pressure, and increases how hard your heart has to work (increases stroke risk two times)

If you quit smoking today, your stroke risk from this factor will decrease significantly within two years. Within five years, your stroke risk from smoking would be the same as someone who's never smoked.

- High cholesterol, being overweight, not getting enough exercise, and drinking too much alcohol—all associated with increased stroke risk

These risk factors are highly responsive to positive changes in diet and activity. A low-fat, low-salt diet combined with limited alcohol intake (less than 3 oz. of hard liquor, such as whiskey OR 8 oz. of wine OR 24 oz. of beer per day) and an exercise plan approved by your doctor—can help bring these factors back within desirable ranges.

Recognizing Symptoms

Very few Americans know the symptoms of stroke. Do you? Learning them—and knowing what to do when they occur—could save your life.

The most common symptoms of a stroke are

- Numbness, weakness, or paralysis of face, arm, or leg—especially on one side of the body
- Sudden blurred or decreased vision in one or both eyes
- Difficulty speaking or understanding simple statements
- Dizziness, loss of balance or loss of coordination, especially when combined with another symptom

Other important but less common symptoms include

- Sudden, unexplainable, and intense headache—often described as "the worst headache ever" and "totally unlike a regular headache"
- Sudden nausea, fever and vomiting—distinguished from a viral illness by the speed of onset (minutes or hours vs. several days)
- Brief loss of consciousness or period of decreased consciousness (fainting, confusion, convulsions, or coma)

> Special note: Sometimes these symptoms may appear for only a very short period of time and then disappear. These episodes are known as TIAs, or *transient ischemic attacks*. Although it might be tempting to ignore them, it's important to call 911 whenever you experience any stroke symptoms. While TIAs are not strokes, they indicate serious underlying stroke risks and are a powerful warning that a full stroke may soon follow. Never ignore stroke symptoms! Call 911.

Stroke is an Emergency!

If you experience any stroke symptoms—or recognize them in someone else—call 911 immediately! Getting emergency medical treatment is important for two reasons:

- Only a doctor can tell for sure if you are having a stroke or a TIA.

  If you are having a stroke, emergency medical treatment could save your life and greatly improve your chances for successful rehabilitation and recovery. If you are having a TIA, your doctor will evaluate and treat the underlying causes. Following your doctor's orders for medication and treatment can help reduce your risk of having a stroke.

- Stroke-related brain damage gets worse the longer a stroke goes untreated. Several drugs currently in the testing phase may soon offer physicians the means to stop—and even reverse—this brain damage when administered immediately after the stroke.

Contact National Stroke Association for more information on

- NSA and Stroke Data
- Prevention
- Acute Care
- Rehabilitation
- Survivor & Caregiver Resources
- Research

■ **Document Source:**
National Stroke Association
8480 E Orchard Rd, Ste 1000
Englewood, CO 80111-5015
(303) 771-1700
FAX (303) 771-1886; TDD (303) 771-1887
1-800-STROKES; (1-800-787-6537)
1994

See also: About Carotid Endarterectomy (page 227); Stroke Prevention: Atrial Fibrillation and Stroke (page 478)

STROKE TREATMENT & RECOVERY

A Message from Jacquelyn Mayer Townsend
Miss America, 1963
Stroke Survivor, 1970

A stroke in the family affects every member of the family. Although it may not seem like it at first, there *is* life after stroke—both for the survivor and the survivor's family.

The road to recovery is difficult at times...but there is a road. This brochure, along with the videotape *Stroke: The Story of Treatment and Recovery,* is for you—the family. The brochure and video are designed to help you

- *Learn* what a stroke is and how it can affect your loved one;
- *Understand* what will be done in the hospital to treat the stroke;
- *Look ahead* to rehabilitation and what will happen once your loved one is released from the hospital;
- *Find out* what you can do to help; and
- *Learn* where to go for help and more information.

In addition, this brochure includes a glossary of some of the most common stroke-related medical terms you may hear from doctors and other health professionals. These terms are displayed in *bold italics* throughout this brochure.

The road to recovery for the stroke survivor and the family may feel like a roller coaster at times. There's no getting around that. But there is a road...and lots of people who will help you along the way.

If you would like more information about stroke and recovery, please contact the National Stroke Association at 1-800-STROKES.

Best wishes to you and your family.

Stroke and Its Effects

What is a stroke?

A stroke affects the brain. A stroke occurs when the normal blood flow to an area of the brain is cut off. Once the blood—and the oxygen it carries—are lost, brain cells stop working and begin to die. If part of the brain dies, it can't be replaced. That's why stroke is permanent.

How is blood flow to the brain interrupted?

In general, there are three ways...*thrombosis, embolism,* and *hemorrhage.*

In a *thrombotic stroke* a blockage forms inside one of the arteries that supplies blood to the brain.

An *embolic stroke* is caused when a blood clot that forms in another part of the body—such as the heart—breaks loose and is carried by the blood stream to the brain.

Hemorrhagic stroke occurs when a blood vessel breaks, causing bleeding in or around the brain, resulting in damage to the brain. Hemorrhagic strokes tend to be more severe, but fortunately, they are less common than the other types of stroke.

How can a stroke affect a person?

The brain controls everything we do—thinking, moving, speaking, and our five senses. The effects of a stroke depend on how large the stroke is and which area of the brain it has injured. When stroke affects a specific brain function, we call this a *neurological deficit* or *impairment.*

The brain is divided into right and left hemispheres. The *right hemisphere* controls the left side of the body, and the *left hemisphere* controls the right side of the body.

A stroke that occurs in the right hemisphere may cause left-body paralysis or an impairment of left-side vision. The right hemisphere also controls sensation for the left side of the body. In addition, damage to a large area of the right hemisphere can cause *left-body neglect,* a condition in which the stroke survivor becomes inattentive to the surroundings on his or her left side or fails to recognize left-body deficits (for example, "forgetting" the food on the left side of the dinner plate unless reminded).

Similarly, the left hemisphere of the brain controls what happens on the right side of the body, including right-body strength, sensation and vision. In addition, the left hemisphere of the brain controls speech and language in most people.

In addition to the right and left hemispheres, your brain has two other parts: the *brain stem* and the *cerebellum.* They are found underneath the hemispheres.

These parts of your brain control a variety of automatic, non-thinking functions like breathing, blood pressure, balance, coordination of eye movement, and swallowing.

In the Hospital

Emergency Care and Diagnosis

Stroke is an emergency, just like a heart attack. So the first thing doctors and nurses will do is provide emergency care—such as stabilizing blood pressure and heart rate and attending to any breathing or other complications.

After the stroke survivor's most immediate medical needs have been met, doctors will try to find out what caused the stroke and which area of the brain has been damaged.

One of the most helpful tools doctors have for this is a *CT or "CAT" scanner.* This machine gives doctors a highly detailed picture of the brain, showing where in the brain the stroke happened and the extent of the damage. Since many strokes are due to problems with blood vessels or blood clots, doctors may also order diagnostic tests to evaluate the blood vessels and blood itself.

Treatment

Once doctors know what caused the stroke, where in the brain it happened, and the extent of the damage, they can decide on the best method of treatment and the best way to prevent possible complications.

In particular, there are some important complications that the doctors and nurses will be watching for. It's important to remember that each stroke is unique—the stroke survivor may have some or none of the following complications.

- *Second or recurrent stroke:* Between 25% and 42% of stroke survivors have second strokes. Fortunately, just like most first strokes, most second strokes are preventable. For instance, if the first stroke was caused by a blood clot, doctors may start the stroke survivor on *blood-thinning medication.* If the stroke was caused by a blocked *carotid artery,* doctors may perform a special surgical procedure called a *carotid endarterectomy* to clear the blockage and help prevent a second stroke.
- *Heart attack:* Heart disease is often an underlying contributor to stroke. Therefore, doctors will carefully monitor the stroke survivor's heart function. A small percentage of stroke survivors suffer a heart attack shortly after the stroke.
- *Aspiration pneumonia:* A stroke may interfere with the survivor's ability to chew and swallow food. This neurological deficit is called *dysphagia.* If the stroke results in dysphagia, these swallowing problems can cause food or fluid to go down into the lungs instead of the stomach. This causes coughing, choking, and—sometimes—aspiration pneumonia, in which the food or fluid causes an infection of the lungs. To help prevent this, hospital staff will position the dysphagic stroke

survivor carefully and observe him or her closely during mealtimes.

- *Cerebral edema:* This term is used to describe the swelling of the brain within the skull in response to an injury such as stroke. Although cerebral edema is a very serious complication of stroke, treatment with medication is often not necessary. Like swelling in other parts of the body, time is usually the best healer. In very severe cases, doctors may prescribe drugs to reduce the increased pressure due to swelling.

- *Pulmonary embolism:* Blood clots forming in other parts of the body may travel through the circulatory system and become lodged in a blood vessel in the lungs. The resulting interruption of blood flow in the lungs is called pulmonary embolism. It can lead to lung damage, heart problems, or even sudden death. Here, again, doctors will monitor the stroke survivor's blood very closely and can prescribe medication to prevent the formation of threatening blood clots.

- *Urinary tract complications:* Stroke survivors may have problems with their urinary tract function because of inadequate fluid intake, loss of bladder sensation, medication side effects, or infection. Hospital staff will closely monitor the stroke survivor and initiate proper treatment for these complications if necessary.

Early Recovery and Rehabilitation

There's still so much we don't know about how the brain compensates for stroke. Some brain cells may be only temporarily damaged—not killed—and can resume functioning. In some cases, the brain can reorganize its own functioning. Sometimes, a region of the brain "takes over" for a region damaged by the stroke. Stroke survivors sometimes experience remarkable and unanticipated recoveries that can't be explained.

There are some general guidelines, however. Statistics tell us that:

- 10% of stroke survivors recover almost completely.
- 25% recover with minor impairments.
- 40% experience moderate to severe impairments requiring special care.
- 10% require care in a nursing home or other long-term care facility.
- 15% die shortly after the stroke.

There are about three million stroke survivors living in America today.

Rehabilitation actually starts in the hospital as soon as possible after the stroke. In patients who are stable, rehabilitation may begin within two days after the stroke has occurred, and should be continued as necessary after release from the hospital.

The goal in rehabilitation is to improve function so that the stroke survivor can become as independent as possible while preserving his or her dignity and motivation to relearn old skills that the stroke may have taken away—skills like eating, dressing, and walking.

Rehabilitation is a team effort, and there are a number of health care professionals who can assist. They include doctors, nurses and speech, physical, recreational and occupational therapists, as well as social workers, counselors and clergy.

After the Stroke Survivor Is Released from the Hospital

Can the stroke survivor go home?

That depends on the severity of the stroke. The stroke survivor might:

- Move to a rehabilitation unit in the hospital;
- Be transferred to a rehabilitation hospital;
- Go home with home therapy; or
- Move to a long-term care facility that provides therapy and skilled nursing care.

How is rehabilitation accomplished?

The primary means of rehabilitation include physical therapy, occupational therapy, and speech therapy.

Physical therapy (PT) is one of the major rehabilitative tools. The purpose is to help restore physical functioning and skills like walking and range of movement. Through PT, work is done on some of the big impairments—like problems caused by partial or one-sided paralysis (called *hemiparesis*) faulty balance, or *foot drop.*

Occupational therapy (OT) is also very important. While the word "occupational" may make you think that this kind of therapy deals with employment or a job, it includes this but is actually something more. It's relearning the very skills needed for everyday living—skills such as eating, toileting, dressing, and taking care of oneself.

Speech and language therapy is another major rehabilitative therapy. Some stroke survivors are left with *aphasia,* an impairment of language and speaking skills in which the stroke survivor can think as well as before the stroke, but is unable to get the right words out or is unable to process words coming in. Aphasia is usually caused by a stroke on the left side of the brain. Speech therapy can teach the aphasic stroke survivor and his or her family members methods for coping with this frustrating impairment.

> Remember...recovery from stroke is a never-ending process. Although a lot of recovery may happen right away, recovery will also continue throughout the stroke survivor's life.

How Family Members Can Help

- **Have confidence that things will get better**...because they will.
- **Encourage, support, and give a great deal of love to the stroke survivor.**
- **Allow the stroke survivor to do things for him or herself,** no matter how painful it is to watch the struggle. As much as you'd like to, you cannot do the work of recovery for your loved one.
- **Be flexible about taking on new or different responsibilities.** One family member may have to take charge.

Similarly, the stroke survivor may have to give up some of his or her previous responsibilities.

- **Be ready to accept changing relationships** in accordance with new responsibilities.
- **Learn how to recognize and deal with *emotional lability*.** Emotional lability means that a stroke survivor may have difficulty controlling emotions and may suddenly start to laugh or cry for no reason at all. These emotional outbursts usually pass by quickly and, in time, may disappear completely.
- **Learn how to recognize and deal with depression.** The changes, the stress and the frustration surrounding stroke can all add up and result in depression. This is normal and in some ways, even healthy—it would almost be abnormal for the survivor and his or her family not to experience occasional depression. Patience, understanding, and humor are vital. In some cases, therapy and medications can also be helpful.
- **Check into joining a stroke support group.** These groups can be a tremendous source of strength to help deal with all of the changes that you will be facing.
- **Schedule a break in the caregiving.** Pace yourself and take some time off. Family members need to recharge their batteries, too.

Where to Go for Help and More Information

For more information about stroke, contact your local chapter of the National Stroke Association or contact National Stroke Association's headquarters at

8480 E Orchard Rd, Ste 1000
Englewood, CO 80111-5015
Toll-free: 1-800-STROKES (1-800-787-6537)
TDD: (303) 771-1886
Fax: (303) 771-1887

Ask your doctor for information about local resources such as stroke support groups, respite care, Meals on Wheels, etc.

Glossary of Stroke-Related Medical Terms

Aphasia: The loss or reduction of the ability to speak, read, write, or understand, due to dysfunction of brain centers.

Aspiration pneumonia: Pneumonia caused by inhaling foreign matter into the lungs. Most aspiration pneumonia in stroke survivors is caused by inhaling food or drink into the lungs, usually as the result of impaired swallowing ability.

Blood-thinning medication: Drugs designed to prevent the formation or further growth of blood clots. These drugs work by interfering with one or more of the blood components or processes essential to the clotting process.

Brain stem: The stemlike part of the brain that connects the brain's right and left hemispheres with the spinal cord. Responsible for non-thinking activities such as breathing, blood pressure, and coordination of eye movements.

Carotid artery: An artery which carries blood from the heart to the brain. You have a carotid artery on each side of your neck. Each artery divides into "internal" and "external" carotid arteries. Each external carotid artery supplies blood to the neck and face. Each internal carotid artery supplies blood to the front part of the brain.

Carotid endarterectomy: The surgical removal of the lining of a carotid artery. Performed when the artery is significantly diseased or blocked.

Cerebellum: The second largest portion of the brain, responsible for coordinating voluntary muscle movements.

Cerebral edema: Swelling of the brain due to an increase in its water content.

CT or "CAT" scanner: A specialized form of X-ray that allows physicians to see the internal structure of the brain in precise detail.

Dysphagia: Inability to or difficulty in swallowing.

Embolic stroke: A stroke resulting from the blockage of an artery by a blood clot (or "embolus").

Embolism: Term used to describe the blockage of a blood vessel by a blood clot.

Embolus: A mass of undissolved matter in a blood vessel, carried there by the bloodstream. In the case of stroke, this undissolved matter is usually a blood clot.

Emotional lability: Instability or changeability of the emotions. In stroke survivors, emotional lability usually takes the form of inappropriate laughing or crying (i.e., for no obvious reason).

Foot drop: Inability to pull the foot and toes up toward the shin. Common in patients who are in bed continuously (especially if comatose). Can usually be prevented through use of a foot board.

Heart attack: Death of heart tissue caused by the blockage of one or more of the arteries supplying blood to the heart. Also called a myocardial infarction.

Hemiparesis: Paralysis affecting only one side of the body.

Hemorrhage: Bleeding.

Hemorrhagic stroke: A stroke caused by a ruptured blood vessel and characterized by bleeding within or surrounding the brain.

Impairment: A difficulty in performing or lack of ability to perform an action. In stroke, an impairment is generally the direct result of damage to an area of the brain controlling a specific action. Sometimes referred to as a "neurological deficit."

Left hemisphere: The left half of the brain. Controls the actions of the right side of the body, as well as analytic abilities, such as calculating, speaking, and writing.

Left-side neglect: A lack of awareness of actions or objects on the left side of the body. For example, a stroke survivor with left-side neglect may ignore or forget about food on the left side of the dinner plate. To help this person, remind him or her about the left side of the plate, or move the food to the right side of the plate.

Neurological deficit: See Impairment.

Occupational therapy: Therapy designed to help stroke survivors become independent in their activities of daily living, such as eating bathing, and using the bathroom.

Physical therapy: Therapy which uses physical agents such as heat, massage, hydrotherapy, radiation, electricity, and exercise to help patients improve or regain muscle function or strength.

Pulmonary embolism: The blockage of a lung artery by a mass of undissolved matter (usually a blood clot).

Recurrent stroke: A second or any subsequent stroke following a first stroke.

Right hemisphere: The right half of the brain. Controls the actions of the left side of the body.

Second stroke: See Recurrent stroke.

Speech and language therapy: Therapy designed to diagnose and treat defects and disorders of the voice and of spoken and written communication.

Thrombosis: The blockage of a blood vessel which is caused by the gradual build-up of deposits within blood vessels. A partial blockage is often made complete when a blood clot develops on top of the deposits, preventing the free flow of blood. Thrombosis occurs most frequently in blood vessels already compromised by atherosclerosis ("hardening of the arteries").

Thrombotic stroke: A stroke resulting from the blockage of a blood vessel by accumulated deposits, with the blockage made complete when a blood clot develops on top of the deposits, preventing the free flow of blood.

Thrombus: A blood clot on the wall of a blood vessel. Can grow large enough to block the blood vessel and cause a thrombotic stroke, particularly if the clot forms on top of previously built-up deposits.

Urinary tract complications: Term used to describe a broad range of problems associated with the elimination of urine from the body. In stroke, most urinary tract complications are the result of brain damage which disrupts the exchange of messages between the brain and the bladder. As a result, stroke survivors may often be unable to control the elimination of urine or may retain too much urine. Physicians and nurses have a variety of ways to help stroke survivors cope with and gain control over urinary tract complications.

Vertebrobasilar artery: Artery which supplies blood to the brain stem and cerebellum.

Contact National Stroke Association for more information on

- NSA and Stroke Data
- Prevention
- Acute Care
- Rehabilitation
- Survivor & Caregiver Resources
- Research

■ **Document Source:**
National Stroke Association
8480 E Orchard Rd, Ste 1000
Englewood, CO 80111-5015
(303) 771-1700
FAX (303) 771-1886;
TDD (303) 771-1887
1-800-STROKES; (1-800-787-6537)
1995

See also: About Carotid Endarterectomy (page 227); Recovering After a Stroke (page 470)

WOMEN'S HEALTH CONCERNS

■ ■ ■

ABOUT CESAREAN CHILDBIRTH

Cesarean (se-sa'-re-an) section refers to the delivery of a baby through a surgical incision in the mother's lower abdominal wall and uterus, rather than through the vagina. This booklet will explain:

- Why you may need to have a cesarean section
- How a cesarean section is performed
- What to expect after the operation

Remember that each individual is different, and the outcome of any operation depends upon the patient's individual condition.

This booklet is not intended to take the place of the professional expertise of a qualified obstetrician who is familiar with your situation. After reading this booklet, you should discuss any questions you may have openly and honestly with your obstetrician.

About Cesarean Section

A cesarean section is performed only after an obstetrician has carefully weighed the factors involved in a woman's pregnancy and has decided that performing cesarean section is necessary. The indication for cesarean section may be evident at any time during the prenatal course. For the most part, the need for a cesarean section is only evident after the onset of labor, either in the early part or late during the course of labor.

Why cesarean section?

The presence of several conditions during pregnancy or labor may necessitate a cesarean section. Some of the most common conditions for which a cesarean section may be advised are:

1. **Prolonged or Ineffective Labor.** When labor is prolonged for various reasons, including insufficient contractions of the uterus, a cesarean section may be necessary to speed the birth process.
2. **Placenta Previa.** This condition exists when the placenta (or afterbirth) becomes positioned abnormally low within the uterus and there is a possibility that it could completely block the cervix. This condition could prevent the baby from advancing through the birth canal and it could also cause hemorrhaging (severe bleeding).
3. **Placenta Abruptia.** Occasionally, the placenta can suddenly separate from the wall of the uterus prior to the delivery of the baby, possibly causing the mother to hemorrhage, and the baby to have heart rate abnormality.
4. **Disproportion.** This condition occurs when the baby's head is too large or the mother's birth canal is too small to allow for a safe vaginal delivery.
5. **Abnormal Presentation.** In some instances, the baby's position in the uterus may make vaginal delivery dangerous. This problem may occur when the baby is in a breech (buttocks or feet first) or traverse (side or shoulder first) position.
6. **Prolapsed Cord.** This condition exists when the umbilical cord precedes the baby through the vagina during labor. This problem could strangle the baby as it is being born or block the baby's progress through the vagina during a vaginal delivery.
7. **Fetal Distress.** If the baby has a slow or very rapid heart rate, deceleration of heart rate, or a heartbeat that does not fluctuate, it may be advisable to speed the delivery by performing a cesarean section.
8. **Medical Problems.** The mother may have medical problems, such as diabetes, genital herpes, hypertension, cardiac disease, toxemia, and ovarian or uterine cysts or tumors that could make labor hazardous to both the mother and the baby.
9. **Multiple Births.** Multiple births, such as twins and triplets, may sometimes be delivered more safely by cesarean section, particularly if one or more of the babies' position in the uterus will result in an abnormal presentation.
10. **Previous Cesarean Delivery.** Previously, women who had one cesarean birth would deliver subsequent births by the same method. Now, however, it is estimated that as many as 60 percent of women who have had a cesarean section may be able to have a successful vaginal delivery. This is an option that must be discussed with a qualified obstetrician.

11. **Birth Defects.** Some babies with birth defects who are diagnosed by ultrasound have a better outcome when delivered by cesarean section. The risks and benefits should be discussed with a qualified obstetrician.

Although any of these conditions may make a cesarean section advisable, they do not necessarily rule out the possibility of a normal vaginal delivery.

About the Operation

It is estimated that cesarean section is performed in approximately one out of every five deliveries in the United States; in most instances, it is not considered a dangerous or risky procedure.

While the type of anesthesia used for a cesarean section is determined by the condition of the mother and baby, in most cases either a spinal or epidural anesthetic is administered to numb the mother's legs and abdomen. Either anesthetic will allow the mother to remain awake without feeling pain. Sometimes, however, a general anesthetic that allows the mother to be asleep during the operation may be preferable.

Two types of abdominal skin incisions can be used for a cesarean section. The vertical or longitudinal incision extends from the navel to the public hair line. The transverse, or horizontal incision (also known as the "bikini cut"), runs across the pubic hair line. After making the first incision, the obstetrician usually makes a horizontal incision on the lower part of the uterus. The obstetrician then gently removes the baby and the placenta from the uterus. The incision in the mother's uterus is then tightly sutured, and the abdomen is closed in the same manner as is used for any other operation.

Recovery from the Operation

The average hospital stay after a cesarean section may be from three to five days. Most patients are encouraged to get out of bed the day after the operation or earlier and are able to return to normal activities in approximately four to six weeks.

Surgery by Surgeons

A fully trained surgeon is a physician who, after medical school, has gone through years of training in an accredited residency program to learn the specialized skills of a surgeon. One good sign of a surgeon's competence is certification by a national surgical board approved by the American Board of Medical Specialties. All board-certified surgeons have satisfactorily completed an approved residency training program and have passed a rigorous specialty examination.

The letters F.A.C.S. (Fellow of the American College of Surgeons) after a surgeon's name are a further indication of a physician's qualifications. Surgeons who become Fellows of the College have passed a comprehensive evaluation of their surgical training and skills; they also have demonstrated their commitment to high standards of ethical conduct. This evaluation is conducted according to national standards that were established to ensure that patients receive the best possible surgical care.

Reviewed by: Byron J. Masterson, MD, FACS, J. Wayne Reitz Professor and Chairman, Department of Obstetrics and Gynecology, University of Florida, College of Medicine, Gainesville, FL; James Howard Maxwell, MD, FACS, Colorado Springs, CO.

■ **Document Source:**
American College of Surgeons
55 E Erie St
Chicago, IL 60611
September 1994

ABOUT HYSTERECTOMY

A hysterectomy is the surgical removal of the uterus or womb. This booklet will explain

- Why you may need to have a hysterectomy
- How a hysterectomy is performed
- What to expect before and after the operation

Remember, no two women undergoing a hysterectomy are alike. The reasons for and the outcome of any surgical procedure depend on your age, the severity of your problem, and your general health. This brochure is not intended to take the place of your surgeon's professional opinion. Rather, it is intended to help you understand the basics of this surgical procedure. Read this information carefully. If you have questions after reading this material, discuss them openly and honestly with your surgeon.

Why are hysterectomies performed?

A hysterectomy, which is an elective procedure 90 percent of the time, may be performed to treat a variety of gynecological (female reproductive system) problems.

For example, today most hysterectomies are done to treat benign fibroid tumors (non-cancerous) of the uterus. These growths, while not life-threatening, cause pelvic pain, excessive bleeding, or pain during sexual intercourse.

Endometriosis is a condition in which pieces of tissue from the lining of the uterus become displaced and move to other parts of the abdomen where the tissue can grow and cause pain. Endometriosis is the second most common reason for a woman to have a hysterectomy. However, the tendency to treat endometriosis by performing a hysterectomy has been declining in the last decade because other treatments have evolved. You should discuss these other options with your surgeon to see if another treatment for endometriosis may be effective for you.

Prolapse of the uterus is another reason why women opt for hysterectomy. In this condition, the uterus descends or sags into the vagina due to stretching of the ligaments and fibrous tissue that usually hold it in place. For women with cancer of the uterine lining or cancer of the cervix, a hysterectomy is necessary to prevent its spread.

Are all hysterectomies the same?

You may hear different names in reference to this type of operation. That is because there are different types of hysterectomies. A true total hysterectomy or *panhysterectomy* applies only to the removal of the uterus and cervix. When the ovaries and fallopian tubes on both sides are also removed, the procedure is called a hysterectomy and *bilateral salpingo-oophorectomy* (*salpingo* is Greek for fallopian tube while *oophor* is Greek for bearing eggs, that is, the ovaries). A *radical hysterectomy* is an operation performed only for certain pelvic cancers and includes removal of the uterus, cervix, upper vagina, and adjacent lymph nodes.

Is hysterectomy mainly for older women?

You may be surprised to know that 42, a relatively young age, is the average age for undergoing a hysterectomy. More than three-fourths of all women who have a hysterectomy are between 20 and 49 years of age.

Is there any reason to avoid or delay hysterectomy?

It is not sensible to have a hysterectomy in order to prevent cancer of the cervix or uterus. In this case, the risks of having a major operation outweigh any supposed cancer-protection benefits. Furthermore, hysterectomy is not considered to be the first choice of sterilization in most healthy women. Another procedure, tubal ligation, is a cheaper, easier, and safer method in most cases.

Sometimes, hysterectomy may not be the answer if your problem has not been adequately diagnosed. For instance, if you have pelvic pain that is not specifically caused by the uterus, a hysterectomy may not relieve your pain. The pain may be due to problems in your digestive, urinary, or skeletal systems. In these cases, your doctor will want to do the proper tests and X rays to locate the exact source of your pain. In addition to the tests and X rays indicated, a diagnostic laparoscopy may be helpful prior to hysterectomy in order to select the appropriate treatment.

Similarly, postmenopausal women who experience bleeding should avoid hysterectomy until a D&C (dilation and curettage) or a hysteroscopy (a surgical procedure in which a gynecologist uses a small lighted telescopic instrument called a hysteroscope to diagnose and treat many uterine disorders, including abnormal bleeding) are done. These procedures may reveal that another form of therapy is needed.

Finally, women who are obese, who have diabetes, high blood pressure, or some other type of chronic condition, are at increased risk during any type of operation. For these women, hysterectomy should only be considered if all reasonable alternatives have been exhausted.

If you have any questions about hysterectomy, ask your doctor. If it would make you feel more confident about your medical treatment, get a second opinion from another physician who is qualified to diagnose and treat your condition. Unless you have cancer, a severe pelvic infection, or uncontrollable bleeding, you do not have to rush into having a hysterectomy.

How do I decide about having a hysterectomy?

Following a hysterectomy, you will not longer be able to get pregnant. Thus, before you choose elective hysterectomy, you must consider both the severity of your problem and your desire to have children in the future. Although this operation may improve your quality of life by relieving chronic symptoms such as pain or bleeding, some women are willing to tolerate these conditions.

Ask yourself:

- Will I want to become pregnant in the future?
- How do I feel about not having a uterus?
- What is my husband's (or my partner's) attitude toward this operation?

Ask your surgeon:

- What will happen if I don't have a hysterectomy?
- What are the risks of hysterectomy in my particular case?
- Is my condition likely to improve on its own, stay the same, or get worse?
- Is hysterectomy medically necessary or recommended to relieve my particular symptoms?

Before your operation, you will be asked to sign a document giving your "informed consent" to the operation. This form lets you know any risks or possible complications that can be caused by the surgical procedure. Some states have specific laws that pertain to hysterectomies. They require surgeons to explain the alternatives and the risks of the procedure and are intended to make sure you understand the potential aftereffects of the operation.

How is a hysterectomy performed?

The surgeon can remove the uterus through a surgical incision made either inside the vagina or in the abdomen. In both the vaginal and abdominal approaches, the surgeon detaches the uterus from the fallopian tubes and ovaries as well as from the upper vagina.

Abdominal Hysterectomy

This type of hysterectomy allows the surgeon to easily see the pelvic organs and gives him or her more operating space than is permitted in a vaginal hysterectomy. Thus, for large pelvic tumors or suspected cancer, your surgeon may opt to do the procedure abdominally. When compared with the vaginal approach, the down-side of an abdominal hysterectomy is a slightly longer hospital stay, greater discomfort immediately following the operation, and a visible scar. However, the surgeon often can make a less-noticeable horizontal incision, called a bikini-cut, that extends along the top of the pubic hairline.

Vaginal Hysterectomy

The vaginal approach is ideal when the uterus is not enlarged or when the uterus has dropped as a result of the weakening of surrounding muscles. This approach is technically more difficult than the abdominal procedure because it offers the surgeon less operating space and less opportunity to view the pelvic organs. However, it may be preferred if the patient has a prolapsed uterus, if the patient is obese, or in cases of cervical cancer that has not spread. In closing the incision, the vagina is slightly shortened, resulting in possible initial pain during intercourse. A vaginal hysterectomy leaves no external scar.

A variation on vaginal hysterectomy is LAVH (laparo-scopic-assisted vaginal hysterectomy). A laparoscope is a device the surgeon can use to examine the inside of the pelvis. LAVH is an alternative for women who have ovarian disease but previously had only one choice: an abdominal hysterectomy that leaves a long incision. With LAVH, much of the procedure is done through tiny incisions using a laparoscope. The rest of the procedure can then be finished vaginally.

Stages of Recovery

After the operation, you will likely remain in the recovery room for one to three hours. You may be given pain medication and possibly antibiotics to prevent infection.

You will probably be able to walk around your room the day after your operation, depending on the type of procedure you underwent. Most patients go home the third day following an abdominal hysterectomy and by the first or second day after a vaginal hysterectomy or LAVH.

Complete recovery from abdominal hysterectomy—because the incision is typically five inches long—usually takes six to eight weeks. During your recovery, you can expect a gradual increase in activities. Avoid all lifting during the first two weeks of your recovery period and get plenty of rest. In the weeks following the surgical procedure, you can begin to do light chores, some driving, and even return to work, provided your occupation does not involve too much physical activity.

Around the sixth week following the operation, you can take tub baths and resume sexual activity. Women who have had vaginal hysterectomies generally recover more quickly.

Risks or Complications?

Hysterectomy is one of the safest operations. Yet no operation is without risk. Fever and infection can occur after vaginal hysterectomies. This condition can usually be treated without complication with antibiotics. More serious complications following this surgical procedure include thrombophlebitis (or blood clots in the legs that may travel through the blood vessels to the lungs) and severe bleeding.

Long-Term Effects

After a hysterectomy, you will become sterile (cannot get pregnant) and will no longer have menstrual periods. If you are premenopausal (before menopause) and have had your fallopian tubes and ovaries removed, you will experience all of the symptoms of menopause as your body gets used to different hormone levels. These symptoms may include hot flashes and perhaps irritability and depression. If the symptoms are severe, your doctor may prescribe hormone medication. A hysterectomy usually has no physical effect on your ability to experience sexual pleasure or orgasm.

Following hysterectomy, the ovaries will continue to function; however, the actual occurrence of menopause will be difficult to determine since the uterus has been removed and the patient will no longer have periods. As the age of menopause, approximately age 50, is approached, symptoms such as hot flashes may warrant testing to see if hormonal therapy is indicated.

If you experience vaginal dryness, it can be remedied by using prescription hormone creams or pills or water-soluble lubricants that you can purchase at the pharmacy.

A sense of loss following the removal of any organ is normal and takes time for adjustment. While depression following hysterectomy does not happen to everyone, it is more common if the operation was done because of cancer or severe illness, rather than as an elective operation. Additionally, if you are under age 40 or the operation interfered with your plans to have children, depression is more likely to occur. This depression can be temporary, depending on your general outlook on life, and the availability of a good support group of family and friends.

Most women experience an improvement of mood and increased sense of well-being following hysterectomy. For many, relief from fear of pregnancy results in heightened sexual enjoyment following the procedure.

Surgery by Surgeons

A fully-trained surgeon is a physician who, after medical school, has gone through years of training in an accredited residency program to learn the specialized skills of a surgeon. One good sign of a surgeon's competence is certification by a national surgical board approved by the American Board of Medical Specialties. All board-certified surgeons have satisfactorily completed an approved residency training program and have passed a rigorous specialty examination.

The letters F.A.C.S. (Fellow of the American College of Surgeons) after a surgeon's name are a further indication of a physician's qualifications. Surgeons who become Fellows of the College have passed a comprehensive evaluation of their surgical training and skills; they also have demonstrated their commitment to high standards of ethical conduct. This evaluation is conducted according to national standards that were established to ensure that patients receive the best possible surgical care.

Reviewed by: Byron J. Masterson, MD, FACS; J. Wayne Reitz, Professor and Chairman, Department of Obstetrics and Gynecology, University of Florida, College of Medicine, Gainesville, FL; James Howard Maxwell, MD, FACS, Colorado Springs, CO.

■ **Document Source:**
American College of Surgeons
55 E Erie St
Chicago, IL 60611
September 1994

Information from PDQ for Patients

ENDOMETRIAL CANCER

Description

What is cancer of the endometrium?

Cancer of the endometrium, a common kind of cancer in women, is a disease in which cancer (malignant) cells are found in the lining of the uterus (endometrium). The uterus is the hollow, pear-shaped organ where a baby grows. Cancer of the endometrium is different from cancer of the muscle of the uterus, which is called sarcoma of the uterus. A separate statement containing information on uterine sarcoma is also available in PDQ.

Like most cancers, cancer of the endometrium is best treated when it is found (diagnosed) early. You should see a doctor if you have any of the following problems: bleeding or discharge not related to your periods (menstruation), difficult or painful urination, pain during intercourse, and pain in the pelvic area.

Endometrial cancer has been found in a few breast cancer patients treated with the hormone, tamoxifen. If you take this hormone, you should go to your doctor for a pelvic exam every year and report any vaginal bleeding other than your menstrual period as soon as possible.

Your doctor may use several tests to see if you have cancer, usually beginning with an internal (pelvic) exam. During the exam, your doctor will feel for any lumps or changes in the shape of the uterus. Your doctor will then do a Pap test, using a piece of cotton, a brush, or a small wooden stick to gently scrape the outside of the cervix (opening of the uterus) and vagina to pick up cells.

Because cancer of the endometrium begins inside the uterus, it does not usually show up on the Pap test. For this reason, your doctor may also do a dilation and curettage (D & C) or similar test to remove pieces of the lining of the uterus. During a D & C, the opening of the cervix is stretched with a spoon-shaped instrument and the walls of the uterus are scraped gently to remove any growths. This tissue is then checked for cancer cells.

Your chance of recovery (prognosis) and choice of treatment depend on the stage of your cancer (whether it is just in the endometrium or has spread to other parts of the uterus or other parts of the body) and your general state of health. Your chance of recovery may also depend on how your cells look under the microscope. If you have early stage cancer, your prognosis may also depend on whether female hormones (progesterones) affect the growth of the cancer.

Stage Explanation

Stages of Cancer of the Endometrium

Once cancer of the endometrium has been found, more tests will be done to find out if the cancer has spread from the endometrium to other parts of the body (staging). Your doctor needs to know the stage of your disease to plan treatment. The following stages are used for cancer of the endometrium:

Stage 0 or Carcinoma In Situ

Stage 0 cancer of the endometrium is a very early cancer. The cancer is found only inside the uterus and is only in the surface layer of the endometrium.

Stage I

Cancer is found only in the main part of the uterus (it is not found in the cervix).

Stage II

Cancer cells have spread to the cervix.

Stage III

Cancer cells have spread outside the uterus but have not spread outside the pelvis.

Stage IV

Cancer cells have spread beyond the pelvis, to other body parts, or into the lining of the bladder (the sac which holds urine) or rectum.

Recurrent

Recurrent disease means the cancer has come back (recurred) after it has been treated.

Treatment Option Overview

How Cancer of the Endometrium is Treated

There are treatments for all patients with cancer of the endometrium. Four kinds of treatment are used:

- surgery (taking out the cancer in an operation)
- radiation therapy (using high-dose x-rays or other high-energy rays to kill cancer cells and shrink tumors)
- chemotherapy (using drugs to kill cancer cells)
- hormone therapy (using female hormones to kill cancer cells).

Surgery is the most common treatment for cancer of the endometrium. Your doctor may take out the cancer using one of the following operations:

- Total abdominal hysterectomy and bilateral salpingo-oophorectomy, taking out the uterus, fallopian tubes, and ovaries through a cut in the abdomen. Lymph nodes in the pelvis may also be taken out (lymph node dissection). (The lymph nodes are small, bean-shaped structures that are found throughout the body. They produce and store infection-fighting cells, but may contain cancer cells.)
- Radical hysterectomy, taking out the cervix, uterus, fallopian tubes, ovaries, and part of the vagina. Lymph nodes in the area may also be taken out (lymph node dissection).

Radiation therapy uses high-dose x-rays to kill cancer cells and shrink tumors. Radiation may come from a machine outside the body (external radiation) or from putting materials that produce radiation (radioisotopes) through thin plastic tubes into the area where the cancer cells are found (internal radiation). Radiation may be used alone or before or after surgery.

Chemotherapy uses drugs to kill cancer cells. Chemotherapy may be taken by pill, or it may be put into the body by a needle in the vein. Chemotherapy is called a systemic treatment because the drugs enter the bloodstream, travel through the body, and can kill cancer cells outside the uterus.

Hormone therapy uses hormones, usually taken by pill, to kill cancer cells.

Treatment by Stage

Treatment for cancer of the endometrium depends on the stage of your disease, the type of disease, your age, and your overall condition.

You may receive treatment that is considered standard based on its effectiveness in a number of patients in past studies, or you may choose to go into a clinical trial. Not all patients are cured with standard therapy and some standard treatments may have more side effects than are desired. For these reasons, clinical trials are designed to find better ways to treat cancer patients and are based on the most up-to-date information. Clinical trials are going on in most parts of the country for most stages of cancer of the endometrium. If you want more information, call the Cancer Information Service at 1-800-4-CANCER (1-800-422-6237).

Stage 0 Endometrial Cancer

Your treatment may be one of the following:
1. Dilation and curettage (D & C) followed by hormone therapy. Your doctor may tell you not to take any more medicine that contains estrogen.
2. Hysterectomy.

Stage I Endometrial Cancer

Your treatment may be one of the following:
1. Surgery to remove the uterus and both ovaries and fallopian tubes (total abdominal hysterectomy and bilateral salpingo-oophorectomy) with removal of some of the lymph nodes in the pelvis and abdomen to see if they contain cancer.

2. Total abdominal hysterectomy and bilateral salpingo-oophorectomy with removal of some of the lymph nodes in the pelvis and abdomen to see if they contain cancer, followed by radiation therapy to the pelvis.
3. Clinical trials of radiation and/or chemotherapy following surgery.
4. Radiation therapy alone for selected patients.

Stage II Endometrial Cancer

Your treatment may be one of the following:
1. Total abdominal hysterectomy, bilateral salpingo-oophorectomy, and removal of some of the lymph nodes in the pelvis and abdomen to see if they contain cancer, followed by radiation therapy.
2. Internal and external beam radiation therapy followed by surgery to remove the uterus and both ovaries and fallopian tubes (total abdominal hysterectomy and bilateral salpingo-oophorectomy). Some of the lymph nodes in the pelvis and abdomen are also removed to see if they contain cancer.
3. Surgery to remove the cervix, uterus, fallopian tubes, ovaries, and part of the vagina (radical hysterectomy). Lymph nodes in the area may also be taken out (lymph node dissection).

Stage III Endometrial Cancer

Your treatment may be one of the following:
1. Surgery to remove the cervix, uterus, fallopian tubes, ovaries, and part of the vagina (radical hysterectomy). Lymph nodes in the area may also be taken out (lymph node dissection). Surgery is usually followed by radiation therapy.
2. Internal and external beam radiation therapy.
3. Hormone therapy.

Stage IV Endometrial Cancer

Your treatment may be one of the following:
1. Internal and external beam radiation therapy.
2. Hormone therapy.
3. Clinical trials of chemotherapy.

Recurrent Endometrial Cancer

If your cancer has come back, your treatment may be one of the following:
1. Radiation therapy to relieve symptoms, such as pain, nausea, and abnormal bowel functions.
2. Hormone therapy.
3. Clinical trials of chemotherapy.

To Learn More

To learn more about cancer of the endometrium, call the National Cancer Institute's Cancer Information Service at 1-800-4-CANCER (1-800-422-6237). By dialing this toll-free number, you can speak with someone who can answer your questions.

The Cancer Information Service can also send you free booklets. The following booklet may be of some help to you:

- What You Need to Know About Cancer of the Uterus

The following general booklets on questions related to cancer may also be helpful:

- What You Need to Know About Cancer
- Taking Time: Support for People with Cancer and the People Who Care About Them
- What Are Clinical Trials All About?
- Chemotherapy and You: A Guide to Self-Help During Treatment
- Radiation Therapy and You: A Guide to Self-Help During Treatment
- Eating Hints for Cancer Patients
- Advanced Cancer: Living Each Day
- When Cancer Recurs: Meeting the Challenge Again

There are many other places you can get material about cancer treatment and services to help you. You can check the social service office at your hospital for local and national agencies that help with your finances, getting to and from treatment, care at home, and dealing with your problems. The American Cancer Society, for example, has many free services. Their local offices are listed in the white pages of the telephone book.

You can also write to the National Cancer Institute at this address:

National Cancer Institute
Office of Cancer Communications
31 Center Dr, MSC 2580
Bethesda, MD 20892-2580

■ **Document Source:**
U.S. Department of Health and Human Services, Public Health Service
National Institutes of Health
National Cancer Institute

HORMONE REPLACEMENT THERAPY: SHOULD YOU TAKE IT?

Menopause is the stage in a woman's life when menstruation stops and she can no longer bear children. During menopause, the body makes less of the female hormones, estrogen and progesterone. After menopause, the lower hormone levels free a woman from concerns about monthly menstrual periods and getting pregnant. But they can also cause troublesome symptoms, such as hot flashes (a sudden flush or warmth, often followed by sweating) and sleep problems. Sometimes women have other physical problems, such as vaginal dryness. While many women have little or no trouble with menopause, others have moderate to severe discomfort. Estrogen loss also raises a woman's risk for other serious health problems. They include heart disease and stroke, lead-

ing causes of death for women over the age of 50. Estrogen loss also can lead to bone loss.

Some bone loss is normal as people age. However, a more serious condition called osteoporosis weakens bones and lets them break easily. It affects 24 million people in this country. Women have a higher risk than men.

Doctors sometimes prescribe hormones to replace those lost during menopause. This treatment, called *hormone replacement therapy* (HRT), can ease symptoms of menopause and protect against risks of heart disease, stroke, and osteoporosis. Although millions of women take HRT, this may not be the right choice for everyone.

What can you do?

Doctors usually prescribe HRT combining estrogen and another female hormone, progestin. They usually prescribe estrogen without progestin for women who have had their uterus removed (hysterectomy). Estrogen can be used in pill or tablet form, vaginal creams, or shots. There are also patches that attach to the skin and release estrogen through the skin. The form of estrogen your doctor chooses may depend on your symptoms. For instance, creams are used for vaginal dryness, while pills or patches are used to ease different menopause symptoms, such as hot flashes, or to prevent bone loss. Progestin usually is taken in pill form.

Doctors may prescribe different schedules for taking HRT. Some women take estrogen for a set number of days, add progestin for a set number of days, and then stop taking one or both for a specific period of time. They repeat the same pattern every month. This pattern often causes regular monthly bleeding like a menstrual period. Some women take HRT every day of the month without any break. This pattern usually stops regular monthly bleeding. Talk with your doctors about the system that is best for you.

Who should take HRT?

Many experts believe that the benefits of HRT may be greater than the risks. But scientists do not yet fully know the risks of long-term HRT. Before you decide about HRT, discuss the possible benefits, risks, and side effects with your doctor.

Risk Factors for Osteoporosis

Women who are at high risk of getting osteoporosis may want to think about taking HRT to prevent it. Risk factors include:

- Having early menopause (natural or due to surgery)
- Being White or Asian
- Being physically inactive
- Taking corticosteriod medicines (prescribed for arthritis or other inflammatory diseases)
- Having a slight build
- Getting too little calcium from diet
- Smoking cigarettes
- Drinking more than a moderate amount of alcohol
- Having thyroid or kidney disease

Your doctor may warn against HRT if you have high blood pressure, diabetes, liver disease, blood clots, seizures, migraine headaches, gallbladder disease, or a history of cancer. Also, daughters of mothers who took DES (diethylstilbestrol) during pregnancy may have changes to their reproductive system that make HRT dangerous.

Side Effects and Risks of HRT

Some women may have side effects from HRT, such as unwanted vaginal bleeding, headaches, nausea, vaginal discharge, fluid retention, swollen breasts, or weight gain. Other health concerns for women taking HRT include:

Cancer of the uterus (endometrial cancer). Research shows that women who have their uterus and use estrogen alone are at risk for endometrial cancer. But today, most doctors prescribe the combination of estrogen and progestin. Progestin protects against endometrial cancer. If a woman who still has a uterus takes estrogen alone, her doctor should take sample tissue from her uterus (endometrial biopsy) to check for cancer every year. Women without a uterus have no risk of endometrial cancer.

Breast cancer. Today, many scientists are studying the possible link between HRT and breast cancer. Some studies have shown that HRT increases the risk of breast cancer.

Heart disease. Estrogen alone or combined with progestin reduces the risk of heart disease. Scientists recently have shown that estrogen lowers risks of heart disease and stroke in women over the age of 50, when they are most at risk for heart disease and stroke.

Abnormal vaginal bleeding. Women taking HRT are more likely than other women to have abnormal vaginal bleeding. When this happens, the doctor may perform a "D and C" (dilation and curettage) to find the cause of bleeding. In more serious cases, the doctor may suggest removing the uterus.

Scientists are still studying the risks of taking estrogen alone or in combination with progestin over a long period of time. Women who have their uterus, are at low risk for stroke, heart disease, or serious bone disease, and have no major menopause symptoms may choose to avoid HRT.

Medical Checkups

If you are taking hormones you should have regular medical checkups. The American College of Obstetricians and Gynecologists recommends that all women taking HRT get a medical checkup every year. At that time, the doctor or nurse should read your blood pressure, give you pelvic and breast exams, and take an xray picture of your breasts (mammogram) to check for breast cancer.

If you don't take HRT

If you decide against HRT, there are other ways to deal with the symptoms of menopause. There are drugs that can reduce hot flashes, and you can apply water soluble surgical jelly (**not** petroleum jelly) to the vagina to reduce dryness. Simply

lowering the room temperature may help you sleep better and ease uncomfortable hot flashes.

To strengthen your bones, good health habits can help, even if you don't start until later in life. Experts suggest that all adult women have 1,000 mg of calcium each day; after menopause, women not using HRT should have 1,500 mg each day. Low-fat milk and dairy foods such as cheese and yogurt are good sources for calcium. If you find it hard to get that amount from your diet, you can take calcium supplements.

Your body also needs vitamin D to absorb calcium. Most people get enough vitamin D just by being out in the sun for at least a short time every day. Supplements or milk fortified with vitamin D are also good sources for this vitamin.

Weight-bearing exercises, which make your muscles work against gravity, help strengthen bones and prevent osteoporosis. Walking, jogging, and playing tennis are all good weight-bearing exercises.

You may also want to ask your doctor about a new drug to treat osteoporosis in women past menopause. The new treatment is safe and effective in increasing bone mass.

Resources

You can get more information on this topic by contacting the organizations listed below.

The American College of Obstetricians and Gynecologists (ACOG) offers the following pamphlets, *Hormone Replacement Therapy, Preventing Osteoporosis,* and *The Menopause Years.* To obtain copies, send a self-addressed envelope to
ACOG
409 12th Street, SW
Washington, DC 20024-2188

The American Association of Retired Persons (AARP) Women's Initiative has a fact sheet, *Hormone Replacement Therapy: Facts to Help You Decide.* To obtain a copy, write:
AARP
601 E Street, NW
Washington, DC 20049
1-800-424-3410

The National Osteoporosis Foundation (NOF) has information for health professionals and the public. Contact:
NOF
1150 17th St, NW, Ste 500
Washington, Dc 20036-4603
1-800-223-9994

The National Resource Center on Osteoporosis and Related Bone Diseases is a national clearinghouse with information on the risks, prevention, and treatment of osteoporosis. For more information, call: 1-800-624-BONE

The North American Menopause Society (NAMS) answers written requests for information. Write:
NAMS
11100 Euclid Ave
7th Ave
McDonald Hospital
Cleveland, OH 44105

The National Women's Health Network distributes educational materials on a variety of women's health topics. Contact:
National Women's Health Network
514 10th St, NW
Washington, DC 20004
202-347-1140

The Older Women's League (OWL) educates the public about problems and issues of concern to middle age and older women.

Contact:
OWL
666 11th St, NW
Suite 700 Washington, DC 20001
202-783-6686

The National Cancer Institute (NCI), part of NIH, funds cancer research and offers information for health professionals and the public. For more information about cancer risks and other related issues, call: 1-800-4-CANCER

The National Heart, Lung, and Blood Institute, part of NIH, carries out research and provides educational information on heart disease, stroke, and other related topics. For more information call: 301-251-1222

National Institute on Aging Information Center has information on menopause, osteoporosis, and a variety of other topics related to health and aging. Contact:
PO Box 8057
Gaithersburg, MD 20898-8057
800-222-2225
800-222-4225 (TTY)

■ Document Source:
**U.S. Department of Health and Human Services, Public Health Service
National Institutes of Health
National Institute on Aging
1995**

A STATUS REPORT ON BREAST IMPLANT SAFETY

by Marian Segal

Recently published studies have shown that women with silicone gel-filled breast implants do not have a greatly increased risk of some well-defined autoimmune diseases, which were among the serious health concerns surrounding the devices. These include potentially fatal connective tissue diseases such as scleroderma and lupus erythematosus.

Widespread reports of adverse reactions to silicone gel-filled implants and a lack of evidence supporting their safety led the Food and Drug Administration to order the devices off the market in April 1992. They remained available only to women in clinical studies, mostly women seeking breast reconstruction after breast cancer surgery. Saline-filled implants were allowed to remain on the market for all uses.

The new studies do not, however, rule out the possibility that a subset of women with implants may have a small increased risk of these conditions, or that some women might develop other immune-related symptoms that don't conform to "classic" disease descriptions.

Nor did the studies address other important safety questions, including implant rupture rates and the incidence of capsular contracture (shrinking of scar tissue around the implant, which can cause painful hardening of the breast or distort its appearance). Answers to these and other questions await the results of new or ongoing studies.

Reasons for New Studies

Breast implants had been marketed since the early 1960s—several years before the first medical device law was enacted in 1976, charging FDA with regulation of medical devices.

Every year, thousands of American women had had implant surgery for augmentation (to enlarge or reshape their breasts) or for reconstruction following mastectomy (removal of the breast) to treat breast cancer. Most of the implants consisted of a rubber silicone envelope filled with silicone gel; about 10 percent were filled with saline (salt water).

Under the 1976 law, implants and many other devices already in use were allowed to remain on the market, with the understanding that the agency would at some time ask manufacturers to submit scientific data showing these "grandfathered" products were safe and effective.

FDA requested this information for silicone gel-filled implants in April 1991 in response to a growing number of adverse reaction reports that raised safety concerns about the devices. The data submitted did not prove the devices safe, as required by law, so the agency restricted their use to clinical trials designed to resolve the safety questions.

Between Jan. 1, 1985, and March 16, 1995, FDA received 91,322 adverse reaction reports associated with silicone breast implants and 19,296 reports involving the saline implants. These reports included risks clearly associated with the devices, as well as adverse effects attributed to the implants, but not proved to be linked to them.

Polyurethane-Coated Implants

About 110,000 women have silicone gel-filled implants with a polyurethane coating, intended to reduce the risk of capsular contracture. In April 1991, an FDA analysis showed that polyurethane foam could break down under human body conditions to form a chemical called TDA, which can cause cancer in animals. As a result, the manufacturer immediately stopped selling the product.

Recently, however, a study to measure TDA in women with polyurethane implants found that a woman's risk of cancer from exposure to TDA released by the implant is negligible—about one in a million over a lifetime. FDA considers it unlikely that even one woman would develop cancer from these implants. The study supports the agency's original recommendation that women who are not having problems should not have the implants removed solely because of concern about cancer from TDA exposure.

Silicone Implant Studies

Some recent studies comparing the rates of immune-related diseases in women with implants versus those without implants have provided reassurance that women with implants are not at a greatly increased risk of these disorders.

The largest of these retrospective, or "look-back," studies is the Harvard Nurses' Health Study. The study used data from 87,501 nurses followed for other research purposes from 1976 through May 31, 1990, before there was widespread media coverage of the possible association between breast implants and connective tissue disease. None of the women had connective tissue disease at the start of the study.

In an article published in the June 22, 1995, *New England Journal of Medicine,* the researchers reported that 516 of the nurses had developed definite connective tissue diseases. Women with breast implants numbered 1,183. The types of implants included 876 silicone gel-filled, 170 saline-filled, 67 double lumen (silicone gel-filled implants with a saline-filled outer envelope), 14 polyurethane-coated, and 56 of unknown type. Only three of the 516 women with definite connective tissue disease had implants (one silicone-gel filled, one saline, and one double lumen).

The authors reported they "did not find an association between silicone breast implants and connective tissue disease, defined according to a variety of standardized criteria, or signs and symptoms of these diseases."

Similarly, a 1994 study conducted at the Mayo Clinic found no increased risk of connective tissue diseases among implant recipients. The investigators based their conclusion on comparison of the medical histories of 749 women with breast implants in Olmsted County, Minn., with a similar group of women who did not have implants.

Immunology Tests

Several laboratories are offering tests that claim to detect levels of antibodies to silicone that presumably indicate a leaking or ruptured implant.

FDA has not cleared or approved these tests for such purposes, and the agency has sent letters to several companies, warning of future regulatory action if they continue to promote the devices without a premarket approval application.

"There are important unresolved issues with these tests," says Peter Maxim, Ph.D., chief of the Center for Devices and Radiological Health's immunology branch of the division of clinical laboratory devices. "For one thing, the very existence of silicone antibodies has not been proven to the satisfaction of all scientists," he says. "Secondly, if antibodies are detected, is there in fact a correlation with the presence or the status of implants, or do they reflect prior environmental exposure? Silicone is in a myriad of products, including foods, medicines, and antiperspirants absorbed by the skin, to name a few."

The next problem, Maxim says, is that there are claims that extremely high antibody levels may indicate a leaking or ruptured implant. This, then, raises the question of what medical intervention, if any, should be taken.

Sahar M. Dawisha, MD, a rheumatologist in FDA's division of general and restorative devices, adds that no one really knows what the clinical significance of an antibody to silicone means or at what level it is harmful.

"Furthermore," she says, "in autoimmune or connective tissue disease—where antibody tests are generally used—the presence of antibodies doesn't define the disease. A disease is defined by clinical signs and symptoms, and antibodies are used as supporting evidence."

Finally, John Nagle, consumer safety officer in the Center for Devices and Radiological Health's diagnostic devices branch, says, "The tests themselves may be harmless, but they sure are expensive, somewhere between $500 and $1,000," adding that "a lot of them are being done for litigation purposes rather than to help the patient medically."

"Because of the limitations in the size and type of the studies, however, the true risk of these diseases is not known," says S. Lori Brown, Ph.D., a research scientist officer in the epidemiology branch of the agency's Center for Devices and Radiological Health. "Although the criteria others may be using to assess those studies show that some concerns are eliminated," Brown says, "unfortunately, they don't rule out a small, but significant, increased risk."

An immunology and epidemiology expert, Brown explains that an inherent problem in the studies is that some connective tissue diseases are extremely rare. "If you have a disease that has an incidence of 1 in 100,000 in the general population, for example, and you do a study of 750 women with implants, like the Mayo Clinic Study, then you wouldn't really expect to see even a single case of that disease," she says, "unless there's an exceedingly high—more than a hundredfold—increase in risk."

Small studies like these can rule out huge risks, but not smaller, yet significant risk increases that would only show up in studies that include several thousand women with implants, Brown says. Nor do the studies fully examine or answer whether the implants might in some women lead to symptoms not typical of classical disease manifestations.

Other Concerns

Brown also stresses that connective tissue diseases are not the only issue of concern, especially since they may affect a much smaller proportion of women with implants. The larger issue, she says, is the local complications that are clearly related to breast implants, such as rupture and migration of the silicone gel, capsular contracture, and infection.

Known Risks of Breast Implants

Surgical Risks

- possible complications of general anesthesia, as well as nausea, vomiting and fever
- infection
- hematoma (collection of blood that may cause swelling, pain and bruising, perhaps requiring surgical draining)
- hemorrhage (abnormal bleeding)
- thrombosis (abnormal clotting)
- skin necrosis—skin tissue death resulting from insufficient blood flow to the skin. The chance of skin necrosis may be increased by radiation treatments, cortisone-like drugs, an implant too large for the available space, or smoking.

Implant Risks

- capsular contracture (hardening of the breast due to scar tissue)
- leak or rupture—silicone implants may leak or rupture slowly, releasing silicone gel into surrounding tissue; saline implants may rupture suddenly and deflate, usually requiring immediate removal or replacement
- temporary or permanent change or loss of sensation in the nipple or breast tissue
- formation of calcium deposits in surrounding tissue, possibly causing pain and hardening
- shifting from the original placement, giving the breast an unnatural look

- interference with mammography readings, possibly delaying breast cancer detection by "hiding" a suspicious lesion. Also, it may be difficult to distinguish calcium deposits formed in the scar tissue from a tumor when interpreting the mammogram. *When making an appointment for a mammogram, the woman should tell the scheduler she has implants to make sure qualified personnel are on-site. At the time of the mammogram she should also remind the technician she has implants before the procedure is done, so the technician can use special techniques to obtain the best mammogram and to avoid rupturing the implant.*

Possible Risks of Breast Implants

- Autoimmune-like disorders—signs include joint pain and swelling; skin tightness, redness or swelling; swelling of hands and feet; rash; swollen glands or lymph nodes; unusual fatigue; general aching; greater chance of getting colds, viruses and flu; unusual hair loss; memory problems; headaches; muscle weakness or burning; nausea or vomiting; and irritable bowel syndrome.
  Recent studies have shown, however, that there is not a large increased risk of traditional autoimmune, or connective tissue disease, from silicone gel implants.
- Fibrositis/fibromyalgia-like disorder (pain, tenderness and stiffness of muscle tendons and ligaments).

"Of the two groups of women who consider getting implants—for breast reconstruction or for augmentation." Brown says, "the larger group wants them for cosmetic purposes. These are healthy women who may go out and get implants without a clear picture of what the possible risks are. They may end up going back in for surgery time and again and never be happy with the cosmetic effect."

In testimony before a congressional subcommittee in August 1995, FDA Commissioner David A. Kessler, MD, stated that "Published studies to date suggest a rupture rate between 5 and 51 percent—an enormous range—and unfortunately, we do not know with any confidence where within that range the real rupture rate lies." He also cited two studies that indicate the risk of rupture increases as the implants age.

Another concern—increased risk of breast cancer—has not been borne out by studies. "Several studies have indicated there is no increased risk of breast cancer in women with implants," Brown says. However, she adds, these women are not yet in the age group that is more prone to breast cancer, and it remains to be seen whether they will eventually have a higher incidence of breast cancer than women without implants. Long-term studies to look at this are under way.

Manufacturers' Studies

The events that led to removal of silicone implants from the market made it clear that prospective, or forward-looking, studies were also needed to answer important safety questions. Implant manufacturers agreed to conduct human trials in three phases: urgent need, adjunct, and core studies.

"The purpose of the first phase [urgent need] actually was simply to quickly provide implants to women who were already in the process of getting them for breast reconstruction or for another medical reason, and to bridge the time until the adjunct studies were begun," says Sahar M. Dawisha, MD, a rheumatologist and medical officer who joined FDA's division of general and restorative devices in April 1993.

The women did, however, have to sign an informed consent form that summarized the risks and benefits of the implants. This form had not previously been required.

"The second phase, or adjunct, studies were intended to follow reconstruction patients for five years to assess short-term safety data, including rates of capsular contracture, rupture, and complications such as infection and hematoma [collection of blood that may cause swelling, pain and bruising]," Dawisha says. "These studies are open to all women wanting breast reconstruction with implants because of mastectomy, traumatic injury to the breast, or a disease or congenital disorder causing a severe breast abnormality. They do not include augmentation patients."

Mentor Corporation of Santa Barbara, Calif., began adjunct studies in 1992. According to Pamela Powell of the company's Clinical Programs Department, as of July 5, 1995, 12,125 patients were enrolled in the studies.

The third phase, or core studies, Dawisha says, were intended to determine the full safety and effectiveness profile of the device, including rupture rates, quality-of-life benefits, extent of interference with mammography, and many more safety concerns—including rheumatologic assessments—that would need a large number of women. They were also to include augmentation patients. The sponsors, however, have not initiated these studies.

Information Packet

To obtain a comprehensive packet of information on breast implant issues, request FDA's publication, "Breast Implants, An Information Update," by calling the agency's breast implant information line at (1-800) 532-4440.

Saline Implants

Although many of the local complications of gel-filled implants are also associated with saline implants, the latter were permitted to remain on the market unrestricted for both reconstruction and augmentation. FDA considers saline-filled implants less risky, because although they have the same silicone rubber envelope as gel-filled implants, leakage or rupture would release only salt water, not silicone gel, into the body.

Nevertheless, FDA is requiring manufacturers to collect data on the saline implants as well, because the incidence of known risks (for example, deflation and capsular contracture) is not well defined. When the Medical Device Amendments were passed, it was determined that these devices would also eventually require premarket approval. In January 1993, FDA notified saline implant manufacturers that they would have to submit safety and effectiveness data for their products. In December 1994, the agency told them what type of safety and effectiveness data were needed, and delineated objectives and time frames for the trials.

Saline implants will stay on the market while the studies are conducted, but the companies must report the laboratory, animal and clinical data in stages, and must provide written information on the known and possible risks of their products.

"Women considering saline implants should ask their doctor for a copy of the manufacturer's information sheet, a copy of the product insert sheet for the specific implant to be used, and a copy of the hospital informed consent form," says Barbara Stellar, FDA's breast implant information and outreach coordinator.

Stellar recommends women be given these documents at least a month before surgery is planned, if possible, so they can thoroughly discuss benefits and possible risks with surgeons, radiologists, and other women. These women should also ask their physicians about participating in the saline breast implant trials.

Brown hopes that further studies will more clearly define risks associated with all types of implants.

"We need to be able to tell women considering breast implants—whether for augmentation or reconstruction—the specific risks on which they can base their decision," she says. "It should be made clear that implants do not last forever, that they may break, and in what time period it is thought they might break. Most women have no idea implants break and there's very little information about rupture rates."

"The same is true for other complications, some of which may require further surgery or may cause the woman to be displeased with the cosmetic effect, which, of course, is the reason she got them," Brown says. "For a product that a person is putting in her body presumably for 20 years or more, we should have this information."

■ **Document Source:**
U.S. Department of Health and Human Services, Public Health Service
Food and Drug Administration
FDA Consumer
November 1995

THINGS TO KNOW ABOUT QUALITY MAMMOGRAMS

What is a mammogram?

A mammogram is a safe, low-dose x-ray picture of the breast.

Mammograms are taken during a mammography exam. There are two kinds of mammography exams—screening and diagnostic.

A screening mammogram is a quick, easy way to detect breast cancer early, when treatment is more effective and survival is high. Usually two x-ray pictures are taken of each breast. A physician trained to read x-ray pictures—a radiologist—examines them later.

It is generally agreed that screening mammography decreases deaths from breast cancer in women 50 and over. There is a range of opinion about the value of screening mammography for women under 50.

Have a screening mammogram as often as your doctor or other health care provider suggests. A screening mammogram often can show breast changes like lumps long before they can be felt.

A diagnostic mammogram is used if there may be a problem. It is also used if it is hard to get a good picture because of special circumstances (for instance, in women with breast implants). Diagnostic mammography takes a little longer than screening mammography because more x-ray pictures usually are taken. A radiologist may check the x-ray pictures while you wait.

Purpose of this Booklet

This booklet can help you learn more about getting the best possible mammogram. Being informed will help you work with members of your health care team before, during, and after your mammogram to get quality, reliable results.

Many types of health care providers can help you with your breast care. Doctors, nurses, nurse practitioners, and physician assistants can examine your breasts, refer you for mammography when appropriate, and help you get more exams if they are needed. In this booklet, the word "doctor" is used for easier reading, but any of these health care providers can provide good care.

At the mammography facility, the person who takes the x-ray pictures (the radiologic technologist), the radiologist, and the people who keep the equipment in top working order have all had special training in mammography. They work as a team to make sure you get the best mammogram possible.

After your mammogram, your doctor receives your mammography results. Make sure you get your results from either your doctor or the mammography facility.

Make sure you understand the results and any recommendations for followup. And never be afraid to ask questions.

Following the seven steps in this booklet can help you maintain your breast health. Stay on top of things every step of the way.

Seven Steps to Breast Health

1. Get regular exams.

This is the most important way you can protect your breast health.

- Get a breast exam from your doctor when you get your regular physical exam.
- Get a mammogram as often as your doctor recommends. Ask your doctor when to schedule your next mammogram.
- Check your breasts each month. Your doctor can show you how.

These three exams can help you and your doctor learn what is normal for your breasts and what may be signs of problems.

Call your doctor if you notice

- A lump or thickening of the breast.
- A discharge from the nipple that stains your bra or bed-clothes.
- Skin changes in the breast.

These changes may be normal, but you should always have them checked as soon as possible.

---

2. Choose a quality facility.

Many hospitals, clinics, and imaging or x-ray centers perform mammography. Mobile units (often vans) offer screening at shopping malls, community centers, and offices. All of these facilities must meet the same quality standards.

Your doctor may refer you to a mammography facility. Or you may select the one that is most convenient for you.

Make sure the mammography facility you choose is certified by the Food and Drug Administration (FDA) unless it is a Veterans Health Administration (VHA) facility.

A new law, called the Mammography Quality Standards Act, requires all mammography facilities except those of VHA to be FDA certified beginning October 1, 1994. To be certified, facilities must meet standards for the equipment they use, the people who work there, and the records they keep. VHA has its own high-quality mammography program, similar to FDA's.

If the facility is not FDA certified, get your mammogram in a facility that is certified.

To find a certified mammography facility, ask your doctor or call the National Cancer Institute's Cancer Information Service toll free at 800-4-CANCER.

---

3. Schedule the mammogram for when your breasts will be least tender.

During mammography, the breast is pressed between two clear plastic plates for a few seconds. This gives a clear picture of the breast with the least amount of x-rays. But it may be uncomfortable, and a few women complain of some pain.

If you have sensitive breasts, try having your mammogram at a time of month when your breasts will be least tender. Try to avoid the week right before your period. This will help to lessen discomfort.

4. Give and get important information when you schedule the mammogram.

When you call for an appointment, be ready to provide information the mammography facility needs to know. The facility may wait until your appointment to ask some questions, so it's a good idea also to take the information with you when you have your mammogram. The information requested may include

- Your name, address, and phone number.
- Your age.
- Name, address, and phone number of any facility where you have had a mammogram.

- Any breast disease in your family.
- Any current problems with your breasts, and how long you have had the problems.
- Past problems with your breasts, breast biopsies, or breast surgeries.
- Whether you have breast implants.
- Other personal information:
  - Whether you are pregnant or nursing.
  - The timing of your menstrual cycle or when menopause began.
  - Anything that might make it harder to do a mammogram (unusually large breasts or inability to stand, for example).
- Name, address, and phone number of your doctor.

Here are some questions for you to ask before your appointment:

- How and when you will find out the results of the exam.
- What you need to do to prepare for the exam.

If you have any other questions before your mammogram, be sure to call your doctor or the mammography facility.

5. Know what to expect.

Understanding what happens during a mammogram will help reduce any anxious feelings you might have. It is important to know that only a small amount of radiation is used in mammography.

When you have a mammogram, you stand in front of a special x-ray machine. The radiologic technologist lifts each breast and places it on a platform that holds the x-ray film. The platform can be raised or lowered to match your height.

The breast is then gradually pressed against the platform by a specially designed clear plastic plate. Some pressure is needed for a few seconds to make sure the x-rays show as much of the breast as possible.

This pressure is not harmful to your breast. In fact, flattening the breast lowers the x-ray dose needed.

Studies show that most women do not find a mammogram painful for the short time needed to take the picture. Try to relax. If the pressure becomes painful, you can tell the radiologic technologist to stop.

If there is an area of your breast that appears to have a problem, the radiologist or radiologic technologist may examine the breast.

6. Come prepared.

- Wear a two-piece outfit so you will have to remove only your top.
- Don't use deodorant, talcum powder, or lotion under your arms or near the breasts that day. These products can show up on the x-ray picture.
- Bring the name, address, and phone number of your doctor or other health care provider.
- Bring a list of the places and dates of mammograms, biopsies, or other breast treatment you have had before.
- Ask the facilities where you had mammograms before to release them to you, and bring them with you if

possible. Your new mammogram can be compared with the earlier ones to see if there have been any changes.

It also may be helpful to

- Bring a list of any questions you may have about mammography and your mammograms.
- If you think you may have trouble hearing or understanding the instructions, consider bringing a friend or family member to help you.
- If you are worried about discomfort, you may want to take a mild over-the-counter pain reliever about an hour before your mammogram. This will not affect the mammogram.

If there is something you do not understand, ask. And keep asking until all your questions are answered.

7. Follow up on your results.

Learning the results of your mammogram is very important.

Chances are your mammogram will be normal. **But do not assume that your mammogram is normal just because you have not received the results.** If you have not received your screening results within 10 days, ask your doctor or call the mammography facility.

If your screening mammogram shows anything unusual, talk to your doctor as soon as possible about what you should do next. Your doctor may schedule a diagnostic mammogram, or you can schedule it yourself—but have it done soon. Discuss the results with your doctor.

When a diagnostic mammogram shows something abnormal, the radiologist may recommend another type of exam. A biopsy is a way to obtain a small piece of breast tissue for study under a microscope. Sometimes a biopsy is needed because of something your doctor found in checking your breast even though the mammogram appears normal.

Whenever a mammogram uncovers a problem or a need to check something further:

- Make sure you understand what you need to do next.
- Always get results of any test that you have.
- Ask questions about your results if something is hard to understand.

If you do not have a doctor or other health care provider, you will need to find one if you have an abnormal mammogram. Ask the mammography facility to help you find a doctor. Then make an appointment right away so you can discuss your results and what should be done next.

Mammography is very effective, but it does not detect all breast problems. If you find something unusual in your breast, see your doctor.

How can I learn more about mammography?

Most mammography facilities have printed information and videotaped instructions on breast care. You can read or watch them when you go for a mammogram.

For general information on breast cancer and mammography, contact

Cancer Information Service (a service of the National Cancer Institute)
800-4-CANCER

Food and Drug Administration (FDA)
MQSA Consumer Inquiries
1350 Piccard (HFZ-240)
Rockville, MD 20850

American Cancer Society
800-227-2345

You're in charge of your breast health:

- Schedule screening mammograms as often as your doctor recommends.
- Always find out the results of your mammogram.
- Follow your doctor's recommendations for follow-up and schedule diagnostic mammography, if needed, as soon as possible.
- Have your doctor check your breasts as part of your regular physical exam, and check your breasts yourself each month.
- If you have a breast lump or change at any time, even if your last mammogram was normal, see a doctor as soon as possible.

For Further Information

The information in this booklet is based on the Clinical Practice Guideline, Quality Determinants of Mammography. The Guideline was developed by a non-federal panel of experts sponsored by the Agency for Health Care Policy and Research. Other guidelines on health issues are available, and more are being developed.

For more information about guidelines or to receive more copies of this booklet, call toll free 800-358-9295, or write to:

Agency for Health Care Policy and Research
Publications Clearinghouse
PO Box 8547
Silver Spring, MD 20907

■ **Document Source:**
  U.S. Department of Health and Human Service, Public Health Service
  Agency for Health Care Policy and Research
  Executive Office Center, Ste 501
  2101 E Jefferson St
  Rockville, MD 20852
  AHCPR Publication No. 95-0634
  October 1994

See also: What You Need to Know About Breast Cancer (page 501)

VAGINITIS: IMPORTANT INFORMATION FOR YOUR GOOD HEALTH

Vaginitis is a medical term that is used to refer to *any* infection or inflammation of the vagina. The symptoms of vaginitis are common and most women will have at least one form of vaginitis in their lifetime. Even though vaginitis is so common, many women know little about it.

The term "yeast infection" is what most women think of when they hear the word vaginitis. However, a yeast infection is only *one kind* of vaginal infection. Vaginitis can be caused by several different organisms, sometimes at the same time, as well as by hormonal changes, allergies, or irritations.

Because vaginitis can have many causes, it is important to see your doctor or other health care professional so that the proper cause can be identified and the correct treatment can be prescribed. Once started, the medication should be used exactly according to your doctor's instructions in order to cure the vaginitis. The symptoms may go away before you finish the medication. Even so, you should complete the therapy to help ensure a cure.

Vaginitis can sometimes be a sign of other health problems. Knowing more about the signs and symptoms of this common condition will help you and your health care provider make a proper diagnosis.

What is vaginitis?

"Vaginitis" is a word that is used to describe disorders that cause infection or inflammation ("itis" means inflammation) of the vagina. Vulvovaginitis refers to inflammation of both the vagina and vulva (the external female genitals). These conditions can result from an infection caused by organisms such as bacteria, yeast, or viruses, as well as by irritations from chemicals in creams, sprays, or even clothing that are in contact with this area. In some cases, vaginitis results from organisms that are passed between sexual partners.

How do I know if I have vaginitis?

The common symptoms of vaginitis are itching, burning, and vaginal discharge that is different from your normal secretions. The itching and burning can be inside the vagina or on the skin or vulva just outside the vagina. Discomfort during urination or sexual intercourse may also occur. If everyone with vaginitis had these symptoms, then the diagnosis would be fairly simple. However, it is important to realize that as many as four out of every 10 women with vaginitis may not have these typical symptoms. Frequently, a routine gynecologic exam will confirm vaginitis even if symptoms are not present. This is one reason why it is important to have a gynecologic exam at least every two years.

Is vaginal discharge normal?

A woman's vagina normally produces a discharge that is usually described as clear or slightly cloudy, nonirritating, and odor-free. During the normal menstrual cycle the amount and consistency of discharge vary. At one time of the month there may be a small amount of a very thin or watery discharge and at another time, a more extensive, thicker discharge may appear. All of these descriptions could be considered normal.

A vaginal discharge that has an odor or that is irritating is usually an abnormal discharge. The irritation might be itching or burning or both. The burning could feel like a bladder infection. The itching may be present at any time of the day but it is often most bothersome at night. Both of these symptoms are usually made worse by sexual intercourse. It is important to see a doctor or clinician if there has been a *change* in the amount, appearance, or smell of the discharge.

What are the most common types of vaginitis?

The six most common types of vaginitis are
- *Candida* or "yeast" vaginitis
- Bacterial vaginosis
- *Trichomoniasis* vaginitis
- *Chlamydia* vaginitis
- Viral vaginitis
- Noninfectious vaginitis

Although each of these causes of vaginal infection can have different symptoms, it is not always easy for a patient to figure out which type of vaginitis she has; in fact, diagnosis can even be tricky for an experienced clinician. Part of the problem is that sometimes more than one type of vaginitis can be present at the same time. Often vaginitis is present without any symptoms at all.

To help you better understand these six major causes of vaginitis, let's look briefly at each one of them and how they are treated.

What are Candida or "yeast" infections?

Yeast infections of the vagina are what most women think of when they hear the term "vaginitis." They are caused by one of the many species of fungus called *Candida*. *Candida* normally live in small numbers in the vagina as well as in the mouth and digestive tract of both men and women.

Yeast infections produce a thick, white vaginal discharge with the consistency of cottage cheese. Although the discharge can be somewhat watery, it is odorless. Yeast infections usually cause the vagina and the vulva to be very itchy and red.

Since yeast is normal in a woman's vagina, what makes it cause an infection? Usually this happens when a change in the delicate balance in a woman's system occurs. For example, a woman may take an antibiotic to treat a urinary tract infection and the antibiotic kills her "friendly" bacteria that normally keep the yeast in balance; as a result the yeast overgrows and causes the infection. Other factors which can upset the delicate balance include pregnancy which changes hormone levels and diabetes which allows too much sugar in the urine and vagina.

Risk Factors for Vaginal Candida Infections

- Recent Course of Antibiotics
- Uncontrolled Diabetes
- Pregnancy
- High Estrogen Contraceptives
- Immunosuppression
- Thyroid or Endocrine Disorders
- Corticosteroid Therapy

What is bacterial vaginosis?

Although "yeast" is the name most women know, bacterial vaginosis is actually the most common vaginal infection in women of reproductive age. Bacterial vaginosis will often cause a vaginal discharge. The discharge is usually thin and milky and is described as having a "fishy" odor. This odor may become more noticeable after intercourse. Redness or itching of the vagina are not common symptoms of bacterial vaginosis. It is important to note that many women with bacterial vaginosis have no symptoms at all and the vaginitis is only discovered during a routine gynecologic exam. Bacterial vaginosis is caused by a combination of several bacteria. These bacteria seem to overgrow much the same way as *Candida* will when the vaginal balance is upset. The exact reason for this overgrowth is not known. Since bacterial vaginosis is caused by bacteria, not by yeast, it is easy to see that different methods are needed to treat the different infections. A medicine that is appropriate for yeast is not effective against the bacteria that causes bacterial vaginosis.

What are trichomoniasis, chlamydia, and viral vaginitis?

Trichomonias, commonly called "trich" (pronounced "trick"), is caused by a tiny single-celled organism known as a "protozoa." When this organism infects the vagina it can cause a frothy, greenish-yellow discharge. Often this discharge will have a foul smell. Women with trichomonal vaginitis may complain of itching and soreness of the vagina and vulva, as well as burning during urination. In addition, there can be discomfort in the lower abdomen and vaginal pain with intercourse. These symptoms may be worse after the menstrual period. Many women, however, do not develop any symptoms. It is important to understand that this type of vaginitis can be transmitted through sexual intercourse. For treatment to be effective, the sexual partner must be treated at the same time as the patient.

Another primarily sexually transmitted form of vaginitis is caused by the germ known as *Chlamydia.* Unfortunately, most women do not have symptoms. This makes diagnosis difficult. A vaginal discharge is sometimes present with this infection but not always. More often a woman might experience light bleeding especially after intercourse. She may have pain in the lower abdomen and pelvis. Chlamydial vaginitis is most common in young women (18 to 35 years) who have multiple sexual partners. If you fit this description, you should request screening for *Chlamydia* during your annual checkup. The best "treatment" for *Chlamydia* is prevention. Use of a condom will decrease your risk of contracting not only *Chlamydia,* but other sexually transmitted diseases as well.

Viruses are a common cause of vaginitis. One form caused by the *herpes simplex virus* (HSV) is often just called "herpes" infection. These infections are also spread by sexual intimacy. The primary symptom of herpes vaginitis is pain associated with lesions or "sores." These sores are usually visible on the vulva or the vagina but occasionally are inside the vagina and can only be seen during a gynecologic exam.

Outbreaks of HSV are often associated with stress or emotional upheaval.

Another source of viral vaginal infection is the human papillomavirus (HPV). HPV can also be transmitted by sexual intercourse. This virus can cause painful warts to grow in the vagina, rectum, vulva, or groin. These warts are usually white to gray in color, but they may be pink or purple. However, visible warts are not always present and the virus may only be detected when a Pap smear is abnormal.

What is noninfectious vaginitis?

Occasionally, a woman can have itching, burning, and even a vaginal discharge without having an infection. The most common cause is an allergic reaction or irritation from vaginal sprays, douches, or spermicidal products. The skin around the vagina can also be sensitive to perfumed soaps, detergents, and fabric softeners.

Another noninfectious form of vaginitis results from a decrease in hormones because of menopause or because of surgery that removes the ovaries. In this form, the vagina becomes dry or "atrophic." The woman may notice pain, especially with sexual intercourse, as well as vaginal itching and burning.

How do you treat vaginitis?

The key to proper treatment of vaginitis is proper diagnosis. This is not always easy since the same symptoms can exist in different forms of vaginitis. You can greatly assist your health care practitioner by paying close attention to exactly which symptoms you have and when they occur, along with a description of the color, consistency, amount, and smell of any abnormal discharge. Do *not* douche before your office or clinic visit; it will make accurate testing difficult or impossible.

Because different types of vaginitis have different causes, the treatment needs to be *specific* to the type of vaginitis present. When a woman has had a yeast infection diagnosed by her doctor, she is usually treated with a prescription for a vaginal cream or suppositories. If the infection clears up for some period of time but then the *exact same* symptoms occur again, a woman can obtain, with her doctor or pharmacist's advice, a vaginal cream or suppository without a prescription that can completely treat the infection. The important thing to understand is that this medication may only cure the most common types of *Candida* associated with vaginal yeast infections and will not cure other yeast infections or any other type of vaginitis. If you are not absolutely sure, see your doctor. You may save the expense of buying the wrong medication and avoid delay in treating your type of vaginitis.

When obtaining these over-the-counter medicines, be sure to read all of the instructions completely before using the product. Be sure to use all of the medicine and don't stop just because your symptoms have gone away. Be sure to see your health care practitioner if:

- All of the symptoms do not go away completely.

- The symptoms return immediately or shortly after you finish treatment. You have any other serious medical problems such as diabetes.
- You might be pregnant.

Other forms of infectious vaginitis are caused by organisms that need to be treated with oral medication and/or a vaginal cream prescribed by your doctor. Products available without a prescription will probably not be effective. As with all medicine, it is important to follow your doctor's instructions as well as the instructions that come with the medication. Do not stop taking the medicine when your symptoms go away. Do not be embarrassed to ask your doctor or health care practitioner questions. Good questions to ask include: Is it okay to douche while on this vaginal cream? Should you abstain from sexual intercourse during treatment? Should your sexual partner(s) be treated at the same time? Will the medication for this vaginitis agree with your other medication(s)? Should you continue the vaginal cream or suppositories during your period? Do you need to be reexamined and if so, when?

"Noninfectious" vaginitis is treated by changing the probable cause. If you have recently changed your soap or laundry detergent or have added a fabric softener, you might consider stopping the new product to see if the symptoms remain. The same instruction would apply to a new vaginal spray, douche, sanitary napkin, or tampon. If the vaginitis is due to hormonal changes, estrogen may be prescribed to help reduce symptoms.

How can I prevent vaginitis?

There are certain things that you can do to decrease the chance of getting vaginitis. If you suffer from yeast infections, it is usually helpful to avoid garments that hold in heat and moisture. The wearing of nylon panties, pantyhose without a cotton panel, and tight jeans can lead to yeast infections. Good hygiene is also important. Many doctors have found that if a woman eats yogurt that contains active cultures (read the label) she will get fewer infections.

Because they can cause vaginal irritation, most doctors do not recommend vaginal sprays or heavily perfumed soaps for cleansing this area. Likewise, repeated douching may cause irritation or, more importantly, may hide a vaginal infection.

Safe sexual practices can help prevent the passing of diseases between partners. The use of condoms is particularly important.

If you are approaching menopause, have had your ovaries removed, or have low levels of estrogen for any reason, discuss with your doctor the use of hormone pills or creams to keep the vagina lubricated and healthy.

Summary

- "Vaginitis" is a medical term that describes an infection or irritation of the vagina and/or vulva by yeast, bacteria, viruses, other organisms, or chemical irritants.
- When present, symptoms of different types of vaginitis overlap which can make diagnosis difficult. In addition, more than one cause of vaginitis can be present at the same time in the same woman.

- Proper diagnosis by your doctor or health care practitioner is the key to proper treatment. Yeast, bacteria, viruses, and other organisms each require a specific type of therapy. Use of the wrong medication will not help and will only delay proper treatment.
- All vaginitis is not caused by yeast. The use of a nonprescription medication or other treatment may make the proper diagnosis more difficult if yeast is not the cause of the infection.
- Some forms of vaginitis are sexually transmitted and can co-exist with other more serious sexually transmitted diseases. The proper use of condoms can be helpful in preventing some forms of vaginitis.
- Follow complete instructions in treating your vaginal infection. If symptoms do not clear completely or if they reoccur, see your doctor or health care practitioner for further instructions.

■ **Document Source:**
U.S. Department of Health and Human Services, Public Health Service
National Institutes of Health
National Institute of Child Health and Human Development
NIH Pub. No. 95-3512
December 1994

WHAT YOU NEED TO KNOW ABOUT BREAST CANCER

Breast cancer is the most common type of cancer among women in the United States. The National Cancer Institute (NCI) has written this booklet to help women with breast cancer and their families and friends better understand this disease. We hope others will read it as well to learn more about breast cancer.

This booklet describes breast cancer symptoms, diagnosis, treatment, and rehabilitation. Other NCI booklets about cancer, its treatment, and living with the disease are listed inside the back cover. We know that booklets like these cannot answer every question about breast cancer. They cannot take the place of talks with doctors, nurses, and other members of the health care team. We hope our booklets will help with those talks.

Our knowledge about breast cancer keeps increasing. For up-to-date information, call the NCI-supported Cancer Information Service (CIS) at 1-800-4-CANCER (1-800-422-6237). The CIS is described later.

What is cancer?

Cancer is a group of diseases. It occurs when cells become abnormal and divide without control or order.

Every organ in the body is made up of various kinds of cells. Cells normally divide in an orderly way to produce more cells only when they are needed. This process helps keeps the body healthy.

If cells divide when new cells are not needed, they form too much *tissue.* The mass of extra tissue, called a *tumor,* can be *benign* or *malignant.*

- Benign tumors are not cancer. They can usually be removed, and in most cases, they don't come back. Most important, the cells in benign tumors do not invade other tissues and do not spread to other parts of the body. Benign breast tumors are not a threat of life.
- Malignant tumors are cancer. They can invade and damage nearby tissues and organs. Also, cancer cells can break away from a malignant tumor and enter the bloodstream or *lymphatic system.* That is how breast cancer spreads and forms secondary tumors in other parts of the body. The spread of cancer is called *metastatis.*

The Breasts

Each breast has 15 to 20 sections, called *lobes,* that are arranged like the petals of a daisy. Each lobe has many smaller *lobules,* which end in dozens of tiny bulbs that can produce milk. The lobes, lobules, and bulbs are all linked by thin tubes called *ducts.* These ducts lead to the nipple in the center of a dark area of skin called the *areola.* Fat fills the spaces between lobules and ducts. There are no muscles in the breast, but muscles lie under each breast and cover the ribs.

Each breast also contains blood vessels and vessels that carry *lymph.* The lymph vessels lead to small bean-shaped organs called *lymph nodes.* Clusters of lymph nodes are found under the arm, above the collarbone, and in the chest. Lymph nodes are also found in many other parts of the body.

Types of Breast Cancer

There are more than 100 different types of cancer, including several types of breast cancer. The most common type of breast cancer begins in the lining of the ducts and is called ductal *carcinoma.* Another type, called lobular carcinoma, arises in the lobules. Cancers that begin in other tissues in the breast are rare and are not discussed in this booklet.

When breast cancer spreads outside the breast, cancer cells are often found in the lymph nodes under the arm. If the cancer has reached these nodes, it may mean that cancer cells have spread to other parts of the body—other lymph nodes and other organs, such as the bones, liver, or lungs.

Cancer that spreads is the same disease and has the same name as the original (primary) cancer. When breast cancer spreads, it is called metastatic breast cancer, even though the secondary tumor is in another organ. Doctors may call this problem "distant" disease.

Early Detection

When breast cancer is found and treated early, a woman has more treatment choices and a good chance of complete recovery. So it is important to detect breast cancer as early as possible. The National Cancer Institute encourages women to take an active part in early detection. They should talk with their doctor about this disease, the symptoms to watch for, and an appropriate schedule of checkups. The doctor's advice will be based on the woman's age, medical history, and other factors.

Women should ask the doctor about

- Mammograms (x-rays of the breast)
- Breast exams by a doctor or nurse
- Breast self-examination (BSE)

A mammogram is a special kind of x-ray. It is different from a chest x-ray or x-rays of other parts of the body.

Mammography involves two x-rays of each breast, one taken from the side and one from the top. The breast must be squeezed between two plates for the pictures to be clear. While this squeezing may be a bit uncomfortable, it lasts only a few seconds. In many cases, mammograms can show breast tumors before they cause symptoms or can be felt. A mammogram can also show small deposits of calcium in the breast. A cluster of very tiny specks of calcium (called *microcalcifications*) may be an early sign of cancer.

Mammography should be done only by specially trained people using machines designed just for taking x-rays of the breasts. The pictures should be checked by a qualified *radiologist.* Women should talk with their doctor or call the Cancer Information Service for help in finding out where to get a mammogram.

Mammography is an excellent tool, but we know that it cannot find every abnormal area in the breast. So another important step in early detection is for women to have their breasts examined regularly by a doctor or nurse.

Between visits to the doctor, women should examine their breasts every month. It's important to remember that every woman's breasts are different. And each woman's breasts change because of age, the *menstrual cycle,* pregnancy, *menopause,* or taking birth control pills or other hormones. It is normal for the breasts to feel lumpy and uneven. Also, it's common for a woman's breasts to be swollen and tender right before or during her menstrual period. These are some of the reasons why many women are not certain what their breasts are supposed to feel like. By doing monthly BSE, a woman learns what is normal for her breasts, and she is more likely to detect a change. Any changes should be reported to the doctor.

Symptoms

Early breast cancer usually does not cause pain. In fact, when it first develops, breast cancer may cause no symptoms at all. But as the cancer grows, it can cause changes that women should watch for:

- A lump or thickening in or near the breast or in the underarm area;
- A change in the size or shape of the breast;
- A discharge from the nipple; or
- A change in the color or feel of the skin of the breast, areola, or nipple (dimpled, puckered, or scaly).

A woman should see her doctor if she notices any of these changes. Most often, they are not cancer, but only a doctor can tell for sure.

Diagnosis

An abnormal area on a mammogram, a lump, or other changes in the breast can be caused by cancer or by other, less serious problems. To find out the cause of any of these signs or symptoms, a woman's doctor does a careful physical exam and asks about her personal and family medical history. In addition to checking general signs of health, the doctor may do one or more of the breast exams described below to help make a diagnosis.

- **Palpation.** The doctor can tell a lot about a lump—its size, its texture, and whether it moves easily—by *palpation,* carefully feeling the lump and the tissue around it. Benign lumps often feel different from cancerous ones.
- **Mammography.** X-rays of the breast can give the doctor important information about a breast lump. If an area on the mammogram looks suspicious or is not clear, additional views may be needed.
- **Ultrasonography.** Sometimes the doctor orders *ultrasonography,* which can often show whether a lump is solid or filled with fluid. This exam uses high-frequency sound waves, which cannot be heard by humans. The sound waves enter the breast and bounce back. The pattern of their echoes produces a picture called a sonogram, which is displayed on a screen. This exam is often used along with mammography.

Based on these exams, the doctor may decide that no further tests are needed and no treatment is necessary. In such cases, the doctor may want to check the woman regularly to watch for any changes. Often, however, the doctor must remove fluid or tissue from the breast to make a diagnosis.

- **Aspiration or needle biopsy.** The doctor uses a needle to remove fluid or a small amount of tissue from a beast lump. This procedure may show whether the lump is a fluid-filled cyst (not cancer) or a solid mass (which may or may not be cancer). The material removed in a needle biopsy goes to a lab to be checked for cancer cells.
- **Surgical biopsy.** The doctor cuts out part or all of a lump or suspicious area. A *pathologist* examines the tissue under a microscope to check for cancer cells.

When a woman needs a biopsy, these are some questions she may want to ask her doctor:

- What type of biopsy will I have? Why?
- How long will the biopsy or aspiration take? Will I be awake? Will it hurt?
- How soon will I know the results?
- If I do have cancer, who will talk with me about treatment? When?

When Cancer is Found

When cancer is present, the pathologist can tell what kind of cancer it is (whether it began in a duct or a lobule) and whether it is invasive (has invaded nearby tissues in the breast).

Special laboratory tests of the tissue help the doctor learn more about the cancer. For example, *hormone receptor tests (estrogen and progesterone* receptor tests) can show whether the cancer is sensitive to hormones. Positive test results mean hormones help the cancer grow and the cancer is likely to respond to hormone treatment. Other lab tests are sometimes done to help the doctor predict whether the cancer is likely to grow slowly or quickly.

If the diagnosis is cancer, the patient may want to ask these questions:

- What kind of breast cancer do I have? Is it invasive?
- What did the hormone receptor test show? What other lab tests were done on the tumor tissue, and what did they show?
- How will this information help the doctor decide what type of treatment or further tests to recommend?

The patient's doctor may refer her to doctors who specialize in treating breast cancer. Treatment generally follows within a few weeks after the diagnosis. The woman will have time to talk with the doctor about her treatment choices, to consider getting a second opinion, and to prepare herself and her loved ones.

Treatment

Many treatment methods are used for breast cancer. Treatment depends on the size and location of the tumor in the breast, the results of lab tests (including hormone receptor tests) done on the cancer cells, and the *stage* (or extent) of the disease. The patient may have further tests to find out whether the cancer has spread. For example, the doctor usually orders x-rays of the lungs and blood tests to check the liver. In some cases, the doctor orders other special exams of the liver, lungs, or bones because breast cancer tends to spread to these areas. To develop a treatment plan to fit each patient's needs, the doctor also considers the woman's age and general health as well as her feelings about the treatment options.

Women with breast cancer are likely to have many questions and concerns about their treatment plan. They want to learn all they can about their disease and their treatment choices so they can take an active part in decisions about their medical care. The doctor is the best person to answer questions about how the disease can be treated, how successful the treatment is expected to be, and how much it is likely to cost. Also, the patient may want to talk with her doctor about taking part in a research study of new treatment methods. Information about such studies, called *clinical trials,* follows.

Many patients find it helps to make a list of questions before seeing the doctor. Taking notes during talks with the doctor can make it easier to remember what the doctor says. Some patients also find that it helps to have a family member or friend with them when they see the doctor—to take part in the discussion, to take notes, or just to listen.

Here are some questions a woman may want to ask the doctor before treatment begins:

- What is the stage of the disease?
- What are my treatment choices? Which do you recommend for me? Why?
- What are the expected benefits of each kind of treatment?
- What are the risks and possible side effects of each treatment?
- Would a clinical trial be appropriate for me?

Most patients also want to know how they will look after treatment and whether they will have to change their normal activities. There's a lot to learn about breast cancer and its treatment. Patients should not feel that they need to ask all their questions or understand all the answers at once. They will have many other chances to ask the doctor to explain things that are not clear and to ask for more information.

Planning Treatment

Before starting treatment, the patient might want a second opinion about the diagnosis and the treatment plan. It may take a week or two to arrange to see another doctor. Studies show that a brief delay between biopsy and treatment does **not** make breast cancer treatment less effective. There are a number of ways to find a doctor for a second opinion:

- The patient's doctor may refer her to a specialist. Specialists who treat breast cancer include surgeons, medical *oncologists,* and radiation oncologists. Sometimes these doctors work together at cancer centers or special centers for breast disease.
- The Cancer Information Service, at 1-800-4-CANCER, can tell callers about cancer centers and other NCI-supported programs in their area.
- Patients can get the names of specialists from their local medical society, a nearby hospital, or a medical school.

Methods of Treatment

Methods of treatment for breast cancer are *local* or *systemic.* Local treatments are used to remove, destroy, or control the cancer cells in a specific area. *Surgery* and *radiation therapy* are local treatments. Systemic treatments are used to destroy or control cancer cells all over the body. *Chemotherapy* and *hormone therapy* are systemic treatment. A patient may have just one form of treatment or a combination, depending on her needs.

Surgery is the most common treatment for breast cancer. An operation to remove the breast is a *mastectomy;* an operation to remove the cancer but not the breast is called breast-sparing surgery. Breast-sparing surgery usually is followed by radiation therapy to destroy any cancer cells that may remain in the area. In most cases, the surgeon also removes lymph nodes under the arm to help determine the stages of the disease.

Several types of surgery are used to treat breast cancer. The doctor can explain them in detail and can tell the patient how each will affect her appearance.

- In *lumpectomy,* the surgeon removes just the breast lump and a margin of normal tissue around it.
- In partial (segmental) mastectomy, the tumor, some of the normal breast tissue around it, and the lining over the chest muscles below the tumor are removed.
- In total (simple) mastectomy, the whole breast is removed.
- In modified radical mastectomy, the surgeon removes the breast, some of the lymph nodes under the arm, and the lining over the chest muscles. Sometimes the smaller of the two chest muscles is removed.
- In radical mastectomy (also called Halsted radical mastectomy), the surgeon removes the breast, the chest muscles, all of the lymph nodes under the arm, and some additional fat and skin. This operation was the standard one for many years, but it is seldom used now.

These are some questions a woman may want to ask her doctor before surgery:

- What kind of operation will it be?
- How will I feel after the operation? If I have pain, how will you help me?
- Where will the scars be? What will they look like?
- If I decide to have plastic surgery to rebuild my breast, when can that be done?
- Will I have to do special exercises?
- When can I get back to my normal activities?

In **radiation therapy** (also called radiotherapy), high-energy rays are used to damage cancer cells and stop them from growing. Radiation may come from a machine outside the body (external radiation). It can also come from radioactive materials placed directly in the breast in thin plastic tubes (implant radiation). Sometimes the patient receives both kinds of radiation therapy.

Patients go to the hospital or clinic each day for external radiation treatments. When this therapy follows breast-sparing surgery, the treatments are given five days week for five to six weeks. At the end of that time, an extra "boost" of radiation is often given to the tumor site. The boost may be either external or internal (using an implant). Patients stay in the hospital for a short time for implant radiation.

Before radiation therapy, a patient may want to ask her doctor these questions:

- Why do I need this treatment?
- When will the treatments begin? When will they end?
- How will I feel during therapy?
- What can I do to take care of myself during therapy?
- Can I continue my normal activities?
- How will my breast look afterward?

Chemotherapy is the use of drugs to kill cancer cells. In most cases, breast cancer is treated with a combination of drugs. The drugs may be given by mouth or by injection into a vein or muscle. Either way, chemotherapy is a systemic therapy, because the drugs enter the bloodstream and travel through the body.

Chemotherapy is given in cycles: a treatment period followed by a recovery period, then another treatment, and so on. Most patients have chemotherapy in an outpatient part of the hospital, at the doctor's office, or at home. Depending on which drugs are given and the woman's general health, however, she may need to stay in the hospital during her treatment.

Hormone therapy is used to keep cancer cells from getting the hormones they need to grow. This treatment may include the use of drugs that change the way hormones work or surgery to remove the *ovaries,* which make hormones. Like chemotherapy, hormone therapy is a systemic treatment; it can affect cancer cells throughout the body.

Patients may want to ask these questions about chemotherapy or hormone therapy:

- Why do I need this treatment?
- If I need hormone treatment, which would be better for me—drugs or an operation?
- What drugs will I be taking? What will they do?
- Will I have side effects? What can I do about them?
- How long will I be on this treatment?

Treatment Choices

Treatment decisions are complex. These decisions are affected by the experience and judgment of the doctor and by the desires of the patient. The choices available for a particular patient depend on a number of factors. These include the woman's age and menopausal status, her general health, the location of the tumor, and the size of her breast. Certain features of the cancer cells (such as whether they depend on hormones and how fast they are growing) are also considered. The most important factor is the stage of the cancer. The stage is based on the size of the tumor and whether the cancer is only in the breast or has spread to other organs.

- **Carcinoma in situ** is very early breast cancer. Cancer cells are found in only a few layers of cells. Because it has not invaded nearby tissue, the cancer is called noninvasive.

    Patients with carcinoma *in situ* may have breast-sparing surgery or mastectomy. The type of surgery depends mainly on whether the cancer developed in a duct (intraductal carcinoma) or a lobule (lobular carcinoma *in situ*). In some cases, some of the underarm lymph nodes are removed, and radiation therapy may be recommended.

- **Stage I** and **stage II** are early stages of breast cancer, but the cancer has invaded nearby tissue. Stage I means that cancer cells have not spread beyond the breast and the tumor is no more than about an inch across. Stage II means that cancer has spread to underarm lymph nodes and/or the tumor in the breast is 1 to 2 inches across.

    Women with early stage breast cancer may have breast-sparing surgery followed by radiation therapy as their primary local treatment, or they may have a mastectomy. These treatments are equally effective. With either approach, lymph nodes under the arm generally are removed.

In addition, some women with stage I and most with stage II breast cancer have chemotherapy and/or hormone therapy in addition to their local treatment. This added treatment is called *adjuvant therapy.* It is given to prevent the cancer from recurring by killing undetected cancer cells that may have begun to spread.

- **Stage III** means the tumor in the breast is more than 2 inches across, the cancer is more extensive in the underarm lymph nodes, or it has spread to other lymph node areas or to other tissues near the breast. This stage of breast cancer is also called locally advanced cancer.

    Patients with stage III breast cancer usually have both local treatment to remove or destroy the cancer in the breast and systemic treatment to stop the disease from spreading. The local treatment may be mastectomy and/or radiation therapy to the breast; also, the lymph nodes under the arm may be removed or treated with radiation. The systemic treatment may be chemotherapy, hormone therapy, or both; it may be given before local treatment.

- **Stage IV** is metastatic cancer. The cancer has spread from the breast to other organs of the body.

    Women who have stage IV breast cancer receive chemotherapy and/or hormone therapy to shrink the tumor or destroy cancer cells. They may have surgery or radiation therapy to control the cancer in the breast. Radiation may also be useful to control tumors in other parts of the body.

- **Recurrent Cancer** means the disease has reappeared, even though the patient's treatment has seemed to be successful. Even when a tumor in a breast seems to have been completely removed or destroyed, the disease sometimes returns because undetected cancer cells have remained in the area after treatment or because the disease had already spread before the treatment.

    When the cancer returns only in the breast area, it is called a local recurrence. If the disease returns in another part of the body, it is called metastatic breast cancer (or distant disease). The doctor will choose one type of treatment or a combination of treatments to meet the woman's needs.

Side Effects of Treatment

It is hard to limit the effects of cancer treatment so that only cancer cells are removed or destroyed. Because healthy cells and tissues may also be damaged, treatment often causes unpleasant side effects.

Removal of a breast can cause a woman's weight to shift and be out of balance—especially if she has large breasts. This imbalance can also cause discomfort in a woman's neck and back. Also, the skin in the breast area may be tight, and the muscles of the arm and shoulder may feel stiff. After a mastectomy, a few women have some permanent loss of strength in these muscles, but for most women, reduced strength and limited movement are temporary. The doctor, nurse, or physical therapist can recommend exercises to help a woman regain movement and strength in her arm and shoulder.

Because nerves are injured or cut during surgery, a woman may have numbness and tingling in the chest, underarm, shoulder, and arm. These feelings usually go away within a few weeks or months, but some numbness may be permanent.

Removing the lymph nodes under the arm slows the flow of lymph. In some women, lymph builds up in the arm and hand and causes swelling (*lymphedema*). Also, it is harder for the body to fight infection after the lymph nodes have been removed, so women need to protect the arm and hand on the treated side from injury—for the rest of their lives. They should ask the doctor how to handle any cuts, scratches, insect bites, or other injuries that may occur. Also, they should contact the doctor if an infection develops.

The radiation oncologist will explain the possible side effects of radiation therapy for breast cancer—including uncommon side effects that may involve the heart, lungs, and ribs—before treatment begins. Some of the more common side effects are described here. For example, during radiation therapy, patients may become very tired, especially in the later weeks of treatment. Resting is important, but doctors usually advise their patients to try to stay reasonably active. Women should match their activities to their energy level. It's common for radiation to cause the skin in the treated area to become red and dry, tender, and itchy. Toward the end of the treatment, the skin may become moist and "weepy." This area should be exposed to the air as much as possible. Patients should avoid wearing a bra or clothes that may rub; loose-fitting cotton clothes are usually best. Good skin care is important at this time, but patients should not use any lotions or creams without the doctor's advice, and they should not use any deodorant on the treated side. The effects of radiation therapy on the skin are temporary. The area will heal when the treatment is over.

Following radiation therapy, the treated breast may be firmer. Also, it may be larger (due to fluid buildup) or smaller (because of tissue changes) than before. For some women, the breast skin is more sensitive after radiation treatment; for others, it is less sensitive.

The side effects of chemotherapy depend mainly on the drugs the patient receives. In addition, as with other types of treatment, side effects vary from person to person. In general, anticancer drugs affect rapidly dividing cells. These include blood cells, which fight infection, cause blood to clot, and carry oxygen to all parts of the body. When blood cells are affected by anticancer drugs, patients are more likely to get infections, bruise or bleed easily, and have less energy. Cells in *hair follicles* and cells that line the digestive tract also divide rapidly. As a result of chemotherapy, patients may lose their hair and may have other side effects, such as loss of appetite, nausea, vomiting, or mouth sores. These generally are short-term side effects. They gradually go away during the recovery part of the chemotherapy cycle or after the treatment is over.

Some anticancer drugs can damage the ovaries. If the ovaries fail to produce hormones, the woman may have symptoms of menopause, such as hot flashes and vaginal dryness. Her periods may become irregular or may stop, and she may not be able to become pregnant. In women over the age of 35 or 40, some of these effects, such as *infertility* are likely to become permanent.

Hormone therapy can cause a number of side effects. They depend largely on the specific drug or type of treatment, and they vary from patient to patient. Tamoxifen is the most commonly used form of hormone treatment. This drug blocks the body's use of estrogen but does not stop estrogen production. Its side effects usually are not severe. Tamoxifen may cause hot flashes, vaginal discharge or irritation, and irregular periods, but it does not cause menopause or infertility. Young women whose ovaries are removed to deprive the cancer cells of estrogen, experience menopause immediately. The side effects they have—including hot flashes and vaginal dryness—are likely to be more severe than those of natural menopause.

Loss of appetite can be a problem for cancer patients. They may not feel hungry when they are uncomfortable or tired. Also, some of the common side effects of cancer treatment, such as nausea and vomiting, can make it hard to eat. The doctor may suggest medicine to help with these problems because good nutrition is important. Patients who eat well often feel better and have more energy. They may also be better able to withstand the side effects of their treatment. Eating well means getting enough calories and protein to help prevent weight loss, regain strength, and rebuild normal tissues. Many patients find that eating several small meals and snacks a day works better than trying to have three large meals.

The side effects of cancer treatment are different for each person, and they may be different from one treatment to the next. Doctors try to plan treatment to keep problems at a minimum. They also watch patients carefully so they can help with any problems that occur. Doctors, nurses, and dietitians can explain the side effects of treatment and can suggest ways to deal with them. The NCI booklets *Radiation Therapy and You, Chemotherapy and You,* and *Eating Hints* have helpful information about cancer treatment and coping with side effects.

After Treatment

Rehabilitation is a very important part of breast cancer treatment. The medical team makes every effort to help women return to their normal activities as soon as possible. Recovery will be different for each woman, depending on the extent of the disease, the treatment she had and other factors.

Exercising after surgery can help a woman regain motion and strength in her arm and shoulder. It can also reduce pain and stiffness in her neck and back. Carefully planned exercises should be started as soon as the doctor says the woman is ready, often within a day or so after surgery. Exercising begins slowly and gently and can even be done in bed. Gradually exercising can be more active, and regular exercise should become part of a woman's normal routine. (Women who have a mastectomy and immediate breast reconstruction-plastic surgery to rebuild the breast, need special exercises, which the doctor or nurse will explain.)

Lymphedema after surgery can be reduced or prevented with certain exercises and by resting with the arm propped up on a pillow. If lymphedema occurs later on, the doctor may suggest exercises and other ways to deal with this problem. For example, some women with lymphedema wear an elastic sleeve or wear an elastic cuff to improve lymph circulation. The doctor also may suggest other approaches—such as medication or use of a machine that compresses the arm.

After a mastectomy, some women decide to wear a breast form (*prosthesis*). Others prefer to have a breast reconstruction—either at the same time as the mastectomy or later on. Each plan has its pros and cons, and what is right for one woman may not be right for another. What's important is that nearly every woman treated for breast cancer has a choice. It may be helpful to talk with a plastic surgeon before the mastectomy, but reconstruction is still possible years later.

Various procedures are used to reconstruct the breast. Some use artificial implants; others use tissue moved from another part of the woman's body. The woman should ask the plastic surgeon to explain the risks and benefits of each type of reconstruction. The Cancer Information Service can suggest sources of printed information about breast reconstruction and can tell callers about breast cancer support groups. Members of such groups are often willing to share their personal experiences with breast reconstruction.

Followup

Regular followup exams are very important after breast cancer treatment. The doctor will continue to check the woman closely to be sure that the cancer has not returned. Regular checkups usually include exams of the chest, underarm, and neck. From time to time, the woman has a complete physical exam, blood and urine tests, mammography, and a chest x-ray. The doctor sometimes orders scans (special x-rays) and other exams as well.

A woman who has had cancer in one breast has a higher-than average risk of developing cancer in her other breast. She should continue to practice breast self-examination, checking both the treated area and her other breast each month. She should report any changes to her doctor right away.

Also, a woman who has had breast cancer should tell her doctor about other physical problems if they come up, such as pain, loss of appetite or weight, changes in menstrual periods, or blurred vision. She should also report dizziness, coughing or hoarseness, headaches, or digestive problems that seem unusual or that don't go away. These symptoms may be a sign that the cancer has returned, but they can also be signs of many other problems. Only the doctor can tell for sure.

Living with Cancer

The diagnosis of cancer can change a woman's life and lives of those close to her. These changes can be hard to handle. It's common for the woman and her family and friends to have many different and sometimes confusing emotions.

At times, patients and their loved ones may be frightened, angry or depressed. These are normal reactions when people face a serious health problem. Most people find it helps to share their thoughts and feelings with loved ones. Sharing can help everyone feel more at ease and can open the way for others to show their concern and offer their support.

Sometimes women who have had breast cancer are afraid that the changes to their body will affect not only how they look but how other people feel about them. They may be concerned that breast cancer and its treatment will affect their sexual relationships. Most couples find that talking about these concerns helps them find ways to express their love during and after treatment.

Cancer patients may worry about holding a job, caring for their families, or starting new relationships. Worries about tests, treatments, hospital stays, and medical bills are also common. Doctors, nurses, or other members of the health team can help calm fears and ease confusion about treatment, working, or daily activities. Also, meeting with a nurse, social worker, counselor, or member of the clergy can be helpful to patients who want to talk about their feelings or discuss their concerns about the future or about personal relationships.

Members of the health care team can provide information and suggest other resources. In addition, the public library is a good source of books and articles on living with cancer. Cancer patients and their families can also find helpful suggestions in the NCI booklets listed on the inside back cover.

Support for Breast Cancer Patients

Finding the strength to deal with the changes brought about by breast cancer can be easier for patients and those who love them when they have appropriate support services.

Many patients find it helpful to talk with others who are facing problems like theirs. Cancer patients often get together in self-help and support groups, where they can share what they have learned about cancer and its treatment and about coping with the disease. Often a social worker or nurse meets with the group.

The American Cancer Society's Reach to Recover program offers special help to breast cancer patients. Trained volunteers, who have had breast cancer themselves, visit patients at the doctor's request and lend emotional support to women before and after treatment. They share their experiences with breast cancer treatment and rehabilitation and with breast reconstruction. Information about the American Cancer Society is listed at the end of this article.

Friends and relatives, especially those who have had cancer themselves, can also be very supportive. It's important to keep in mind, however, that each patient is different. Treatments and ways of dealing with cancer that work for one person may not be right for another—even if they both have the same kind of cancer. It is always a good idea to discuss the advice of friends and family members with the doctor.

Often, the doctor's staff or social worker at the hospital or clinic can suggest local and national groups that can help with emotional support, rehabilitation, financial aid, transportation, or home care. Information about programs and services for breast cancer patients and their families is also available through the Cancer Information Service.

What the Future Holds

Researchers are finding better ways to detect and treat breast cancer, and the chances of recovery keep improving. Still, it is natural for patients to be concerned about their future.

Sometimes patients use statistics they have heard to figure out their own chances of being cured. It is important to remember, however, that statistics are averages based on large numbers of patients. They can't be used to predict what will happen to a particular woman because no two cancer patients are alike. The doctor who takes care of the patient and knows her medical history is in the best position to talk with her about the chance of recovery (*prognosis*). Women should feel free to ask the doctor about their prognosis, but they should keep in mind that not even the doctor knows exactly what will happen. Doctors often talk about surviving cancer, or they may use the term *remission*. Doctors use these terms because, although many breast cancer patients are cured, the disease can recur.

The Promise of Cancer Research

Scientists at hospitals and medical centers all across the country are studying breast cancer. They are trying to learn more about what causes the disease and how to prevent it. They are also looking for better ways to diagnose and treat it.

Causes and Prevention

Each year, more than 180,000 women in the United States find out they have breast cancer. Although this disease also occurs in about 1,000 men in this country each year, more than 99 percent of all breast cancer patients are women.

Scientists do not know what causes breast cancer, and doctors can seldom explain why one person gets this disease and another doesn't. It is clear, however, that breast cancer is **not** caused by bumping, bruising, or touching the breast. And this disease is **not** contagious; no one can "catch" breast cancer from another person.

By studying large numbers of women all over the world, researchers have found certain *risk factors* that increase a woman's chance of developing breast cancer. Women with these risk factors have a higher-than-average chance of getting this disease. However, studies also show that most women with these risk factors do not get breast cancer. And many women who get breast cancer have none of the risk factors we know about.

The following are some of the known risk factors for this disease:

- **Age.** The risk of breast cancer increases as a woman gets older. Most breast cancers occur in women over the age of 50; the risk is especially high for women over 60. This disease is uncommon in women under the age of 35.
- **Family history.** The risk of getting breast cancer increases for a woman whose mother, sister, or daughter has had the disease. The woman's risk increases more if her relative's cancer developed before menopause or if it affected both breasts.

- **Personal history.** Women who have had breast cancer face an increased risk of getting breast cancer again. About 15 percent of women treated for breast cancer get a second breast cancer later on. The risk is greater for women who have had lobular carcinoma *in situ.*

Other risk factors for breast cancer include starting to menstruate at an early age (before 12) or having a late menopause (after 55). The risk is also greater in women who had their first child after the age of 30 and those who never had children. Because these factors are all related to a woman's natural hormones, many people are concerned about medicines that contain hormones (either for birth control or as estrogen replacement therapy to control symptoms of menopause), especially if women take them for many years. At this time, no one knows for sure whether taking hormones affects the risk of breast cancer. Scientists hope to find the answer to this important question by studying a large number of women taking part in hormone-related research.

Research suggests that a person's diet may affect the chances of getting some types of cancer. Breast cancer appears more likely to develop in women whose diet is high in fat. Older women who are overweight also seem to have greater risk. Although the possible link between diet and breast cancer is still under study, some scientists believe that choosing a low-fat diet, eating well-balanced meals with plenty of fruits and vegetables, and maintaining ideal weight can lower a woman's risk.

Some studies suggest a slightly higher risk of breast cancer among women who drink alcohol. The risk appears to go up with the amount of alcohol consumed, so women who drink should only do so in moderation.

Many women are concerned about benign breast conditions. For most women, the ordinary "lumpiness" they feel in their breasts does not increase their risk of breast cancer. However, women who have had breast biopsies that show certain benign changes in breast tissues, such as *atypical hyperplasia*, do have an increased risk of breast cancer.

Women who are at high risk for breast cancer are taking part in a study of the drug Tamoxifen, which is often used to treat breast cancer patients. This nationwide study is designed to help doctors learn whether tamoxifen can prevent breast cancer in these women. The Cancer Information Service can provide information about this study.

Detection

When breast cancer is found early, patients have more treatment choices and their chance of complete recovery is better. Because breast cancer often occurs in women with none of the known risk factors (mentioned above), it is important for all women to ask their doctor about mammography, breast exams by a doctor or nurse, and breast self-examination.

Unfortunately, the test we have now cannot reveal every breast cancer at an early stage. Scientists are trying to find better ways to detect breast cancers when they are very small. For example, they are looking for ways to make mammography more accurate. They are also exploring new techniques to produce detailed pictures of the tissues in the breasts.

In addition, researchers are studying tumor markers, substances that may be present in abnormal amounts in the blood or urine of a woman who has breast cancer. Several markers have been studied, and this research is continuing. At this time, however, no blood or urine test is reliable enough to reveal early breast cancer.

Treatment

Researchers also are looking for more effective ways to treat breast cancer. In addition, they are exploring ways to reduce the side effects of treatment and improve the quality of patients' lives. When laboratory research shows that a new treatment method has promise, cancer patients receive the treatment in clinical trials. These trials are designed to answer scientific questions and to find out whether the new approach is both safe and effective. Often, clinical trials compare a new treatment with a standard approach. Patients who take part in clinicals trials make an important contribution to medical science and may have the first chance to benefit from improved treatment methods.

Trials to study new treatments for patients with all stages of breast cancer are under way. Researchers are testing new treatment methods, new doses and treatment schedules, and new ways of combining treatments. They are working with various anticancer drugs and drug combinations as well as several types of hormone therapy. They are also exploring new ways to combine chemotherapy with hormone therapy and radiation therapy. Some trials include *biological therapy*, treatment with substances that boost the immune system's response to cancer.

In a number of trials, doctors are trying to learn whether very high doses of anticancer drugs are more effective than the usual doses in destroying breast cancer cells. Because these higher doses seriously damage the patients' *bone marrow*, where blood cells are formed, researchers are testing ways to replace the bone marrow or to help it recover. These new approaches (*bone marrow transplantation, peripheral stem cell support,* and the use of *colony-stimulating factors*) are described in "Definition of Terms" section.

Cancer patients may want to read an NCI booklet called *What are Clinical Trials All About?*, which explains some of the possible benefits and risks of treatment studies. Those who are interested in taking part in a trial should discuss this option with their doctor.

One way to learn about clinical trials is through PDQ, a computerized resource developed by NCI. PDQ contains information about cancer treatment and an up-to-date list of trials all over the country. Doctors can also obtain an access code and use a personal computer to get PDQ information. Also, the Cancer Information Service can provide PDQ information to doctors, patients, and the public.

Definitions of Terms

Adjuvant therapy (AD-ju-vant): Treatment given in addition to the primary treatment.

Areola (a-REE-oe-la): The area of dark-colored skin that surrounds the nipple.

Aspiration (as-per-AY-shun): Removal of fluid from a lump, often a cyst, with a needle.

Atypical hyperplasia (hy-per-PLAY-zha): A benign (noncancerous) condition in which breast tissue has certain abnormal features. This condition increases the risk of breast cancer.

Axilla (ak-SIL-a): The underarm.

Benign (bee-NINE): Not cancerous; does not invade nearby tissue or spread to other parts of the body.

Biological therapy (by-o-LOJ-i-kal): Treatment to stimulate or restore the ability of the immune system to fight infection and disease. Also called immunotherapy.

Biopsy (BY-op-see): The removal of a sample of tissue, which is then examined under a microscope to check for cancer cells. Excisional biopsy is surgery to remove an entire lump and a margin of normal tissue around it. In incisional biopsy, which is done less often for breast tumors, the surgeon removes part of the tumor. Removal of tissue with a needle is called biopsy.

Bone marrow: The soft, sponge-like material inside some bones. Blood cells are produced in bone marrow.

Bone marrow transplantation (trans-plan-TAY-shun): A procedure in which doctors replace marrow destroyed by high doses of anticancer drugs or radiation. The replacement marrow may be taken from the patient before treatment or may be donated by another person. When the patient's own marrow is used, the procedure is called autologous (aw-TAHL-o-gus) bone marrow transplantation.

Cancer: A term for more than 100 disease in which abnormal cells divide without control. Cancer cells can spread through the bloodstream and lymphatic system to other parts of the body.

Carcinoma (kar-sin-OE-ma): Cancer that begins in the lining or covering of an organ.

Carcinoma in situ (kar-sin-OE-ma in SY-too): Cancer that involves only the tissue in which it began; it has not spread to other tissues. Lobular carcinoma *in situ* develops in the lobules of the breast. Ductal carcinoma *in situ* (also called intraductal carcinoma) arises in the ducts.

Chemotherapy (kee-moe-THER-a-pee): Treatment with anticancer drugs.

Clinical trials: Research studies that involve patients. Each study is designed to answer scientific questions and to find better ways to prevent or treat cancer.

Colony-stimulating factors: Laboratory-made substances similar to substances in the body that stimulate the production of blood cells. Treatment with colony-stimulating factors can help cells in the bone marrow recover from the effects of chemotherapy and radiation therapy.

Cyst (sist): A closed sac or capsule filled with fluid.

Diaphanography (dy-a-fan-OG-ra-fee): An exam that involves shining a bright light through the breast to reveal features of the tissues inside. This technique is under study; its value in detecting breast cancer has not been proven. Also called transillumination.

Duct: A tube in the breast through which milk passes from the lobules to the nipple. Cancer that begins in a duct is called ductal carcinoma.

Estrogen (ES-troe-jin): A female hormone.

Gynecologist (guy-ni-KOL-o-jist): A doctor who specializes in treating diseases of the female reproductive organs.

Hair follicle (FOL-i-kul): A sac from which a hair grows.

Hormones: Chemicals reproduced by glands in the body. Hormones control the actions of certain cells or organs.

Hormone receptor test: A test to measure the amount of certain proteins, called hormone receptors, in breast cancer tissue. Hormones can attach to these proteins. A high level of hormone receptors means hormones probably help the cancer grow.

Hormone therapy: Treatment of cancer by removing, blocking, or adding hormones.

Infertility: The inability to have children.

Lobe: A part of the breast; each breast contains 15 to 20 lobes.

Lobule (LOB-yool): A subdivision of the lobes of the breast. Cancer that begins in a lobule is called lobular carcinoma.

Local therapy: Treatment that affects cells in the tumor and the area close to it.

Lumpectomy (lump-EK-toe-mee): Surgery to remove only the cancerous breast lump; usually followed by radiation therapy.

Lymph (limf): The almost colorless fluid that travels through the lymphatic system and carries cells that help fight infection and disease.

Lymph nodes: Small, bean-shaped organs located along the channels of the lymphatic system. Bacteria or cancer cells that enter the lymphatic system may be found in the nodes. Also called lymph glands.

Lymphatic system (lim-FAT-ik): The tissues and organs (including bone marrow, spleen, thymus, and lymph nodes) that produce and store cells that fight infection and disease. The channels that carry lymph are also part of this system.

Lymphedema (lim-fa-DEE-ma): Swelling of the hand and arm caused by extra fluid that may collect in tissues when underarm lymph nodes are removed or blocked, sometimes called "milk arm."

Malignant (ma-LIG-nant): Cancerous; can spread to other parts of the body.

Mammogram (MAM-o-gram): An x-ray of the breast.

Mammography (mam-OG-ra-fee): The use of x-rays to create a picture of the breast.

Mastectomy (mas-TEK-to-mee): Surgery to remove the breast.

Menopause: The time of a woman's life when menstrual periods stop; also called "change of life."

Menstrual cycle (MEN-stroo-al): The hormone changes that lead up to a woman's having a period. For most women, one cycle takes 28 days.

Metastasis (meh-TAS-ta-sis): The spread of cancer from one part of the body to another. Cells in the metastatic (secondary) tumor are like those in the original (primary) tumor.

Microcalcifications (MY-krow-kal-si-fi-KA-shun): Tiny deposits of calcium in the breast that cannot be felt but can be detected on a mammogram. A cluster of these very small specks of calcium may indicate that cancer is present.

Oncologist (on-KOL-o-jist): A doctor who specializes in treating cancer.

Ovaries (OE-va-reez): The pair of female reproductive organs that produce eggs and hormones.

Palpation (pal-PAY-shun): A simple technique in which a doctor presses on the surface of the body to feel the organs or tissues underneath.

Pathologist (path-OL-o-jist): A doctor who identifies diseases by studying cells and tissues under a microscope.

Peripheral stem cell support (per-IF-er-al): A method for replacing bone marrow destroyed by cancer treatment. Certain cells (*stem cells*) in the blood that are similar to those in bone marrow are removed from the patient's blood before treatment. The cells are given back to the patient after treatment to help the bone marrow recover and continue producing healthy blood cells.

Progesterone (proe-JES-ter-own): A female hormone.

Prognosis (prog-NOE-sis): The probable outcome or course of a disease; the chance of recovery.

Prosthesis (pros-THEE-sis): An artificial replacement of a part of the body. A breast prosthesis is a breast form worn under clothing.

Radiation therapy (ray-dee-AY-shun): Treatment with high-energy rays to kill cancer cells. Radiation therapy that uses a machine located outside the body to aim high-energy rays at the cancer is called external radiation. When radioactive material is placed in the breast in thin plastic tubes, the treatment is called implant radiation.

Radiologist: A doctor who specializes in creating and interpreting pictures of areas inside the body. The pictures are produced with x-rays, sound waves, or other types of energy.

Remission: Disappearance of the signs and symptoms of cancer. When this happens, the disease is said to be "in remission." A remission can be temporary or permanent.

Risk factor: Something that increases a person's chance of developing a disease.

Stage: The extent of the cancer. The stage of breast cancer depends on the size of the cancer and whether it has spread from its original site to other parts of the body.

Stem cells: Cells that produce new cells that become specialized.

Surgery: An operation.

Systemic therapy (sis-TEM-ik): Treatment that reaches and affects cells all over the body.

Thermography (ther-MOG-ra-fee): A test to measure and display heat patterns of tissues near the surface of the breast. Abnormal tissue generally is warmer than healthy tissue. This technique is under study; its value in detecting breast cancer has not been proven.

Tissue (TISH-oo): A group or layer of cells that performs a specific function.

Tumor: An abnormal mass of tissue.

Ultrasonography (ul-tra-son-OG-ra-fee): A test in which sound waves are bounced off tissues and the echoes are converted into a picture (sonogram). These pictures are shown on a monitor like a TV screen. Tissues of different densities look different in the picture because they reflect sound waves differently. A sonogram can show whether a breast lump is a fluid-filled cyst or a solid mass.

Xeroradiography (ZEE-roe-ray-dee-OG-ra-fee): A type of mammography in which a picture of the breast is recorded on paper rather than film.

X-ray: High energy radiation. It is used in low doses to diagnose diseases and in high doses to treat cancer.

Resources

Information about cancer is available from several sources, including the ones listed below. You may wish to check for additional information at your local library or bookstore or from support groups in your community.

Cancer Information Service (CIS)

The Cancer Information Service, a program of the National Cancer Institute, provides a nationwide telephone service for cancer patients and their families and friends, the public, and health professionals. The staff can answer questions and can send booklets about cancer. They also know about local resources and services. One toll-free number, 1-800-4-CAN-CER (1-800-422-6237), connects callers all over the country to the office that serves their area. Spanish-speaking staff members are available.

American Cancer Society (ACS)

The American Cancer Society is a voluntary organization with a national office and local units all over the country. It supports research, conducts educational programs, and offers many services to patients and their families. It provides free booklets on breast cancer and on sexuality. To obtain booklets or to learn about Reach and Recovery or other services and activities in local areas, call the Society's toll-free number, 1-800-ACS-2345 (1-800-227-2345), or the number listed under American Cancer Society in the white pages of the local telephone book.

Breast Self-Examination (BSE) Instructions

Do breast self-examination (BSE) once a month. Become familiar with how your breasts look and feel. Do BSE to look for any change from what looks and feels normal for you.

If you still menstruate, the best time to do BSE is 2 or 3 days after your period ends. These are the days when your breasts are least likely to be tender or swollen.

If you no longer menstruate, pick a certain day—such as the first day of each month—to remind yourself to do BSE.

If you are taking hormones, talk with your doctor about when to do BSE.

1. Stand in front of a mirror that is large enough for you to see your breasts clearly. Check each breast for anything unusual. Check the skin for puckering, dimpling, or scaliness. Look for a discharge from the nipples.

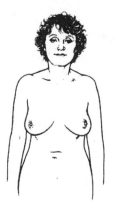

Do steps 2 and 3 to check for any change in the shape or contour of your breasts. As you do these steps, you should feel your chest muscles tighten.

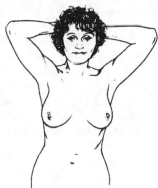

2. Watching closely in the mirror, clasp your hands behind your head and press your hands forward.

3. Next, press your hands firmly on your hips and bend slightly toward the mirror as you pull your shoulder and elbows forward.

4. Gently squeeze each nipple and look for a discharge.

5. Raise one arm. Use the pads of the fingers of your other hand to check the breast and the surrounding area—firmly, carefully, and thoroughly. Some women like to use lotion or powder to help their fingers glide easily over the skin. Feel for any unusual lump or mass under the skin.

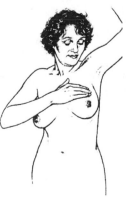

Feel the tissue by pressing your fingers in small, overlapping areas about the size of a dime. To be sure you cover your whole breast, take your time and follow a definite pattern: lines, circles, or wedges.

Some research suggest that many women do BSE more thoroughly when they use a pattern of up-and-down lines or strips. Other women feel more comfortable with another pattern. The important thing is to cover the whole breast and to pay special attention to the area between the breast and the underarm, including the underarm itself. Check the area above the breast, up to the collarbone and all the way over to your shoulder.

Lines: Start in the underarm area and move your fingers downward little by little until they are below the breast. Then move your fingers slightly toward the middle and slowly move back up. Go up and down until you cover the whole area.

Circles: Beginning at the outer edge of your breasts, move your fingers slowly around the whole breast in a circle. Move around the breast in smaller and smaller circles, gradually working toward the nipple. Don't forget to check the underarm and upper chest areas, too.

Wedges: Starting at the outer edge of the breast, move your fingers toward the nipple and back to the edge. Check your whole breast, covering one small wedge-shaped section at a time. Be sure to check the underarm area and the upper chest.

6. It's important to repeat step 5 while you are lying down. Lie flat on your back, with one arm over your head and a pillow or folded towel under the shoulder. This position flattens the breast and makes it easier to check. Check each breast and the area around it very carefully using one of the patterns described above.

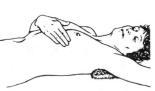

7. Some women repeat step 5 in the shower. Your fingers will glide easily over soapy skin, so you can concentrate on feeling for changes underneath.

> If you notice a lump, a discharge, or any other change during the month—whether or not it is during BSE—contact your doctor.

Other Booklets

The National Cancer Institute booklets listed below and others that deal with breast cancer are available free of charge by calling 1-800-4-CANCER.

Booklets about Cancer Treatment

- Radiation Therapy and You: A Guide to Self-Help During Treatment
- Chemotherapy and You: A Guide to Self-Help During Treatment
- Eating Hints: Recipes and Tips for Better Nutrition During Cancer Treatment
- Questions and Answers about Pain Control (also available from the American Cancer Society)
- What are Clinical Trials All About?

Booklets about Living with Cancer

- Taking Time: Support for People with Cancer and the People Who Care about Them
- Facing Forward: A Guide for Cancer Survivors
- When Cancer Recurs: Meeting the Challenge Again
- Advanced Cancer: Living each Day

■ **Document Source:**
U.S. Department of Health and Human Services, Public Health Service
National Institutes of Health
National Cancer Institute
NIH Publication No. 94-1556
Revised July 1993

See also: Things to Know about Quality Mammograms (page 496)

MISCELLANEOUS

∎∎∎

BE INFORMED: QUESTIONS TO ASK YOUR DOCTOR BEFORE YOU HAVE SURGERY

Are you facing surgery? You are not alone. Millions of Americans have surgery each year. Most operations are not emergencies. This means you have time to ask your surgeon questions about the operation and time to decide whether to have it, and if so, when and where. This brochure does **not** apply to emergency surgery.

The most important questions to ask about elective surgery are why the procedure is necessary for you and what alternatives there are to surgery. If you do not need to have the operation, then you can avoid any risks that might result. All surgeries and alternative treatments have risks and benefits. They are only worth doing if the benefits are greater than the risks.

Your primary care doctor—that is, your regular doctor—may be the one who suggests that you have surgery and may recommend a surgeon. You may want to identify another independent surgeon to get a second opinion. Check to see if your health insurance will pay for the operation and the second opinion. If you are eligible for Medicare, it will pay for a second opinion. You should discuss your insurance questions with your health insurance company or your employee benefits office.

Overview

This booklet provides 12 questions to ask your primary care doctor and surgeon before you have surgery—and the reasons for asking them. The answers to these questions will help you be informed and help you make the best decision. Sources are listed at the end of this booklet to help you get more information from other places.

Your doctors should welcome questions. If you do not understand the answers, ask the doctors to explain them clearly. Patients who are well informed about their treatment tend to be more satisfied with the outcome or results of their treatment.

What operation are you recommending?

Ask your surgeon to explain the surgical procedure. For example, if something is going to be repaired or removed, find out why it is necessary to do so. Your surgeon can draw a picture or a diagram and explain to you the steps involved in the procedure.

Are there different ways of doing the operation? One way may require more extensive surgery than another. Ask why your surgeon wants to do the operation one way or another.

Why do I need the operation?

There are many reasons to have surgery. Some operations can relieve or prevent pain. Others can reduce a symptom of a problem or improve some body function. Some surgeries are performed to diagnose a problem. Surgery also can save your life. Your surgeon will tell you the purpose of the procedure. Make sure you understand how the proposed operation fits in with the diagnosis of your medical condition.

Are there alternatives to surgery?

Sometimes, surgery is not the only answer to a medical problem. Medicines or other nonsurgical treatments, such as a change in diet or special exercises, might help you just as well—or more. Ask your surgeon or primary care doctor about the benefits and risks of these other choices. You need to know as much as possible about these benefits and risks to make the best decision.

One alternative may be "watchful waiting," in which your doctor and you check to see if your problem gets better or worse. If it gets worse, you may need surgery right away. If it gets better, you may be able to postpone surgery, perhaps indefinitely.

What are the benefits of having the operation?

Ask your surgeon what you will gain by having the operation. For example, a hip replacement may mean that you can walk again with ease.

Ask how long the benefits are likely to last. For some procedures, it is not unusual for the benefits to last for a short time only. There might be a need for a second operation at a later date. For other procedures, the benefits may last a lifetime.

When finding out about the benefits of the operation, be realistic. Sometimes patients expect too much and are disappointed with the outcome, or results. Ask your doctor if there is any published information about the outcomes of the procedure.

What are the risks of having the operation?

All operations carry some risk. This is why you need to weigh the benefits of the operation against the risks of complications or side effects.

Complications can occur around the time of the operation. Complications are unplanned events, such as infection, too much bleeding, reaction to anesthesia, or accidental injury. Some people have an increased risk of complications because of other medical conditions.

In addition, there may be **side effects** after the operation. For the most part, side effects can be anticipated. For example, your surgeon knows that there will be swelling and some soreness at the site of the operation.

Ask your surgeon about the possible complications and side effects of the operation. There is almost always some pain with surgery. Ask how much there will be and what the doctors and nurses will do to reduce the pain. Controlling the pain will help you be more comfortable while you heal, get well faster, and improve the results of your operation.

What if I don't have this operation?

Based on what you learn about the benefits and risks of the operation, you might decide not to have it. Ask your surgeon what you will gain—or lose—by not having the operation now. Could you be in more pain? Could the problem go away?

Where can I get a second opinion?

Getting a second opinion from another doctor is a very good way to make sure having the operation is the best alternative for you. Many health insurance plans require patients to get a second opinion before they have certain non-emergency operations. If your plan does not require a second opinion, you may still ask to have one. Check with your insurance company to see if it will pay for a second opinion. If you get one, make sure to get your records from the first doctor so that the second one does not have to repeat tests.

What has been your experience in doing the operation?

One way to reduce the risks of surgery is to choose a surgeon who has been thoroughly trained to do the procedure and has plenty of experience doing it. You can ask your surgeon about his or her recent record of successes and complications with the procedure. If it is more comfortable for you, you can discuss the topic of surgeons' qualifications with your regular or primary care doctor.

Where will the operation be done?

Most surgeons practice at one or two local hospitals. Find out where your operation will be performed. Have many of the operations you are thinking about having been done in this hospital? Some operations have higher success rates if they are done in hospitals that do many of those procedures. Ask your doctor about the success rate at this hospital. If the hospital has a low success rate for the operation in question, you should ask to have it at another hospital.

Until recently, most surgery was performed on an inpatient basis—patients stayed in the hospital for one or more days. Today, a lot of surgery is done on an outpatient basis in a doctor's office, a special surgical center, or a day surgery unit of a hospital. Outpatient surgery is less expensive because you do not have to pay for staying in a hospital room.

Ask whether your operation will be done in the hospital or in an outpatient setting. If your doctor recommends inpatient surgery for a procedure that is usually done as outpatient surgery—or just the opposite, recommends outpatient surgery that is usually done as inpatient surgery—ask why. You want to be in the right place for your operation.

What kind of anesthesia will I need?

Anesthesia is used so that surgery can be performed without unnecessary pain. Your surgeon can tell you whether the operation calls for local, regional, or general anesthesia, and why this form of anesthesia is recommended for your procedure.

Local anesthesia numbs only a part of your body for a short period of time—for example, a tooth and the surrounding gum. Not all procedures done with local anesthesia are painless. *Regional anesthesia* numbs a larger portion of your body—for example, the lower part of your body—for a few hours. In most cases, you will be awake with regional anesthesia. *General anesthesia* numbs your entire body for the entire time of the surgery. You will be unconscious if you have general anesthesia.

Anesthesia is quite safe for most patients and is usually administered by a specialized physician (anesthesiologist) or nurse anesthetist. Both are highly skilled and have been specially trained to give anesthesia.

If you decide to have an operation, ask to meet with the person who will give you anesthesia. Find out what his or her qualifications are. Ask what the side effects and risks of having anesthesia are in your case. Be sure to tell him or her what medical problems you have—including allergies—and any medications you have been taking, since they may affect your response to the anesthesia.

How long will it take me to recover?

Your surgeon can tell you how you might feel and what you will be able to do—or not do—the first few days, weeks, or months after surgery. Ask how long you will be in the hospital. Find out what kind of supplies, equipment, and any other help you will need when you go home. Knowing what to expect can help you cope better with recovery.

Ask when you can start regular exercise again and go back to work. You do not want to do anything that will slow down the recovery process. Lifting a 10-pound bag of potatoes may not seem to be "too much" a week after your operation, but it could be. You should follow your surgeons advice to make sure you recover fully as soon as possible.

How much will the operation cost?

Health insurance coverage for surgery can vary, and there may be some costs you will have to pay. Before you have the operation, call your insurance company to find out how much of these costs it will pay and how much you will have to pay yourself.

Ask what your surgeon's fee is and what it covers. Surgical fees often also include several visits after the operation. You also will be billed by the hospital for inpatient or outpatient care and by the anesthesiologist and others providing care related to your operation.

Surgeon's Qualifications

You will want to know that your surgeon is experienced and qualified to perform the operation. Many surgeons have taken special training and passed exams given by a national board of surgeons. Ask if your surgeon is "board certified" in surgery. Some surgeons also have the letters F.A.C.S. after their name. This means they are Fellows of the American College of Surgeons and have passed another review by surgeons of their surgical practices.

For More Information

Surgery. The American College of Surgeons (ACS) has a free series of pamphlets on "When You Need an Operation." For copies, write to the ACS, Office of Public Information, 55 E Erie St, Chicago, IL 60611, or call 312-664-4050. Pamphlets in this series range from those providing general information about surgery to those explaining specific surgical procedures.

Second Opinion. For a free brochure on "Medicare Coverage for Second Surgical Opinions: Your Choice Facing Elective Surgery," write to Health Care Financing Administration, Room 555, East High Rise Building, 6325 Security Blvd, Baltimore, MD 21207. Ask for Publication No. HCFA 02173.

To get the name of a specialist in your area who can give you a second opinion, ask your primary doctor or surgeon, the local medical society, or your health insurance company. Medicare beneficiaries may also obtain information from the U.S. Department of Health and Human Services' Medicare Hotline: call toll-free 800-638-6833.

Anesthesia. Free booklets on what you should know about anesthesia are available from the American Society of Anesthesiologists (ASA) or the American Association of Nurse Anesthetists (AANA). For copies, write to ASA at 520 N Northwest Highway, Park Ridge, IL 60608, or call 708-825-5586; or AANA at 222 S Prospect Ave, Park Ridge, IL 60068-4001, or call 708-692-7050.

Pain Control. "Pain Control After Surgery: A Patient's Guide" is available free from the Agency for Health Care Policy and Research (AHCPR). For a copy of this consumer version of the AHCPR-supported clinical practice guideline and for information on other patient guides, write to the AHCPR Publication Clearinghouse, PO Box 8547, Silver Spring, MD 20907, or call toll-free 800-358-9295.

General. For almost every disease, there is a national or local association or society that publishes consumer information. Check your local telephone directory. There are also organized groups of patients with certain illnesses that can often provide information about a condition, alternative treatments, and experience with local doctors and hospitals. Ask your hospital or doctors if they know of any patient groups related to your condition. Also, your local public library has medical reference materials about health care treatments.

Some of the issues discussed in this booklet are covered in greater detail in a guidebook and video program, "PREPARED for Health Care: A Consumer's Guide to Better Medical Decisions," by J.C. Gambone, DO, and R.C. Reiter, MD, copyright 1993, Great Performance, Beaverton, Oregon. For information on obtaining copies, write to Great Performance, Inc. at PO Box 91400, Portland, OR 97291-0400.

For further information you may also wish to see "The Savvy Patient: How to Be an Active Participant in Your Medical Care," by David R. Stutz, MD, Bernard Feder, PhD, and the Editors of Consumer Reports Books, copyright 1990, published by Consumers Union of U.S., Inc, Yonkers, NY, 10703.

Reference to these materials does not constitute endorsement by the Public Health Service or the U.S. Department of Health and Human Services.

Take this list of questions with you when you go to your doctor to discuss your surgery.

1. What operation are you recommending?
2. Why do I need the operation?
3. Are there alternatives to surgery?
4. What are the benefits of having the operation?
5. What are the risks of having the operation?
6. What if I don't have this operation?
7. Where can I get a second opinion?
8. What has been your experience in doing the operation?
9. Where will the operation be done?
10. What kind of anesthesia will I need?
11. How long will it take me to recover?
12. How much will the operation cost?

■ Document Source:
U.S. Department of Health and Human Services, Public Health Service
Agency for Health Care Policy and Research
Executive Office Center, Ste 501
2101 East Jefferson St
Rockville, MD 20852
AHCPR Pub. No. 95-0027
January 1995

See also: Talking with Your Doctor: A Guide for Older People (page 530)

FACT SHEET: REYE'S SYNDROME

Reye's Syndrome is a very serious disease that you should know about. Some people develop Reye's Syndrome as they are getting over a viral illness, such as the flu or chicken pox. Reye's Syndrome usually affects people from infancy through young adulthood; however, no age group is immune. Although Reye's generally occurs when someone is recovering from a viral illness, it can develop three to five days after the onset of the illness. Its main targets are the liver and brain, it is noncontagious, and too often is misdiagnosed as encephalitis, meningitis, diabetes, poisoning, drug overdose, or sudden infant death.

Early diagnosis is crucial. An individual should be watched during the next two to three weeks following a viral illness for these symptoms, usually occurring in this order:

- **Relentless or continuous vomiting**
- **Listlessness** (loss of pep and energy with little interest in their environment)
- **Drowsiness** (excessive sleepiness)
- **Personality change** (such as irritability, slurred speech, sensitivity to touch)
- **Disorientation or confusion** (unable to identify whereabouts, family members, or answer questions)
- **Combativeness** (striking out at those trying to help them)
- **Delirium, convulsions, or loss of consciousness**

Reye's Syndrome should be suspected in anyone who vomits repeatedly. Phone your doctor immediately if these symptoms develop. Voice your concern about Reye's Syndrome. If your physician is unavailable, take the person to an Emergency Room promptly. Two liver function tests (SGOT, SGPT) can be done to determine the possibility of Reye's Syndrome. There is a 90% chance of recovery when the syndrome is treated in its earliest stages by physicians and nurses experienced in the treatment of Reye's.

Studies have shown that using aspirin or aspirin-containing medications to treat the symptoms of viral illnesses increases the chance of developing Reye's Syndrome. If you or a member of your family have a viral illness, **do not use aspirin or aspirin-containing medications.** In fact, you should consult your physician before you take any drugs to treat the flu or chicken pox, particularly aspirin or anti-nausea

medicines. Anti-nausea medicines may mask the symptoms of Reye's Syndrome.

The National Reye's Syndrome Foundation (NRSF), the U.S. Surgeon General, the Food and Drug Administration, and the Centers for Disease Control recommend that aspirin and combination products containing aspirin not be taken by anyone under 19 years of age during fever-causing illnesses.

Aspirin is a part of the salicylate family of medicines. Another name for aspirin is acetylsalicylate; some drug labels may use the words acetylsalicylate, acetylsalicylic acid, salicylic acid, salicylate, etc., instead of the word aspirin. Currently, there is no conclusive data as to whether other forms of salicylates are associated with the development of Reye's Syndrome. Until further research has answered this question, the NRSF recommends that products containing any of these substances not be taken during episodes of viral infections.

The NRSF is a nonprofit, tax-exempt organization with affiliates located in 43 states. The NRSF has pioneered the movement to disseminate knowledge about the disease in an effort to aid in early diagnosis and also provides funds for research into the cause, cure, care, treatment, and prevention of Reye's Syndrome.

For additional information, please contact:

National Reye's Syndrome Foundation
426 N Lewis, PO Box 829
Bryan, OH 43506
1-800-233-7393 or 419-636-2679
Fax: 419-636-3366
e-mail: reyessyn@bright.net
http://www.bright.net/~reyessyn

■ Document Source:
National Reye's Syndrome Foundation
426 N Lewis St, PO Box 829
Bryan, OH 43506

See also: Medications Containing Aspirin (Acetylsalicylate) (page 523); Reye's Syndrome: Because You Need to Know (page 528)

LEAD POISONING AND YOUR CHILDREN

Lead Awareness and Your Children

About one in six children in America have high levels of lead in their blood, according to the Agency for Toxic Substances and Disease Registry. You may have lead around your building without knowing it because you can't see, taste, or smell lead. You may have lead in the dust, paint, or soil in and around your home or in your drinking water or food. Because it does not break down naturally, lead can remain a problem until it is removed.

Before we knew how harmful it could be, lead was used in paint, gasoline, water pipes, and many other products. Now that we know the dangers of lead, house paint is almost lead-free. Leaded gasoline is being phased out, and household plumbing is no longer made with lead materials.

How Lead Affects Your Child's Health

The long term effects of lead in a child can be severe. They include learning disabilities, decreased growth, hyperactivity, impaired hearing, and even brain damage. If caught early, these effects can be limited by reducing exposure to lead or by medical treatment. If you are pregnant avoid exposing yourself to lead. Lead can pass through your body to your baby. The good news is that there are simple things you can do to help protect your family.

1. Get your child tested.

Even children who appear healthy may have high levels of lead. You can't tell if a child has lead poisoning unless you have him or her tested. A blood test takes only ten minutes, and results should be ready within a week.

- The Centers for Disease Control recommend that children be tested for the first time when they are a year old, or at six months if you think your home has lead in it or if you live in an older building.
- Children older than one year should have a blood test every couple of years—every year if your house or apartment contains lead paint, or if you use lead in your job or hobby.

To find out where to have your child tested, call your doctor or local health clinic.

2. Keep it clean.

Ordinary dust and dirt may contain lead. Children can swallow lead or breathe lead contaminated dust if they play in dust or dirt and then put their fingers or toys in their mouths, or if they eat without washing their hands first.

- Keep the areas where your children play as dust free and clean as possible.
- Wash pacifiers and bottles after they fall on the floor. Keep extras handy.
- Mop floors and wipe window ledges and chewable surfaces such as cribs with a solution of powdered automatic dishwasher detergent in warm water. Do this twice each week. Wear gloves to avoid possible skin irritation. (Dishwasher detergents are recommended because of their high-phosphate content. Most multipurpose cleaners do not contain phosphates and are not effective in cleaning lead dust.)
- Wash toys and stuffed animals regularly.
- Make sure your children wash their hands before meals, naptime, and bedtime.

3. Reduce the risk from lead paint.

Most homes built before 1960 contain heavily leaded paint. Some homes built as recently as 1978 may also contain lead paint. This paint could be on window frames, walls, the outside of your house, or other surfaces. Tiny pieces of peeling or chipping lead paint are dangerous if eaten. Lead paint in good condition is not usually a problem except ill places where painted surfaces rub against each other and create dust. (For example, when you open a window, the painted surfaces rub against each other.)

- Make sure your child does not chew on anything covered with lead paint, such as painted window sills, cribs, or playpens.
- Don't burn painted wood. It may contain lead.

4. Don't remove lead paint yourself.

Families have been poisoned by scraping or sanding lead paint because these activities generate large amounts of lead dust. Lead dust from repairs or renovations of older buildings can remain in the building long after the work is completed. Heating lead paint may release lead into the air.

- Ask your local or state health department if they will test your home for lead paint. Some will test for free. Home test kits cannot detect small amounts of lead under some conditions.
- Hire a person with special training for correcting lead paint problems to remove lead paint from your home, someone who knows how to do this work safely and has the proper equipment to clean up thoroughly. Don't try to remove lead paint yourself.
- All occupants, especially children and pregnant women should leave the building until all work is finished and a thorough cleanup is done.

5. Don't bring lead dust into your home.

If you work in construction demolition or painting, with batteries, or in a radiator repair shop or lead factory, or if your hobby involves lead you may unknowingly bring lead into your home on your hands or clothes. You may also be tracking in lead from the soil around your home. Soil very close to homes may be contaminated from lead paint on the outside of the building. Soil by roads or highways may be contaminated from years of exhaust fumes from cars and trucks that used leaded gas.

- If you work with lead on your job or a hobby, change your clothes before you go home.
- Encourage your children to play in sand or grassy areas instead of dirt which sticks to fingers and toys. Try to keep your children from eating dirt, and make sure they wash their hands when they come inside.

6. Get lead out of your drinking water.

Most well or city water does not naturally contain lead. Water usually picks up lead inside your home from household plumbing that is made with lead materials. Boiling the water will not reduce the amount of lead. Bathing is not a problem because lead does not enter the body through the skin.

- The only way to know if you have lead in your water is to have it tested. Call your local health department or your water supplier to see how to get it tested. Testing your water is easy and cheap ($15-$25).

- Household water will contain more lead if it has sat for a long time in the pipes, is hot, or is naturally acidic.
- If your water has not been tested or has high levels of lead:
  1. Do not drink, cook, or make baby formula with water from the hot water tap.
  2. If the cold water hasn't been used for more than two hours run it for 30 to 60 seconds before drinking it or using it for cooking.
  3. Consider buying a filter certified for lead removal. Call EPA's Sate Drinking Water Hotline for more information.

7. Eat right.

A child who gets enough iron and calcium will absorb less lead. Foods rich in iron include eggs, lean red meat, and beans. Dairy products are high in calcium.

- Don't store food or liquid in lead crystal glassware or imported or old pottery.
- If you reuse plastic bags to store or carry food, keep the printing on the outside of the bag.

For Further Information

EPA's Safe Drinking Water Hotline at 1-800-426-4791

For information on laboratories certified to test for lead in water and for filter information:

National Lead Information Center at 1-800-LEADFYI

Funded by the Environmental Protection Agency, Centers for Disease Control, Department of Housing and Urban Development, and Department of Defense.

■ Document Source:
   U.S. Environmental Protection Agency
   Office of Pollution Prevention and Toxics
   Office of Ground Water and Drinking Water

MARIJUANA: FACTS PARENTS NEED TO KNOW

A Letter to Parents

Marijuana is the illegal drug most often used in this country. During the last three years, we have seen a doubling in marijuana use among 8th graders, and significant increases among 10th and 12th graders. Our research shows that accompanying this upward pattern of use is a significant erosion in antidrug perceptions and knowledge among young people today. While current marijuana use among high school seniors has increased by 38 percent, the proportion of those who believe marijuana use is harmful has dropped by 22 percent in the past three years.

These changes in perception and knowledge may be due to a decrease in antidrug messages in the media, an increase in prodrug messages through the pop culture, and a lack of awareness among parents about this resurgence in drug use—most thinking, perhaps, that this threat to their children had diminished.

In December 1994, HHS Secretary Donna E. Shalala, PhD called for an Initiative to alert the public—particularly parents—to the rise in marijuana use, its potential health consequences to young people, and the need for parents to take action to prevent the return of a full-blown epidemic of teenage drug use.

Because many parents of this generation of teenagers experimented with marijuana when they were in college, they often find it difficult to talk about marijuana use with their children and to set strict ground rules against drug use. But marijuana use today starts at a younger age—the average age of first use is about 13.5 years old—and more potent forms of the drug are available to these young children. Parents need to recognize that marijuana use is a serious threat - and they need to tell their children not to use it.

We at the National Institute on Drug Abuse (NIDA) are pleased to offer these two short booklets, Marijuana: Facts for Teens and Marijuana: Facts Parents Need to Know, for parents and their children to review the scientific facts about marijuana. While it is best to talk about drugs when children are young, it is never too late to talk about the dangers of drug use.

Talking to our children about drug abuse is not always easy, but it is very important. I hope these booklets can help.

Alan I. Leshner, PhD
Director, National Institute on Drug Abuse

Fact: There are stronger forms of marijuana available to adolescents today than in the 1960's. Stronger marijuana means stronger effects.

Q: What is marijuana? Are there different kinds?
A: Marijuana is a green, brown, or gray mixture of dried, shredded flowers and leaves of the hemp plant (Cannabis sativa). Before the 1960s, many Americans had never heard of marijuana, but today it is the most often used illegal drug in this country.

Cannabis is a term that refers to marijuana and other drugs made from the same plant. Stronger forms of cannabis include sinsemilla (sin-seh-me-yah), hashish ("hash" for short), and hash oil.

All forms of cannabis are mind-altering (psychoactive) drugs; they all contain THC (delta9-tetrahydrocannabinol), the main active chemical in marijuana. There are about 400 chemicals in a cannabis plant, but THC is the one that affects the brain the most.

There are stronger forms of marijuana available today than there were in the 1960s. The strength of the drug is measured by the amount of average THC in test samples confiscated by law enforcement agencies.

- Most ordinary marijuana has an average of 3 percent THC.

- Sinsemilla (made from just the buds and flowering tops of female plants) has an average of 7.5 percent THC, with a range as high as 24 percent.
- Hashish (the sticky resin from the female plant flowers) has an average of 3.6 percent, with a range as high as 28 percent.
- Hash oil, a tar-like liquid distilled from hashish, has an average of 16 percent, with a range as high as 43 percent.

Q: What are the current slang terms for marijuana?
A: There are many different names for marijuana. Slang terms for drugs change quickly, and they vary from one part of the country to another. They may even differ across sections of a large city.

Terms from years ago, such as pot, herb, grass, weed, Mary Jane, and reefer, are still used. You might also hear the names Aunt Mary, skunk, boom, gangster, kif, or ganja.

There are also street names for different strains or "brands" of marijuana, such as "Texas tea," "Maui wowie," and "Chronic." A recent book of American slang lists more than 200 terms for various kinds of marijuana.

Q: How is marijuana used?
A: Most users roll loose marijuana into a cigarette (called a joint or a nail). The drug can also be smoked in a pipe. One well-known type of water pipe is the bong. Some users mix marijuana into foods or use it to brew a tea.

Lately, young people have a new method: They slice open cigars and replace the tobacco with marijuana, making what's called a blunt. When the blunt is smoked with a 40 oz. bottle of malt liquor, it is called a "B40."

Q: How many people smoke marijuana? At what age do children generally start?
A: A recent government survey tells us

- Over 70 million Americans over the age of 12 have tried marijuana at least once.
- About 10 million had used the drug in the month before the survey.
- More than 5 million Americans smoke marijuana at least once a week.
- Among teens aged 12 to 17, the average age of first trying marijuana was 13.5 years old.

A yearly survey of students in grades 8 through 12 shows that by 10th grade, nearly 16 percent are "current" users (that is, used within the past month). Among 12th-graders, nearly 40 percent have tried marijuana/hash at least once, and 19 percent were current users.

Other researchers have found that use of marijuana and other drugs usually peaks in the late teens and early twenties, then goes down in later years.

> Fact: Research shows that nearly 40 percent of teenagers try marijuana before they graduate high school.

Q: How can I tell if my child has been using marijuana?
A: There are some signs you might be able to see. If someone is high on marijuana, he or she might

- seem dizzy and have trouble walking;
- seem silly and giggly for no reason;
- have very red, bloodshot eyes; and
- have a hard time remembering things that just happened.

When the early effects fade, over a few hours, the user can become very sleepy.

Parents should be aware of changes in their child's behavior, although this may be difficult with teenagers. Parents should look for withdrawal, depression, fatigue, carelessness with grooming, hostility, and deteriorating relationships with family members and friends. In addition, changes in academic performance, increased absenteeism or truancy, lost interest in sports or other favorite activities, and changes in eating or sleeping habits could be related to drug use. However, these signs may also indicate problems other than use of drugs.

In addition, parents should be aware of

- signs of drugs and drug paraphernalia, including pipes and rolling papers
- odor on clothes and in the bedroom
- use of incense and other deodorizers
- use of eye drops
- clothing, posters, jewelry, etc., promoting drug use

Q: Why do young people use marijuana?
A: Children and young teens start using marijuana for many reasons. Curiosity and the desire to fit into a social group are common reasons. Certainly, youngsters who have already begun to smoke cigarettes and/or use alcohol are at high risk for marijuana use.

Also, research suggests that the use of alcohol and drugs by other family members plays a strong role in whether children start using drugs. Parents, grandparents, and older brothers and sisters in the home are models for children to follow.

Some young people who take drugs do not get along with their parents. Some have a network of friends who use drugs and urge them to do the same (peer pressure). All aspects of a child's environment—home, school, neighborhood—help to determine whether the child will try drugs.

Children who become more heavily involved with marijuana can become dependent and that is their prime reason for using the drug. Others mention psychological coping as a reason for their use—to deal with anxiety, anger, depression, boredom, and so forth. But marijuana use is not an effective method for coping with life's problems, and staying high can be a way of simply not dealing with the problems and challenges of growing up.

Q: Does using marijuana lead to other drugs?
A: Long-term studies of high school students and their patterns of drug use show that very few young people use other illegal drugs without first trying marijuana. Using marijuana puts children and teens in contact with people who are users and sellers of other drugs. So there is more of a chance for a marijuana user to be exposed to and urged to try more drugs. However, most marijuana users do not go on to use other illegal drugs.

Q: What are the effects of marijuana?
A: The effects of marijuana on each person depend on the

- type of cannabis and how much THC it contains;
- way the drug is taken (by smoking or eating);
- experience and expectations of the user;
- setting where the drug is used; and
- whether drinking or other drug use is also going on.

Some people feel nothing at all when they first try marijuana. Others may feel high (intoxicated and/or euphoric).

It's common for marijuana users to become engrossed with ordinary sights, sounds, or tastes, and trivial events may seem extremely interesting or funny. Time seems to pass very slowly, so minutes feel like hours. Sometimes the drug causes users to feel thirsty and very hungry—an effect called "the munchies."

Q: What happens after a person smokes marijuana?
A: Within a few minutes of inhaling marijuana smoke, the user will likely feel, along with intoxication, a dry mouth, rapid heartbeat, some loss of coordination and poor sense of balance, and decreased reaction time. Blood vessels in the eye expand, so the user's eyes look red.

For some people, marijuana raises blood pressure slightly and can double the normal heart rate. This effect can be greater when other drugs are mixed with the marijuana; but users do not always know when that happens.

As the immediate effects fade, usually after 2 to 3 hours, the user may become sleepy.

Q: How long does marijuana stay in the user's body?
A: THC in marijuana is strongly absorbed by fatty tissues in various organs. Generally, traces (metabolites) of THC can be detected by standard urine testing methods several days after a smoking session. However, in heavy chronic users, traces can sometimes be detected for weeks after they have stopped using marijuana.

Q: Can a user have a bad reaction?
A: Yes. Some users, especially someone new to the drug or in a strange setting, may suffer acute anxiety and have paranoid thoughts. This is more likely to happen with high doses of THC. These scary feelings will fade as the drug's effects wear off.

In rare cases, a user who has taken a very high dose of the drug can have severe psychotic symptoms and need emergency medical treatment.

Other kinds of bad reactions can occur when marijuana is mixed with other drugs, such as PCP or cocaine.

> Fact: Marijuana has adverse effects on many of the skills for driving a car. Driving while high leads to car accidents.

Q: How is marijuana harmful?
A: Marijuana can be harmful in a number of ways, through both immediate effects and damage to health over time.

Marijuana hinders the user's short-term memory (memory for recent events), and he or she may have trouble handling complex tasks. With the use of more potent varieties of marijuana, even simple tasks can be difficult.

Because of the drug's effects on perceptions and reaction time, users could be involved in auto crashes. Drug users also may become involved in risky sex. There is a strong link between drug use and unsafe sex and the spread of HIV, the virus that causes AIDS.

Under the influence of marijuana, students may find it hard to study and learn. Young athletes could find their performance is off; both timing and coordination are affected by THC.

Some of the more long-range effects of marijuana use are described later in this document.

Q: How does marijuana affect driving?
A: Marijuana has adverse effects on many of the skills needed for driving a car. These effects may include difficulty in judging distances and delayed reactions to sights and sounds that drivers need to notice.

There are data showing that marijuana plays a role in crashes. When users combine marijuana with alcohol, as they often do, the hazards of driving can be more severe than with either drug alone.

A study of patients in a shock-trauma unit who had been in traffic accidents revealed that 15 percent of those who had been driving a car or motorcycle had been smoking marijuana, and another 17 percent had both THC and alcohol in their blood.

In Memphis, Tennessee, researchers found that, of 150 reckless drivers who were tested for drugs at the arrest scene, 33 percent showed signs of marijuana use, and 12 percent tested positive for both marijuana and cocaine.

> Fact: Marijuana users may have many of the same respiratory problems that tobacco smokers have, such as chronic bronchitis and inflamed sinuses.

Q: What are the long-term effects of marijuana?
A: While all of the long-term effects of marijuana use are not yet known, there are studies showing serious health concerns. For example, a group of scientists in California examined the health status of 450 daily smokers of marijuana but not tobacco. They found that the marijuana smokers had more sick days and more doctor visits for respiratory problems and other types of illness than did a similar group who did not smoke either substance.

Findings so far show that the regular use of marijuana or THC may play a role in cancer and problems in the respiratory, immune, and reproductive systems.

Cancer

It is hard to find out whether marijuana alone causes cancer because many people who smoke marijuana also smoke cigarettes and use other drugs. Marijuana smoke contains some of the same cancer-causing compounds as tobacco, sometimes in higher concentrations. Studies show that someone who smokes five joints per week may be taking in as many cancer-causing chemicals as someone who smokes a full pack of cigarettes every day.

Tobacco smoke and marijuana smoke may work together to change the tissues lining the respiratory tract. Marijuana smoking could contribute to early development of head and neck cancer in some people.

Reproductive System

Heavy marijuana use can affect hormones in both males and females, so it can affect sexual characteristics and reproductive function. Heavy doses of the drug may delay the onset of puberty in young men. Marijuana also can have adverse effects on sperm production.

Among women, regular marijuana use can disrupt the normal monthly menstrual cycle and inhibit the discharge of eggs from the ovaries (ovulation).

Immune System

The immune system protects the body from many agents that cause disease. It is not certain whether marijuana damages the immune system of people. But both animal and human studies have shown that marijuana impairs the ability of T-cells in the lungs' immune defense system to fight off some infections. People with HIV and others whose immune system is impaired should avoid marijuana use.

Respiratory system

Someone who smokes marijuana regularly may have many of the same respiratory problems that tobacco smokers have. They have symptoms of daily cough and phlegm (chronic bronchitis) and more frequent chest colds. Continuing marijuana smoking can lead to abnormal function of the lungs and airways. Scientists have found signs of lung tissue injured or destroyed by marijuana smoke.

Q: What about pregnancy: Will smoking marijuana hurt the baby?
A: Doctors advise pregnant women not to use any drugs because they might harm the growing fetus.

Some scientific studies have found that babies born to marijuana users were shorter, weighed less, and had smaller head sizes than those born to mothers who did not use the drug. Smaller babies are more likely to develop health problems. Other scientists have found effects of marijuana that resemble the features of fetal alcohol syndrome. There are also research findings that show nervous system problems in children of mothers who smoked marijuana.

Researchers are not certain whether a newborn baby's health problems, if they are caused by marijuana, will continue as the child grows.

Q: What happens if a nursing mother uses marijuana?
A: When a nursing mother uses marijuana, some of the THC is passed to the baby in her breast milk. This is a matter for concern, since the THC in the mother's milk is much more concentrated than that in the mother's blood. One study has shown that the use of marijuana by a mother during the first month of breastfeeding can impair the infant's motor development (control of muscle movement).

> Fact: Marijuana smoking affects the brain and leads to impaired short-term memory, perception, judgment and motor skills.

Q: How does marijuana affect the brain?
A: THC disrupts the nerve cells in the part of the brain where memories are formed. This makes it hard for the user to recall recent events (such as what happened a few minutes ago), and so it is hard to learn while high. A working short-term memory is required for learning and performing tasks that call for more than one or two steps.

Some studies show that when people have smoked large amounts of marijuana for many years, the drug takes its toll on mental functions. Among a group of long-time heavy marijuana users in Costa Rica, researchers found that the people had great trouble when asked to recall a short list of words (a standard test of memory). People in that study group also found it very hard to focus their attention on the tests given to them.

It may be that marijuana kills some brain cells. In laboratory research, some scientists found that high doses of THC given to young rats caused a loss of brain cells such as that seen with aging. At 11 or 12 months of age (about half their normal life span), the rats' brains looked like those of animals in old age.

Researchers are still learning about the many ways that marijuana could affect the brain.

Q: Can the drug cause mental illness?
A: Scientists do not yet know how the use of marijuana relates to mental illness. Some researchers in Sweden report that regular, long-term intake of THC (from cannabis) can increase the risk of developing certain mental diseases, such as schizophrenia.

Still others maintain that regular marijuana use can lead to chronic anxiety, personality disturbances, and depression.

Q: Do marijuana users lose their motivation?
A: Some frequent, long-term marijuana users show signs of a lack of motivation (amotivational syndrome). Their problems include not caring about what happens in their lives; no desire to work regularly; fatigue; and lack of concern about how they look. As a result of these symptoms, most users tend to perform poorly in school or at work. Scientists are still studying these problems.

Q: Can a person become addicted to marijuana?
A: Yes. While not everyone who uses marijuana becomes addicted, when a user begins to feel that he or she needs to take the drug to feel well, that person is said to be dependent on the drug or addicted to it. In 1993, over 100,000 people entering drug treatment programs reported marijuana as their primary drug of abuse, showing they need help to stop using.

Some heavy users of marijuana show signs of dependence because when they do not use the drug, they develop withdrawal symptoms. Some subjects in an experiment on marijuana withdrawal had such symptoms as restlessness, loss of appetite, trouble with sleeping, weight loss, and shaky hands.

Q: What is "tolerance" for marijuana?
A: "Tolerance" means that the user needs increasingly larger doses of the drug to get the same desired results that he or she previously got from smaller amounts. Some frequent, heavy users of marijuana may develop tolerance for it.

Q: Are there treatments to help marijuana users?

A: Up until a few years ago, it was hard to find treatment programs specifically for marijuana users. Treatments for marijuana dependence were much the same as therapies for other drug abuse problems. These include detoxification, behavioral therapies, and regular attendance at meetings of support groups, such as Narcotics Anonymous.

Recently, researchers have been testing different ways to attract marijuana users to treatment and help them abstain from drug use. There are currently no medications for treating marijuana dependence. Treatment programs focus on counseling and group support systems. From these studies, drug treatment professionals are learning what characteristics of users are predictors of success in treatment and which approaches to treatment can be most helpful.

Further progress in treatment to help marijuana users includes a number of programs set up to help adolescents in particular. Some of these programs are in university research centers, where most of the young clients report marijuana as their drug of choice. Others are in independent adolescent treatment facilities. Family physicians are also a good source for information and help in dealing with adolescent marijuana problems.

Q: Can marijuana be used as medicine?

A: No. Under U.S. law since 1970, marijuana is a Schedule I controlled substance. This means that the drug, at least in its smoked form, has no commonly accepted medical use in this country.

In considering possible medical uses of marijuana, it is important to distinguish between whole marijuana and pure THC or other specific chemicals derived from cannabis. Whole marijuana contains hundreds of chemicals, some of which are clearly harmful to health.

THC, manufactured into a pill that is taken by mouth, not smoked, can be used for treating the nausea and vomiting that go along with certain cancer treatments. Another chemical related to THC (nabilone) has also been approved by the Food and Drug Administration for treating cancer patients who suffer nausea. The oral THC is also used to help AIDS patients eat more to keep up their weight.

Scientists are studying whether THC and related chemicals in marijuana (called cannabinoids) may have other medical uses. Some think that these chemicals could be useful for treating severe pain. But further research is needed before such compounds can be recommended for treatment of medical problems.

Q: How can I prevent my child from getting involved with marijuana?

A: There is no magic bullet for preventing teenage drug use. But parents can be influential by talking to their children about the dangers in using marijuana and other drugs, and remain actively engaged in their children's lives. Even after teenage children enter high school, parents can stay involved in schoolwork, recreation, and social activities with their children's friends. Research shows that appropriate parental monitoring can reduce future drug use, even among those adolescents who may be prone to marijuana use, such as those who are rebellious, cannot control their emotions, and experience internal distress.

Talking to Your Children About Marijuana

As this booklet has shown, marijuana is clearly a dangerous drug which poses a particular threat to the health and well-being of children and adolescents at a critical point in their lives—when they are growing, learning, maturing, and laying the foundation for their adult years. As a parent, your children look to you for help and guidance in working out problems and in making decisions, including the decision not to use drugs. As a role model, your decision to not use marijuana and other illegal drugs will reinforce your message to your children.

There are numerous resources, many right in your own community, to obtain information so that you can talk to your children about drugs. To find these, you can consult your local library, school, or community service organization.

The National Clearinghouse for Alcohol and Drug Information (NCADI) offers an extensive collection of publications, videotapes, and educational materials to help parents talk to their children about drug use. For more information on marijuana and other drugs, contact

National Clearinghouse on Alcohol and Drug Information,
PO Box 2345,
Rockville, MD 20847
(800) 729-6686

Resources

Fried, P.A., Prenatal exposure to tobacco and marijuana: effects during pregnancy, infancy, and early childhood. *Clinical Obstetrics and Gynecology* 36:319-337, 1993.

Growing Up Drug Free: A Parent's Guide to Prevention, U.S. Department of Education, Washington, DC, NCADI Publication No. PHD533 (also in Spanish PHD541), 1993.

Hermes, W.J., and Galperin, A. *The Encyclopedia of Psychoactive Drugs: Marijuana, Its Effects on Mind and Body,* Chelsea House Publishers, 1992.

Jaffe, J.H., Drug abuse and addiction. In: Gilman, A.G.; Rall, T.W.; Nies, A.S.; Taylor, P., eds. *The Pharmacological Bases of Therapeutics,* 8th ed. New York: Macmillan, 522-573, 1990.

Johnston, L.D.; O'Malley, P.M.; and Bachman, J.G. *National Survey Results on Drug Use From the Monitoring the Future Study, 1975-1993* (Vol. I and II). National Institute on Drug Abuse. Washington, DC: BKD 149 and BKD 150, 1994.

Keeping Youth Drug Free: A Guide for Parents, Grandparents, ...and other Caregivers, Center for Substance Abuse Prevention, U.S. Department of Health and Human Services, In Press, 1995.

Marijuana: Facts for Teens, National Institute on Drug Abuse, U.S. Department of Health and Human Services, NCADI Publication No. PHD713, 1995.

Marijuana: Facts Parents Need to Know, National Institute on Drug Abuse, U.S. Department of Health and Human Services, NCADI Publication No. PHD712, 1995.

Marijuana: What Can Parents Do? Videotape, National Institute on Drug Abuse, U.S. Department of Health and Human Services, NCADI Stock No. VHS82, 1995. Cost: $8.50

O'Brien, C.P., Drug Abuse and Dependence. In: Syngaarden, J.B., et al. (eds.) *Cecil Textbook of Medicine.* 19th ed. Philadelphia: W.B. Saunders Co., 1992.

Schwartz, R.H.; Gruenewald, P.J.; Klitzner, M.; and Fedio, P. Short-term memory impairment in cannabis-dependent adolescents. *American J. of Diseases of the Child* 143:1214-1219, 1989.

Tashkin, D.P.; Coulson, A.H.; Clark, V.A.; et al. Respiratory system and lung function in habitual, heavy smokers of marijuana alone, smokers of marijuana and tobacco, smokers of tobacco alone, and nonsmokers. *Am Rev Respir Dis* 135:209-216, 1987.

Tips for Parents

- Be a good listener
- Give clear no-use messages about drugs and alcohol
- Help your child deal with peer pressure to use drugs
- Get to know your child's friends and parents
- Monitor your child's whereabouts
- Supervise teen activities
- Maintain an open and honest dialogue with your child

■ Document Source:
U.S. Department of Health and Human Services, Public Health Service
National Institutes of Health
National Institute on Drug Abuse
NIH Publication No. 95-4036
Printed 1995

MEDICATIONS CONTAINING ASPIRIN (ACETYLSALICYLATE) AND ASPIRIN-LIKE PRODUCTS

Epidemiologic research has shown an association between the development of Reye's Syndrome and the use of aspirin-type products for treating the symptoms of influenza-like illnesses, chicken pox, and colds. The National Reye's Syndrome Foundation, the U.S. Surgeon General, the Food and Drug Administration, and the Centers for Disease Control recommend that aspirin and combination products containing aspirin not be given to children or teenagers who are suffering from one of these illnesses. The following pages display products which contain aspirin or salicylate compounds. This is **NOT** a complete list. Some medication labels may use the words acetylsalicylate, acetylsalicylic acid, salicylsalicylic, salicylamide, phenyl salicylate, etc., instead of the word aspirin. While there is no data as to whether other forms of salicylate other than aspirin may be associated with the development of Reye's Syndrome and until further research has answered this question, we recommend that products listing any of these substances not be taken by individuals during an episode of a viral illness. Products may be reformulated from time to time to add or remove ingredients. Always ask your doctor or pharmacist before taking any medication and be sure to **NEVER** exceed the recommended dosage.

Non-prescription Products

Alka-Seltzer Effervescent Antacid Regular, Extra Strength, & Lemon Lime Pain Reliever (Miles)

Alka-Seltzer Plus Cold Medicine, Cold & Cough Medicine, and Night-Time Cold Medicine (Miles)
Alka-Seltzer Plus Sinus Medicine (Miles)
Anacin Tablets & Caplets (Whitehall)
Arthritis Foundation Safety Coated Aspirin Tablets (McNeil)
Ascriptin Arthritis Pain, Maximum Strength, and Regular Strength Tablets (CIBA)
Aspirin Tablets (Warner Chilcott)
Backache Caplets (Bristol-Myers)
Bayer Aspirin Regimen Adult Low Strength 81 mg Tablets, Regular Strength 325 mg Caplets, and Arthritis Pain Formula (Bayer)
Bayer Children's Chewable Aspirin (Bayer)
Bayer Extended-Release and Extra Strength 8-Hour Aspirin (Bayer)
Bayer Extra Strength, PM, and Plus Aspirin Tablets & Caplets (Bayer)
Bayer Genuine Aspirin Tablets & Caplets (Bayer)
Bayer Select Backache Pain Relief Formula (Bayer)
BC Cold Powder, Multi-Symptom Formula and Non-Drowsy Formula (Block)
Buffaprin (Buffington)
Buffasal (Dover)
Bufferin Analgesic, Arthritis Strength, and Extra Strength Tablets & Caplets (Bristol-Myers)
Buffinol (Otis Clapp)
Cama Arthritis Pain Reliever (Sandoz)
Doan's Regular, Extra Strength, and PM (CIBA)
Ecotrin Enteric Coated Aspirin Regular, Maximum Strength, and Adult Low Strength Tablets & Caplets (SK Beecham)
Empirin Aspirin Tablets (Warner Wellcome)
Excedrin Extra-Strength Analgesic Tablets & Caplets (Bristol-Myers)
Genprin (Goldline)
Goody's Extra Strength (Goody's)
Goody's Headache Powders (Goody's)
Halfprin (Kramer)
Healthprin Aspirin (Smart)
Mobigesic Tablets (Ascher)
Norwich Aspirin (Chattem)
Pepto-Bismol Regular & Maximum Strength Liquid, Tablets, & Caplets (Procter & Gamble)
St. Joseph Adult Chewable Aspirin (Schering-Plough)
Ursinus Inlay-Tabs (Sandoz)
Vanquish Analgesic Caplets (Miles)

Prescription Products

Acuprin 81 Adult Low Dose Aspirin (Richwood)
Ascol Delayed-Release Tablets (Procter & Gamble)
Aspirin 15 gr Delayed Release Tablets (Duramed)
Axotal (Savage)
Azdone Tablets (Central)
Carisoprodol and Aspirin Tablets (Par)
Damason-P (Mason)
Darvon Compound-65 (Lilly)
Disalcid Capsules & Tablets (3M)
Easprin (Parke-Davis)
Empirin with Codeine Tablets (Burroughs Wellcome)

Equagesic Tablets (Wyeth-Ayerst)
Fiorinal Capsules & Tablets (Sandoz)
Fiorinal with Codeine Capsules (Sandoz)
Gelpirin Tablets (Alra)
Lortab ASA Tablets (Whitby)
Magsal Tablets (U.S.)
Methocarbamol and Aspirin Tablets (Robins)
Mono-Gesic Tablets (Central)
Norgesic Forte Tablets (3M)
Norgesic Tablets (3M)
PC-CAP Propoxyphene Hydrochloride Compound, USP (Alra)
Panasal 5/500 Tablets (ECR)
Pentasa (Marion Merrell Dow)
Percodan Tablets (DuPont)
Prosed/DS (Star)
Quadrinal Tablets (Knoll)
Robaxisal Tablets (Robins)
ROWASA Rectal Suppositories (Solvay)
ROWASA Rectal Suspension Enema (Solvay)
Roxiprin Tablets (Roxane)
Salflex Tablets (Carnrick)
Salsalate Tablets (Duramed)
Salsitab Tablets (Upsher-Smith)
Soma Compound Tablets (Wallace)
Soma Compound with Codeine Tablets (Wallace)
Synalgos-DC Capsules (Wyeth-Ayerst)
Talwin Compound (Sanofi Winthrop)
Tricosal Tablets (Duramed)
Trilisate Liquid & Tablets (Purdue Frederick)
Urised Tablets (PolyMedica)

For additional information, please contact

National Reye's Syndrome Foundation
426 N Lewis St, PO Box 829
Bryan, OH 43506
1-800-233-7393 or 1-419-636-2679
e-mail: reyessyn@bright.net
http://www.bright.net/~reyessyn

■ **Document Source:**
   National Reye's Syndrome Foundation
   426 N Lewis St, PO Box 829
   Bryan, OH 43506

See also: Fact Sheet: Reye's Syndrome (page 516); Reye's Syndrome: Because You Need to Know (page 528)

PREVENTING CHILDHOOD POISONING

by Audrey T. Hingley

Most people regard their home as a safe haven, a calming oasis in an often stormy world.

But home can be a dangerous place when it comes to accidental poisoning, especially accidental poisoning of children. One tablet of some medicines can wreak havoc in or kill a child.

Childhood poisonings caused by accidental overdoses of iron-containing supplements are the biggest concern of poison control experts, consumer protection groups, and health-care providers. Iron-containing supplements are the leading cause of pediatric poisoning deaths for children under six in the United States. According to the American Association of Poison Control Centers, from 1986 to 1994, 38 children between the ages of nine months and three years died from accidentally swallowing iron-containing products. The number of pills consumed by these children varied from as few as five to as many as 98.

FDA is taking steps to protect children from iron poisoning by proposing regulations that will make it harder for small children to gain access to high-potency iron products (30 milligrams of iron or more per tablet). FDA is also taking steps to ensure that health-care providers and consumers are alerted to the dangers associated with accidental overdoses of iron-containing products, including pediatric multivitamin supplements that contain iron.

Although iron poisoning is the biggest concern when it comes to childhood poisoning, there is also concern about other drugs.

"Over-the-counter diet pills have the potential to be lethal to children, as do OTC stimulants used to keep you awake and decongestant tablets," says George C. Rodgers, MD, PhD, medical director of the Kentucky Regional Poisoning Center. "Tofranil [imipramine], an antidepressant drug also used for childhood bedwetting, and Catapres [clonidine], a high blood pressure medicine, can be very hazardous because it takes very little to produce life-threatening problems in children. One tablet may do it.

"Antidepressant drugs have a high degree of toxicity," he continues. "They are cardiac and central nervous system toxins, and it doesn't take much of them to do harm, particularly in children. They are prescribed fairly ubiquitously. One of the things we look at when we get kids' poisonings is who had the medicine, and why."

Rodgers also urges extra caution when antidepressant drugs are prescribed for teenage patients who may have behavioral or emotional problems.

"Antidepressant drugs are commonly given to adolescents with behavioral problems, and often a month or two-month supply is prescribed. Teens should not be given more than a week's supply to begin with, and parents need to monitor their usage," he says.

The marketing of pediatric vitamins is also a cause of concern for Rodgers.

"Because they're marketed to look like candy or cartoon characters, it looks like candy and doesn't seem like medicine," he explains.

In addition, children frequently mimic the behavior of their parents. Children who watch their parents take pills may want to do it, too—with potentially fatal results.

Poison-Proofing Your Home

Poison-proofing your home is the key to preventing childhood poisonings. In the case of iron-containing pills or any medicine:

- Always close the container as soon as you've finished using it. Properly secure the child-resistant packaging, and put it away immediately in a place where children can't reach it.
- Keep pills in their original container.
- Keep iron-containing tablets, and all medicines, out of reach—and out of sight—of children.
- Never keep medicines on a countertop or bedside table.
- Follow medicine label directions carefully to avoid accidental overdoses or misdoses that could result in accidental poisoning.

For other substances, buy the least hazardous products that will serve your purposes. When buying art supplies, for example, look for products that are safe for children. For hazardous products such as gasoline, kerosene, and paint thinners that are often kept on hand indefinitely, buy only as much as you need and safely get rid of what you don't use. Never transfer these substances to other containers. People often use cups, soft-drink bottles, or milk cartons to store leftover paint thinner or turpentine. This is a bad idea because children associate cups and bottles with food and drink.

The kitchen and bathroom are the most likely unsafe areas. (Medicines should never be stored in the bathroom for another reason: a bathroom's warm, moist environment tends to cause changes or disintegration of the product in these rooms.) Any cabinet containing a potentially poisonous item should be locked.

"Bathrooms with medicines, kitchens with cleaning products, even cigarette butts left out, can be toxic to kids," Rodgers explains. "And remember that child-resistant caps are child-resistant, not childproof. The legal definition is that it takes greater than five minutes for 80 percent of 5-year-olds to get into it: that means 20 percent can get in in less time! Kids are inventive, and can often figure it out. And leftover liquor in glasses on the counter after parties? Don't do it!"

Alcohol can cause drunkenness as well as serious poisoning leading to seizures, coma, and even death in young children. Children are more sensitive to the toxic effects of alcohol than are adults, and it doesn't take much alcohol to produce such effects. Alcohol-laced products, such as some mouthwashes, aftershaves or colognes, can cause the same problems.

Garages and utility rooms should also be checked for potential poison hazards. Antifreeze, windshield washing fluid, and other products should be stored out of children's reach in a locked cabinet. Childproof safety latches can be purchased at your local hardware store.

In the living room or family room, know your plants' names and their poison potential. Although most houseplants are not poisonous, some are. To be on the safe side, keep houseplants out of the reach of young children. Although much has been made of problems with poinsettias (blamed for a death as early as 1919), recent studies indicate it is not as highly toxic as was once believed. Although ingesting it may cause some stomach irritation and burning in the mouth, it's unlikely to be fatal.

"Plants are mostly a problem for children, since it's a natural response for children to taste things. Few adults eat houseplants," Rodgers points out. "Plants have a high capacity for making you sick, but they are usually low risk for producing life-threatening symptoms." After poison-proofing your home, prepare for emergencies. Post the numbers of your regional poison control center (which can be found on the inside cover of the Yellow Pages or in the white pages of your phone directory) and your doctor by the phone. Keep syrup of ipecac on hand—safely locked away, of course. (See "Antidotes.") Never administer any antidote without first checking with your doctor or poison control center.

Lead Poisoning

Although lead levels in food and drink are the lowest in history, concern remains about lead leaching into food from ceramic ware. Improperly fired or formulated glazes on ceramic ware can allow lead to leach into food or drink.

Long recognized as a toxic substance, adverse health effects can result from exposure to lead over months or years.

After a California family suffered acute lead poisoning in 1969 from drinking orange juice stored in a pitcher bought in Mexico, FDA established "action levels" for lead in ceramic ware used to serve food. Over the years, these original action levels have been revised as research has shown that exposure to even small amounts of lead can be hazardous. The last revision for ceramic foodware was in 1991. On Jan. 12, 1994, FDA published a regulation for decorative ceramic ware not intended for food use, requiring a permanently affixed label on high-lead-leaching products.

"Most lead toxicity comes from multiple exposure and is a slow accumulation over time," says Robert Mueller, a nurse and poison information specialist at the Virginia Poison Center, headquartered at The Medical College of Virginia Hospitals in Richmond. "Refusing to eat, vomiting, convulsions, and malaise can all be symptoms of lead poisoning." Because lead poisoning occurs over time, such symptoms may not show up right away. A blood test is the surest way to determine that your child has not been exposed to significant amounts of lead.

"In general, if a consumer purchases ceramic ware in the US marketplace today, it meets the new action levels," says Julia Hewgley, public affairs specialist with FDA's Center for Food Safety and Applied Nutrition. "But if you travel abroad and buy ceramic ware, be aware that each country has its own safety regulations. Safety can be terribly variable depending on the type of quality control and whether the piece is made by a hobbyist." To guard against poisonings, Hewgley advises that ceramic ware not be used to store foods. Acidic foods—such as orange, tomato and other fruit juices, tomato sauces, vinegar, and wine—stored in improperly glazed containers are potentially the most dangerous. Frequently used products, like cups or pitchers, are also potentially dangerous, especially when used to hold hot, acidic foods.

"Stop using any item if the glaze shows a dusty or chalky gray residue after washing. Limit your use of antique or collectible housewares for food and beverages," she says.

"Buy one of the quick lead tests available at hardware stores and do a screening on inherited pieces."

Iron Poisoning

Iron-containing products remain the biggest problem by far when it comes to childhood poisoning. In October 1994, FDA proposed regulations for unit-dose packaging requirements for iron-containing products with 30 milligrams or more of iron per dosage unit. The agency also proposed requiring warning labels about the adverse effects of high-dose iron ingestion by children for all iron-containing products taken in solid oral dosage forms. Because of the time and effort needed to open unit-dose products, FDA believes unit-dose packaging will discourage a youngster, or at least limit the number of tablets a child would swallow, reducing the potential for serious illness or death.

FDA's proposed requirements would be in addition to existing U.S. Consumer Product Safety Commission regulations, which require child-resistant packaging for most iron-containing products. FDA issued a supplementary proposed rule in February 1995. At press time, a final rule regarding iron-containing products was expected soon.

Iron is an essential nutrient sometimes lacking in people's diets, which is why iron is often recommended for people with conditions such as iron-deficiency anemia. Taken as indicated, iron is safe. But when tablets are taken beyond the proper dose in a short period, especially by toddlers or infants, serious injury or death may result.

Children poisoned with iron face immediate and long-term problems. Within minutes or hours of swallowing iron tablets, nausea, vomiting, diarrhea, and gastrointestinal bleeding can occur. These problems can progress to shock, coma, seizures, and death. Even if a child appears to have no symptoms after accidentally swallowing iron, or appears to be recovering, medical evaluation should still be sought since successful treatment is difficult once iron is absorbed from the small intestine into the bloodstream. And children who survive iron poisoning can experience other problems, such as gastrointestinal obstruction and liver damage, up to four weeks after the ingested poisoning.

FDA regulates iron-containing products as either drugs or foods, depending on the product formulation and on intended use, as defined by labeling and other information sources. Iron products are regulated as drugs if they are intended to affect the structure or function of the body, or are used in the diagnosis, cure, treatment, or prevention of disease and are listed in the U.S. Pharmacopoeia. All other products are regulated as foods.

Some iron-containing products have been regulated as prescription drugs because they included pharmacologic doses of folic acid and usually were prescribed to meet high nutritional requirements during pregnancy.

Between June 1992 and January 1993, five toddlers died after eating iron supplement tablets, according to the National Centers for Disease Control and Prevention's Morbidity and Mortality Weekly Report of Feb. 19, 1993. All tablets involved in the reported deaths were prenatal iron supplements. The incidents occurred in a variety of ways: Children ate tablets from uncapped or loosely capped bottles, swallowed tablets found spilled on the floor, and, in one case, a 2-year-old fed an 11-month-old sibling tablets from a box found on the floor.

Iron is always included in prenatal vitamins prescribed for pregnant women, and is sometimes included in multivitamin formulas. Often available without prescription, iron supplements can be found in grocery stores, drugstores, and health food stores in a wide variety of potencies, ranging from 18 milligrams (mg) to 150 mg per pill. For a small child, as little as 600 mg of iron can be fatal.

Because iron supplements are typically brightly colored and may look like candy, they are particularly attractive to children. In 1993, the Nonprescription Drug Manufacturers Association (NDMA), which manufactures about 95 percent of nonprescription OTC medicines available to Americans today, adopted formulation provisions for iron products containing 30 mg or more of elemental iron per solid dosage form. These provisions also stipulated that such products would not be made with sweet coatings. That same year, NDMA manufacturers also independently agreed to develop new voluntary warning labels for these products. The voluntary labels read: "Warning: Close tightly and keep out of reach of children. Contains iron, which can be harmful or fatal to children in large doses. In case of accidental overdose, seek professional assistance or contact a poison control center immediately."

Signs of Poisoning

How can you tell if your child has ingested something poisonous? "Most poisons, with the exception of lead, work fairly quickly. A key is when the child was otherwise well and in a space of hours develops unusual symptoms: They can't follow you with their eyes, they're sleepy before it's their nap time, their eyes go around in circles. Any unusual or new symptoms should make you think of poisoning as a possibility," Rodgers advises. "Poisonings typically affect the stomach and central nervous system. If a child suddenly throws up, that can be more difficult to diagnose."

Other signs of poison ingestion can be burns around the lips or mouth, stains of the substance around the child's mouth, or the smell of a child's breath. Suspect a possible poisoning if you find an opened or spilled bottle of pills.

If you suspect poisoning, remain calm. For medicines, call the nearest poison control center or your physician. For household chemical ingestion, follow first-aid instructions on the label, and then call the poison control center or your doctor. When you call, tell them your child's age, height and weight, existing health conditions, as much as you know about the substance involved, the exposure route (swallowed? inhaled? splashed in the eyes?), and if your child has vomited. If you know what substance the child has ingested, take the remaining solution or bottle with you to the phone when you call. Follow the instructions of the poison control center precisely.

Progress Against Poisonings

The nation's first poison control center opened in Chicago in 1953, after a study of accidental deaths in childhood reported a large number were due to poisoning. Since that time, a combination of public education, the use of child-resistant caps, help through poison control centers, and increased sophistication in medical care have lowered overall death rates.

Often, calling a poison center simply reassures parents that the product ingested is not poisonous. In other cases, following phone instructions prevents an emergency room trip.

Children are not the only victims of accidental poisonings: Older people in particular are at risk because they generally take more medicines, may have problems reading labels correctly, or may take a friend's or spouse's medicine.

In June 1995, the U.S. Consumer Product Safety Commission voted unanimously to require that child-resistant caps be made so adults—especially senior citizens—will have a less frustrating time getting them off. Because many adults who had trouble with child-resistant caps left them off, or transferred their contents to less secure packaging that endangers children, officials say the new caps will be safer for children.

"Childhood poisoning will always be a focus, because children are so vulnerable, especially children under age five," says Ken Giles, public affairs spokesman for the Consumer Product Safety Commission. "The first two or three years of a child's life are the highest-risk time for all kinds of injuries, so there is a special need to educate new parents. It's essential we keep raising these safety messages that medicines and chemicals can be poisonous."

Protect Yourself Against Tampering

With FDA's new proposed regulations regarding packaging of high-dose, iron-containing pills in mind, it's important to remember that no packaging or warnings can protect without your involvement. Nonprescription OTC drugs sold in the United States are among the most safely packaged consumer products in the world, but "child-resistant" and "tamper-resistant" do not mean "childproof" and "tamperproof."

FDA adopted "tamper-resistant" packaging requirements after seven people in the Chicago area died from taking cyanide-laced Extra-Strength Tylenol capsules in 1982. Although the product met all FDA requirements at the time, it wasn't designed so tampering would leave visible evidence. FDA swiftly enacted new regulations requiring most OTC drug products to be packaged in "tamper-resistant" packaging, defined as "packaging having an indicator or barrier to entry that could reasonably be expected to provide visible evidence that tampering had occurred," and required OTC product labeling to alert consumers to tamper-resistant packaging. In 1989, FDA regulations were amended to require two-piece hard gelatin capsules to be packaged using at least two tamper-resistant features unless sealed with a tamper-resistant technology.

"Consumer vigilance is part of the equation," says Lana Ragazinsky, consumer safety officer with FDA's Center for Drug Evaluation and Research, Division of Drug Quality Evaluation, Office of Compliance. "The consumer is being led into a false sense of security because they see 'tamper-resistant'...'tamper evident' means you, the consumer, need to look for evidence of tampering."

FDA has proposed changing the term "tamper-resistant" to "tamper-evident" to underscore the fact that no package design is tamperproof. The most important tool to detect tampering is you! Here are a few tips to help protect against tampering:

- Read the label. OTC medicines with tamper-evident packages tell you what seals and features to look for.
- Inspect the outer packaging before you buy.
- Inspect the medicine when you open the package, and look again before you take it. If it looks suspicious: be suspicious.
- Look for capsules or tablets different in any way from others in the package.
- Don't use any medicine from a package with cuts, tears, slices, or other imperfections.
- Never take medicine in the dark. Read the label and look at the medicine every time you take a dose.

Antidotes

If you suspect childhood poisoning, call the nearest poison control center or your physician first, and follow their instructions precisely.

To induce vomiting in case of accidental poisoning, experts recommend keeping on hand syrup of ipecac—safely stored away from children, of course! Syrup of ipecac induces vomiting, thus ridding the body of the swallowed poison. It usually works within a half-hour of ingestion.

Some medical experts also recommend that parents keep activated charcoal on hand as well: You may have to ask your druggist for it, because it may not be on store shelves. Although some poison control experts recommend having activated charcoal on hand, there is a difference of opinion on its use by consumers. The U.S. Consumer Product Safety Commission, for example, does not recommend that consumers use activated charcoal because it is less palatable to young children.

Activated charcoal (or charcoal treated with substances that increase its absorption abilities) absorbs poison, preventing it from spreading throughout the body. One advantage of activated charcoal is that it can be effective for a considerable time after the poison is swallowed. But activated charcoal should never be used at the same time you administer syrup of ipecac: The charcoal will absorb the ipecac.

For children ages one to 12, give one tablespoon of syrup of ipecac followed by one or two glasses of water. Children ages 12 and over should get two tablespoons, followed by one or two glasses of water.

Activated charcoal is usually found in drugstores in liquid form in 30-gram doses. For children under five, give one gram per every two pounds of body weight. Older children and adults may require much higher doses.

Both antidotes should only be used on conscious poison victims; an unconscious victim should always be treated by professionals.

"Remember to call your local poison control center first before giving your child any at-home antidote," says Robert

Mueller, poison information specialist at the Virginia Poison Center in Richmond, VA.

■ **Document Source:**
U.S. Department of Health and Human Services, Public Health Service
Food and Drug Administration
FDA Consumer
March 1996

REYE'S SYNDROME: BECAUSE YOU NEED TO KNOW

What is Reye's Syndrome?

Reye's Syndrome is a disease which affects all organs of the body, but **most lethally the liver and the brain.**

Is Reye's Syndrome a common disease?

The number of recognized cases of Reye's Syndrome has decreased in recent years as a result of greater awareness. There is a need to be informed; no need for panic. Statistical data remains uncertain and the exact incidence of the disease are not known since:

1) Reye's Syndrome can be, and is, **misdiagnosed.**
2) It is not, by law, a reportable disease in many states.
3) Cases are not always reported to health officials.

What age groups are affected?

No age group is immune; however, the disease usually affects children from infancy to about 19 years of age.

The disease strikes all races. Both sexes are affected equally. In black children less than one year of age, the incidence is higher.

The largest number of **reported** cases have occurred in the 10-14 year-old age group. Increasing numbers of cases have been reported in adolescents. This may be due to the fact that they are unaware of the Reye's/aspirin link before taking over-the-counter medicines.

How does a person get Reye's Syndrome?

It is defined as a two-phase illness because it is almost always associated with a previous viral infection, such as influenza or chicken pox. Scientists do know that Reye's Syndrome is **not contagious and the cause is unknown.** Clusters of cases have occurred in some areas.

Reye's Syndrome is often misdiagnosed as encephalitis, meningitis, diabetes, drug overdose, poisoning, Sudden Infant Death Syndrome or psychiatric illness.

Is Reye's Syndrome seasonal?

It appears with greatest frequency during January, February and March *when influenza is most common.* Cases have been reported in **every** month of the year.

An epidemic of flu or chicken pox is commonly followed by an increase in the number of cases of Reye's Syndrome.

Why is early diagnosis so important?

A person's life can depend on early diagnosis.

Statistics indicate an excellent chance of recovery when Reye's Syndrome is diagnosed and treated **in its earliest stages.**

The later the diagnosis and treatment, the more severely reduced are chances for successful recovery and survival.

What does Reye's Syndrome do to the body?

Abnormal accumulations of fat develop in the liver and other organs of the body, along with a severe increase of pressure in the brain.

> **Unless diagnosed and treated successfully, death is common often within a few days.**

What is the role of aspirin?

Epidemiologic research has shown an association between the development of Reye's Syndrome and the use of aspirin (a salicylate) for treating the symptoms of influenza-like illnesses, chicken pox and colds. The U.S. Surgeon General, the Food and Drug Administration and the Centers for Disease Control recommend that aspirin and combination products containing aspirin not be given to children under 19 years of age during episodes of fever-causing illnesses. *Acetylsalicylate is another word for aspirin; some drug labels may use the words acetylsalicylate, acetylsalicylic acid, salicylic acid, or salicylate instead of the word aspirin.* Always ask your doctor or pharmacist before taking any medication.

Is it possible to develop Reye's Syndrome without taking aspirin?

Yes! Reye's Syndrome can develop without taking aspirin. However, the chances of developing Reye's Syndrome can be reduced by not giving aspirin to children and teenagers for relief of discomfort or fever without first consulting a physician for each specific use.

What are the early stages of Reye's Syndrome?

Stage I

*   Persistent or continuous vomiting
*   Signs of brain dysfunction:

Listlessness
Loss of pep and energy
Drowsiness

Stage II

- Personality changes:
    Irritability
    Aggressive behavior
- Disorientation:
    Confusion
    Irrational behavior
- Delirium, convulsions

Reye's Syndrome should be suspected in a person if this pattern of symptoms appear during or, most commonly, after a viral illness such as "flu" or chicken pox. Fever is not usually present. Many diseases have symptoms in common. Physicians and medical staff in emergency rooms who have not had experience in treating Reye's Syndrome may misdiagnose the disease. The symptoms of Reye's Syndrome in infants do not follow a typical pattern. For example, vomiting does not always occur.

Under these circumstances, two liver function tests should be done immediately:

- SGOT(SAT)
- SGPT(ACT)

The results of these tests are commonly available within two to three hours.

Abnormal SGOT and SGPT strongly suggest a diagnosis of Reye's Syndrome. **Immediate** further diagnostic testing will give a definite diagnosis.

How is Reye's Syndrome treated?

Reye's Syndrome is a medical emergency and time is of the utmost importance. The chance of recovery is greatly increased when it is treated in its earliest stages. There is to date no cure for the disease. **Successful management** depends on early diagnosis. Therapy is primarily directed to protect the brain against irreversible damage by reducing the brain swelling.

People with Reye's Syndrome **require** the services of an intensive care unit and physicians and nurses **experienced** in the treatment of the disease. A person with Reye's Syndrome should be transferred to a **known** treatment center. If this is not possible, immediate phone consultation with a treatment center should be made.

Are there lasting effects?

Recovery is related to the severity of the swelling of the brain. Some people recover completely. Others may sustain brain damage, extending from slight to severe brain dysfunction. Those who progress rapidly through the stages and lapse into a coma have a poorer prognosis than those with a less severe disease. All people surviving Reye's Syndrome should be evaluated using quantitative psychological and neuropsychological test measures.

Are there referral resources for survivors left with disabilities?

The National Reye's Syndrome Foundation has affiliates in almost every state. Other resources include Crippled Children's Services, State Developmental Disabilities Agencies, child development clinics, local school systems and health departments. Parents should familiarize themselves with Public Law 94-142, available through public libraries.

What needs to be done to help prevent Reye's Syndrome?

Research is needed to

- Find the cause of Reye's Syndrome
- Improve treatment methods
- Develop improved means for early detection

The National Reye's Syndrome Foundation was formed in 1974. It is the **only** citizen group to generate a concerted organized lay movement to eradicate the disease and provide funds for research in the cause, treatment, cure and prevention of Reye's Syndrome.

An audio-visual slide/tape on Reye's Syndrome is available for the general public. Two additional programs for in-service hospital programs are technical in nature and are designed for members of the health profession. A VHS documentary is also available for the general public. Inquiries regarding their use should be directed to the Bryan office.

The Foundation needs your help. Funds for our work are also needed and can be sent to your local affiliate or the National Reye's Syndrome Foundation, PO Box 829, Bryan, OH 43506.

Remember . . .

- Reye's Syndrome usually appears soon after a flu-like infection or chicken pox.
- Early signs of Reye's Syndrome are continuous vomiting, listlessness, loss of energy, drowsiness, irritability, aggressiveness, confusion and irrational behavior.
- Medicines, at the very least, can mask symptoms. Therefore, if any of the symptoms of Reye's Syndrome develop, **do not** use aspirin or anti-nausea medicine.
- Phone your physician immediately.
- Abnormal SGOT and SGPT tests strongly suggest a diagnosis of Reye's Syndrome.
- Early diagnosis is vital. Current statistics of recorded cases show
    - 90 percent recovery if diagnosed early
    - 10 percent recovery if diagnosed late
    - 52 percent fatalities overall (1995)

■ **Document Source:**
National Reye's Syndrome Foundation

426 N Lewis St, PO Box 829
Bryan, OH 43506
(419)636-2679 or 800/233-7393
e-mail: reyessyn@bright.net
http://www.bright.net/~reyessyn

See also: Fact Sheet: Reye's Syndrome (page 516); Medications Containing Aspirin (Acetylsolicylete) (page 523)

TALKING WITH YOUR DOCTOR: A GUIDE FOR OLDER PEOPLE

Opening Thoughts

How well you and your doctor talk to each other is one of the most important parts of getting good health care. Unfortunately, this isn't always easy. It takes time and effort on your part as well as your doctor's.

In the past, the doctor typically took the lead and the patient followed.

Today, a good patient-doctor relationship is more of a partnership, with both patient and doctor working together to solve medical problems and maintain the patient's good health.

This means asking questions if the doctor's explanations or instructions are unclear, bringing up problems even if the doctor doesn't ask, and letting the doctor know when a treatment isn't working. Taking an active role in your health care puts the responsibility for good communication on both you and your doctor.

Why does it matter? Choosing a doctor you can talk to.

The first step in good communication is finding a doctor with whom you can talk. Having a main doctor (often called your primary doctor) is one of the best ways to ensure your good health. This doctor knows you and what your health normally is like. He or she can help you make medical decisions that suit your values and daily habits and can keep in touch with other medical specialists and health care providers you may need.

If you don t have a primary doctor or are not at ease with the doctor you currently see, now may be the time to find a new doctor. The suggestions below can help you find a doctor who meets your needs.

1. Decide what you are looking for in a doctor.

A good first step to make a list of qualities that are important to you. Then, go back over the list and decide which are most important and which are nice, but not essential.

2. Identify several possible doctors.

After you have a general sense of what you are looking for, ask friends and relatives, medical specialists, and other health professionals for the names of doctors with whom they have had good experiences. A doctor whose name comes up often may be a strong possibility. Rather than just getting a name, ask about the person's experiences. For example, say "What do you like about Dr. Smith?" It may be helpful to come up with a few names to choose from, in case the doctor you select is not currently taking new patients.

3. Consult reference sources.

The Directory of Physicians in the United States and the Official American Board of Medical Specialties Directory of Board Certified Medical Specialists are available at many libraries. These references won't recommend individual doctors, but they will provide a list to choose from. Doctors who are "board certified" have had training after regular medical school and have passed an exam certifying them as specialists in certain fields of medicine. This includes the primary care fields of general internal medicine, family medicine, and geriatrics. Board certification is one way to tell about a doctor's expertise, but it doesn't address the doctor's communication skills.

4. Learn more about the doctors you are considering.

Once you have selected two or three doctors, call their offices. The office staff can be a good source of information about the doctor's education and qualifications, office policies, and payment procedures. Pay attention to the office staff—you will have to deal with them often! You may want to set up an appointment to talk with a doctor. He or she is likely to charge you for such a visit.

5. Make a choice.

After choosing a doctor, make the first appointment. This visit may include a medical history and a physical examination. Be sure to bring your medical records and a list of your current medicines with you. If you haven't interviewed the doctor, take time during this visit to ask any questions you have about the doctor and his or her practice. After the appointment, ask yourself whether this doctor is a person with whom you could work well. If you are not satisfied, schedule a visit with one of your other candidates.

Summary: Choosing a Doctor You Can Talk To

- Decide what you are looking for in a doctor.
- Identify several possible doctors.
- Consult reference sources, current patients, and colleagues.
- Learn more about the doctors you are considering.
- Make a choice.

What Can I Do?

Tips for Good Communication

A basic plan can help you communicate better with your doctor, whether you are starting with a new doctor or continuing with the doctor you've been visiting. The following tips can help you and your doctor build a partnership.

Getting Ready for Your Appointment

Be prepared: make a list of your concerns—Before going to the doctor, make a list of what you want to discuss. For example, are you having a new symptom you want to tell the doctor about? Did you want to get a flu shot or pneumonia vaccine? If you have more than a few items to discuss, put them in order so you are sure to ask about the most important ones first. Take along any information the doctor or staff may need such as insurance cards, names of your other doctors, or your medical records. Some doctors suggest you put all your medicines in a bag and bring them with you, others recommend bringing a list of medications you take.

Make sure you can see and hear as well as possible—Many older people use glasses or need aids for hearing. Remember to take your eyeglasses to the doctor's visit. If you have a hearing aid, make sure that it is working well, and wear it. Let the doctor and staff know if you have a hard time seeing or hearing. For example, you may want to say, "My hearing makes it hard to understand everything you're saying. It helps a lot when you speak slowly."

Consider bringing a family member or friend—Sometimes it is helpful to bring a family member or close friend with you. Let your family member or friend know in advance what you want from your visit. The person can remind you what you planned to discuss with the doctor if you forget, and can help you remember what the doctor said.

Plan to update the doctor—Think of any important information you need to share with your doctor about things that have happened since your last visit. If you have been treated in the emergency room, tell the doctor right away. Mention any changes you have noticed in your appetite, weight, sleep, or energy level. Also tell the doctor about any recent changes in the medication you take or the effect it has had on you.

Your doctor may ask you how your life is going. This isn't just polite talk or an attempt to be nosy. Information about what's happening in your life may be useful medically. Let the doctor know about any major changes or stresses in your life, such as a divorce or the death of a loved one. You don't have to go into detail; you may just want to say something like, "I thought it might be helpful for you to know that my sister passed away since my last visit with you," or "I had to sell my home and move in with my daughter."

Summary: Getting Ready for Your Appointment

- Be prepared: make a list of concerns.
- Make sure you can see and hear as well as possible.
- Consider bringing a family member or friend.
- Plan to update the doctor.

Sharing Information With Your Doctor

Be honest—It is tempting to say what you think the doctor wants to hear; for example, that you smoke less or eat a more balanced diet than you really do. While this is natural, it's not in your best interest. Your doctor can give you the best treatment only if you say what is really going on.

Stick to the point—Although your doctor might like to talk with you at length, each patient is given a limited amount of time. To make the best use of your time, stick to the point. Give the doctor a brief description of the symptom, when it started, how often it happens, and if it is getting worse or better.

Ask questions—Asking questions is key to getting what you want from the visit. If you don't ask questions, your doctor may think that you understand why he or she is sending you for a test or that you don't want more information. Ask questions when you don't know the meaning of a word (like aneurysm, hypertension, or infarct) or when instructions aren't clear (e.g., does taking medicine with food mean before, during, or after a meal?). You might say, "I want to make sure I understand. Could you explain that a little further?" It may help to repeat what you think the doctor means back in your own words and ask, "Is this correct?" If you are worried about cost, say so.

Share your point of view—Your doctor needs to know what's working and what's not. He or she can't read your mind, so it is important for you to share your point of view. Say if you feel rushed, worried, or uncomfortable. Try to voice your feelings in a positive way. For example, "I know you have many patients to see, but I'm really worried about this. I'd feel much better if we could talk about it a little more." If necessary, you can offer to return for a second visit to discuss your concerns.

Summary: Sharing Information With Your Doctor

- Be honest.
- Stick to the point.
- Ask questions.
- Share your point of view.

Getting Information From Your Doctor and Other Health Professionals

Take notes—It can be difficult to remember what the doctor says, so take along a note pad and pencil and write down the main points, or ask the doctor to write them down for you. If you can't write while the doctor is talking to you, make notes in the waiting room after the visit. Or, bring a tape recorder along, and (with the doctor's permission) record what is said. Recording is especially helpful if you want to share the details of the visit with others.

Get written or recorded information—Whenever possible, have the doctor or staff provide written advice and instructions. Ask if your doctor has any brochures, cassette tapes, or videotapes about your health conditions or treatments. For example, if your doctor says that your blood pressure is high, he or she may give you brochures explaining what causes high blood pressure and what you can do about it. Some doctors have videocassette recorders for viewing tapes in their offices. Ask the doctor to recommend other sources, such as public libraries, nonprofit organizations, and government agencies, which may have written or recorded materials you can use.

Remember that doctors don't know everything—Even the best doctor may be unable to answer some questions. There still is much we don't know about the human body, the aging process, and disease. Most doctors will tell you when they don't have answers. They also may help you find the information you need or refer you to a specialist. If a doctor regularly brushes off your questions or symptoms as simply part of aging, think about looking for another doctor.

Talk to other members of the health care team—Today, health care is a team effort. Other professionals, including nurses, physician assistants, pharmacists, and occupational or physical therapists, play an active role in your health care. These professionals may be able to take more time with you.

Summary: Getting Information From Your Doctor and Other Health Professionals

- Take notes.
- Get written or recorded information.
- Remember that doctors don't know everything.
- Talk to other members of the health care team.

Where do I begin? Getting started with a new doctor.

Your first meeting is the best time to begin communicating positively with your new doctor. When you see the doctor and office staff, introduce yourself and let them know how you like to be addressed. The first few appointments with your new doctor also are the best times to:

Learn the basics of the office—Ask the office staff how the office runs. Learn what days are busiest and what times. Ask what to do if there is an emergency, or when the office is closed.

Share your medical history—Tell the doctor about your illnesses or operations, medical conditions that run in your family, and other doctors you see. You may want to ask for a copy of the medical history form before your visit so you have all the time and information you need to complete it. Your new doctor may ask you to sign a medical release form to get copies of your medical records from doctors you have had before. Be prepared to give the new doctor your former doctors' names and addresses, especially if they are in a different city.

Give information about your medications—Many people take several medicines. It is possible for medicines to interact, causing unpleasant and sometimes dangerous side effects. Your doctor needs to know about ALL of the medicines you take, including over-the-counter (nonprescription) drugs, so bring everything with you to your first visit, including eye drops, vitamins, and laxatives. Tell the doctor how often you take each and describe any drug allergies or reactions you have had and which medications work best for you. Be sure your doctor has the phone number of your regular drugstore.

Tell the doctor about your habits—To provide the best care, your doctor must understand you as a person and know what your life is like. The doctor may ask about where you live, what you eat, how you sleep, what you do each day, what activities you enjoy, your sex life, and if you smoke or drink. Be open and honest with your doctor. It will help him or her to understand your medical conditions fully and recommend the best treatment choices for you.

Summary: Getting Started with a New Doctor

- Learn the basics of how the office runs.
- Share your medical history.
- Give information about your medications.
- Tell the doctor about your habits.

What should I say? Talking about your health.

Talking about your health means sharing information about how you feel both physically and emotionally. Knowing how to describe your symptoms, discuss treatments, and talk with specialists will help you become a partner in your health care. Here are some issues that may be important to you when you talk with your doctor.

Preventing Disease and Disability

Until recently, preventing disease in older people received little attention. But things are changing. It's never too late to stop smoking, improve your diet, or start exercising. Getting regular checkups and seeing other health professionals such as dentists and eye specialists help promote good health. Even people who have chronic diseases, like arthritis or diabetes, can prevent further disability and in some cases, control the progress of the disease.

If a certain disease or health condition runs in your family, ask your doctor if there are steps you can take to help prevent it. If you have a chronic condition, ask how you can manage it and if there are things you can do to prevent it from getting worse. If you want to discuss health and disease prevention with your doctor, say so when you make your next appointment. This lets the doctor plan to spend more time with you as well as to prepare for the discussion.

Sharing Any Symptoms

It is very important for you to be clear and concise when describing your symptoms. Your description helps the doctor identify the problem. A physical exam and medical tests provide valuable information, but it is your symptoms that point the doctor in the right direction.

Tell the doctor when your symptoms started, what time of day they happen, how long they last (seconds? days?), how often they occur, if they seem to be getting worse or better, and if they keep you from going out or doing your usual activities. Take the time to make some notes about your symptoms before you call or visit the doctor. Concern about your symptoms is not a sign of weakness. It is not necessarily complaining to be honest about what you are experiencing.

Learning More About Medical Tests

Sometimes doctors need to do blood tests, x-rays, or other procedures to find out what is wrong or to learn more about your medical condition. Some tests, such as Pap smears, mammograms, glaucoma tests, and screenings for prostate and colorectal cancer, are done on a regular basis to check for hidden medical problems.

Before having a medical test, ask your doctor to explain why it is important and what it will cost, and, if possible, to give you something to read about it. Ask how long the results of the test will take to come in.

When the results are ready, make sure the doctor tells you what they are and explains what they mean. You may want to ask your doctor for a written copy of the test results. If the test is done by a specialist, ask to have the results sent to your primary doctor.

Discussing Your Diagnosis and What You Can Expect

If you understand your medical condition, you can help make better decisions about treatment. If you know what to expect it may be easier for you to deal with the condition.

Ask the doctor to tell you the name of the condition and why he or she thinks you have it. Ask how it may affect your body, and how long it might last. Some medical problems never go away completely. They can't be cured, but they can be treated or managed. You may want to write down what the doctor says to help you remember.

It is not unusual to be surprised or upset by hearing you have a new medical problem. Questions may occur to you later. When they do, make a note of them for your next appointment.

Sometimes the doctor may want you to talk with other health professionals who can help you understand how to manage your condition. If you have the chance to work with other health professionals, take advantage of it. Also, find out how you can reach them if you have questions later.

Talking About Treatments

Although some medical conditions do not require treatment, most can be helped by medicine, surgery, changes in daily habits, or a combination of these. You will benefit most from treatment when you know what is happening and are involved in making decisions. If your doctor suggests a treatment, be sure you understand what it will and won't do and what it involves. Have the doctor give you directions in writing, and feel free to ask questions.

If your doctor suggests a treatment that makes you uncomfortable, ask if there are other treatments to consider. For example, if the doctor recommends medicine for your blood pressure, you may want to ask if you can try lowering it through diet and exercise first. If cost is a concern, ask the doctor if less expensive choices are available. The doctor can work with you to develop a treatment plan that meets your needs.

Making the Most of Medications

Your doctor may prescribe a drug for your condition. Make sure you know the name of the drug and understand why it has been prescribed for you. Ask the doctor to write down how often and how long you should take it. Make notes about any other special instructions such as foods or drinks you should avoid. If you are taking other medications, make sure your doctor knows, so he or she can prevent harmful drug interactions.

Sometimes medicines affect older people differently than younger people. Let the doctor know if your medicine doesn't seem to be working or if it is causing problems. Don't stop taking it on your own. If another doctor (for example, a specialist) prescribes a medication for you, call your primary doctor to let him or her know. Also call to check with your doctor before taking any over-the-counter medications. You may find it helpful to keep a chart of all the medicines you take and when you take them.

The pharmacist also is a good source of information about your medicines. In addition to answering questions, the pharmacist keeps records of all the prescriptions you get filled at that drugstore. Because your pharmacist keeps these records, it is helpful to use a regular drugstore.

A pharmacist also can help you select over-the-counter medicines that are best for you. At your request, the pharmacist can fill your prescriptions in easy-to-open containers and may be able to provide large print prescription labels.

Changing Your Daily Habits

Doctors and other health professionals may suggest you change your diet, activity level, or other aspects of your life to help you deal with medical conditions. Sometimes the doctor's suggestions may not be acceptable to you. For example, the doctor might recommend a diet that includes foods you cannot eat or do not like. Tell your doctor if you don't feel a plan will work for you and explain why. There may be other choices. Keep talking with your doctor to come up with a plan that works.

Seeing Specialists

Your doctor may send you to a specialist for further evaluation. You also may request to see one yourself, although your insurance company may require that you have a referral from your primary doctor.

When you see a specialist, ask that he or she send information about further diagnosis or treatment to your primary doctor. This allows your primary doctor to keep track of your medical care. You also should let your primary doctor know at your next visit about any treatments or medications the specialist recommended.

A visit to the specialist may be short. Often, the specialist already has seen your medical records or test results and is familiar with your case. If you are unclear about what the specialist tells you, ask him or her questions. For example, if the specialist says that you have a medical condition that you aren't familiar with, you may want to say, "I don't know very much about that condition. Could you explain what it is and how it might affect me?" or, "I've heard it's painful. What can be done to prevent or manage the pain?" You also may ask for written materials to read or call your primary doctor to clarify anything you haven't understood.

Surgery

In some cases, surgery may be the best treatment for your condition. If so, your doctor will refer you to a surgeon. Knowing more about the operation will help you make an informed decision. It also will help you get ready for the surgery, which, in turn, makes for a better recovery. Ask the surgeon to explain what will be done during the operation and what reading material or videotapes you can look at before the operation. Find out if you will have to stay overnight in the hospital to have the surgery, or if it can be done on an outpatient basis. Minor surgeries that don't require an overnight stay can sometimes be done at medical centers called "ambulatory surgical centers."

When surgery is recommended, it is common for the patient to seek a second opinion. In fact, your insurance company may require it. Doctors are used to this practice, and most will not be insulted by your request for a second opinion. Your doctor may even be able to suggest other doctors who can review your case. Hearing the views of two different doctors can help you decide what's best for you.

If You Are Hospitalized

If you have to go to the hospital, some extra guidelines may help you. First, most hospitals have a daily schedule. Knowing the hospital routine can make your stay more comfortable. Find out how much choice you have about your daily routine, and express any preferences you have about your schedule. Doctors generally visit patients during specific times each day. Find out when the doctor is likely to visit so you can have your questions ready.

In the hospital, you may meet with your primary doctor and various medical specialists, as well as nurses and other health professionals. If you are in a teaching hospital, doctors-in-training, known as medical students, interns, residents, and fellows, also may examine you. Many of these doctors-in-training already have a lot of knowledge. They may be able to take more time to talk with you than other staff. Nurses also can be an important source of information, especially since you will see them on a regular basis.

If You Have to Go to the Emergency Room

A visit to the emergency room is always stressful. If possible, take along the following items: your health insurance card or policy number, a list of your medications, a list of your medical problems, and the names and phone numbers of your doctor and one or two family members or close friends. Some people find it helpful to keep this information on a card in their wallets or purses.

While in the emergency room, ask questions if you don't understand tests or procedures that are being done. Before leaving, make sure you understand what the doctor told you. For example, if you have bandages that need to be changed, be sure you understand how and when it is to be done. Tell your primary doctor as soon as possible about your emergency room care.

Can I really talk about that? Discussing sensitive subjects.

Much of the communication between doctor and patient is personal. To have a good partnership with your doctor, it is important to talk about sensitive subjects, like sex or memory problems, even if you are embarrassed or uncomfortable. Doctors are used to talking about personal matters and will try to ease your discomfort. Keep in mind that these topics concern many older people. For more information on the topics discussed below, see the resource list at the end of this book.

It is important to understand that problems with memory, depression, sexual function, and incontinence are not normal parts of aging. If your doctor doesn't take your concerns about these topics seriously or brushes them off as being part of normal aging, you may want to consider looking for a new doctor.

Sexuality—Most health professionals now understand that sexuality remains important in later life. If you are not satisfied with your sex life, don't automatically assume it's due to your age. In addition to talking about age-related changes, you can ask your doctor about the effects of an illness or a disability on sexual function. Also, ask your doctor what influence medications or surgery may have on your sexual life. If you aren't sure how to bring the topic up, try saying, "I have a personal question I would like to ask you..." or, "I understand that this condition can affect my body in many ways. Will it affect my sex life at all?"

Incontinence—About 15 to 30 percent of older people living at home have problems controlling their bladder—this is called urinary incontinence. Often, certain exercises or other measures are helpful in correcting or improving the problem. If you have trouble with control of your bladder or bowels, it is important to let the doctor know. In many cases, incontinence is the result of a treatable medical condition. When discussing incontinence with your doctor, you may want to say something like, "Since my last visit there have been several times that I couldn't control my bladder. I'm concerned, because this has never happened to me before."

Grief, mourning, and depression—As people grow older, they experience losses of significant people in their lives, including spouses and cherished friends. A doctor who knows about your losses is better able to understand how you are feeling. He or she can make suggestions that may be helpful to you.

Although it is normal to feel grief and mourning when you have a loss, later life does not have to be a time of ongoing sadness. If you feel down all the time or for more than a few weeks, let your doctor know. Also tell your doctor about symptoms such as lack of energy, poor appetite, trouble sleeping, or lack of interest in life. These could be signs of medical depression. If you feel sad and withdrawn and are having trouble sleeping, give your doctor a call. Depression can be a side effect of medications or a sign of a medical condition that needs attention. It often can be treated successfully—but only if your doctor knows about it.

Memory problems—One of the greatest fears of older people is problems with their ability to think and remember. For most older people, thinking and memory remain good throughout the later years. If you seem to have problems remembering recent events or thinking clearly, let your doctor know. Try to be specific about the changes you have noticed, for example, "I've always been able to balance my checkbook without any problems, but lately I'm finding that I get very confused." The doctor will probably want you to undergo a thorough checkup to see what might be causing your symptoms.

In many cases, these symptoms are caused by a passing, treatable condition such as depression, infection, or a side effect of medication. In other cases, the problem may be Alzheimer's disease or a related condition that causes ongoing loss of skills such as learning, thinking, and remembering. While there currently is no way to determine for sure if a person has Alzheimer's disease, a careful history, physical evaluation, and mental status examination are still important. They help the doctor rule out any other, perhaps treatable, causes of your symptoms and determine the best plan of care for you.

Care in the event of a serious illness—You may have some concerns or wishes about your care if you become seriously ill. If you have questions about what choices you have, ask your doctor. You can specify your desires through documents called advance directives such as a living will or durable power of attorney for health care. Advance directives allow you to say what you'd prefer if you were too ill to make your wishes known. In an advance directive you can name a family member or other person to make decisions about your care if you aren't able.

In general, the best time to talk with your doctor about these issues is when you are still relatively healthy. If you are admitted to the hospital or a nursing home, you will be asked if you have any advance directives. If the doctor doesn't raise the topic, do so yourself. To make sure that your wishes are carried out, write them down. You also should talk with family members so that they understand your wishes.

Problems with family—Even strong and loving families can have problems, especially under the stress of illness. Although family problems can be painful to discuss, talking about them can help your doctor help you. Your doctor may be able to suggest steps to improve the situation for you and other family members. If you feel you are being mistreated in some way, let your doctor know. Some older people are subjected to abuse by family members or others. Abuse can be physical, verbal, psychological, or even financial in nature. Your doctor may be able to provide resources or referrals to other services that can help you if you are being mistreated.

Feeling unhappy with your doctor—Misunderstandings can come up in any relationship, including between a patient and his or her doctor. If you feel uncomfortable with something your doctor or the doctor's staff has said or done, be direct. For example, if the doctor does not return your telephone calls, you may want to say something like, "I realize that you care for a lot of patients and are very busy, but I feel frustrated when I have to wait for days for you to return my call. Is there a way we can work together to improve this?" Being honest is much better for your health than avoiding the doctor. If you have a longstanding relationship with your doctor, working out the problem may be more useful than looking for a new doctor.

Summary

If you have questions or worries about a subject that your doctor does not talk about with you, bring them up yourself. Practice with family or friends what you will tell or ask the doctor. If there are brochures or pamphlets about the subject in the doctor's waiting room, use them as a way to begin to talk. Talking with your doctor about sensitive subjects is important. Although talking about these subjects may be awkward for both you and your doctor, don't avoid it. If you feel the doctor doesn't take your concerns seriously, remember that you can always change doctors.

Who else will help? Involving your family and friends.

It can be helpful to take a family member or friend with you when you go to the doctor's office. You may feel more confident if someone else is with you. Also, a friend or relative can help you remember what you planned to tell or ask the doctor. He or she also can help you remember what the doctor says. But don't let your companion take too strong a role. The visit is between you and the doctor. You may want some time alone with the doctor to discuss personal matters. For best results, let your companion know in advance how he or she can be most helpful.

If a relative or friend helps with your care at home, having that person along when you visit the doctor may be useful. In addition to the questions you have, your caregiver may have concerns he or she wants to discuss with the doctor. Some things caregivers may find especially helpful to discuss are: what to expect in the future, sources of information and support, community services, and ways they can maintain their own well-being.

Even if a family member or friend can't go with you to your appointment, he or she can still help. For example, the person can serve as your sounding board, helping you to practice what you want to say to the doctor before the visit. And after the visit, talking about what the doctor said can remind you about the important points and help you come up with questions to ask next time.

What's next? Some closing thoughts.

Good health care always depends on good communication with your doctor and other health professionals. We hope this book will help you take an active role in your health care.

If you have suggestions to add to future editions of this book or other ideas for making it more helpful, please write to Freddi Karp, Editor, National Institute on Aging, Public Information Office, Building 31, Room 5C27, 31 Center Drive MSC 2292, Bethesda, MD 20892-2292.

Getting More Information

You can make the best use of your time with your doctor by being informed. This often includes drawing on other sources of health information such as home medical guides, books and articles available at libraries, organizations such as the American Heart Association and the Arthritis Foundation, other institutes within the National Institutes of Health, and self-help groups.

The National Institute on Aging (NIA) has information about a variety of issues relating to aging, including menopause, incontinence, and pneumonia. Large-print *Age Pages* are available on topics such as depression, stroke, safe use of medications, and types of doctors you may see.

To order publications or to request a publications list, call the NIA Information Center at 1-800-222-2225; TTY 1-800-222-4225.

For a fact sheet and other publications about Alzheimer's disease, contact the NIA Alzheimer's Disease Education and Referral (ADEAR) Center at 1-800-438-4380.

Additional Resources

Sexuality

Sexuality Information and Education Council of the United States
130 W 42nd St, Ste 2500
New York, NY 10036
1-212-819-9770

Incontinence

Help for Incontinent People (HIP)
PO Box 544
Union, SC 29379
1-800-BLADDER

The Simon Foundation
PO Box 835
Wilmette, IL 60091
1-800-237-4666

Grief, Mourning, and Depression

NIMH Depression Awareness, Recognition and Treatment Program
5600 Fishers Ln, Rm 10-85
Rockville, MD 20857
1-800-421-4211

Memory Problems

Alzheimer's Association
919 N Michigan Ave, Ste 1000
Chicago, IL 60611
1-800-272-3900

Alzheimer's Disease Education and Referral (ADEAR) Center
PO Box 8250
Silver Spring, MD 20907-8250
1-800-438-4380

National Stroke Association
8480 E Orchard Rd, Ste 1000
Englewood, CO 80111-5015
1-800-367-1990

Care in the Event of a Terminal Illness

National Hospice Organization
1901 N Moore St, Ste 901
Arlington, VA 22209

Problems with Family

Children of Aging Parents
1609 Woodbourne Rd, Ste 302-A
Levittown, PA 19057-1511
1-215-945-6900

Eldercare Locator Service
1112 16th St NW, Ste 100
Washington, DC 20036
1-800-677-1116

National Center on Elder Abuse
810 First St NE, Ste 500
Washington, DC 20002
1-202-682-2470

■ **Document Source:**
U.S. Department of Health and Human Services, Public Health Service
National Institutes of Health
National Institute on Aging
NIH Publication No. 94-3452
December 1994

See also: Be Informed: Questions to Ask Your Doctor Before You Have Surgery (page 513)

APPENDIX A

■ ■ ■

OVERVIEW OF PHYSICIAN DATA QUERY (PDQ)

What is PDQ?

PDQ is a computer system that gives up-to-date information on cancer treatment. It is a service of the National Cancer Institute (NCI) for people with cancer and their families, and for doctors, nurses, and other health care professionals.

PDQ tells about the current treatments for most cancers. The information in PDQ is reviewed each month by cancer experts. It is updated when there is new information. The patient information in PDQ also tells about warning signs and how the cancer is found. PDQ also lists information about research on new treatments (clinical trials), doctors who treat cancer, and hospitals with cancer programs.

How to Use PDQ

You can use PDQ to learn more about current treatment for your kind of cancer. Bring this material from PDQ with you when you see your doctor. You can talk with your doctor, who knows you and has the facts about your disease, about which treatment would be best for you. Before you start your treatment, you might also want to seek a second opinion from a doctor who treats cancer.

Before you start treatment, you also may want to think about taking part in a clinical trial. A clinical trial is a study that uses new treatments to care for patients. Each study is based on past studies and what has been learned in the laboratory. Each trial answers certain scientific questions in order to find new and better ways to help cancer patients. During clinical trials, more and more information is collected about new treatments, their risks, and how well they do or do not work. If clinical trials show that the new treatment is better than the treatment currently being used, the new treatment may become the "standard" treatment. Listings of clinical trials are a part of PDQ. Many cancer doctors who take part in clinical trials are listed in PDQ.

If you want to know more about cancer and how it is treated, or if you wish to learn about clinical trials for your kind of cancer, you can call the National Cancer Institute's Cancer Information Service. The number is 1-800-4-CAN-CER (1-800-422-6237). The call is free and a trained information specialist will talk with you and answer your questions.

PDQ may change when there is new information. Check with the Cancer Information Service to be sure that you have the most up-to-date information.

■ Document Source:
U.S. Department of Health and Human Services, Public Health Service
National Institutes of Health
National Cancer Institute
1996

APPENDIX B

■ ■ ■

TOLL-FREE NUMBERS FOR HEALTH INFORMATION (BY SUBJECT)

This Healthfinder lists selected toll-free numbers and describes organizations that provide health-related information. The numbers do not diagnose or recommend treatment for any disease. Some offer recorded information; others provide personalized counseling, referrals, and/or written materials. Unless otherwise stated, numbers can be reached within the continental United States Monday through Friday, and hours of operation are Eastern time. Numbers that operate 24 hours a day can be reached seven days a week unless otherwise noted.

This Healthfinder is one in a series of publications, on a variety of topics, prepared by the National Health Information Center (NHIC). NHIC is a service of the Office of Disease Prevention and Health Promotion, Public Health Service, U.S. Department of Health and Human Services. The information contained on the following pages in no way should be construed as an endorsement, real or implied, by the U.S. Department of Health and Human Services.

Adoption

A-1. Bethany Christian Services
(800) 238-4269

Services for women considering adoption as an option. Free counseling. Housing is available. 8 a.m.-12 midnight, every day.

A-2. National Adoption Center
(800) TO-ADOPT
(215) 735-9988

Expands adoption opportunities throughout the United States, particularly for children with special needs. Links all state adoption agencies through a telecommunication network. Addresses adoption and child welfare issues. 9 a.m.-5 p.m.

Aging

Eldercare Locator
(800) 677 1116

Provides referrals to local resources nationwide. 9 a.m. 11 p.m. (Eastern)

A-3. National Institute on Aging Information Center
(800) 222-2225
(800) 222-4225 (TTY)
(301) 589-3014 (Fax)

Provides publications on health topics of interest to older adults, to the public, and to doctors, nurses, social activities directors, and health educators. 8:30 a.m.-5 p.m. (See also A-16, A-17, A-18, A-81, B-1)

AIDS/HIV

A-4. AIDS Clinical Trials Information Service
(800) 874-2572
(800) 243-7012 (TTY/TDD)
(301) 217-0023
(301) 738-6616 (Fax)

Sponsored by the Centers for Disease Control and Prevention, the Food and Drug Administration, the National Institute of Allergy and Infectious Diseases, and the National Library of Medicine. Provides current information on federally and privately sponsored clinical trials for AIDS patients and others with HIV infection and on the drugs used in those trials. All calls are confidential. Spanish-speaking operators available. 9 a.m.-7 p.m.

A-5. CDC National AIDS Clearinghouse
(800) 458-5231
(800) 243-7012 (TDD)
(301) 217-0023
(301) 738-6616 (Fax)
(800) 458-5231 (NAC Fax-Back Service)
aidsinfo@cdcnac.aspensys.com

Sponsored by the Centers for Disease Control and Prevention. A national reference, referral, and distribution service for HIV/AIDS-related information. Answers questions and provides technical assistance; distributes published HIV-related materials including current information on scientific findings, CDC guidelines, and trends in the HIV epidemic;

and provides specific information on AIDS-related organizations, educational materials, funding opportunities, and other topics. Services include a 24-hour fax-back service for HIV/AIDS-related information and the Business and Labor Resource Service for resources, technical assistance, publications, and referrals concerning managing AIDS in the workplace. Provides information and publications in English and Spanish. 9 a.m.-7 p.m. (See also B-3)

A-6. CDC National AIDS Hotline
(800) 342-2437 (English)
(800) 344-7432 (Spanish)
(800) 243-7889 (TDD)

Sponsored by the Centers for Disease Control and Prevention. Provides information to the public on the prevention and spread of HIV/AIDS. The first toll-free number provides 24-hour service; the second number provides service in Spanish 8 a.m.-2 a.m., everyday except holidays. The third toll-free number is available 10 a.m.-10 p.m., Monday-Friday.

HIV/AIDS Treatment Information Service
(800) HIV-0440
(800) 243-7012 (TDD)
(301) 217-0023
(301) 738-6616 (Fax)

Sponsored by the CDC National AIDS Clearinghouse. Provides timely, accurate treatment information on HIV and AIDS. Answers questions about treatment of HIV disease; distributes copies of federally-approved HIV/AIDS treatment guidelines and information; provides services in Spanish and English. 9 a.m. 7 p.m. All calls are confidential.

A-7. National Indian AIDS Hotline
(800) 283-2437
(510) 444-2051
(510) 444-1593 (Fax)

Sponsored by the National Native American AIDS Prevention Center. Provides technical assistance, printed materials and information about AIDS and AIDS prevention in the Native American community. 8:30 a.m.-12 p.m. and 1 p.m.-5 p.m. (Pacific). Leave recorded message after hours.

A-8. Project Inform HIV/AIDS Treatment Hotline
(800) 822-7422
(415) 558-9051

Provides treatment information and referral for HIV-infected individuals. Information on clinical trials. No diagnosis. 10 a.m.-4 p.m., Monday-Saturday (Pacific).

Alcohol Abuse

See also **Drug Abuse**

A-9. ADCARE Hospital Helpline
(800) ALCOHOL

Provides information and referral for alcohol and other drug concerns. Operates 24 hours.

A-10. Al-Anon Family Group Headquarters
(800) 356-9996

Al-Anon and Alateen provide help for families and friends of alcoholics. The headquarters provides literature and refers people who need assistance to local meetings. 9 a.m.-4:30 p.m.

A-11. Alcohol and Drug Helpline
(800) 821-4357
(801) 272-4357

Sponsored by Pioneer Health Care. Provides referrals to local facilities where adolescents and adults can seek help. Operates 24 hours.

A-12. American Council on Alcoholism
(800) 527-5344
(410) 889-0297 (Fax)

Offers information and sources for alcoholism treatment to callers concerned about excessive drinking of someone close to them. 9 a.m.-5 p.m.

A-13. National Clearinghouse for Alcohol and Drug Information
(800) 729-6686
(301) 468-2600
(800) 487-4889 (TTY/TDD)
(301) 230-2867 (TTY/TDD)
(301) 468-6433 (Fax)

Sponsored by the Center for Substance Abuse Prevention, Substance Abuse and Mental Health Services Administration. Gathers and disseminates information on alcohol and other drug-related subjects, including tobacco. Distributes publications. Services include subject searches and provision of statistics and other information. Operates the Regional Alcohol and Drug Awareness Resource Network, a nationwide linkage of alcohol and other drug information centers. Maintains a library open to the public. 8 a.m.-7 p.m.

A-15. National Council on Alcoholism and Drug Dependence, Inc.
(800) 622-2255
(212) 206-6770
(212) 645-1690 (Fax)

Refers to local affiliates for counseling and provides written information on alcoholism and drug dependence. The toll-free number operates 24 hours; the other number is staffed 9 a.m.-5 p.m.

Allergy/Asthma

See **Lung Disease/Asthma/Allergy**

Alzheimer's Disease

See also **Aging**

A-16. Alzheimer's Association
(800) 272-3900
(312) 335-8882 (TDD)
(312) 335-1110 (Fax)
http://www.alz.org

Refers to local chapters and support groups. Offers basic information about Alzheimer's disease and related disorders including research, drug treatments and clinical trials, warning signs of the disease, and caregiving information. Printed materials are available in English and Spanish. Spanish-speaking operators are available. The information and referral line is available 24 hours; operators staff the line 8:30 a.m.-5 p.m. Central, M-F. Leave message after hours.

A-17. Alzheimer's Disease Education and Referral Center
(800) 438-4380
(301) 495-3334 (Fax)
adear@alzheimers.org

Sponsored by the National Institute on Aging. Provides information and publications on Alzheimer's disease. 8:30 a.m.-5 p.m.

Arthritis

A-18. Arthritis Foundation Information Line
(800) 283-7800

Provides information about arthritis and referrals to local chapters. 24 hours. (See also B-7)

Lyme Disease Foundation, Inc.
(800) 886-5963

Services include public education; supporting research relating to the condition; guiding and supporting self-help groups; and providing medical referrals. Distributes brochures on Lyme disease and reprints of scientific articles.

Audiovisuals

See **Library Services**

Autism

See **Child Development**

Bone Marrow

See **Cancer**

Cancer

A-19. American Cancer Society Response Line
(800) 227-2345 (Voice/TDD/TT)

Provides information and publications about cancer and pain management. Offers support services to cancer patients. Through the One-Day Memorial Response Service, donors can make contributions, during or after hours, in memory of a friend or loved one to help American Cancer Society Programs. 8:30 a.m. 4:30 p.m.

A-20. Cancer Information Service
(800) 422-6237

Provides information about cancer and cancer-related resources to patients, the public, and health professionals. Inquiries are handled by trained information specialists.

Spanish-speaking staff members are available. Distributes free publications from the National Cancer Institute. Operates 9 a.m.-7 p.m.

A-21. National Marrow Donor Program
(800) MARROW-2

Sponsored by the National Heart, Lung, and Blood Institute and the Department of the Navy. Provides multilingual information on donating marrow and the transplant process. Also provides information on donor centers in the caller's area. Professional staff answer questions from 8 a.m.-6 p.m. (Central); recorded message at all other times. (See also A-117)

Susan G. Komen Breast Cancer Foundation
(800) IM AWARE

Organizes breast health seminars throughout the country and provides education material about breast cancer, mammography, and breast self-examination.

A-22. Y-Me National Breast Cancer Organization
(800) 221-2141
(312) 986-8228

Provides breast cancer patients with presurgery counseling, treatment information, peer support, self-help counseling, and patient literature. Also provides information to any and all women concerned about breast health and breast cancer. Y-ME has a matching caller program for men whose partners have been diagnosed with breast cancer. 9 a.m.-5 p.m. (Central). Local number operates 24 hours.

Cerebral Palsy

See **Rare Disorders**

Chemical Products/Pesticides

See also **Housing**

A-23. Chemtrec Non-Emergency Services Hotline
(800) 262-8200

Provides non-emergency referrals to companies that manufacture chemicals and to federal and state agencies for health and safety information and information regarding chemical regulations. 9 a.m.-6 p.m.

A-24. National Pesticide Telecommunications Network
(800) 858-7378

Sponsored by the U.S. Environmental Protection Agency and Oregon State University. Provides information about a variety of pesticide-related subjects, including: pesticide product information; information on the recognition and management of pesticide poisonings; toxicology; environmental chemistry; referrals for laboratory analyses, investigation of pesticide incidents, and emergency treatment information; safety information; health and environmental effects; clean-up and disposal procedures. TDD capability. 6:30 a.m.-4:30 p.m. (Pacific); voice mail provided for off-hours calls.

Child Abuse/Missing Children/Mental Health

A-25. Boys Town National Hotline
(800) 448-3000
(800) 448-1833 (TDD)

Provides short-term intervention and counseling and refers callers to local community resources. Counsels on parent-child conflicts, family issues, suicide, pregnancy, runaway youth, physical and sexual abuse, and other issues that impact children and families. Spanish-speaking operators are available. TDD capability. Operates 24 hours.

A-26. Child Find of America, Inc.
(800) 426-5678 (I-AM-LOST)

Searches for missing children under age 18 who are victims of parental abduction, stranger abduction, or who have run away. Provides safety prevention information. Operates 24 hours.

(800) 292-9688 (A-WAY-OUT)

Provides unique crisis mediation program for parents contemplating abduction of their children, or who have already abducted their children and want to use Child Find Volunteer Family Mediators to resolve their custody dispute. Operates 24 hours.

A-27. CHILDHELP/IOF Foresters
National Child Abuse Hotline
(800) 4-A-CHILD
(800) 2-A-CHILD (TDD)

Provides multilingual crisis intervention and professional counseling on child abuse and domestic violence issues. Gives referrals to local agencies offering counseling and other services related to child abuse, adult survivor issues, and domestic violence. Provides literature on child abuse in English and Spanish. Operates 24 hours.

A-28. Covenant House Nineline
(800) 999-9999

Crisis line for youth, teens, and families. Locally based referrals throughout the United States. Help for youth and parents regarding drugs, abuse, homelessness, runaway children, and message relays. Operates 24 hours.

A-31. National Center for Missing and Exploited Children
(800) 843-5678
(703) 235-3900
(800) 826-7653 (TDD)
(703) 235-4067 (Fax)

Operates a hotline for reporting missing children and sightings of missing children. Offers assistance and training to law enforcement agents. Takes reports of sexually exploited children. Serves as the National Child Porn TipLine. Provides books and other publications on prevention and issues related to missing and sexually exploited children. Ability to serve callers in over 140 languages. Operates 24 hours.

A-29. National Child Safety Council Childwatch
(800) 222-1464

Answers questions and distributes literature on safety, including drug abuse, household dangers, and electricity. Provides safety information to local police departments. Sponsor of the missing kids milk carton program. Operates 24 hours.

A-30. National Clearinghouse on Child Abuse and Neglect Information
(800) 394-3366
(703) 385-7565
(703) 385-3206 (Fax)
nccanch@clark.net

Serves as a national resource for the acquisition and dissemination of child abuse and neglect materials and distributes a free publications catalog upon request. Maintains bibliographic databases of documents, audiovisuals, and national organizations. Services include searches of databases and annotated bibliographies on frequently requested topics. CD-ROM containing Clearinghouse databases is available free to qualified institutions. 8:30 a.m.-5 p.m.

A-32. National Resource Center on Child Abuse and Neglect
(800) 227-5242

Sponsored by the American Humane Association. Provides general information and statistics about child abuse. 8:30 a.m.-4:30 p.m., Monday Friday (Mountain).

A-33. National Runaway Switchboard
(800) 621-4000
(800) 621-0394 (TDD)
(312) 929-5150 (Fax)

Provides crisis intervention and travel assistance information to runaways. Gives referrals to shelters nationwide. Also relays messages to, or sets up conference calls with parents at the request of the child. Has access to AT&T Language Line. Operates 24 hours.

A-34. National Youth Crisis Hotline
(800) 448-4663

Provides counseling and referrals to local drug treatment centers, shelters, and counseling services. Responds to youth dealing with pregnancy, molestation, suicide, and child abuse. Operates 24 hours.

Child Development

Autism Society of America
(800) 3AUTISM
(301) 657-0869 (Fax)

Educates parents, professionals, and the public regarding autism; improves the welfare of people with autism; supports research regarding autism; and oversees over 200 local chapters nationwide.

A-36. Human Growth Foundation
(800) 451-6434
(703) 883-1773

Provides parent education and mutual support, funds research, and promotes public awareness of the physical and emotional problems of short-statured people. Offers brochures on child growth abnormalities. 8:30 a.m.-5 p.m.

Child Education

A-37. National Association for the Education of Young Children
(800) 424-2460
(202) 232-8777
(202) 328-1846 (Fax)

The National Association for the Education of Young Children is neither a helpline nor hotline. The association publishes books, posters, and brochures for teachers and parents of young children, birth through age 8. Sponsors conferences and public awareness activities concerning quality programs for the education of young children. 9 a.m.-5 p.m.

Cleft Palate

See **Rare Disorders**

Cystic Fibrosis

See **Rare Disorders**

Diabetes/Digestive Diseases

A-38. American Diabetes Association
(800) 232-3472
(703) 549-1500
(703) 549-6995 (Fax, Customer Service)
(800) ADA-ORDER (Fax, Order Fulfillment)

Offers patient assistance in many areas, including general information about diabetes, nutrition, exercise, treatment, and referrals to diabetes medical professionals. For people with diabetes facing discrimination, the association offers referrals from a nationwide attorney's network and information on how to influence public leaders. The association also conducts a variety of patient activities, including educational seminars and workshops, culturally diverse programs, support groups, and youth programs. Spanish-speaking operators available. 8:30 a.m.-5 p.m.

A-39. Crohn's and Colitis Foundation of America, Inc.
(800) 932-2423
(800) 343-3637 (Warehouse)

Provides educational materials on Crohn's disease and ulcerative colitis. Refers to local support groups and physicians. 9 a.m.-5 p.m. Recording after hours. Warehouse is open 8 a.m.-5 p.m.

A-40. Juvenile Diabetes Foundation International Hotline
(800) 223-1138
(212) 785-9500

Answers questions and provides brochures on diabetes. Refers to local chapters, physicians, and clinics. Chapters located worldwide. 9 a.m.-5 p.m.

Disabling Conditions

See also **Hearing and Speech**

Americans with Disabilities Act Hotline
(800) 514-0301
(800) 514-0383 (TTY)
(202) 514-6193 (Electronic Bulletin Board)

Sponsored by the U.S. Department of Justice. Provides a 24-hour recording of information on the Americans with Disabilities Act. The recording also allows callers to request publications. ADA specialists available 10 a.m.-6 p.m. on Monday, Tuesday, Wednesday, and Friday and 1 p.m.-6 p.m. on Thursday.

A-41. Handicapped Media, Inc.
(800) 321-8708 (Voice/TDD)

Provides information, referral on services, and advocacy. Operates 8 a.m.-5 p.m. (Mountain).

A-42. Heath Resource Center
(800) 544-3284
(202) 939-9320

Operates the national clearinghouse on postsecondary education for individuals with disabilities and on learning disabilities. 9 a.m.-5 p.m.

A-43. Job Accommodation Network
(800) ADA-Work (Voice/TDD)
(800) 526-7234 (Voice/TDD)
(800) 526-2262 (in Canada)
(800) DIAL-JAN (Electronic Bulletin Board)
(304) 293-5407 (Fax)

Sponsored by the President's Commission on the Employment of People with Disabilities. Offers ideas for accommodating disabled persons in the workplace and information on the availability of accommodation aids and procedures. Services available in English, Spanish, and French. 8 a.m.-8 p.m., Monday-Thursday; 8 a.m.-5 p.m., Friday.

A-44. Medical Rehabilitation Education Foundation
(800) 438-7342

Provides medical rehabilitation information and a referral service for help in locating rehabilitation facilities throughout the country. 8 a.m.-5 p.m.

A-45. National Center for Youth with Disabilities: Adolescent Health Program: University of Minnesota
(800) 333-6293
(612) 626-2825
(612) 626-2134 (Fax)
(612) 624-3939 (TDD)

NCYD is an information, policy, and resource center focusing on adolescents with chronic illnesses and disabilities and the issues surrounding their transition to adult life. Offers a number of publications, including a newsletter, Connections, and a series of annotated bibliographies, CYDLINE Reviews. Maintains the National Resource Library, a database containing abstracts of current research literature, information about model programs, training/educational materials, and a list of consultants. 8 a.m.-4:30 p.m. (Central).

A-46. National Clearinghouse on Family Support and Children's Mental Health
(800) 628-1696
(503) 725-4040
(503) 725-4165 (Fax)
(503) 725-4180 (TDD)

Sponsored by the National Institute on Disability and Rehabilitation Research, U.S. Department of Education, and the Center for Mental Health Services, U.S. Department of Health and Human Services. Provides publications on parent/family support groups, financing, early intervention, various mental disorders, and other topics concerning children's mental health. Also offers a computerized data bank and a state by state resource file. Recording is operated 24 hours.

A-47. National Easter Seal Society
(800) 221-6827
(312) 726-6200
(312) 726-1494 (Fax)
(312) 726-4258 (TDD)

Through its 160 affiliates nationwide, provides rehabilitative and other support services to assist children and adults with disabilities to achieve their maximum independence. 8:30 a.m.-5 p.m. (Central).

A-48. National Information Center for Children and Youth with Disabilities
(800) 695-0285 (Voice/TT)
(202) 884-8200 (Voice/TT)
(202) 884-8441 (Fax)
nichcy@capcon.net

Sponsored by the US Department of Education. Information and referral service dedicated to disabled children. 9 a.m.-5 p.m. or leave recorded message after hours.

A-49. National Information Clearinghouse for Infants with Disabilities and Life Threatening Conditions
(800) 922-9234, ext. 201

Sponsored by the National Center for Child Abuse and Neglect, Administration on Children and Families, U.S. Department of Health and Human Services. Makes referrals to support groups and sources of financial, medical, and educational assistance for families having infants with disabilities (birth to age 3). Spanish-speaking operators available. 9 a.m.-5 p.m.

A-50. National Information System for Vietnam Veterans and their Families
(800) 922-9234, ext. 401 (Voice/TDD)

Provides information and referral for Vietnam veterans having children with disabilities or special health care needs. Produces and disseminates fact sheets on health conditions common to Vietnam veterans' children and on advocacy topics. 9 a.m.-5 p.m.

A-51. National Rehabilitation Information Center (NARIC)
(800) 346-2742 (Voice/TDD)
(301) 588-9284 (Voice/TDD)
(301) 587-1967 (Fax)

Sponsored by the National Institute on Disability and Rehabilitation Research. Collects and disseminates the results of federally funded research projects. The collection includes commercially published books, journal articles, and audiovisuals. Spanish-speaking operators available. 8 a.m.-6 p.m.

Scoliosis Association
(800) 800-0669
(407) 994-4435 (Fax)

Provides information on scoliosis and related spinal deformities.

Down Syndrome

See **Rare Disorders**

Drinking Water Safety

A-52. Safe Drinking Water Hotline
(800) 426-4791
(202) 260-8072 (Fax)
sdwa@epamail.epa.gov

Sponsored by the U.S. Environmental Protection Agency. Provides general and technical information on the federal drinking water program and referrals to other organizations when appropriate. Does not provide site-specific information on local water quality, bottled water, or home water treatment units. Has the ability to communicate in English, Spanish, French, Lebanese, and Persian. 9 a.m.-5:30 p.m., weekdays, except Federal holidays.

Drug Abuse

See also **Alcohol Abuse and Substance Abuse**

A-53. CSAP Workplace Helpline
(800) 843-4971

Sponsored by the Center for Substance Abuse Prevention, Substance Abuse and Mental Health Services Administration. Offers information, publications, and referrals to corporations, businesses, industry, and national organizations on assessing drug abuse within an organization and developing and implementing drug abuse policy and programs. 9 a.m.-8 p.m.

A-54. Housing and Urban Development Drug Information and Strategy Clearinghouse
(800) 578-3472

Promotes strategies for eradicating drugs and drug trafficking from public housing. Provides housing officials, residents, and community leaders a source for information and assistance on drug abuse prevention and trafficking control techniques. Maintains a database system consisting of national and community program descriptions, publications, research, and news articles. Provides resource lists. 8 a.m.-5 p.m.

A-55. "Just Say No" International
(800) 258-2766
(510) 451-6666

Thirteen thousand clubs. Founded in 1985. Provides materials, technical assistance, and training to help children and teenagers lead healthy, productive, drug-free lives. The New Youth Power program builds on young people's resiliency, drawing on and encouraging the skills and attributes that allow young people to cope with challenges and adversity. Youth Power empowers youth to discover and hone their assets to succeed in all areas of their lives. 7 a.m.-5 p.m. (Pacific).

A-56. National Cocaine Hotline
(800) 262-2463

Sponsored by the Phoenix House Foundation. Answers questions on cocaine, alcohol, and other drugs from users, their friends, and families. Provides referrals to drug rehabilitation centers. Operates 24 hours.

A-57. National Federation TARGET Resource Center
(800) 366-6667
(816) 464-5400

Sponsored by the National Federation of State High School Associations. Provides education and prevention materials on tobacco, alcohol, and other drugs, including steroids and other performance-enhancing drugs, and on other healthy lifestyle issues surrounding high school athletics and activities. Catalog available. 8 a.m.-4:30 p.m. (Central).

Dyslexia

See **Learning Disorders**

Endometriosis

See **Women**

Environment

A-58. Indoor Air Quality Information Clearinghouse
(800) 438-4318

Provides information on indoor air quality, including the health effects of passive smoke, formaldehyde, and various indoor air pollutants. 9 a.m.-5 p.m.

Epilepsy

See **Rare Disorders**

Ethics

A-59. Joseph and Rose Kennedy Institute of Ethics
National Reference Center for Bioethics Literature
Georgetown University
(800) 633-3849
(202) 687-3885
(202) 687-6770 (Fax)
medethx@guvm.ccf.georgetown.edu

Provides reference assistance and conducts free searches on bioethical topics. Produces a variety of publications, as well as the BIOETHICSLINE database on the MEDLARS information system. 9 a.m.-5 p.m., Monday, Wednesday, Thursday, Friday; 9 a.m.-9 p.m., Tuesday; 10 a.m.-3 p.m., Saturday, except summers and holidays.

Fire Prevention

A-60. National Fire Protection Association
(800) 344-3555 (Customer Service)
(617) 770-3000
(617) 984-7880 (TDD)
(617) 770-0200 (Fax)

Develops fire protection codes and standards, fire safety education materials, and provides technical information on fire prevention, firefighting procedures, and the fire loss experience. 8:30 a.m.-5 p.m.

Fitness

A-61. Aerobics and Fitness Foundation of America
(800) 446-2322 (For Professionals)
(800) YOUR-BODY (Consumer Hotline)

Answers questions regarding safe and effective exercise programs and practices. Written health and fitness guidelines also available (shipping and handling charges may apply). 7:30 a.m.-5:30 p.m. (Pacific).

Consumer Fitness Hotline
(800) 529-8227

Sponsored by the American Council on Exercise. Provides information on health and fitness, including information on how to start an exercise program. Answers specific questions concerning a variety of fitness topics. 8 a.m.-5 p.m. (Pacific)

A-62. YMCA of the USA
(800) 872-9622
(312) 977-9063 (Fax)

Provides information about YMCA services and locations of Ys in residential areas. 8 a.m.-5 p.m. (Central).

Food Safety

A-63. Food Labeling Hotline
Meat and Poultry Hotline
(800) 535-4555

Sponsored by the U.S. Department of Agriculture. Provides information on safe handling, preparation, and storage of meat, poultry, and eggs. Also provides tips on buying a turkey, holiday food safety, and understanding labels on meat and poultry. 10 a.m.-4 p.m.

A-64. Seafood Hotline
(800) FDA-4010
(202) 205-4314
http://vm.cfsan.fda.gov/list.html

Sponsored by the Food and Drug Administration. Provides information on seafood buying, handling, and storage for home consumption. Also provides seafood publications and prerecorded seafood safety messages. Information available on food safety, chemicals and contaminants, food and color additives, biotechnology, food labeling, nutrition, health and disease, and women's health. Messages and publications available in Spanish. Staff are available for assistance 12 p.m.-4 p.m. (Eastern). Automated Hotline operates 24 hours.

Foot Health

American Podiatric Medical Association, Inc.
(800) FOOTCARE
(301) 571-9200
(301) 530-2752 (Fax)

Provides a variety of patient education literature on topics including specific foot problems and diseases, sports and fitness activities, and systemic disease manifestations in the foot and ankle. Operates 24 hours.

General Health

A-65. Agency for Health Care Policy and Research Clearing-
house
(800) 358-9295
(301) 495-3453

Distributes lay and scientific publications produced by the agency, including clinical practice guidelines on a variety of topics, reports from the National Medical Expenditure Survey, and health care technology assessment reports. 9 a.m.-5 p.m.

American Osteopathic Association
(800) 621-1773

Provides materials on osteopathic medicine and patient education materials. Directories of osteopathic physicians and specialists are also available.

A-66. MedicAlert Foundation
(800) 432-5378
(800) 344-3226
(209) 669-2495 (Fax)

Provides emergency service for people who cannot speak for themselves by means of a unique member number on a Medic-Alert bracelet or necklace. Operates 24 hours.

A-67. National Health Information Center
(800) 336-4797
(301) 565-4167
(301) 984-4256 (Fax)
nhicinfo@health.org
http://nhic-nt.health.org

Helps the public and health professionals locate health information through identification of health information resources, an information and referral system, and publications. Uses a database containing descriptions of health-related organizations to refer inquirers to the most appropriate resources. Does not diagnose medical conditions or give medical advice. Prepares and distributes publications and directories on health promotion and disease prevention topics.

Grief

A-68. Grief Recovery Helpline
(800) 445-4808

Provides educational services on recovering from loss. 9 a.m.-5 p.m., Monday- Friday (Pacific).

Headache/Head Injury

A-70. Brain Injury Association, Inc.
(800) 444-6443 (Family Helpline)
(202) 296-6443 (Business office)
(202) 296-8850 (Fax)

Formerly the National Head Injury Foundation. Dedicated to improving the quality of life of people with brain injuries and promoting prevention of brain injury. Provides information and resources for people with brain injury, their families, and professionals. Offers educational materials on the impact of brain injury, location of rehabilitative facilities, and availability of community services. 9 a.m.-5 p.m. (Eastern).

A-69. National Headache Foundation
(800) 843-2256
(312) 907-6278 (Fax)

Disseminates free information on headache causes and treatments, funds research, and sponsors public and professional education programs nationwide. Offers audio and videotapes, brochures, and other helpful materials for purchase. Organized a nationwide network of local support groups. 9 a.m.-5 p.m. (Central) Monday-Friday.

Hearing and Speech

A-71. American Speech-Language-Hearing Association
(800) 638-8255
(301) 897-5700

Offers information on speech, language, and hearing disabilities. Also provides referrals to speech language pathologists and audiologists certified by the American Speech-Language-Hearing Association. 8:30 a.m.-5 p.m.

A-72. Deafness Research Foundation
(800) 535-3323
(212) 684-6556 (Voice/TDD)
(212) 779-2125 (Fax)

Funds research into causes, treatment, and prevention of hearing loss and other ear disorders. Also offers resource and referral information on ear-related problems. 9 a.m.-5 p.m. (Eastern).

A-73. Dial A Hearing Screening Test
(800) 222-3277 (Voice/TDD)
(610) 543-2802 (Fax)

Sponsored by Occupational Hearing Services. Answers questions on hearing problems and makes referrals to local numbers for a 2-minute telephone hearing screening test, as well as for ear, nose, and throat specialists. Also makes referrals to organizations that have information on ear-related problems, including broken hearing aids. 9 a.m.-5 p.m. (Eastern).

A-74. The Ear Foundation at Baptist Hospital
(800) 545-4327
(615) 329-7849
(615) 329-7935 (Fax)

Committed to integration of hearing and balance impaired people into the mainstream of society through public awareness and medical education. Includes the Meniere's Network and Young EAR's Program. Provides brochure about Meniere's disease and other literature, including newsletters. 8:30 a.m.-4:30 p.m. (Central) or leave recorded message after hours.

A-75. Hear Now
(800) 648-4327 (Voice/TDD)
(303) 695-7797 (Voice/TDD)
(303) 695-7789 (Fax)

Provides hearing aids and cochlear implants for deaf and hard of hearing individuals with limited financial resources. Collects used hearing aids. Applications for assistance available. 8 a.m.-4 p.m. (Mountain).

A-76. Hearing HelpLine
(800) EAR-WELL
(703) 642-0580
(703) 750-9302 (Fax)

Sponsored by the Better Hearing Institute. Implements national public information programs on hearing loss and available medical, surgical, hearing aid, and rehabilitation assistance for millions with uncorrected hearing problems. Provides information on hearing loss and hearing help. 9 a.m.-5 p.m.

A-78. International Hearing Society
(800) 521-5247
(810) 478-4520 (Fax)

Provides general information on hearing aids and a listing of local hearing aid specialists. 9 a.m.-5 p.m.

A-77. John Tracy Clinic
(800) 522-4582 (Voice/TTY)
(213) 749-1651 (Fax)

Provides free diagnostic, habilitative, and educational services to preschool deaf children and their families through onsite services and to the preschool deaf and deaf-blind children through worldwide correspondence courses in Spanish and English. 8 a.m.-4 p.m. (Pacific). Leave recorded message after hours.

National Family Association for Deaf-Blind
(800) 255-0411, ext. 275

Provides information and resources; facilitates family organizations in each state; and develops family/professional partnerships to benefit people with deaf-blindness.

A-79. National Institute on Deafness and Other Communication Disorders Information Clearinghouse
(800) 241-1044
(800) 241-1055 (TT)

Collects and disseminates information on hearing, balance, smell, taste, voice, speech, and language for health professionals, patients, people in industry, and the public. Maintains a database of references to brochures, books, articles, fact sheets, organizations, and educational materials, which is a subfile on the Combined Health Information Database (CHID). Develops publications. 8:30 a.m.-5 p.m.

A-80. TRIPOD GRAPEVINE
(800) 352-8888 (Voice/TDD in the US)
(800) 287-4763 (Voice/TDD in Canada)
(818) 972-2090 (Fax)
tripodla@aol

Offers information on deafness, including raising and educating a deaf child. Refers callers to parents, professionals, and other resources in their own communities nationwide. 8 a.m.-5 p.m. (Pacific) or leave recorded message after hours.

Heart Disease

A-81. American Heart Association
(800) 242-8721

Provides English and Spanish publications and information about heart and blood vessel diseases, exercise, nutrition, and smoking cessation. Additional information is available for minority and senior citizen audiences. Callers are routed to local AHA offices for additional local information. 9 a.m.-5 p.m.

National Heart, Lung, and Blood Institute's High Blood Pressure Program
(800) 575-WELL

Provides a 24-hour recording of information on high blood pressure and high blood cholesterol in English and Spanish.

Histiocytosis

See **Rare Disorders**

Homelessness

A-82. National Resource Center on Homelessness and Mental Illness
(800) 444-7415

Sponsored by the Center for Mental Health Services, Substance Abuse and Mental Health Services Administration. Provides technical assistance and information about services and housing for the homeless and mentally ill population. 8 a.m.-5 p.m.

Hormonal Disorders

Thyroid Foundation of America, Inc.
(800) 832-8321

Provides health education and support for thyroid patients and health professionals. Responds to inquiries on all aspects of thyroid dysfunction. Provides information on genetically related autoimmune diseases including vitiligo, diabetes mellitus, and pernicious anemia.

Hospital/Hospice Care

A-83. Children's Hospice International
(800) 242-4453
(703) 684-0330

Provides support system and information for health care professionals, families, and the network of organizations that offer hospice care to terminally ill children. Distributes educational materials. 9:30 a.m.-5:30 p.m.

A-84. Hill-Burton Hospital Free Care
(800) 638-0742
(800) 492-0359 (in MD)

Sponsored by the Bureau of Health Resources Development, Health Resources and Services Administration. Provides information on hospitals and other health facilities participating in the Hill-Burton Hospital Free Care Program. 9:30 a.m.-5:30 p.m. or leave recorded message after hours.

A-85. Hospice Education Institute "Hospice Link"
(800) 331-1620
(860) 767-2746 (Fax)

Offers information and advice about hospice and palliative care, makes referrals to local hospice and palliative care programs nationwide, and offers information and advice on grief support programs. Maintains a current database of hospices and palliative care units, publishes books and pamphlets, offers continuing education. No medical advice or psychological counseling offered, but "sympathetic listening" is available to patients and families coping with advanced illness and loss. 9 a.m.-4 p.m.

A-86. Shriners Hospital Referral Line
(800) 237-5055

Gives information on free hospital care available to children under 18 who need orthopedic care or burn treatment. Sends application forms to requesters who meet eligibility requirements for treatment provided by 22 Shriners Hospitals in the United States, Mexico, and Canada. 8 a.m.-5 p.m.

Housing

See also **Chemical Products/Pesticides; Lead**

A-87. Housing and Urban Development User
(800) 245-2691

Disseminates publications for U.S. Department of Housing and Urban Development's Office of Policy Development and Research. Offers database searches on housing research. Provides reports on housing safety, housing for elderly and handicapped persons, and lcad-based paint. 8:30 a.m.-5:15 p.m.

Huntington's Disease

See **Rare Disorders**

Immunization

CDC Immunization Hotline
(800) 232-SHOT

Provides information on childhood immunizations and specific vaccinations.

Impotence

A-88. Impotence Information Center
(800) 843-4315
(800) 543-9632

Provides free information to prospective patients regarding the causes of and treatments for impotence. Provides referrals to local physicians. 8:30 a.m.-5 p.m. (Central) or leave recorded message after hours.

Insurance/Medicare/Medicaid

A-90. DHHS Inspector General's Hotline
(800) HHS-TIPS

Handles complaints regarding fraud, employee misconduct, and waste and abuse of U.S. Department of Health and Human Services' funds, including Medicare, and Medicaid. 9 a.m.-8 p.m.

A-91. Medicare Issues Hotline
(800) 638-6833
(800) 820-1202 (TDD/TTY)

Sponsored by the Health Care Financing Administration. Gives information on Medicare/Medigap insurance and policies, answers general questions on Medicare problems, and sends free Medicare publications. Publications include: Your Medicare Handbook, The Guide to Health Insurance for People with Medicare, and publications related to Mammograms, HMOs, Low Income Beneficiaries, Hospice Benefits, and Nursing Homes. 8 a.m.-8 p.m.

A-92. National Insurance Consumer Helpline
(800) 942-4242

Provides general information and answers questions regarding life, health, and home and automobile insurance. Free consumer publications available. Spanish-speaking operators available. 8 a.m.-8 p.m. (Eastern).

Social Security Administration
(800) 772-1213

Provides public information materials about the Social Security and supplemental security income (SSI) programs, as well as information on entitlement to Medicare. Free pamphlets on Social Security benefits, disability benefits, and supplemental security income are available.

Justice

A-93. National Criminal Justice Reference Service (NCJRS)
(800) 851-3420
(301) 738-8895 (Electronic Bulletin Board)

Provides criminal justice research findings and documents from bureaus within the Office of Justice Programs, U.S. Department of Justice. The NCJRS library collection contains more than 130,000 documents and is accessible online. Clearinghouse resources and activities also can be accessed via the NCJRS electronic bulletin board. 8:30 a.m.-7 p.m. Leave recorded message after hours.

Kidney Disease

See **Urological Disorders**

Lead

See also **Housing**

A-94. National Lead Information Hotline
(800) LEAD-FYI (Hotline)
(800) 424-LEAD (Clearinghouse)
(800) 526-5456 (TDD)
EHC@cais.com (E-mail)
cais.com (Internet gopher)

Hotline supplies a basic information packet to the public in English or Spanish on lead poisoning and prevention through a 24-hour automated response system. Clearing-

house provides technical information and answers in English or Spanish to specific lead-related questions for private citizens and professionals. 8:30 a.m.-5 p.m.

Learning Disorders

See also **Handicapping Conditions**

Children and Adults with Attention Deficit Disorders (CH.A.D.D.)
(800) 233-4050

Provides an information packet on attention deficit disorders and information on joining CH.A.D.D.

A-95. The Orton Dyslexia Society
(800) 222-3123
(410) 296-0232

Clearinghouse that provides information on testing tutoring and computers used to aid people with dyslexia and related disorders and general information. Operates 24 hours a day.

Library Services

See also **Handicapping Conditions**

A-96. Modern Talking Picture Service, Inc. Captioned Films/Videos
(800) 237-6213 (Voice/TDD)
(800) 538-5636 (Fax)

Provides free loan of captioned films and videos for deaf and hearing impaired people. 9 a.m.-5 p.m.

A-99. National Library Service for the Blind and Physically Handicapped
(800) 424-8567
(202) 707-5100
(202) 707-0744 (TDD)
(202) 707-0712 (Fax)

A total of over 140 network libraries that work in cooperation with the Library of Congress to provide free library service to anyone who is unable to read standard print because of visual or physical impairment. Provides both audio and Braille formats through a network of regional libraries. 8 a.m.-4:30 p.m.

A-100. Recording for the Blind and Dyslexic
(800) 221-4792

Serves people who cannot read standard print because of a visual, perceptual or other physical disability. Service includes free lending library of academic textbooks on audio cassette and sale of books on computer diskette and specially adapted tape players and recorders. Provides information on becoming a registered borrower.

Liver Diseases

A-101. American Liver Foundation
(800) 223-0179
(201) 256-2550

Provides information, including fact sheets, and makes physician and support group referrals. Liver disease information brochures and information sheets available upon request. 9 a.m.-5 p.m.

Hepatitis Foundation International
(800) 891-0707
(201) 857-5044 (Fax)

Educates the public about the prevention, diagnosis and treatment of viral hepatitis. Disseminates a variety of materials on viral hepatitis.

Lung Disease/Asthma/Allergy

American Lung Association
(800) 586-4872

Provides information on such topics as air pollution, smoking, tuberculosis, lung hazards on the job, marijuana, asthma, emphysema, and other lung diseases. Some materials are available in Spanish.

A-102. Asthma and Allergy Foundation of America
(800) 7-ASTHMA (727-8462)

Provides a 24-hour recording for callers to request general information, publications and videotapes.

A-103. Asthma Information Line
(800) 822-2762
(414) 276-3349 (Fax)

Sponsored by the American Academy of Allergy, Asthma, and Immunology. Provides written materials on asthma and allergies and offers a printed listing of physician referrals. Operates 24 hours.

A-104. Lung Line National Jewish Center for Immunology
    and Respiratory Medicine
(800) 222-5864
(303) 355-5864
(800) 552-LUNG (LUNG FACTS)
(303) 270-2150 (Fax)
http://www.njc.org (Internet)

Answers questions about asthma, emphysema, chronic bronchitis, allergies, juvenile rheumatoid arthritis, smoking, and other respiratory and immune system disorders. Questions answered by registered nurses. 8 a.m.-5 p.m. (Mountain). LUNG FACTS, a companion to LUNG LINE, is a 24-hour, 7-days-a-week automated information service. Using a touch-tone telephone, callers can choose among a selection of recorded topics on lung disease and immunological disorders.

Maternal and Infant Health

A-105. La Leche League International
(800) LA-LECHE
(708) 519-7730
(708) 519-0035 (Fax)

Provides breastfeeding information and mother-to-mother support for women who wish to breastfeed. Distributes and sells a wide variety of materials on breastfeeding and parent-

ing. Also organizes training for health professionals and provides a reliable source for current breastfeeding research information through the Center for Breastfeeding Information. Catalogue free of charge upon request. 9 a.m.-5 p.m. (Central).

Medicare/Medicaid

See **Insurance/Medicare/Medicaid**

Mental Health

See also **Child Abuse/Missing Children/Mental Health**

American Academy of Child and Adolescent Psychiatry
(800) 333-7636

Distributes fact sheets on mental illnesses affecting youngsters.

A-106. Depression Awareness, Recognition, and Treatment
    (D/ART)
(800) 421-4211

Sponsored by the National Institute of Mental Health. Provides a 24-hour recording for callers to request free brochures on clinical depression. Foreign language materials available upon request.

National Alliance for the Mentally Ill
(800) 950-6264

Provides information on severe mental illness and its effects on families, support for the rights of patients and families, and help in starting local groups.

A-107. National Clearinghouse on Family Support and Children's Mental Health
(800) 628-1696
(503) 725-4040
(503) 725-4165 (TTD)
(503) 725-4180 (Fax)

Sponsored by the National Institute on Disability and Rehabilitation Research, U.S. Department of Education, and the Center for Mental Health Services, U.S. Department of Health and Human Services. Provides publications on parent/family support groups, financing, early intervention, various mental disorders, and other topics concerning children's mental health. Also offers a computerized databank and a state by state resource file. Recording operates 24 hours a day.

A-108. National Foundation for Depressive Illness
(800) 248-4344
(212) 268-4434 (Fax)
NAFDI@pipeline.com (E-mail)

A 24-hour recorded message describes symptoms of depression and manic depression and gives an address for more information and physician and support group referrals by state.

A-109. National Mental Health Association
(800) 969-6642
(703) 684-5968 (Fax)

Provides public education, direct services and advocacy for mental health and mental illness concerns in communities across the nation. Distributes information on various mental health topics and provides referrals to other organizations.

National Mental Health Services Clearinghouse
(800) 789-2647

Provides referrals to individuals requesting mental health services within their communities. 9 a.m. 5:30 p.m. (Pacific)

National Mental Illness Screening Project
(800) 262-4444

A-110. National Resource Center on Homelessness and Mental Illness
(800) 444-7415

See **Homelessness**

A-111. Panic Disorder Information Line
(800) 64-PANIC

Sponsored by the National Institute of Mental Health. Provides educational materials on panic disorder symptoms, diagnosis, referral, and treatment to health care and mental health professionals and the public. Also disseminates lists of additional resource materials and organizations that can help callers locate a treatment professional. Spanish-speaking operators available. Operates 24 hours a day.

Minority Health

A-112. Office of Minority Health Resource Center
(800) 444-6472

Responds to consumer and professional inquiries on minority health-related topics by distributing materials, providing referrals, and identifying sources of technical assistance. Spanish- and Asian-speaking operators available. 9 a.m.-5 p.m.

Nutrition

A-113. American Dietetic Association's Consumer Nutrition Hotline
(800) 366-1655

Provides consumers with direct and immediate access to reliable food and nutrition information. Callers may listen to recorded nutrition messages in English or Spanish, 8 a.m.-8 p.m. (Central). Registered dietitians (RDs) answer food and nutrition questions and provide referrals to RDs in the caller's area 9 a.m.-4 p.m. (Central). TDD available.

A-114. American Institute for Cancer Research
(800) 843-8114

Provides free educational publications about diet, nutrition, and cancer prevention, as well as a Nutrition Hotline staffed by registered dietitians. 9 a.m.-5 p.m.

A-115. National Dairy Council
(800) 426-8271
(800) 974-6455 (Fax)
(708) 803-2077 (Fax)

Develops and provides educational materials on nutrition. 8:30 a.m.-4:30 p.m. (Central).

Oral Health

American Dental Association
(800) 947-4746

Distributes educational materials on dental health topics such as dentures, tooth decay, smoking, diet, oral care, and fluoridation.

Organ Donation

See also **Urological Disorders; Vision**

A-116. The Living Bank
(800) 528-2971
(713) 961-0979 (Fax)

The Living Bank is a nonprofit organization established in 1969 to promote organ, tissue, and body donations through public education and registration of donors. Assistance is available in English and Spanish. Operates 24 hours.

A-117. National Marrow Donor Program
(800) MARROW-2

See **Cancer**

A-118. United Network for Organ Sharing
(800) 243-6667
(804) 330-8507 (Fax)
http://www.infi.net/~shreorg/unos.html

Offers information and referrals for organ donation and transplantation. Answers requests for organ donor cards. Operates 24 hours.

Paralysis and Spinal Cord Injury

See also **Handicapping Conditions; Stroke**

A-119. American Paralysis Association
(800) 225-0292
(201) 912-9433 (Fax)

Raises money to fund worldwide research to find a cure for paralysis caused by spinal injuries and other central nervous system disorders. Provides information about spinal cord research. 9 a.m.-5 p.m.

A-120. National Rehabilitation Information Center
(800) 346-2742 (Voice/TDD)
(301) 588-9284 (Voice/TDD)
(301) 587-1967 (Fax)

Provides research referrals and information on rehabilitation issues and concerns. Spanish-speaking interpreters available upon request. 8 a.m.-6 p.m.

A-121. National Spinal Cord Injury Association
(800) 962-9629 (Members and individuals with spinal cord in-
juries; no vendors)
(617) 441-8500 (Nonmembers, public, professionals)

Provides peer counseling to those with spinal cord injuries through local chapters and organizations. Provides information and referral service. 9 a.m.-5 p.m.

A-122. National Spinal Cord Injury Hotline
(800) 526-3456
(410) 366-2325 (Fax)

Financially supported by the Paralyzed Veterans of America. Offers information on spinal cord injuries and peer support to those with spinal cord injuries and their families. 24-hour answering service will page for emergency. 9 a.m.-5 p.m.

A-123. National Stroke Association
(800) STROKES
(303) 771-1700
(303) 771-1887 (TDD)

Provides both written and referral information to individuals, including stroke survivors, families, and health care providers on prevention, treatment, and rehabilitation. 8 a.m.-4:30 p.m., Monday-Thursday; 8 a.m.-4 p.m., Friday (Mountain).

Paralyzed Veterans of America
(800) 424-8200
(800) 795-4327 (TDD)

An organization for veterans of the armed forces who have experienced spinal cord injury or dysfunction. Advocates for quality health care and civil rights and opportunities for its members. Conducts research and disseminates information addressing spinal cord injury and dysfunction.

Parkinson's Disease

A-124. American Parkinson's Disease Association
(800) 223-2732
(718) 981-4399 (Fax)

Operates 51 information and referral centers throughout the United States. Raises funds for Parkinson's disease research and education. Provides information and referrals to patients and families. Multilingual educational literature available. 9 a.m.-5 p.m. (Eastern). Leave recorded message after hours.

A-125. National Parkinson Foundation, Inc.
(800) 327-4545
(800) 433-7022 (in FL)
(305) 548-4403 (Fax)

A worldwide research, clinical, and therapeutic organization. Also provides physician references, support group systems, and educational materials in both English and Spanish. Professional staff answer questions about the disease from 9 a.m.-5 p.m., Monday-Friday; recorded messages at all other times.

Pesticides

See **Chemical Products/Pesticides**

Physicians

A-127. American Board of Medical Specialties
(800) 776-2378

The ABMS is the umbrella organization for the 24 medical specialty boards authorized and recognized to certify physician specialists in the United States. As a service to the public, a toll-free number is provided to verify board certification of physicians certified by the Member Boards of ABMS from 9 a.m.-6 p.m.

Practitioner Reporting

A-128. USP Practitioners Reporting Network
(800) 4-USP-PRN (487-7776)
(800) 23-ERROR (Medication error)

Offers a service for health professionals to report problems with drugs, medical devices, radiopharmaceuticals, animal drugs, and actual or potential medication errors. Recording operates 24 hours a day; staff available 9 a.m.-4:30 p.m., Monday-Friday. Medication error telephone number records information 24 hours a day.

Pregnancy/Miscarriage

A-129. American Academy of Husband-Coached Childbirth
(800) 4-ABIRTH
Provides free listing of teachers of the Bradley Method, including package of information and referral for local classes in natural childbirth. Books and videotapes may be ordered also. 9 a.m. 5 p.m. (Pacific). Leave recorded message after hours.

A-130. ASPO/Lamaze (American Society for Psychoprophy-
laxis in Obstetrics)
(800) 368-4404
(202) 857-1128
(202) 223-4579 (Fax)
MThompso@SBA.Com

Operates a toll-free telephone service to provide consumers with information about prepared childbirth and how to locate a local ASPO-Certified Childbirth Educator. 9 a.m.-5 p.m. (Eastern).

A-131. International Childbirth Education Association
(800) 624-4934 (Book Center orders)
(612) 854-8660 (General information)

Provides referrals to local chapters and support groups, membership information, certification, and mail-order service. 7 a.m.-4:30 p.m. (Central).

A-132. Liberty Godparent Home
(800) 542-4453

Provides a residential program for unwed mothers. Provides counseling referrals to local and national organizations and distributes brochures on request. An adoption agency is also on site. Operates 24 hours.

Radon

A-133. Radon Hotline
(800) SOS-RADON
(800) 526-5456 (TDD)

Operated by the National Safety Council. Provides a 24-hour recording for callers to request a brochure on reducing radon risks in the home and a listing of local contacts.

Rare Disorders*

*A rare disorder is defined as a disorder that affects less than 1 percent of the population at any given time.

A-134. American Leprosy Missions (Hansen's Disease)
(800) 543-3131
(803) 271-7040
(803) 271-7062 (Fax)

Answers questions and distributes materials on the disease. Also assists in raising funds for people with this disease. 8 a.m.-5 p.m.

A-135. The American Lupus Society
(800) 331-1802
(805) 339-0467 (Fax)

Provides a 24-hour recording for callers to leave their names and addresses to receive information on services provided.

A-136. American SIDS Institute
(800) 232-7437
(800) 847-7437 (in GA)

Answers inquiries from families and physicians, distributes literature, and makes referrals to other organizations. 8 a.m.-5 p.m. Leave recorded message after hours.

A-137. Amyotrophic Lateral Sclerosis Association (ALS, Lou Gehrig's Disease)
(800) 782-4747
(818) 340-2060 (Fax)

Provides names of support groups and locations of clinics and distributes literature. 8 a.m.-5 p.m. (Pacific). Leave recorded message after hours.

A-138. Batten's Disease Support and Research Association
(800) 448-4570

Provides a 24 hour recording for callers to request information on Batten's Disease.

The CFIDS Association of America
(800) 442 3437

Provides information on chronic Epstein-Barr Virus, myalgic encephalomyelitis, HBLV, and related disorders, such as interstitial cystitis, mitral valve prolapse, and vestibular problems.

A-139. Cleft Palate Foundation
(800) 242-5338 (CLEFTLINE)
(412) 481-1376
(412) 481-0847 (Fax)

Provides information and referral to individuals and families affected by cleft lip, cleft palate, or other craniofacial birth defects. Referrals are made to local cleft palate/craniofacial teams for treatment and to parent/patient support groups. Free information on various aspects of clefting is available; some available in Spanish. CLEFTLINE operates 24 hours. Spanish-speaking operators available 8:30 a.m.-4:30 p.m., Monday-Friday.

A-140. Cooley's Anemia Foundation
(800) 522-7222
(718) 321-CURE
(718) 321-3340 (Fax)

Provides information on patient care, research, fundraising, patient-support groups, and research grants. Makes referrals to local chapters and screening centers. 9 a.m.-5 p.m.

A-141. Cornelia de Lange Syndrome Foundation, Inc.
(800) 223-8355
(800) 753-2357
(203) 693-0159
(203) 693-6819 (Fax)

Promotes research and provides a variety of materials for families, friends, and professionals about this syndrome. Services include an international professional network, a newsletter, Family Support Program, and a Scientific Advisory Committee. 9 a.m.-4:30 p.m. (Eastern). Leave recorded message after hours.

A-142. Crohn's and Colitis Foundation of America, Inc.
(800) 932-2423
(800) 343-3637 (Warehouse)

See **Diabetes/Digestive Diseases**

A-143. Cystic Fibrosis Foundation
(800) 344-4823
(301) 951-6378 (Fax)

Responds to patient and family questions, offers literature, and provides referrals to local clinics. 8:30 a.m.-5:30 p.m.

A-144. Epilepsy Foundation of America
(800) 332-1000
(800) 213 5821 (Publications)
(301) 459-3700
(301) 577-2684 or 4941 (Fax)

Provides information on epilepsy and makes referrals to local chapters. Spanish-speaking operators available. 9 a.m.-5 p.m.

Epilepsy Information Service
(800) 642-0500

Provides general information on epilepsy. Distributes pamphlets on epilepsy free of charge. 8 a.m. 5 p.m. (Eastern).

Fibromyalgia Network
(800) 853-2929
(520) 290-5550 (Fax)

Provides information on Fibromyalgia, Chronic Fatigue Syndrome, and Myofascial Pain Syndrome. Maintains state-by-state listings for support group and health professional referrals. 8 a.m. 5 p.m. (Mountain).

A-145. Histiocytosis Association
(800) 548-2758
(609) 589-6614 (Fax)

Provides patient and family support to those affected with any of the histiocytoses. Quarterly newsletter, information, brochures, networking directory, regional meetings, and funds research. Operates 8:30 a.m.-4 p.m., Monday-Friday. Voice mail at all other times.

A-146. Huntington's Disease Society of America, Inc.
(800) 345-4372
(212) 242-1968
(212) 243-2443 (Fax)

Provides written and audiovisual materials pertaining to all aspects of Huntington's Disease; information and referral to local support groups, chapter social workers, physicians, nursing homes and a variety of other resources via local representatives; and support for research into the causes, treatment and cure of Huntington's Disease.

A-147. Lupus Foundation of America
(800) 558-0121 (English)
(800) 558 0231 (Spanish)
(301) 670-9292
(301) 670-9486 (Fax)

Answers basic questions about the disease and provides health professionals and patients and their families with information and literature. Refers to local affiliates. 9 a.m.-5 p.m. Recording 24 hours a day.

A-148. Meniere's Network
(800) 545-4327

See **Ear Foundation at Baptist Hospital; Hearing and Speech**

Muscular Dystrophy Association
(800) 572-1717
(520) 529-5300 (Fax)

Provides information on 40 neuromuscular diseases, including the muscular dystrophies, motor neuron diseases, inflammatory myopathies, diseases of the neuromuscular junction, diseases of the peripheral nerve, metabolic diseases of the muscles, myopathies due to endocrine abnormalities, and certain other myopathies.

A-149. Myasthenia Gravis Foundation
(800) 541-5454
(312) 258-0461 (Fax)

Provides information regarding services for myasthenia patients, and patient and medical literature. Promotes public awareness. Funds research. 8:45 a.m.-4:45 p.m. (Central).

A-150. National Down Syndrome Congress
(800) 232-6372
(404) 633-2817 (Fax)
ndsc@charitiesusa.com

Responds to questions concerning all aspects of Down syndrome. Refers to local organizations. Information available in Spanish. 9 a.m.-5 p.m. (Eastern). Recording after hours.

A-151. National Down Syndrome Society Hotline
(800) 221-4602
(212) 460-9330

Sponsors internationally renowned scientific symposia. Advocates on behalf of families and individuals affected by this condition. Provides information and referral services through its toll-free hotline staffed by English and Spanish speakers. Develops educational materials, many of which are distributed free of charge.

A-153. National Lymphedema Network
(800) 541-3259

Provides information on the prevention and management of primary and secondary lymphedema to the general public as well as health care professionals. Offers referrals to health care professionals and treatment centers, local support groups, and exercise programs. Provides a quarterly newsletter, resource guide, and information on support groups, conferences, and professional training courses. Leave recorded message.

A-154. National Multiple Sclerosis Society
(800) FIGHT-MS
(212) 986-7981 (Fax)

Offers a 24-hour telephone message line. Staff members available to answer questions 11 a.m.-5 p.m., Monday-Thursday.

A-155. National Neurofibromatosis Foundation
(800) 323-7938
(212) 344-6633
(212) 747-0004 (Fax)

Responds to inquiries from health professionals and patients and families. Makes referrals to physicians on clinical advisory board. 9 a.m.-5 p.m.

A-156. National Organization for Rare Disorders
(800) 999-6673
(203) 746-6518
(203) 746-6481 (Fax)
(203) 746-6927 (TDD)

A clearinghouse for information on over 3,000 rare diseases, offers networking programs linking patients and family members together, and administers several medication assistance programs for indigent patients. Fees charged for some services. 9 a.m.-5 p.m. (Eastern) Monday-Friday. Leave recorded message after hours.

A-157. National Reye's Syndrome Foundation
(800) 233-7393
(419) 636-2679
(419) 636-3366 (Fax)

Provides awareness materials to the public and medical community, raises funds for research, and offers guidance and counseling to victims. 8 a.m.-5 p.m. Leave recorded message after hours.

A-159. National Sarcoidosis Foundation
(800) 223-6429

Provides a 24 hour recording for callers to request information on sarcoidosis.

A-158. National Tuberous Sclerosis Association
(800) 225-6872
(301) 459-9888
(301) 459-0394 (Fax)
ntsa@aol.com
Answers questions about the disease and makes parent-to-parent contact referrals. Literature is provided to families and professionals. 8:30 a.m.-5 p.m.

Office of Orphan Products Development
Food and Drug Administration
(800) 300-7469

Disseminates information on orphan drugs and rare diseases; responds to inquiries from patients, health professionals, and pharmaceutical manufacturers, as well as the general public.

The Paget Foundation for Paget's Disease of Bone and Related Disorders
(800) 23-PAGET
(212) 229-1582
(212) 229-1502 (Fax)

Provides educational literature on Paget's disease of bone, primary hyperparathyroidism and other disorders to patients and the medical community. Gives physician referrals. 9 a.m.-5 p.m. (Eastern).

A-167. Scleroderma Foundation, United
(800) 722-HOPE
(408) 728-2202
(408) 728-3328 (Fax)
outreach@scleroderma.com

Develops chapter and support groups, distributes printed materials, and provides patient support and information and medical reference lists. 8 a.m.-5 p.m. (Pacific).

A-160. Sickle Cell Disease Association of America, Inc.
(800) 421-8453

Offers educational materials, referrals for client services, research support, and public awareness. 8:30 a.m.-5 p.m. (Pacific). Recording after hours and weekends.

A-161. SIDS Alliance
(800) 221-SIDS (7437)
(410) 653-8226
(410) 653-8709 (Fax)

Hotline is available for parents who wish to discuss their concerns with a SIDS counselor, request additional information, and/or be connected to the local SIDS Affiliate for support services in their area. 9 a.m.-5 p.m. (Eastern). Phoneline available 24 hours.

A-162. Spina Bifida Association of America
(800) 621-3141
(202) 944-3285
(202) 944-3295 (Fax)

Provides information to consumers and health professionals and referrals to local chapters. 9 a.m.-5 p.m.

A-163. Spondylitis Association of America (formerly the Ankylosing Spondylitis Association)
(800) 777-8189
(818) 981-1616
(818) 981-9826 (Fax)

Provides information on ankylosing spondylitis, psoriatic arthritis, and Reiter's syndrome. 9 a.m.-5 p.m. (Pacific). Leave recorded message after hours.

A-164. Sturge-Weber Foundation
(800) 627-5482

Provides list of publications, long-distance support groups, and referrals for families, friends, and professionals. 9 a.m.-3 p.m., Monday-Friday.

A-165. Tourette Syndrome Association, Inc.
(800) 237-0717
(718) 224-2999
(718) 279-9596 (Fax)

Provides a 24-hour recording for callers to request information and leave name and address. To speak with a staff member, call the local number between 9 a.m.-5 p.m.

A-166. United Cerebral Palsy Association
(800) 872-5827
(202) 776-0406
(202) 776-0414 (Fax)

Provides literature about cerebral palsy and related disorders. Responds to inquiries from people with cerebral palsy and related disorders, their families, and the public. Makes referrals to local affiliates. 8:30 a.m.-5:30 p.m.

Rehabilitation

See **Disabling Conditions; Paralysis and Spinal Cord Injury**

Retinitis Pigmentosa

See **Vision**

Rural

A-168. Rural Information Center Health Service (RICHS)
(800) 633-7701
(301) 504-5547
(301) 504-6856 (TTY/TDD)
(301) 504-5181 (Fax)
ric@nalusda.gov
gopher://gopher.nalusda.gov

Provides information and referrals to the public and to professionals on rural health issues. Performs brief, complimentary literature searches. 8 a.m.-4:30 p.m.

Safety

See also **Chemical Products/Pesticides**

A-169. National Child Safety Council Childwatch
(800) 222-1464

See **Child Abuse/Missing Children/Mental Health**

A-170. National Highway Traffic Safety Administration Auto Safety Hotline
(800) 424-9393
(202) 366-0123

Provides information and referral on the effectiveness of occupant protection, such as safety belt use, child safety seats, and automobile recalls. Gives referrals to other government agencies for consumer questions on warranties, service, automobile safety regulations, and reporting safety problems. 8 a.m.-4 p.m.

A-171. National Institute for Occupational Safety and Health Technical Information Branch
(800) 356-4674

Provides information on chemical and physical hazards in the workplace, training courses, publications, and the health hazard evaluation program. 9 a.m.-4 p.m.

National Safety Council
(800) 621-7615

Offers a safety-training institute, a child safety club, home study courses in safety, and traffic and transportation safety services. Provides materials on all aspects of safety, accident prevention, and prevention of occupational illnesses.

A-172. Office of Navigation Safety and Waterway Services U.S. Coast Guard Customer Infoline
(800) 368-5647
(202) 267-0780
(800) 689-0816 (TDD/TT)
(202) 267-6707 (TDD/TT)
Modem #703313591 (Navigation Center Bulletin Board)
http://www.dot.gov/affairs/index.htm

Provides information on boating safety, including a kit for consumers, recalls on boating products, makes referrals to other organizations, and other Coast Guard missions. 8 a.m.-4 p.m.

A-173. US Consumer Product Safety Commission Hotline
(800) 638-2772
(800) 638-8270 (TDD)
info@cpsc.gov

Provides 24-hour messages on consumer product safety, including product hazards and product recalls. Covers only products used in and around the home, excluding automobiles, child safety seats, health care products, warranties, foods, drugs, cosmetics, boats, and firearms.

Sexual Education

A-174. Planned Parenthood Federation of America, Inc.
(800) 669-0156

Provides family planning, reproductive, and sexual health care information

(800) 230-PLAN

Callers will reach the nearest Planned Parenthood center for clinical appointments or education staff.

Sexually Transmitted Diseases

A-175. Centers for Disease Control and Prevention National STD Hotline
(800) 227-8922

Information regarding all sexually transmitted diseases. Referral to community clinics offering free or low-cost examination and treatment. 8 a.m.-11 p.m. Free written information available.

Herpes Resource Center
(800) 230-6039
(800) 478-3227 (Canada)

Provides information and support services to persons who suffer from herpes. Sponsors local support groups nationwide, telephone counseling services, information, research and education projects. 9 a.m. 7 p.m.

Spinal Cord Injury

See **Paralysis and Spinal Cord Injury**

Stroke

See also **Paralysis and Spinal Cord Injury**

A-176. American Heart Association Stroke Connection
(800) 553-6321
(214) 696-5211 (Fax)

Maintains a listing of more than 1000 groups across the nation for referral to stroke survivors, their families, caregivers, and interested professionals. Publishes Stroke Connection magazine, a forum for stroke survivors and their families to share information about coping with stroke. Provides information and referral and carries stroke-related books, videotapes, and literature available for purchase. 8:30 a.m.-5 p.m. (Central).

National Institute of Neurological Disorders and Stroke
(800) 352-9424

Conducts and supports research on the causes, prevention, diagnosis, and treatment of neurological disorders and stroke. Consumer publications are available on the brain and nervous system and a variety of neurological disorders.

Stuttering

A-177. National Center for Stuttering
(800) 221-2483

Provides treatment for older children (age 7 and above) and adults, training for professionals, and information for parents with young children (below age 7). 9 a.m.-6 p.m.

A-178. Stuttering Foundation of America
(800) 992-9392
(901) 452-7343
(901) 452-3931 (Fax)
stuttersfa@aol.com

Provides materials and makes referrals to speech-language pathologists. 9 a.m.-5 p.m.

Substance Abuse

See also **Alcohol Abuse and Drug Abuse**

National Inhalant Prevention Coalition
(800) 269-4237

Provides a free information packet on inhalant abuse. Distributes videotapes and posters on inhalant abuse (a fee is charged for this material when sent to states other than Texas).

Sudden Infant Death Syndrome

See **Rare Disorders**

Surgery/Facial Plastic Surgery

A-179. American Society for Dermatologic Surgery, Inc.
(800) 441-2737

Provides information about various dermatologic surgical procedures, as well as referrals to dermatologic surgeons in local areas. 8:30 a.m.-5 p.m. (Central).

A-180. American Society of Plastic and Reconstructive Surgeons, Inc.
(800) 635-0635

Provides referrals to board-certified plastic surgeons nationwide and in Canada. 8:30 a.m.-4:30 p.m. (Central). Leave recorded message after hours.

A-181. Facial Plastic Surgery Information Service
(800) 332-3223
(202) 842-4500

Provides physician referral list and brochures. 24 hours.

Trauma

A-182. American Trauma Society (ATS)
(800) 556-7890
(301) 420-4189
(301) 420-0617 (Fax)

Offers information to health professionals and the public; answers questions about trauma prevention and trauma systems. 9 a.m.-5 p.m.

Urological Disorders

A-183. American Association of Kidney Patients
(800) 749-2257
(813) 223-0001 (Fax)

Helps renal patients and their families to deal with the physical and emotional impact of kidney disease. Supplies information on renal conditions. 9 a.m.-5 p.m.

A-184. American Foundation for Urologic Disease
(800) 242-2383
(410) 528-0550 (Fax)

Provides a 24 hour recording for callers seeking patient information on urologic diseases and dysfunctions.

A-185. American Kidney Fund
(800) 638-8299

Offers financial assistance to kidney patients who are unable to pay treatment-related costs. Also provides information on organ donations and kidney-related diseases. 8 a.m.-5 p.m.

Incontinence Information Center
(800) 843-4315
(800) 543-9632

Provides free information to prospective patients regarding the causes and treatments for incontinence. Provides referrals to local physicians. 8:30 a.m.-5 p.m. (Central) or leave recorded message after hours.

A-186. National Kidney Foundation
(800) 622-9010
(212) 689-9261 (Fax)

Provides information and referrals to the public and health professionals regarding kidney disorders. 9 a.m.-5 p.m.

A-187. The Simon Foundation for Continence
(800) 237-4666 (Patient information)
(708) 864-3913
(708) 864-9758 (Fax)

Provides information on continence and ordering a quarterly newsletter and other publications. Also has a community-based education program/self-help group and informational videotape. Toll-free number operates 24 hours; second number is staffed 9 a.m.-5 p.m. (Central).

Venereal Diseases

See **Sexually Transmitted Diseases**

Vision

See also **Library Services**

A-188. American Council of the Blind
(800) 424-8666 (Live operators available 3 p.m.-5:30 p.m. Eastern)
(202) 467-5081 (9 a.m.-5:30 p.m. Eastern)
(202) 467-5085 (Fax)
(202) 331-1058 (Electronic Bulletin Board)
hcraff@ACCESS.DIGEX.NET

Offers information on blindness and referrals to rehabilitation organizations, research centers, and chapters. Publishes resource lists. Leave recorded message after hours.

A-189. Blind Children's Center
(800) 222-3566
(800) 222-3567
(213) 665-3828 (Fax)
info@blindcntr.org
http://www.blindcntr.org/bcc

Nonprofit early intervention program and educational preschool. Family support services. Information and referral line. Educational booklets for parents, educators, and specialists. 7:30 a.m.-5 p.m. (Pacific).

A-199. The Foundation Fighting Blindness
(800) 683-5555
(800) 683-5551 (TDD)
(410) 771-9470 (Fax)

Funds medical research and provides information on retinitis pigmentosa and other inherited retinal degenerations. Scope of information includes current research, genetics, retina donor program, and practical resources available throughout the United States. 8:30 a.m.-5 p.m.

A-190. Guide Dog Foundation for the Blind, Inc.
(800) 548-4337
(516) 265-2121
(516) 361-5192 (Fax)
(516) 366-4462 (Electronic Bulletin Board)

School for blind individuals requiring guide dogs. Operates a computer bulletin board system. Operates 24 hours.

A-191. The Lighthouse National Center for Education
(800) 334-5497
(212) 821-9200
(212) 821-9705 (Fax)
(212) 821-9713 (TDD)

Provides educational materials and information on vision and child development and age-related vision loss to professionals and consumers. Provides information nationwide on local resources such as low vision centers, support groups, and vision rehabilitation agencies. Some materials in Spanish. 9 a.m.-5 p.m. Leave recorded message after hours.

A-192. Louisiana Center for the Blind
(800) 234-4166
(318) 251-2891
(318) 251-0109 (Fax)

Private, residential training program for legally blind adults and children. 8 a.m.-5 p.m. (Central).

A-193. National Association for Parents of the Visually Impaired
(800) 562-6265
(617) 972-7444 (Fax)

Provides support and information to parents of visually impaired, blind, deaf-blind, and blind multi-handicapped children. 9 a.m.-5 p.m. (Central).

A-194. National Eye Care Project Helpline
(800) 222-EYES (3937)

Provides medical and surgical eye care to disadvantaged elderly people who can no longer access the ophthalmologists they have visited in the past. 8 a.m.-4 p.m. (Pacific).

A-195. National Eye Research Foundation
(800) 621-2258
(708) 564-4652
(708) 564-0807 (Fax)

Recording provides patient and membership information. Publishes the Green Directory, an international listing of member optometrists for patient referrals. 8:30 a.m.-5 p.m. Leave recorded message after hours.

A-196. The National Eye Research Foundation's Memorial Eye Clinic
(800) 621-2258

Provides low-vision care, orthokeratology, and problem contact lens care. 9 a.m. 5 p.m., Monday, Tuesday, Wednesday; 9 a.m.-2 p.m., Friday. Leave recorded message after hours.

National Family Association for Deaf-Blind
(800) 255-0411, ext. 275

See **Hearing and Speech**

A-197. National Federation of the Blind: Job Opportunities for the Blind (JOB)
(800) 638-7518

Offers support and factual information to blind individuals seeking jobs, employers, parents, and teachers. Also provides a free sample package and job magazine on cassette. 12:30 p.m.-5 p.m.

A-198. Prevent Blindness Center for Sight
(800) 331-2020

Sponsored by Prevent Blindness America. Provides information on a broad range of eye health and safety topics. 8 a.m.-5 p.m. (Central).

Violence

A-200. Family Violence Prevention Fund
(800) 313-1310

Provides information and resources on how to diagnose, treat, and prevent domestic violence. Materials available include a Primary Care Information Packet and an Emergency Department Information Packet, as well as research studies and a variety of other publications. Technical assistance available through a program specialist.

Rape, Abuse, and Incest National Network
(800) 656-4673

Connects caller to the nearest counseling center which provides counseling for rape, abuse, and incest victims.

Women

Breast Implant Hotline
(800) 532-4440

Sponsored by the Food and Drug Administration. Provides a 24-hour recording of general information on breast implants. Distributes a breast implant information packet.

A-201. Endometriosis Association
(800) 992-3636
(414) 355-6065 (Fax)

Provides a 24-hour recording for callers to request information and leave name and address.

National Osteoporosis Foundation
(800) 464-6700
(202) 223-2237 (Fax)

Provides women with information on bone density testing, advice on how to talk to physicians about osteoporosis, and location of bone density testing facilities.

A-202. PMS Access
(800) 222-4767
(608) 833-7412 (Fax)

Sponsored by Madison Pharmacy Associates, Inc. Provides information, literature, and counseling on premenstrual syndrome (PMS). Gives referrals to physicians and clinics in the caller's area. 9 a.m.-5 p.m. (Central).

A-203. Women's Sports Foundation
(800) 227-3988
(516) 542-4716 (Fax)

A national, nonprofit, educational organization that promotes and enhances sports and fitness opportunities for all girls and women.

Alphabetical Listing (all numbers add 1-800)

ADCARE Hospital Helpline, 252-6465
Aerobics and Fitness Foundation of America, 968-7263 (Consumers); 446-2322 (Professionals)
Agency for Health Care Policy and Research Clearinghouse, 358-9295
AIDS Clinical Trials Information Service, 874-2572, 243-7012 (TTY/TDD)
Al-Anon Family Group Headquarters, 356-9996
Alcohol and Drug Helpline, 821-4357
Alzheimer's Association, 272-3900
Alzheimer's Disease Education and Referral Center, 438-4380
American Academy of Child and Adolescent Psychiatry, 333-7636
American Academy of Husband-Coached Childbirth, 422-4784
American Association of Kidney Patients, 749-2257
American Board of Medical Specialties, 776-2378
American Cancer Society Response Line, 227-2345 (Voice/TDD/TT)

American Council on Alcoholism, 527-5344
American Council of the Blind, 424-8666
American Dental Association, 947-4746
American Diabetes Association, 232-3472, 232-6733 (Fax/Order Fulfillment)
American Dietetic Association's Consumer Nutrition Hotline, 366-1655
American Foundation for Urologic Disease, 242-2383
American Heart Association, 242-8721
American Heart Association Stroke Connection, 553-6321
American Institute for Cancer Research, 843-8114
American Kidney Fund, 638-8299
American Leprosy Missions (Hansen's Disease), 543-3131
American Liver Foundation, 223-0179
American Lung Association, 586-4872
American Lupus Society, The, 331-1802
American Osteopathic Association, 621-1773
American Paralysis Association, 225-0292
American Parkinson's Disease Association, 223-2732
American Podiatric Medical Association, Inc., 366-8227
American SIDS Institute, 232-7437; 847-7437
American Society for Dermatologic Surgery, Inc., 441-2737
American Society of Plastic and Reconstructive Surgeons, Inc., 635-0635
American Speech-Language-Hearing Association, 638-8255
American Trauma Society, 556-7890
Americans with Disabilities Act Hotline, 514-0301; 514-0383 (TTY)
Amyotrophic Lateral Sclerosis Association, 782-4747
Arthritis Foundation Information Hotline, 283-7800
ASPO/Lamaze, 368-4404
Asthma and Allergy Foundation of America, 727-8462
Asthma Information Line, 822-2762
Autism Society of America, 328-8476
Batten's Disease Support and Research Association, 448-4570
Bethany Christian Services, 238-4269
Blind Children's Center, 222-3566; 222-3567
Boys Town National Hotline, 448-3000; 448-1833 (TDD)
Brain Injury Association, 444-6443
Breast Implant Hotline, 532-4440
Cancer Information Service, 422-6237
CDC Immunization Hotline, 232-7468
CDC National AIDS Clearinghouse, 458-5231; 243-7012 (TDD)
CDC National AIDS Hotline, 342-2437 (English); 344-7432 (Spanish); 243-7889 (TDD)
Centers for Disease Control National STD Hotline, 227-8922
CFIDS Association of America, The, 442-3437
Chemtrec Non-Emergency Services Hotline, 262-8200
Child Find of America, Inc., 426-5678; 292-9688
CHILDHELP/IOF Foresters National Child Abuse Hotline, 422-4453; 222-4453 (TDD)
Children and Adults with Attention Deficit Disorder, 233-4050
Children's Hospice International, 242-4453
Cleft Palate Foundation, 242-5338
Consumer Fitness Hotline, 529-8227
Cooley's Anemia Foundation, 522-7222
Cornelia de Lange Syndrome Foundation, 223-8355; 753-2357
Covenant House Nineline, 999-9999
Crohn's and Colitis Foundation of America, Inc., 932-2423; 343-3637 (Warehouse)
CSAP Workplace Helpline, 843-4971
Cystic Fibrosis Foundation, 344-4823
Deafness Research Foundation, 535-3323
Depression Awareness, Recognition, and Treatment (D/ART), 421-4211
DHHS Inspector General's Hotline, 447-8477
Dial A Hearing Screening Test, 222-3277 (Voice/TDD)

National Rehabilitation Information Center, 346-2742 (Voice/TDD)

National Resource Center on Child Abuse and Neglect, 227-5242

National Resource Center on Homelessness and Mental Illness, 444-7415

National Reye's Syndrome Foundation, 233-7393

National Runaway Switchboard, 621-4000; 621-0394 (TDD)

National Safety Council, 621-7615

National Sarcoidosis Foundation, 223-6429

National Spinal Cord Injury Association, 962-9629

National Spinal Cord Injury Hotline, 526-3456

National Stroke Association, STROKES

National Tuberous Sclerosis Association, 225-6872

National Youth Crisis Hotline, 448-4663

Office of Minority Health Resource Center, 444-6472

Office of Navigation Safety and Waterway Services, U.S. Coast Guard Customer InfoLine, 368-5647

Office of Orphan Products Development, Food and Drug Administration, 300-7469

Orton Dyslexia Society, The, 222-3123

Paget Foundation for Paget's Disease of Bone and Related Disorders, 237-2438

Panic Disorder Information Line, 647-2642

Paralyzed Veterans of America, 424 8200; 795-4327 (TDD)

Planned Parenthood, 230-7526; 669-0156

PMS Access, 222-4767

Prevent Blindness Center for Sight, 331-2020

Project Inform HIV/AIDS Treatment Hotline, 822-7422

Radon Hotline, 767-7236; 526-5456 (TDD)

Rape, Abuse, and Incest National Network, 656-4673

Recording for the Blind and Dyslexic, 221-4792

Rural Information Center Health Service, 633-7701

Safe Drinking Water Hotline, 426-4791

Scleroderma Foundation, United, 722-4673

Scoliosis Association, 800-0669

Seafood Hotline, 332-4010

Shriners Hospital Referral Line, 237-5055

Sickle Cell Disease Association of America, Inc., 421-8453

SIDS Alliance, 221-7437

Simon Foundation for Continence, The, 237-4666

Social Security Administration, 772-1213

Spina Bifida Association of America, 621-3141

Spondylitis Association of America, 777-8189

Sturge-Weber Foundation, 627-5482

Stuttering Foundation of America, 992-9392

Susan G. Komen Breast Cancer Foundation, 462-9273

Thyroid Foundation of America, Inc., 832-8321

Tourette Syndrome Association, Inc., 237-0717

TRIPOD GRAPEVINE, 352-8888 (Voice/TDD); 287-4763 (Voice/TDD in Canada)

United Cerebral Palsy Association, 872-5827

United Network for Organ Sharing, 243-6667

U.S. Consumer Product Safety Commission Hotline, 638-2772; 638-8270 (TDD)

USP Practitioners Reporting Network, 487-7776; 233-7767 (Medication Error)

Women's Sports Foundation, 227-3988

YMCA of the USA, 872-9622

Y-ME National Organization for Breast Cancer Information Support Program, 221-2141.

■ **Document Source:**
U.S. Department of Health and Human Services, Public Health Service
National Health Information Centers

DOCUMENT SOURCE INDEX

■■■

TITLE INDEX

■ ■ ■

SUBJECT INDEX

■■■

by Kay Banning